act

VITREORETINAL SURGICAL TECHNIQUES

VITREORETINAL SURGICAL TECHNIQUES

Edited by

Gholam A Peyman MD
Professor of Ophthalmology and Co-Director of the Vitreoretinal Service
Department of Ophthalmology
Tulane University Medical School
New Orleans, LA
USA

Stephen A Meffert MD
North Bay Vitreoretinal Consultants, Santa Rosa, and
Consultant, Retina Service, Department of Ophthalmology,
California Pacific Medical Center,
San Francisco, CA
USA

Mandi D Conway MD, FACS
Professor of Ophthalmology, Vitreoretinal Surgeon, and
Director, Medical Retina and Uveitis Service Department of Ophthalmology
Tulane University Medical School
New Orleans, LA
USA

Famin Chou MD
Jervey Eye Group
Greenville, SC
USA

with the assistance of

Trisha Chiasson
Editorial consultant

MARTIN DUNITZ

First published in the United Kingdom in 2001 by
Martin Dunitz Ltd
The Livery House
7–9 Pratt Street
London NW1 0AE

Tel: +44 (0)20 7482 2202
Fax: +44 (0)20 7267 0159
E-mail: info@mdunitz.globalnet.co.uk
Website: http://www.dunitz.co.uk

A CIP catalogue record for this book is available from the British Library

ISBN 1-85317-585-4

Distributed in the United States by:
Blackwell Science Inc.
Commerce Place, 350 Main Street
Malden MA 02148, USA
Tel: 1 800 215 1000

Distributed in Canada by:
Login Brothers Book Company
324 Salteaux Crescent
Winnipeg, Manitoba R3J 3T2
Canada
Tel: 1 204 224 4068

Distributed in Brazil by:
Ernesto Reichmann Distribuidora de Livros, Ltda
Rua Coronel Marques 335
03440-000 São Paulo–SP
Brazil

The front cover illustration shows a fundus photograph of a cat taken approximately 3 months after implantation surgery of a microphotodiode array (Figure 53.2). The back cover illustrations show, from the left, bimanual pars plana vitrectomy with infusion endoilluminator and suction cutter (Figure 22.12), intraocular scissors being used to create a retinotomy within the margins of a previously applied diathermy (Figure 29.3), exposing a tumor by dissecting a retinal flap (Figure 36.13) and a silicone-tipped flute needle being used to separate the retina along the row of diathermy in posterior relaxing retinotomy (Figure 29.5b).

Composition by Scribe Design, Gillingham, Kent
Printed and bound in Singapore by Kyodo Pte Ltd

Contents

Contributors

Thomas M Aaberg Jr MD
Assistant Professor of Ophthalmology, Emory University School of Medicine, Atlanta, GA, USA

Gary W Abrams MD
Chairman and Professor, Kresge Eye Institute, Wayne State University, Detroit, MI, USA

Everett Ai MD
Assistant Clinical Professor, University of California, Berkeley, and Director, Retina Unit, California Pacific Medical Center, San Francisco, CA, USA

Levent Akduman MD
The Retina Center of St Louis County, St Louis, MO, USA

Abdulrahman A Alghadyan MD
Professor and Chairman, Department of Ophthalmology, King Faisal University, Alkhober, Saudi Arabia

Charles C Barr MD
Professor of Ophthalmology, Department of Ophthalmology and Visual Sciences, University of Louisville School of Medicine, Louisville, KY, USA

Michael D Bennett MD
Retina Consultants of Hawaii, Honolulu, HI, USA

Brian B Berger MD
Clinical Professor of Ophthalmology, University of Texas Health Sciences at San Antonio, TX, USA (Office in Austin, Texas)

Kevin J Blinder MD
Barnes Retina Institute, St Louis, and Assistant Clinical Professor, Department of Ophthalmology and Visual Sciences, Washington University School of Medicine, St Louis, MO, USA

Gary C Brown MD
Professor of Ophthalmology, Thomas Jefferson University, Wills Eye Hospital, Philadelphia, PA, USA

Rizwan A Cheema MD, FRCOphth.
Louisiana State University Eye Center, Louisiana State University Health Sciences Center School of Medicine, New Orleans, LA, USA

Famin Chou MD
Jervey Eye Group, Greenville, SC, USA

Alan Y Chow MD
Optobionics Corporation, and Adjunct Assistant Professor, Louisiana State University Eye Center, Louisiana State University Health Sciences Center School of Medicine, New Orleans, LA, USA

Mandi D Conway MD, FACS
Professor of Ophthalmology, Vitreoretinal Surgeon, and Director, Medical Retina and Uveitis Service Department of Ophthalmology, Tulane University Medical School, New Orleans, LA, USA

Paul G DeGregorio MD
Retina Associates of Florida, Tampa, FL, USA

Eugene de Juan Jr MD
Professor of Ophthalmology, The Wilmer Eye Institute, The Johns Hopkins University School of Medicine, Baltimore, MD, USA

Uday R Desai MD
Henry Ford Hospital, Department of Ophthalmology, Detroit, MI, USA

Sundeep Dev MD
Fellow in Vitreoretinal Diseases, Medical College of Wisconsin Eye Institute, Milwaukee, WI, USA

Jay S Duker MD
Director, Vitreoretinal Service, and Associate Professor of Ophthalmology, New England Eye Center, Tufts University School of Medicine, Boston, MA, USA

Andrew W Eller MD
Associate Professor of Ophthalmology, The Eye and Ear Institute, University of Pittsburgh School of Medicine, Pittsburgh, PA, USA

Ting Fang MD
Louisiana State University Eye Center, Louisiana State University Health Sciences Center School of Medicine, New Orleans, LA, USA

John Fenton MD
Vitreoretinal Fellow, Louisiana State University Eye Center, Louisiana State University Health Sciences Center School of Medicine, New Orleans, LA, USA

Paul T Finger MD
Associate Professor of Ophthalmology, New York University School of Medicine, and Director, Ocular Tumor Service, The New York Eye and Ear Infirmary, North Shore-LIJ Health System, New York, NY, USA

Yale L Fisher MD
Assistant Clinical Professor, Department of Ophthalmology, The New York Hospital, Cornell Medical Center, and Surgeon Director, Manhattan Eye, Ear and Throat Hospital, New York, NY, USA

Harry W Flynn Jr MD
Professor of Ophthalmology, Bascom Palmer Eye Institute, University of Miami School of Medicine, Miami, FL, USA

Jorge Freire MD
Department of Radiation Oncology, Alleghany Hospital, Hahneman University, Philadelphia, PA, USA

Dwain Fuller MD
Texas Retina Associates, Dallas, and Associate Clinical Professor of Ophthalmology, University of Texas-Southwestern, TX, USA

Mark DJ Greve MD, FRCS(C)
Assistant Clinical Professor of Ophthalmology, University of Alberta, Edmonton, Alberta, Canada

W Sanderson Grizzard MD
Clinical Professor of Ophthalmology, University of South Florida, Tampa, FL, USA

Julia A Haller MD
Associate Professor of Ophthalmology, The Wilmer Eye Institute, Johns Hopkins University School of Medicine, Baltimore, MD, USA

Mark E Hammer MD
Associate Clinical Professor, University of South Florida, Tampa, FL, USA

Dennis P Han MD
Professor of Ophthalmology, Medical College of Wisconsin Eye Institute, Milwaukee, WI, USA

April Harris MD
Ophthalmology Chief Resident, Louisiana State University Eye Center, Louisiana State University Health Sciences Center School of Medicine, New Orleans, LA, USA

Gustavo C Heringer MD
International Fellow, Manhattan Eye, Ear and Throat Hospital, New York, NY, USA

Nancy M Holekamp MD
Barnes Retina Institute, St Louis, and Assistant Clinical Professor, Department of Ophthalmology and Visual Sciences, Washington University School of Medicine, St Louis, MO, USA

Mark S Humayun MD, PhD
Assistant Professor of Medicine, The Wilmer Eye Institute, The Johns Hopkins University School of Medicine, Baltimore, MD, USA

Ilkka Immonen MD
Department of Ophthalmology, Helsinki University Eye Clinic, Helsinki, Finland

Michael Ip MD
Vitreoretinal Fellow, New England Eye Center, Boston, MA, USA

Robert N Johnson MD
Assistant Clinical Professor of Ophthalmology, University of California, San Francisco, CA, USA

Peter K Kaiser MD
Division of Ophthalmology, Cleveland Clinic Foundation Eye Institute, Cleveland, OH, USA

Peter J Kertes MD, FRCS(C)
Assistant Professor, University of Ottawa Eye Institute, Ottawa, Canada

Alan E Kimura MD
Retina Consultants of Colorado, Denver, CO, USA

Kamal Kishore MD
Bond Eye Associates, Peoria, IL, USA

Robert J Kraut MD
Florida Eye Clinic, Altamonte Springs, FL, USA

Ingrid Kreissig MD
Chairman, Department of Ophthalmology (Retina and Vitreous), University of Tübingen, Germany, and Adjunct Professor of Clinical Ophthalmology, New York Hospital, Cornell Medical Center, New York, NY, USA

Maurice B Landers III MD, FACS
Houston, TX, USA

Michael S Lee MD
Associate Instructor and Vitreoretinal Fellow, Kresge Eye Institute, Wayne State University, Detroit, MI, USA

Hilel Lewis MD
Professor and Chairman, and Director, Division of Ophthalmology, Cleveland Clinic Foundation Eye Institute, Cleveland, OH, USA

Jennifer I Lim MD
Associate Professor of Ophthalmology, Doheny Eye Institute, University of Southern California School of Medicine, Los Angeles, CA, USA

Harvey A Lincoff MD
Professor of Ophthalmology, Department of Ophthalmology, The New York Hospital, Cornell Medical Center, New York, NY, USA

Anat Loewenstein MD
The Wilmer Eye Institute, Johns Hopkins University School of Medicine, Baltimore, MD, USA

Patrick E Ma MD, FRCS(C)
University of British Columbia/VGH Eye Care Centre, Vancouver, BC, Canada

Cathleen M McCabe MD
Bascom Palmer Eye Institute, University of Miami School of Medicine, Miami, FL, USA

H Richard McDonald MD
Associate Clinical Professor of Ophthalmology, University of California, San Francisco, CA, USA

Stephen A Meffert MD
North Bay Vitreoretinal Consultants, Santa Rosa, and Consultant, Retina Service, Department of Ophthalmology, California Pacific Medical Center, San Francisco, CA, USA

William F Mieler MD
Professor of Ophthalmology, Cullen Eye Institute, Baylor College of Medicine, Houston, TX, USA

Darius M Moshfeghi MD
Fellow, Department of Ophthalmology, University of Tennessee Memphis College of Medicine, Memphis, TN, USA

A Linn Murphree MD
Professor of Ophthalmology and Pediatrics, University of Southern California School of Medicine, and Director, Ocular Oncology Service, Children's Hospital of Los Angeles, The Kenneth T Norris Jr Cancer Hospital and Tumor Institute, Estelle Doheny Eye Foundation, Los Angeles, CA, USA

R Joseph Olk MD, FACS
The Retina Center of St Louis County, St Louis, MO, USA

Machelle T Pardue PhD
Research Associate, Hines VA Hospital, Hines, IL, and Research Fellow, Department of Neurology, Loyola University Medical Center, Chicago, IL, USA

Neal S Peachey PhD
Research Health Scientist, Hines VA Hospital, Hines, IL, and Associate Professor, Departments of Neurology and Ophthalmology, Loyola University Medical Center, Chicago, IL, USA

Gholam A Peyman MD
Professor of Ophthalmology and Co-Director of the Vitreoretinal Service, Department of Ophthalmology, Tulane University Medical School, New Orleans, LA, USA

Marta A Recasens MD
Vitreoretinal Fellow, Louisiana State University Eye Center, Louisiana State University Health Sciences Center School of Medicine, New Orleans, LA, USA

Elias Reichel MD
Associate Professor of Ophthalmology, New England Eye Center, Tufts University School of Medicine, Boston, MA, USA

Mark Rivellese MD
Fellow, New England Eye Center, Tufts University School of Medicine, Boston, MA, USA

Patrick E Rubsamen MD
Coral Gables, FL, USA

Alan J Ruby MD
Associated Retinal Consultants, P.C., Royal Oak, MI, USA

William E Smiddy MD
Associate Professor of Ophthalmology, Bascom Palmer Eye Institute, University of Miami School of Medicine, Miami, FL, USA

Paul Sternberg Jr MD
Thomas M Aaberg Professor of Ophthalmology, and Director, Vitreoretinal Service, Emory University School of Medicine, Atlanta, GA, USA

Matthew A Thomas MD
Barnes Retina Institute, St Louis, and Associate Clinical Professor, Department of Ophthalmology and Visual Sciences, Washington University School of Medicine, St Louis, MO, USA

John T Thompson MD
Retina Specialists, Towson, Baltimore, MD, USA

Paul E Tornambe MD
Retina Consultants, LaJolla, CA, USA

Michael T Trese MD
Associated Retinal Consultants, P.C., Royal Oak, MI, USA

James D Weiland PhD
The Wilmer Eye Institute, The Johns Hopkins University School of Medicine, Baltimore, MD, USA

Robert T Wendel MD
Retinal Consultants, Sacramento, CA, USA

George A Williams MD
Associated Retinal Consultants, P.C., Royal Oak, MI, USA

Steven M Williams MD
Utica, New York, NY, USA

William J Wirostko MD
Vitreoretinal Fellow, Medical College of Wisconsin, Milwaukee, WI, USA

Preface

In the steady evolution of vitreoretinal surgical techniques, new methods appear and traditional techniques evolve. Vitreoretinal surgeons practicing today rely on the foundation of knowledge provided by early workers in the field such as Gonin, Custodis, Schepens, Machemer, and Lincoff as well as contributions by the many innovators who have followed them. Recent additions to the vitreoretinal surgeon's armamentarium include the perfluorocarbon liquids, wide-angle viewing systems, endoscopy of the vitreous cavity, transscleral diode laser, and retinal translocation. We have compiled a comprehensive array of current vitreoretinal techniques as they are applied in the 'state of the art' today by the pioneers and innovators of vitreoretinal surgery.

Authors were asked to describe the details of the surgical techniques that they currently use, not in broad strokes but in detail useful to others interested in vitreoretinal surgery. Because many equally viable approaches to similar surgical problems exist, no attempt was made to standardize techniques among chapters; in fact, we feel the variation enhances the value of this volume. We feel that this variation in surgical methods should flourish as it may provide the raw material for further evolution in the techniques. A vitreoretinal problem may often be approached by any number of different surgical techniques and the surgeon selects the method with which he or she has had the greatest success or highest comfort level. We have endeavored to present a full array of current vitreoretinal techniques, without bias, so that the reader may understand the merits of each and use this knowledge in serving patients.

This book begins with the least invasive procedures and progresses to the more invasive; anterior approaches are followed by more posterior techniques. The book begins with surgical anatomy followed by discussions of laser retinopexy, cryopexy, and diathermy. Pneumatic retinopexy and scleral buckling are then discussed, followed by multiple chapters covering the latest techniques in vitreoretinal surgery. Sections are devoted to visualization systems for vitreoretinal surgery, complications of cataract surgery, diabetic retinopathy, proliferative vitreoretinopathy, trauma, choroidal tumors, subretinal surgery, and vitrectomy in infants and children. Selected narrow topics are discussed in single chapters. The book concludes with a section describing promising new surgical techniques and some devices that are not yet routine but which may be of great benefit to patients in the future.

The value of this book lies in the quality of the authors of the selected subjects. Many of the finest surgeons in vitreoretinal surgery today have contributed chapters emphasizing their research and clinical interests. The compiling of this volume represents many lifetimes of experience and dedication to the evolution of modern vitreoretinal surgery. We are grateful for the knowledge the authors have imparted by describing their current surgical techniques.

Acknowledgments

The completion of this volume required the endurance and dedication of many people. The individual contributors purposefully form the heart and soul of this text and it is to them and their staffs that we are most deeply indebted. We have greatly enjoyed the collegiality and opportunity for exchange of ideas provided by working with such an intelligent and accomplished group of people.

Trisha Chiasson provided organization and long hours of dedicated work as our in-house medical editor. Mike Meakin, the Editor, and Susan Grant, the Production Manager, at Martin Dunitz Ltd also did a fine job of editing the book and kept the work flowing across the Atlantic. Marion Tasker, the medical illustrator, turned our rough sketches into professional artwork. We would also like to thank Alan Burgess at Martin Dunitz Ltd, the Commissioning Editor who oversaw this project.

Part I Surgical Techniques for the Treatment of Retinal Tears and Complicated Retinal Detachment

Chapter 1 Vitreoretinal surgical anatomy

Mark DJ Greve

EXTERNAL ANATOMY

ANTERIOR VIEW

Each of the extraocular muscles inserts at a different distance from the corneal limbus (Fig. 1.1a). These muscle insertions form a spiral known as the spiral of Tillaux. This is important for surgical landmarking and scleral buckling surgery.

SUPERIOR OBLIQUE INSERTION

The superior oblique muscle travels temporally under the superior rectus to its insertion 12–14 mm posterior to the limbus (Fig. 1.1b).[1] Muscle hooks should be inserted temporal to nasal to avoid engaging the superior oblique tendon.

POSTERIOR VIEW

The inferior oblique originates from the anteronasal orbital wall and courses temporally and posteriorly beneath the inferior rectus and inserts in the inferotemporal quadrant 10 mm posterior to the lateral rectus insertion (Fig. 1.1c). The ophthalmic artery gives rise to roughly 20 short posterior ciliary arteries; these along with 10 short posterior ciliary nerves enter the sclera in a ring around the optic nerve to supply the uvea. There are also two long posterior ciliary arteries and nerves that enter the sclera on either side of the optic nerve at the horizontal meridians. They run anteriorly to anastomose with short anterior ciliary arteries to form the arterial circle of the iris and ciliary body. These are often used surgically to mark the 3 and 9 o'clock meridians. There are usually seven vortex veins with at least one in each quadrant. The ampulla of the vortex vein is located just posterior to the equator and the veins exit 14–18 mm posterior to the limbus. Care must be taken to avoid damaging a vortex vein by sutures or scleral buckling material.

GLOBE ANATOMY

The adult globe is a slightly asymmetric sphere with an average axial length of 24 mm (Fig. 1.2).[1] The vertical and horizontal diameters are slightly smaller at 23 and 23.5 mm, respectively.[2,3] The radius of curvature of the cornea is steeper (8 mm) compared to the sclera (12 mm). The average corneal diameter is 10.6 mm and the depth of the anterior chamber is 3.15 mm. The pars plana, which meets the retina at the ora serrata, has a width of 4–4.5 mm.

The anatomic equator of the globe is 4.8 mm posterior to the ora serrata perpendicularly and 5.5 mm in chord length along the external scleral surface.[4,5]

The circumference of the average adult globe at the equator is 74 mm (see Fig. 1.2). The scleral arc distance from the limbus to the equator is 9–12 mm and the distance from the limbus to the posterior pole is 29–32 mm.[6]

Scleral thickness varies throughout the globe, being thinnest (0.3 mm) just posterior to the extraocular muscle insertions and thickest (1.2 mm) adjacent to the optic nerve. At the equator, the average thickness is approximately 1 mm.

VITREOUS ANATOMY

The vitreous is a clear fluid-like substance composed of greater than 99% water.[7] The viscosity and rigidity of the vitreous are the result of a mixture of type II

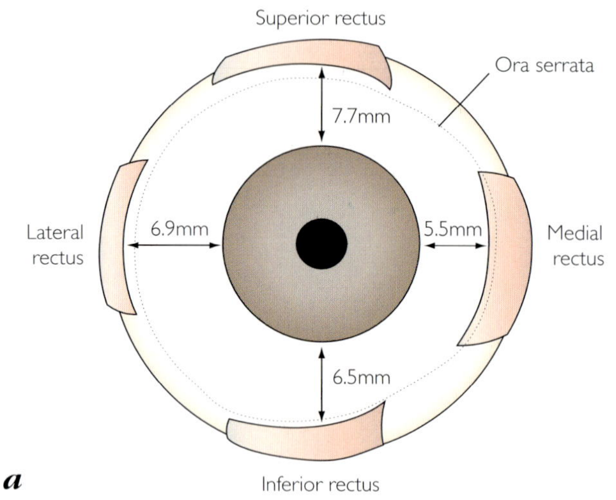

a

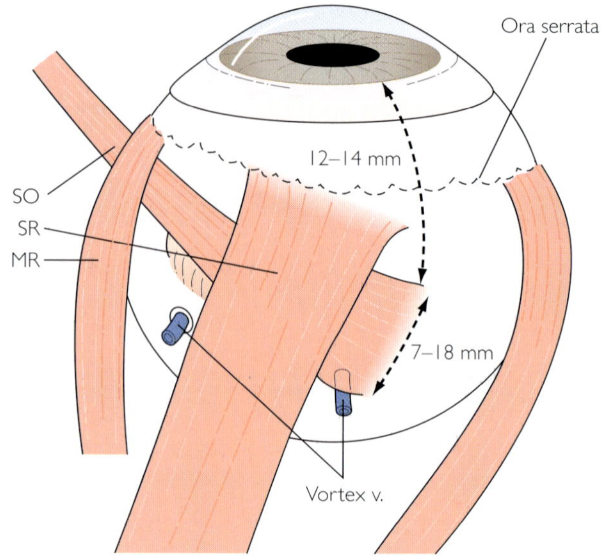

b

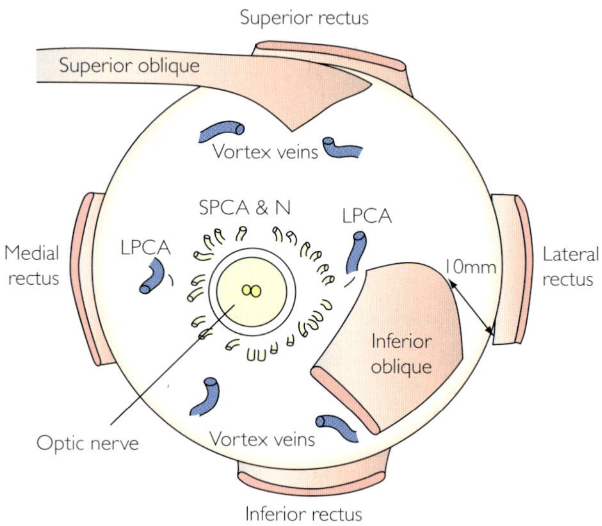

c

Figure 1.1 *(a) Anterior view of right globe demonstrating the location of the ora serrata and the spiral of Tillaux. (b) Superior view of right globe demonstrating the course and insertion of the superior oblique muscle (SO) and its relationship to the superior rectus muscle (SR); medial rectus (MR). (c) Posterior view of right globe demonstrating the scleral entry point of the short posterior ciliary arteries (SPCA) and nerves (SPCN), the long posterior ciliary arteries (LPCA), and vortex veins. The inferior oblique also inserts approximately 10 mm posterior to the lateral rectus muscle insertion.*

collagen with hyaluronic acid, glycoproteins and proteoglycans to form a delicate fibrillar meshwork.[8,9] The volume of the vitreous is approximately 4.0 ml,[10] which represents 70–80% of the volume of the globe.[7,11]

The outer, denser portion of the vitreous body is termed cortical vitreous and measures approximately 100 μm in thickness (Fig. 1.3a). The anterior hyaloid face or membrane is cortical vitreous extending anterior to the ora serrata. The anterior hyaloid is fixed firmly to the posterior peripheral lens surface by Weigert's ligament (hyaloideocapsular ligament, ligamentum pectinatum).[8,12] The potential space between the posterior lens surface and the anterior hyaloid face is termed Berger's space. The condensed posterior cortical vitreous forms the posterior hyaloidal membrane, which merges with and is indistinguishable from the internal limiting membrane.[7] The posterior hyaloid does not adhere to the optic nerve and this potential space is called the area of Martegiani. Cloquet's canal is a central tubular structure derived from primary vitreous that previously housed the hyaloidal artery.

The strongest point of attachment of the vitreous to the retina and pars plana is at the vitreous base located anteriorly (Fig. 1.3b). It extends 1.5–2 mm anterior and 2–3 mm posterior to the ora serrata. Clinically, traction of the vitreous often is exerted at the posterior margin of the vitreous base, resulting in retinal tears at this site.

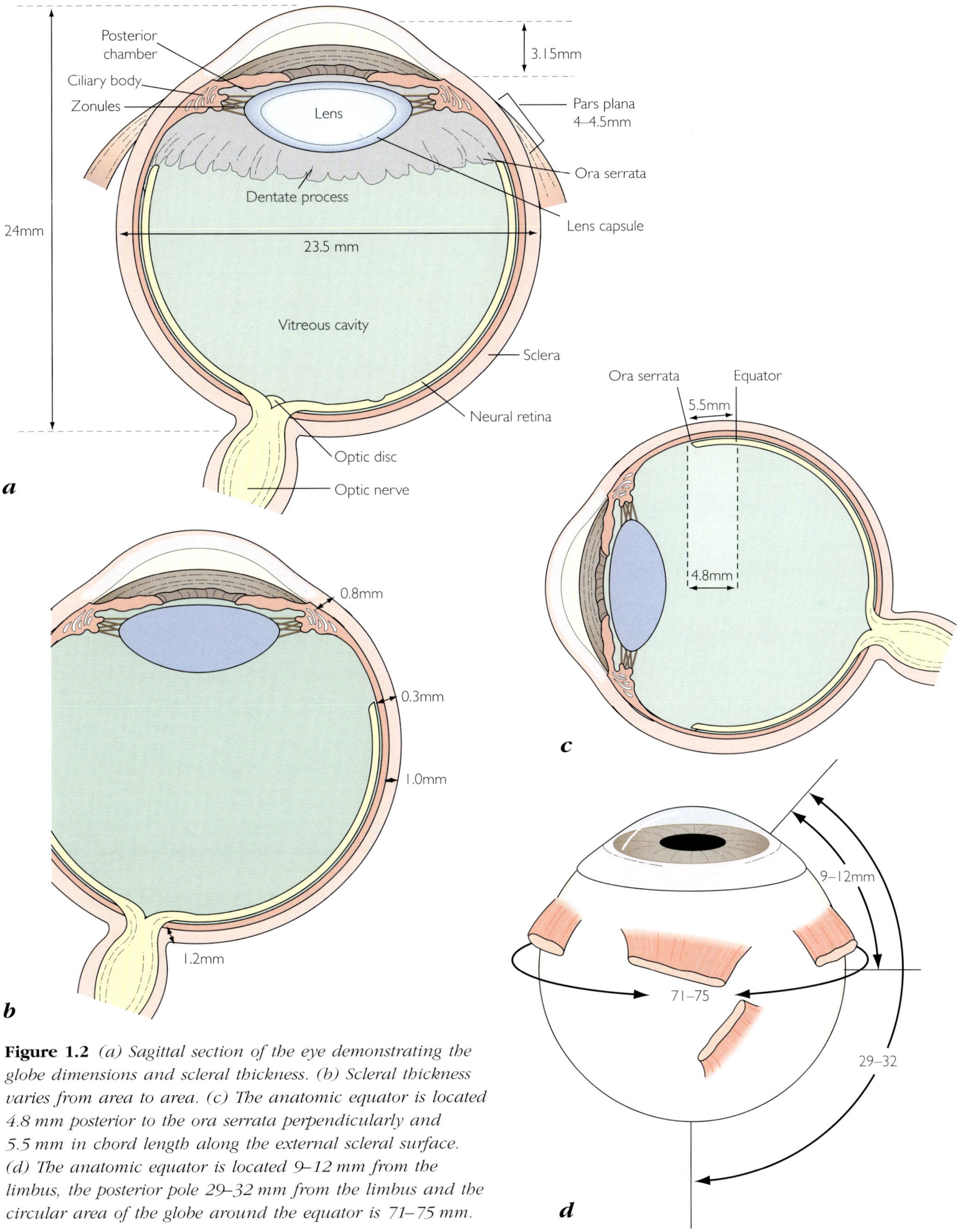

Figure 1.2 *(a) Sagittal section of the eye demonstrating the globe dimensions and scleral thickness. (b) Scleral thickness varies from area to area. (c) The anatomic equator is located 4.8 mm posterior to the ora serrata perpendicularly and 5.5 mm in chord length along the external scleral surface. (d) The anatomic equator is located 9–12 mm from the limbus, the posterior pole 29–32 mm from the limbus and the circular area of the globe around the equator is 71–75 mm.*

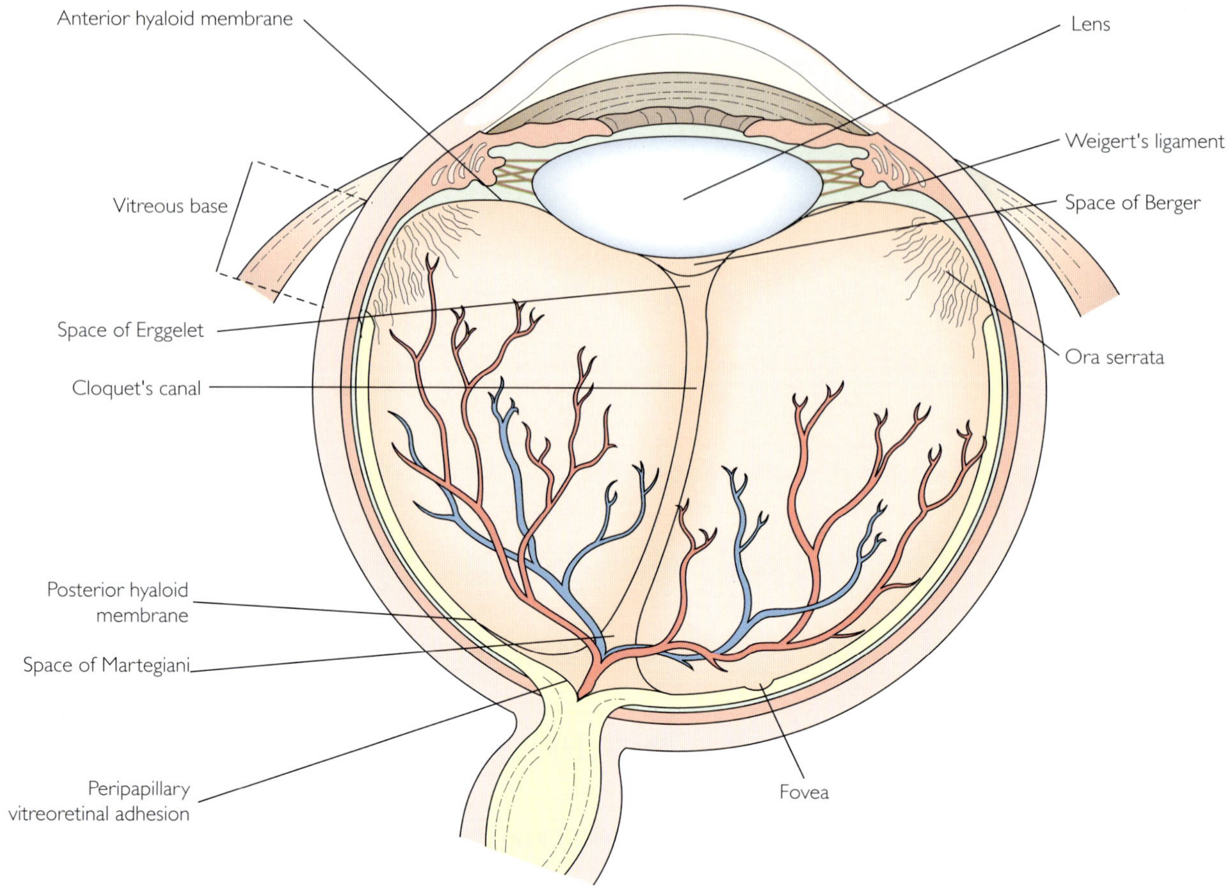

a

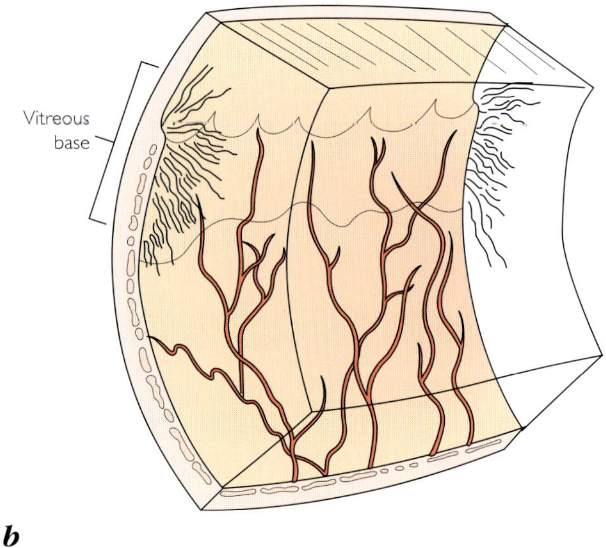

b

Figure 1.3 *(a) Sagittal section demonstrating vitreous anatomy. (b) The vitreous base extends 1.5–2 mm anterior and 2–3 mm posterior to the ora serrata and is firmly attached to the retina and pars plana.*

RETINAL ANATOMY

The neurosensory retina is composed of multiple layers of cells that sense light, partially process that information and then send it out through the optic nerve (Fig. 1.4a). The thickness of the retina varies from 0.23 mm in the paramacular region with the majority of the rest of the retina 0.1 mm thick.

Controversy exists regarding retinal nomenclature. Clinicians refer to the 6 mm area within the arcades as the posterior pole, whereas anatomists refer to it as the area centralis (Fig. 1.4b). The clinical macula or anatomic fovea is a central circular area 1.5 mm in diameter. It is centered 3.4 mm temporal to the optic disc margin and 0.8 mm below the center of the nerve head.[13] The center of the macula is the clinical fovea or anatomic foveola, measuring 350 μm in diameter. It appears in profile as a pit because of the absence of inner retinal layers.

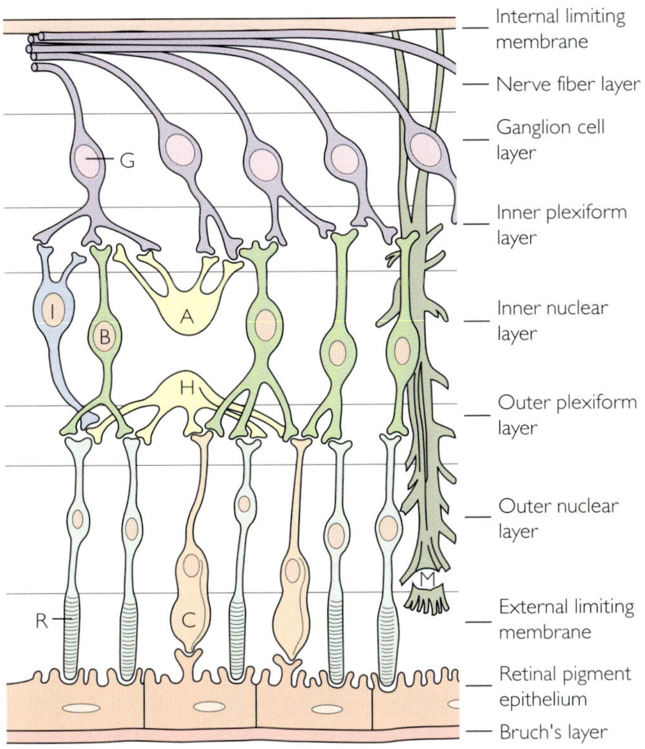

a

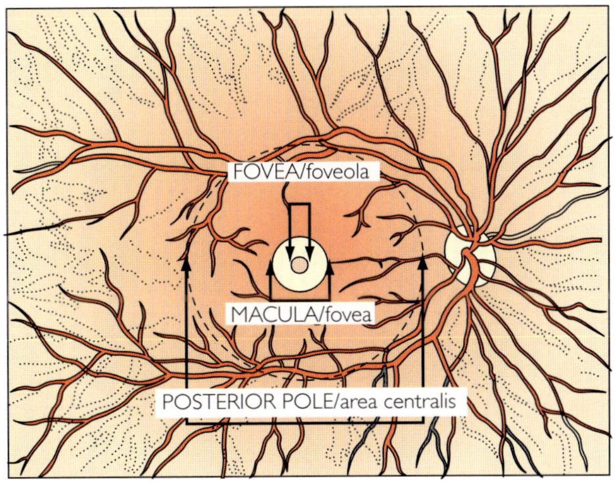

b

Figure 1.4 *(a) Cross-sectional diagram of retinal layers. The cellular components of the retina include the ganglion (G), amacrine (A), bipolar (B), inner plexiform (I), horizontal (H), Müller's cells (M), rods (R), and cones (C). (b) Anatomy of the posterior retina. Clinical terms are capitalized, anatomic terms are in lower case. Adapted with permission from Wilkinson CP, Rice TA.* Michels Retinal Detachment, *2nd edn (CV Mosby: St Louis, 1997): 21.*[6]

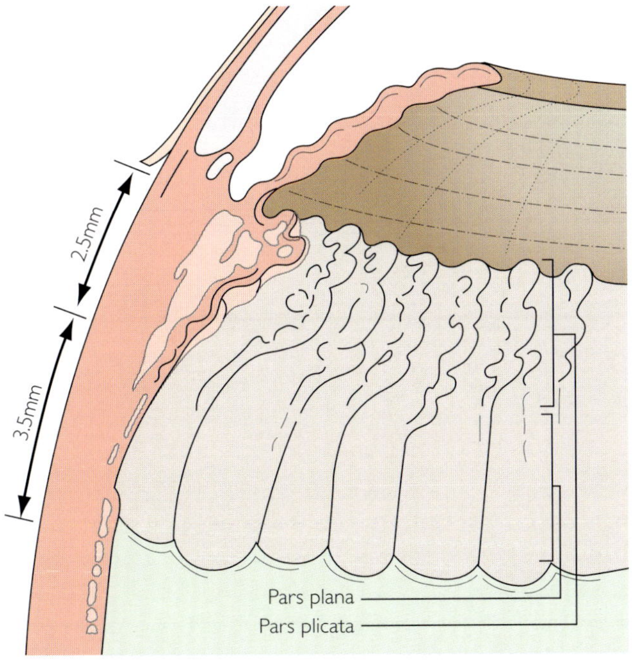

a

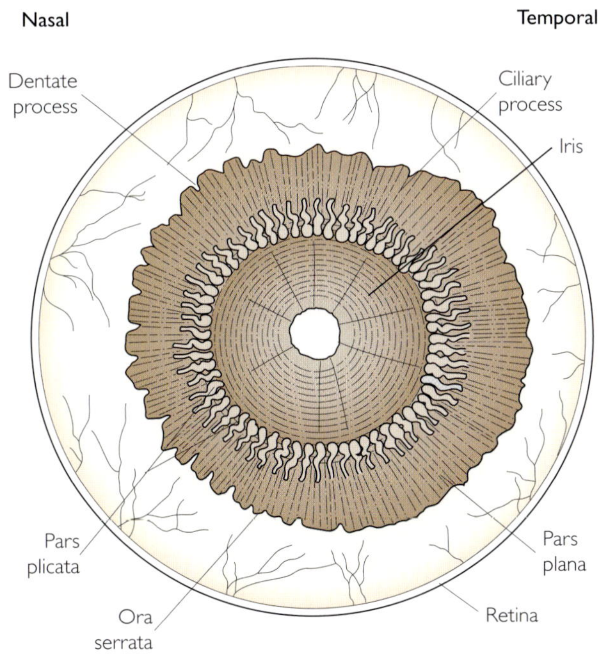

b

Figure 1.5 *(a) Ciliary body comprised of anterior pars plicata 2.5 mm in width and pars plana 3.5 mm in length. (b) Posterior view of ora serrata and ciliary body. Nasally there are 17 to 34 prominent dentate processes. Temporally the pars plicata is broader and the dentate processes less prominent. Ora bays of retina extend between the dentate processes.*

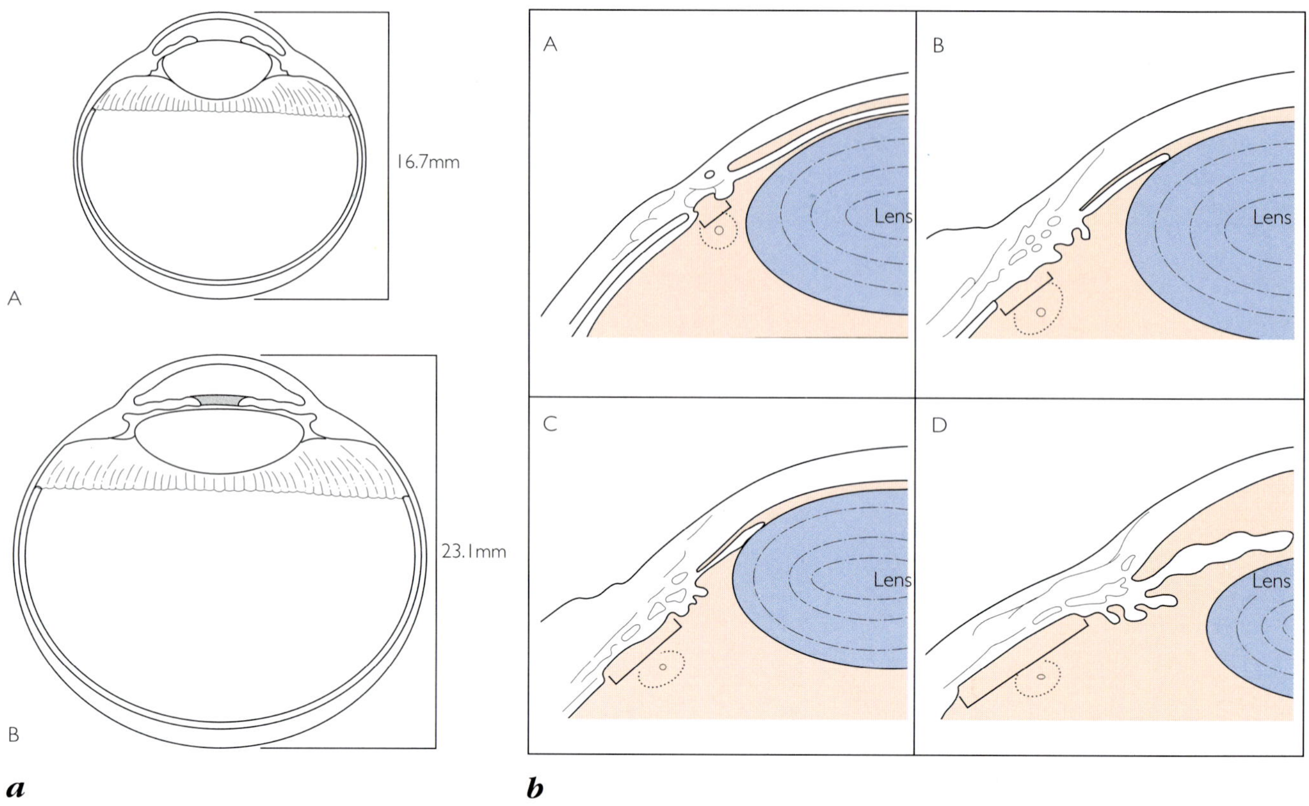

Figure 1.6 *(a) Sagittal section of infant eye (A) compared to adult eye (B). (b) Development of the pars plana. (A) Birth. (B) 6 Months. (C) 2–3 Years. (D) 6 Years.*

PARS PLANA ANATOMY

The ciliary body is composed of two parts: the pars plicata and the pars plana (Fig. 1.5a). The pars plicata extends from the iris root posteriorly approximately 2.5 mm and contains 70–80 ciliary processes that secrete aqueous humor. The pars plana portion of the ciliary body is 3 mm in width nasally and 4.5 mm temporally. The posterior portion of the pars plana meets the ora serrata and is overlapped by the vitreous base more temporally than nasally.

Sclerotomies for vitrectomy surgery or intravitreal injections are safest when placed 4.0 mm posterior to the limbus in phakic eyes and 3.5 mm posterior to the limbus in aphakic or pseudophakic eyes.[14] This allows instruments to pass through the pars plana, avoiding the pars plicata anteriorly and the vitreous base insertion posteriorly.

The ora serrata meets the pars plana with a scalloped margin (Fig. 1.5b). Nasally there are 17–34 ora bays extending between prominent dentate processes; temporally these processes are less developed.[15]

DEVELOPMENTAL AND PEDIATRIC ANATOMY

The axial length of the eye increases from 16.5 mm in a full-term infant to 24.5 mm in an adult (Fig. 1.6a). Three varying exponential growth curves are noted: from birth to 1.5 years, the axial length increases 3.8 mm; by 5 years, the axial length increases another 1.2 mm; and by age 13 years the axial length has increased another 1.44 mm to reach adult size.[16] Between 30 and 40 weeks' gestation the eye does not grow very much and is virtually the proportion of that of a full-term infant.[7]

The ciliary body at birth is fairly flat with a short pars plana and ciliary processes that are anteriorly displaced (Fig. 1.6b). The ciliary body, pars plana and retina do not attain adult proportions until age 7 years.[17]

The volume of the eye at birth is 2.4 ml, increasing to 6.9 ml in adulthood. The vitreous volume increases from 1.5 ml at birth to 4.6 ml in adulthood.[18]

The sclerotomies in a pediatric vitrectomy are placed through the pars plicata[19] to avoid the anterior insertion of the retina[17] and the creation of iatrogenic retinal breaks. The lens in an infant occupies a larger portion of the posterior segment[20] and therefore may restrict intraocular manipulation and increase the risk of mechanical damage to the lens by intraocular instruments.[7]

REFERENCES

1. Hogan MJ, Alvarado JA, Weddell JE. *Histology of the Human Eye: an Atlas and Textbook* (WB Saunders: Philadelphia, 1971): 49.
2. Last RJ, ed. *Wolff's Anatomy of the Eye and Orbit Including the Central Connections, Development, and Comparative Anatomy of the Visual Apparatus*, 6th edn (WB Saunders: Philadelphia, 1968): 30.
3. Salzmann M. *Anatomy and Histology of the Human Eyeball in its Normal State, its Development and Senescense*, Brown EVL translation (University of Chicago Press: Chicago, 1912): 3–10.
4. Straatsma BR, Landers MB, Kreiger AE. The ora serrata in the adult human eye, *Arch Ophthalmol* (1968) **80**:3–20.
5. Duke-Elder WS. *System of Ophthalmology*, Vol. II. *The Anatomy of the Visual System*. (Mosby: St Louis, 1961): 269.
6. Wilkinson CP, Rice TA. *Michels Retinal Detachment*, 2nd edn (CV Mosby: St Louis, 1997): 2, 21.
7. Peyman GA, Schulman JA. *Intravitreal Surgery: Principles and Practice*, 2nd edn (Appleton & Lange: Norwalk, CT, 1994): 1.
8. Sebag J. Structure, function, and age-related changes of the human vitreous. In: Schepens CL, Neetens A, eds, *The Vitreous and Vitreoretinal Interface* (Springer-Verlag: New York, 1987): 37–57.
9. Swann DA. Biochemistry of the vitreous. In: Schepens CL, Neetens A, eds, *The Vitreous and Vitreoretinal Interface* (Springer-Verlag: New York, 1987): 59–72.
10. Tolentino FI, Schepens CL, Freeman HM. *Vitreoretinal Disorders: Diagnosis and Management* (WB Saunders: Philadelphia, 1976): 25–109.
11. Reeser FH, Aaberg TM. Vitreous humor. In: Records RE, ed, *Physiology of the Human Eye and Visual System* (Harper & Row: Hagerstown, MD, 1979): 261.
12. Spencer WH. Vitreous. In: Spencer WH, ed, *Ophthalmic Pathology: an Atlas and Textbook*, Vol. 2, 3rd edn (WB Saunders: Philadelphia, 1985–86): 548–88.
13. Sigelman J, Ozamis V. Retina. In: Duane TD, Jaeger EA, eds, *Biomedical Foundations of Ophthalmology*, Vol. 1 (JB Lippincott: Philadelphia, 1988): 5.
14. Gross JG, Freeman WR, Goldbaum MH, Mendez TL. Useful adjuncts for vitreoretinal surgery, *Br J Ophthalmol* (1989) **73**:435–9.
15. Duke-Elder S. *System of Ophthalmology*, Vol.II, *The Anatomy of the Visual System* (Mosby: St Louis, 1961): 223.
16. Larsen JS. The sagittal growth of the eye. IV. Ultrasonic measurement of the axial length of the eye from birth to puberty, *Acta Ophthalmol* (1971) **49**:873–86.
17. Peyman GA, Raichand M, Goldberg MF. Surgery of congenital and juvenile cataracts: a pars plicata approach with the vitrophage. *Br J Ophthalmol* (1978) **62**:780–3.
18. Mann I. *The Development of the Human Eye* (Grune & Stratton: New York, 1964): 150, 201.
19. Maguire AM, Trese MT. Lens-sparing vitreoretinal surgery in infants, *Arch Ophthalmol* (1992) **110**:284–6.
20. Apple DJ, Nauman GOH. General anatomy and development of the eye: Techniques of investigation. In: Nauman GOH, ed, *Pathology of the Eye* (Springer-Verlag: New York, 1986): 1–18.

Chapter 2 Retinal breaks

Charles C Barr

INTRODUCTION

A retinal break may be defined as any full-thickness defect in the retina. When retinal breaks occur in the presence of vitreous traction, retinal detachment may result, making identification of retinal breaks associated with vitreous traction important. In the peripheral retina, tears, holes and dialyses are the most commonly observed retinal breaks. A flap or horseshoe tear is almost always the result of vitreous traction. The horseshoe points toward the optic disc; the vitreous is attached to the elevated flap. Round holes may be either atrophic or operculated. An operculum is a piece of retinal tissue that has been pulled free from the retina by vitreous traction and usually can be seen in the vitreous cavity over the resultant defect. Even though the operculum is free, there may still be traction around the hole. Round atrophic holes are felt to be the result of dissolution of retinal tissue, rather than the result of vitreous traction, and thus differ from operculated holes and flaps or horseshoe retinal tears (Fig. 2.1). Retinal dialyses are often the result of blunt trauma. Lattice degeneration (Fig. 2.2) is an atrophic change in the peripheral retina, often associated with both atrophic retinal holes and retinal traction.[1]

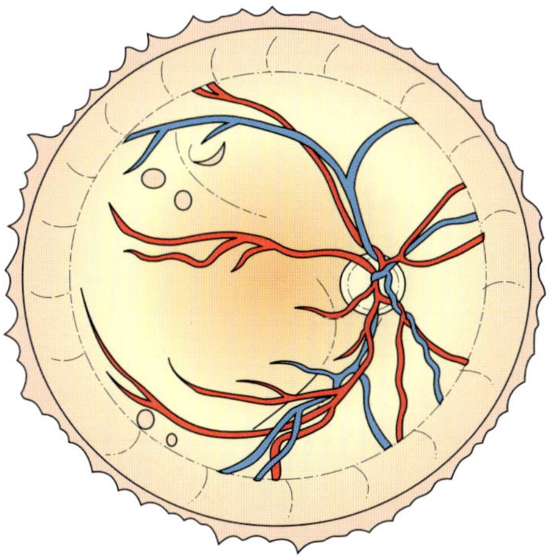

Figure 2.1 *Flap tear and operculated retinal break superiorly. Atrophic round holes inferiorly.*

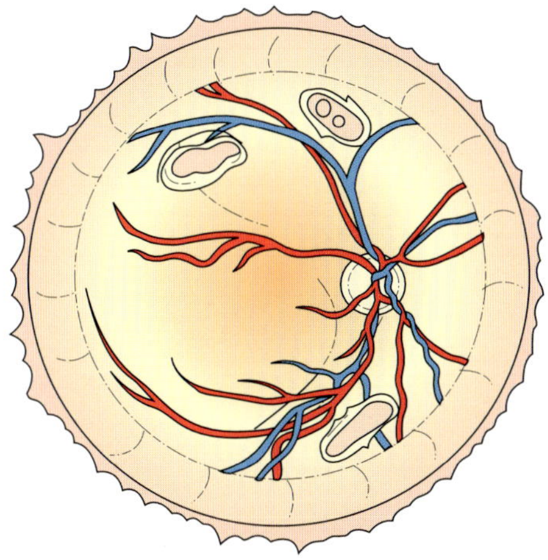

a

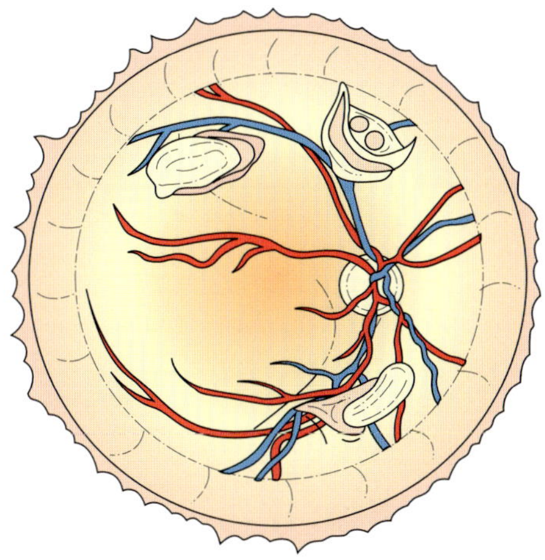

b

Figure 2.2 *(a) Peripheral lattice degeneration which often appears as white lines anterior to the equator. (b) Retinal breaks associated with lattice degeneration also occur at the edges of lattice degeneration where the retina is thinnest.*

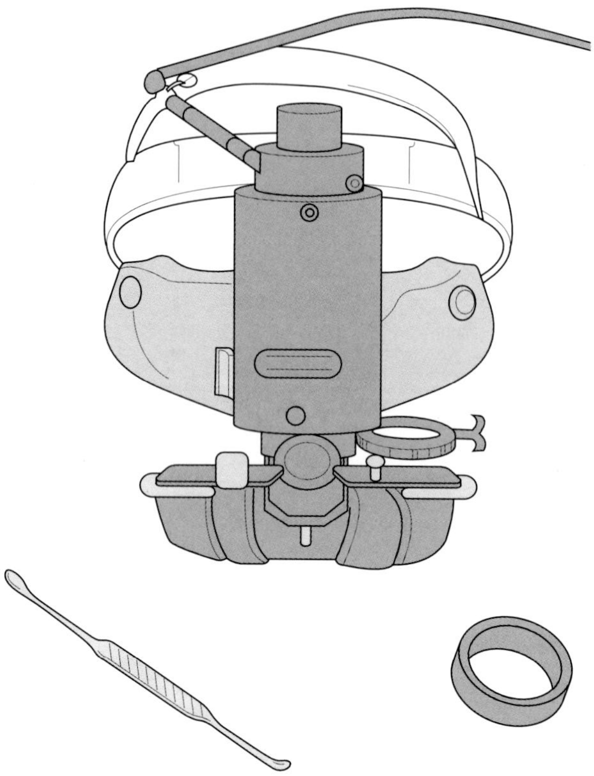

Figure 2.3 *The indirect ophthalmoscope (top) as popularized by Schepens. Scleral indentor (left) and condensing lens (right).*

Prophylactic treatment of retinal breaks to prevent retinal detachment was rarely performed until Schepens popularized the use of the indirect ophthalmoscope more than 40 years ago. The use of the indirect ophthalmoscope (Fig. 2.3) led to better examination of the peripheral retina and increased detection of retinal breaks in the attached retina. With the subsequent development of cryotherapy and photocoagulation, treatment of retinal breaks in the absence of retinal detachment became more widespread.

However, studies of the natural history of retinal breaks in attached retina have demonstrated that only a minority of these lesions require treatment. Clinical and autopsy studies have shown that retinal breaks and lattice degeneration are common, occurring in 5–10% of the general population.[2] However, retinal detachment is uncommon; in a French study, only 0.005% of the general population developed retinal detachment.[3] The prevalence of retinal breaks is obviously much greater than the incidence of retinal detachment, and because the treatment of retinal breaks may be associated with complications, only those breaks more likely to result in retinal detachment should be treated prophylactically.

INDICATIONS

Asymptomatic retinal breaks have a different prognosis than symptomatic retinal breaks. The best studies of asymptomatic retinal breaks have been performed by Byer.[4–8] In separate reports, he described the natural history of both asymptomatic retinal breaks and lattice degeneration. He followed 235 eyes of 196 patients with asymptomatic retinal breaks for 1–33 years; almost 60% had more than 10 years of follow-up. Of 172 eyes with round holes without an operculum, only one progressed to a clinical retinal detachment, and of 32 eyes with asymptomatic operculated breaks, none developed retinal detachment. Also, most eyes with asymptomatic flap tears did not progress, but most of these patients were young and did not have posterior vitreous detachment (PVD). If PVD did occur, there was no tendency for pre-existing breaks to lead to retinal detachment, but several of the patients developed new flap tears at the time of PVD, which were treated. Byer also followed 423 eyes of 276 patients with asymptomatic lattice degeneration and found that less than 1% progressed, indicating that this lesion does not require prophylactic treatment to prevent retinal detachment.[5]

Several studies have demonstrated that symptomatic retinal breaks are more likely to lead to retinal detachment than asymptomatic breaks detected during a routine examination.[7,9,10] Symptomatic retinal breaks are often the result of vitreoretinal traction (Fig. 2.4). The two most important symptoms associated with vitreoretinal traction are photopsia or 'flashing lights' and entopsia or 'floaters'. Photopsia is caused by the discharge of neural impulses from the peripheral retina as the result of the mechanical force of the vitreous gel on the anterior retina. Entopsia may result from either PVD or bleeding into the vitreous cavity from retinal tears. All patients with photopsia or entopsia should undergo dilated examination of the peripheral fundus to rule out the presence of retinal breaks. Of patients with symptomatic posterior vitreous detachment 8–10% will develop retinal tears, so a thorough vitreoretinal examination should be performed on all these patients.[11]

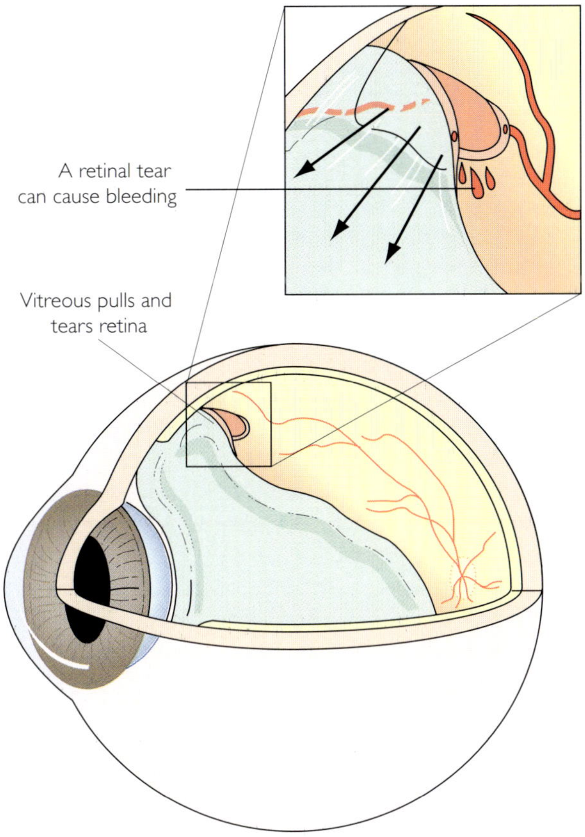

Figure 2.4 *Vitreous traction on the peripheral retina results in tearing of the retina and often intraocular bleeding. The traction is on the flap of the horseshoe retinal tear.*

In general, symptomatic retinal breaks should be treated prophylactically to prevent retinal detachment, whereas asymptomatic retinal breaks may be observed safely. Guidelines for treatment in different clinical situations can be found in Table 2.1.

Certain conditions may increase the asymptomatic patient's risk of developing retinal detachment. The family history is positive in 4% of patients with retinal detachment.[12] If a patient has more than 6 diopters of myopia, there is a 2% incidence of retinal detachment, and 35% of patients with retinal detachment are myopic.[13–15] Aphakia and pseudophakia are also associated with retinal detachment.[10] In the days before intraocular lenses, up to 5% of aphakic patients developed retinal detachment. In pseudophakic patients with an intact posterior capsule, the rate of retinal detachment is much less, of the order of 0.3–0.5%. However, if the posterior capsule is ruptured, or if the patient undergoes YAG-laser capsulotomy, the rate rises to 1–2%. Although definitive data are lacking, I recommend that patients with asymptomatic flap or horseshoe tears receive prophylactic treatment before cataract surgery or YAG-laser capsulotomy. Asymptomatic round or operculated holes may be observed safely in these patients.

The natural history study of Davis et al[16] demonstrated that fellow eyes of patients who have had a retinal detachment in one eye also have an increased risk of developing retinal detachment. A more recent study by Folk and associates[17] found that untreated fellow eyes with lattice degeneration had a 5% risk of retinal detachment, whereas treated eyes had a 2%

Table 2.1 Treatment guideline for retinal breaks

Type of break	*Phakic*	*Aphakic/ pseudophakic*	*Highly myopic*	*Fellow eye*
Horseshoe, symptomatic	Treat all	Treat all	Treat all	Treat all
Horseshoe, asymptomatic	Observe	Treat some	Treat some	Treat all
Operculated, symptomatic	Treat some	Treat all	Treat all	Treat all
Operculated, asymptomatic	Observe	Observe	Treat few	Observe
Round hole, asymptomatic	Observe	Observe	Observe	Treat some?
Lattice	Observe	Observe	Observe	Treat some unless lattice
Lattice with round holes	Observe	Observe	Observe	>6 clock-hours
References	*4–11*	*10*	*13–15*	*16,17*

Table 2.2 Risk factors for retinal detachment (RD)

Condition	*Risk*
Fellow eye	10% Incidence of RD
Lattice	Cause of 20% of all RD
High myopia	2–4% Develop RD
Cataract surgery	1–2% Develop RD
Family history	Positive in 4% of patients with RD
Marfan's syndrome	9% Will develop RD
Trauma	Increased risk of RD in boxers
Glaucoma	4–7% Of patients with a RD have open-angle glaucoma

risk. Although they did not recommend either treatment or observation of fellow eyes, they did find that eyes with more than 6 clock-hours of lattice degeneration or more than 6 diopters of myopia may fare worse with treatment.

Eyes that have suffered blunt or sharp trauma are at increased risk for retinal detachment, as are eyes with glaucoma. Once again, prospective data are lacking, but 4–7% of patients with retinal detachment have glaucoma.[12] Miotic therapy also is associated anecdotally with retinal detachment. For these reasons, I recommend treatment of asymptomatic flap tears in glaucoma patients, but asymptomatic round holes, operculated holes and lattice degeneration may be observed safely in the reliable patient.

Conditions that may increase the patient's risk of retinal detachment are listed in Table 2.2. If any patients with the conditions in Table 2.2 develop a *symptomatic* break, they should be treated promptly, as indicated in the preceding paragraphs. Patients with risk factors for retinal detachment listed in Table 2.2 should be educated about symptoms of vitreoretinal traction and the need for prompt vitreoretinal examination if symptoms of photopsia and/or entopsia should occur.

Some patients with peripheral vitreoretinal pathology may develop subclinical retinal detachments as a result of retinal breaks and vitreoretinal traction. Subclinical retinal detachments are defined as the presence of subretinal fluid extending more than one disc diameter from the retinal break but no more than two disc diameters posterior to the equator. Although Davis found that 30% of these patients developed clinical detachment,[9] Byer feels that they may be observed safely.[6] I recommend prophylactic treatment of all symptomatic subclinical retinal detachments, and I am more likely to treat the more extensive asymptomatic ones. If patients develop recurrent subretinal fluid following otherwise successful scleral buckling surgery no greater in extent than described above for subclinical retinal detachments, timely photocoagulation is often effective in limiting the spread of this fluid. Treatment is performed in the same manner as treatment of retinal breaks without detachment (see below).

Other clinical conditions, such as cytomegalic inclusion retinitis and acute retinal necrosis, are associated with a high incidence of retinal detachment. In these patients, small areas of retinal detachment may be 'walled off' with photocoagulation or cryotherapy. Alternatively, panretinal photocoagulation, applied in a manner similar to that used for proliferative diabetic retinopathy, may be used in an attempt to prevent retinal detachment from encroaching on the macular area.[18]

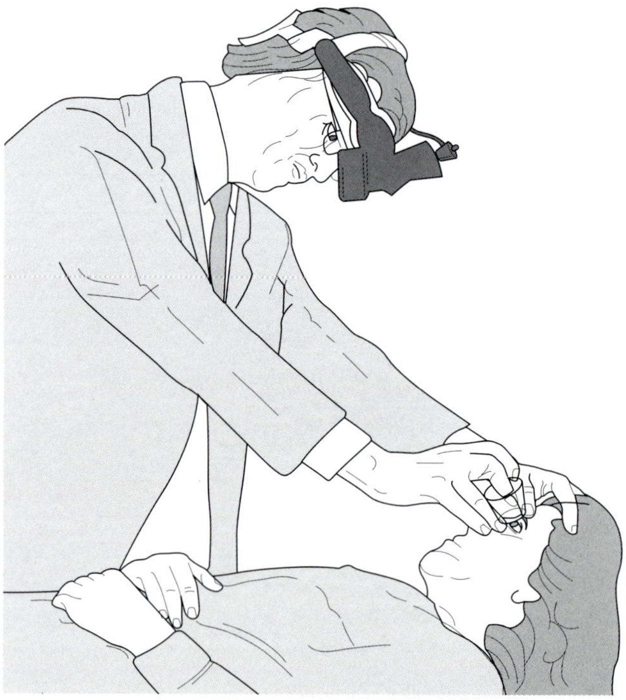

Figure 2.5 *The examiner uses the indirect ophthalmoscope at a good working distance. Scleral depression is usually performed with a cotton-tipped applicator.*

PREOPERATIVE EVALUATION

Careful ophthalmoscopic examination of the patient at risk will ensure that all retinal breaks are identified. The patient should be educated as to the importance of the examination of the peripheral retina, and the pupil must be fully dilated. Although superior breaks are more common, the entire fundus, both superior and inferior, must be inspected. The examination room must be darkened, and effort should be made to make both the patient and the doctor as comfortable as possible. I prefer to use the indirect ophthalmoscope with scleral depression to identify peripheral retinal breaks (Fig. 2.5). The use of a three-mirror lens or other panfunduscopic lens is acceptable, but the entire peripheral retina from equator to ora serrata should be visualized. The examination may take 20–45 minutes, and cannot be rushed.

SURGICAL TECHNIQUE

The purpose of prophylactic treatment of retinal breaks is to prevent retinal detachment and is usually accomplished by creating a chorioretinal scar around the peripheral retinal pathology so that the retina will not separate from the underlying pigment epithelium. Once a retinal break or breaks in attached retina that need treatment have been identified, cryotherapy or photocoagulation in an outpatient setting is usually most appropriate. I prefer laser photocoagulation at the slit lamp to treat most retinal breaks. Although there is little difference in the final result from different wavelengths of laser light (blue-green, green, dye yellow, krypton or diode), I prefer argon green because of its lower potential for interaction with the lens and xanthochromic tissues. Topical anesthesia is generally sufficient but I do not hesitate to use retrobulbar anesthesia if the patient requires it. I prefer the Rodenstock lens, but three-mirror and quadraspheric lenses are equally acceptable. The surgeon should use the lens with which he or she is most comfortable, and which allows visualization of the peripheral retinal break. It is often useful to identify a retinal landmark, such as a retinal vessel or pigment spot, with the indirect ophthalmoscope before photocoagulation.

I start with a 200 µm spot size with the Rodenstock lens, because this gives me a retinal burn of approximately 400 µm. With the Goldmann three-mirror lens, I use a 500 µm spot size. I usually start at 200 mW of power for 0.1 second, and then adjust the power to produce a gray-white burn. The patient will often experience mild pain with this peripheral photocoagulation. Peripheral retinal breaks should be treated with two or three rows of burns placed 1–2 burn-widths apart (Figs 2.6, 2.7 and 2.8). Confluent burns are not necessary. Care should be taken to use

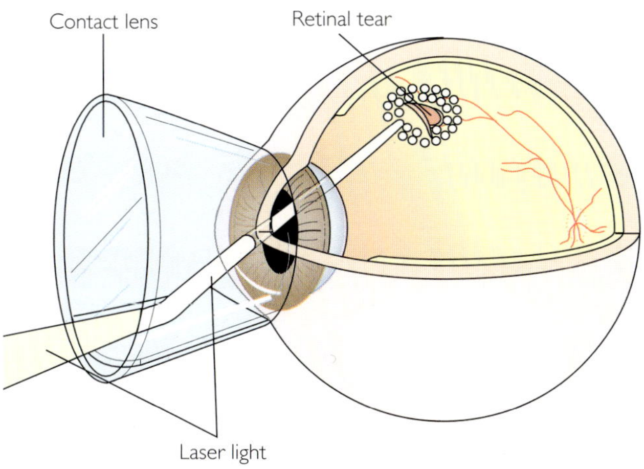

Figure 2.6 *The three-mirror lens or other panfunduscopic lens is used to photocoagulate the retina around a peripheral retinal break.*

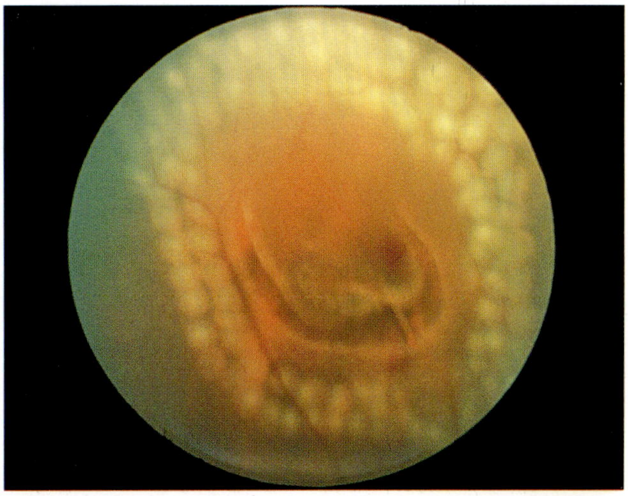

Figure 2.7 *Appearance of a retinal break immediately after photocoagulation treatment.*

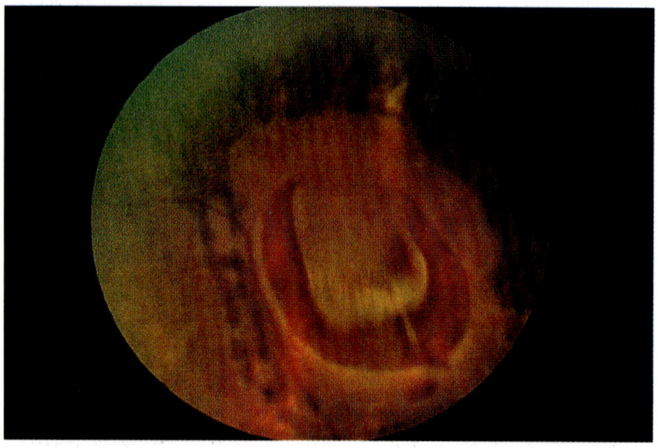

Figure 2.8 *Appearance of the same retinal break two weeks after photocoagulation treatment. Note pigmentation of the photocoagulation burns.*

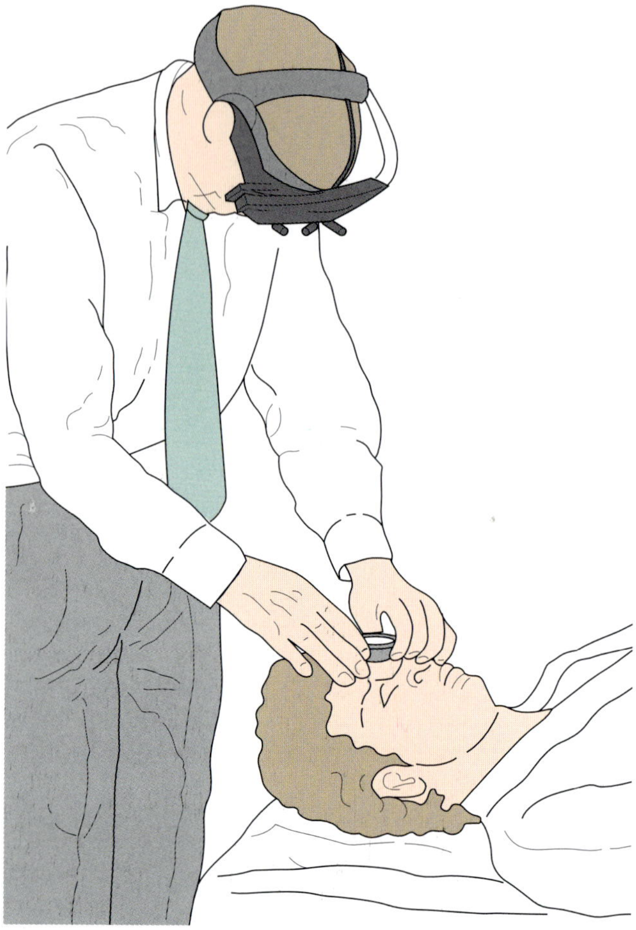

Figure 2.9 *The laser indirect ophthalmoscope is used in a manner very similar to the use of the indirect ophthalmoscope with scleral depression. The intensity of the photocoagulation burns depends on head position, working distance, and laser power.*

the least amount of power necessary, because excessive power can lead to complications such as hemorrhage, rupture of Bruch's membrane and macular pucker. Scleral depression may be necessary for more peripheral breaks. At completion of photocoagulation at the slit lamp, I frequently check the peripheral retina with the indirect ophthalmoscope to ensure that the treatment is adequate. Most patients will tolerate this procedure quite well, and postoperative medications are rarely necessary.

If the retinal breaks are too peripheral for photocoagulation at the slit lamp, the ophthalmic surgeon may employ the alternatives of photocoagulation with the laser indirect ophthalmoscope (LIO) or cryotherapy. In using the LIO, topical anesthesia is usually adequate and the same power settings are used initially. The power density of the laser burns will depend to a large degree on the variables of head position, condensing lens, working distance and lens tilt. As with the slit-lamp delivery system, treatment becomes easier with experience. The photocoagulation should completely surround the break or extend to the ora serrata. It is easier to perform scleral depression with the LIO than at the slit lamp (Fig. 2.9).

Cryotherapy is an alternative method of treating retinal breaks. Laboratory studies have shown that there is little difference in the strength of the chorioretinal scar created by laser photocoagulation and that created by cryotherapy.[19] Because cryotherapy does not have to pass through the ocular media in the same way that a laser beam does, it is particularly useful in patients with hazy media or cataracts. It is also useful in treating more peripheral retinal breaks that cannot be visualized easily at the slit lamp with contact lenses. A variety of probe tips and cryotherapy machines are available; most are gas operated. The surgeon should be certain that the shaft of the probe is insulated, and that it is freezing well before usage (Fig. 2.10).

The majority of retinal surgeons use the indirect ophthalmoscope to visualize the location of the probe tip in relation to the retinal break (Fig. 2.11),

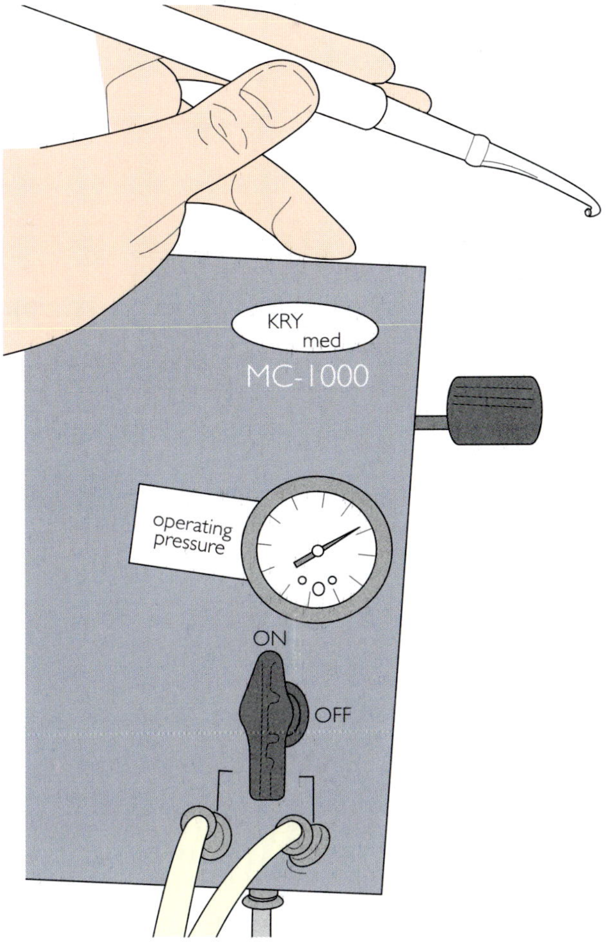

Figure 2.10 *The cryoprobe should be checked before use to make certain that there is sufficient gas pressure in the cryo tanks to perform treatment.*

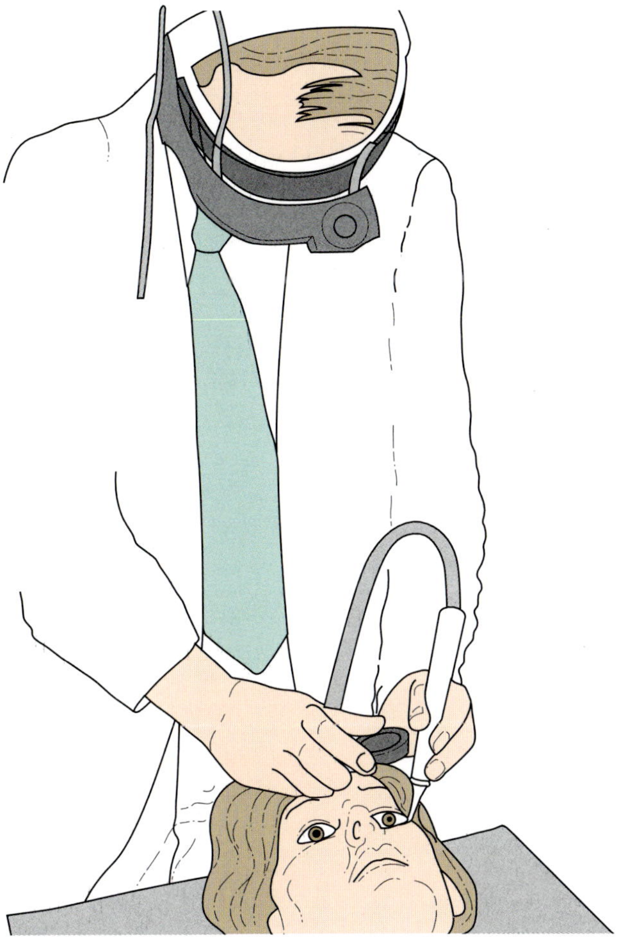

Figure 2.11 *The indirect ophthalmoscope is used to visualize the retinal break while the cryo probe is used to depress the peripheral retina.*

but many European surgeons use a three-mirror lens with the operating microscope or slit lamp to localize the probe tip (Fig. 2.12).

In general, patients require subconjunctival anesthesia for cryotherapy. I usually try to inject 0.2–0.3 ml of 2% or 4% Xylocaine into the subconjunctival space over the retinal break with a 30-gauge needle and a tuberculin syringe before commencing cryotherapy (Fig. 2.13). After a period of 10–15 minutes, sufficient anesthesia is achieved and treatment may proceed.

The probe is positioned over the retinal break by placing it on the external ocular surface; conjunctival incisions are rarely necessary (Fig. 2.14). Breaks that are two disc diameters or smaller may be treated by placing the probe tip directly under the break. The probe is activated, and then deactivated when all of the retina around the break has been frozen. Prolonged freezing is to be avoided, because this disperses pigment epithelial cells into the vitreous cavity and may lead to preretinal fibrosis and traction. For larger breaks, the probe is placed to the side of the break and a series of freezes are placed around the circumference of the break, care being taken to avoid over-freezing. It is not necessary to treat in the center of the break itself as long as the healthy tissue

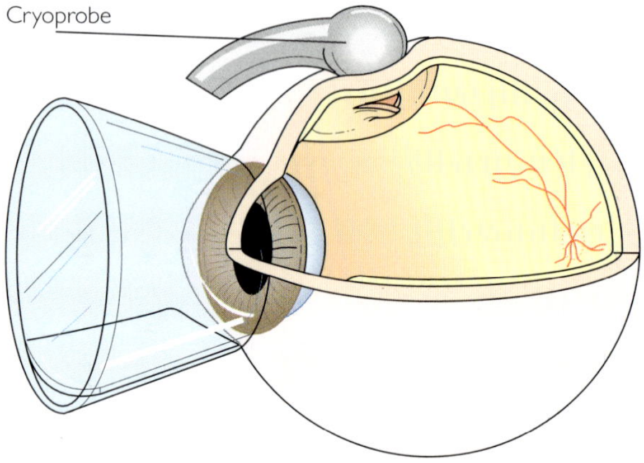

Figure 2.12 *Instead of the indirect ophthalmoscope, a three-mirror lens may also be used either at the slit lamp or at the operating microscope.*

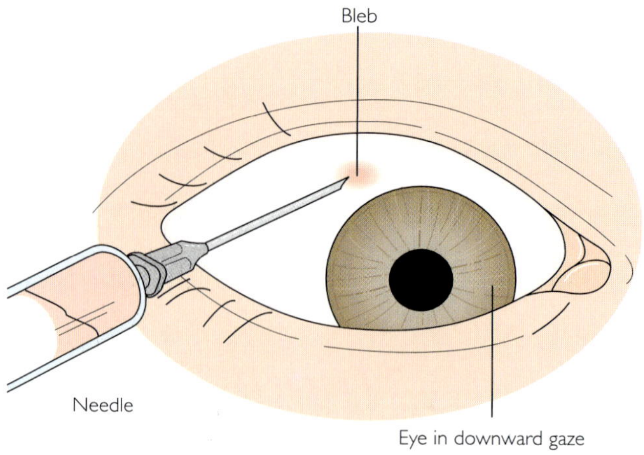

Figure 2.13 *A small bleb of subconjunctival anesthesia is injected with a 30-gauge needle over the region of the retinal break.*

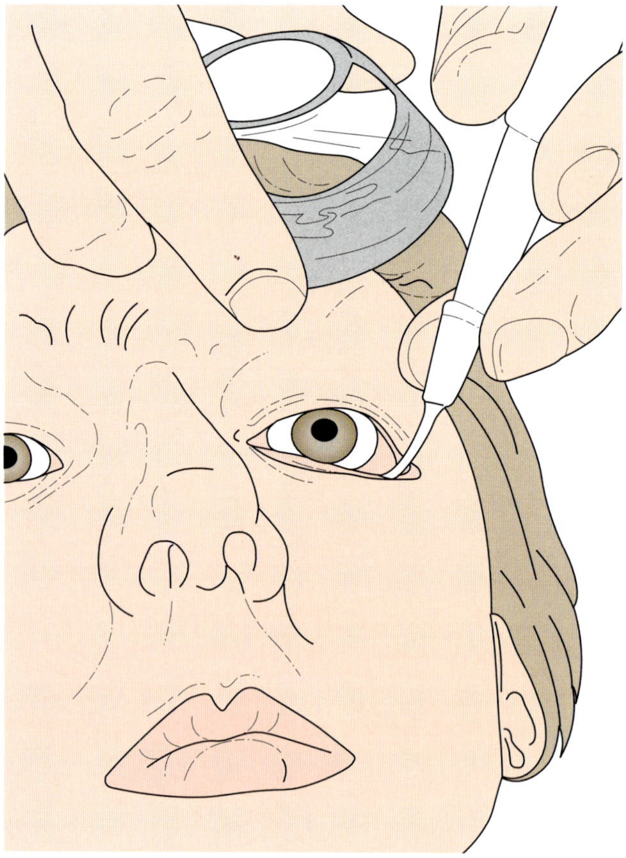

Figure 2.14 *The cryoprobe is placed in the conjunctival cul de sac. The shaft of the cryoprobe may be used to retract the lid if it is well insulated. However, the use of a lid speculum is preferred.*

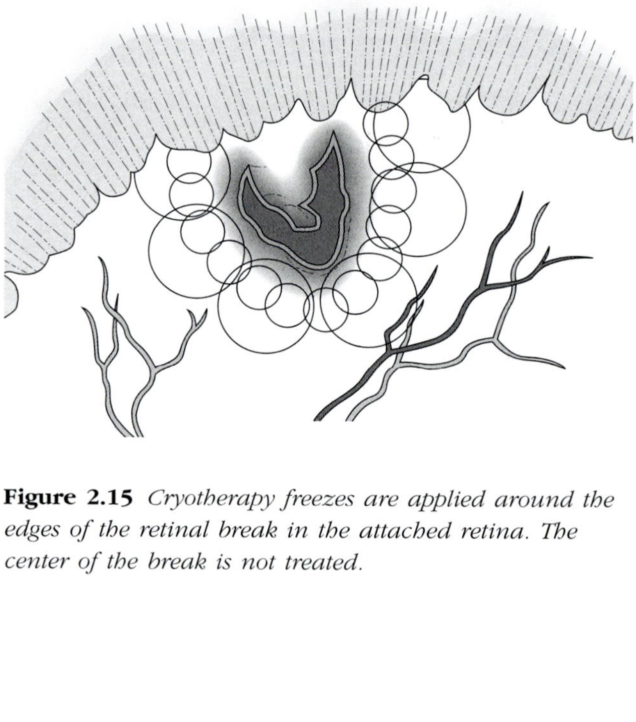

Figure 2.15 *Cryotherapy freezes are applied around the edges of the retinal break in the attached retina. The center of the break is not treated.*

around the break has been treated (Fig. 2.15). Cryotherapy in the center of larger breaks serves no useful purpose and, once again, leads to dispersion of pigment epithelial cells into the vitreous cavity. Postoperative medications are rarely necessary, but I often apply antibiotic ointment and patch the treated eye for 24 hours.

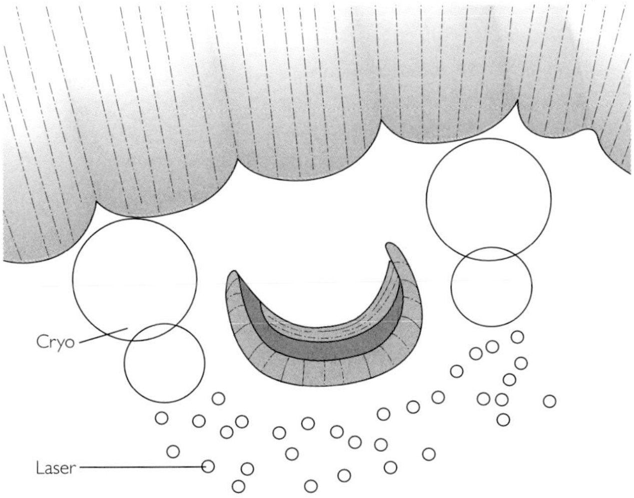

Figure 2.16 *A combination of cryotherapy freezes anteriorly and photocoagulation burns posteriorly may be used if a laser indirect ophthalmoscope is not available to complete photocoagulation therapy.*

Although most retinal breaks can be treated with either photocoagulation or cryotherapy, some breaks will require a combination of these two treatment modalities. I often treat the posterior portion of these breaks with photocoagulation, and then finish the treatment by placing cryotherapy freezes at the anterior edges of the photocoagulation (Fig. 2.16). This combination of laser and cryotherapy is particularly useful if the LIO is not available.

COMPLICATIONS AND POSTOPERATIVE CARE

Complications of treatment itself, such as corneal abrasion, subconjunctival hemorrhage and intraocular hemorrhage are rare, but require recognition and management. If intraocular hemorrhage occurs during treatment, whether from the choroid or retina, the surgeon should apply pressure to the eye by pushing on the eye with the contact lens or scleral depressor. Once the bleeding has stopped, photocoagulation may be applied around the area of bleeding or to the retinal vessel. Complications that occur after photocoagulation or cryotherapy of retinal breaks are not infrequent, and both the ophthalmologist and the patient must be aware of the need for continued follow-up care. New tears occur in approximately 10% of patients, and 5% will progress to clinical retinal detachment.[20,21] Macular pucker and epiretinal membranes occur in up to 5% of patients. In the recent study by Smiddy and associates, 22% of 171 patients who underwent prophylactic treatment of retinal breaks needed further treatment.[22] The reasons for further treatment included inadequate closure of the original retinal break, new breaks without detachment and retinal detachment caused by either the original retinal break or a new break. These authors emphasized the need for continued follow-up in all patients undergoing prophylactic therapy of retinal breaks. I routinely see uncomplicated patients at 1 week, 3 weeks, 3 months and 1 year after treatment. If new symptoms arise, or if rctreatment becomes necessary, more frequent visits are warranted.

EQUIPMENT NEEDS

- Cryoprobe
- Laser and slit lamp or laser indirect ophthalmoscope
- Indirect ophthalmoscope
- Condensing (20- and 28-diopter) lenses for indirect ophthalmoscope
- Lid speculum
- Topical anesthetic
- Local anesthetic for injection (2 or 4% Xylocaine without epinephrine)
  - Tuberculin syringe
  - 30-Gauge needles
- Mydriatic drops (Tropicamide 1% or Cyclopentolate 1%)
- Contact lenses for use with laser
  - Rodenstock
  - Goldmann three-mirror
  - Panfunduscopic
- Scleral depressor
- Eye pads, steroid–antibiotic ointment, adhesive tape.

REFERENCES

1. Foos RY. Retinal holes, *Am J Ophthalmol* (1978) **86**:354–8.
2. Foos RY. Tears of the peripheral retina: pathogenesis, incidence, and classification in autopsy eyes, *Mod Prob Ophthalmol* (1975) **15**:68–81.
3. Haut J, Massin M. Fréquence des decollements de retine dans la population française: pourcentage des decollements bilateraux, *Arch Ophtalmol (Paris)* (1975) **35**:533–6.
4. Byer NE. Prognosis of asymptomatic retinal breaks, *Arch Ophthalmol* (1974) **92**:208–10.
5. Byer NE. Long-term natural history of lattice degeneration of the retina, *Ophthalmology* (1989) **96**:1396–402.
6. Byer NE. The natural history of asymptomatic retinal breaks, *Ophthalmology* (1982) **89**:1033–9.
7. Byer NE. Natural history of posterior vitreous detachment with early management as the premier line of defense against retinal detachment, *Ophthalmology* (1994) **101**:1503–14.
8. Byer NE. What happens to asymptomatic retinal breaks?, *Ophthalmology* (1998) **105**:1045–50.
9. Davis MD. Natural history of retinal breaks without detachment, *Arch Ophthalmol* (1974) **92**:183–94.
10. Friedman Z, Neumann E, Hyams S. Vitreous and peripheral retina in aphakia: a study of 200 non-myopic aphakic eyes, *Br J Ophthalmol* (1973) **57**:52–7.
11. Lindner B. Acute posterior vitreous detachment and its retinal complications, *Acta Ophthalmol* (1977) **87** (Suppl):1.
12. Duke-Elder A, Dobree JH. *System of Ophthalmology*, Vol. X, *Diseases of the Retina* (Mosby: St Louis, 1967): 778–856.
13. Neumann E, Hyams S, Barkai S et al. The natural history of retinal holes with special reference to the development of retinal detachment and the time factor involved. In: Michaelson IC, Berman ER, eds. *Causes and Prevention of Blindness* (Academic Press: New York, 1972): 404–8.
14. *Preferred Practice Patterns: Retinal Detachment.* (American Academy of Ophthalmology). Publication #110022, San Francisco (1998), 10–13.
15. Barraquer C, Cavelier C, Mejia LF. Incidence of retinal detachment following clear-lens extraction in myopic patients, *Arch Ophthalmol* (1994) **112**:336–9.
16. Davis MD, Segal PP, MacCormack A. The natural course followed by the fellow eye in patients with rhegmatogenous retinal detachment. In: Preutt RC, Regan CDJ, eds, *Retina Congress* (Appleton-Century Crofts: New York, 1972): 643–60.
17. Folk JC, Arrindell EL, Klugman MR. The fellow eye of patients with phakic lattice retinal detachment, *Ophthalmology* (1989) **96**:72–9.
18. Sternberg P Jr, Han DP, Yeo JH, et al. Photocoagulation to prevent retinal detachment in acute retinal necrosis, *Ophthalmology* (1988) **95**:1389–93.
19. Zauberman H. Tensile strength of chorioretinal lesions produced by photocoagulation, diathermy, and cryopexy, *Br J Ophthalmol* (1969) **53**:749–52.
20. Kanski JJ, Daniel R. Prophylaxis of retinal detachment, *Am J Ophthalmol* (1975) **79**:197–205.
21. Goldberg RE, Boyer DS, Sequential retinal breaks following a spontaneous initial retinal break, *Ophthalmology* (1981) **88**:10–12.
22. Smiddy WE, Flynn HW, Nicholson DH, et al. Results and complications in treated retinal breaks, *Am J Ophthalmol* (1991) **112**:623–31.

Chapter 3 Laser indirect ophthalmoscopy

Famin Chou, Mandi D Conway and Gholam A Peyman

INTRODUCTION

The binocular indirect laser photocoagulation system, developed by Mizuno and Takaku[1,2] in 1981, uses an indirect ophthalmoscope coupled with a fiberoptic cable to a laser optic (Figs 3.1 and 3.2). Argon and infrared diode lasers are currently used with laser indirect ophthalmoscope (LIO) delivery systems. The binocular ophthalmoscope permits visualization of the entire fundus with ease.

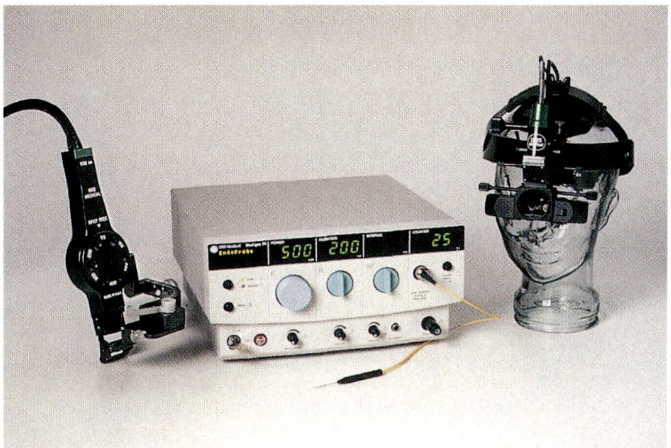

Figure 3.1 *TruFocus™ laser indirect ophthalmoscope. (Courtesy of Iris Medical Instruments, Mountain View, CA.)*

CLINICAL USES

The LIO is widely used now in treating various clinical problems, including retinopathy of prematurity,

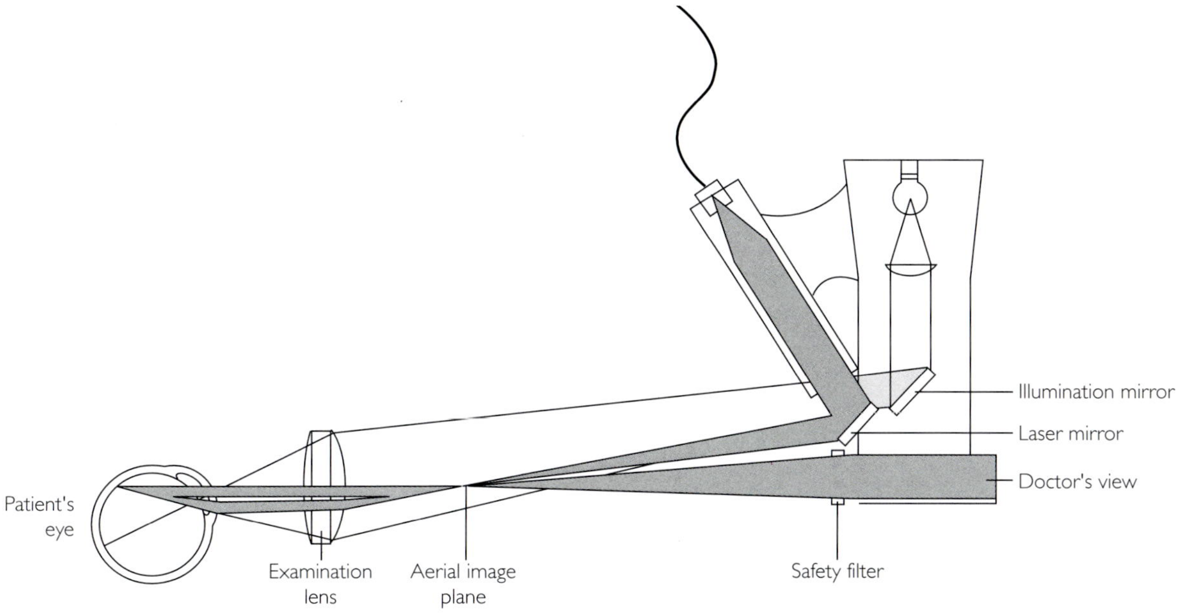

Figure 3.2 *Diagram of laser pathway through the Coherent laser indirect ophthalmoscope. (Courtesy of Coherent Radiation Co., Palo Alto, CA.)*

diabetic retinopathy, proliferative vitreoretinopathy, retinal breaks, pneumatic retinopexy, Coats' disease, intraocular tumors and pars planitis. This chapter discusses the indications, instrumentation and complications of the LIO delivery system.

INDICATIONS

The LIO is used to supplement panretinal photocoagulation to the anterior retina in eyes with diabetic retinopathy, venous occlusive disease and carotid occlusive disease. Peripheral retinal photocoagulation, with or without scleral indentation, is easier to perform with the LIO delivery system than with a slit-lamp delivery system. Anterior retinal pathologies such as retinal tears, holes, dialysis or tumors (melanoma, angioma, retinoblastoma) are all accessible to coagulation with LIO. Initial or supplemental laser photocoagulation also can be administered with the LIO in children and uncooperative adults under general anesthetic. The LIO is also useful in patients with orthopedic conditions or head tremor who are unable to be positioned comfortably at the slit lamp.

Other indications for the use of the LIO are cases with decreased media clarity, small pupils, lenticular opacities, vitreous hemorrhage, post-traumatic corneal irregularities, corneal scars and postoperative corneal edema or striae. The LIO enables viewing of the retina through vitreous substitutes such as gas or silicone oil. The LIO is also better tolerated than a contact lens (for laser treatment at the slit lamp) in the immediate postoperative period because of ocular tenderness and edema.

The LIO may be required in certain intraoperative and postoperative situations. Peripheral retinal pathology can be treated with or without scleral indentation in phakic eyes intraoperatively. It is also useful postoperatively because contact lens placement at the slit lamp may be difficult in eyes with a large trabeculectomy bleb, a shallow anterior chamber or in a patient who requires supine postoperative positioning.

INSTRUMENTATION

The LIO consists of a coaxial illuminating light and laser beam. This provides the surgeon with greater flexibility in moving around the patient and achieving an adequate view of the fundus pathology. The condensing lenses used most frequently are the 14-, 20- and 28-diopter lenses. However,

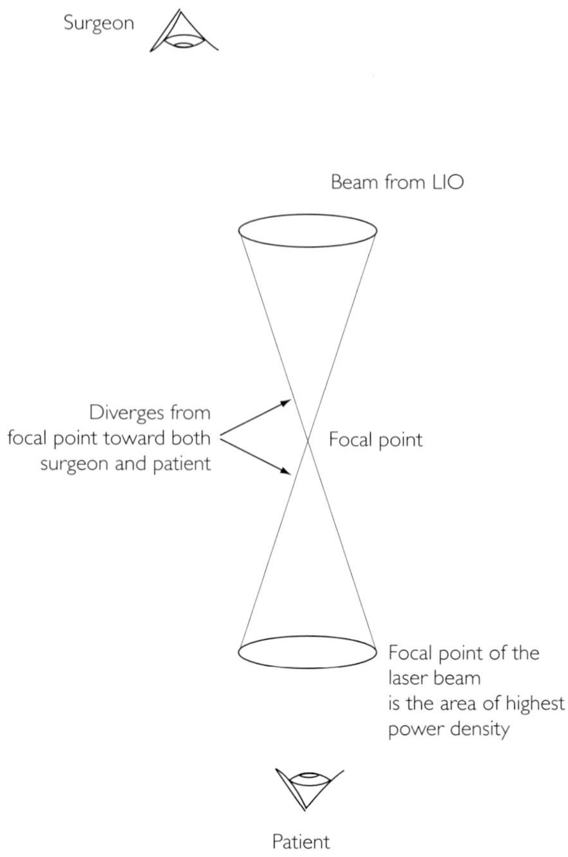

Figure 3.3 *Diagram of laser beam showing focal point divergence. (Adapted with permission from Conway MD, Olk RJ.* A Retina Video Series: Laser and Cryopexy Techniques. *Copyright © Lippincott Williams & Wilkins: Media, Philadelphia, PA, 1995.*[4]*)*

the 40-diopter lens is particularly useful in retinopathy of prematurity and in eyes with small pupils or with vitreous substitutes. Most LIOs are equipped with either a permanently fixed safety filter or an electrically operated filter to minimize the laser exposure to the surgeon's retina.

Because the LIO laser beam is not columnated but is cone shaped, the highest power density is at the focal point of the laser beam (Fig. 3.3). This is critical in focusing and achieving uniform burns. The diameter of the laser beam at the focal point usually ranges from 850 to 1000 μm. The spot size of the laser beam depends on the following variables: the power of the condensing lenses, the eye's refractive status and the focal point position in reference to the aerial image (formed by the condensing lens and the distance between the surgeon and the patient's eye).

Table 3.1 Effect of condensing lens on LIO spot size Altering the power of the hand-held condensing lens

Rule to remember
Retinal spot size increases as power of hand-held condensing lens increases

$$\text{Spot size at image plane} \times \frac{\text{Power of hand-held lens}}{\text{Refractive power of average eye}} = \text{Spot size at retina}$$

Examples
900 µm × 20 D/60 D = 300 µm
900 µm × 30 D/60 D = 450 µm

For a rough estimate of retinal spot size, use an optic disc of 1500–1800 µm and compare spot size to size of optic disc

Table 3.2 Effect of refractive status of eye on retinal spot size

Rule to remember
Retinal spot size increases as plus power of eye increases

- Minus refraction (–) means decreased spot size
- Plus refraction (+) means increased spot size

Explanation
Myopic eye
Compared to an emmetropic eye, a myopic retinal image appears magnified at the image plane. A laser spot of a given size will cover less area of the magnified retinal image of the myopic eye than it will on the unmagnified retinal image of an emmetropic eye. Therefore, the final spot size is smaller on the myopic fundus image than an identical spot placed on an emmetropic eye's retinal image

Hyperopic eye
Compared to an emmetropic eye, a hyperopic retinal image appears 'minified' at the image plane. A laser spot of a given size will cover more area of the minified retinal image of the hyperopic eye than it will on the 'unminified' retinal image of an emmetropic eye. Therefore, the final spot size is larger on the hyperopic fundus image than an identical spot placed on an emmetropic eye's retinal image

Essential equipment required, in addition to the condensing lenses, are a lid speculum, balanced salt solution, topical anesthetic and a scleral depressor. Safety goggles for assistants and observers also are necessary. The patient's contralateral eye is patched to avoid laser light inadvertently entering it if the patient or surgeon moves unexpectedly.

EFFECT OF CONDENSING LENS ON SPOT SIZE

The laser beam spot size increases when the power of the condensing lens increases and in hyperopes (Tables 3.1 and 3.2). The reverse is true for lower power condensing lenses and myopes. Therefore, a 28-diopter lens will give a larger burn than a 20-diopter lens because the spot will cover a greater area of the 'minified' retinal image. With a 20-diopter lens, the same area of retina is relatively 'magnified' and the spot will cover less area. The same reasoning applies to the relatively 'minified' images of a hyperopic fundus compared with the magnified image of a myopic fundus created with the eye's optics.

EFFECT OF VITREOUS SUBSTITUTES ON SPOT SIZE

The laser beam spot size also varies with different vitreous substitutes. Both silicone and perfluorocarbon liquids create a hyperopic shift in the eye's refraction, thus increasing the laser beam's spot size (Table 3.3). In contrast, air and gas cause a myopic shift in the eye's refraction, thus decreasing laser beam spot size.

EFFECT OF FOCUSING ON LASER BEAM SPOT SIZE

The laser beam converges at the focal point, but it also diverges on either side of it (toward both the surgeon and the patient) (Fig. 3.3). With this concept in mind, it is intuitive that the closer the retinal image is to the focal point, the smaller the laser beam spot size will be and the higher energy the laser beam will deliver. Hence, it is much easier to create intense burns in the peripheral fundus and more difficult to produce equally intense burns in the posterior pole due to focusing differences. In addition, the difference in thickness between thin peripheral retina and

Table 3.3 Effect of vitreous substitutes on LIO spot size

- Key point: memorize what myopic (–) and hyperopic (+) refractive status does to spot size
- Then view the retina with the vitreous substitute in place and decide if the substance renders the eye myopic or hyperopic
- Then apply the rules for myopia or hyperopia to predict the spot size on the retina with a particular vitreous substitute

Vitreous substitute	Effect on LIO spot size
Air (myopic)	Decreased spot size
Gas (myopic)	Decreased spot size
Silicone (hyperopic)	Increased spot size
Perfluorocarbon (hyperopic)	Increased spot size

thicker posterior pole retina accentuates the laser energy delivery in the periphery even further.

The retinal spot size can be estimated roughly with the following equation:[3,4]

Spot size or beam diameter at aerial image plane × (Condensing lens power used ÷ Refractive power of average eye) = Final spot size at retina.

Because the working distance for the LIO is not fixed (like the slit-lamp delivery system is), the spot size is quite variable because of the factors mentioned above (condensing lens, refractive status of eye, length of surgeon's arms). Consequently, laser spots can only be approximated to ±200 μm accuracy, necessitating a longer duration of burn to achieve a desired spot intensity and to minimize damage to neighboring tissues.

During the LIO laser treatment, the simplest way to change the effective tissue treatment and laser spot size is to change the distance between the focal point and aerial image generated by the condensing lens. When the focal point coincides with the aerial image, the laser beam spot size will be the smallest and the highest energy power will be delivered. The authors recommend that treatment is carried out away from the focal point of the beam. By treating slightly anterior or posterior to the focal point, the surgeon can easily titrate the 'effective burn' by altering the spot size and energy density. This is particularly helpful in creating burns in the posterior pole retina, where more power density is required, compared to the peripheral fundus, where less laser energy is needed.

Table 3.4 Anesthesia for panretinal photocoagulation (PRP) with LIO

Topical — prior to retrobulbar
Peribulbar — if monocular
Retrobulbar — some surgeons prefer peribulbar to allow eye rotation by patient to assist in viewing the peripheral retina

Recommended retrobulbar 50:50 mixture: 0.75% bupivacaine and 2.0% xylocaine
Suggest adding 150 IU of hyaluronidase (Wydase™)

General — LIO useful during surgical procedures when patient is asleep

Safety features for personnel and patient
- Safety filter for surgeon (built into LIO)
- Safety goggles for assistants and observers
- Patch opposite eye of patient (contralateral from treated eye)

Condensing lenses needed
- 14-diopter
- 20-diopter
- 28-diopter

Other supplies needed
- Lid speculum
- Balanced salt solution
- Topical anesthetic
- Scleral depressor

ANESTHESIA

Topical, peribulbar or retrobulbar anesthesia can be used with the LIO delivery system (Table 3.4). With diode or argon red laser photocoagulation, and any treatment in the anterior half of the eye, retrobulbar or peribulbar anesthesia is desirable.

TIPS FOR USING THE LIO WITH THE CONDENSING LENS (Table 3.5)

- Set duration of laser treatment at least at 0.2 seconds or higher.
- Locate the focal point by finding the smallest laser beam spot size on the aerial image (Fig. 3.2).

Table 3.5 Tips for focusing spot and choosing condensing lenses

Line up three points of light: • Laser beam coming from indirect source • Purkinje images of condensing lens • Retinal target point
Use central two-thirds of condensing lens for ideal optical effect. Peripheral lens causes elliptical burns
Use 28-diopter lens to magnify spot size in highly myopic eyes or eyes rendered myopic by vitreous substitutes (phakic gas-filled eye)
Use 20- or 14-diopter lens to minify spot size in hyperopic eyes or eyes rendered hyperopic by vitreous substitutes (aphakic gas-filled eye, phakic silicone-filled eye)
Aids to placing spots: • Move patient's eye with scleral depressor • Move retinal image with prismatic (base-in) effect of hand-held condensing lens • Move spot by gentle movement of surgeon's head[a] • Use combination of all techniques (most commonly done)

[a] Least desirable because this causes neck fatigue

- Titrate the laser power and treat at a position slightly anterior or posterior to the focal point (Fig. 3.3).
- Use the central two-thirds of the condensing lens to obtain an ideal optical effect and to decrease peripheral lens aberrations (to form a round laser spot).
- Use the 28-diopter lens in myopic and phakic air- or gas-filled eyes.
- Use the 20-diopter or smaller lens in hyperopic or aphakic air- or gas-filled and silicone oil-filled eyes.
- Use the scleral depressor to move the patient's eye and place the laser aiming beam in the area of retinal pathology.
- Use the 'base-in' prismatic effect of the 'plus' condensing lens to move the retinal image and to avoid vitreous opacities, retinal traction bands and lenticular opacities.
- Keep both the surgeon and the patient comfortable.

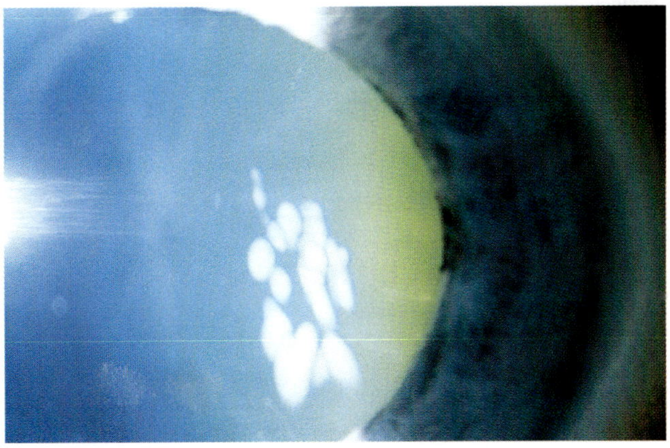

Fig. 3.4 *Photograph of the crystalline lens of an eye with proliferative diabetic retinopathy showing cataractous changes and gray-white photocoagulation lesions that were inadvertently created during panretinal photocoagulation using the laser indirect ophthalmoscope. The argon green wavelength was used.*

COMPLICATIONS

Because of the less-controlled aiming, focusing and alignment with the LIO laser delivery system, accidental macular burns may occur; thus, the use of this system in the treatment of macular disease is contraindicated and must be avoided carefully.[1–4] Other potential complications are: anterior segment burns (cornea, iris, lens) (Fig. 3.4); perforation of Bruch's membrane with choroidal hemorrhage and subsequent choroidal neovascularization; retinal hole formation and late-onset retinal detachment; vascular occlusion or spasm; preretinal or retinal hemorrhage; and epiretinal membrane formation.

REFERENCES

1. Mizuno K. Binocular indirect argon laser photocoagulator, *Br J Ophthalmol* (1981) **65**:425–8.
2. Mizuno K, Takaku Y. Dual delivery system for argon laser photocoagulation: improved techniques of the binocular indirect argon laser photocoagulator, *Arch Ophthalmol* (1983) **101**:648–52.
3. Friberg TR. Clinical experience with a binocular indirect ophthalmoscope laser delivery system, *Retina* (1987) **7**:28–31.
4. Conway MD, Olk RJ. *A Retina Video Series: Laser and Cryopexy Techniques* (Lippincott Williams & Wilkins: Media, Philadelphia, PA, 1995).

Chapter 4 Transscleral diode laser retinopexy in the treatment of retinal detachment

Anat Loewenstein and Julia A Haller

INTRODUCTION

Successful repair of retinal detachments is achieved by closure of retinal breaks with a scleral buckle or gas tamponade and creation of a chorioretinal adhesion, or retinopexy, to seal the breaks. Cryotherapy has been the standard modality for achieving retinopexy since it largely supplanted the use of diathermy in the 1970s. Cryopexy, however, has certain disadvantages, including breakdown of the blood–retinal barrier, with its increased potential to cause cystoid macular edema, macular pucker and proliferative vitreoretinopathy.[1–3] There are also some situations in which transscleral cryotherapy cannot be delivered to the retina, e.g. through an existing scleral buckle. Laser photocoagulation for retinopexy has some potential advantages over both diathermy and cryotherapy, but the development of a transscleral delivery system required a number of technologic advances before it became practical.[4–10]

A variety of laser sources and delivery systems have been investigated; one is currently FDA approved, using near-infrared (810 nm) light transmitted through a fiberoptic probe with a prism tip. The solid-state construction of the diode laser has the additional practical advantages of portability, use of standard 110-V electrical outlets, solid-state circuitry with no cooling system needed and adaptability for multiple delivery modes.

The diode laser wavelength (810 nm) is well transmitted through the sclera with minimal scleral interaction. The energy not transmitted is lost to scattering, with insufficient irradiance to produce toxicity. Melanin in the target tissues (the retinal pigment epithelium (RPE) and choroid) absorbs about 20% of the transmitted energy, which is sufficient to create a laser burn.[5–9] The chorioretinal adhesion obtained with the diode laser has been shown to be clinically and histologically similar to that produced with cryotherapy, and with similar adhesive properties.[11,12]

Experimental and clinical evidence suggests that, as opposed to other modalities for retinopexy, transscleral diode laser retinopexy may be associated with fewer side-effects[3,13] and is a safe and effective means of creating chorioretinal adhesion during retinal reattachment surgery.[14–16]

INDICATIONS AND TECHNICAL ADVANTAGES

Transscleral diode laser retinopexy is used to produce a chorioretinal adhesion around a retinal break or breaks. Specific situations exist in which transscleral laser retinopexy may offer advantages over cryotherapy.

- Unlike cryotherapy, laser energy can be delivered through silicone elements, such as existing scleral buckling hardware or glaucoma drainage devices/reservoirs.
- The aiming beam of the transscleral diode laser is projected coaxially with the treatment beam. It can be seen on the retina when the surgeon observes the retina through the pupil using an indirect ophthalmoscope. Because the localized tissue reaction to the laser is under direct observation by the treating physician at all times, the precise placement of the intended burn can be pinpointed accurately and the size and intensity of the burn can be titrated with the laser foot switch. This is an advantage over cryotherapy, during which the surgeon may mistake the

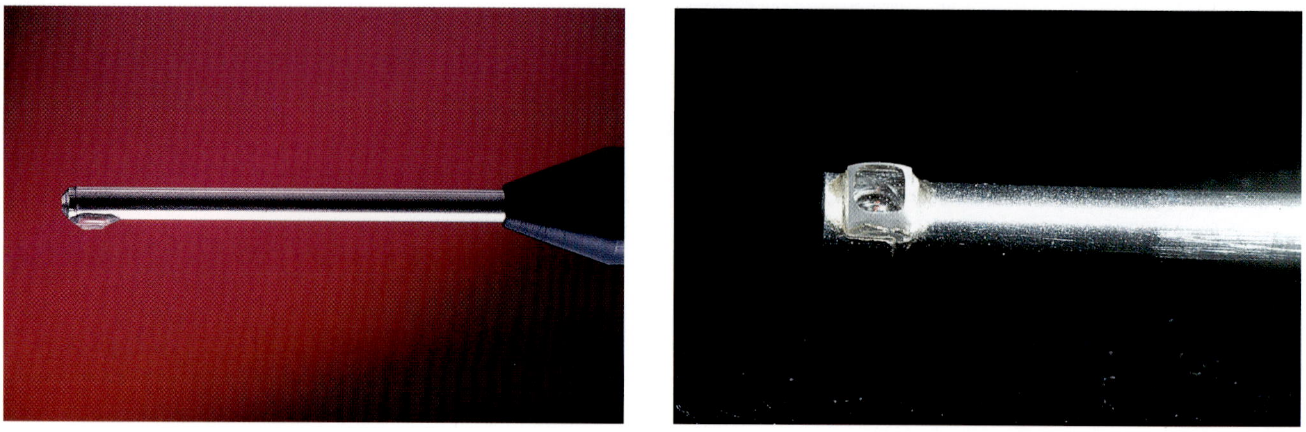

a *b*

Figure 4.1 *(a) A multiple-use fiberoptic diode laser probe designed for transscleral retinopexy. (b) The prism tip of the diode laser probe deflects the laser energy 90° from the axis of the shaft and functions as a scleral depressor.*

indentation of the probe shaft for the cryoprobe tip and unintentionally administer posterior (even macular) freezes.

- Research suggests that transscleral diode laser may result in a reduced breakdown of the blood–ocular barrier and therefore, potentially result in a lower incidence of proliferative vitreoretinopathy compared to cryopexy treatment. Its use may be ideal in high-risk eyes, such as those with large tears and/or rolled posterior edges, although this has yet to be proven clinically.

OPERATIVE PROCEDURE

The standard surgical procedure sequence is: conjunctival peritomy, rectus muscle isolation, retinal break localization, scleral suture placement, diode laser transscleral retinopexy, drainage of subretinal fluid (if required), placement of buckling material and conjunctival closure.

FOR LASER RETINOPEXY

The diode laser probe is a multiple-use fiberoptic laser delivery device with integral optics that terminates in a contact prism tip. The prism tip is designed to be used simultaneously to deflect laser energy 90° from the axis of the shaft and as a scleral depressor (Fig. 4.1).

After retinal break localization and scleral suture placement, the laser probe is placed against the external surface of the sclera. The probe is kept at right angles to the sclera and the contact site is well irrigated. While viewing through the indirect ophthalmoscope, the treatment site is located by observing the scleral indentation and the transscleral red aiming beam on the retinal target area (Fig. 4.2). An effort is made to indent the eye wall as much as possible, to allow the RPE and choroid to come into near apposition with the retina.[17]

The laser is initially set at 200 mW power and 1000 ms duration. If no reaction is observed, power and duration are increased gradually. Typical power and duration used differ with ocular pigmentation. Eyes of darkly pigmented patients require substantially less power to obtain similar lesions than eyes of more lightly pigmented patients. The treatment effect observed is retinal whitening, analogous to that seen with laser photocoagulation or diathermy but with a lighter, almost gray endpoint (Fig. 4.3). Whitening of the underlying RPE and choroid (and not the sensory retina) is considered adequate if significant subretinal fluid is present.

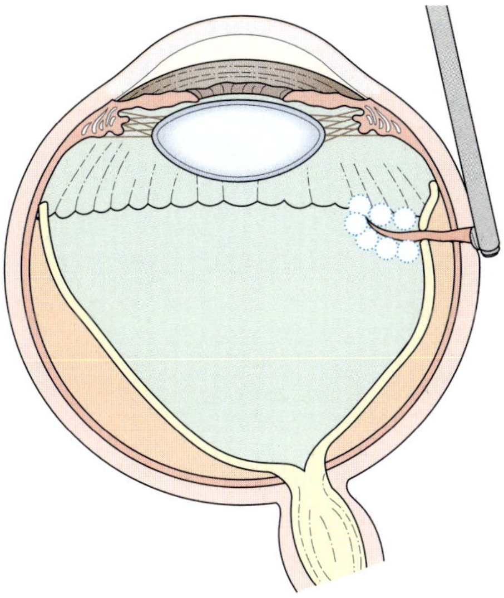

Figure 4.2 *The laser probe is used as a scleral depressor and the red aiming beam allows precise placement of retinal burns.*

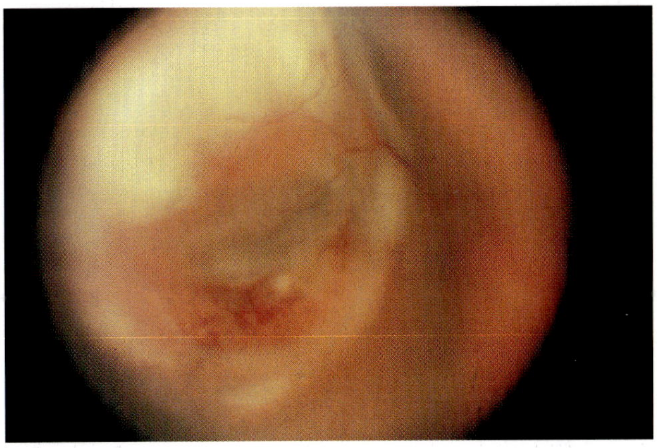

Figure 4.3 *Retinal burns applied by the diode laser probe at the appropriate light-gray endpoint.*

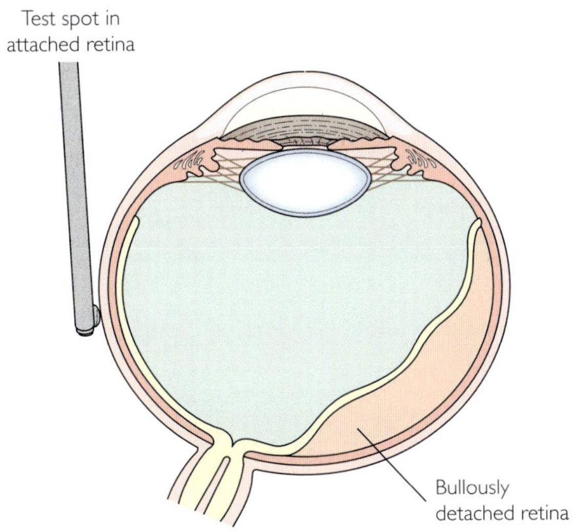

Figure 4.4 *A test spot may be applied in peripheral attached retina to determine the appropriate laser setting for treatment of a retinal break in detached retina.*

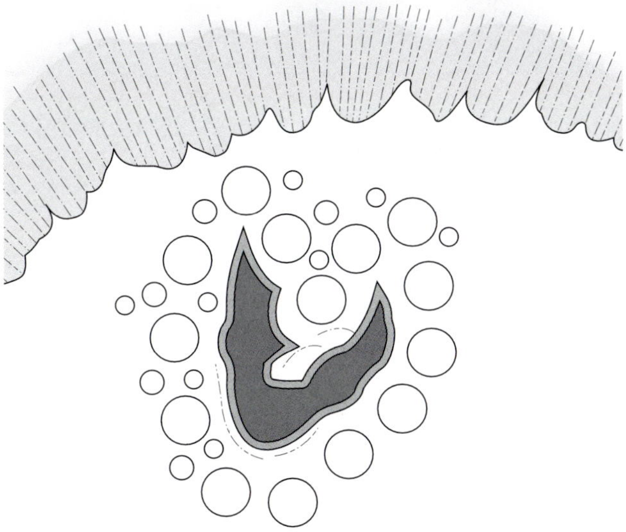

Figure 4.5 *Laser burns applied to surround a retinal break completely.*

If the retina is quite elevated and no uptake is seen at the level of the neuroretina, RPE color change beneath it is sufficient. Another strategy is to place a test spot in an area of attached retina, obtain good uptake and then use these power settings to treat the break in the area of detached retina (Fig. 4.4). Caution must be observed in areas where pigmentation becomes more intense, because more absorption (and greater tissue uptake) is encountered. Less energy is required to obtain a clinical lesion when it

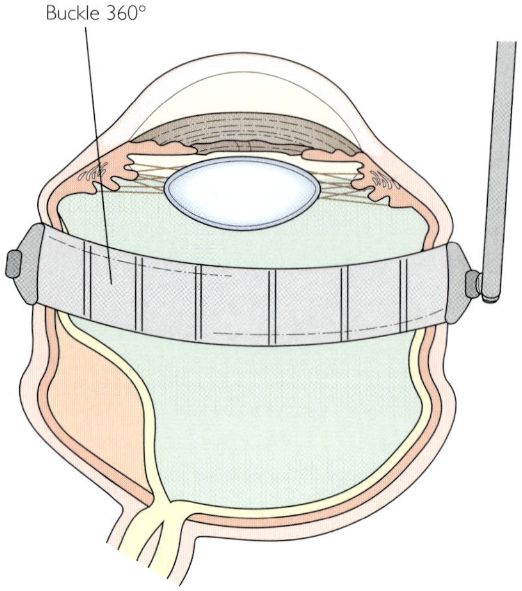

Figure 4.6 *The diode laser probe may be used to treat the retina beneath a scleral buckle.*

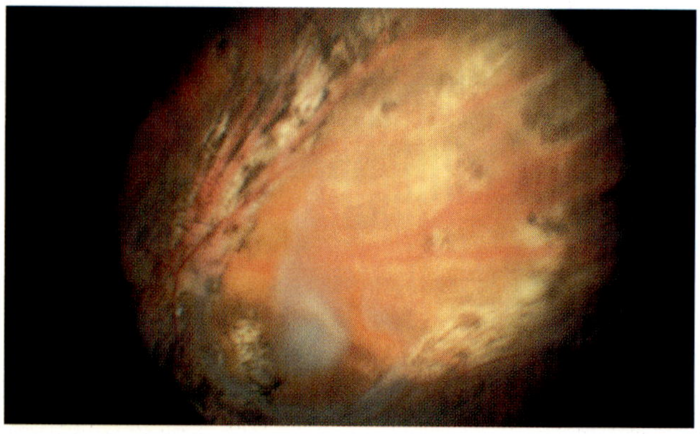

Figure 4.7 *Mature laser scars created by transscleral diode laser retinopexy surround a retinal flap tear completely.*

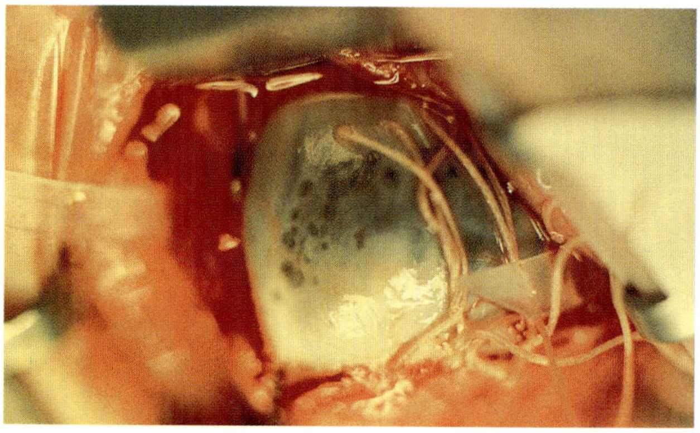

Figure 4.8 *Focal scleral discoloration where high energy settings were used over thinned sclera. (Reprinted with permission from* Arch Ophthalmol *1993;* ***111****:952–6. Copyright © 1993 American Medical Association.*[15]*)*

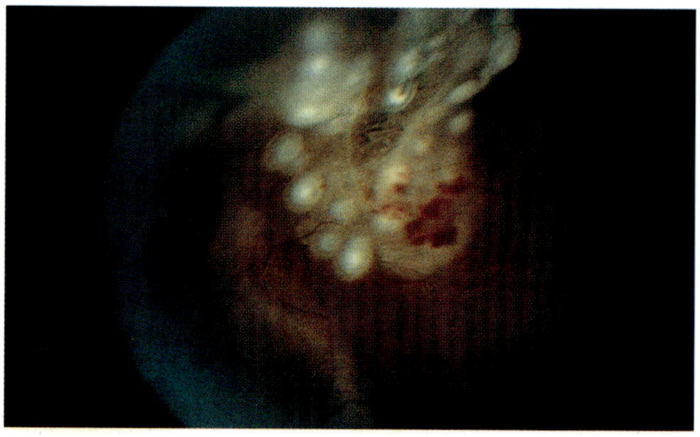

Figure 4.9 *Retinal hemorrhage associated with a presumed rupture in Bruch's membrane and an audible pop following an intense laser application. (Reprinted with permission from* Arch Ophthalmol *1993;* ***111****:952–6. Copyright © 1993 American Medical Association.*[15]*)*

is delivered anteriorly near the ora serrata, where the sclera is thinner and chorioretinal pigmentation is often greater. The foot switch can be released easily to terminate the delivery of laser energy instantly when adequate retinal reaction is observed.

An appropriate number of spots are delivered to surround the retinal break(s) adequately (Fig. 4.5).

Transscleral diode laser can be applied to the retina beneath an existing scleral buckle (Fig. 4.6).

Mature laser scars created by transscleral diode laser retinopexy completely surrounding a retinal flap tear are seen in Fig. 4.7.

COMPLICATIONS

Approximately 20% of the energy is attenuated when treatment is delivered through silicone exoplants and hardware.[14] Power is increased gradually until a mild tissue effect is seen.

Thermal injury to the sclera is seen as a color change at the treatment sites on the sclera (Fig. 4.8). To avoid this complication, after delivering 10 pulses at any one setting, the sclera is inspected to ensure that there is no thermal effect, especially in areas of scleral thinning and/or pigmentation.

Tissue 'pops' resulting from apparent rupture of Bruch's membrane are associated with excessive energy delivery and are seen as focal, deep areas of tissue disruption exactly like those produced by overly hot burns with the transpupillary laser. These burns can be avoided by gradually increasing the energy delivery and aiming for an endpoint of a small, gray-white burn. These factors are correlated significantly with the surgeon's experience using the transscleral diode probe.

Choroidal, retinal (Fig. 4.9) and (very rarely) vitreous hemorrhages can occur when local delivery of energy is too high. These hemorrhages can be minimized by starting at low powers and slowly increasing the power and the duration of burns. This complication is associated significantly with the surgeon's experience.

SUMMARY

Transscleral diode laser retinopexy serves as a safe and effective means of creating a chorioretinal adhesion during retinal reattachment surgery. In certain instances, such as when treatment is needed through existing scleral buckling or glaucoma drainage device hardware, it may be the only available modality for achieving transscleral retinopexy. Complications are self limited and significantly associated with the surgeon's experience. Its other advantages include precise localization of the burn with the aiming beam and a decreased breakdown of the blood–ocular barrier when compared to cryopexy.

REFERENCES

1. Campochiaro PA, Kaden IH, Vidaurri-Leal J, Glaser BM. Cryotherapy enhances intravitreal dispersion of viable retinal pigment epithelial cells, *Arch Ophthalmol* (1985) **103**:434–6.
2. Jaccoma EH, Conway BP, Campochiaro PA. Cryotherapy causes extensive breakdown of the blood retinal barrier: a comparison with argon laser coagulation, *Arch Ophthalmol* (1985) **103**:1728–30.
3. Bonnet M, Fleury J, Guenoun S, et al. Cryopexy in rhegmatogenous retinal detachment: a risk factor for postoperative proliferative vitreoretinopathy? *Graefes Arch Clin Exp Ophthalmol* (1996) **234**:739–43.
4. Peyman GA, Conway MD, Raichand M, Lin J. Histopathological studies on transscleral argon–krypton laser coagulation with an exolaser probe, *Ophthalmic Surg* (1984) **15**:496–501.
5. Peyman GA, Naguib KS, Gaasterland D. Transscleral application of semiconductor diode laser, *Lasers Surg Med* (1990) **10**:569–75.
6. Okamato S, Takahasi H, Fukado Y, Ozawa T. Laser diode application of transscleral photocoagulation, *Lasers Light Ophthalmol* (1990) **3**:29–37.
7. Jennings T, Fuller T, Vukich JA, et al. Transscleral contact retinal photocoagulation with a 810 nm semiconductor diode laser, *Ophthalmic Surg* (1990) **21**:492–6.
8. Rol P, Niederer P, Durr U, et al. Experimental investigations of the light scattering properties of the human sclera, *Lasers Light Ophthalmol* (1990) **3**:201–12.
9. Vogel A, Glugos C, Nuffer R, Birngruber R. Optical properties of human sclera and their consequences for transscleral laser applications, *Laser Surg Med* (1991) **11**:311–40.
10. Benner JD, Galustian JC, Lim M, et al. Comparison of techniques for transscleral diode photocoagulation in the rabbit, *Retina* (1995) **15**:253–60.
11. Smiddy WE, Hernandez E. Histologic results of retinal diode laser photocoagulation in rabbit eyes, *Arch Ophthalmol* (1992) **110**:693–8.
12. Han D, Nash R, Blair J, O'Brien W, Medina R. Comparison of tensile strength after transscleral retinal cryotherapy, diathermy, and diode laser photocoagulation, *Arch Ophthalmol* (1995) **113**:1195–9.
13. Arrindell E, Wu J, Wolf M, et al. High-resolution magnetic resonance imaging evaluation of blood–retinal barrier integrity following transscleral diode laser treatment, *Arch Ophthalmol* (1995) **113**:96–102.
14. Nanda S, Han D. Experimental transconjunctival diode laser retinal photocoagulation through silicone scleral exoplants, *Arch Ophthalmol* (1995) **113**:926–31.
15. Haller JA, Lim JI, Goldberg MF. Pilot trial of transscleral diode laser retinopexy in retinal detachment surgery, *Arch Ophthalmol* (1993) **111**:952–6.
16. Haller JA, Blair N, de Juan E Jr, et al. Transscleral diode laser retinopexy in retinal detachment surgery: results of a multicenter trial, *Retina* (1998) **18**:399–404.
17. Loewenstein A, Lamborne AN, Haller JA, de Juan E Jr. Effect of scleral indentation on diode transscleral retinal photocoagulation, *Ophthalmic Surg Lasers* (1998) **29**:658–62.

Chapter 5 Cryosurgery of the retina

Ingrid Kreissig and Harvey A Lincoff

INTRODUCTION

Freezing the eye to create inflammation in the area of application began early in the 20th century. In 1918, Schöler described chorioretinal inflammation after the application of solid carbon dioxide to the sclera.[1]

In 1931 Gonin[2] presented his original concept, that retinal detachment is caused by a retinal break and reattachment could be achieved by inducing inflammation around the break with diathermy and by simultaneous draining of subretinal fluid. In 1933 Deutschmann[3] and Bietti[4] reported freezing the break with solid carbon dioxide to obtain adhesion. At that time, the instruments for diathermy application were more satisfactory and retinal adhesion was more effective. Cryosurgery of the retina was an idea whose time had not yet arrived.

Things changed 20 years later when an extraocular detachment technique appeared. In 1953, Custodis introduced a revolutionary technique[5] for retinal detachment surgery that eliminated three major hazards: scleral perforation for the drainage of subretinal fluid; intravitreal injection to restore vitreous volume; and scleral dissection to preserve part of the scleral wall from diathermy necrosis. The Custodis operation compressed an elastic (polyviol) explant precisely over the retinal hole. The hole was treated with surface transscleral diathermy. This technique was nearly abandoned because of an unacceptable rate of extraocular infection (scleral abscess in 6 of 25 eyes) and endophthalmitis (in 4 of the 6 infected eyes) reported by Schepens et al 1960.[6]

Lincoff (who adopted the Custodis operation) experienced similar complications (but much less frequently).[7] Convinced of the correctness of the operation, he looked for a way to avoid diathermy-induced scleral necrosis and the toxic effects of the polyviol (which he thought was the root of the problem). In 1963 Lincoff[8] created experimental lesions in animal eyes using carbon dioxide applicators that he borrowed from dermatology. In the same year the Cooper–Linde Neurosurgical Unit (which used liquid nitrogen to cool a brain probe) was developed.

Lincoff and McLean modified the device to make it suitable for the eye. They designed a small maneuverable instrument that provided controlled temperatures from +37°C to –180°C at the tip of an insulated probe. The first liquid nitrogen instrument was complicated, but was an excellent research tool and provided extensive data (to be described later). In subsequent years the Linde instrument was supplanted by more dependable devices that employed carbon dioxide or nitrous oxide gas, both cryogenic agents that are easier to handle than liquid nitrogen.

The primary advantage of cryosurgery is the ability to penetrate the sclera and to create a retinal adhesion without causing scleral necrosis. This facilitated a new retinal detachment technique of primarily full-thickness scleral buckling without the need for a lamellar scleral dissection.[9] Thus, cryosurgery provided Lincoff with the means he was seeking to retain the Custodis concept. In addition to replacing diathermy by cryosurgery, Lincoff and McLean substituted the silicone sponge for the irritative polyviol explant.[10] Cryosurgery and silicone sponges made local buckling popular. Subsequently, the Schepens technique, in which solid silicone structures were buried in lamellar scleral dissections, with cryopexy changed to a full-thickness scleral operation.[11] Cryosurgery also allowed transconjunctival prophylactic coagulation of peripheral lesions without causing necrosis of the intervening tissues.[12]

At its inception in the 1960s, cryosurgery, now called cryopexy, was generally reserved for simple detachments where there was little traction; diathermy remained the standard method of choice.

The reluctance to employ cryosurgery was the uncertainty of the strength of the cryopexy-induced adhesion.

These doubts persisted through other animal experiments by Bellows,[13] Böke and Hollwich,[14] Curtin et al,[15] Oosterhuis et al[16] and Törnquist.[17]

To rescue this new thermal modality (for the newly developed local buckling technique without drainage), the cryosurgical adhesion was studied more extensively in additional animal experiments at the end of the 1960s by Lincoff et al;[18,19] also, Kreissig[20,21] addressed the problem in her postdoctoral thesis for habilitation entitled 'The strength and ultrastructure of the cryopexy adhesion in retinal surgery.'[22] In collaboration with Bloch, a biomathematician, extensive animal experiments were undertaken.

Answers to the following questions were sought:

- How does the strength of the cryopexy-induced adhesion compare to that produced by diathermy?
- Is there a difference in strength of an adhesion produced by light, medium and heavy applications of cryopexy or diathermy?
- On what day is maximum adhesion obtained?

This extensive research project, which was supported by the National Institute of Health (USA) and the Heinrich Hertz Foundation (Germany), provided data to clinicians that cryopexy was a suitable alternative to the time-tested diathermy modality. A summary of the study follows.

DOSAGE OF THERMAL APPLICATIONS

The experimental applications were created in animal eyes under ophthalmoscopic control. A more objective quantification such as temperature and time, although considered, was rejected because it did not imitate the clinical situation. Thermal lesions ($n = 640$) were applied transconjunctivally in 336 eyes.[22–24]

DOSAGE OF CRYOSURGERY

Light cryosurgical application is an application in which the choroid blanches and the lesion is barely perceptible after removing the cryoprobe.

Medium cryosurgical application involves sustained freezing until the retina first turns white. With removal of the cryoprobe, the white area of the retina fades, leaving a faint gray area representing intraretinal edema.

A **heavy cryosurgical application** involves sustained freezing for 3 seconds after the retina first turns white. When the probe is removed, an opaque lesion persists.

DOSAGE OF DIATHERMY

The light diathermy application caused the faintest gray response in the retina. The medium application was stopped when the retina turned white. The heavy lesion continued the application for 3 seconds after the retina turned white.

ADHESIVE STRENGTH OF THERMAL LESIONS

We found in earlier experiments[19] that a normal retina will tear when subjected to a force of 300 mg. Thermal lesions were placed at the ends of the myelinated fibers of rabbit retina; then with the myelinated bundle, it was pulled upon the retina to test the strength of adhesion created by the thermal lesion. The myelinated bundle withstood a force of 1850 mg. The 640 thermal lesions were tested at various time intervals by the pulling mechanism depicted in Fig. 5.1. We tested 328 diathermy and 312 cryosurgical lesions.

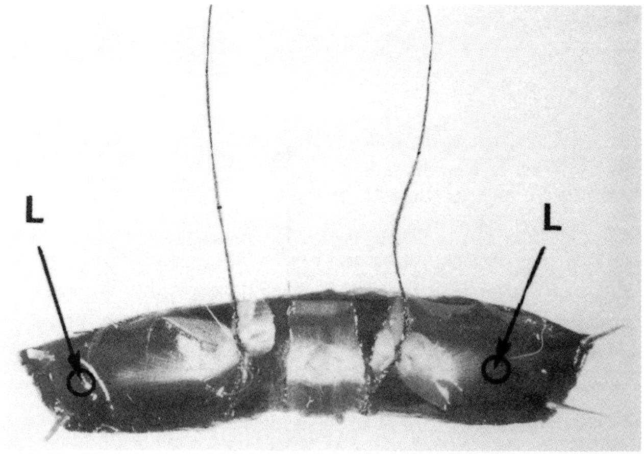

Figure 5.1 *Flat preparation of rabbit retina: lesions (L pointing at encircled lesion) have been placed at peripheral ends of myelinated fibers. Proximal ends have been severed at the disc and seized with a silk suture in preparation for pulling. (Reproduced with permission from Kreissig I, Lincoff H. Cryosurgery of the retina,* Int Ophthalmol Clin *(1976)* ***16****:63–81.*[9]*)*

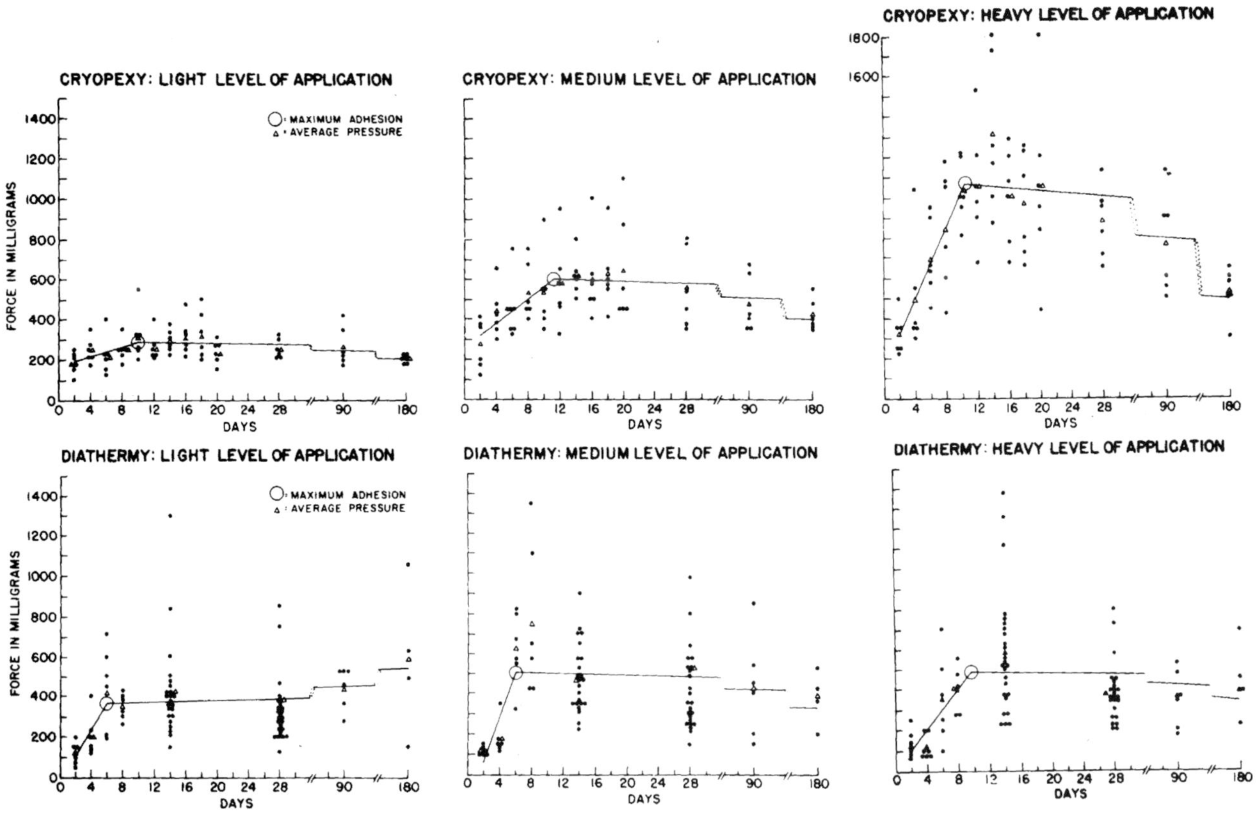

Figure 5.2 *Graphic depiction of the relative adhesiveness of cryopexy (n = 312) and diathermy lesions (n = 328): Solid dots represent lesions; circled points represent joined points (days of maximum adhesion) of the two straight lines fitted to the data; triangles represent average adhesiveness of each group. The abscissa represents time in days between application and experimental separation. The ordinate represents milligrams of force required to separate the lesion. (Reproduced with permission from Kreissig I. Ultrastructure of the cryopexy adhesion in retinal surgery.* Postdoctoral Thesis for Habilitation. *Rheinische Friedrich-Wilhelms-Universität: Bonn, 1972: 1–172. Copyright © Lippincott Williams & Wilkins, 1972.*[22]*)*

CRYOSURGICAL LESIONS

Cryosurgical lesions increased in strength with increasing intensity of application. Three distinct levels of adhesive strength corresponded to light, medium and heavy applications. A light cryosurgical lesion resisted an average pull of 300 mg, a medium lesion resisted 575 mg and a heavy lesion resisted 1175 mg (Fig. 5.2).

DIATHERMY LESIONS

No such stratification of lesion strength was observed with diathermy applications. The adhesive strength ranged from 50 to 1550 mg but was poorly correlated to the intensity of diathermy application. A light diathermy application occasionally yielded a strong adhesion. The average adhesive strength of the diathermy lesions was approximately 500 mg, regardless of the application intensity (light, medium or heavy). This approximates to the adhesive strength of a medium cryosurgical lesion (Fig. 5.2).

DEVELOPMENT OF ADHESIVE STRENGTH OVER TIME

The cryosurgical adhesion gained strength rapidly after the second day and the diathermy lesion after the fourth day. Diathermy lesions reached their maximum adhesive strength by the tenth day and cryosurgery by the twelfth day.

OPHTHALMOSCOPIC APPEARANCE OF CRYOSURGICAL LESIONS

The early ophthalmoscopic appearance of a cryosurgical lesion is a function of the retinal transparency.

Light cryosurgical lesion

On the first postoperative day, the pigment epithelium is damaged, creating a pale patch of pigment epithelial edema. On day 2, a thin, white, outer ring combined with a thin, black, inner ring becomes apparent at the edge of the lesion. The outer white ring defines the edge of the untreated retina. The pigment epithelium appears less dense in the center of the lesion. During the third and fourth days, some pigment aggregates and the lesion develops a fine stippled appearance. By the fifth day, coarse pigment clumping is evident and the peripheral rings of the lesion are no longer apparent. Subsequently, there are small changes in the distribution of clumps of retinal pigment epithelium (RPE) and choroidal pigment in the background.

Medium cryosurgical lesion

On day 1, the lesion has a grayish-white appearance with a velvet-like character and the retina is semiopaque. This limits the view of the changes occurring in the RPE and choroid. By day 2, a thin white line appears in the periphery defining untreated retina. The retinal edema decreases over the next 5 days and by the sixth day marked pigment clumps on a yellowish-white background become evident. The entire lesion appears paler than the untreated retina. Large choroidal vessels become visible in the center of the lesion.

Heavy cryosurgical lesion

Opaque retinal edema persists for 1 week. The edema regresses slowly, beginning at the periphery of the lesion and progressing centrally. A thin white line appears at the periphery, followed by pigment clumping at the center. At the fourteenth day, the lesion is characterized by large pigment clumps on a very pale, white-to-yellow background. The retina appears reduced to a thin shiny membrane.

HISTOLOGY OF CRYOSURGICAL LESIONS

The strength of cryosurgically induced retinal adhesions demonstrated an adhesive strength proportional to the intensity of the cryosurgical application (Fig. 5.2).

To correlate the anatomic changes occurring at these three levels of cryopexy-induced adhesive strength, another animal experiment was done.[22] Light, medium and heavy cryosurgical applications were made in 68 rabbit eyes under ophthalmoscopic control. The Linde instrument was set at –30°C. The same three intensities of application were used, similar to the previous animal experiments. Lesions were placed at both ends of the nerve fibers (two lesions for each animal eye). The animals were sacrificed at time points between 4 days to 3 years.

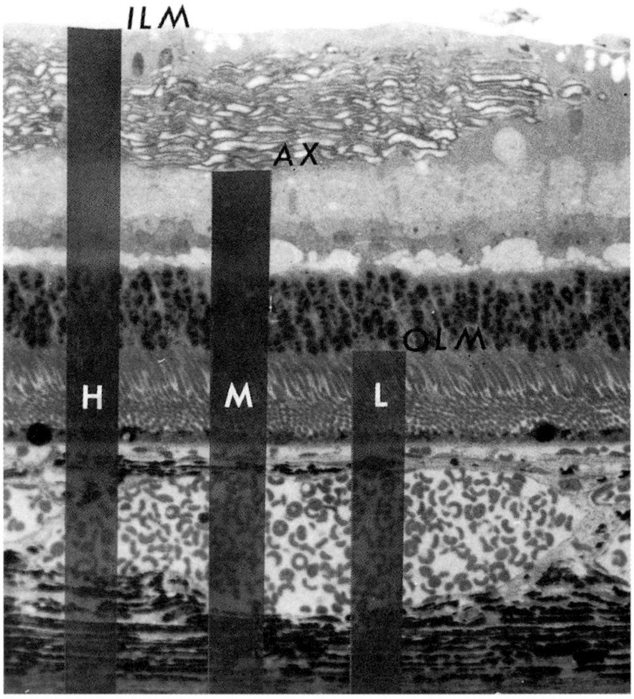

Figure 5.3 *Photograph of normal retina section to demonstrate penetration of cryogenic necrosis (represented by columns): to the outer limiting membrane (OLM) after a light (L) application; to the nerve fiber layer (AX) after a medium (M) application; and to the internal limiting membrane (ILM) after a heavy (H) application.*

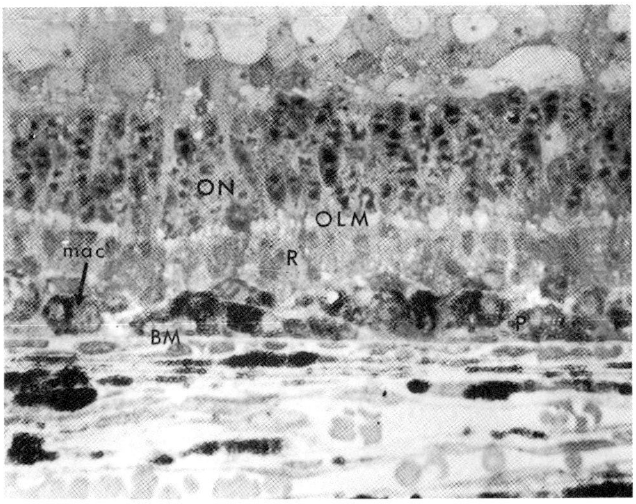

Figure 5.4 *Retina 4 days after light cryopexy: section reveals retinal necrosis to the level of the outer limiting membrane (OLM); the outer nuclei (ON), above, look normal. Basement membrane (BM) of pigment epithelium (P) survives. There are many macrophages (mac) above. Photoreceptor elements (R) are necrotic. (Reproduced with permission from Kreissig I, Lincoff H. Cryosurgery of the retina,* Int Ophthalmol Clin *(1976)* ***16****:63–81.*[9]*)*

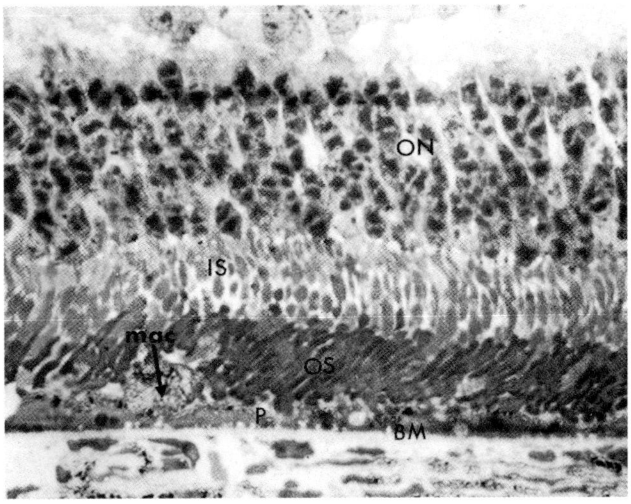

Figure 5.5 *Retina 14 days after light cryopexy: section shows recovery of photoreceptor elements. Inner (IS) and outer (OS) segments are again in parallel columns and interdigitating with retinal pigment epithelium (P). A large macrophage (mac) among the outer segments is the most striking evidence of previous injury. Basement membrane (BM) of pigment epithelium is intact. ON = Outer nuclei. (Reproduced with permission from Kreissig I, Lincoff H. Cryosurgery of the retina,* Int Ophthalmol Clin *(1976)* ***16****:63–81.*[9]*)*

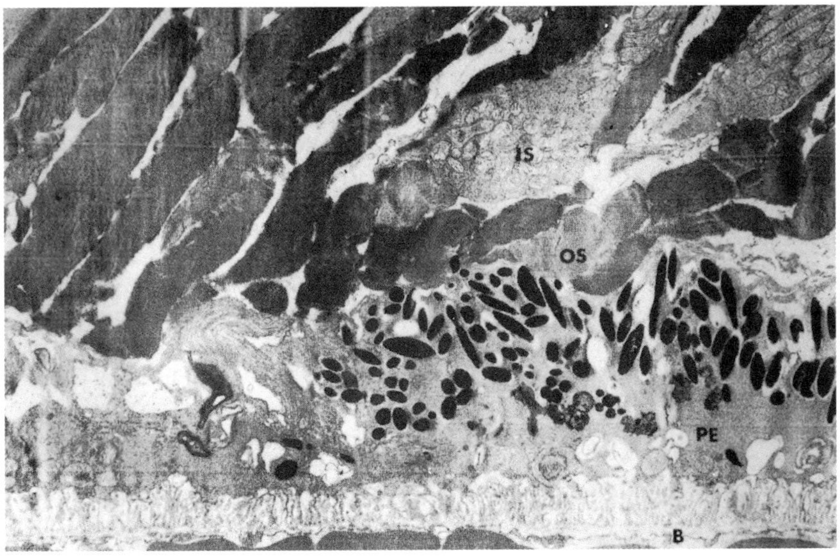

Figure 5.6 *Retina 14 days after light cryopexy: electron micrograph of outer segments (OS) shows rods* ***interdigitating*** *with villi of pigment epithelium (PE). Outer segment discs are again in horizontal order. IS = Inner segment. (Reproduced with permission from Kreissig I, Lincoff H. Cryosurgery of the retina,* Int Ophthalmol Clin *(1976)* ***16****:63–81.*[9]*)*

All lesions were studied with electron microscopy. Three anatomic patterns were discerned and characterized as **interdigital**, **desmosomal** and **infiltrative**.[20,22]

The pattern of the healed retinal cryosurgical lesion depends on the depth of thermal necrosis created by the cryopexy application and the extent of the basement membrane interruption (Fig. 5.3). If the freezing-induced retinal necrosis progresses to the level of the outer limiting membrane (Fig. 5.4), but the outer nuclei survive, the rods regenerate and again interdigitate with villi of regenerated RPE (Figs 5.5 and 5.6). This new adhesion is stronger than the natural adhesion.

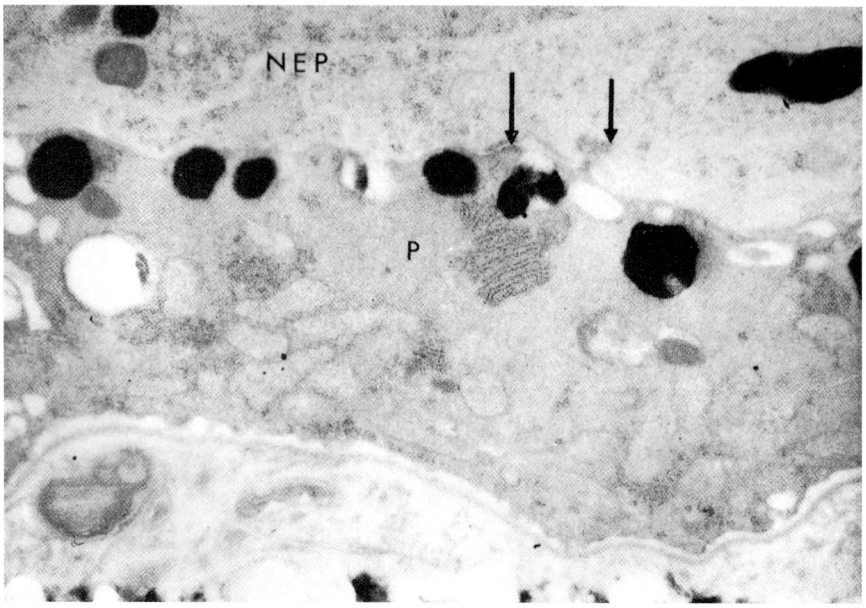

Figure 5.7 *Retina 28 days after medium cryopexy: electron micrograph shows* ***desmosomal*** *connection (arrows) between smooth membranes of adjacent neuroepithelial cells, i.e. the less-specialized neuroepithelium (Nep) without finger processes and the new pigment epithelium (P) without villus processes. (Reproduced with permission from Kreissig I, Lincoff H. Cryosurgery of the retina,* Int Ophthalmol Clin *(1976)* ***16****:63–81.*[9]*)*

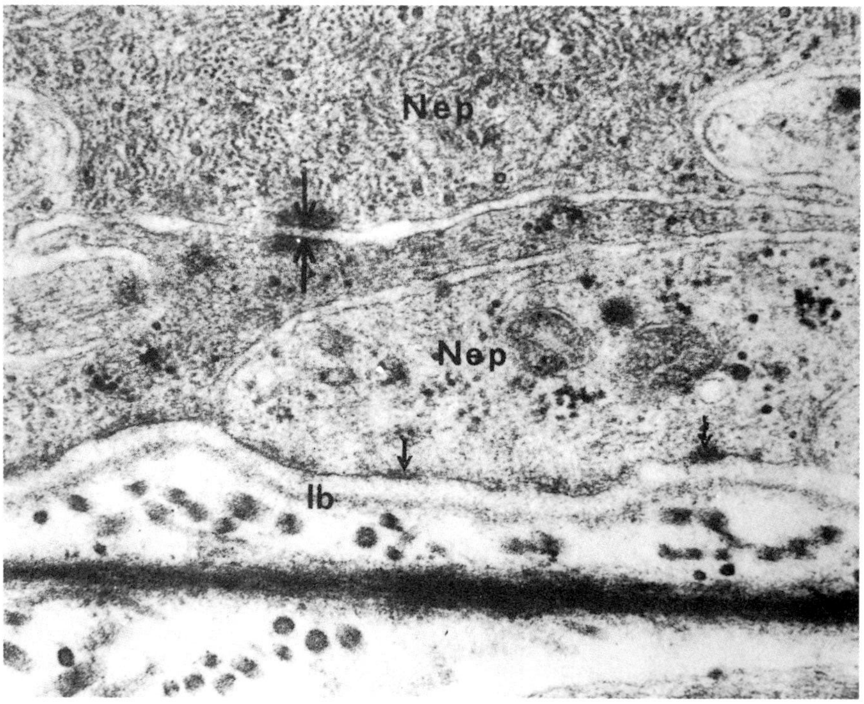

Figure 5.8 *Retina 28 days after medium cryopexy: electron micrograph shows undifferentiated neuroepithelial cells (Nep) of retina. They are connected to each other by desmosomes (double arrow), spread along the basement membrane (Ib) and attached to it with* ***hemidesmosomal-like*** *structures (single arrow). (Reproduced with permission from Kreissig I, Lincoff H. Cryosurgery of the retina,* Int Ophthalmol Clin *(1976)* ***16****:63–81.*[9]*)*

When the thermal injury penetrates to the nerve fiber layer, the outer nuclei and the rods do not regenerate. An adhesion develops between regenerating RPE (without villus processes) and the processes of Müller cells. The adhesion is desmosomal (Fig. 5.7).

If the recovery of RPE is delayed, undifferentiated retinal neuroepithelial cells may spread directly along the basement membrane and attach to it with hemidesmosomal-like structures (Fig. 5.8). The residual retina becomes a thin band of neuroepithelium between the inner limiting membrane and the

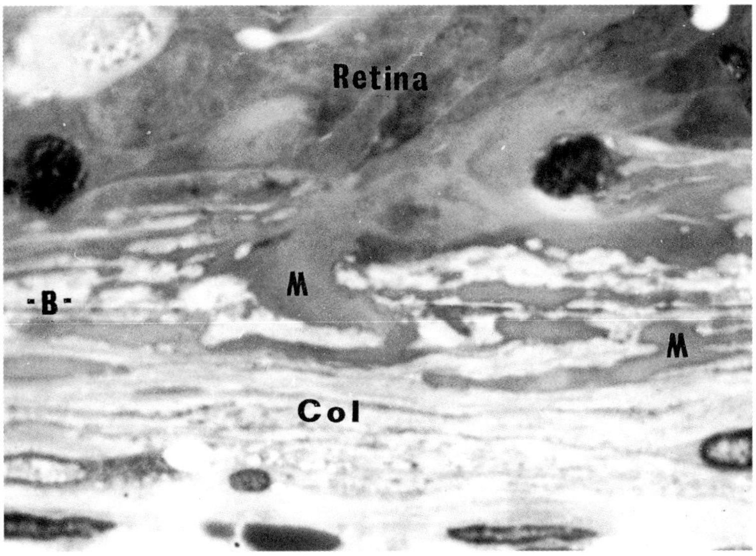

a

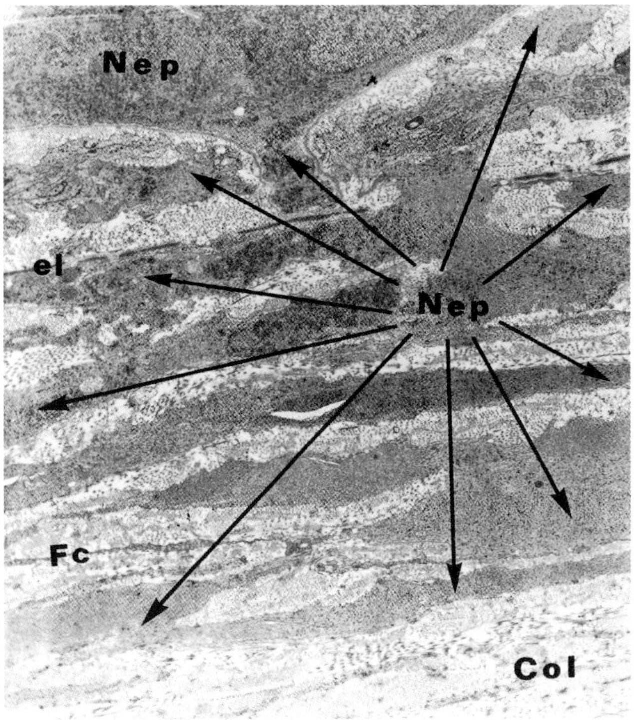

b

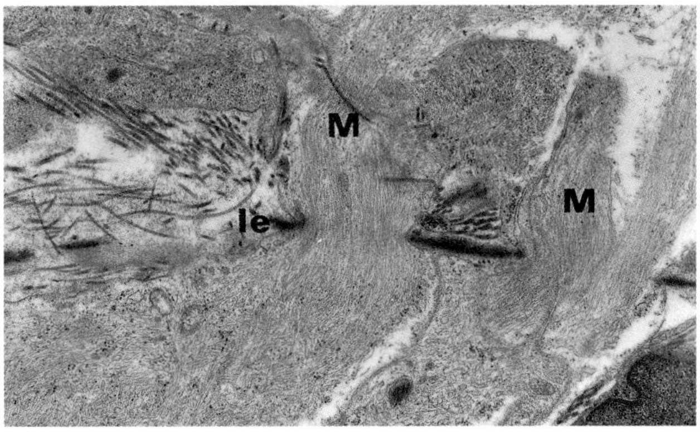

c

Figure 5.9 *Retina and Bruch's membrane 2 years after heavy cryopexy. (a) Light microscopic section shows* ***chorioretinal*** *scar by* ***infiltration****. Thermal injury necrosed the basement membrane of pigment epithelium. Therefore, regenerating Müller cells (M) of neuroepithelium infiltrate the collagen lamellae of Bruch's membrane (B), cross the level of elastic lamina and penetrate into the collagen (COL) of choroid. (Reproduced with permission from Kreissig I. Ultrastructure of the cryopexy adhesion in retinal surgery.* Postdoctoral Thesis for Habilitation. *Rheinische Friedrich-Wilhelms-Universität: Bonn, 1972: 1–172. Copyright © Lippincott Williams & Wilkins, 1972.*[22]*) (b) Electron micrograph shows area in which regenerated neuroepithelium (Nep) has infiltrated the layers of Bruch's membrane and crosses its elastic lamina (el). Fc = Fibrocyte, Col = collagen lamellae. (Reproduced with permission from Kreissig I, Lincoff H. Cryosurgery of the retina,* Int Ophthalmol Clin *(1976)* ***16****:63–81.*[9]*) (c) Electron micrograph of higher magnification also depicts area of Bruch's membrane in which Müller cells (M) have crossed the elastic lamina (le) toward the choroid. (Reproduced with permission from Kreissig I. Ultrastructure of the cryopexy adhesion in retinal surgery.* Postdoctoral Thesis for Habilitation. *Rheinische Friedrich-Wilhelms-Universität: Bonn, 1972: 1–172. Copyright © Lippincott Williams & Wilkins, 1972.*[22]*)*

RPE basement membrane. Finally, if the cryocoagulation is severe enough to cause necrosis of the basement membrane of RPE, surviving neuroepithelium may infiltrate the collagen lamellae of Bruch's membrane[24] and cause a chorioretinal scar (Figs 5.9 and 5.10).

An excessively heavy cryopexy application that penetrates the inner limiting membrane may induce vitreoretinal adhesions, therefore overfreezing should be avoided.

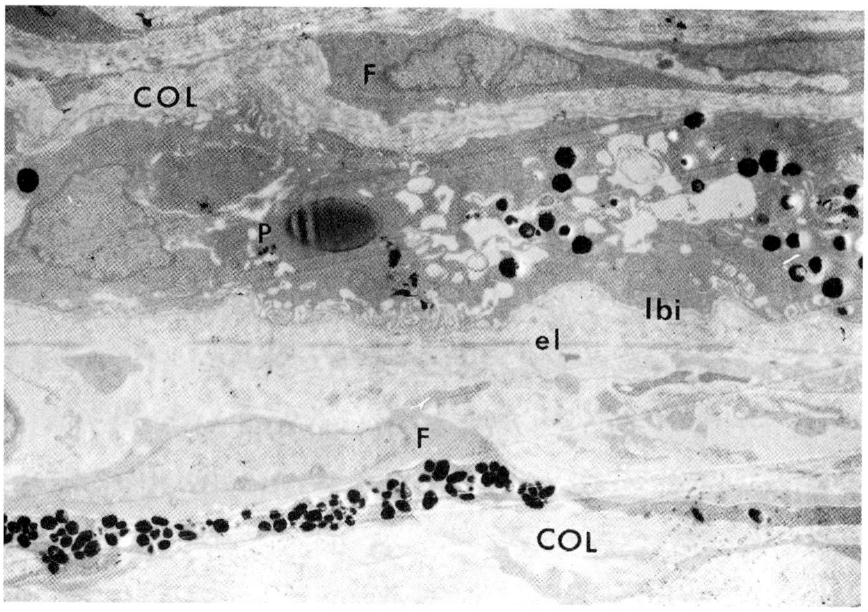

Figure 5.10 *Retina 28 days after heavy cryopexy: electron micrograph also shows a* ***chorioretinal*** *scar, yet here collagen fibers (COL) and fibroblasts (F) penetrate by a defect in the basement membrane (lbi = lamina basalis interna) of the pigment epithelium (P) into the overlying retinal tissue. el = Elastic lamina of Bruch's membrane. (Reproduced with permission from Kreissig I. Ultrastructure of the cryopexy adhesion in retinal surgery.* Postdoctoral Thesis for Habilitation. *Rheinische Friedrich-Wilhelms-Universität: Bonn, 1972: 1–172. Copyright © Lippincott Williams & Wilkins, 1972.*[22]*)*

SUMMARY

There are at least three distinct anatomic mechanisms that produce retinal adhesions after cryosurgery:

- **Interdigitation** of newly formed rods with villi of the RPE, producing a mild adhesion.
- **Desmosomal connection** between the Müller cells and the smooth surface of new RPE or the basement membrane of RPE, resulting in a strong adhesion.
- **Infiltrative or chorioretinal adhesion** in which processes of Müller cells infiltrate the collagen lamellae of Bruch's membrane to yield a very strong adhesion with a thin fragile retina.[25]

These varied ultrastructural changes result in different strengths of cryosurgery-induced adhesion, therefore a different adhesive strength is produced by light, medium and heavy cryopexy applications (but not by diathermy). The cryosurgical adhesive strength is predictable and can be controlled by ophthalmoscopic observation during application. The adhesive strength of the cryosurgical adhesion increases for 12 days to:

- 300 mg for the light cryopexy application.
- 575 mg for the medium application.
- 1175 mg for the heavy application.

REMODELING OF THE CRYOSURGICAL ADHESION

The maximum adhesion obtained by the medium cryopexy application at 12 days is mediated by depolarized cells and is unstable.[26] Repolarization of the RPE begins as early as 1 month. Basal infoldings of RPE and apical processes become evident. Initially the villus processes are disoriented and located between adjacent RPE cells. The apical surfaces exhibit stretches of blunt cell membranes adjacent to Müller cells (Fig. 5.11).

Intercellular organization of the RPE also becomes apparent. Pigment granules reappear with stacks of rough-surfaced endoplasmic reticulum. The actin-like filaments typical of the earlier migrating RPE cells are no longer conspicuous. From 2 months to 3 years, the cells remodel their relationship. The blunt cell apposition of adjacent plasma membranes of RPE and processes of Müller cells progressively develop an interdigitating villus architecture. The RPE cells display a myriad of delicate apical processes (villi), which mesh with shorter processes elaborated by Müller cells (Fig. 5.12). The desmosomes found between adjacent Müller cells simulate an external limiting membrane but no desmosomes are seen between RPE and Müller cells because of the interposition of their respective villus differentiation (Fig. 5.13). The entire evolution of the medium cryosurgical lesion is shown in Fig. 5.14.

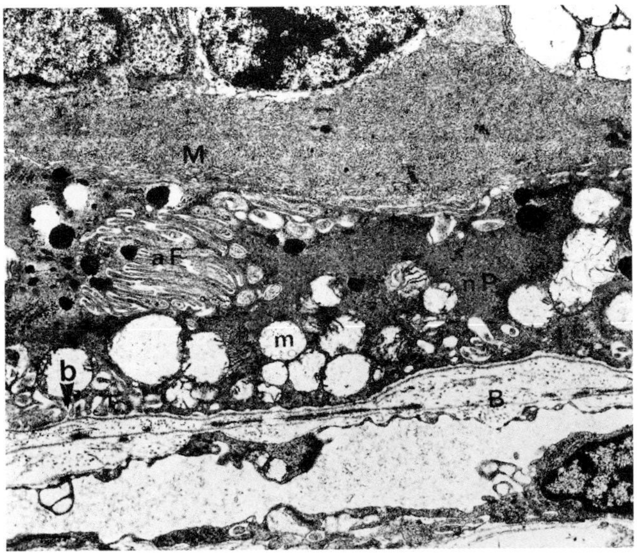

Figure 5.11 *At 3 weeks, pigment epithelial cells (nP) show signs of repolarization and differentiation: lateral villous processes (aF), basal infoldings (b) and pigment granules. Note: the apical surface abuts adjacent Müller cell (M) and still remains blunt and straight. B = Bruch's membrane. (Reproduced with permission from Kreissig I. Ultrastructure of the cryopexy adhesion in retinal surgery.* Postdoctoral Thesis for Habilitation. *Rheinische Friedrich-Wilhelms-Universität: Bonn, 1972: 1–172. Copyright © Lippincott Williams & Wilkins, 1972.[22])*

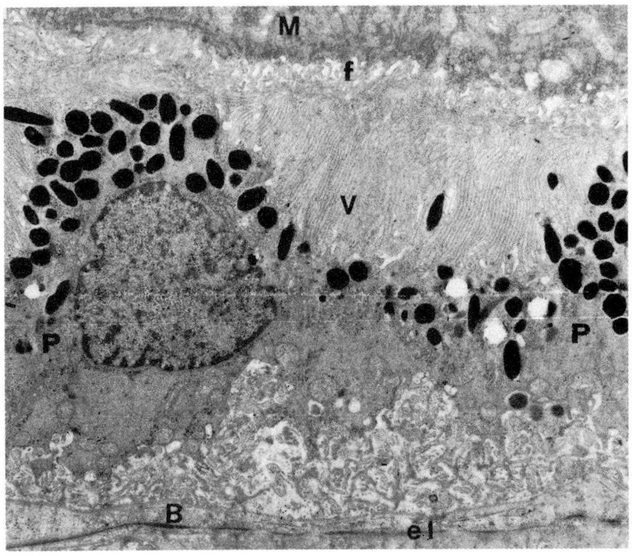

Figure 5.12 *At 18 months, remodeling of interface between pigment epithelial cells (P) and Müller cells (M) has resulted in exclusive intervillous adhesion (V). Müller cells have shorter villi that are finger-like (f). B = Bruch's membrane; el = elastic lamina. (Reproduced with permission from Kreissig I. Ultrastructure of the cryopexy adhesion in retinal surgery.* Postdoctoral Thesis for Habilitation. *Rheinische Friedrich-Wilhelms-Universität: Bonn, 1972: 1–172. Copyright © Lippincott Williams & Wilkins, 1972.[22])*

The correlation between the maximum adhesion of the cryosurgical lesion (at 12 days) with the development of desmosomal connections between the smooth surfaces of RPE and proliferating processes of Müller cells suggests that remodeling of the lesion with the displacement of desmosomal connections might correlate with a late weakening of the adhesion.[27] However, this conclusion is not justified with the present evidence because of the lack of uniformity of the lesions and the long-term clinical experience (see later section on cryosurgery with a temporary balloon buckle, p. 46).

It should be pointed out that the cryosurgical application causes a deeper and more profound necrosis of tissue in the center of the lesion than in the periphery.[19] Remodeling with villous proliferation is limited to those areas in the adhesion in which RPE has regenerated and recovered Bruch's membrane. In the center of moderate cryopexy lesions, there are sometimes areas in which RPE fails to recover Bruch's membrane before Müller cell

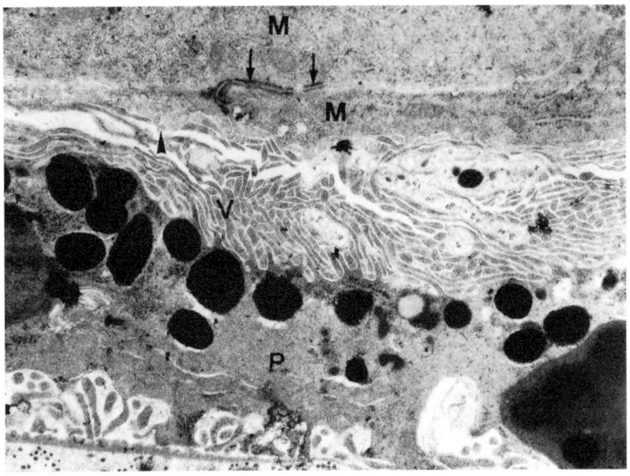

Figure 5.13 *At 2.5 years, desmosomes (arrows) are formed only between adjacent Müller cells (M). Thin long villi (V) of pigment epithelium (P) contrast with short finger-like villi (arrowhead) of Müller cells. (Reproduced with permission from Kreissig I. Ultrastructure of the cryopexy adhesion in retinal surgery.* Postdoctoral Thesis for Habilitation. *Rheinische Friedrich-Wilhelms-Universität: Bonn, 1972: 1–172. Copyright © Lippincott Williams & Wilkins, 1972.[22])*

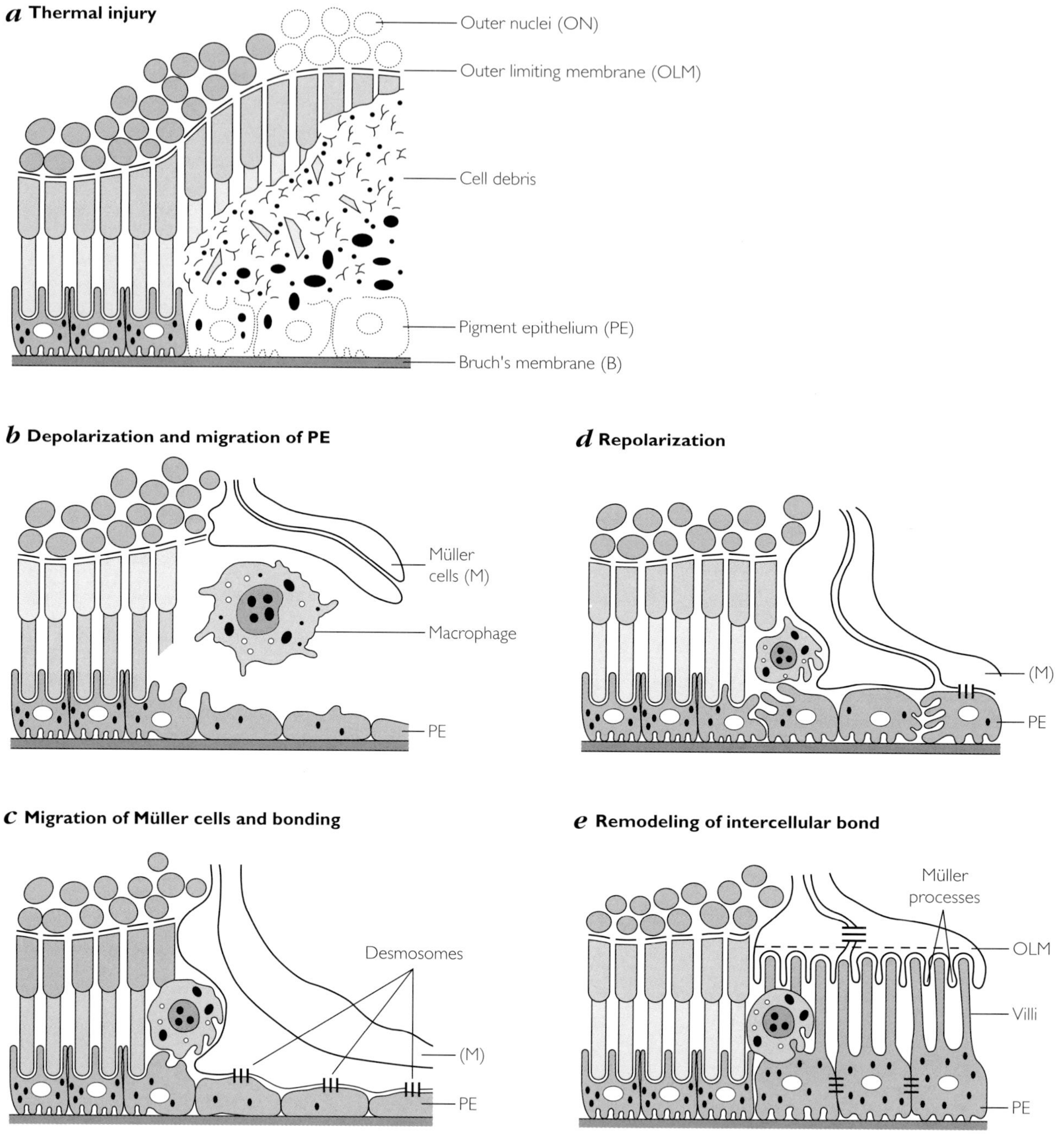

Figure 5.14 *Five stages of repair and remodeling of cryosurgical adhesion. (a) One day after medium cryopexy application: center of lesion is at right. Retinal pigment epithelium (PE), rods and outer nuclei (ON) are necrotic with cellular debris. Bruch's membrane (B) is intact. OLM = Outer limiting membrane. (b) At 4 days: depolarized PE cells are sliding across Bruch's membrane. Macrophage swollen with cellular debris lies above PE. Outer nuclei are gone and processes of Müller cells (M) descend from retina. (c) At 2 weeks: processes of Müller cells (M) have filled the defect and attached with desmosomes to the smooth surface of PE. Macrophages filled with phagosomes collect at periphery of lesion. (d) At 4 weeks: PE repolarizes. Basal infoldings are present. Disoriented villous processes appear at lateral edges. Subcellular reorganization (not shown) also occurs (see Fig. 5.11). (e) At 2 months: villi of PE reorient to apex of cell and interdigitate with short processes from Müller cell processes that protrude through restructured OLM (see Figs 5.12 and 5.13).*

processes come into contact with it. In these areas, Müller cell processes secrete a basement membrane and adhere to it with hemidesmosomes.[24] At some points, the surface of Bruch's membrane is penetrated by processes of Müller cells; these processes distribute in the collagen lamellae of the membrane. There is no evidence of late remodeling in these areas.

Even after 3 years, the hemidesmosomal attachments and infiltrations of collagen lamellae appeared to be unchanged. It is difficult in morphologic terms to conceive of any weakening in this portion of the adhesion.

SUMMARY OF THERMAL EXPERIMENTS

The experiments confirm the clinical impression that cryosurgery produces an adhesion sufficient for the treatment of retinal detachment. The reservations about the reliability of the cryosurgical adhesion in cases of retinal detachment with traction are not justified. Only the light cryosurgical lesion was occasionally weaker than diathermy; for medium-intensity lesions, there was no difference. Heavy cryosurgical lesions were stronger than all diathermy lesions.

More valuable to the clinicians is the fact that the adhesiveness of the cryosurgical lesions varies directly with the intensity of the applications. Furthermore, it is within the surgeon's ability to select a light, medium or heavy application by ophthalmoscopic control.

The predictability of the cryosurgical lesion provides the surgeon with the ability to select an appropriate application for various problems in retinal detachment surgery. A light application is probably sufficient for prophylactic treatment of round holes and areas of degeneration. Operculated tears and holes in retinal detachments are best treated at the medium level.

Heavy applications are to be avoided because the residual retina is fragile and subject to tearing if redetachment should occur.

The rapid rise in the adhesive strength of the cryosurgical lesions justifies early mobilization of the patient with retinal detachment, early hospital discharge and return to full activity in the second week.

Knowledge of the strength of the cryosurgical adhesion at 7 days has provided the basis for the temporary scleral buckle for treating a retinal detachment. The balloon buckle, a temporary device, represents another step toward minimal extraocular surgery for retinal detachment.[28]

CLINICAL APPLICATION OF CRYOSURGERY (CRYOPEXY)

PROCEDURE INSTRUMENTATION

The cryoprobe is a plastic insulated pencil-like device with a metallic tip that diverges from the end of the shaft at 90°. Nitrous oxide gas is transferred to the probe and recovered through channels encased in a flexible tube. The cooling effect is obtained by expansion of the gas in the probe tip (Joules–Thompson effect). The temperature at the tip varies with the pressure of N_2O released from the gas cylinder (which is attached to the console). Pressure is regulated by a knob on the console. Working pressures vary between 400 and 625 psi and yield temperatures at the tip between –30°C and –60°C. The flow is activated by a foot pedal.

TECHNIQUE

For treating retinal detachments, the cryoprobe is applied to the sclera after opening the conjunctiva and dissecting Tenon's tissue in the quadrant(s) of intended treatment. Indirect ophthalmoscopic visualization of the tip allows localization of the break by indenting and moving the probe from the ora serrata radially toward the break (to avoid parallactic displacement of the detached break). Care must be taken to keep the shaft from also indenting the sclera. 'Only the tip should touch the sclera' should be the frequent cautionary advice given to the assistant.

Freezing (cryocoagulation) is controlled by the pressure setting on the console and the duration of the application. The working temperature for most adult eyes is –60°C, which is obtained with a pressure setting of 625 psi. The duration of the freeze varies between 2 and 4 seconds. The freezing effect varies with the thickness of the sclera and, to a lesser extent, with the vascularity of the choroid. The choroid is largely exsanguinated by the indentation. To obtain the optimal lesion (medium) it is necessary to monitor each application ophthalmoscopically.

Do not rely on the appearance of the freeze on the surface of the sclera.

In the presence of opaque vitreous precluding the view of the peripheral retina (caused by hemorrhage), cryopexy is not advised. However, in most eyes with vitreous hemorrhage the anterior retina can be visualized by indirect ophthalmoscopy and sufficient scleral depression.

CRYOPEXY OF RETINAL BREAKS

The cryoprobe is the optimal instrument for localizing breaks in detached retina. A freeze mark in the retina eliminates parallax and provides an absolute localization of the break on the sclera. In practice it is expedient to localize the anterior extent and then the posterior extent of the break and to mark them with ink (methylene blue) on the sclera. Interrupted cryopexy then can be applied to the remaining edges of the break. The space between each cryopexy-induced adhesion remodels to form a water-tight interdigital adhesion between villi of pigment epithelium and the outer segments, so contiguous cryopexy is never indicated.

Anterior breaks tend to be in more shallowly detached retina. The indentation of the probe usually can bring the RPE into contact or close to the retina so that a moderate freeze appears as a white spot in the retina.

Posterior breaks in bullous retina often cannot be reached by the cryoprobe. A whitening in the choroid and RPE must be accepted for localization of the break. This requires the surgeon to correct for anterior–posterior parallax.

In this situation, do not maintain the application and overfreeze in an attempt to obtain retinal whitening. Instead, buckle the break on the basis of the choroidal localization and photocoagulate the edges of the break the day after the retina has become attached. Freezing RPE alone may provide some adhesion, but a more effective adhesion requires coagulation of the outer retina as well.

When localizing, do not try to keep the defrosted probe in contact with the sclera when rotating the eye into a position for marking the sclera. The probe is likely to slip during the rotation and the apparent indentation mark on the sclera when the probe is lifted will be incorrect. Faulty marking is a frequent cause of buckle failure.

The marking error can be prevented by training an assistant to move the probe as directed by the ophthalmoscopist and to do the marking.

TRANSCONJUNCTIVAL CRYOPEXY

Transconjunctival cryopexy can be optimal for prophylactic treatment of anterior retinal tears and to supplement a panretinal photocoagulation (PRP) in a diabetic eye. Each lesion must be monitored ophthalmoscopically. The freezing time at –60°C will be only slightly longer because of the intact conjunctiva. The conjunctiva will be edematous for 1–2 days after cryopexy. Topical or subconjunctival corticosteroids will diminish the edema. Breaks as posterior as the equator sometimes can be treated with cryopexy without opening the conjunctiva, by pushing the probe into the conjunctival fornix.

It is necessary to keep the fornix dry, otherwise the freezing effect is absorbed by the lake of fluid surrounding the tip of the probe.

COMPLICATIONS OF CRYOPEXY

Complications of cryopexy are rare. The probe can perforate thin (blue) sclera. This is an effect of pressure, not of freezing. It is to be avoided by examining the area of the sclera before treating it. The best technique again is to have the assistant move the probe while he/she observes the sclera. Breakdown of the blood–aqueous barrier and dispersion of RPE results from excessive freezing. The therapeutic freeze is produced by the medium application (first whitening in the retina). Multiple applications are separated by at least half of the diameter of the freeze. The mean number of applications for a detachment operation is 6 (4–10).

Avoid random freezing of peripheral areas of retina in search of a break.

Reserve exploratory freezing for the few spots that look suspicious when depressed by the probe.

ANESTHESIA

The conjunctiva, sclera and choroid are moderately sensitive to freezing. The pain response varies from patient to patient; thus, transconjunctival cryopexy can be accomplished with topical tetracaine 1% or with subconjunctival injection of lidocaine 1%. More extensive surgery, e.g. pancryopexy in the diabetic or transscleral cryopexy in a buckle operation, requires parabulbar anesthesia with lidocaine 2%.

CLINICAL EXPERIENCE WITH CRYOSURGERY (CRYOPEXY)

In the last 25 years, the indications for cryosurgery have increased. Cryosurgery has been applied for:

- Prophylactic treatment of retinal breaks.
- Retinal breaks combined with segmental buckling.

- A retinal break combined with a temporary balloon buckle.
- Supplemental peripheral retinal ablation (pancryocoagulation) in the photocoagulated diabetic eye.
- Treatment of threshold retinopathy of prematurity.
- Destruction of selected intraocular tumors, e.g. retinoblastoma and angioma.

The first four topics will be discussed.

PROPHYLACTIC TREATMENT OF RETINAL BREAKS

In recent years, the indications for prophylactic treatment of retinal breaks have changed. This was influenced largely by the long-term observations of Byer.[29] Today we are less inclined to treat asymptomatic retinal breaks and more inclined to practice '**passive prophylaxis**', i.e. to explain to the patient the symptoms of a retinal tear and to instruct on how to test for a visual field defect.

For '**active prophylaxis**', i.e. to seal a retinal break, cryopexy may be preferred in the presence of hazy optic media or a narrow pupil if either preclude photocoagulation.

CLINICAL STUDY OF PROPHYLACTIC CRYOPEXY

In a prospective study, 161 eyes with retinal breaks were sealed prophylactically with cryopexy.[22,30] Each cryopexy lesion was monitored by ophthalmoscopy; an interrupted pattern of medium lesions was applied to the margin of the breaks.

Complications

In one eye, a small detachment at the anterior edge of the break did not appear confined and was supplemented by an episcleral plomb on the fourth day. There was no hemorrhage (neither intraoperatively nor postoperatively) or postoperative decrease of visual function.

Long-term results

All of the 161 patients had a follow-up of between 1 and 4 years (a mean of 2.4 years). No eye developed proliferative changes, e.g. star folds. Six eyes developed a new break between 2 weeks and 1 year postoperatively. The new breaks were treated with cryopexy. A detachment occurred in two eyes after 2 and 17 months, respectively. The retinas in both eyes were attached with additional cryopexy to the break and segmental buckling.[30]

Conclusion

Cryopexy has proved to be a reliable method for prophylactic treatment of retinal breaks. In the presence of hazy media, it is the optimal method for retinal coagulation.

CRYOPEXY OF RETINAL BREAKS COMBINED WITH SEGMENTAL BUCKLING WITHOUT DRAINAGE OF SUBRETINAL FLUID

The minimal procedure for a retinal detachment, i.e. a local buckle without drainage, was made feasible by the introduction of cryosurgery in 1963.[8] This entirely extraocular procedure minimizes the inflicted surgical trauma and is accompanied by a very low morbidity.[31] The absence of scleral necrosis has virtually eliminated buckle-related infections.

Clinical studies

Between 1970 and 1977, a series of 1000 consecutive retinal detachments was treated prospectively with a medium application of cryopexy and segmental buckles without drainage of subretinal fluid. Eyes had an average follow-up of 32 months.[32] After one operation, reattachment was obtained in 83% and after reoperation in 91%.

A second series of detachments was treated prospectively with segmental buckles and cryopexy between August 1979 and January 1980 and followed for 15 years in order to answer the following questions:

- Does cryopexy induce proliferative vitreoretinopathy (PVR)?
- Does the absence of a cerclage jeopardize long-term results obtained with segmental buckling and cryopexy?
- Does the postoperative vision deteriorate in comparison to the fellow eye during a 15–year follow-up?

After one operation, the retina was reattached in 92.6% and after reoperation in 97%.[33,34]

Complications

In one eye, the buckle had to be removed because of infection (the retina remained attached). A highly myopic eye developed a massive choroidal effusion. Four eyes (3.7%) failed to attach because of progressive PVR.

Long-term anatomic results

The 104 (97%) attached retinas were followed for 15 years. Early redetachment (2–6 months) occurred in six eyes. Late redetachment (>6 months–15 years) occurred in seven eyes. After reoperation with another segmental buckle without cerclage or vitrectomy, the retina was attached in 99 eyes (92.6%) during long-term follow-up.

Long-term functional results

All of the eyes were observed periodically during the 15-year follow-up.[34] The mean visual acuity was 20/40 after 6 months and 20/30 at 1 year. Thereafter, there was a linear decrease of 0.07 lines in Snellen's chart per year in all eyes. The decrease over time was not significantly different from the decrease in the fellow eye and was consistent with aging.[35]

Conclusion

The long-term anatomic and visual results demonstrated a low morbidity of cryopexy in combination with segmental buckling, and answered the three questions:

- The rate of PVR was 3.7%, which is relatively low.
- The absence of a cerclage did not jeopardize long-term results after minimal extraocular surgery with cryopexy.
- The postoperative vision did not deteriorate in comparison to the fellow eye during a 15-year follow-up.

CRYOPEXY OF A RETINAL BREAK COMBINED WITH A TEMPORARY BALLOON BUCKLE WITHOUT DRAINAGE OF SUBRETINAL FLUID

Cryopexy of the break was combined with a temporary buckle that was left in place for 1 week. After removal of the balloon, retinal attachment depended solely on the strength of the cryosurgical adhesions around the break.

Clinical study

A series of 500 retinal detachments (with one break or a group of breaks within 1 clock-hour) were treated with medium applications of cryopexy and a temporary balloon buckle[28] without drainage of subretinal fluid. Follow-up ranged between 6 months and 7.5 years (a mean of 25 months).

Complications

There were no intraoperative complications and no postoperative infections.

Results

After one balloon insertion, the retina was reattached in 465 (93%) eyes. After removal of the balloon, the retina detached in 12 (2.4%) eyes. After reoperation, the retina was attached in 495 (99%) eyes. Sustained retinal attachment after the balloon is deflated and removed is solely dependent on the strength of the mature cryosurgical adhesions around the break.

The balloon operation provided a clinical experiment to confirm the results of the animal experiments done 25 years earlier, investigating the strength of the cryosurgical adhesion. The sustained retinal attachment after withdrawal of the balloon buckle attested to the strength of the cryosurgical adhesion.

Even during long-term follow-up, there was no evidence of late weakening of the cryosurgical adhesion.

Another investigation was performed to answer the question: Is the adhesion after cryopexy as strong as after laser surgery?

Clinical study

One-hundred aphakic detachments were treated with a temporary balloon buckle: in 55 eyes the break was treated with laser on postoperative day 1 or 2; in 45 eyes the break was treated intraoperatively with cryopexy.[36] After removal of the balloon the retina started to detach in two eyes treated with laser coagulation. The difference is not statistically significant.

Conclusion

This study confirms that the retinal adhesion after cryopexy is comparable to that obtained after laser surgery; both are strong enough to secure the edges of a retinal break, even after removal of a temporary balloon buckle.

PANCRYOCOAGULATION IN THE DIABETIC EYE

Pancryocoagulation can be applied in the diabetic eye to enhance the clearing of an intravitreal hemorrhage or to induce regression of persistent retinal neovascularization or rubeosis iridis. Schöler[1] demonstrated that transscleral cryopexy applications accelerated the clearing of vitreous hemorrhage. Additional reports by Haut et al[37] and Oosterhuis and Bijlmer-Gorter[38] confirmed this.

In the presence of a vitreous hemorrhage, cryopexy is a rational substitute for laser coagulation to induce regression of neovascularization.

Clinical study

From July 1989 to June 1990, there were 27 diabetic eyes with a persistent vitreous hemorrhage treated with pancryocoagulation.[39] A vitreous hemorrhage suitable for cryopexy was one in which the blood did not settle inferiorly despite double patching and elevation of the patient's head, maneuvers to enhance settling to make the retina visible for laser treatment. Preoperative visual acuity ranged between light perception and finger counting. In 17 of the 27 eyes a rubeosis iridis grade II–IV was present.

Surgical procedure

Transconjunctival anterior pancryocoagulation was applied in an interrupted manner. One treatment consisted of 8–12 lesions in the superior or inferior circumference 10–13 mm from the limbus. Indentation with the cryoprobe allowed visualization of freezing applications in the retina. They were monitored ophthalmoscopically and applied to a medium level. Pancryocoagulation in the superior circumference is prophylactic against retinal detachment that might emanate from subsequent vitrectomy ports.

After one to three pancryopexy treatments in 23 eyes, laser supplementation was possible. In two eyes, despite cryopexy, a vitrectomy was necessary to clear the media. The mean follow-up for all patients was 32 months.

Results

The visual acuity improved in 25 of the 27 patients: in 23 patients it was between 20/200 and 20/50. Rubeosis iridis decreased significantly after pancryocoagulation and there was no evidence of recurrence after a mean of 32 months.

DISCUSSION

After 30 years, cryosurgery still maintains an important place in posterior segment surgery.

It can induce strong retinal adhesions comparable to those obtained by laser coagulation.[36] Cryosurgery allows retinal coagulation through full-thickness sclera without scleral damage and thus allows a minimal extraocular procedure for retinal detachment that employs an elastic explant to buckle the area limited to the retinal break. The procedure obtains attachment without drainage of subretinal fluid.[31] This type of minimal operation represents a realization of Gonin's postulate:[2] the retinal break is the cause of the detachment and closing it is the solution. Applying cryopexy at a medium intensity in combination with segmental buckling has yielded a primary reattachment rate of >90% and has reduced the rate of PVR in scleral buckling to <4%,[33] which may be the natural incidence of the complication without surgical augmentation. In diabetic patients, the medium cryosurgical lesions can augment retinal laser coagulation and induce a regression of rubeosis iridis.[39]

Thirty years of favorable clinical experience with cryosurgery support its continued use.

REFERENCES

1. Schöler F. Experimentelle Erzeugung von Aderhaut-Netzhautentzündung durch Kohlensäureschnee, *Klin Monatsbl Augenheilk* (1918) **60**:1.

2. Gonin J. La thermoponction oblitérante des déchirures dans le décollement de la rétine, *Ann Oculist (Paris)* (1931) **168**:1–29.

3. Deutschmann R. Über zwei Verfahren bei Behandlung der Netzhautablösung (eines davon der Diathermie scheinbar entgegengesetzt) nebst Bemerkungen zur Genese des Netzhautrisses und seines Verhältnisses zur Entstehung der Ablösung, *Klin Monatsbl Augenheilk* (1933) **91**:450–6.
4. Bietti GB. Criocausticazioni episclerali come mezzo di terapia nel distacco retinico, *Boll Ocul* (1934) **13**:576–617.
5. Custodis E. Bedeutet die Plombenaufnähung auf die Sklera einen Fortschritt in der operativen Behandlung der Netzhautablösung? *Ber Dtsch Ophthalmol Ges* (1953) **58**:102–5.
6. Schepens CL, Okamura ID, Brockhurst RJ, Regan CDJ. Scleral buckling procedures: V. Synthetic sutures and silicone implants, *Arch Ophthalmol* (1960) **64**:868–81.
7. Lincoff HA, McLean JM, Nano H. Scleral abscess, I. A complication of retinal detachment buckling procedures, *Arch Ophthalmol* (1965) **74**:641–8.
8. Lincoff HA, McLean JM, Nano H. Cryosurgical treatment of retinal detachment, *Trans Am Acad Ophthalmol Otolaryngol* (1964) **68**:412–32.
9. Kreissig I, Lincoff H. Cryosurgery of the retina, *Int Ophthalmol Clin* (1976) **16**:63–81.
10. Lincoff H, McLean JM. Modifications to the Custodis-procedure: II. A new silicone implant for large tears, *Am J Ophthalmol* (1967) **64**:877–9.
11. McPherson A, Girard L. Cryosurgery in the prophylaxis and management of retinal detachment, *Bibl Ophthalmol* (1967) **72**:381–97.
12. Kreissig I, Sbaiti A. Cryopexy in the prophylaxis of retinal detachment, *Klin Monatsbl Augenheilk* (1971) **159**:588–96.
13. Bellows JG. The application of cryogenic techniques in ophthalmology, *Am J Ophthalmol* (1964) **57**:29–33.
14. Böke W, Hollwich F. Zur Kryochirurgie am Auge. In: Jaeger W, ed., *Deutsche Ophthalmologische Gesellschaft* (Verlag Bergmann: Munich, 1965): 212–18.
15. Curtin VT, Fujino T, Norton EWD. Comparative histopathology of cryosurgery and photocoagulation: observations on the advantages of cryosurgery in retinal detachment operations, *Arch Ophthalmol* (1966) **75**:674–82.
16. Oosterhuis JA, Brihaye M, de Haan AB. A comparative study of experimental transscleral cryocoagulation by solid carbon dioxide and diathermocoagulation of the retina, *Ophthalmologica* (1968) **156**:38–76.
17. Törnquist R. Cryosurgery for retinal detachment, *Acta Ophthalmol* (1968) **46**:529–34.
18. Lincoff H, O'Connor P, Bloch D, et al. The cryosurgical adhesion: Part II, *Trans Am Acad Ophthalmol Otolaryngol* (1970) **74**:98–107.
19. Lincoff H, Kreissig I. The mechanism of the cryosurgical adhesion: Part IV. Electron microscopy, *Am J Ophthalmol* (1971) **71**:674–89.
20. Kreissig I, Lincoff H. Ultrastructure of cryopexy adhesion, (Ultrastruktur der Kryopexieadhäsion). In: Jaeger W, ed., *Symposion der Deutschen Ophthalmologischen Gesellschaft, Die Prophylaxe der idiopathischen Netzhautabhebung* (Verlag Bergmann: Munich, 1971): 191–205.
21. Kreissig I, Lincoff H. Animal experiments about retinal scarring, *Graefes Arch Clin Exp Ophthalmol* (1974) **190**:165–82.
22. Kreissig I. Ultrastructure of the cryopexy adhesion in retinal surgery (Ultrastruktur der Kryopexie-Adhäsion in der Netzhautchirurgie). *Postdoctoral Thesis for Habilitation.* (Rheinische Friedrich-Wilhelms-Universität: Bonn, 1972): 1–172.
23. Kreissig I, Lincoff H. Mechanism of retinal attachment after cryosurgery, *Trans Ophthalmol Soc UK* (1975) **95**:148–57.
24. Kreissig I, Lincoff H. Bruch's membrane and its structural changes after cryopexy, *Klin Monatsbl Augenheilk* (1974) **164**:71–89.
25. Kreissig I, Lincoff H. Cryosurgery of the retina, *Int Ophthalmol Clin* (1976) **16**:63–81.
26. Lincoff H, Kreissig I, Jakobiec F, Iwamoto T. Remodeling of the cryosurgical adhesion, *Arch Ophthalmol* (1981) **99**:1845–9.
27. Lincoff H, Kreissig I, Jakobiec FA, Iwamoto T. Morphologic features of the possible weakening of the cryosurgical adhesion (summary), *Dev Ophthalmol* (1981) **2**:302.
28. Kreissig I, Failer J, Lincoff H, Ferrari F. Results of a temporary balloon buckle in the treatment of 500 retinal detachments and a comparison with pneumatic retinopexy, *Am J Ophthalmol* (1989) **107**:381–9.
29. Byer NE. Long-term natural history of lattice degeneration of the retina, *Ophthalmology* (1989) **96**:1396–402.
30. Kreissig I, Ruge I, Lippert U. Cryopexy in retinal detachment prophylaxis: Part II (Kryopexie in der Ablatio-Prophylaxe: II. Mitteilung), *Sitzungsber Vers Rheinisch-Westfälische Augenärzte* (1975) **130**:41–7.
31. Kreissig I. Minimalizing of detachment surgery, *Klin Monatsbl Augenheilk* (1989) **195**:126–34.
32. Kreissig I. Detachment surgery without drainage, *Klin Monatsbl Augenheilkd* (1978) **173**:140–9.
33. Kreissig I, Rose D, Jost B. Minimized surgery for retinal detachments with segmental buckling and nondrainage: an 11–year follow-up, *Retina* (1992) **12**:224–31.
34. Kreissig I, Simader E, Fahle M, Lincoff H. Visual acuity after segmental buckling and non-drainage: a 15–year follow-up, *Eur J Ophthalmol* (1995) **5**:240–6.
35. Slataper FJ. Age norms of refraction and vision, *Arch Ophthalmol* (1950) **43**:466–81.
36. Lincoff H, Kreissig I, Farber M. Results of 100 aphakic detachments treated with a temporary balloon buckle: a case against routine encircling operations, *Br J Ophthalmol* (1985) **69**:798–804.
37. Haut J, Robert P, Chatellier P, Leon MC. Place de la cryothérapie dans le traitement de la rétinopathie diabétique, *Bull Mem Soc Fr Ophthalmol* (1978) **90**:124–8.
38. Oosterhuis JA, Bijlmer-Gorter H. Cryotreatment in proliferative diabetic retinopathy: long-term results, *Ophthalmologica* (1980) **181**:81–7.
39. Kreissig I, Hipp E, Schneider U. Persistent massive vitreous hemorrhage in diabetic retinopathy: conservative management with pancryopexy and longterm follow-up, *Spektrum Augenheilkd* (1995) **9**:1–6.

Chapter 6 Pneumatic retinopexy

Paul E Tornambe

INTRODUCTION

The first injection of gas for repair of retinal detachment was probably performed by Ohm in 1911.[1] Intravitreal injection of air with drainage of subretinal fluid and diathermy was used for retinal reattachment by Rosengren in 1937.[2] Pneumatic retinopexy (as an office-based, outpatient treatment for retinal detachment) has become a recognized alternative to scleral buckling since its introduction in 1985 by Hilton and Grizzard[3] in the USA and by Dominguez[4] in Spain. The Pneumatic Retinopexy Clinical Trial (PRCT) (Tables 6.1–6.3) showed that the overall anatomic success is similar between pneumatic retinopexy and scleral buckling (99% vs 98%), and eyes treated with pneumatic retinopexy attained better visual acuity (20/50 or better in macula-off eyes; pneumatic retinopexy vs scleral buckling, 89% vs 67%).[5,6] Morbidity was lower with pneumatic retinopexy, patients returned to work sooner and pneumatic retinopexy is approximately half as costly as scleral buckling because the operating room is avoided. The PRCT also proved that a failed pneumatic procedure does not compromise anatomic reattachment or visual recovery, making it reasonable to try pneumatic retinopexy first.

The following approach has evolved over the past 13 years, with experience gained by treating and following more than 300 eyes. Pneumatic retinopexy appears deceptively simple but it is not. It should be performed by those familiar with retinal disease who

Table 6.1 Surgical results

Feature	*Pneumatic retinopexy 13-year review*	*Pneumatic Retinopexy Clinical Trial*
No. of eyes treated with pneumatic retinopexy	302	103
Meet CTG[a]	64%	100%
Male	61%	62%
Phakic	45%	55%
>50% retinal detachment	41%	57%

[a] CTG Meets Pneumatic Retinopexy Clinical Trial group criteria (see Table 6.2)

Note: This table and Tables 6.3 and 6.4 summarize and compare the salient features of the Pneumatic Retinopexy Clinical Trial (103 eyes) with the author's 13-year experience (302 eyes) of consecutive cases treated with pneumatic retinopexy. Although many eyes exceeded the inclusion criteria of the Pneumatic Retinopexy Clinical Trial, outcomes were similar. Special attention should be given to visual outcomes in eyes with the macula detached for 2 weeks or less.

Table 6.2 Admission criteria for the Pneumatic Retinopexy Clinical Trial

Inclusion criteria

- A single break no larger than 1 clock-hour located in the superior 8 clock-hours of the ocular fundus, or a group of small breaks within 1 clock-hour
- Media sufficiently clear to: rule out the presence of other retinal breaks; determine macula attachments; and not significantly reduce visual acuity
- Patient willingness to enter into the randomized study
- Stated availability for at least 6 months' follow-up
- Eye is judged suitable for treatment by either procedure
- All eyes must have a history of good vision before retinal detachment (to facilitate statistical evaluation of postoperative visual acuity)
- Macula-on eyes must have a corrected visual acuity of 20/50 or better (at least 35 letters on the ETDRS[a] chart)
- Macula-off eyes must have a corrected visual acuity worse than 20/50 (< 35 letters on the ETDRS[a] chart)
- The shortest diameter of the detached area must be at least six disc diameters.

Exclusion criteria

- Proliferative vitreoretinopathy, grade C or D_3
- Glaucoma that is medically controlled or where the cup/disc ratio exceeds 0.6
- Retinal breaks in the inferior 4 clock-hours of the fundus
- Inadequate physical or mental competence to maintain the required postoperative head position

[a] ETDRS Early Treatment Diabetic Retinopathy Study

Table 6.3 Surgical results

Feature	*Pneumatic retinopexy 13-year review of 302 eyes*	*Pneumatic Retinopexy Clinical Trial*
C_3F_8/C_2F_6	31%/11%	83%/0%
SF_6	57%	17%
New/missed break	33%	23%
Proliferative vitreoretinopathy	10%	3%
SOS pneumatic retinopexy	68%	73%
SOS pneumatic retinopexy + L/C	78%	81%
SOS pneumatic retinopexy + PPV/SB	95%	99%
Visual acuity ≥ 20/50 at 24 months if macula-off ≤ 14 days	82%	89%

SOS Single-operation success
L/C Laser or cryoretinopexy
PPV/SB Pars plana vitrectomy and/or scleral buckle
Note: See Table 6.1 footnote

have an understanding of vitreoretinal relationships and can handle possible complications. Over the past 5 years, approximately 80% of all retinal detachments encountered in my practice were treated with pneumatic retinopexy. A review of these eyes indicated that the single-operation success rate varied from 60% to 97% (Table 6.4), and was dependent upon:

Table 6.4 Retinal detachment characteristics vs probability of single-operation success

	Probability of single-operation success > 90%	81–90%	71–80%	51–70%
No. of breaks	1	2	3	>4
Extent of retinal detachment	< 25%	26–100%	26–100%	26–100%
Phakic status	Phakic	Pseudophakic	Pseudophakic	Pseudophakic
CTG[a]	Meets	Meets	Exceeds	Exceeds

[a] CTG Meets Pneumatic Retinopexy Clinical Trial group criteria
Note: This table was generated using data from the 13-year review of 302 eyes. It can be used, in general, to give the patient and surgeon an idea of the success rate for a relatively specific set of circumstances and may help in making an informed decision regarding the chances for success.

- The surgeon's ability to recognize retinal pathology.
- Appropriate case selection.
- The surgical technique.
- The surgeon's experience.

The following is my approach to an eye with a retinal detachment.

INDICATIONS FOR PNEUMATIC RETINOPEXY

Pneumatic retinopexy may be used to repair retinal detachments caused by retinal break(s) located in the upper two-thirds of the fundus with proliferative vitreoretinopathy (PVR) of grade B or less. Patients must be capable of postoperative positioning.

The following variables may decrease the success rate of pneumatic retinopexy:

- Pseudophakia.
- Multiple breaks.
- Detachment of 20 or more retinal quadrants.

Pneumatic retinopexy has been used in the following clinical situations with less than one-operation success:

- Multiple breaks in multiple quadrants.
- Extensive lattice degeneration.
- PVR up to grade C if the starfold does not exert traction on the retinal break.

Pneumatic retinopexy has not been evaluated thoroughly but has been successful in the following clinical situations:

- Hypotony.
- Posterior retinal breaks, including macular holes.
- High myopia.
- Dialysis.
- Selected giant tears.

CONTRAINDICATIONS FOR PNEUMATIC RETINOPEXY

The contraindications for pneumatic retinopexy are:

- Inferior breaks between the 4 and 8 o'clock positions.
- Inability to find the retinal break(s).
- Inability to evaluate the peripheral retina.
- Visualization-limiting media change.
- Poor patient cooperation.
- Limited expertise with indirect ophthalmoscopy.

- Excessive vitreoretinal adhesions.
- Inability of the patient to position self postoperatively for 3–5 days.
- Inability to follow the patient closely during the first two postoperative weeks.
- Inability of the surgeon to manage potential retinal complications.
- Necessity for the patient to fly or visit an area with a rise in altitude above 4000 feet while gas bubble is present.

Pneumatic retinopexy may be applied in eyes with a broad range of retinal findings that influence surgical outcome. Eyes in which pneumatic retinopexy may be indicated can be grouped into higher, intermediate and lower predicted success rate categories based on ocular findings at initial examination. Eyes with the highest predicted success rate would have a normal axial length, small holes or less than 1 clock-hour horseshoe tear, breaks within 1 clock-hour of 12 o'clock or at the horizontal meridian, detachment of only the superior quadrants, a crystalline lens or posterior chamber implant with a clear intact capsule, and clear media. Eyes with intermediate predicted success rate would have a long axial length, horseshoe tears of 1–2 clock-hours, tears just below the horizontal meridian, detachment of one inferior quadrant, aphakia, an anterior chamber lens or posterior capsule haze, and mild-to-moderate vitreous opacity. Those eyes with the lowest predicted success rate would have a very long axial length, large horseshoe tears more than 3 clock-hours apart, inferior retinal breaks, detachment of both inferior quadrants, an iris plane lens or open capsule with peripheral haze, and fixed retinal folds.

ADVANTAGES OF PNEUMATIC RETINOPEXY

The advantages provided by pneumatic retinopexy are:

- Better postoperative vision.
- Less perioperative morbidity.
- Less discomfort than scleral buckling procedures.
- No diplopia.
- No refractive error changes (induced astigmatism, or anisometropia).
- No scleral buckling material-related complications.
- Faster visual recovery.
- Similar overall success.
- Less costly: 50–75% less expensive than scleral buckling.
- No ultimate compromise of reattachment or visual return if pneumatic retinopexy fails.

REASONS WHY PNEUMATIC RETINOPEXY IS NOT PERFORMED MORE FREQUENTLY

Some of the reasons why pneumatic retinopexy is not performed more frequently are:

- Surgeon's inexperience.
- Surgeon's bad experience.
- Poor case selection.
- Poor surgical technique.
- Unwillingness to change if another procedure works.
- Pneumatic retinopexy requires more preoperative and postoperative time.
- Pneumatic retinopexy requires more patient cooperation.
- Pneumatic retinopexy requires closer follow-up.

PREOPERATIVE EVALUATION AND CONSIDERATIONS

The patient must be cooperative and physically and mentally capable of positioning postoperatively. Frequent follow-up must be possible, with consideration given to geographic, transportation and compliance issues. The patient cannot fly in an airplane or ascend to greater than 4000 feet in elevation. Preoperatively, drawings, models and videos can be used to educate the patient about the procedure.

Larger eyes require larger bubbles to subtend similar arcs of retinal contact. Additionally, recent ocular surgery mandates a paracentesis before gas introduction in order to avoid iris incarceration. Eyes with advanced glaucomatous optic neuropathy may not tolerate even a brief, modest elevation of intraocular pressure and must be managed accordingly. In eyes with filtering blebs, cryopexy must be avoided in those areas. Media clarity is important because cataract, opacified capsule, pseudophakia or vitreous opacities may prevent an adequate evaluation of the peripheral retina.

All retinal detachment repairs require all retinal breaks to be located, and pneumatic retinopexy is no exception. Importantly, posterior breaks and those at the 4 and 8 o'clock positions are difficult to close by pneumatic retinopexy. Breaks may be overlooked in eyes with total detachment, media opacities and intraocular lenses. Inferior breaks in attached retina may be problematic if the gas displaces subretinal fluid beneath them. Multiple retinal breaks suggest more extensive vitreoretinal interface pathology.

INSTRUMENTATION AND MEDICATION

The required instrumentation and medication include the following:

- Gloves, Betadine solution (10%).
- Xylocaine 1%, Marcaine 0.5%, gentamicin.
- Antibiotic/steroid ointment.
- Lid speculum, conjunctival forceps, cotton-tipped applicators.
- One eye patch.
- Two tuberculin syringes, two 27-gauge half-inch needles.
- Sulfur hexafluoride (SF_6), perfluoroethane (C_2F_6), or perfluoropropane (C_3F_8) gas.
- One Millipore filter.
- Cryopexy instruments.
- Laser indirect ophthalmoscope delivery system.
- Escalon 'Pneumo Level' (recommended).

GAS SELECTION

Although the gas having the shortest duration should be selected, it is also important to inject the smallest bubble possible; SF_6 lasts 7–10 days and expands twofold, C_2F_6 lasts 21 days and expands threefold and C_3F_8 has a duration of 6–8 weeks and expands fourfold.

OPERATIVE PROCEDURE

STEP 1 – SET-UP (Fig. 6.1)

The procedure is done in the office examination chair with the patient in the supine position. Topical

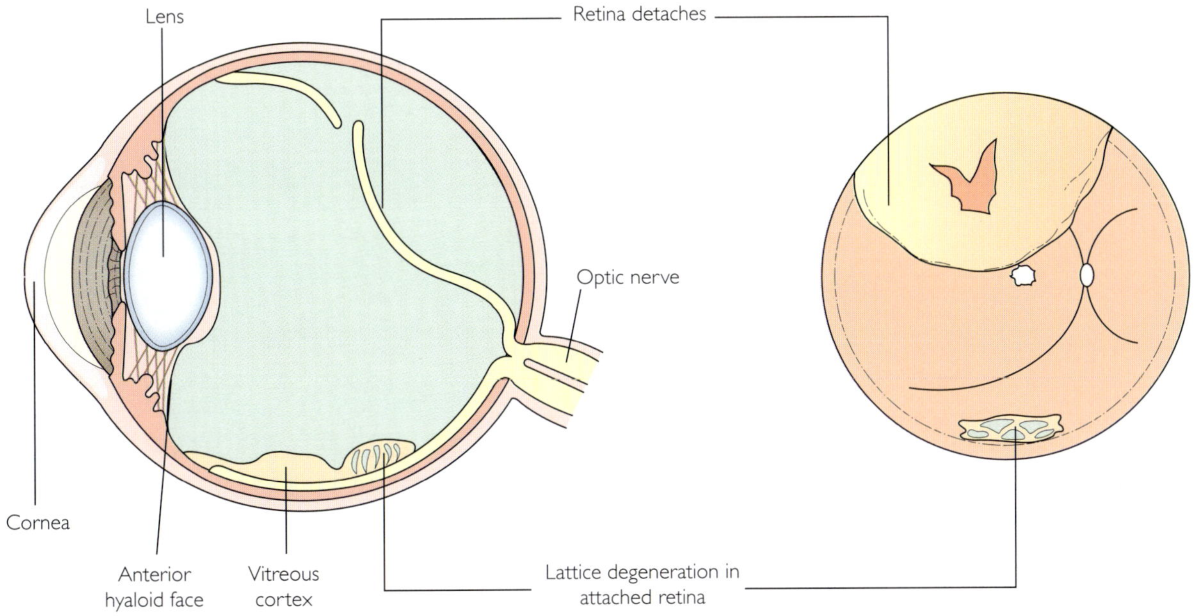

Figure 6.1 *Example of a candidate for pneumatic retinopexy.*

anesthetic drops (proparacaine 0.5%) are applied to the cornea and subconjunctival anesthesia (lidocaine 2%) is applied over the area of the pars plana at the gas injection and cryopexy site. Retrobulbar anesthesia is rarely required.

STEP 2A – PHOTOCOAGULATION (Fig. 6.2)

Apply photocoagulation to areas of attached retina with and without pathology. Low-intensity photocoagulation should be applied between the ora serrata

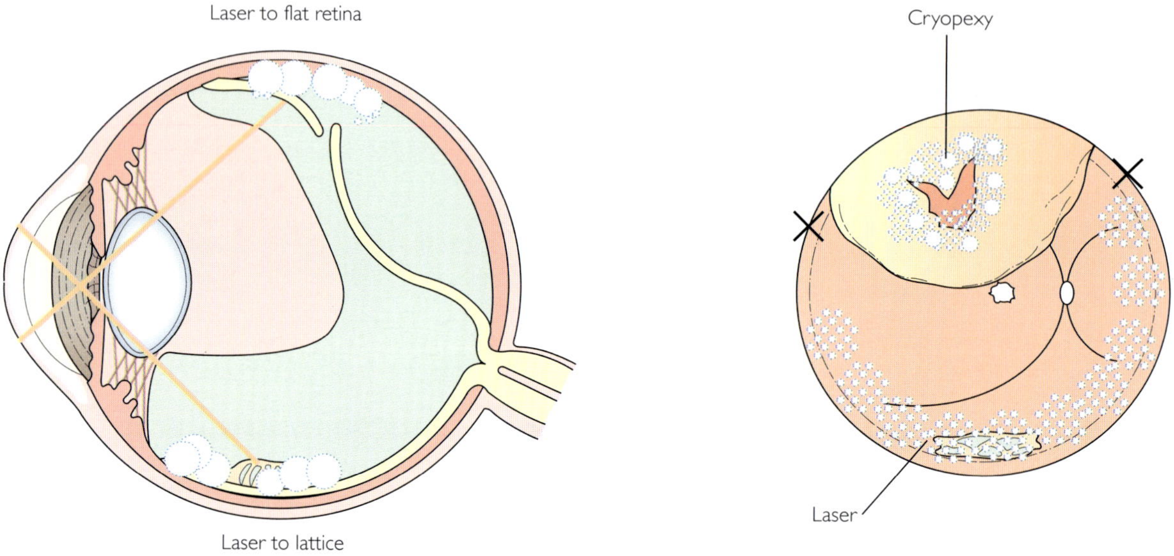

Figure 6.2 *Step 2A – photocoagulation.*

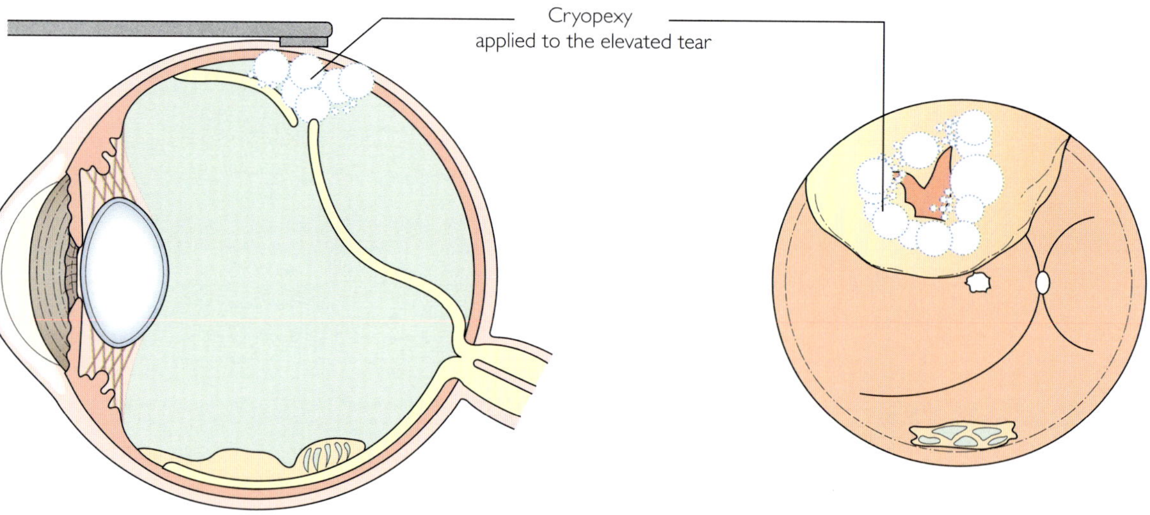

Figure 6.3 *Step 2B – cryopexy. Apply cryopexy to the elevated retinal pathology (but if the breaks are highly elevated, avoid cryopexy at this time).*

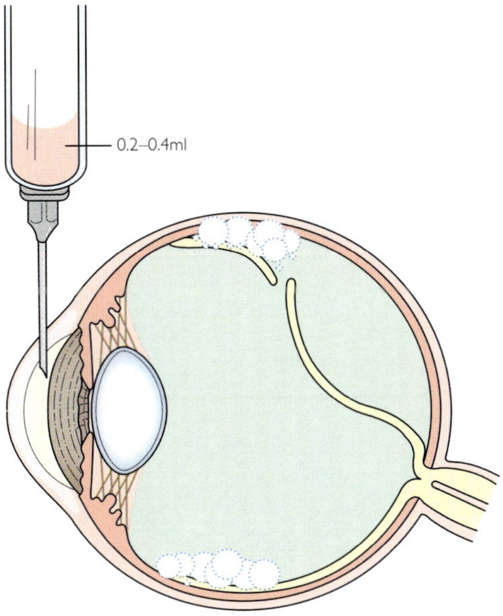

Figure 6.4 *Step 4 – paracentesis. Attach a 27-gauge needle to a tuberculin syringe and remove the plunger. Dry excess Betadine from the conjunctiva with a cotton-tipped applicator. Perform a limbal paracentesis using conjunctival forceps to stabilize the eye. Let 0.2–0.4 ml of aqueous fill the syringe.*

and the insertion of the vitreous base (equator) in all quadrants of attached retina. Laser should not be applied to detached retina, no matter how shallow; nor should it be placed within 1 clock-hour of detached retina.

STEP 2B – CRYOPEXY (Fig. 6.3)

Apply cryopexy to the elevated retinal pathology. However, if the breaks are highly elevated, avoid cryopexy initially.

STEP 3 – FILL SYRINGE WITH GAS

A 10% Betadine solution should be applied full strength to the cornea and left for 3 minutes. After filling the dead space in the tubing and the syringe twice, the gas should be drawn into a tuberculin syringe with a Millipore filter, leaving the exact amount to be injected in the syringe and capping it with a 27-gauge needle.

STEP 4 – PARACENTESIS (Fig. 6.4)

A 27-gauge needle is attached to another tuberculin syringe and the plunger is removed. Excess Betadine solution should be removed from the conjunctiva with a cotton-tipped applicator. A limbal paracentesis is performed, using conjunctival forceps to stabilize the eye. Approximately 0.2–0.4 ml of aqueous is removed.

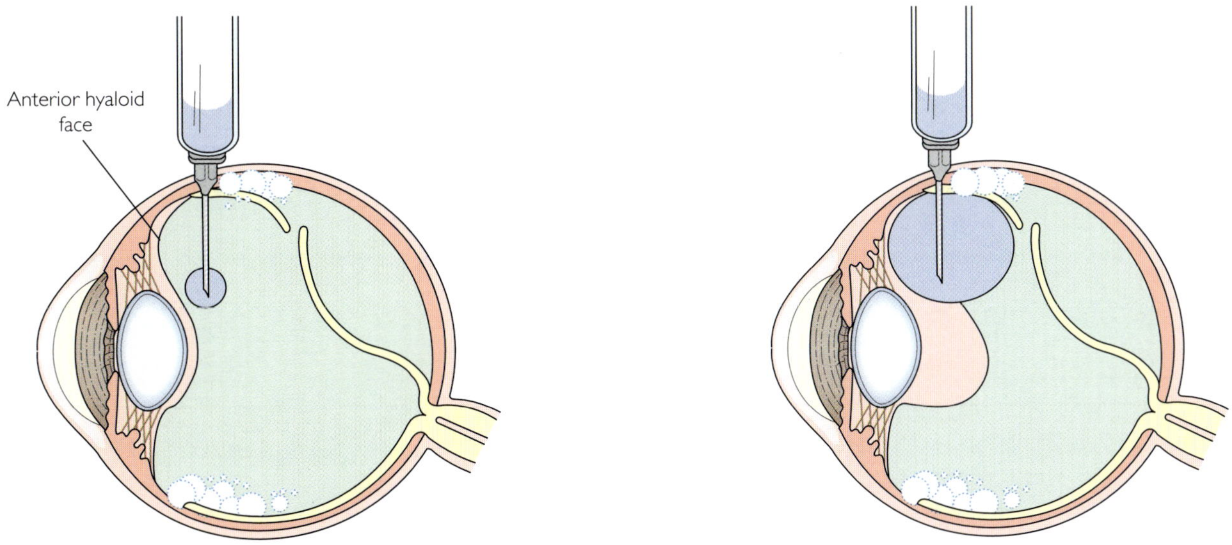

Figure 6.5 *Step 5 – single bubble gas injection.*

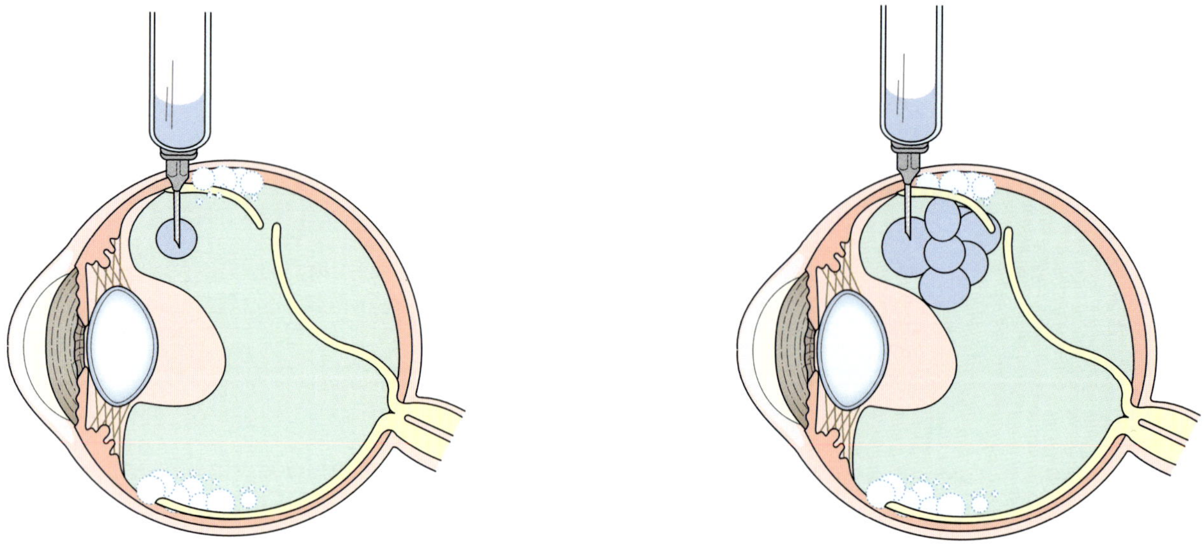

Figure 6.6 *Step 5 – fish eggs. Inject slowly; too rapid an injection forces the bubbles away from the needle tip and creates fish eggs.*

STEP 5 – GAS INJECTION (Fig. 6.5)

With the patient supine, the head is turned so that the pars plana injection site is uppermost. The injection should be performed in an area distant from large, elevated breaks in order to avoid subretinal gas. The injection site is chosen 3.5–4 mm from the limbus. Conveniently, the needle cap may be used to estimate this distance. The safest injection site is just above or below the 3 or 9 o'clock position, to avoid the long posterior ciliary nerves or vessels. The needle is inserted perpendicular to the eye wall. With the patient supine and ideally positioned, the eye wall also should be perpendicular to the floor. The needle is inserted into the midvitreous cavity and pulled back so that 3–4 mm of the needle tip remains in the eye. The indirect ophthalmoscope light may aid in visualizing the needle tip. Care must be used in eyes with bullous detachments in order to avoid the retina.

The gas should be injected at a moderate speed; an injection that is too rapid or too deep in the vitreous cavity forces bubbles away from the needle tip and creates fish eggs (Fig. 6.6). Should fish eggs occur, the surgeon may 'thump' the eye with a cotton-tip applicator to cause coalescence of the gas. Should fish eggs persist, it is prudent to position the patient with the gas away from large retinal breaks until the fish eggs resolve (usually 24 hours). If the needle does not penetrate the anterior hyaloid, loculated gas in the Space of Petit will result (sausage sign) (Fig. 6.7).

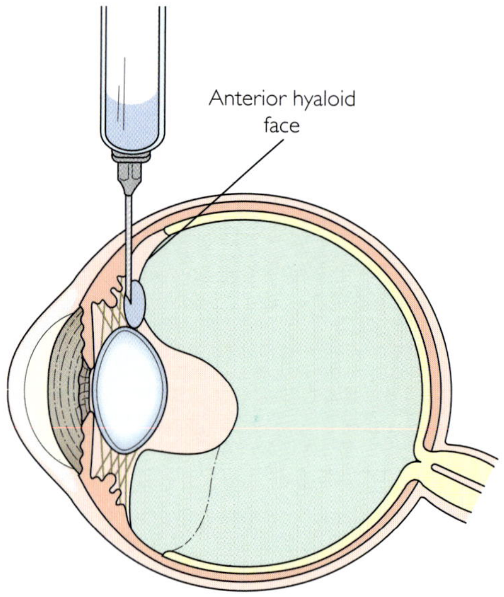

Figure 6.7 *Step 5 – anterior hyaloid gas. If the needle does not penetrate the anterior hyaloid, loculated gas in the Space of Petit will expand (sausage sign).*

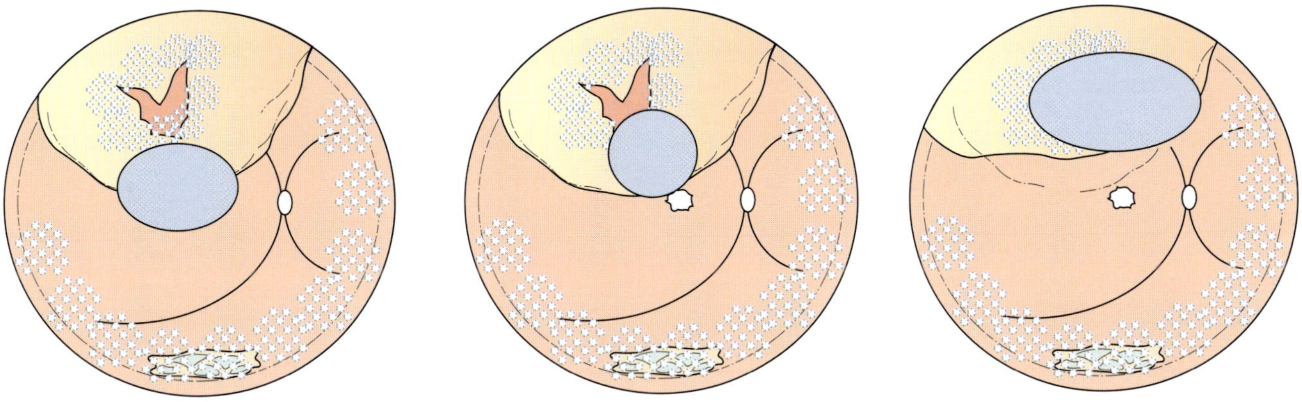

Figure 6.8 *Step 7 – steamroller maneuver.*

STEP 6

Always check the location of the bubble with the indirect ophthalmoscope. If the bubble moves, it is in the vitreous cavity; if not, it is in the Space of Petit.

The patency of the central retinal artery must be evaluated. If the artery is not pulsatile after 10 minutes, perform another paracentesis or remove some gas. The patient's vision must also be checked and if it is not light perception or better, the pressure is too high and must be lowered promptly. It must be emphasized that no patient is allowed to leave the office until the central retinal artery is patent and the visual acuity is at least light perception.

STEP 7 – THE STEAMROLLER MANEUVER (Fig. 6.8)

Indications

The steamroller maneuver is indicated if:

- The detachment is too bullous to see the central retinal artery at the nerve head.
- The attached macula is threatened by displacing subretinal fluid beneath it.
- Inferior breaks in the attached retina are threatened by possibly displacing subretinal fluid beneath them.

Steamroller technique

Place the patient face down and inject the gas. Over 10 minutes, slowly rotate the head to roll the bubble toward the largest, elevated break. If the breaks are small, the steamroller maneuver may not be effective.

STEP 8 – CRYOPEXY

If the breaks are not highly elevated, cryopexy may be applied or may be deferred for 1 or 2 days, until the breaks flatten. Alternatively, laser retinopexy may be applied in 1 or 2 days when the retina is flat. Once the breaks flatten, they may be difficult to find.

STEP 9

An antibiotic is injected subconjunctivally and a steroid antibiotic ointment is applied topically. Patients with a history of glaucoma are treated with topical drugs to lower intraocular pressure. A patch is placed over the eye after it has been determined that the patient has light perception. The Escalon Pneumo Level is then applied. Alternatively, an arrow may be drawn on the eye patch that points to the ceiling when the patient is in the correct position.

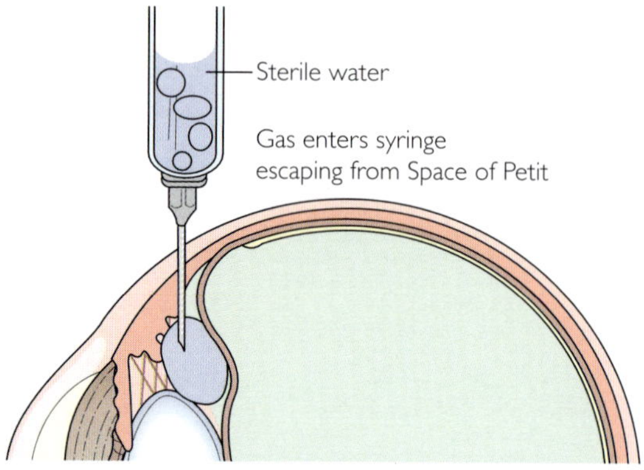

Figure 6.9 *Anterior hyaloidal gas.*

STEP 10 – FINAL DISCUSSION

The proper positioning and its importance should be discussed with the patient; I also give written instructions. A follow-up appointment is scheduled for the next day and the patient is given a prescription for antibiotic/steroid drops for 10 days.

OPERATIVE COMPLICATIONS AND HOW TO AVOID AND MANAGE THEM

ANTERIOR HYALOIDAL GAS (Fig. 6.9)

Anterior hyaloidal gas is caused by the needle not penetrating the anterior hyaloid face, either because it is inserted too anteriorly or not deeply enough. The situation is managed by placing the patient face down for 24–48 hours. As the gas expands, it usually will break through the anterior hyaloid. If this fails to occur in 24–48 hours, a 27–gauge needle on a plungerless 3–cc syringe (with 1 cc of sterile water) is reinserted into the previous gas insertion site. Gas bubbles are aspirated from the Space of Petit in a controlled manner. Reinjection of gas with proper needle placement may be necessary to close the break.

SUBRETINAL GAS

Fish eggs may enter the subretinal space because the injection site was chosen too close to the break or the gas was injected incorrectly under the retina. Subretinal gas is treated by attempting to 'massage' the gas back into the vitreous cavity through the break while the patient lies supine.

A small amount of subretinal gas can be resorbed and may not need positioning. However, there should be enough gas in the vitreous cavity to close the original break.

GAS IN THE ANTERIOR CHAMBER

Fish eggs (gas) may enter the anterior chamber if there is little or no lens capsule or if zonules have been torn. This usually happens in eyes with an anterior chamber intraocular lens. The gas can expand and seclude the pupil. This is managed by dilating the pupil to allow the bubbles to return to the vitreous compartment, and by placing the patient face down. In this position, constricting the pupil will keep the bubbles in the vitreous cavity. However, the pupil should be dilated subsequently to prevent pupillary block glaucoma.

FOLLOW-UP EXAMINATIONS

The patient is examined daily until the macula is attached. Peripheral inferior subretinal fluid may last for weeks to months. Once the macula is completely attached, the patient should be seen weekly for 2 weeks and then monthly for a total follow-up period of 3 months. Most postoperative complications are seen within the first postoperative month. The patient should be examined promptly if new flashes, floaters or decreased vision develop, because secondary tears occur.

When the retina is completely reattached, I now routinely apply light laser burns from the posterior margin of the vitreous base to the ora serrata in the area previously detached and not treated with cryopexy. Thus, combined with laser performed before gas injection, the eye has 360° of peripheral retinopexy. An analysis of the last 100 patients treated with this technique reveals an improved single-operation success rate of 97% in the phakic group and 87% in pseudophakes. Although I apply 360° laser in all pneumatic retinopexy patients, the most marked benefit is seen in pseudophakic eyes.

POSTOPERATIVE COMPLICATIONS

If the retinal tear does not close or the retina does not attach, the following should be re-examined:

- Is positioning correct?
- Is the bubble size adequate?
- Is there another break?
- Is there delayed resorption of subretinal fluid?

NEW BREAKS

If a new break develops, it may be managed with the gas bubble already present in the eye or supplemental gas may be injected. If the break is located inferiorly, it may be treated with a Lincoff balloon, a scleral buckle or a vitrectomy.

SUBRETINAL GAS

A small amount of subretinal gas is tolerated and resorbs quickly. Conservative management is recommended if the break is closed.

OTHER POSTOPERATIVE COMPLICATIONS

Endophthalmitis and central retinal artery occlusion are seen rarely. Neither complication occurred in our series of more than 300 patients. Other causes of reduced visual acuity are pre-existing age-related macular degeneration or amblyopia. Unlike scleral buckling, cystoid macular edema or a visually significant epiretinal membrane rarely occur.

Postoperative glaucoma is rare and seldom occurs because of the expanding gas bubble. However, it may occur if the pupil is secluded in the presence of an anterior chamber intraocular lens.

SURGICAL RESULTS

The surgical outcome depends upon preoperative pathology and the surgical technique. Although the literature describes a wide range of single-operation success rates, the reason for this variable success is usually the differing preoperative conditions, including the number of aphakic or pseudophakic eyes, the number of breaks and the extent of the retinal detachment.

SINGLE-OPERATION SUCCESS RATE

The rate of success with a single operation is:

A. 97% If phakic eye, one quadrant detached, one break.
B. 87% If 'A' but also includes pseudophakia.
C. 77% If 'B' but also includes three or more quadrants detached.
D. 67% If, 'C' but also includes two or more breaks.
E. Subtract 10–20% from the above if only focal retinopexy is used.

REFERENCES

1. Ohm J. Über die Behandlung der Netzhautablösung durch operative Entleerung der subretinalen Flüssigkeit und Einspritzung von Luft in den Glaskörpor, *Albrecht von Graefes Arch Ophthalmol* (1911) **79**:442–50.
2. Rosengren B. Results of treatment of detachment of the retina with diathermy and injection of air into the vitreous, *Acta Ophthalmol* (1938) **16**:573–9.
3. Hilton GF, Grizzard WS. Pneumatic retinopexy: a two-step outpatient operation without conjunctival incision, *Ophthalmology* (1986) **93**:626–41.
4. Dominguez DA. Cirugia precoz y ambulatoria del desprendimento de retina, *Arch Soc Esp Oftalmol* (1985) **48**:47–54.
5. Tornambe PE, Hilton GF. Pneumatic retinopexy: a multicenter randomized controlled clinical trial comparing pneumatic retinopexy with scleral buckling, The Retinal Detachment Study Group, *Ophthalmology* (1989) **96**:772–83.
6. Tornambe PE, Hilton GF, Brinton DA, et al. Pneumatic retinopexy: a two-year follow-up study of the multicenter clinical trial comparing pneumatic retinopexy with scleral buckling, *Ophthalmology* (1991) **98**:1115–23.

Chapter 7 Balloon buckles for the repair of retinal detachment

Harvey A Lincoff and Ingrid Kreissig

INTRODUCTION

In 1979, Lincoff et al[1] described a balloon-tipped catheter to treat retinal detachments. The deflated balloon is inserted between Tenon's capsule and the sclera to a position overlying the retinal break and then inflated. The inflated balloon creates a buckle effect that is readily perceived and confirms its location. A balloon catheter that accepts a fiberoptic stylette to aid in localization has also been developed.[2] The fiberoptic element enters the inflated balloon and its illuminated form can be seen when the fundus is viewed through a darkened ophthalmoscope.

The balloon catheter (Grieshaber & Co. AG, Schaffhausen, Switzerland) consists of a soft plastic tube with a siliconized latex balloon at the distal end. The proximal end has a plastic adapter that accepts a steel stylette to facilitate insertion and a self-sealing valve for inflation. The balloon is inflated by inserting a 1 ml syringe into the valve device and injecting sterile water (Fig. 7.1). The balloon catheter is made in two lengths: 90 mm and 125 mm.

PATHOPHYSIOLOGY

Initially upon insertion and expansion, the balloon is compressed between the eye and the bony orbit. This raises the intraocular pressure and produces a shallow buckle (Fig. 7.2). During the next hour, as the eye decompresses, the balloon becomes more spherical and sinks into an increasing scleral indentation from which it has little tendency to become dislodged with ocular rotations. The balloon buckle looks and acts like a 7.5 × 5.5 mm silicone sponge explant (Fig. 7.3). Subretinal fluid is absorbed once the indentation of the balloon is of sufficient height to close the retinal break.

OPERATIVE TECHNIQUE

The procedure can be performed with parabulbar, subconjunctival or topical anesthesia. The retinal break is localized transconjunctivally by depression. The

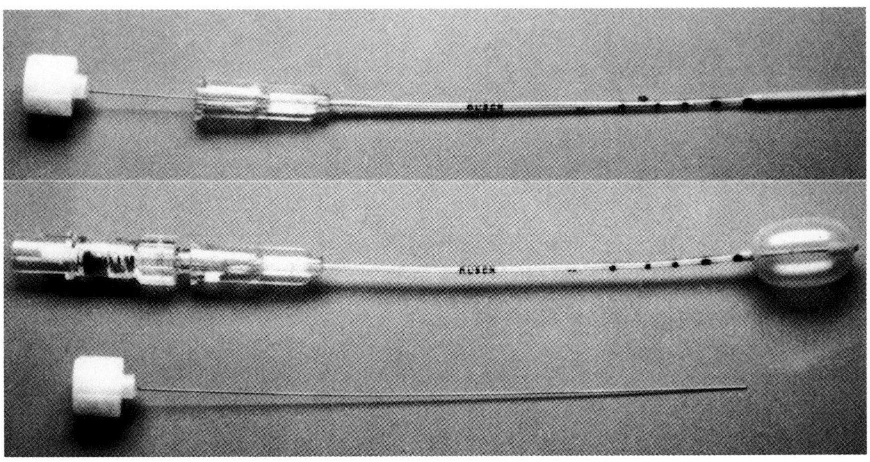

Figure 7.1 *Lincoff–Kreissig balloon catheter with stylette in place. The tube is calibrated in millimeters (top). Balloon is inflated with 1 ml of water and closed with an adapter that has a self-sealing valve (middle). The steel stylette (bottom). (Reproduced with permission from Kreissig I, Lincoff H. Treating detachments with a temporary balloon buckle without fixating sutures and without drainage,* Int Ophthalmol Clin *(1992)* ***32****:43–60.*[5]*)*

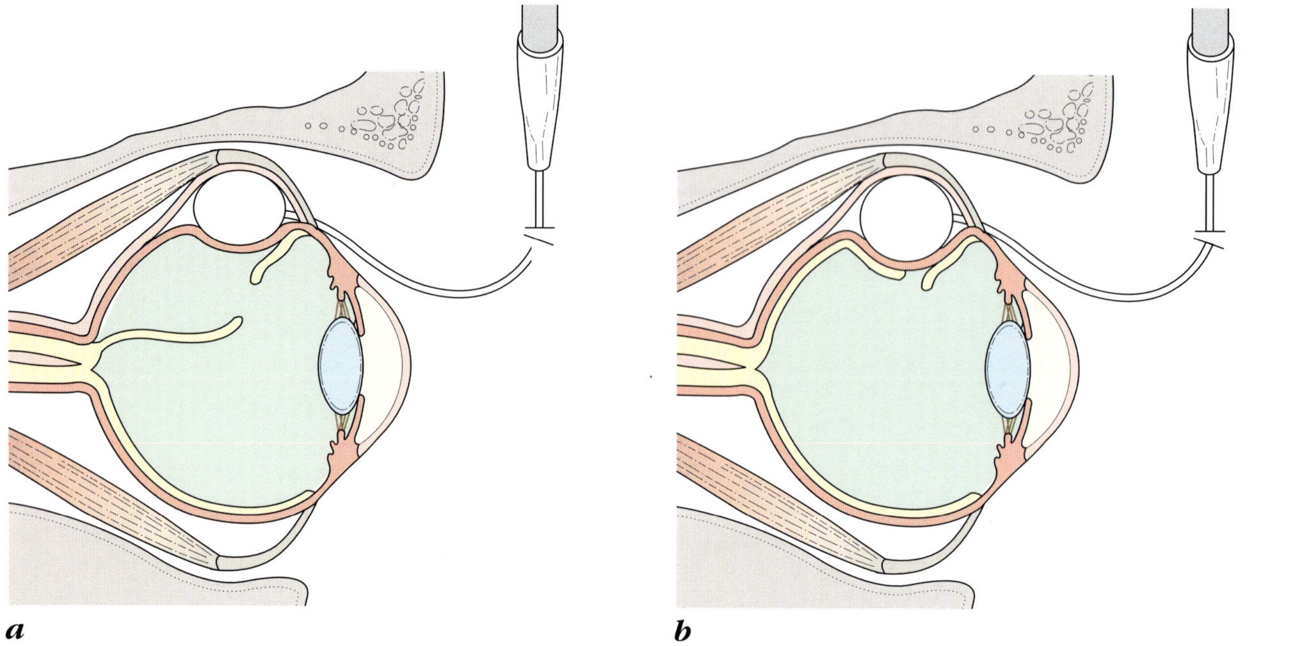

Figure 7.2 *(a) Balloon is compressed between orbital wall and eye. The intraocular pressure is increased. (b) The eye is normotensive and the balloon has expanded, increasing the buckle height and closing the retinal break. (Reproduced with permission from Kreissig I, Lincoff H. Treating detachments with a temporary balloon buckle without fixating sutures and without drainage,* Int Ophthalmol Clin *(1992)* ***32****:43–60.*[5]*)*

position of the break is marked with ink on the conjunctiva and its distance from the limbus is measured. Localization is best achieved by placing the depressor in the correct clock-hour at the ora serrata and then moving it posteriorly in the radian of the break. The radian of the break is also marked on the conjunctiva anteriorly at the ora serrata (Fig. 7.4a). If the break is beyond the limits of the conjunctival cul-de-sac, only the radian of the break is marked and the antero-posterior distance is estimated. Transconjunctival marking of the break can be compromised by the mobility of the posterior conjunctiva. To avert dislocation of the conjunctiva, rotation of the eye is to be avoided during localization and marking.

After localization, a 2-mm incision is made through the conjunctiva and Tenon's tissue at the mark on the ora. The deflated balloon with stylette in place is inserted into Tenon's space and advanced to the location of the break. The stylette is withdrawn, the self-sealing valve is inserted and the balloon is inflated with 0.5 ml of sterile water (Fig. 7.4b). Its position is checked with an ophthalmoscopic examination. If the location of the balloon is not optimal, it can be moved by manipulating the tube transconjunctivally with a wet cotton-tipped swab or by

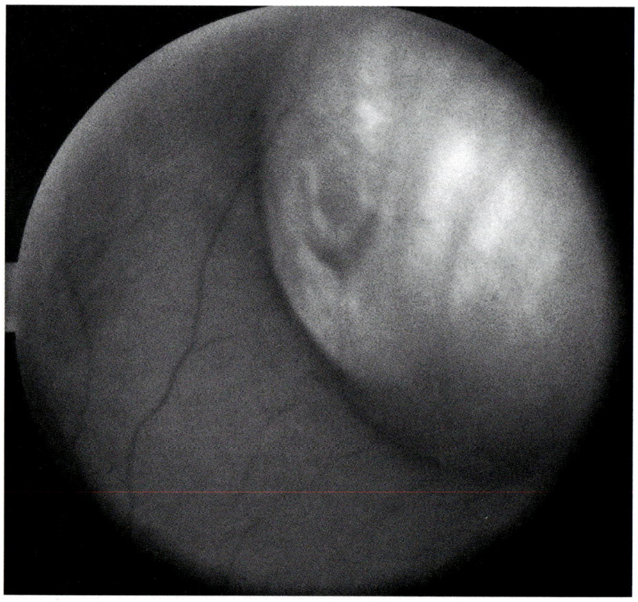

Figure 7.3 *Retinal photograph of balloon buckle under a horseshoe tear. (Reproduced with permission from Kreissig I, Lincoff H. Treating detachments with a temporary balloon buckle without fixating sutures and without drainage,* Int Ophthalmol Clin *(1992)* ***32****:43–60.*[5]*)*

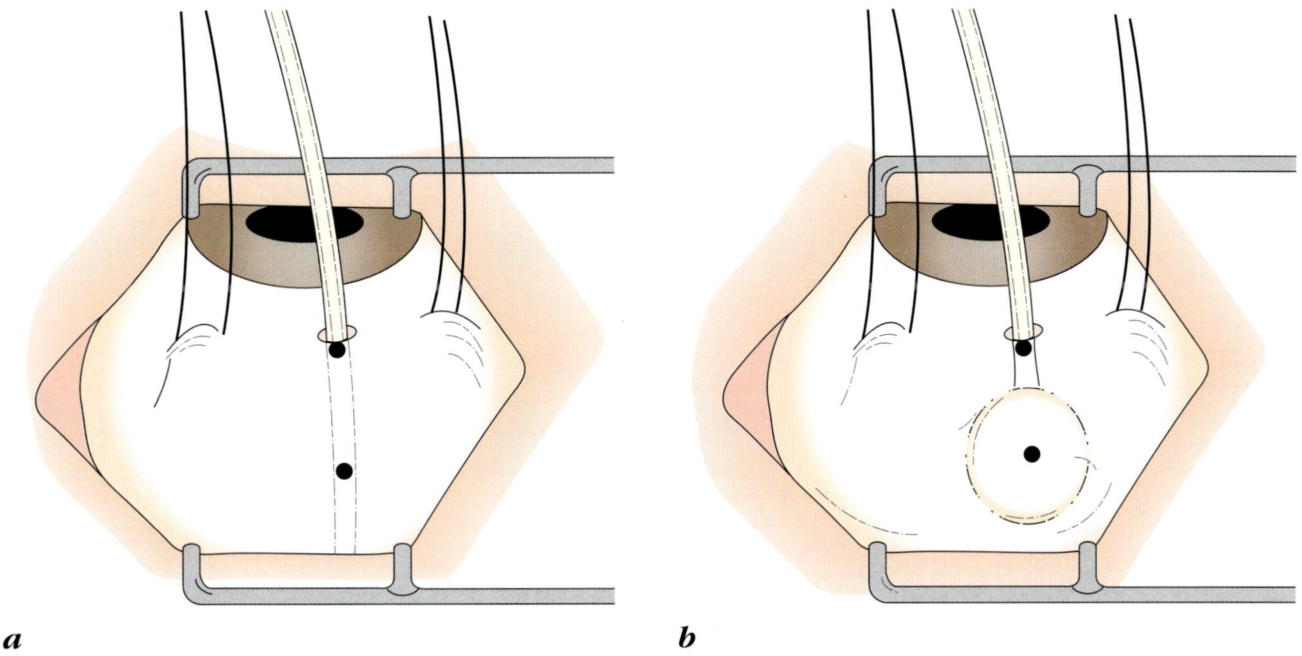

Figure 7.4 *(a) The location of the break and the radian (anterior) have been marked on the conjunctiva with ink. (b) The balloon catheter has been inserted into Tenon's space at the anterior mark and inflated.*

reinsertion. When the balloon appears in the correct position, it is additionally inflated, under ophthalmoscopic control, to a volume appropriate to the height and size of the break. This usually requires adding 0.5–1.0 ml of water. A balloon inflated with 1 ml of water has a diameter of 1.25 cm. The expansion of the balloon and the rise in intraocular pressure make it necessary to check the patency of the central retinal artery. If the artery is closed, water from the balloon is withdrawn until patency is restored.

No sutures are required to secure the balloon. The external portion of the catheter and the valve are taped to the patient's temple or forehead. Antibiotic ointment is applied to the lid margins and the eye is patched. The following day, the balloon buckle is checked for placement and height. If a higher or wider buckle is indicated, the balloon can be enlarged by injecting additional water. The edges of the retinal break can either be cryopexied transconjunctivally at the time of localization or photocoagulated the next day after the retina has reattached.

The balloon buckle is well tolerated. Patients report little or no discomfort. It is usually removed after 7 days when retinal adhesion has developed.[3,4] The balloon is deflated by half its volume on the day before its removal in order to test the adhesion. If the retina remains attached, the balloon is completely deflated and withdrawn under topical anesthesia. The small conjunctival wound closes without a suture.

The balloon buckle is suitable for retinal detachments caused by a single break or a group of breaks that subtend less than 1 clock-hour or 6 mm at the equator[1,5] (Fig. 7.5). The extent of the detachment is not a factor in patient selection. The balloon procedure has been employed successfully in retinal detachments that vary in extent from one to four quadrants.[1,6–14]

A retinal break located beneath a rectus muscle is a special indication for the balloon procedure. A sponge exoplant placed beneath a muscle, particularly a vertical one, is prone to cause postoperative diplopia.[15] Permanent muscle imbalance does not occur with the balloon buckle. To buckle a break that is located in the meridian of a rectus muscle, incise the conjunctiva over the tendon, separate the tendon fibers for 2 mm and insert the balloon catheter through the tendon to a position beneath the muscle. Muscle dysfunction and diplopia can be expected while the balloon is in place; however, diplopia recedes and disappears within hours after the balloon is deflated and withdrawn (Fig. 7.6).[16,17]

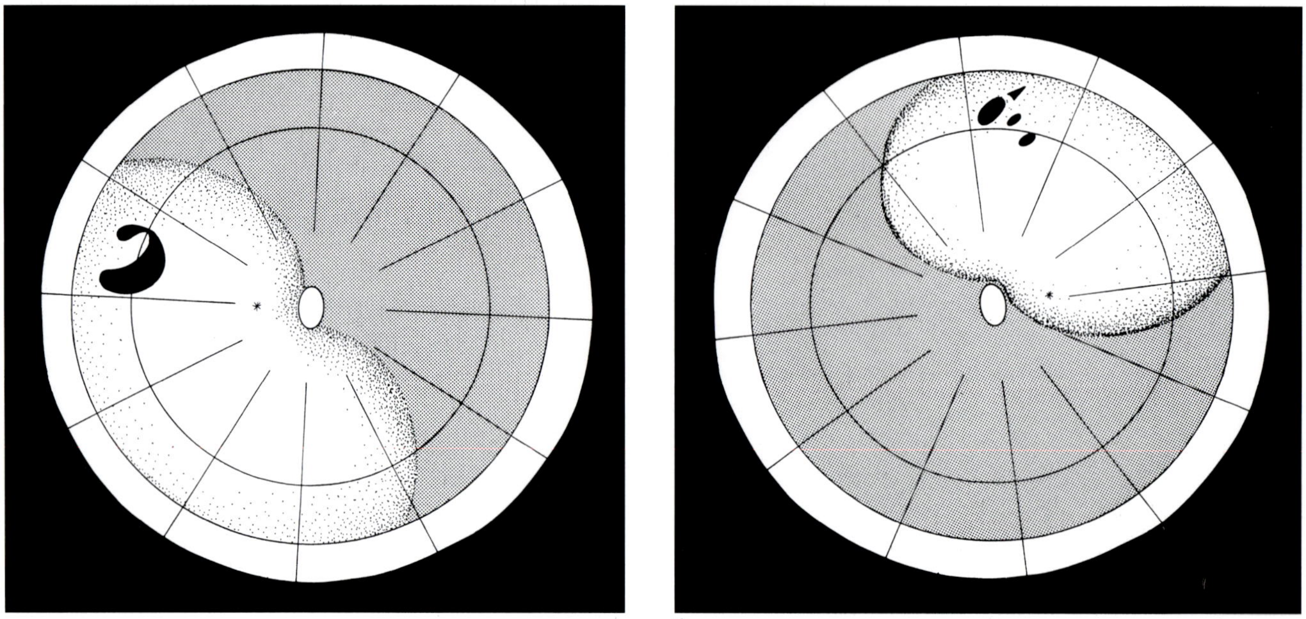

a *b*

Figure 7.5 *The balloon will buckle a break or group of breaks that subtend 1 clock-hour (6 mm at the equator). (Reproduced with permission from Kreissig I, Lincoff H. Treating detachments with a temporary balloon buckle without fixating sutures and without drainage,* Int Ophthalmol Clin *(1992)* ***32****:43–60.*[5]*)*

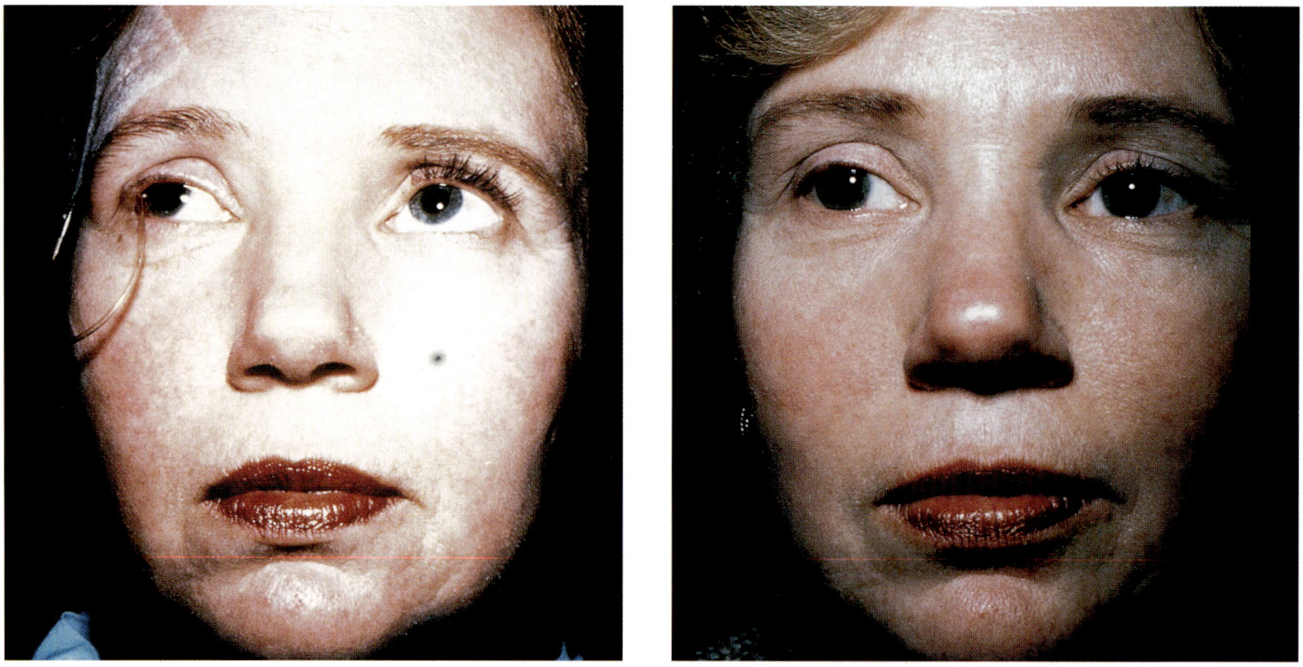

a *b*

Figure 7.6 *(a) Patient with a balloon beneath the superior rectus has limited elevation and experiences diplopia. (b) Three hours after the balloon was deflated and withdrawn, ocular rotations are normal. (Reproduced with permission from Kreissig I, Lincoff H. Treating detachments with a temporary balloon buckle without fixating sutures and without drainage,* Int Ophthalmol Clin *(1992)* ***32****:43–60.*[5]*)*

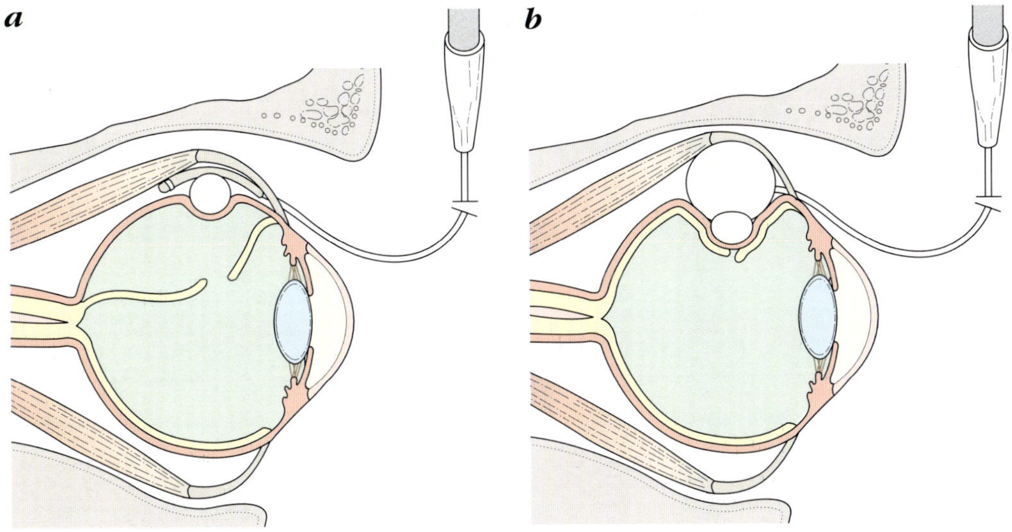

Figure 7.7
(a) The balloon is inserted and expanded external to a sponge buckle, as depicted in Fig. 7.8. (b) The balloon increases the height and width of the buckle and closes the break. (Reproduced with permission from Kreissig I, Lincoff H. Treating detachments with a temporary balloon buckle without fixating sutures and without drainage, Int Ophthalmol Clin *(1992)* ***32****:43–60.*[5]*)*

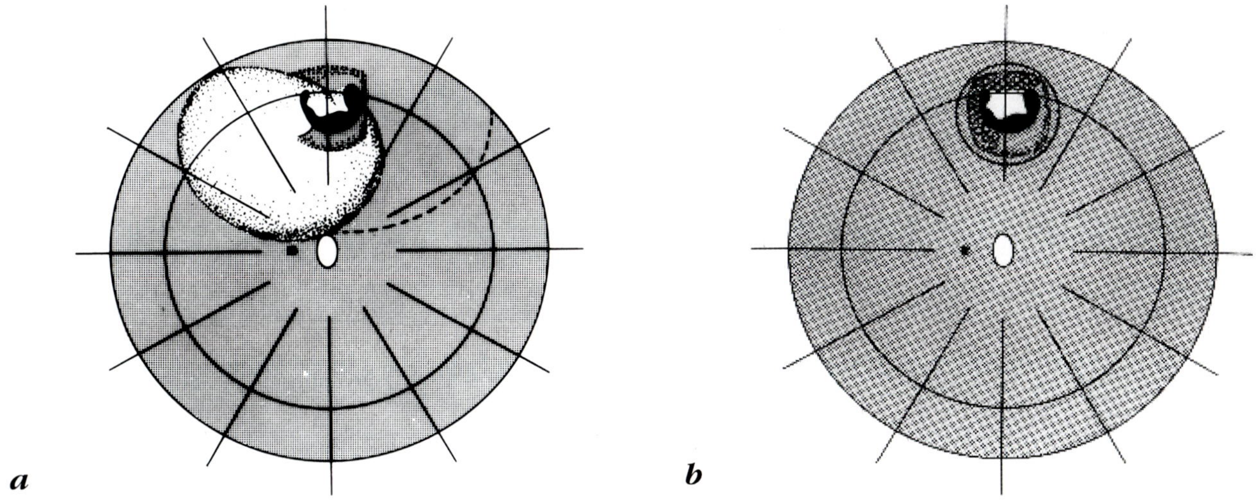

Figure 7.8 *(a) Rescuing a failing buckle: a superior detachment caused by a horseshoe tear at 12 o'clock responded incompletely to a radial sponge. It continues to leak from the temporal side. Dotted line represents former extent of detachment. (b) A balloon augments the buckle and closes the leaking edge, making it suitable for laser coagulation. (Reproduced with permission from Kreissig I, Lincoff H. Treating detachments with a temporary balloon buckle without fixating sutures and without drainage,* Int Ophthalmol Clin *(1992)* ***32****:43–60.*[5]*)*

The balloon procedure can be used to augment a failing scleral buckle.[18] The existing sponge explant interferes with scleral depression to localize the break, but the buckle usually can be seen beneath the conjunctiva and its distance from the limbus can be measured. The radian of the break is determined by scleral depression anterior to the buckle and is marked on the conjunctiva. The conjunctiva and Tenon's capsule are incised for 2 mm near the ora serrata and a path to the external surface of the explant is made by sharp dissection with a scarifier blade. The balloon catheter is inserted to the estimated distance of the break from the limbus and inflated. The balloon increases the height and width of the existing buckle (Fig. 7.7). If the addition of the balloon closes the retinal break, subretinal fluid will be absorbed and the leaking edges of the break can be sealed with laser photocoagulation (Fig. 7.8). The

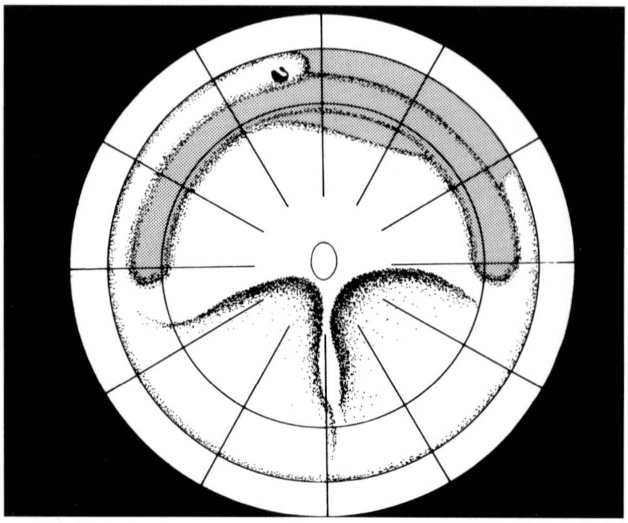

a

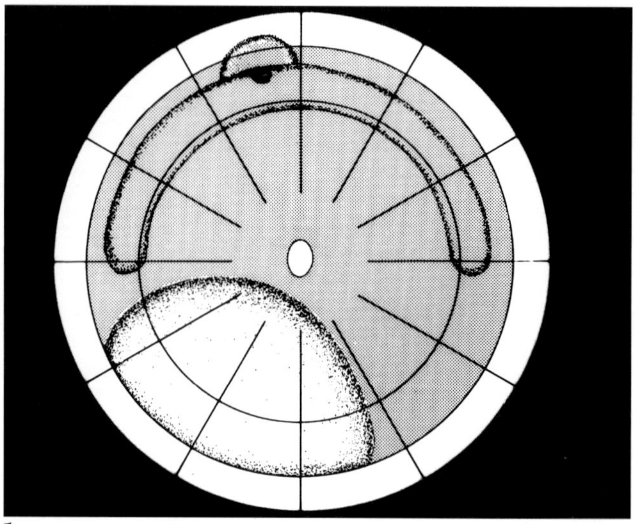

b

Figure 7.9 *(a) Late reoperation: an almost total redetachment 22 years after diathermy and an intrascleral silicone rod implant in the superior periphery. A break was found at 11:45 on the anterior edge of the buckle. (b) The balloon was inserted external to the existing buckle under topical anesthesia (retro- or parabulbar). One day later, the subretinal fluid was absorbed except for some residual fluid below, and the break could be sealed with laser. The residual fluid was absorbed after 1 week. (Reproduced with permission from Kreissig I, Lincoff H. Treating detachments with a temporary balloon buckle without fixating sutures and without drainage,* Int Ophthalmol Clin *(1992)* ***32****:43–60.*[5]*)*

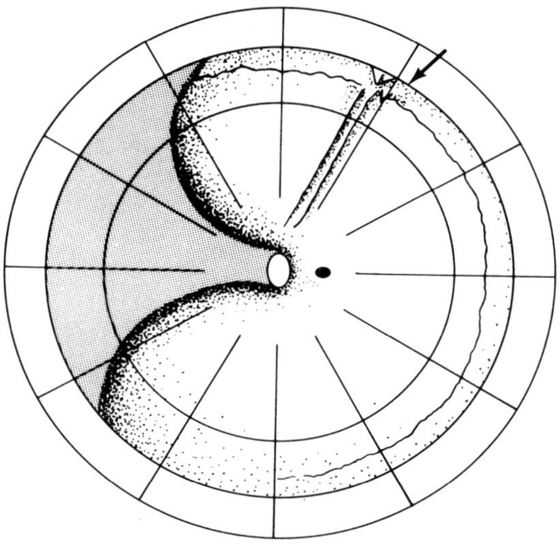

a

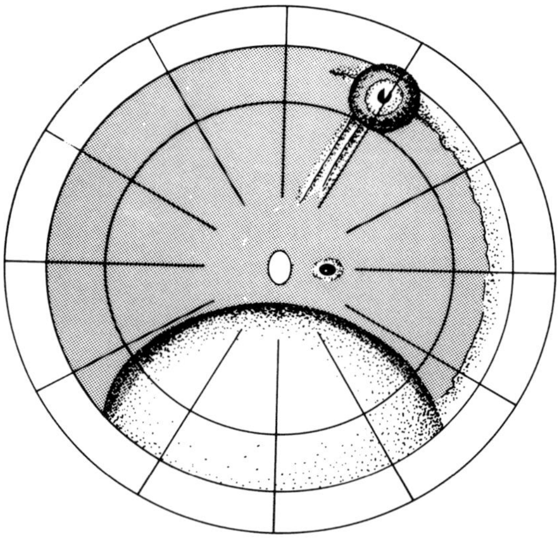

b

Figure 7.10 *(a) Diagnostic balloon: an aphakic detachment with no discernible break but an area of suspicion at 1 o'clock where a radial traction line intersects the insertion of the anterior hyaloidal membrane. (b) The retina reattached when the intersection was buckled with a balloon. The ballooned area was lasered, the residual fluid was absorbed after 2 days and the balloon was withdrawn after 1 week. The retina remained attached.*

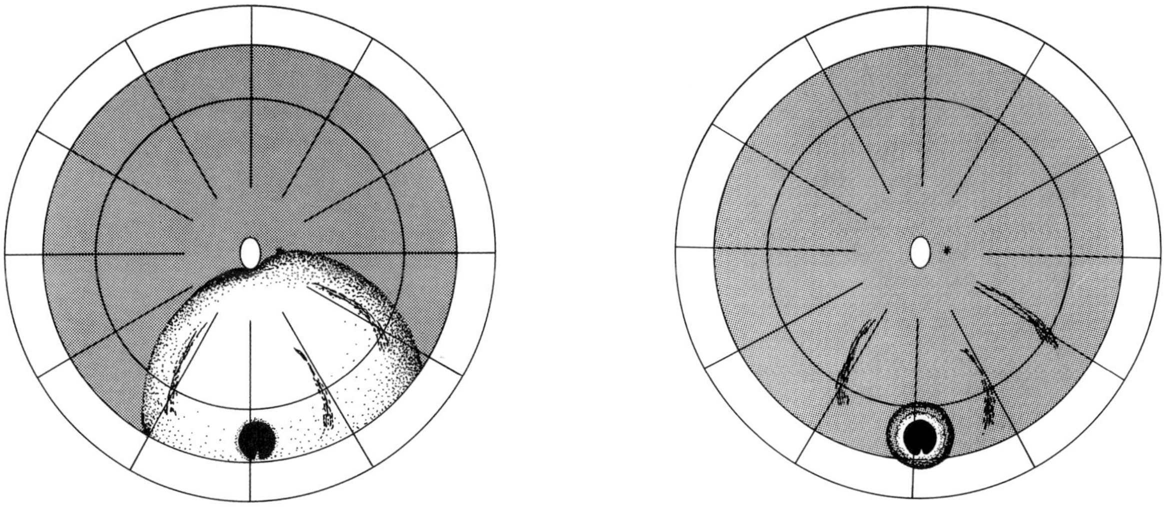

a *b*

Figure 7.11 *(a) Old detachment: an inferior detachment of long standing, evidenced by pigment demarcation lines. (b) The retina reattached overnight after a balloon was expanded beneath the break at 6 o'clock.*

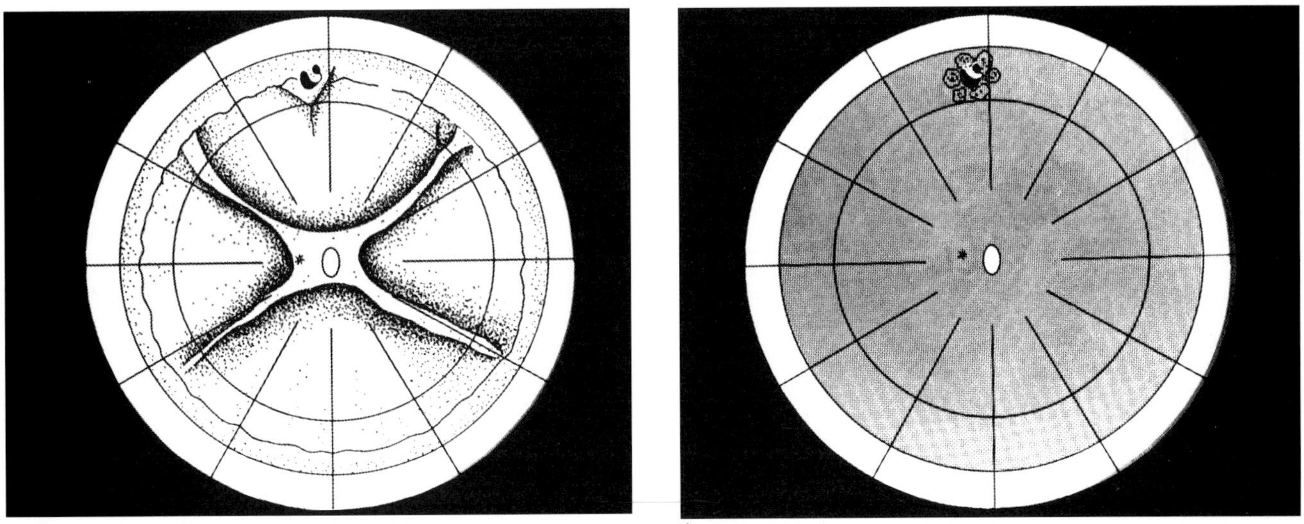

a *b*

Figure 7.12 *(a) Total aphakic detachment with a break at 11:50 beneath the superior rectus. (b) The retina reattached after the break was buckled with a balloon beneath the rectus muscle. The balloon was withdrawn after 1 week. (Reproduced with permission from Kreissig I, Lincoff H. Treating detachments with a temporary balloon buckle without fixating sutures and without drainage,* Int Ophthalmol Clin *(1992)* ***32****:43–60.[5])*

balloon also can be used for a late reoperation, either to close a break that has reopened or to tamponade a new break at the edge of a buckle (Fig. 7.9). Although these cases can be managed by repositioning or replacing the sponge explant, the advantage of managing them with a balloon insertion lies in the minimization of surgical trauma.

The balloon buckle has been used as a diagnostic probe to search for a break. The balloon can be inserted beneath an area of a suspected break (Fig. 7.10). If the detachment fails to regress by the next day, the balloon can be withdrawn and repositioned beneath another area of suspicion. This is an attractive alternative to extensive prospective buckling, drainage of subretinal fluid, gas injection or vitrectomy, all of which carry a higher degree of morbidity.

A longstanding retinal detachment with multiple pigment lines is not a contraindication for a balloon buckle; old subretinal fluid absorbs as rapidly as new fluid when the retinal break is closed (Fig. 7.11).

Aphakic and pseudophakic detachments respond to the balloon procedure (Fig. 7.12). The brevity of the procedure and the minimum trauma that it inflicts make it a desirable operation for elderly or infirm patients. In a report contrasting the balloon procedure with encirclement, 79 of 100 aphakic eyes were completely attached with a balloon procedure.[11] An additional 10 were partially attached. Ten detached after deflation, but were reattached with a sponge explant. The balloon procedure did not adversely affect the second procedure; on the contrary, it confirmed that the break that had responded to the balloon buckle was the sole cause of the aphakic detachment.

RESULTS

In 1989 the results of a prospective study of the balloon buckle operation were published.[13] Five-hundred retinal detachments caused by a single break or a group of breaks that did not subtend more than 6 mm (1 clock-hour) at the equator were buckled with balloons and followed for 6 months to 7.5 years (mean 25 months). The cases included 63 aphakic eyes and 30 eyes for reoperation. The detachments varied in their extent (Table 7.1) and in the character of the breaks (Table 7.2). In 16 eyes the balloon was used to test an area containing an unconfirmed break.

Table 7.1 Extent of 500 detachments

No. of quadrants	*No. of detachments*	*Percentage*
1	366	73
2	91	18
3	28	6
4	15	3

Adapted with permission from Kreissig I, Failer J, Lincoff H, Ferrari F. Results of a temporary balloon buckle in the treatment of 500 retinal detachments and a comparison with pneumatic retinopexy, Am J Ophthalmol *(1989)* ***107****:381–9.*[13]

Table 7.2 Type of retinal breaks treated in 500 detachments

Type of retinal break	*No. of breaks*	*Percentage*
Horseshoe tear	351	70
Round hole	127	26
Oral disinsertion	6	1
Uncertain	16	3

Adapted with permission from Kreissig I, Failer J, Lincoff H, Ferrari F. Results of a temporary balloon buckle in the treatment of 500 retinal detachments and a comparison with pneumatic retinopexy, Am J Ophthalmol *(1989)* ***107****:381–9.*[13]

Table 7.3 Redetachment after deflation of balloon and secondary reattachment

Reasons	*Redetached (n = 12)*	*Secondary repair*	*Reattached (n = 11)*
Additional break	7	Sponge Balloon	5 2
Insufficient cryopexy or excessive traction	4	Sponge Balloon Vitrectomy	1 1 1
Leaking balloon	1	Sponge	1

Adapted with permission from Kreissig I, Failer J, Lincoff H, Ferrari F. Results of a temporary balloon buckle in the treatment of 500 retinal detachments and a comparison with pneumatic retinopexy, Am J Ophthalmol *(1989)* ***107****:381–9.*[13]

The balloon completely attached the retina in 93% of eyes and partially attached the retina in another 2%. After removal of the balloon, the retina redetached in 2.4% (Table 7.3). A second procedure

Table 7.4 Anatomic results of 500 detachments

Attachment	*With balloon insertion (n = 500)*	*After balloon removal (n = 500)*	*After first reoperation (n = 42)*	*After second reoperation (n = 4)*
Complete	466 (93%)	454 (91%)	490 (98%)	493 (98.6%)
Partially	11 (2%)	11 (2%)	3 (0.6%)	2 (0.4%)
None	23 (5%)	35 (7%)	7 (1.4%)	5 (1.0%)

Adapted with permission from Kreissig I, Failer J, Lincoff H, Ferrari F. Results of a temporary balloon buckle in the treatment of 500 retinal detachments and a comparison with pneumatic retinopexy, Am J Ophthalmol *(1989)* ***107****:381–9.*[13]

with another balloon, a silicone sponge, pneumatic retinopexy or vitrectomy raised the attachment rate to 99% (Table 7.4).

COMPLICATIONS

Complications from the balloon buckle operation are infrequent. Superficial corneal erosion occurred in 5% of eyes because of improper placement of the emerging end of the catheter.[13] This complication can be avoided if care is taken to lead the catheter away from the cornea. Choroidal effusion was an infrequent complication in elderly patients.[6,11] Infection occurred once in the first 1000 cases.[24] It presented as pain and a purulent discharge around the catheter on the fourth postoperative day. The infection responded promptly to removal of the catheter and application of topical antibiotics. The retina remained attached.

CONCLUSIONS

The balloon catheter is a versatile instrument for the repair of retinal detachments. The attachment rate is comparable to that obtained with conventional buckling, but there are fewer complications. The balloon can be inserted under local anesthesia and causes minimal surgical trauma. The operation does not require scleral suturing and so eliminates the risk of scleral perforation. Postoperative infection is rare because the balloon is only a temporary foreign body and because topical antibiotics and lysozymes sterilize the conjunctival opening. Changes in refractive error do not occur, because the contour of the eye is not permanently altered. Persistent muscle imbalance also does not occur. The balloon technique represents an additional instrument in the armamentarium of the retinal surgeon. One in four cases of retinal detachment can benefit from the procedure.

REFERENCES

1. Lincoff HA, Kreissig I, Hahn YS. A temporary balloon buckle for the treatment of small retinal detachments, *Ophthalmology* (1979) **86**:586–96.
2. Lincoff H, Stergiu P, Kreissig I. A fiberoptic stylette for localizing the balloon buckle, *Arch Ophthalmol* (1990) **108**:607.
3. Lincoff H, O'Connor P, Bloch D, et al. The cryosurgical adhesion. II, *Trans Am Acad Ophthalmol Otolaryngol* (1970) **74**:98–107.
4. Kreissig I, Lincoff H. Cryosurgery of the retina, *Int Ophthalmol Clin* (1976) **16**:63–81.
5. Kreissig I, Lincoff H. Treating detachments with a temporary balloon buckle without fixating sutures and without drainage, *Int Ophthalmol Clin* (1992) **32**:43–60.
6. Lincoff H, Kreissig I. Results with a temporary balloon buckle for the repair of retinal detachment, *Am J Ophthalmol* (1981) **92**:245–51.
7. Kreissig I, Lincoff H. The balloon operation: a follow-up study, *Fortschr Ophthalmol* (1982) **79**:229–32.
8. Kreissig I. Die Ballon-Operation und ihre Anwendungsmöglichkeiten, *Klin Monatsbl Augenheilkd* (1983) **183**:229–30.
9. Lincoff H, Kreissig I, Richard G, et al. A multicentred trial of the balloon buckle. In: Henkind P, ed, *Acta XXIV International Congress of Ophthalmology* (JB Lippincott: Philadelphia, 1983): 1–3.
10. Lincoff H, Kreissig I, Richard G, Zimmerman N. The repair of aphakic detachments with a temporary balloon buckle

and without drainage, *Fortschr Ophthalmol* (1983) **80**:318–21.

11. Lincoff H, Kreissig I, Farber M. Results of 100 aphakic detachments treated with a temporary balloon buckle: a case against routine encircling operations, *Br J Ophthalmol* (1985) **69**:798–804.
12. Kreissig I, Haustrate F. La technique du ballon avec indentation temporaire et sans drainage, *Bull Soc Belge Ophtalmol* (1986) **218**:13–34.
13. Kreissig I, Failer J, Lincoff H, Ferrari F. Results of a temporary balloon buckle in the treatment of 500 retinal detachments and a comparison with pneumatic retinopexy, *Am J Ophthalmol* (1989) **107**:381–9.
14. Kreissig I. Two new possibilities for using the balloon procedure: different uses of its indentation of the globe, *Klin Monatsbl Augenheilkd* (1989) **194**:27–31.
15. Davies MS, Elkington AR, Kanski JJ. Diplopia following retinal detachment surgery, *Mod Probl Ophthalmol* (1974) **12**:470–5.
16. Lincoff H, Kreissig I. Additional indications for a temporary balloon buckle, *Trans Ophthalmol Soc UK* (1980) **100**:550–2.
17. Schoch LH, Olk RJ, Arribas NP, et al. The Lincoff temporary balloon buckle, *Am J Ophthalmol* (1986) **101**:646–9.
18. Lincoff H, Kreissig I. Parabulbar balloon to augment a failing scleral buckle, *Am J Ophthalmol* (1981) **92**:647–52.
19. Lincoff H, Kreissig I. Diagnostic uses for an unsecured balloon buckle, *Mod Probl Ophthalmol* (1979) **20**:157–63.
20. Lincoff H, Kreissig I. Exploratory buckling with a temporary balloon. In: Blodi F et al, eds, *Acta XXV International Congress of Ophthalmology* (Kugler & Ghedini: Amsterdam, (1987): 2125–7.
21. Lincoff H, Kreissig I. The treatment of retinal detachment without the drainage of subretinal fluid: modifications of the Custodis procedure, VI, *Trans Am Acad Ophthalmol Otolaryngol* (1972) **76**:1121–33.
22. Kreissig I, Rose D, Jost B. Minimized surgery for retinal detachments with segmental buckling and nondrainage: an 11–year follow-up, *Retina* (1992) **12**:224–31.
23. Kreissig I. Zehn Jahre Erfahrungen mit der Ballon-Operation: Anfängliche Skepsis, Weiterentwicklung der Methode, praktische Hinweise für den Ballon-Operateur, *Klin Monatsbl Augenheilkd* (1989) **194**:145–51.
24. Kreissig I. Bemerkungen zur Publikation von S. Leuenberger, J. Faulborn: Beginnende Orbitalphlegmone bei einer Ballonplombe nach Lincoff-Kreissig, *Klin Monatsbl Augenheilkd* (1987) **191**:163–4.

Chapter 8 Technique of scleral buckling for retinal detachment repair

Kamal Kishore and Gholam A Peyman

INTRODUCTION

Our understanding of the pathogenesis of rhegmatogenous retinal detachments evolved from the work of Leber, who was the first to implicate vitreous traction in the development of retinal tears and subsequent detachment. Jules Gonin (1870–1935) performed the first successful retinal detachment repair with accurate pre- and intraoperative localization of retinal breaks, drainage of subretinal fluid and thermocautery applied through a drainage sclerotomy. His first surgical series was presented to the Swiss Ophthalmological Society in 1919, and laid the foundation for modern retinal detachment surgery. Ernst Custodis performed the first scleral buckling procedure in 1949 with an episcleral polyviol exoplant, utilizing a nondrainage technique in most cases. Schepens introduced scleral buckling in the USA in 1951, which he modified in 1960 by substituting soft silicone rubber for the polyethylene tube. In 1965, Lincoff modified the original Custodis procedure by replacing the polyviol exoplant with a silicone sponge, developing a spatula needle for safe passage of scleral sutures and substituting cryotherapy for diathermy to create a chorioretinal adhesion. He also performed a nondrainage procedure in the majority of his cases.

The fundamental concept of scleral buckling has changed little over the last three decades. Buckling is used successfully to treat the majority of cases with rhegmatogenous retinal detachment without significant proliferative vitreoretinopathy (PVR, less than grade C_1). The approach to buckling is highly individualized, but universally accepted components include identification and accurate localization of all retinal breaks, creation of a chorioretinal adhesion and appositional closure of all retinal breaks by indentation of retinal pigment epithelium (RPE) and choroid. Several excellent references are available on the subject.[1–3] By adopting a flexible approach that incorporates the advantages and benefits of different techniques, the surgeon can maximize the rate of anatomic success in reattaching the retina, while minimizing failures and potential complications. Alternative techniques of retinal detachment repair, such as the Lincoff balloon, pneumatic retinopexy and pars plana vitrectomy, are presented elsewhere in this book. Special situations such as scleral buckling for prophylactic treatment of retinal breaks and in fellow eyes with giant retinal tears will not be addressed here but may be approached with the same surgical principles and technique.

ANESTHESIA AND SURGICAL PREPARATION

Whether scleral buckling is performed under local or general anesthesia depends on the surgeon's preference and the community standard of care. The advantages of local anesthesia include shorter operating time, quicker postoperative recovery and decreased systemic morbidity. Potential risks include perforation of the globe by the retrobulbar needle (especially in myopic eyes), retrobulbar hemorrhage, retinal vascular occlusion, optic nerve injury, brainstem anesthesia (leading to respiratory arrest) and grand-mal seizures.[4] Peribulbar anesthesia may reduce these complications. The major disadvantage of local anesthesia is inadequate analgesia, which occurs in 10% of cases even with a mixture of bupivacaine and lidocaine. If a two-injection technique is used for peribulbar anesthesia, the superior injection should be given first, to reduce the risk of globe perforation.[5]

Our technique of peribulbar anesthesia consists of a single injection of an equal volume of 2% lidocaine and 0.75% bupivacaine and 150 units of hyaluronidase given through the lower lid at the

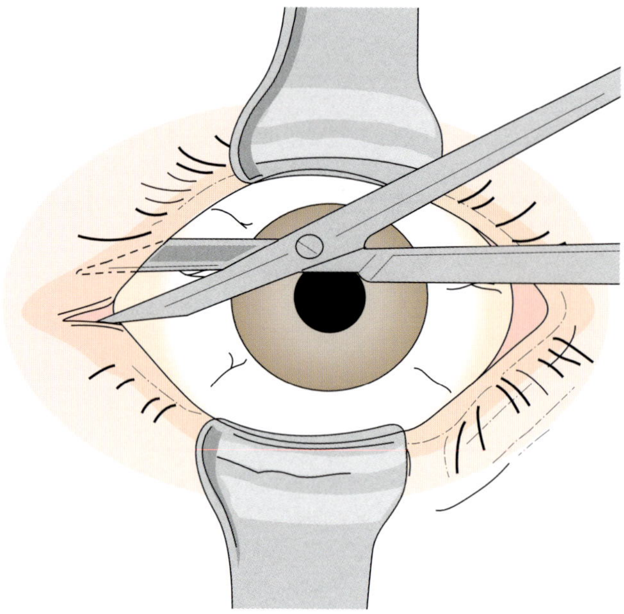

Figure 8.1 *Lateral canthotomy: lateral canthal tissues are clamped with a hemostat and a horizontal incision is made with blunt-tipped scissors.*

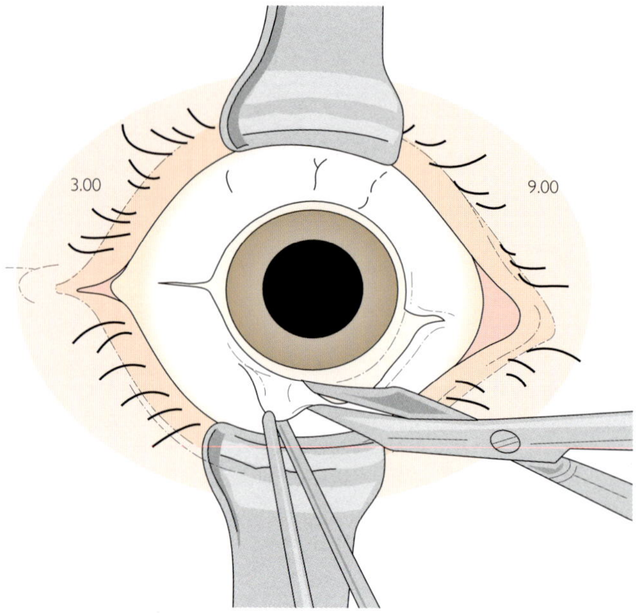

Figure 8.2 *Peritomy with blunt-tipped scissors and nontoothed forceps: radial relaxing incisions at 3 and 9 o'clock meridians improve exposure and minimize later tearing.*

junction of the medial two-thirds and lateral one-third.[6] A 25-gauge ⅝-inch needle is directed toward the orbital apex while the patient looks up to make the orbital septum taut. Constant pressure is applied with the hub of the needle to cause mild eversion of the lid margin during injection. Six milliliters of solution is injected, followed by 10 minutes of gentle ocular massage. Fullness of the upper lid and ptosis, noted in the majority of the eyes during the injection, are signs of a satisfactory injection. Good akinesia and analgesia are obtained in about 90% of eyes with a single injection. Mild conjunctival chemosis is present in about 20% of cases but this does not interfere with the surgical procedure. If necessary, supplemental local anesthesia may be given intraoperatively by injecting additional anesthetic in sub-Tenon's space with a 19-gauge cannula.

The lid margins and periocular skin are prepped with 10% povidone–iodine solution followed by irrigation of the ocular surface with 5% povidone–iodine solution. The lashes may be trimmed preoperatively or isolated by adhesive drapes. Other antiseptics, such as alcohol, soaps and hexachlorophene, are also effective but should be avoided because they are toxic to the corneal epithelium. Frequent administration of broad-spectrum antibiotic drops starting a few hours before surgery reduces the bacterial count from the ocular surface, and is optional.

PERITOMY AND ISOLATION OF MUSCLES

A lateral canthotomy may be considered only in patients with narrow palpebral fissures. To perform this, canthal tissues are clamped with a straight hemostat and cut with straight tenotomy scissors (Fig. 8.1). Cautery may be required to control bleeding. A Jaffe lid speculum is secured with hemostats to the drapes to provide exposure. A 360° peritomy is performed with nontoothed conjunctival forceps and blunt-tipped Wescott scissors. Relaxing incisions in the 3 and 9 o'clock meridians maintain the integrity of the conjunctival edges for easier closure (Fig. 8.2). A limited peritomy is used when planned surgery is

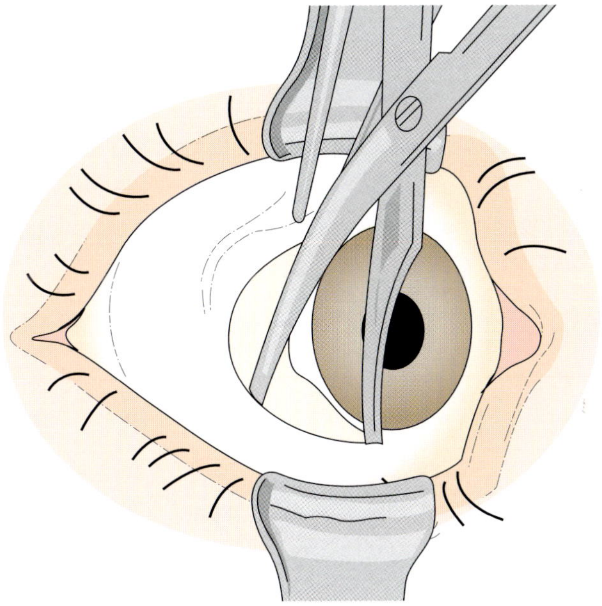

Figure 8.3 *Blunt-tipped curved tenotomy scissors are spread in sub-Tenon's space between rectus muscles to expose the sclera.*

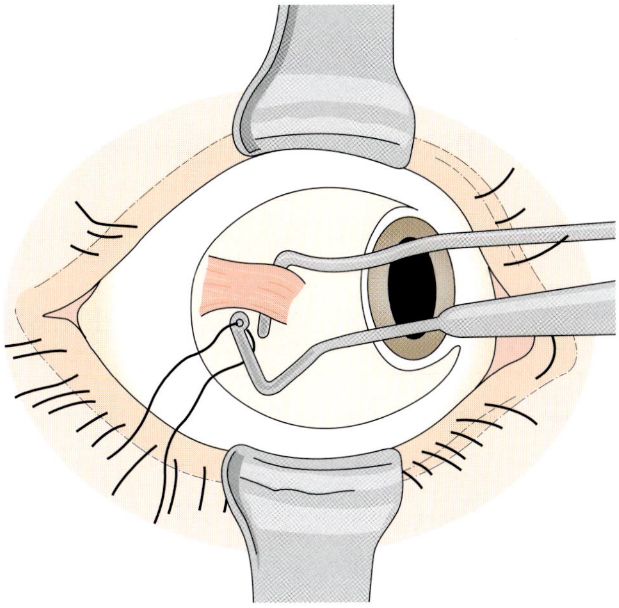

Figure 8.4 *Fenestrated muscle hook used to pass 3-0 silk suture beneath rectus muscle.*

confined to a single quadrant. Blunt-tipped Stevens' tenotomy scissors are inserted in the sub-Tenon's space in each quadrant and spread to expose the sclera (Fig. 8.3). The muscle insertion then is engaged with a muscle hook, which is placed on the sclera posterior to insertion and passed in a circumferential direction. It is then brought anteriorly to engage the muscle tendon. When properly placed, the muscle hook should glide along the sclera with ease. Significant resistance usually means improper placement of the muscle hook. By engaging the muscle anterior to the equator, damage to the vortex veins is avoided. Once the muscle insertion is engaged, attachments of overlying Tenon's fascia are stripped from the muscle with a cotton-tipped applicator. Care should be taken not to strip too posteriorly while isolating vertical recti to avoid damaging the levator muscle superiorly or the inferior oblique muscle and Lockwood's ligament inferiorly. After isolation of each muscle, a 3-0 black-silk traction suture is placed around the muscle using either a fenestrated muscle hook or a reversed needle (Fig. 8.4). Horizontal recti are isolated first and traction sutures around these muscles are used to rotate the globe during isolation of the vertical recti.

Isolation of the superior rectus requires additional care to avoid engaging the superior oblique tendon, which inserts 3–5 mm posterior to the lateral margin of the superior rectus insertion. Passing the muscle hook from the nasal side anterior to the oblique muscle insertion avoids the superior oblique insertion (Fig. 8.5a). Inferior rotation of the globe with traction sutures around medial and lateral recti often brings the insertion of the superior rectus into view, to allow safe passage of a muscle hook. The muscle insertion may be grasped with a pair of toothed forceps to rotate the globe inferiorly, while a muscle hook is passed just posterior to the forceps (Fig. 8.5b). If a limited peritomy is performed, muscles in the exposed segment are isolated first. A transconjunctival traction suture then may be passed under the remaining muscles after grasping and elevating them with forceps (Fig. 8.6).

When disinsertion of a muscle is necessary, it is elevated on a muscle hook and a double-armed 5-0 Vicryl suture is passed through the body of the tendon at half-thickness just posterior to the insertion. Full-thickness bites then are taken at either end of the muscle and a suture is locked to occlude the anterior ciliary arteries (Fig. 8.7). The muscle is cut

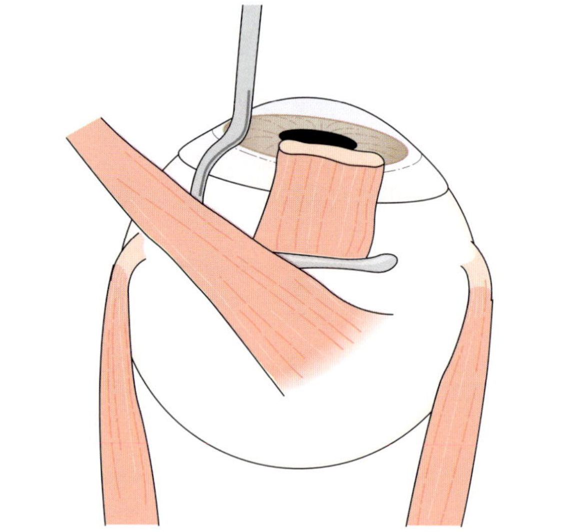

a

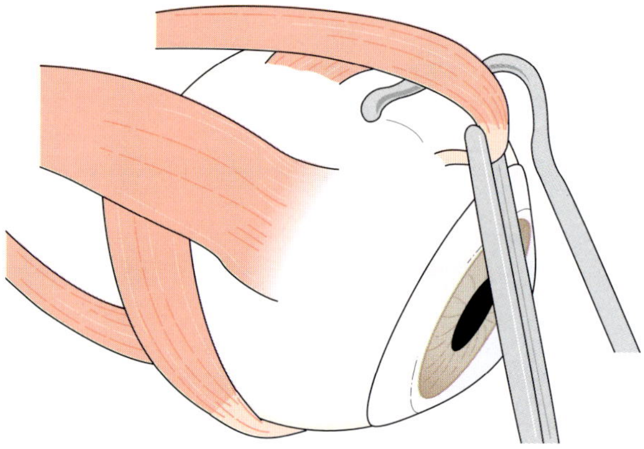

b

Figure 8.5 *(a) Correct position of muscle hook for securing superior rectus from nasal side. (b) Alternative technique: globe is rotated inferiorly, a pair of toothed forceps grasps insertion of superior rectus and the muscle hook is slid just behind the insertion.*

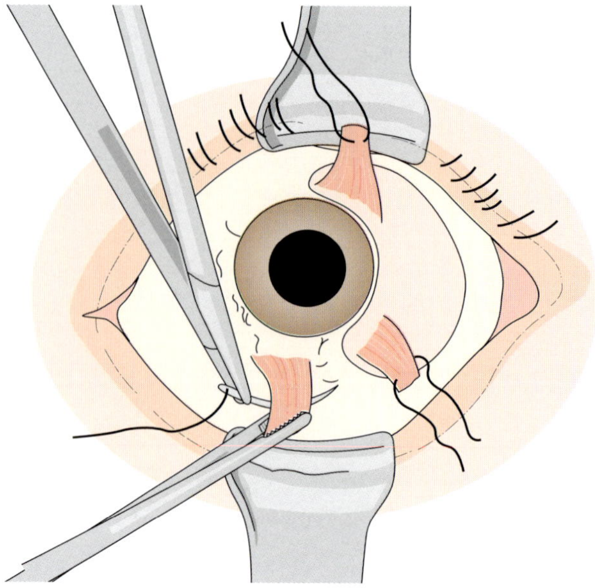

Figure 8.6 *Transconjunctival traction suture: the muscle is grasped and elevated with forceps and a suture is passed beneath its tendon.*

then, leaving a small stump. The insertion may be secured with two or more passes of a 4-0 silk suture. The muscle is repositioned to the insertion at the end of the procedure with the preplaced double-armed 5-0 Vicryl suture.

After isolation of all muscles, the sclera is inspected in each quadrant for evidence of thinning, staphyloma or anomalous vortex veins, and the location of each abnormality is noted. Scleral thinning is noted most commonly in the superotemporal quadrant and appears as a gray-blue area or as radial gray lines.

INDIRECT OPHTHALMOSCOPY AND LOCALIZATION OF BREAKS

No aspect of scleral buckling is more critical to the success of the procedure than accurate placement of the buckle to support the retinal breaks. In order to achieve this, accurate localization of all retinal breaks is necessary. Binocular indirect ophthalmoscopy with scleral depression is performed meticulously to identify all retinal breaks, suspicious lesions, lattice degeneration and any other pathology. The eye is stabilized and rotated by the assistant with the traction sutures held 180° apart. The cornea is moistened periodically with balanced salt solution (BSS). The extent and height of the detachment, the presence or absence of macular detachment, any vitreoretinal traction and all changes of PVR are evaluated and compared with those recorded preoperatively. A significant decrease in the height of subretinal fluid from the preoperative examination usually indicates good RPE function and suggests that a nondrainage procedure probably will be successful.

The position of each retinal break then is marked externally on the sclera. Scleral depression is performed beneath each break to identify the precise

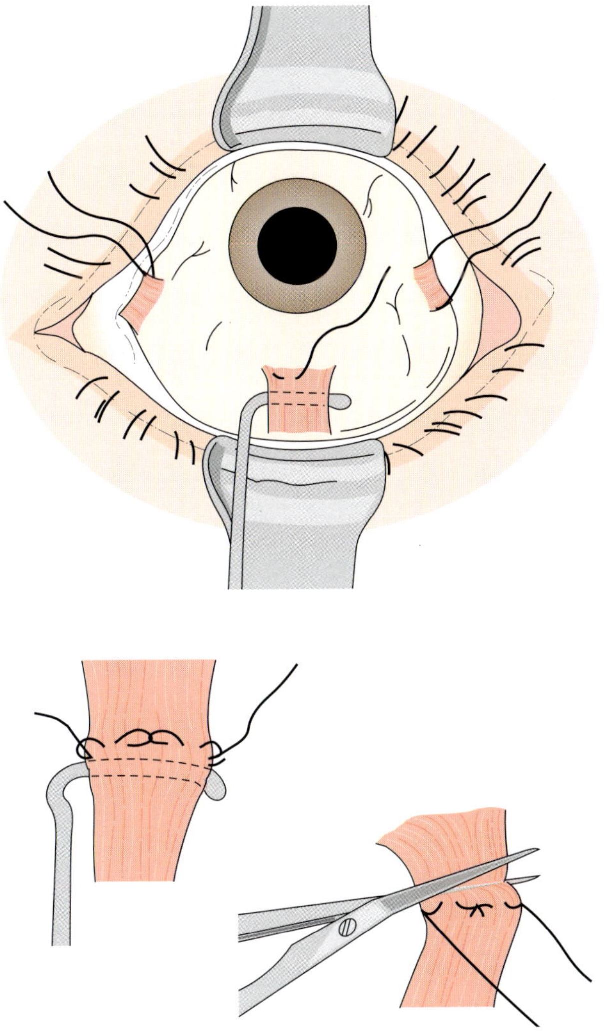

Figure 8.7 *Disinsertion of rectus muscle: a 5-0 Vicryl suture is secured to the central portion of the tendon with a partial-thickness bite; full-thickness bites are taken at each end and the suture is locked; the muscle is then disinserted with scissors leaving a small stump.*

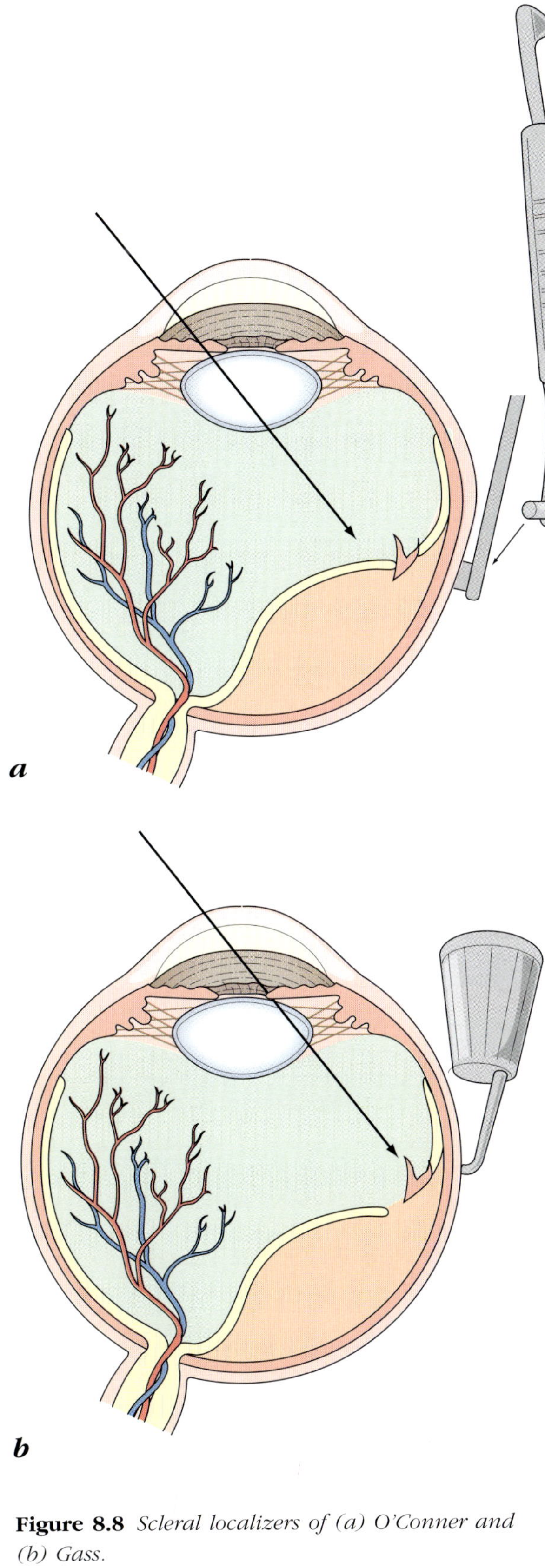

Figure 8.8 *Scleral localizers of (a) O'Conner and (b) Gass.*

location of the central posterior edge of the break, and the sclera is marked with diathermy, dye or cautery. Diathermy and cautery are not used if the sclera is thin, to avoid scleral perforation.

Gass and O'Conner each designed instruments for localization that make a 1-mm circular ring on the sclera with mild indentation (Fig. 8.8). We prefer the O'Conner localizer. This instrument has a smooth surface 90° from the marking surface to allow preliminary exploration without damaging the sclera. Once

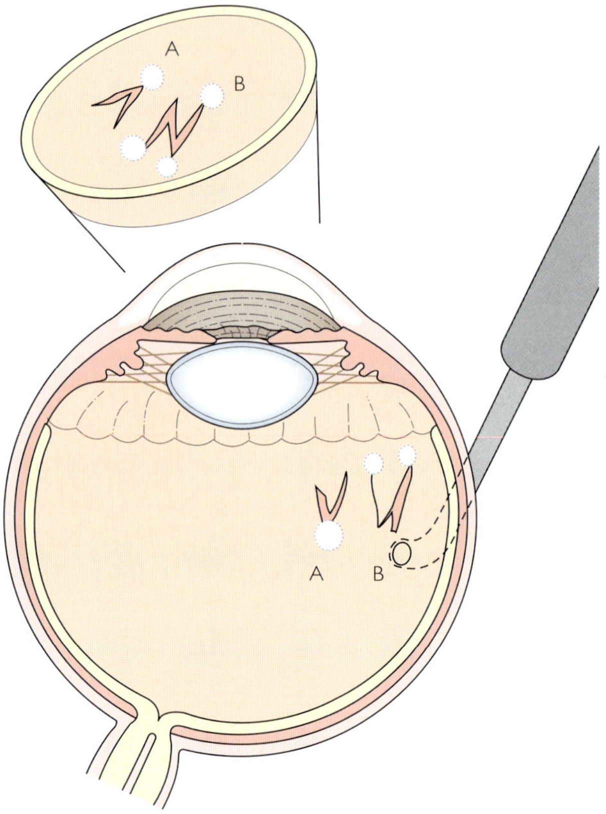

Figure 8.9 *Localization: (a) small flap tears and atrophic holes may be marked at their posterior edge; (b) large flap tears should be marked at central posterior edge and anterior horns.*

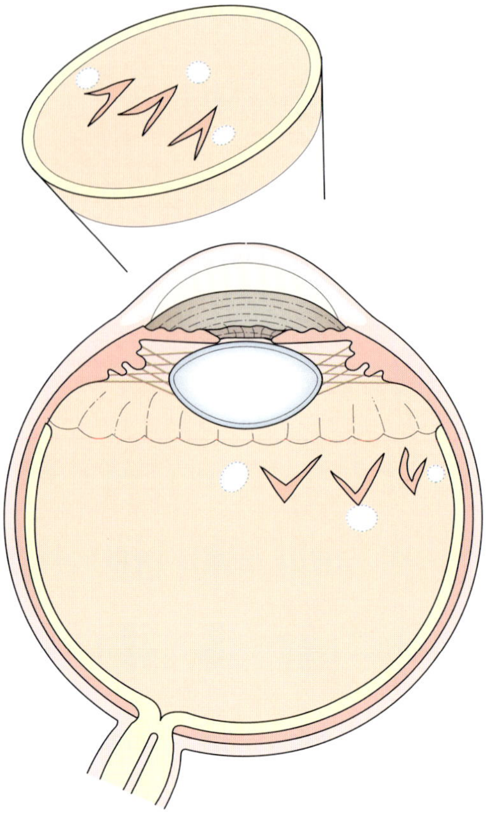

Figure 8.10 *When multiple breaks are present close together, mark the lateral extent of the breaks and the most posterior edge.*

the break is located, the marker is rotated and gentle pressure is applied to the sclera for approximately 5 seconds. The resultant mark then is indicated permanently with a pen. A flat-tip diathermy electrode also may be used for indentation. Once correct localization is achieved, a burn marks the sclera and the retina, provided that the retinal detachment is not very elevated. An alternative technique involves grasping the sclera with a fine-toothed forceps (0.12 mm, Castroviejo) to indent it and primarily is used to confirm placement of previously applied scleral marks.

Small retinal breaks are marked with a single spot. Large flap tears are marked with three spots, including the most posterior extent and the most anterior location of the horns (Fig. 8.9). When multiple retinal breaks are present and a circumferential buckle is planned, the location of the most posterior break in each quadrant is marked (Fig. 8.10). Dialyses at the ora are marked to indicate the location of the two ends and the posterior extent of the midpoint of the dialysis (Fig. 8.11).

Marking may be difficult if the retina is highly elevated or if a break is located far posteriorly. A break may appear farther posterior than its true location because of parallax in high retinal detachments (Fig. 8.12). In such cases, indentation is begun anteriorly in the meridian of the retinal break where the retina is closest to the choroid. As indentation is moved posteriorly, it is usually possible to mark the anterior margins of the break accurately. Other edges of the break are marked subsequently. Alternatively, subretinal fluid may be partially drained. The intraocular pressure (IOP) is

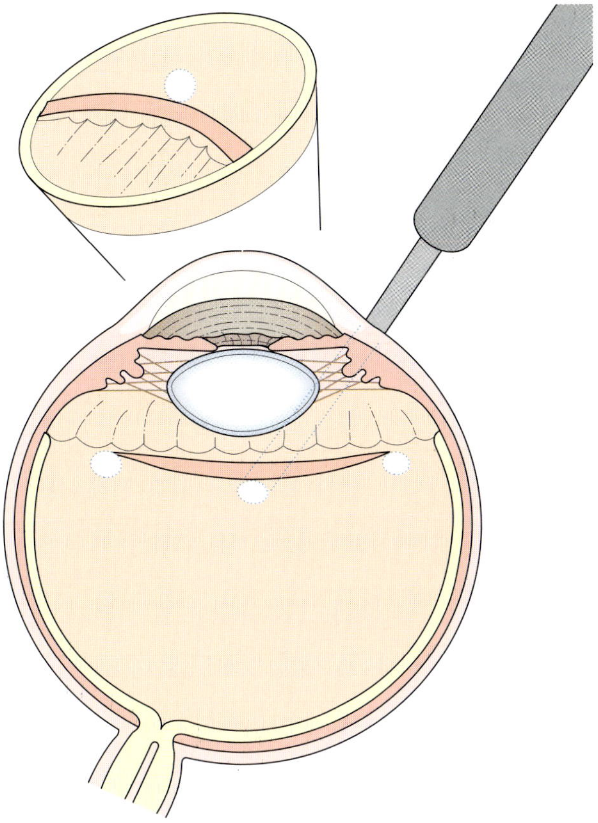

Figure 8.11 *Dialysis is marked by localizing lateral ends and the most posterior extent.*

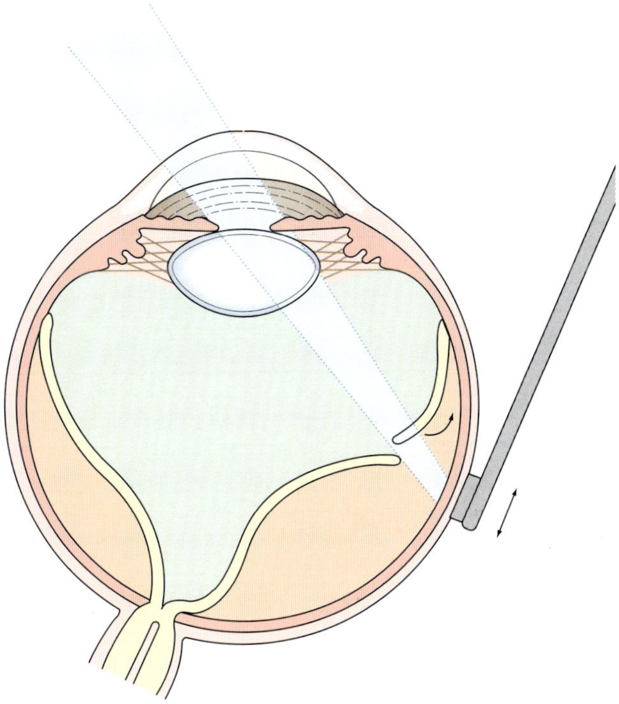

Figure 8.12 *Retinal breaks appear farther posterior than their true location because of parallax if the retina is highly elevated.*

maintained by injection of air or BSS and localization of breaks is continued.

TREATMENT OF RETINAL BREAKS

The rationale for the treatment of retinal breaks is to form an adhesion between the RPE and retina. This is accomplished by using diathermy, cryotherapy or laser. Each technique is capable of producing an effective chorioretinal adhesion but differs in the means of application and the response of surrounding tissues. Each technique also has significant advantages and disadvantages when compared to the other. Selection of a treatment modality may be influenced by the experience and preference of the surgeon and by individual features of the eye.

DIATHERMY

Diathermy, produced by delivering 13.56 MHz of radiofrequency current through the tissues, generates heat because of impedance of the tissue through which it is passed. Diathermy is used infrequently on intact sclera because it causes shrinkage and necrosis of the sclera and often results in elevated IOP. Other disadvantages include penetration of the globe, with resultant retinal hole and intraocular hemorrhage with intense application of diathermy. For optimal diathermy application, a lamellar scleral dissection is required to place diathermy burns in a grid pattern in the bed of the scleral dissection with a blunt-tipped electrode. Diathermy should be avoided in the horizontal meridian to prevent damage to the long posterior artery and nerves. The potential advantages of diathermy over cryotherapy

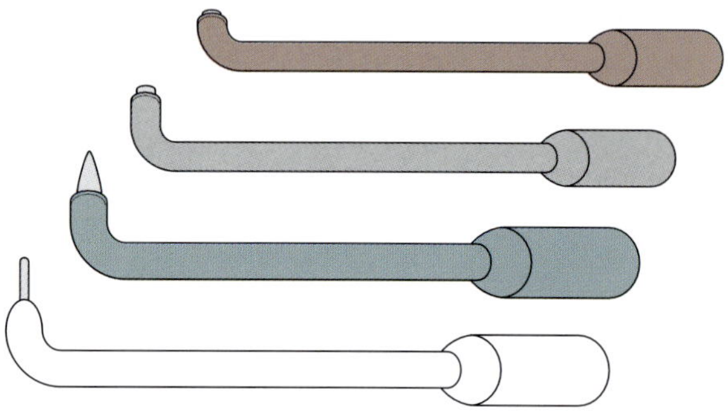

Figure 8.13 *Diathermy electrodes. White: 2.0-mm fine tip for drainage of subretinal fluid. Green: conical tip for surface diathermy and diathermy to choroid. Gray: flat tip for localization posterior to equator. Brown: flat tip for localization anterior to equator.*

include less breakdown of the blood–ocular barrier and less dispersion of RPE cells. Other uses of diathermy in scleral buckling surgery include localization of retinal breaks with a flat-tipped electrode, closure of choroidal vessels before performing drainage with a blunt-tipped electrode and drainage of subretinal fluid with a pin electrode (Fig. 8.13).

CRYOTHERAPY

Cryotherapy has gained popularity because it can be applied through full-thickness sclera without causing significant damage. It is also less likely to cause injury to the long posterior ciliary artery, nerve and vortex veins. Modern cryosurgical units use either carbon dioxide or nitrous oxide gas and are based on the Joule–Thompson principle that a sudden drop in temperature occurs when a pressurized gas is allowed to expand through a narrow aperture. The tube is defrosted by passage of another warm gas, or the same gas under low pressure. A silicone sleeve confines the transfer of the cooling effect to the tip of the probe. When nitrous oxide gas is used, a pressure of 600 psi is usually sufficient to produce cooling up to –89°C.

A probe 2.0–2.5 mm in diameter usually is used for retinal treatment. Two probe shapes, curved and straight, are available. A curved probe may be less

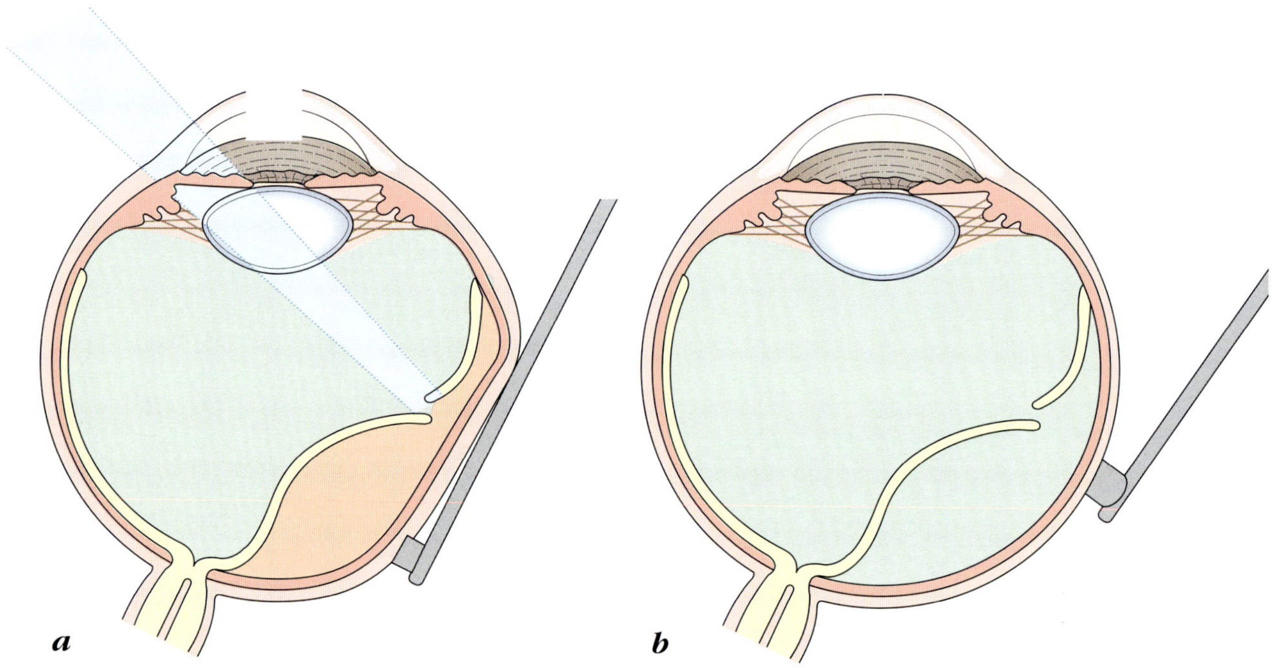

Figure 8.14 *(a) Inadvertent posterior freeze resulting from visualization of depression caused by the shaft of the cryoprobe. (b) Inadvertent posterior freeze is prevented by depressing with the tip alone. The posterior extent of depression must be clearly visible before initiating freezing.*

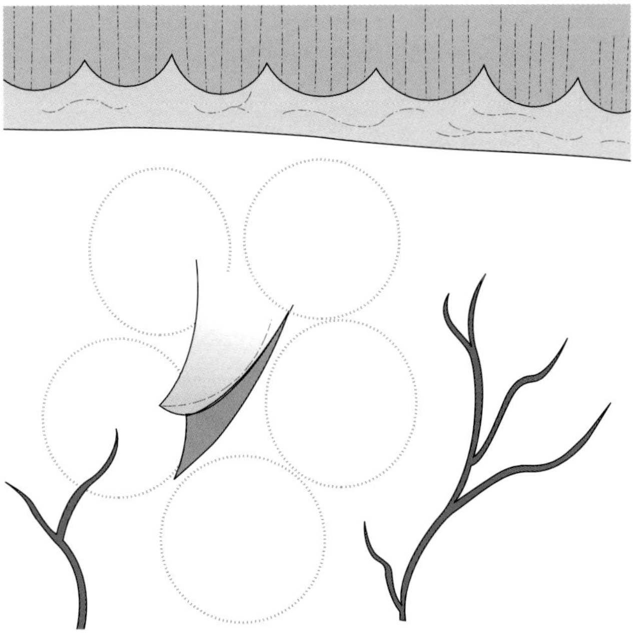

Figure 8.15 *Cryotherapy to surround a large flap tear. Avoid treating the base. Applications should be contiguous but should not overlap significantly.*

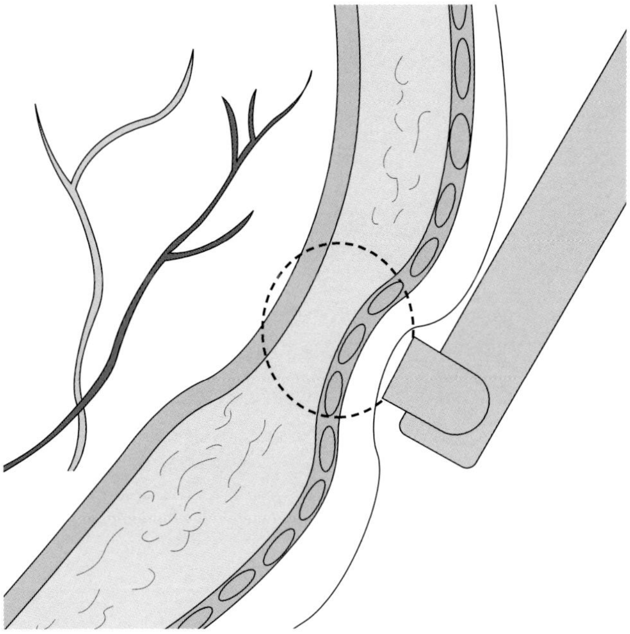

Figure 8.16 *Cryotherapy. When possible, the ice ball should be enlarged to incorporate overlying detached retina, because this results in a stronger chorioretinal adhesion.*

likely to cause an inadvertent posterior freeze with improper technique but slips sideways along the globe easily. The straight probe is less prone to slippage but 'shafting' may occur when the shaft is visually misinterpreted as the tip; when the freeze is initiated, the tip is more posterior than intended. To avoid this, one must ensure that indentation is caused by the tip alone, visualize the posterior limit of the indentation before initiating the freeze and treat the anterior part of the break first (Fig. 8.14).

The goal of cryotherapy is to apply contiguous lesions to surround each retinal break completely (Fig. 8.15). To prevent damage caused by refreezing, applications should not overlap significantly. Treatment should be performed while observing the fundus with the indirect ophthalmoscope, and freezing is terminated soon after the surgeon observes a distinct whitening of the neurosensory retina. Whenever possible, treatment should include both retina and choroid because it creates a stronger adhesion (Fig. 8.16). Initially treating the anterior, shallow part of the detachment may sometimes displace a significant amount of subretinal fluid through the retinal break into the vitreous cavity and permit apposition of the remainder of the break to the pigment epithelium with the indentation of the cryoprobe and allow treatment of both layers.

Mild whitening of the retina is noted several minutes after cryotherapy and is a useful sign to evaluate adequacy of treatment. If, however, the pigment epithelium freezes, as evidenced by an orange hue within the indented choroid, but the overlying highly detached retina does not freeze shortly thereafter, then freezing should be terminated to avoid excessive choroidal damage. Occasionally, localization and cryotherapy are delayed until after drainage of subretinal fluid and normalization of IOP with injection of air or gas. This technique was described initially by Peyman and associates in 1980 (Fig. 8.17),[7] and was popularized subsequently by Gilbert and McLeod as the D–ACE sequence (drainage–air cryo and encirclege).[8] The bare RPE within the base of a large tear should not be treated to prevent dispersion of viable RPE cells into the vitreous cavity. Freezing of the vitreous should be avoided. The tip should be irrigated thoroughly with

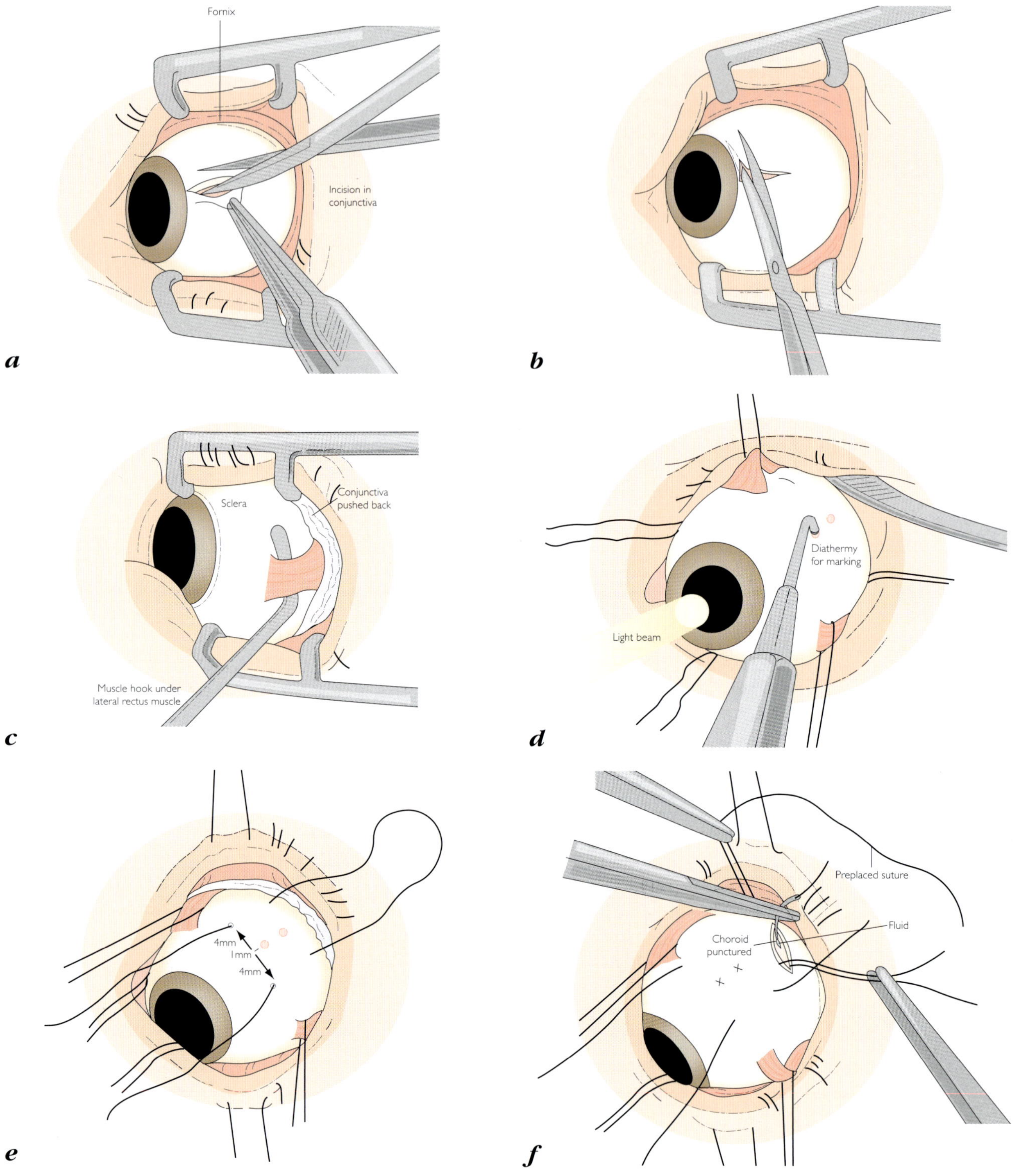

Figure 8.17 *Peyman's (D-ACE) modified exoplant technique of retinal detachment repair. (a) A meridianal conjunctival relaxing incision is made at the 3 o'clock position, beginning 3 mm posterior to limbus. (b) A 360° limbal peritomy is performed with Westcott scissors. (c) Isolation of lateral rectus muscle. (d) Diathermy marking of retinal breaks. (e) A U-shaped mattress suture is placed around the retinal break to accommodate a 5-mm silicone sponge. (f) Sclerotomy is performed and choroid is penetrated at the site of most bullous area of detachment.*

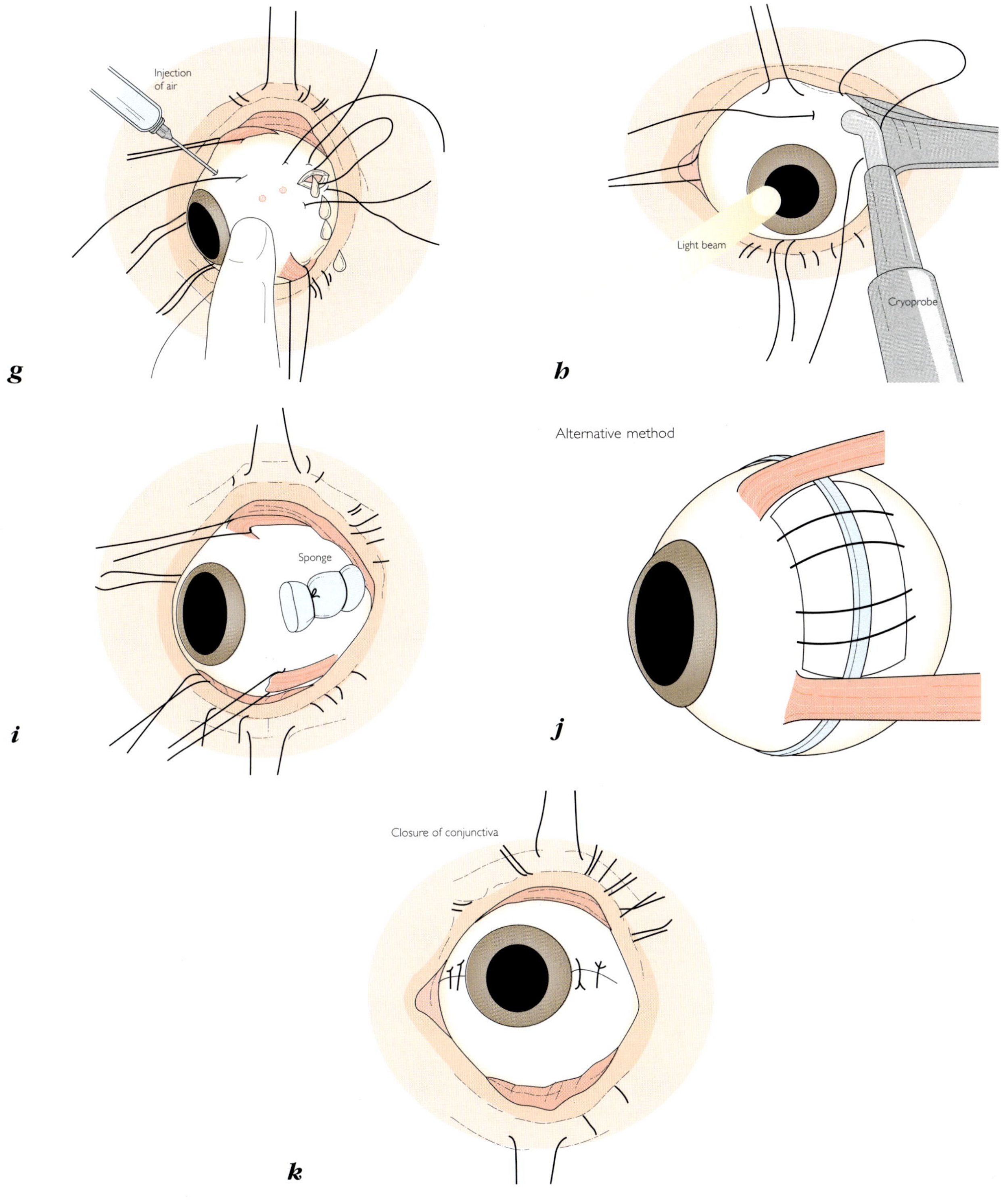

(g) Air is injected into vitreous cavity, and intraocular pressure is monitored by digital palpation. (h) Cryopexy is performed around each break under direct visualization. (i) Silicone sponge is placed meridionally over retinal break and tied with preplaced mattress suture. (j) Aphakic retinal detachments and detachments larger than two quadrants are treated by an encircling band and limbus-parallel silicone plate. (k) Conjunctiva is closed. (Adapted with permission from Goldbaum MH, Joondeph H, Huamonte FU, Peyman GA. Retinal examination and surgery. In: Peyman GA, Sanders DR, Goldberg MF, eds, Principles and Practice of Ophthalmology, *Vol. 2, 1066–8: 1980. Copyright © WB Saunders Co., 1980.[7])*

saline to facilitate thawing of tissues and to prevent complications caused by movement of the probe while still adherent to tissues.

Suspicious areas of the retina also may be treated by cryotherapy. Sometimes a retinal break is identified by the appearance of the freeze. A true retinal break is highlighted and appears red as the surrounding retina turns white during the cryotherapy. If visualization is poor, the cryoprobe is applied to the dried surface of the sclera and freezing is terminated when the tip is surrounded by a 1-mm ring of ice ball or the temperature at the tip drops to –60°C. Cryotherapy may be used to surround areas of abnormal vitreoretinal adhesion, such as lattice degeneration, but laser treatment may be preferable if the retina is attached.

Disadvantages of cryotherapy include breakdown of the blood–ocular barrier, which has been implicated in creating cystoid macular edema, choroidal detachment and exudative retinal detachment. Subretinal fluid should not be drained in the area treated with cryotherapy because resultant choroidal congestion may increase the likelihood of a choroidal hemorrhage.

PHOTOCOAGULATION

Laser treatment is our preferred technique to induce chorioretinal adhesion in attached retina. Compared to cryotherapy, laser causes less inflammation and does not cause dispersion of RPE cells into the vitreous cavity. Sufficient clarity of media is required for successful application of laser. Confluent treatment around retinal breaks with medium-intensity gray-white burns should be applied and should be advanced to the ora whenever possible. Intense white burns may cause retinal hole formation and are not recommended.

Transscleral diode laser treatment to the ciliary body and retina using a specially designed 'exolaser' probe was described originally by Peyman and associates in 1984.[9] A DioPexy® probe is available commercially to administer transscleral diode laser to achieve chorioretinal adhesion in retinal detachment surgery.[10,11] The probe is held like a scleral depressor, perpendicular to the surface of the sclera, and medium-gray lesions are created while monitoring the treatment with the indirect ophthalmoscope. Treatment should be started in attached retina to establish power and duration settings before treating the detached retina. An initial setting of 200 mW power and 1000 ms duration is used and adjusted based on the response. Even if the lesion does not involve overlying detached retina, treatment of pigment epithelium alone may provide adequate chorioretinal adhesion. The foot switch should be released at the first appearance of a lesion in order to avoid creating burns that are too intense. Less power is needed if the sclera is dry, in areas of thin sclera and in areas with increased pigmentation. Unlike cryotherapy, transscleral diode laser can be applied through a pre-existing silicone material, such as a scleral buckle or glaucoma drainage implant.[12]

SCLERAL BUCKLING

The purpose of scleral buckling is to close retinal holes and relieve vitreous traction. Various materials have been used to create a scleral buckling effect, but hard silicone rubber and silicone sponges are the most commonly used materials. The buckling material may be sutured to the surface of the sclera (exoplant) or be placed beneath scleral flaps after lamellar scleral dissection (implant). Absorbable sheets of gelatin are sometimes used as an exoplant or implant to treat retinal detachment. Gelatin is predominantly hydrolyzed collagen. It is supplied as thin, dehydrated sheets, which require hydration for 5–10 minutes at room temperature to make them pliable, although excessive hydration of gelatin may result in marked softening of the material and may make subsequent handling difficult. These sheets then are cut to the desired size and sutured to the sclera, with or without an encircling element. Multiple sheets may have to be used in order to achieve the desired buckling effect. Strips of dry gelatin may be used to fill scleral pockets, which are subsequently closed with nonabsorbable sutures. This technique has been recommended for retinal detachments caused by a single retinal break and those caused by dialysis in children.[13]

Various kinds and shapes of solid silicone rubber and silicone sponges are available for scleral buckling (Fig. 8.18). Silicone rubber is available as symmetric or asymmetric tires, bands, strips and wedges of different shapes and sizes. They are often grooved to permit placement of an encircling band. Tires have radii of curvature that approximate to that of the globe. Asymmetric tires provide increased buckle height posteriorly, decrease the likelihood of erosion anteriorly and permit more equatorial placement of an encircling element.

Sponges are predominantly used for radial buckles but can be used also for encircling the globe when

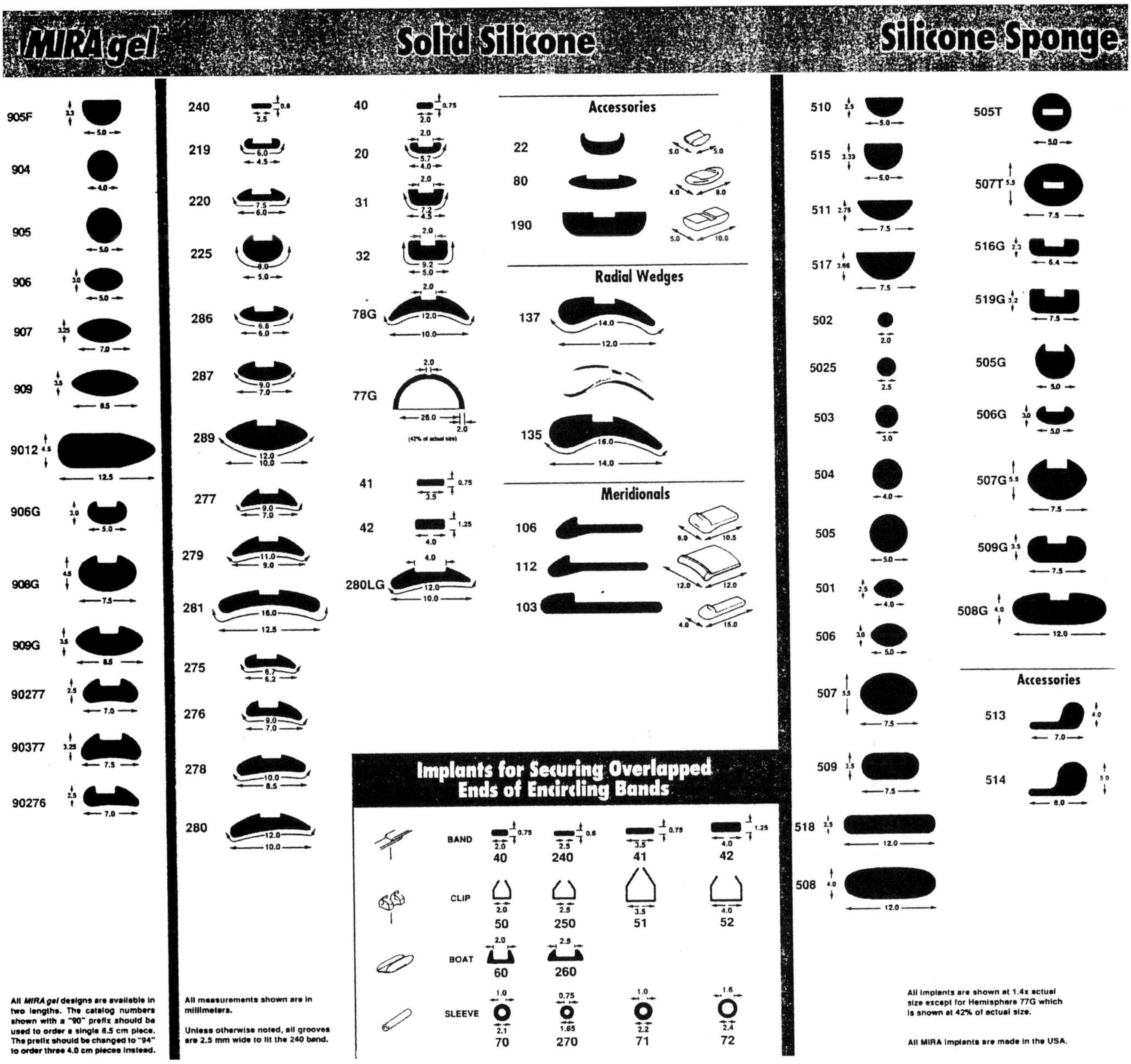

Figure 8.18 *Implants and exoplants for scleral buckling. All measurements are in millimeters. (Courtesy of MIRA, Inc.)*

either a high buckle is needed or when breaks are at varying distances from the ora. Disadvantages of sponges include uneven indentation when used for encircling the globe, increased risk of infection because of air pockets and greater likelihood of erosion through the conjunctiva.[14] Cutting a cylindrical sponge lengthwise to half-thickness and suturing it to the sclera with the convex side facing the globe provides proper indentation of the sclera while avoiding an external bulge above the contour of the globe (Fig. 8.19).

SEGMENTAL BUCKLE

A segmental buckle is appropriate for localized retinal detachments caused by a single break or breaks limited to 1–2 clock-hours without significant PVR in phakic

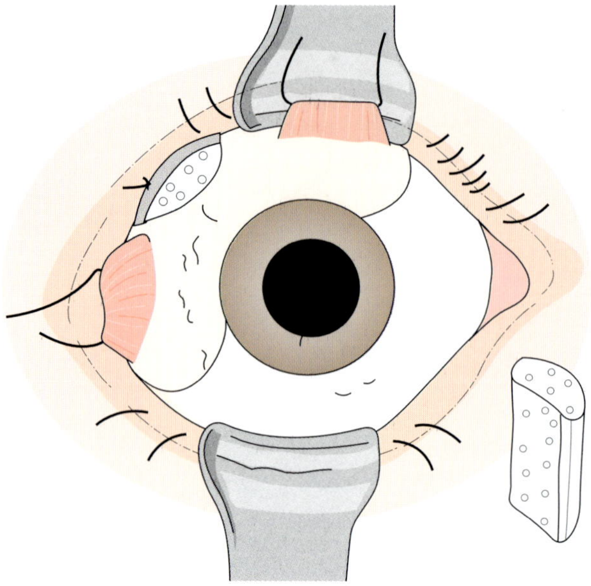

Figure 8.19 *Half-thickness cylindrical sponge minimizes external bulk of the scleral buckle. The convex side is placed facing the sclera.*

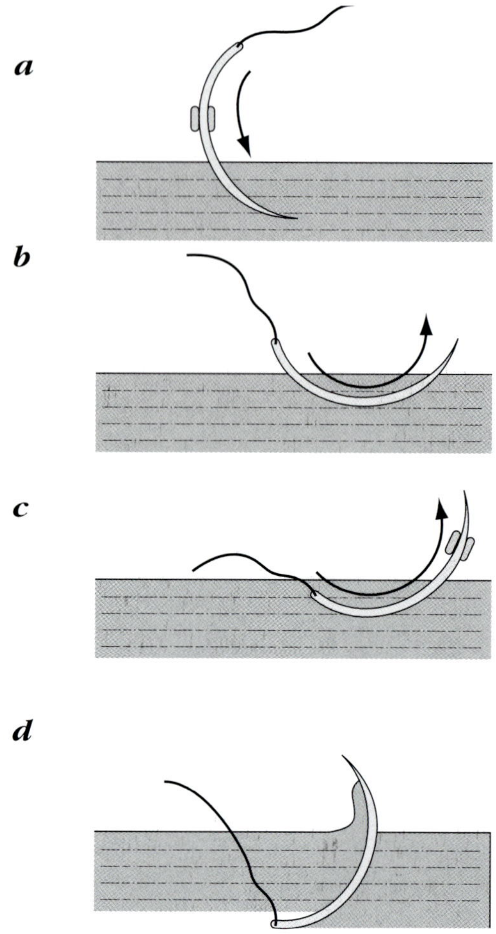

Figure 8.20 *Passage of spatula needle through the sclera. (a) Needle is grasped at the junction of posterior one-third and anterior two-thirds. It is introduced at a 45° angle to obtain adequate depth. (b) Needle is advanced along its arc. (c) Needle is withdrawn following its curvature. (d) Avoid posterior pressure with the hub to prevent inadvertent perforation.*

eyes. Other possible indications for segmental buckling include detachment caused by dialysis, detachment with minimal subretinal fluid and in selected eyes with glaucoma where a segmental buckle may preserve the conjunctiva for future filtration surgery or avoid the area of a previous filtering bleb.

A segmental buckle may be circumferential or radial, depending on the orientation of retinal pathology. A radial buckle is preferred for large flap tears to counter the tendency for the tear to gape open posteriorly if a circumferential buckle is employed, and is particularly suitable for large posterior tears. Segmental buckling can be accomplished by suturing a piece of solid silicone to the surface of the sclera, but the most popular material is silicone sponge. This type of surgery is often done without drainage of the subretinal fluid. The sponge is secured to the sclera with mattress sutures of 5-0 polyester. The assistant holds the sponge with a cotton-tipped applicator or applies moderate stretch with forceps while sutures are being tied so that the sponge is under moderate tension. The IOP may rise considerably if drainage of subretinal fluid is not performed but may rapidly fall to normal levels in a nonglaucomatous eye. In eyes with poor aqueous outflow, such as those with primary open-angle glaucoma, normal IOP should be restored by removing the aqueous, subretinal fluid or fluid vitreous. The central retinal artery should be inspected; pulsation indicates that the blood is entering the retinal circulation, and the patient may be sent safely to the recovery room.

SUTURE PLACEMENT

For a radially oriented buckle, the suture arms should be 2–3 mm farther apart than the diameter of the

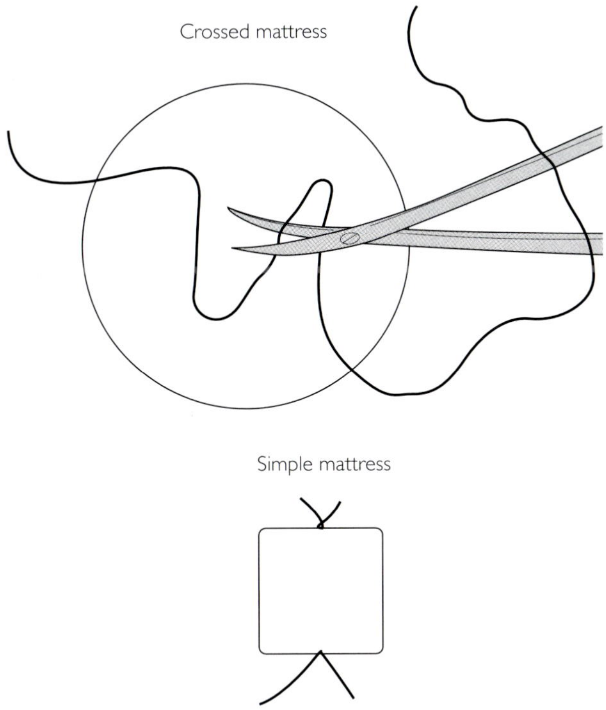

Figure 8.21 *Converting a crossed mattress suture to a simple mattress suture.*

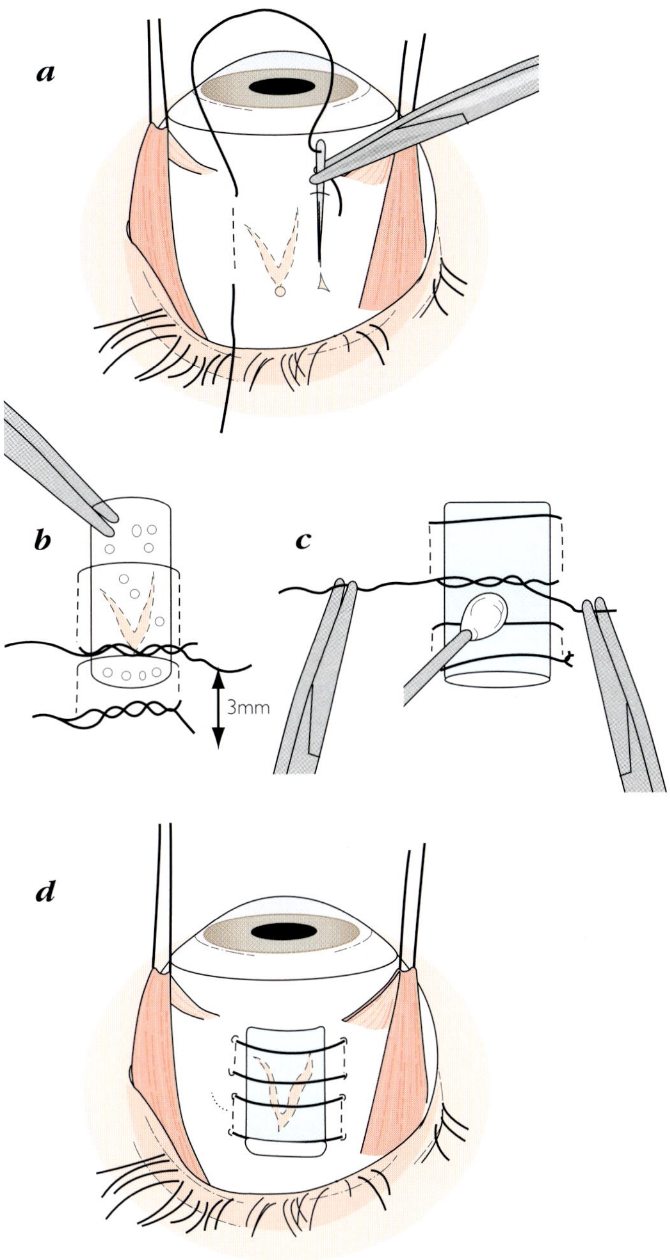

Figure 8.22 *Technique for radial sponge: mattress sutures are placed straddling the break. (a) Initial pass is made in anterior-to-posterior direction and is begun near the muscle insertion. (b) Posterior bite extends 3 mm posterior to the break; triple throws are made and sponge is placed beneath sutures. (c) Pressure with cotton-tipped applicator is applied while sutures are tied. (d) Correct position of a radial sponge for a flap tear.*

buckling material. A good rule is to place sutures 1.5 times the width of the implant apart. For a 5-mm sponge, sutures are placed 7.5 mm apart to close a retinal break 3 mm wide. We prefer 5-0 polyester suture on a spatula needle. Each bite should be approximately half the scleral thickness in depth and 3–4 mm long, to provide secure fixation. The assistant stabilizes the eye by holding adjacent traction sutures at a divergent angle. The surgeon grasps the muscle insertion with a toothed forceps for stability. The needle tip should be visualized at all times as it is passed through the sclera. Once the needle has been brought out, it is important to complete passage of the needle along its arc, avoiding posterior pressure, which may perforate through the remaining underlying sclera and choroid (Fig. 8.20). The posterior bite should be at least 3 mm posterior to the break.

It is often helpful to use a double-armed suture and pass needles in an anterior-to-posterior direction while working posterior to the equator. Alternatively, a crossed mattress suture may be used, which may be converted to a simple mattress suture (Fig. 8.21). Anterior mattress sutures should be placed to provide a buckling effect to the ora (Fig. 8.22).

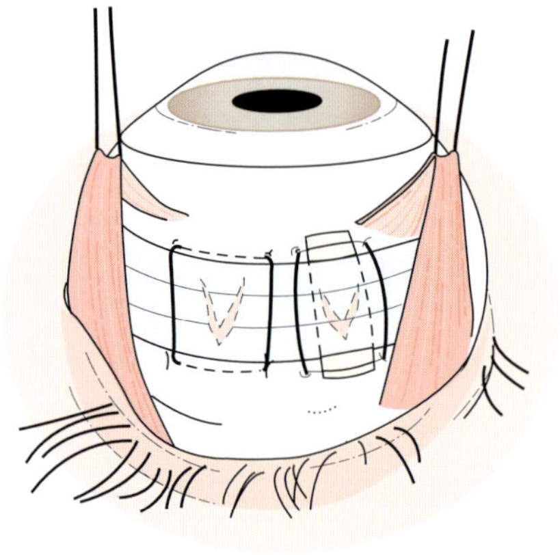

Figure 8.23 *Suture technique to secure a radial sponge extending posterior to a circumferential exoplant: short posterior suture bites provide a loop to indent the radial element.*

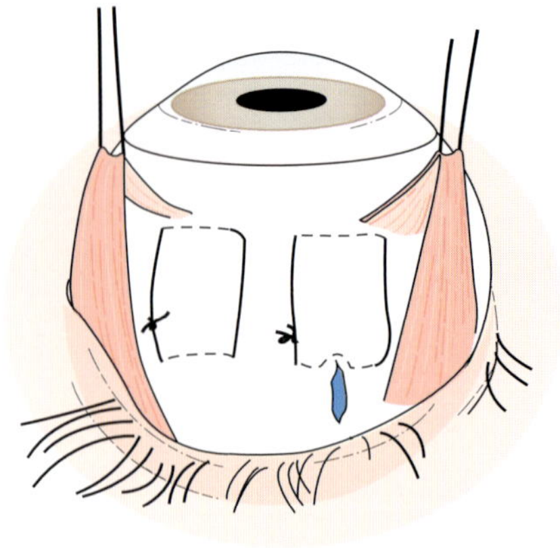

Figure 8.24 *Mattress suture technique to avoid damage to the vortex vein: short scleral bites are taken at either side of the vein to avoid damage to the intrascleral portion.*

Another modification may be used when a radial sponge is placed beneath a broad circumferential buckle. The anterior pass is made parallel to the limbus. Posteriorly, two short scleral bites are taken so that the radially oriented sponge may extend posterior to the circumferential buckle and be covered by the posterior suture loop (Fig. 8.23).

For circumferentially oriented scleral buckles, the mattress sutures are passed parallel to the limbus 2–3 mm farther apart than the width of the buckle. The posterior pass should be at least 3 mm posterior to the retinal break. The anterior sutures are usually taken along the line of the ora, to reduce the risk of leakage of subretinal fluid through the break anteriorly. As with a radial buckle, sutures are placed 1.5 times the width of the sponge apart. The posterior edge of the break is placed on the center of the buckle. Many surgeons like to place the break on the anterior crest of the buckle, especially if a circumferential sponge is used. If this is desired, the posterior suture is passed 4 mm behind the posterior edge of the tear and the anterior suture is only slightly anterior to the anterior edge of the break. The suturing technique may be modified to avoid damage to the intrascleral portion of the vortex vein by taking short bites posteriorly at the corners on either side of the vein (Fig. 8.24). A similar technique may be employed in a very soft eye, where making a long intrascleral pass may be difficult.

ENCIRCLING ELEMENT

Encircling buckles are used commonly in cases with multiple breaks in different quadrants, aphakia, pseudophakia, high myopia and in eyes with diffuse vitreoretinal pathology, such as extensive lattice degeneration and vitreoretinal degeneration. They are also indicated in patients with PVR greater than grade B, retinal detachment caused by trauma, eyes without a recognizable retinal break and giant retinal tears. An encircling element provides a permanent 360° buckle and can be placed over a radial or circumferential segmental element (Figs 8.25 and 8.26). Disadvantages of an encircling buckle include a need for a 360° peritomy, a myopic shift of –2 to –3 diopters and a need to drain subretinal fluid in most eyes. Encircling elements should be avoided in patients with sickle-cell disease to avoid anterior segment ischemia.

Either a sponge or solid silicone can be used for an encircling buckle. An encircling sponge may be preferred if retinal breaks are located at varying distance from the ora. Most surgeons use solid silicone for encircling the globe, securing it to the globe either with horizontal mattress sutures or with belt loops (Fig. 8.27). The necessary width and location of the encircling element depends on the pathology. If a flap tear is being supported with a circumferential segmental buckle beneath an encircling element, its posterior edge should lie on the

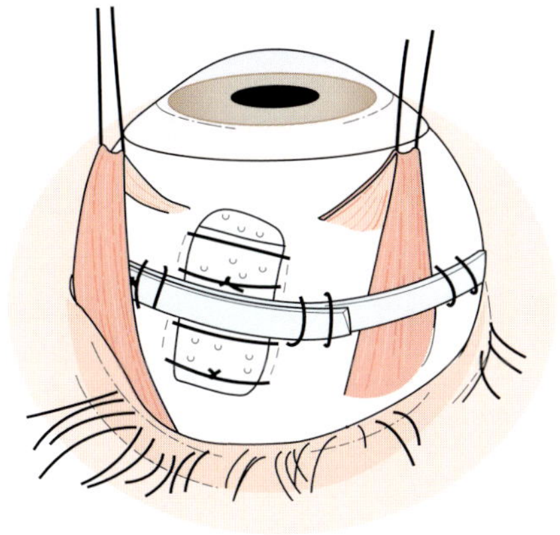

Figure 8.25 *Radial sponge beneath an encircling band: one horizontal mattress suture should be placed on either side of the sponge to secure the encircling band; only one suture per quadrant is needed in other areas.*

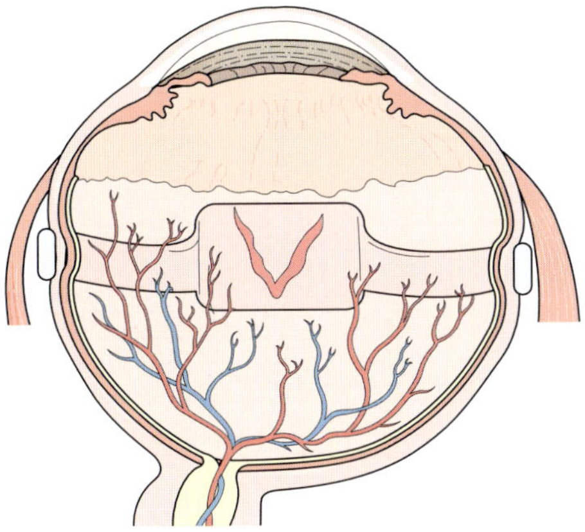

Figure 8.26 *Correct position of circumferential buckle for a flap retinal tear.*

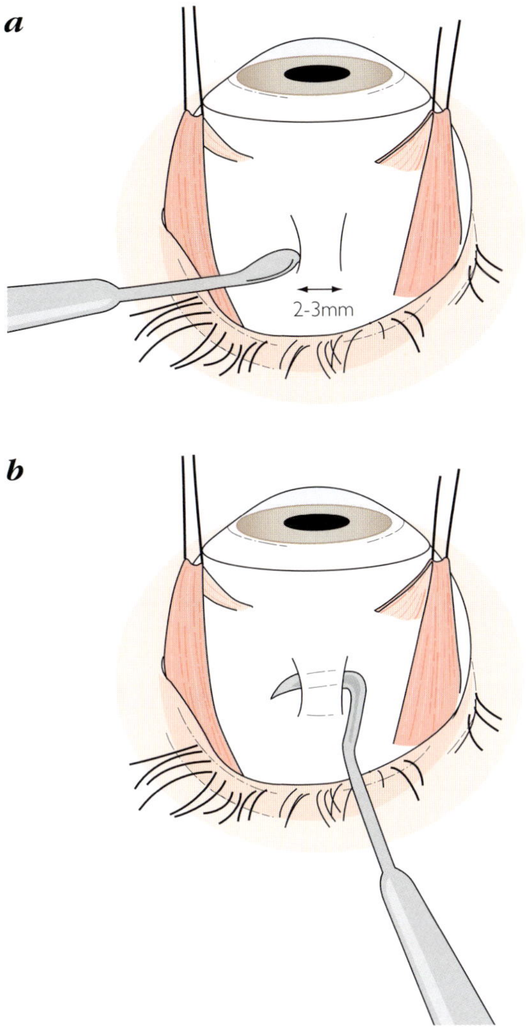

Figure 8.27 *(a) Belt loops are prepared by making two partial-thickness radial incisions starting 2.5 mm posterior to rectus muscle insertion. (b) A crescent blade is used to complete the tunnel.*

center of the crest of the buckle (middle to anterior portion). Buckling should extend to the ora anteriorly and at least 1 clock-hour on either side of its lateral margins (Fig. 8.26). The posterior edge of vitreoretinal pathology, such as lattice degeneration or vitreoretinal adhesion, should be supported on the crest of the encircling element. If the vitreous base requires support, its posterior edge (approximately 3 mm posterior to the ora nasally and 2 mm posterior to the ora temporally) should be placed on the crest of the buckle. It is not necessary to place the encircling element around the greatest curvature of the eye. A 2.5-mm band (no. 240) is often used to support the vitreous base, with its ends secured by a silicone sleeve (no. 70) (Fig. 8.28), a clove-hitch suture of 5-0 polyester (Fig. 8.29) or tantalum clips. Other elements may be secured with a 5-0 polyester suture. A no. 41 band is commonly used to buckle retinal detachments in aphakic and pseudophakic eyes and in eyes without a recognizable break.

When an encircling element is used, the buckle height may be increased by tightening the band. This

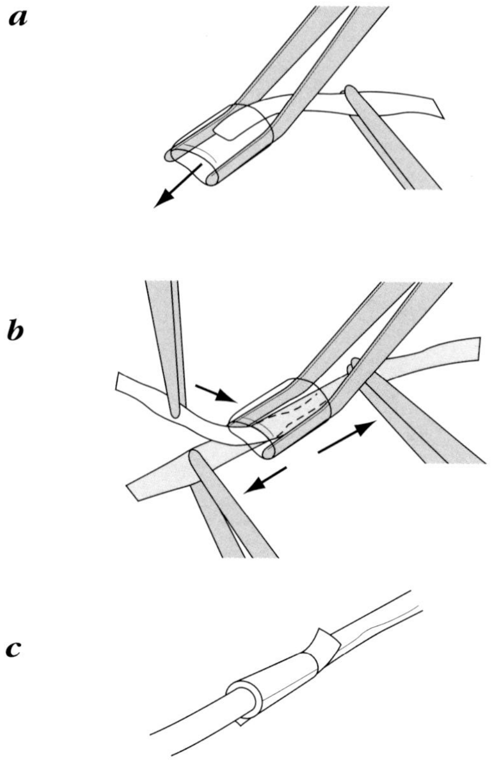

Figure 8.28 *Technique for placement of silicone sleeve.*

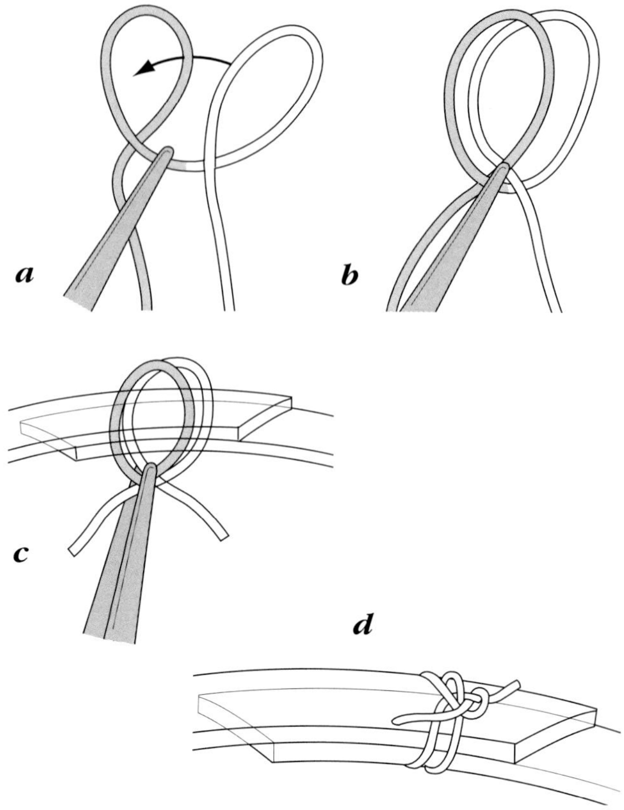

Figure 8.29 *The clove hitch knot: the second loop (white) is placed behind the first loop (black); the clove hitch is held in a straight hemostat; it is placed around one end of the encircling element and the other end is threaded through the loop; the clove hitch is then tightened and secured with a surgeon's knot.*

method leads to circumferential shortening of the sclera in relation to the retina, causing radial fold formation in the retina that may predispose retinal breaks to the fish-mouth phenomenon. Axial elongation of the globe also occurs. Excessive tightening may cause anterior segment ischemia and should be avoided. The second method of increasing the buckle height involves increasing the spread of suture bites. This causes anteroposterior shortening of the sclera and provides excellent control of the buckle height. The axial length may shorten from this procedure but will lengthen as a result of elongation of the eye by the encircling element.

INTRASCLERAL IMPLANT TECHNIQUES

A lamellar scleral dissection is done to create a bed extending 3 mm posteriorly, 2 mm anteriorly and 3 mm circumferentially beyond the retinal break. The initial incision is created parallel to the limbus along the posterior edge of the retinal break. The dissection is continued using a blunt dissector while the scleral flaps are kept stretched. Damage to the vortex veins must be avoided. Diathermy is applied to the dried scleral surface with a blunt-tipped electrode, placing medium-intensity burns approximately 2 mm apart in staggered rows parallel to the limbus. A suitable silicone implant is placed in the bed and an encircling band is passed around the globe, securing it to the sclera with mattress sutures or scleral belt loops. Drainage is usually performed within the bed, after which the scleral flaps are closed with 5-0 nonabsorbable sutures (Fig. 8.30). Reported benefits of scleral dissection include:

- Decreased chance of infection or extrusion of the implant.

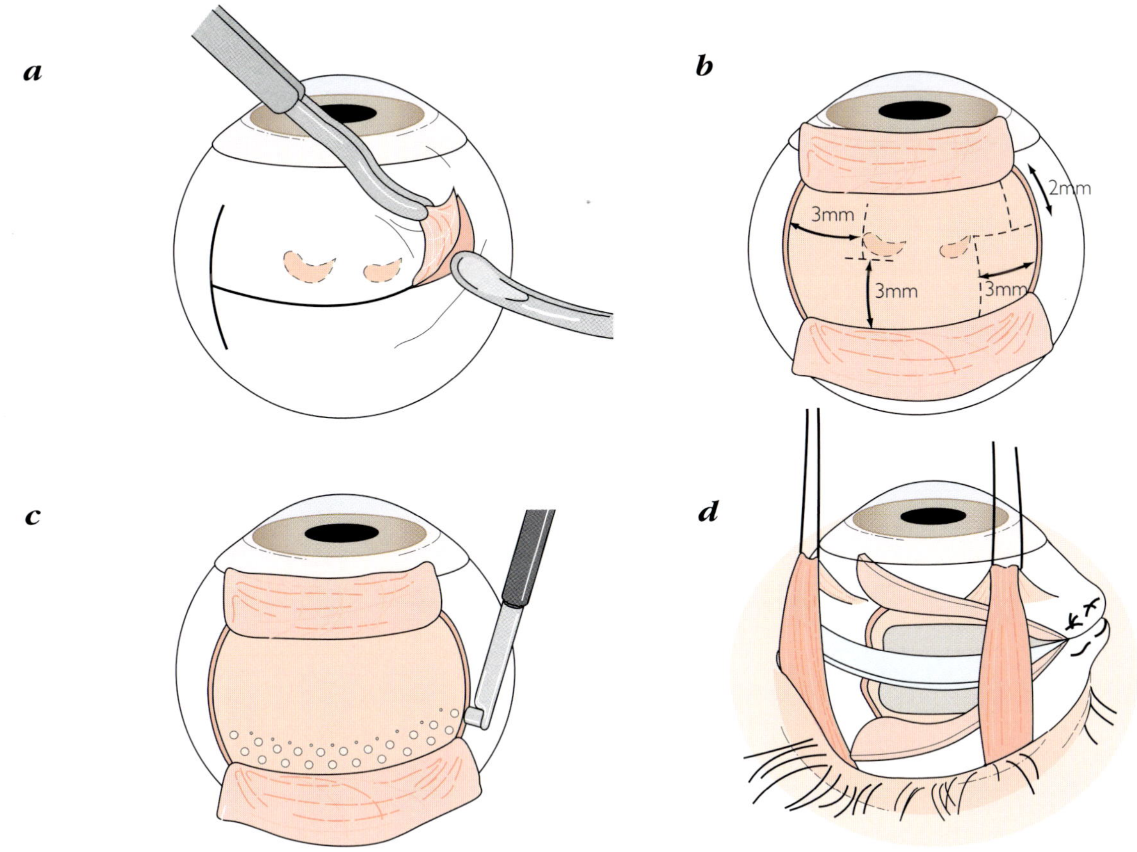

Figure 8.30 *Technique for intrascleral implants: (a) technique of lamellar dissection; (b) desired extent of scleral dissection; (c) diathermy to scleral bed; (d) placement of implant and closure.*

- Diathermy may cause less inflammation compared to cryotherapy, and is less likely to disperse viable RPE cells.
- Drainage is performed in an area already treated with diathermy.

Disadvantages of the implant technique include:

- The need for scleral dissection.
- Permanent scleral damage from diathermy and dissection, making reoperations difficult.
- Elevated IOP caused by scleral shrinkage from diathermy, necessitating drainage of subretinal fluid.
- Increased risk of intrusion of the implant.

DRAINAGE OF SUBRETINAL FLUID

Drainage of subretinal fluid is the most controversial part of the operation and is most likely to cause serious complications. Removal of subretinal fluid brings the retinal break closer to the RPE and removes intraocular volume to allow room for the buckling element. It is usually performed after cryotherapy and placement of buckling material but before the sutures are tied. Attempting to drain the subretinal fluid dry is neither necessary nor recommended. External drainage is ineffective in eyes that have undergone prior vitrectomy, because fluid inside the eye readily gains access to the subretinal space through the retinal break. Internal drainage may be preferable in such cases. Generally accepted indications for drainage are:

- Highly elevated detachments: drainage promotes settling of the break on the buckle and, if performed initially during the operation, may aid in accurate localization of the break and allow more effective cryotherapy (D–ACE sequence).
- Chronic inferior detachments: viscous subretinal

fluid in these cases absorbs slowly after nondrainage surgery. Additionally, inferior breaks may settle less readily on the buckle because of the influence of gravity.

- Proliferative vitreoretinopathy: stiff retina and epiretinal membranes in PVR may cause the break to remain open. We like to drain all cases of PVR grade B or above.
- Aphakic detachments and those in highly myopic eyes: syneretic vitreous may not effectively plug the retinal break and may allow persistent passage of fluid from the vitreous cavity.
- Glaucomatous eyes and eyes with recent intraocular surgery are intolerant of high IOP associated with nondrainage procedures.
- Giant retinal tear.
- Eyes in which no apparent retinal break is found.
- Elderly eyes, because the RPE pump is likely to take a longer time to absorb fluid.
- Eyes with multiple breaks.

SELECTION OF DRAINAGE SITE

Drainage should be performed in an area where there is sufficient subretinal fluid to enter the subretinal space safely. It should be avoided in areas treated with cryotherapy, because choroidal congestion induced by cryotherapy may predispose to hemorrhage. Indirect ophthalmoscopy is performed before drainage, to make sure that subretinal fluid has not shifted and that there are no vortex veins near the proposed site of drainage. Draining just above or below the horizontal meridian is preferable because the choroid is less vascular in these areas. Nasal quadrants may be preferred whenever possible because if subretinal bleeding were to occur, it would be less likely to reach the macula. We attempt to drain beneath a scleral buckle as much as possible, because the drainage site can be supported immediately in the event of retinal incarceration.

TECHNIQUE OF DRAINAGE

Once a proper drainage site has been selected, the globe should be positioned such that the proposed drainage site is easily accessible externally and can be viewed by indirect ophthalmoscopy without significant manipulation. All sources of external pressure on the globe should be removed before making a cutdown. A radial incision 3 mm in length is made with a no. 57 or no. 69 Beaver blade, keeping the

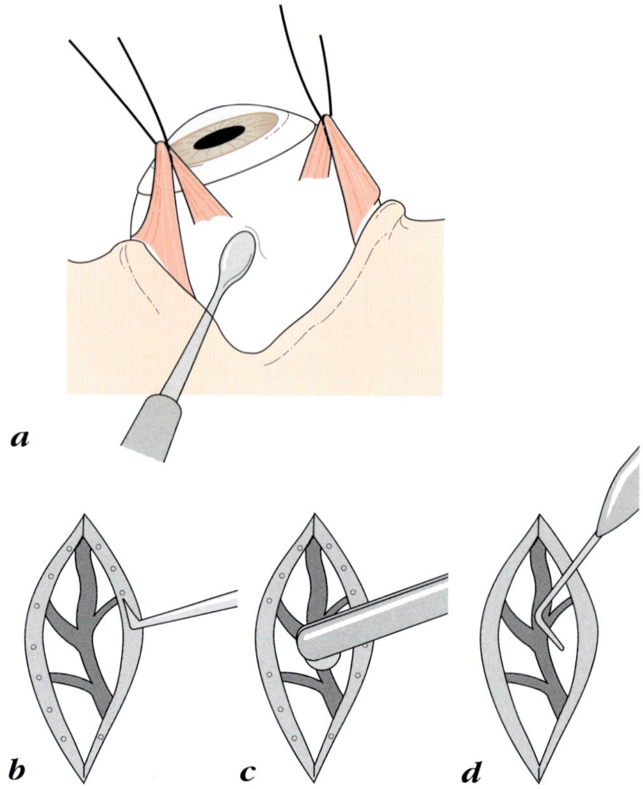

Figure 8.31 *Drainage of subretinal fluid; (a) radial sclerotomy; (b) diathermy to wound edges; (c) diathermy to choroid; (d) entry into subretinal space.*

blade perpendicular to the sclera to prevent shelving of the edges. Light diathermy is applied with a blunt-tipped electrode to cause the edges of the wound to gape. The incision is continued until black choroid bulges into the incision. Magnification provided by a 20-diopter lens or binocular loupes helps in the identification of residual scleral fibers, which must be cut; otherwise, they may swell during drainage, prematurely closing the drainage site.

Diathermy is applied to the choroid to close vessels and to cause shrinkage. The tip should be moved gently to prevent it from sticking to the choroid. A preplaced 5-0 polyester suture is passed in mattress configuration if a sclerotomy is not under the buckle. The choroid is reinspected under magnification for major vessels, which should be avoided during choroidotomy. A fiberoptic light source, placed against the sclera across from the drainage site, helps in the identification of choroidal vessels.

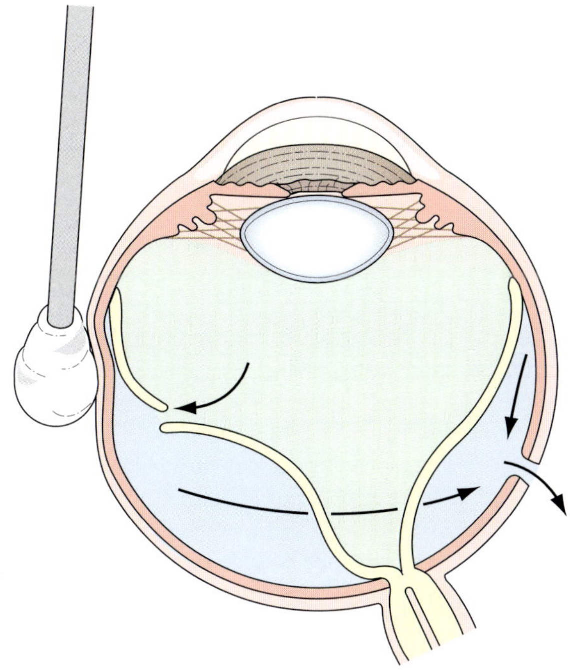

Figure 8.32 *Passage of fluid vitreous is prevented by closing the break with a cotton-tipped applicator during drainage.*

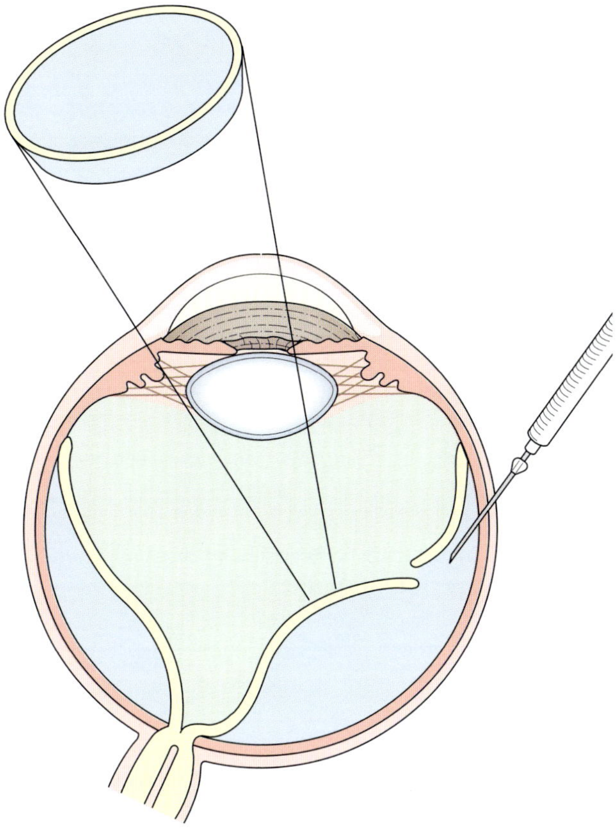

Figure 8.33 *Technique of needle drainage.*

The choroid is penetrated with a 2.0-mm diathermy needle, a suture needle (5-0) or a bent 30-gauge needle to a depth of approximately 2 mm at an angle to avoid injury to the retina. The needle is withdrawn immediately (Fig. 8.31). In most cases, subretinal fluid follows withdrawal of the needle and is allowed to drain spontaneously. As subretinal fluid continues to drain, cotton-tipped applicators are placed to indent the sclera 180° away from the drainage site in order to maintain relatively normal IOP.

As the subretinal fluid drainage slows, pigment particles may be seen in the fluid. This usually means that the drainage is nearing completion. Once drainage stops, indirect ophthalmoscopy is performed to examine the drainage site and residual subretinal fluid. If the drainage was adequate, buckle sutures are tied. If additional drainage is necessary, the lips of the sclerotomy may be manipulated with a 0.12-mm forceps. This will often reopen the site and re-establish the flow. Pressure may be applied anterior to the drainage site with a cotton-tipped applicator to promote flow of subretinal fluid through the drainage site. If drainage stops prematurely because of flattening of the retina over the drainage site, the first site should be closed with a mattress suture and another sclerotomy made. This procedure, however, is rarely necessary.

Occasionally, excessive drainage results in eyes with liquefied vitreous caused by loss of the fluid vitreous through the break. Such an event should be anticipated in patients with aphakia and those with high myopia, particularly if the break is large. In such cases, the drainage site should be selected away from the break, if possible. The retinal break may be closed with a cotton-tipped applicator during drainage to prevent passage of liquid vitreous (Fig. 8.32). If excessive drainage results in hypotony, the IOP may have to be restored by tightening the buckle or, if this is not adequate, by injection of air, gas or BSS through the pars plana.

VARIATIONS

The endolaser probe may be used with the argon laser and a power setting of 800 mW–2 W at 0.2–0.5

seconds to perform choroidotomy.[15,16] The probe is held close to, but not touching, the choroid. Usually only a single burn is needed to enter the subretinal space. This technique may avoid retinal injury from a sharp needle tip but may result in an excessively large hole in the choroid and is difficult to control.

External drainage with a ⅝-inch 25-gauge needle mounted on a tuberculin syringe with its plunger removed under indirect ophthalmoscopic visualization has been described (Fig. 8.33).[17] This technique virtually eliminates the possibility of retinal incarceration, but may result in bleeding or retinal hole formation with improper technique. A randomized study found a slightly higher incidence of subretinal hemorrhage with needle drainage compared with conventional two-step drainage. Damage to the retina was rare with either technique.[18]

Another modification of needle drainage involves introduction of a 26-gauge needle attached to a 2-ml syringe with its plunger depressed. The needle is gradually advanced perpendicular to the sclera until subretinal fluid is seen in the hub. The needle then is withdrawn and the subretinal fluid is allowed to drain spontaneously.[19]

After successful completion of drainage, the buckle sutures adjacent to the drainage site are tied first, followed by those supporting the retinal break. The remaining sutures are tied and the band is adjusted. The perfusion of the central retinal artery is assessed by indirect ophthalmoscopy. If the artery is closed, the buckle may be loosened or fluid removed from the anterior chamber or vitreous, as indicated. If the globe is hypotonus, the volume may be restored by injection of air or gas with a 30-gauge needle through the pars plana.

CLOSURE OF CONJUNCTIVA

After final adjustment of the buckle, suture knots should be rotated posteriorly. Tenon's capsule and the conjunctiva should be irrigated with BSS containing a broad-spectrum antibiotic, such as gentamicin 2 mg/ml. The edges of the conjunctiva and Tenon's capsule are identified and the wound is closed in one or two layers. Subconjunctival injections of antibiotic and steroid are administered.

SPECIAL SITUATIONS

- No break identified. These are usually aphakic or pseudophakic eyes and the break is usually located just posterior to the ora. The breaks may be very small and difficult to visualize. Capsular opacification or inadequate pupillary dilation may also impair visualization. Cryotherapy should be applied to the suspected sites of retinal breaks, based on the configuration of the detachment. An encircling element such as a no. 41 band is used after draining the fluid. Consideration may be given to laser treatment for 360° on the buckle.
- Patients with prior glaucoma-filtering surgery. Careful attention should be paid to the bleb in order to avoid inadvertent injury and leakage. These cases are best managed with a segmental buckle. Excessive elevation of the IOP should be avoided by draining subretinal fluid, the anterior chamber or fluid vitreous as necessary.
- Patients with recent cataract surgery. The cataract wound should be inspected for leaks and reinforced with sutures, if necessary, before proceeding.
- Patients with an anterior chamber intraocular lens or an iris-supported lens. Anterior chamber paracentesis to remove aqueous should be avoided, because it may result in contact between the intraocular lens and the corneal endothelium. Sodium hyaluronate may be injected if the anterior chamber becomes shallow after gas is injected in the vitreous.
- Giant retinal tear. An encircling buckle on a giant retinal tear leads to further anteroposterior opening of the break, which may lead to persistent leakage of fluid posteriorly (Fig. 8.34a). A low, broad buckle should be used in these cases to provide adequate support posteriorly (Fig. 8.34b). Cryotherapy should be performed to seal edges of the giant retinal tear in order to prevent anterior leakage of fluid beneath the anterior flap, which often remains elevated.

INTRAOPERATIVE COMPLICATIONS

CORNEAL CLOUDING

Corneal clouding usually results from epithelial edema or by desiccation. Mild edema may be reversed by rolling a dry cotton-tipped applicator over the cornea. Severe epithelial edema usually requires epithelial removal, which may be accomplished with a rounded blade or Paton's spatula. Care

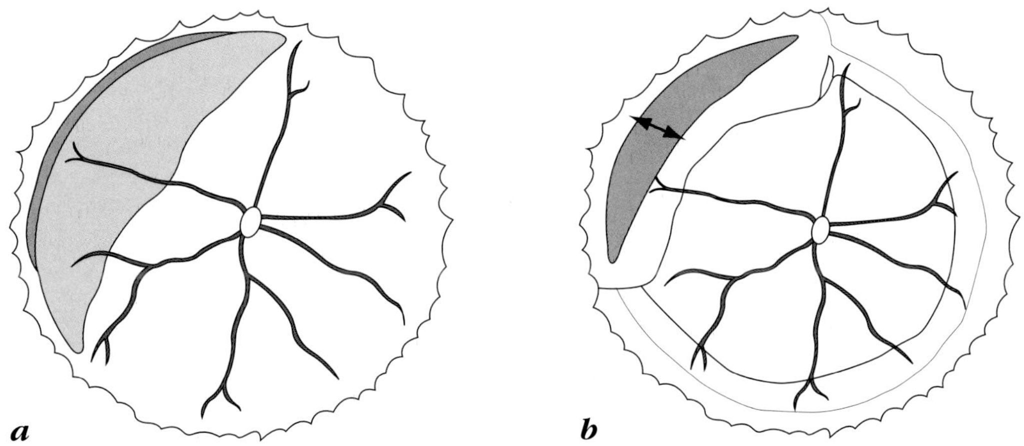

Figure 8.34 *Scleral buckle for a giant retinal tear results in anteroposterior opening of the tear (a), therefore a low, broad scleral buckle (b) is used, extending at least 4 mm posterior to the posterior edge of the tear.*

should be taken to leave a 2-mm rim of epithelium at the periphery to promote faster healing postoperatively.

MIOSIS

Miosis may result from hypotony, trauma to the iris during paracentesis or excessive inflammation from cryotherapy. Preoperative instillation of 0.3% flurbiprofen may diminish intraoperative miosis. Additional mydriatic–cycloplegic drops should be instilled to dilate the pupil. If unsuccessful, intracameral administration of 0.1 ml of epinephrine (1:10 000) may cause prompt dilation of the pupil. Iris hooks may be used as a last resort in one to four quadrants.

SCLERAL PERFORATION

Scleral perforation during suture placement is evidenced by the presentation of blood, pigment, subretinal fluid or vitreous through the site of perforation. The retina should be examined immediately to determine the depth of perforation. If a retinal break has resulted, it should be treated by cryotherapy and supported by extending the buckle. If bleeding occurs, immediate pressure should be applied to the site of perforation to tamponade the bleeding, and the eye should be positioned to prevent migration of blood beneath the fovea. If massive subretinal bleeding occurs, immediate vitrectomy with internal drainage of subretinal blood should be considered.

COMPLICATIONS ASSOCIATED WITH DRAINAGE

A dry tap usually indicates incomplete penetration of the choroid. It is avoided by steadily advancing the needle until fluid is present around the needle. Inspecting the retina just before drainage can minimize the possibility of the shifting of subretinal fluid.

If a retinal break results from the needle striking the retina, it should be treated with cryotherapy and supported on a buckle. Retinal incarceration is identified by characteristic dimpled appearance of the retina and folds leading to the incarceration site. A retinal incarceration should be supported on a buckle. No attempt should be made to free the retina from the incarceration site. Such attempts are futile and may result in further retinal injury.

Choroidal hemorrhage is marked by the appearance of dark blood at the drainage site. If this occurs, the drainage site should be closed immediately with either a buckle or a suture and the IOP elevated above systolic pressure for 5 minutes. The eye should be positioned to place the drainage site as inferiorly

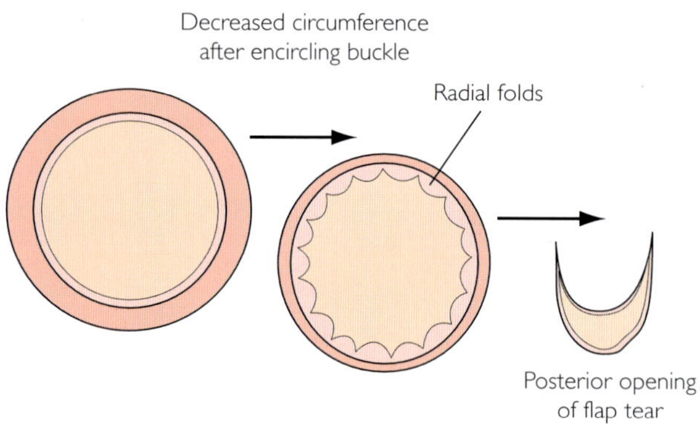

Figure 8.35 *Geometric basis of fish-mouth phenomenon.*

as possible in order to prevent migration of blood beneath the fovea. If massive bleeding occurs, or substantial blood accumulates beneath the fovea, vitrectomy with internal drainage of blood should be considered.

PERSISTENTLY OPEN BREAK: THE FISH-MOUTH PHENOMENON

When an encircling buckle is used, the circumference of the globe is reduced, often causing the retina to become pleated and to develop radial folds. These folds tend to occur at the site of the retinal tear, which may gape open posteriorly, particularly with a large flap tear (Fig. 8.35). The fish-mouth phenomenon can be treated with a radially oriented buckle (Fig. 8.36). Other acceptable techniques for managing the fish-mouth phenomenon include decreasing the buckle height, increasing the width of the buckle and injection of air or gas followed by appropriate postoperative positioning to keep the break uppermost, where the air can flatten it.

POSTOPERATIVE COMPLICATIONS

GLAUCOMA

The IOP should be monitored carefully in the postoperative period to detect and treat significant rises. Antiglaucoma medications should be administered as needed. Angle-closure glaucoma usually results from a shallow detachment of the ciliary body and should be treated with hourly administration of steroid drops, antiglaucoma and cycloplegic medications and a short course of systemic steroids. If the chamber does not reform within 7 days, drainage of choroidals with reformation of the anterior chamber should be performed to prevent permanent damage to the angle.

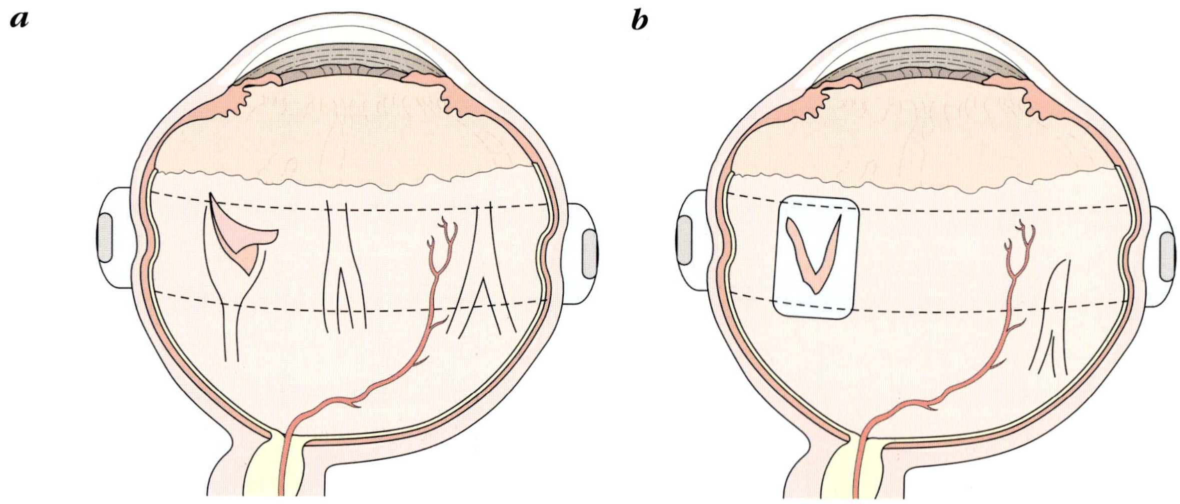

Figure 8.36 *(a) Persistently open flap tear caused by radial folding (fish-mouth phenomenon). (b) Treated by radial element beneath flap tear.*

ANTERIOR SEGMENT ISCHEMIA

High buckles with an encircling element and the disinsertion of more than one rectus muscle may predispose the eye to anterior segment ischemia. Patients with sickle cell disease or trait are particularly susceptible to anterior segment ischemia and should not be treated with an encircling element. The signs of anterior segment ischemia include stromal edema, marked uveitis with fibrin in the anterior chamber, a mid-dilated pupil, elevated IOP, cataract and a shallow anterior chamber. Mild cases may respond to topical steroids and cycloplegics; severe cases require release of the encircling band.

CILIOCHOROIDAL DETACHMENT

Excessive cryotherapy or laser, hypotony, damage to vortex veins, high buckles and advanced age may all predispose a patient to choroidal detachment. Most detachments are serous in nature and are caused by transudation of fluid. Most choroidal detachments are minor and resolve spontaneously. Drainage is indicated for 'kissing choroidals' and those causing a shallow anterior chamber for more than 7 days. Hemorrhagic choroidals are less common but have a poorer prognosis.

PERSISTENT RETINAL DETACHMENT

Sometimes subretinal fluid may persist for up to 3 months, especially with a nondrainage operation. As long as there are no open breaks and the macula is attached, observation may be justified. A concave contour of the subretinal fluid indicates good prognosis. The patient should be seen frequently, to monitor resorption of subretinal fluid. A short course of acetazolamide may promote absorption of subretinal fluid. Persistent detachment caused by open breaks superiorly may require air or gas injection followed by appropriate positioning. The break may be sealed by laser once the retina flattens. In other cases, a buckle revision or vitrectomy may be needed to reattach the retina.

PROLIFERATIVE VITREORETINOPATHY

Proliferative vitreoretinopathy is a serious complication seen in 10–15% of patients after retinal detachment surgery. This is discussed in Chapter 27.

INFECTION OF THE BUCKLE AND EXTRUSION

Most buckle infections are caused by coagulase-negative staphylococci. The presenting signs and symptoms include pain, conjunctival congestion, subconjunctival hemorrhage, purulent discharge, point tenderness and occasionally a draining sinus tract through the conjunctiva. Buckle infections caused by silicone sponges tend to occur sooner (less than 3 months) than those caused by solid silicone.[14] If buckle infection is diagnosed within the first postoperative month, topical and systemic antibiotics should be given to gain sufficient time for the retina to attach firmly. Most buckle infections necessitate removal of the offending material. If the infection does not appear serious, removal of the buckle may be delayed until the end of the first postoperative month. Extrusion of the buckle requires removal of a segment or the entire element.

MISCELLANEOUS COMPLICATIONS

Other complications of scleral buckling procedures include epiretinal membrane formation, migration and intrusion of the buckling material, conjunctival symblepharon formation, diplopia, refractive changes, ptosis, retinal vascular occlusion, pigment migration under the fovea, cystoid macular edema and optic atrophy.

RESULTS OF SCLERAL BUCKLING

A surgical cure is defined as reattachment of the retina for a minimum of 6 months and can be expected in 75–95% of cases with a single scleral buckling operation.[20] The success rate of the scleral buckling procedure is greater than that achieved with pneumatic retinopexy, primarily because the latter is associated with new or missed breaks in about 20% of the eyes.[21] The success rate of scleral buckling is reduced in cases with giant retinal tear, previously failed scleral buckle surgery, trauma, PVR, aphakia and in cases with no apparent retinal breaks. The visual results are less satisfactory than the anatomic results. If the macula was detached preoperatively, only 38% of eyes regained a visual acuity of 20/50 or better. In eyes with 'macula-on' detachment and excellent preoperative visual acuity, 90% achieved an acuity of 20/30 or better at 6 months but 10% suffered decreased visual acuity despite an anatomically successful operation.

SUMMARY

In general, one should do the least amount of surgery necessary to accomplish the surgical goal. The surgeon should plan the steps of surgery based on a careful preoperative evaluation, but should be flexible in modifying the procedure based on intraoperative developments.

REFERENCES

1. Williams GA, Aaberg TM. Techniques of scleral buckling. In: Ryan SJ, Glaser BM, Michels RG, eds, *Retina*, Vol. 3 (Mosby: St Louis, 1989): 111–49.
2. Hilton GF, McLean JB, Bronton DA. *Retinal Detachment: Principles and Practice*, 2nd edn. (American Academy of Ophthalmology: San Francisco, 1995).
3. Wilkinson CP, Rice TA. *Michels Retinal Detachment*, 2nd edn (Mosby: St Louis, 1997): 537–94.
4. Feibel RM. Current concepts in retrobulbar anesthesia, *Surv Ophthalmol* (1985) **30**:102–10.
5. Feibel RM. Ocular explosion after peribulbar anesthesia (letter), *Ophthalmology* (1997) **104**:1727.
6. Kishore K, Agarwal HC, Sood NN, et al. Evaluation of peribulbar anesthesia in eye camps, *Ophthalmic Surg* (1990) **21**:566–70.
7. Goldbaum MH, Joondeph H, Huamonte FU, Peyman GA. Retinal examination and surgery. In: Peyman GA, Sanders DR, Goldberg MF, eds, *Principles and Practice of Ophthalmology*, Vol. 2 (WB Saunders: Philadelphia, 1980): 1066–8.
8. Gilbert C, McLeod D. D-ACE surgical sequence for selected bullous retinal detachments, *Br J Ophthalmol* (1985) **69**:733–6.
9. Peyman GA, Conway MD, Raichand M, Lin J. Histopathologic studies on transscleral argon–krypton photocoagulation with an exolaser probe, *Ophthalmic Surg* (1984) **15**:496–501.
10. Haller JA, Lim JI, Goldberg MF. Pilot trial of transscleral diode laser retinopexy in retinal detachment surgery, *Arch Ophthalmol* (1993) **111**:952–6.
11. Haller JA, Blair N, de Juan E Jr, et al. Multicenter trial of transscleral diode laser retinopexy in retinal detachment surgery, *Trans Am Ophthalmol Soc* (1997) **95**:221–30.
12. Nanda SK, Han DP. Experimental transconjunctival diode laser retinal photocoagulation through silicone scleral exoplants, *Arch Ophthalmol* (1995) **113**:926–31.
13. Borras A, Meerhoff A. Ten years' experience with intrascleral gelatin implants in retinal detachment, *Am J Ophthalmol* (1972) **73**:390–3.
14. Roldán-Pallarés M, del Castillo Sanz JL, Awad-El Susi S, Refojo MF. Long term complications of silicone and hydrogel explants in retinal reattachment surgery, *Arch Ophthalmol* (1999) **117**:197–201.
15. Bovino JA, Marcus DF, Nelsen PT. Argon laser choroidotomy for drainage of subretinal fluid, *Arch Ophthalmol* (1985) **103**:443–4.
16. Fitzpatrick EP, Abbott D. Drainage of subretinal fluid with the argon laser, *Am J Ophthalmol* (1993) **115**:755–7.
17. Charles ST. Controlled drainage of subretinal and choroidal fluid, *Retina* (1985) **5**:233–4.
18. Burton RL, Cairns JD, Campbell WG, Heriot WJ, Heinze JB. Needle drainage of subretinal fluid. A randomized clinical trial, *Retina* (1993) **13**:13–16.
19. Azad RV, Talwar D, Pai A. Modified needle drainage of subretinal fluid for conventional scleral buckling procedures, *Ophthalmic Surg Lasers* (1997) **28**:165–7.
20. Grizzard WS, Hilton GF, Hammer ME, Taren D. A multivariate analysis of anatomic success of retinal detachments treated with scleral buckling, *Graefes Arch Clin Exp Ophthalmol* (1994) **232**:1–7.
21. Tornambe PE, Hilton GF. Pneumatic retinopexy: a multicenter randomized controlled clinical trial comparing pneumatic retinopexy with scleral buckling, *Ophthalmology* (1989) **96**:772–83.

Part II Visualization Techniques During Vitrectomy

Chapter 9 Wide-angle viewing systems for vitreoretinal surgeries

Paul G DeGregorio, Mark E Hammer and W Sanderson Grizzard

INTRODUCTION

WIDE-ANGLE OPHTHALMIC SURGICAL SYSTEMS

Initially, visualization for posterior segment vitrectomy surgery was accomplished with hand-held, plano-concave contact lenses. The lenses neutralize the high convergence effect of the corneal curvature, permitting the operating microscope to focus on the central vitreous and posterior retina. Visualization of the equatorial retina can be accomplished by using the prismatic effect created by tilting the surgical lens on the cornea. This requires a skilled assistant who can anticipate the needs of the surgeon as he/she moves throughout the fundus. Intraocular pressure fluctuates as the pressure on the cornea by the hand-held lens varies. Sewn-on retaining rings avoid the absolute need for a trained assistant and they add to the stability of the contact lens; they also solve the problem of fluctuating intraocular pressure but require a series of special prismatic lenses to view the periphery.[1]

The viewing angle can be increased from 20° to 35° by using a biconcave lens. The Lander's biconcave lens allows visualization of the fundus in the gas-filled pseudophakic or phakic eye.

Indirect contact lens systems, such as the Rodenstock Pan Funduscope, were developed for panretinal photocoagulation and allow a wide view of the retina through a small pupil. However, the image from the panfunduscope is inverted, making surgery difficult. Development of the stereoscopic diagonal inverter (SDI) by Spitznas and Reiver in 1987[1] allowed the use of the wide-field lenses by reinverting the stereoscopic image. The development of the binocular indirect ophthalmomicroscope (BIOM) allowed noncontact imaging of the retina.[2]

The wide-angle viewing systems currently used include:

- The BIOM/SDI noncontact system with or without a miniature, indirect viewing contact lens (field of view 70°, 90°, or 110°).
- The EIBOS noncontact system (100° field with 90-diopter lens, 125° field with 60-diopter lens).
- The Volk reinverting operating lens system (ROLS); Volk miniature indirect contact lenses with both standard lenses and the new self-stabilizing lenses (58, 85 or 156 diopters) for visualization up to the vitreous base and ora serrata, respectively.
- The AVI inverter with miniature indirect contact lenses (68 and 130 diopters).
- The Iris Medical contact wide-angle system.

Common properties of all contact and noncontact wide-angle systems are an inverted fundus view and a device to convert the image to a normally oriented view of the field. The SDI is such a system. In the EIBOS, the indirect and reinversion devices are consolidated and cannot be separated.

Tables 9.1 and 9.2 compare advantages and disadvantages of regular viewing systems, wide-field systems and noncontact and contact wide-angle systems.

COMPARISON OF BIOM VERSUS EIBOS (BOTH NONCONTACT WIDE-ANGLE SYSTEMS)

The BIOM can adapt to many microscopes and can be used with wide-angle contact lenses; the BIOM can be flipped up and out of use during surgery.

Table 9.1 Advantages and disadvantages of contact lenses and wide-field systems used for visualization of the fundus

Advantages	*Disadvantages*
Contact lenses	
• Readily available	• Corneal trauma
• Relatively inexpensive	• Can change the intraocular pressure
• Low maintenance	• Limited access to limbus
• Adaptable to all surgical microscopes	• Blood can obscure the image
• Noninverted view	• Requires good pupil dilation
	• Poor view in gas–fluid exchanges (must change lens)
	• Poor view with lens or corneal opacity
	• May require multiple lenses
	• May require skilled assistance
Wide-field systems	
• Ease of operation	• Higher initial cost
• Gives overall picture of pathology	• Learning curve
• Great depth of field	
• Easy view in gas–fluid exchanges	
• Can use contact lenses, BIOM or no lens	
• May need skilled assistant	
• Facilitates silicone oil–perfluorocarbon exchange	

Table 9.2 Advantages and disadvantages of noncontact and contact wide-angle systems

Advantages	*Disadvantages*
Noncontact wide-angle systems	
• No assistant needed	• Learning curve
• No corneal trauma	• Expensive
• Good with fluid–air exchange	• Adaptability to microscopes
• Good in pediatric cases or with steep corneas easily accessible to limbus	• May require modification of microscope
• Great depth of focus	• Less optical resolution than contact system
• Can move eye and maintain a good image	
• Can be used in conjunction with contact lens	
Contact wide-angle systems	
• Can attain up to 150° field of view	• Very skilled assistant required with hand-held lens
• New self-stabilizing lenses (Volk, SSV) may require less-skilled assistant	• Can change the intraocular pressure
	• Image lost if eye rotated
	• Lens and corneal opacities problematic
	• Corneal trauma
	• Poor access to limbus
	• Poor with steep corneal curvature

The EIBOS can be used only with the Moeller–Wedel microscope and some models of Zeiss and Wild microscopes. The EIBOS cannot be used in conjunction with wide-angle contact lenses because the stereo inverter is integrated into the system. The EIBOS makes it difficult to maintain a sterile field.

INDICATIONS FOR THE USE OF WIDE-ANGLE VIEWING SYSTEMS

Wide-angle viewing systems are used for all intraocular procedures involving vitrectomy and diagnostic inspection of the peripheral and posterior retina and surgery. The wide-angle system can be converted to a conventionally focused contact system when high magnification is required.

Retained lens material is an example of a situation when a wide-angle viewing system can be used. The vitrectomy can be performed with or without scleral depression. If the lenticular material falls posteriorly, the wide-angle viewing system with its increased depth of field allows fragmentation and aspiration of lens material. The peripheral retina then is inspected thoroughly for any lens fragments adherent to the peripheral vitreous.

Similarly, a wide-angle surgical system can be used to remove a posteriorly displaced intraocular lens. The system can be combined with chandelier lighting systems to liberate the operator's hand for an additional instrument for removal of the lens through the limbus or its repositioning in the sulcus.

Complex surgery for diabetic vitreous hemorrhage and traction retinal detachment can be simplified with the use of a wide-angle viewing system. Panretinal endophotocoagulation, dissection of tightly adherent membranes and gas–fluid exchange are all facilitated. Wide-angle systems can be used with phakic, aphakic and pseudophakic patients. When working on a specific area, the surgeon can observe remote traction with impending development of tears or hemorrhages. This global appreciation of complex retinal detachments simplifies and expedites surgical maneuvers (Fig. 9.1).

Wide-angle viewing facilitates dissection of anterior proliferative vitreoretinopathy, gas–fluid exchanges

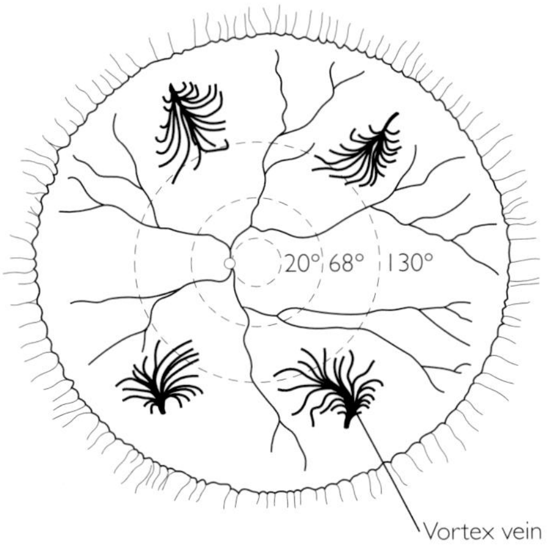

Figure 9.1 *Concentric degree fields centered on the fovea, demonstrating anatomic fundus correlation.*

and silicone oil instillation, either with a gas–silicone exchange or perfluorocarbon liquid–silicone exchange. The indirect systems stay in focus with minimal adjustment when the index of refraction of the vitreous substitute is changed from balanced salt solution (BSS) to air or from perfluorocarbon liquid to silicone oil.

Other specific indications for the use of a wide-angle viewing system include: traumatic eye injuries with or without foreign body removal; cases requiring retinotomy for severe proliferative vitreoretinopathy, subretinal fibrosis or subretinal hemorrhage; and retinopathy of prematurity. Surgery for retinopathy of prematurity is best performed using the noncontact systems, e.g. BIOM or EIBOS, because of the decreased scleral rigidity of the infant eye and the small size of the cornea with a steep corneal curvature.[3]

CASE SELECTION

A clear visual axis with a pupil of at least 2.5 mm usually is required. Should visualization continue to be a problem, other procedures, such as iris retraction with iris hooks, lensectomy, cyclitic membrane dissection, synechiolysis, penetrating keratoplasty or temporary keratoprosthesis combined with keratoplasty, may improve visualization.

It is best to select a case initially where the patient is cooperative and is either pseudophakic or aphakic. As one feels more at ease with the wide-angle system, the complexity of the cases may be increased along with the speed and comfort level of the surgeon.

PREOPERATIVE EVALUATION

The pupil size and clarity of lens and cornea must be evaluated and a determination made of whether adjunctive cornea, iris or lens surgery will be necessary.

PREOPERATIVE PROCEDURES

Setting up the microscope is much the same as for any other routine vitrectomy. The SDI combined with

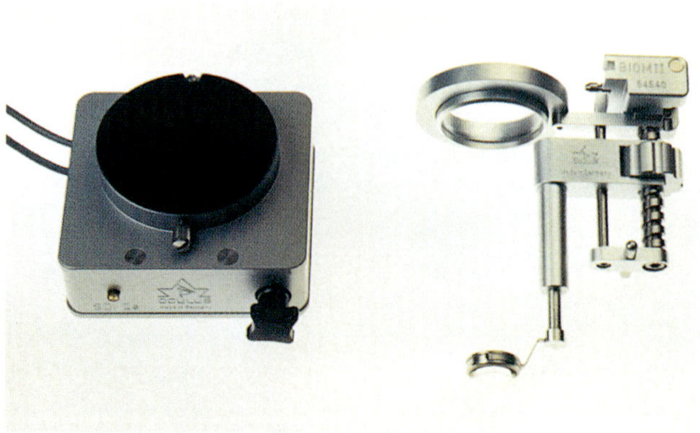

a

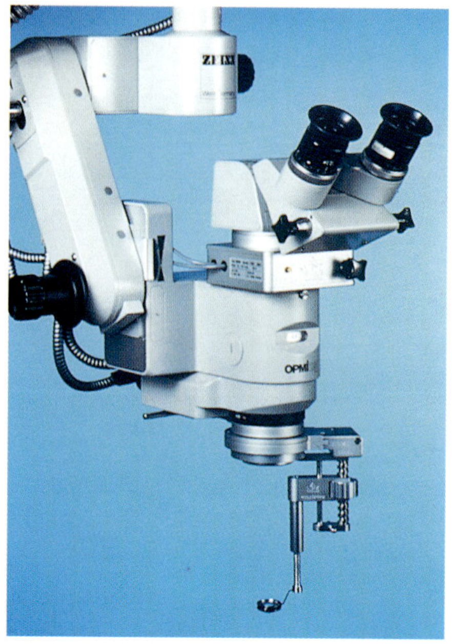

b

Figure 9.2 *The stereoscopic diagonal inverter (SDI) (a) and binocular indirect ophthalmomicroscope (BIOM) (b). (Photographs courtesy of Insight Instruments, Inc., Lake Mary, FL.)*

various laser filters on the microscope increases the distance of the oculars to the patient by as much as 3 inches. Therefore, the operating table should be as low as possible, permitting good leg position for the surgeon.

BIOM/SDI INSTRUMENTATION

There are two models of the BIOM: model 1, which is a closed cone device, and model 2, which is an open arm device that extends from a dovetailed plate screwed onto the bottom of a microscope (Figs 9.2–9.4). There is a condensing lens on the top of the small indirect viewing tower on both models, as well as a smaller objective lens that is combined with the SDI in the stack on the microscope. A foot pedal allows the surgeon to switch between the BIOM wide-angle intraocular system and regular viewing.

Intermittent corneal wetting is required with a noncontact viewing system using BSS or a hydroxypropylmethylcellulose solution diluted with BSS.

The BIOM can be used alternately with a conventional visualization system, because of its flip-up design that permits its removal from the visual axis.

The BIOM can be sterilized with gas or autoclaved. The lenses can be either sterilized with ethylene oxide or Cidex. The SDI is incorporated into the scope and is not sterile.

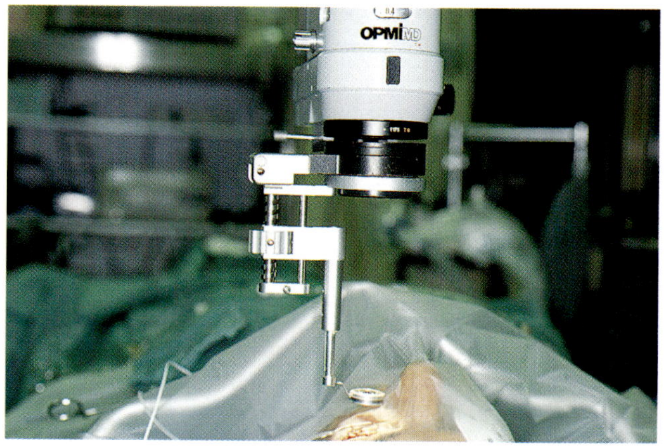

Figure 9.3 *The BIOM and SDI mounted on a Zeiss operating microscope.*

The SDI has an internalized prismatic system with near-zero light escape to achieve maximal illumination and light intensity. The SDI inverts the indirect image from the BIOM or high-convex contact lens to a conventional upright image.

Endoillumination must be used in conjunction with the BIOM. Light is provided by a conventional light

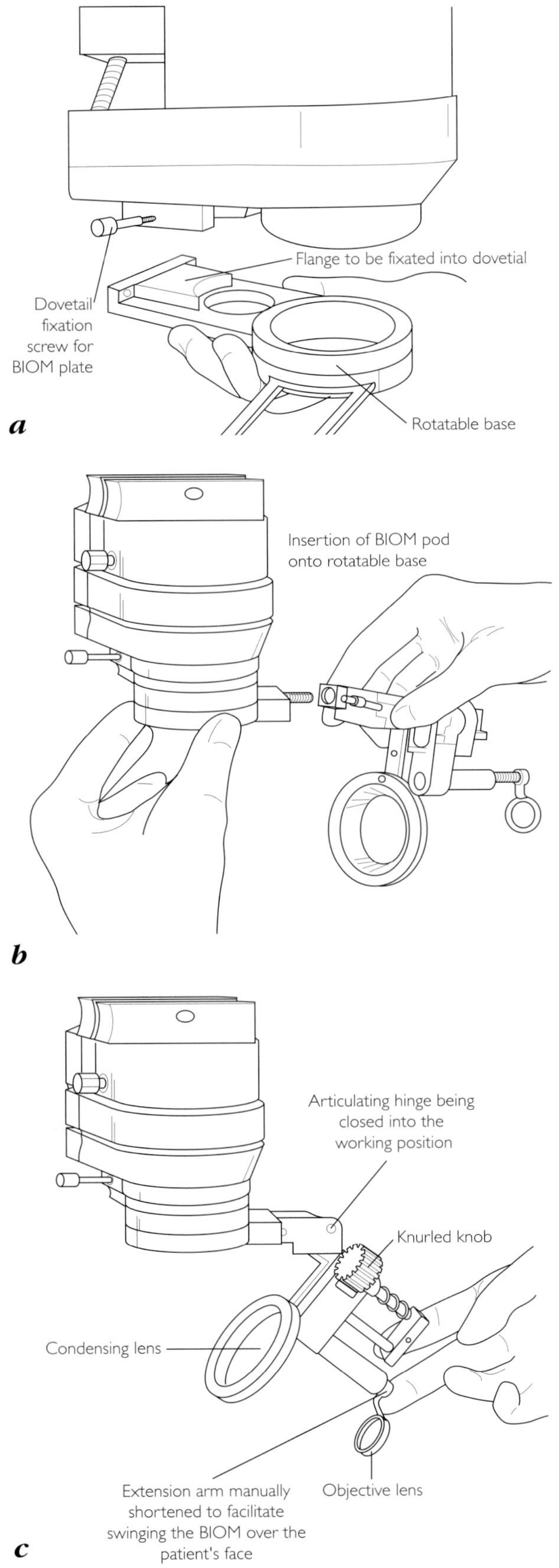

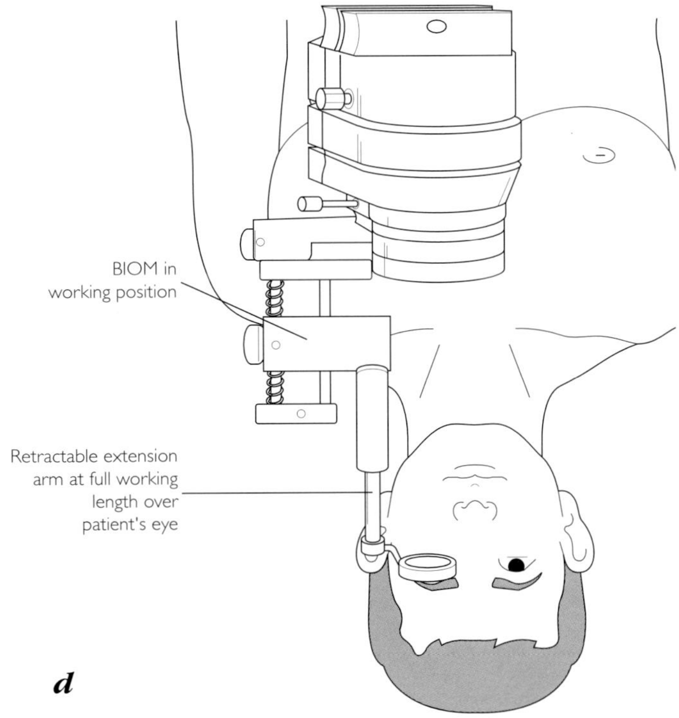

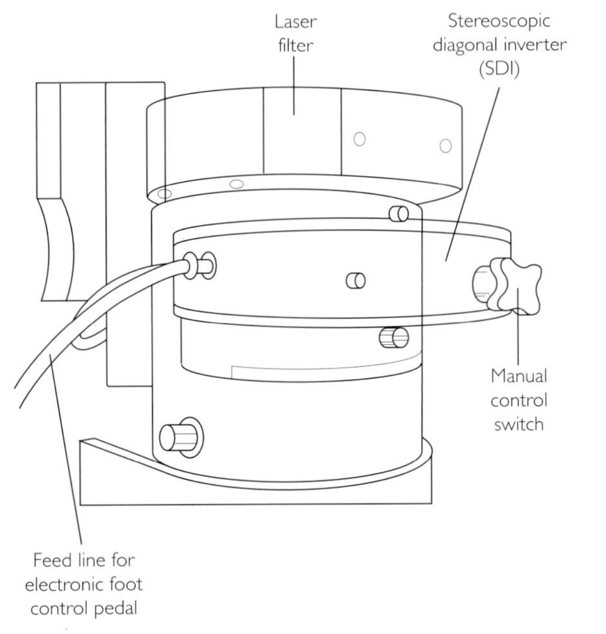

Figure 9.4 *(a) The BIOM mounting plate is secured to the lower surface of the operating microscope by a flange and a dovetail. (b) The BIOM optical system is attached to a rotatable base on the mounting plate. (c) The BIOM optics may be pivoted in and out of the optical axis of the microscope. (d) The BIOM in working position over the patient's eye. (e) The SDI as mounted in the microscope stack, with manual and electronic remote inverter controls.*

pipe, a wide-angle illuminator, lighted instruments, the multiport illumination system (MIS) or a chandelier illumination system.

The microscope light is turned off when endoillumination is used. The SDI pedal is activated. The microscope is slowly lowered using the coarse and then the fine vertical movement. The knurled knob on the BIOM device should be started approximately 0.5–1 inch below its highest setting for most eyes. Turning the knob counterclockwise so that the objective lens elevates will focus down, whereas turning the knob clockwise lowers the objective lens closer to the cornea and focuses upward. Focusing should be practiced with endoillumination aimed at the disc. Maneuvering to see the periphery requires that the globe be tilted slightly in the direction of *X–Y* movement to gain maximum visualization. Globe integrity in these extreme positions can be enhanced further by elevating the height of the bottle. In general, we recommend a low bottle height for most portions of the surgical procedure, because this decreases the risk of corneal edema and vascular compromise. Magnification is achieved by using the zoom system of the operating microscope or by lowering the microscope so that the objective lens is closer to the cornea.

To achieve the initial focus with the system, place the endoillumination probe in the vitreous cavity while viewing the posterior pole. After the posterior pole is in focus, view the periphery by manipulating the eye and the *X–Y* movement of the microscope. The surgeon will quickly develop an intuitive understanding and 'feel' for the system.

The interaction between the surgical microscope and the wide-angle system has the following variables:

- Power of the BIOM objective lens.
- Distance of the BIOM lens from the microscope.
- Distance of the BIOM lens from the cornea.
- When using a contact lens system, only the distance from the microscope to the contact lens changes.

The BIOM can be used in phakic, pseudophakic or aphakic patients. As with any other system in the phakic patient, it is crucial to ensure that no air bubbles enter the vitreous cavity in the infusion fluid. These bubbles can enter the anterior chamber through the zonules and obscure the view of the retina. Pseudophakic eyes can also develop condensation on the intraocular lens during gas–fluid exchange. Aphakic eyes can develop corneal striae, which degrade image quality when gas is in the anterior chamber. In the pseudophakic as well as aphakic cases, we find that a small amount of Healon placed on the intraocular lens or on the corneal endothelium alleviates this problem.

When using gas, one can encounter a bothersome glare factor when the fluid level is below the tip of the endoilluminator. In this situation, we prefer to use a conventional light pipe and to keep the light pipe within the fluid as the fluid level goes down and is replaced with gas. This method provides maximum illumination of the optic disc and posterior pole details, and decreases the amount of glare.

When performing gas–fluid exchange in aphakic and pseudophakic eyes, only slight adjustments need to be made to the knurled knob of the BIOM. In the phakic eye, owing to the posterior curvature of the lens, the knurled knob must be rotated counterclockwise to lift the objective lens toward the microscope. Simultaneously, the objective lens of the BIOM should be brought closer to the cornea using the vertical motor of the microscope. This maneuver will produce a clear image of the disc and posterior pole.

The BIOM is readily adaptable for use with various lighting systems. It is used most often with a straight light pipe that generally comes as part of the vitrectomy package. This light pipe is excellent for visualization of the macula for detailed work, for air–fluid exchange and in cases where the patient is aphakic or pseudophakic. The bullet light pipe produces wide-angle illumination that further enhances wide-angle visualization. Its disadvantages are the increased glare during gas–fluid exchange and the light directed upward toward the surgeon's eyes with some probes.

Supplemental lighting systems may be provided by an illuminated infusion port. The illuminated infusion port does not have enough light to perform surgery under all conditions. True bimanual vitreoretinal surgery can be attained using the MIS. One to three self-sealing illuminated ports can be sewn into the eye to provide lighted instrumentation. The MIS requires a small amount of additional time for securing surgically to the globe. It proves to be invaluable for membrane dissection in diabetic retinopathy.

Lensectomy, if necessary, should be performed through a sclerotomy before placing the MIS port for more posterior work. The utility of bimanual surgery far outweighs these inconveniences. An additional advantage of the MIS is that the surgeon may operate with one hand while depressing the sclera with the

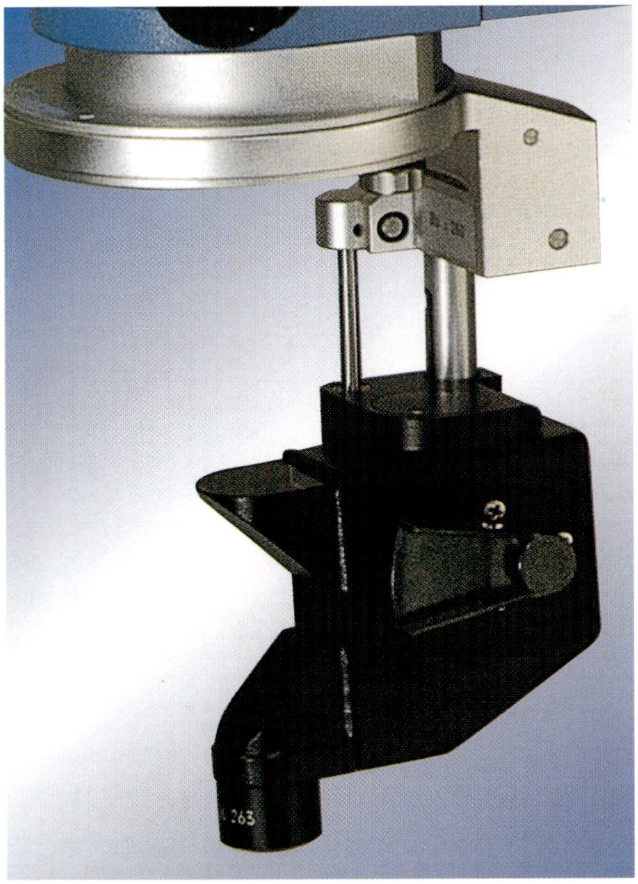

Figure 9.5 *The EIBOS wide-angle viewing system. Reinversion is performed internally without an accessory stereoscopic diagonal inverter. This system allows simultaneous viewing through the wide-angle fundus optics and of sclerotomy sites by looking around the narrow optical system. The EIBOS also may be pivoted to perform anterior segment surgery.*

other hand because the lighted cannula provides sufficient light without endoillumination.

EIBOS INSTRUMENTATION

The EIBOS noncontact lens system is similar to the combined BIOM/SDI system. The EIBOS also can be flipped up and out of the way; however, because the inverter and indirect system are one piece (Fig. 9.5), the inverter cannot be used independently with miniature indirect contact lenses.

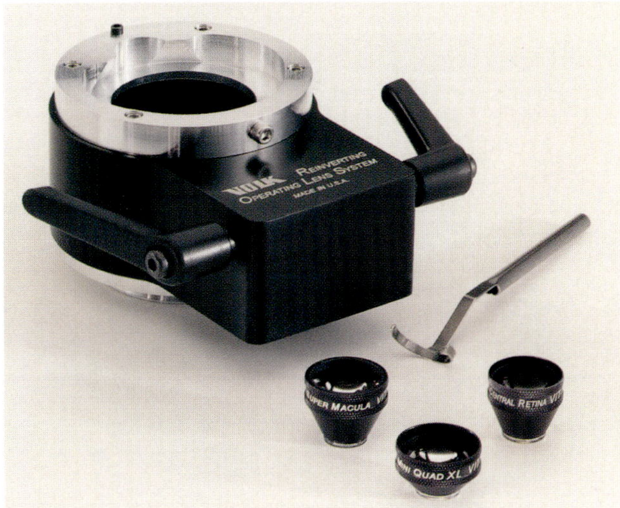

Figure 9.6 *The Volk reinverting operating lens system (ROLS), pictured with miniature fundus contact lenses of differing magnifications and the lens handle. (Courtesy of Volk Optical, Inc., Mentor, OH.)*

The one-piece design does not allow sterilization of the entire unit, which must be draped with a sterile covering. The objective lens can be sterilized to prevent contamination of the surgical field. The unit is spring balanced as a safety feature so that if the objective lens does contact the eye, the unit elevates.

The focusing is done with a sterile lever mounted on the unit. The lever changes only the internal lens distances without changing the distance from the lens to the patient's eye. The scleral ports will appear in the conventional orientation. The retinal and scleral images will be oriented conventionally for facilitation of instrument entry. The combined system means a shorter microscope stack for better ergonomics. This system allows the use of direct contact lenses for posterior work if the EIBOS is tipped up and out of the way.

INDIRECT SURGICAL CONTACT LENS SYSTEMS

The SDI can be used with any indirect surgical contact lens because it is mounted in the stack of the scope. Similar systems would incorporate the reinverting operating lens system (ROLS) or the AVI image inverter combined with any miniature indirect wide-angle surgical contact lens. The SDI can be

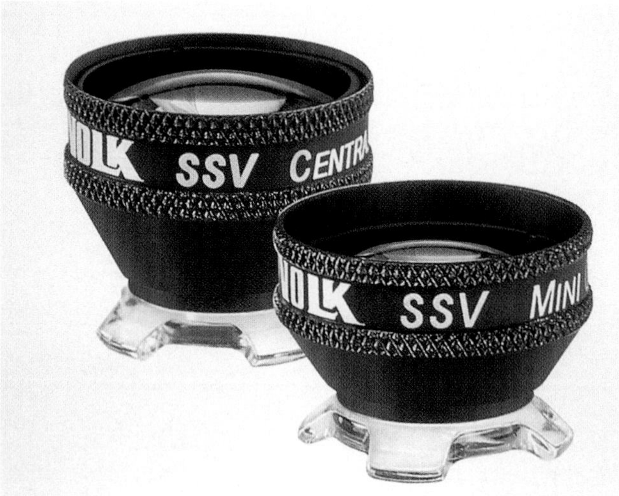

Figure 9.7 *The Volk self-stabilizing vitrectomy (SSV) lens set, which reduces the need for an assistant to center the lens during surgery. (Courtesy of Volk Optical, Inc., Mentor, OH.)*

changed automatically from inverted to noninverted with a foot pedal, whereas the ROLS and AVI require manual engagement for inversion. It is possible to use any inverter system with any objective lens.

The ROLS inverter by Volk uses a single-element image-erecting prism with only four optical surfaces shared by both the right and left eye systems (Fig. 9.6). The ROLS provides excellent transparency and stereopsis with minimal light loss. It is offered in a 'Zeiss style' that fits Zeiss, Topcon, Moeller and Inami microscopes that accept Zeiss accessories. The 'Wild style' will only fit Leica/Wild microscopes. A diode laser safety filter is built in. The ROLS does not contact the eye and needs no sterilization. The Volk wide-angle contact lenses can be sterilized with ethylene oxide gas at 130°F. Sterrad, Steris and glutaraldehyde disinfection will also work. Autoclaving will ruin lenses. Volk now offers self-stabilizing vitrectomy (SSV) lenses in the three different powers (58, 85 and 156 diopters), which decreases the need for skilled assistance (Fig. 9.7).

The AVI system also sits in the stack of the microscope, is less than 1.5 inches thick, weighs one pound and is compatible with Wild, Zeiss and Moeller microscopes. With the miniature indirect contact lens, the AVI system offers either 68° or 130° of viewing.

REFERENCES

1. Spitznas M, Reiver J. A stereoscopic diagonal inverter (SDI) for wide-angle vitreous surgery, *Graefes Arch Clin Exp Ophthalmol* (1987) **225**:9–12.
2. Spitznas M. A binocular indirect ophthalmomicroscope (BIOM) for wide-angle vitreous surgery, *Graefes Arch Clin Exp Ophthalmol* (1987) **225**:13–15.
3. Hammer ME. Stage 4 and 5 acute and cicatricial retinopathy of prematurity: surgical results. Presented at the *International Conference on Retinopathy of Prematurity*, University of Illinois at Chicago, 1 November, 1996.

Chapter 10 Endoscopy for vitreoretinal surgery

Yale L Fisher and Gustavo C Heringer

INTRODUCTION

Microendoscopy is useful in vitreoretinal surgery whenever microscopic imaging is limited or impossible. Ophthalmic endoscopes were introduced in 1934 by Thorpe for extraction of nonmagnetic intraocular foreign bodies.[1] The instrument was rigid and bulky. Over the past 60 years, many individuals have contributed to the development of miniaturized optics and fused flexible fibers, as well as GRIN (gradient index of refraction) lenses to create small, hand-held devices.[2–18] These changes, coupled with brilliant light sources and microminiaturized color cameras, have led to current instrumentation. While stereopsis is not available and resolution not yet comparable to the operating microscope, these new microendoscopes have sufficient viewing capacity to enhance and extend surgical control during vitreoretinal surgery, especially in the retroiridal area and elsewhere when standard microscopic viewing becomes limited.

INDICATIONS

SURGICAL CRITERIA

Endoscopy during vitreoretinal surgery is divided into planned and unplanned usage. Planned endoscopy is determined by preoperative ophthalmic examination that demonstrates sufficient visual axis opacities to prevent or limit microscopic imaging. The most common findings include:

- Corneal scars, edema or bloodstaining.
- Anterior chamber fibrocellular reaction.
- Small, fixed pupils with or without neovascularization and synechiae.
- Mild-to-moderate cataract formation not requiring immediate extraction.
- Viewing of the retroiridal space:
  - residual cortical lens material;
  - imaging haptic placement or suture position for haptic stabilization;
  - imaging and treating anterior neovascularization at the pars plana;
  - confirming correct pars plana infusion placement when not visible microscopically.
- Imaging and treating the peripheral retina when microscopic imaging is limited or impossible.

Unplanned endoscopy is defined as the need for endoscopic imaging to complete surgical maneuvers that suddenly occur during 'routine' procedures when microscopic imaging becomes limited or impossible. Common events include:

- Acute intraoperative corneal edema.
- Anterior chamber obstructions of view, such as blood or air bubbles, that are not easily removed.
- Sudden miosis, especially during fluid–air exchanges.
- Mild-to-moderate intraoperative cataract formation.
- Lenticular capsular haze, and/or visually obstructive light reflections occurring during fluid–air exchanges.

PREOPERATIVE EVALUATION

All preoperative vitreoretinal surgical patients are evaluated for possible need of endoscopy by screening for visual axis obstructions using routine slit-lamp and diagnostic ultrasonic techniques. If endoscopy is required or seems strongly possible, the operating room staff are notified in advance of surgery.

INSTRUMENTATION

The endoscopic system includes:

- Light source, usually xenon.
- Microendoscopic color camera: one- or three-chip (Fig. 10.1).
- Microendoscope: flexible fused-fiber or GRIN lens design—19- or 20-gauge with or without a channel for laser fiber or cautery.
- High-resolution television monitor (700–750 lines).

ENDOSCOPIC OPTICAL QUALITIES

Endoscopic images are more limited in quality than microscopic views. Most differences relate to lens minification or fused-fiber and camera limitations. However, even with these limitations, endoscopic images are sufficient to permit surgical observation and many common vitreoretinal instrument manipulations. In the operating room, a simple, sterilizable test card (Fig. 10.2) is used to maximize instrument performance: by evaluating image quality for the surgeon and ancillary personnel during set-up, use and cleaning; and by comparing new endoscopes or manufacturers. Endoscopes are delicate, optical devices with finite life spans requiring careful monitoring to ensure optimal performance.

Two types of microendoscopes are currently useful in vitreoretinal surgery, both 19- and 20-gauge. The first is a fused-fiber instrument that has 'wide-angle' imaging (up to 50° in water and 70° in air) with depth of field in the range 3–35 mm. The surgical handpiece is small and similar in weight to a standard vitreoretinal endoilluminator (Fig. 10.3).

The second type of endoscope employs a GRIN lens system that provides close focus and a depth of field 0–5 mm (Fig. 10.4). The handpiece is larger and more cumbersome because of the need for close magnification with a narrower field of view.

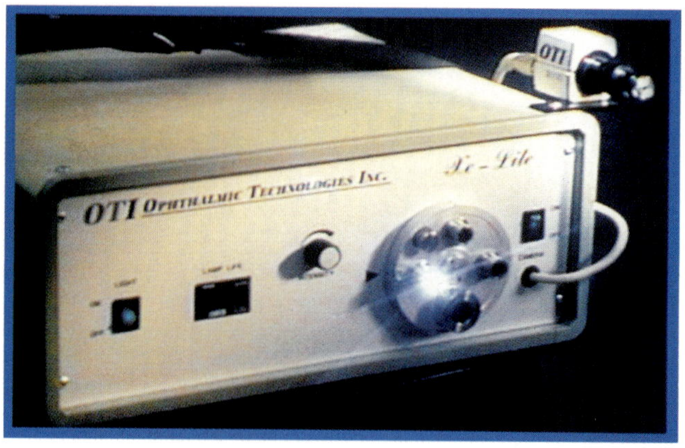

Figure 10.1 *Fused-fiber endoscopic system (Courtesy of Ophthalmic Technologies, Inc., Toronto, Canada).*

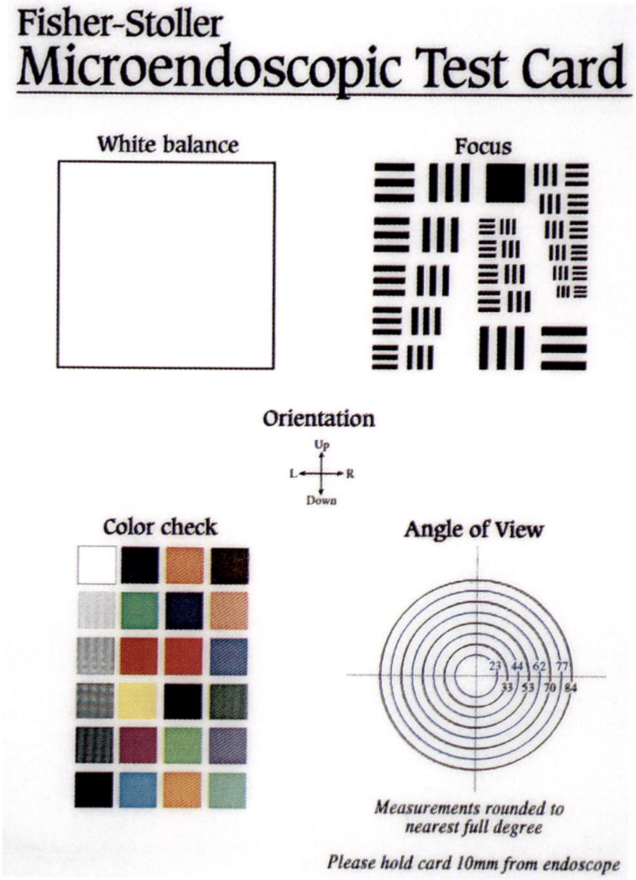

Figure 10.2 *Endoscopic test card. Test card includes targets for: (a) white balance; (b) focus/resolution; (c) image orientation; (d) color fidelity; (e) angle of view.*

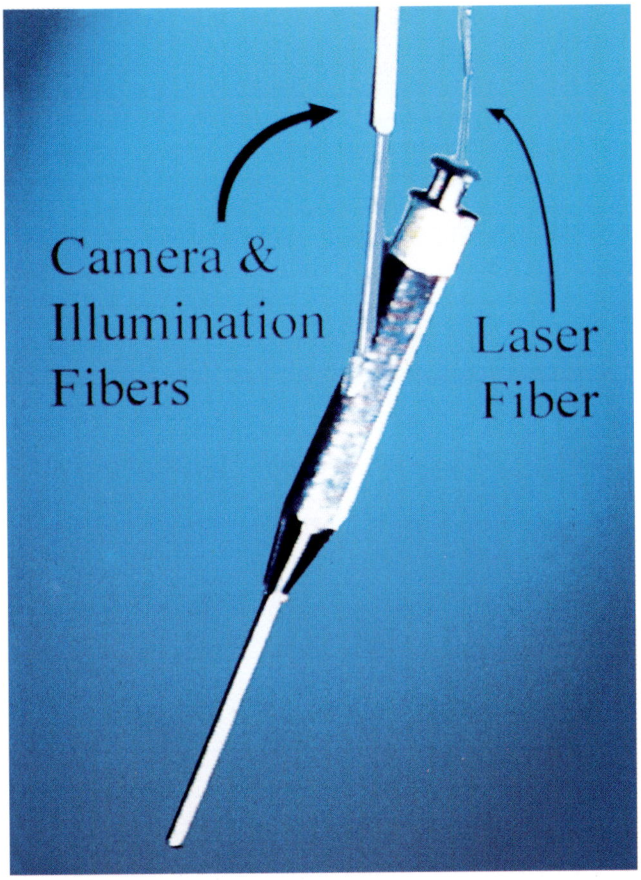

Figure 10.3 *Endoscope. Fused-fiber endoscopic handpiece with working channel, laser fiber (Courtesy of OTI, Toronto, Canada).*

Both types can be manufactured with working channels for laser fibers.

ENDOSCOPIC TECHNIQUE AND TRAINING

For the surgeon and ancillary personnel, endoscopic surgery requires some changes in operating room procedures. Training for set-up, instrument arrangement and cleaning procedures is provided by instrument manufacturers. Because stereopsis is lacking, practice on model eyes prior to operating room experience is recommended for the surgeon to gain confidence with monocular cues for imaging and surgical manipulations under endoscopic control (Fig. 10.5).

In the operating room, the endoscope is introduced through a standard pars plana incision. The 19-gauge scopes require slight enlargement of the standard 20-gauge sclerotomy opening. Initial experience is best obtained in cases with good microscopic control while the illuminating system of the endoscope is used as an endoilluminator. The endoscopic image can be viewed intermittently by the surgeon throughout routine vitrectomy techniques by simply glancing away from the microscope at the monitor with intraocular instruments already safely positioned under microscopic control.

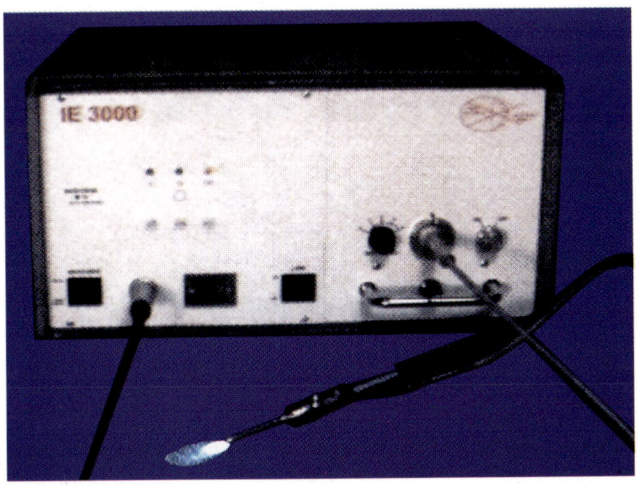

Figure 10.4 *Insight endoscope. Gradient index refraction endoscopic system (GRIN lens). The GRIN lens endoscope is capable of high magnification at short working distance.*

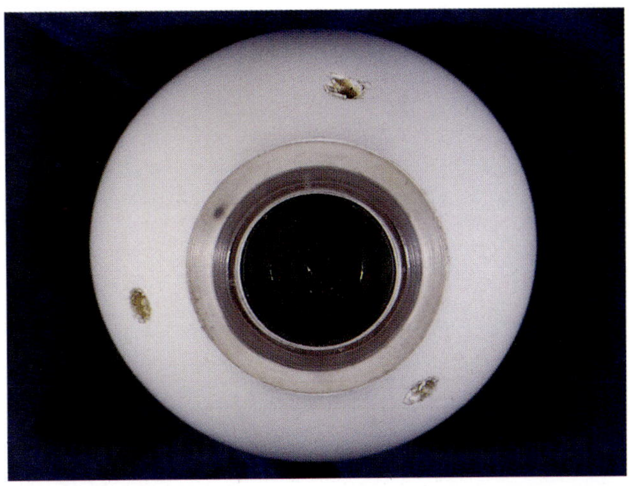

Figure 10.5 *Model eye. Practice model eye for endoscopy with unimanual and bimanual techniques.*

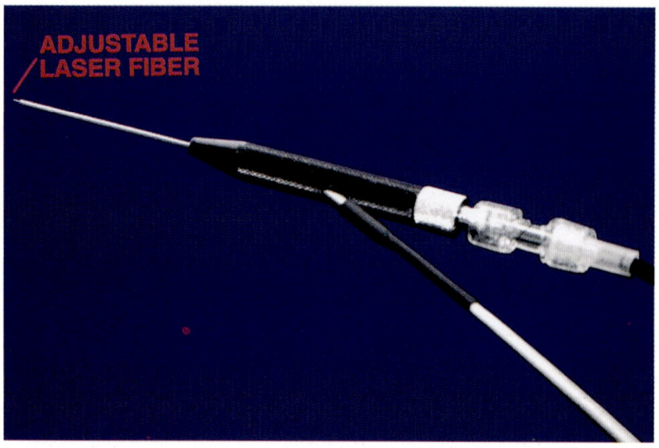

Figure 10.6 *Endoscope with laser fiber in working channel.*

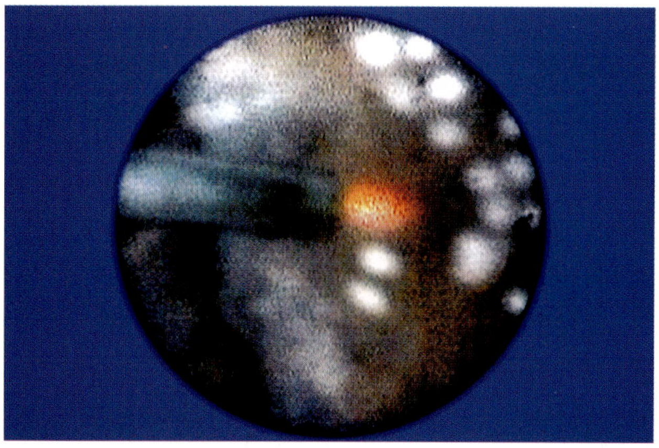

Figure 10.7 *Endoscopic imaging for laser application utilizing lighted laser probe.*

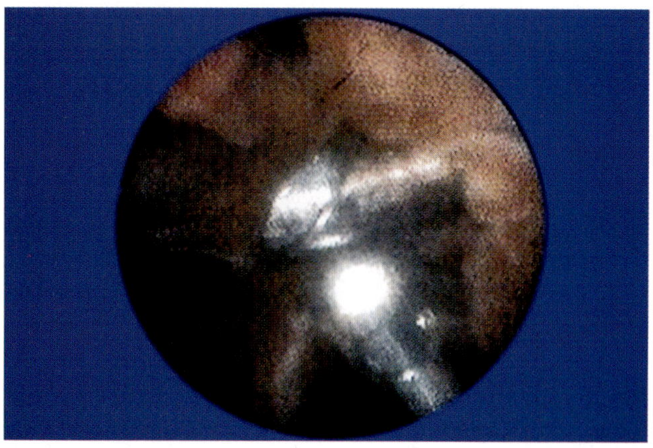

Figure 10.8 *Endoscopic imaging of infusion cannula at pars plana.*

For the novice, image orientation is always the first hurdle. Imaging the optic nerve and macular region quickly permits rotation of the endoscope handpiece or adjustment of the rotation control located on the camera until the monitor image orientation is similar to microscopic views. Once adjusted, the surgeon prevents any axial rotation of the endoscopic handpiece so that image orientation is maintained during movements to the periphery of the eye. Most surgeons rapidly adjust to movements and endoscopic imaging within the vitreous space.

Once imaging is achieved and the surgeon gains confidence, surgical maneuvers become possible. Initial experience is usually easiest with endoscopic laser application using the working channel of the endoscope (Fig. 10.6). Bimanual maneuvers are more difficult but can be facilitated by the use of illuminated accessory instruments such as lighted endolaser probes (Fig. 10.7). The lighted accessory instrument is placed through a second pars plana incision in a similar fashion to microscope-controlled surgery. However, in endoscopically controlled surgery, the light of the accessory instrument is used to determine instrument position and provide a monocular cue for judging proximity to surgical sites, such as the surface of the retina.

As the lighted instrument is brought close to a surface, the diameter of the beacon of light emitted from the accessory instrument diminishes. The surgeon quickly learns to judge distances by noting the change in the beam diameter and adapts to a 'viewing hand' (the endoscope) and an 'instrument hand' (the lighted instrument), making tandem movements that permit surgical manipulations.

A wide variety of vitreoretinal accessory instruments can be fiberoptic light-adapted, including vitreous cutters, picks, forceps and fluid–air exchange cannulas, among others (Fig. 10.8). With experience, many surgeons learn to work easily without lighted accessory instruments.

SURGICAL EXPERIENCE

PATIENTS

From January 1994 to April 1996, 401 consecutive patients underwent pars plana vitreoretinal surgery. Each patient was evaluated preoperatively for possible limited or obstructed microscopic imaging. Examinations included slit-lamp biomicroscopy,

Table 10.1 Distribution of endoscopic cases

Planned endoscopy (72%)		*Unplanned endoscopy (28%)*	
Cases	*No. of cases*	*Cases*	*No. of cases*
Retroiridal imaging	24	Retroiridal imaging	1
Lens fragments	(20)	Lens fragments	(1)
Haptic position	(3)		
Cannula position	(1)		
Corneal opacification	2	Corneal opacification	4
Pupillary miosis	1	Pupillary miosis	2
Lens opacification	1	Lens/intraocular lens opacification	4
Total	28	Total	11

contact lens biomicroscopy (triple-mirror and wide-angle lens), indirect ophthalmoscopy and contact B-scan ultrasonography.

Patients requiring endoscopic imaging during surgery were divided into two groups: planned endoscopy cases expected to require endoscopic imaging preoperatively, and unplanned endoscopy cases with intraoperative, unexpected ocular media opacification causing microscopic visual limitations or obstructions.

Endoscopy was utilized in 39 cases (10%): 28 (72%) in the 'planned' endoscopy group and 11 (28%) in the 'unplanned' group. Within the 'planned' endoscopy cases, the most common reason for endoscopic imaging was the need for retroiridal imaging (24 cases, 86%). Four others had preoperative, predictable visual axis obstruction sufficient to require endoscopy because of corneal blood staining (1), corneal transplant opacity (1), lens opacity (1) and irreversible pilocarpine-induced miosis (1) (Table 10.1).

Within the 'unplanned' endoscopy group, microscopic visual obstruction occurred during surgery because of corneal opacification in four cases (epithelial/stromal edema associated with Descemet's folds), phakic or pseudophakic lens opacification in four cases, intraoperative pupillary miosis in two cases and residual retroiridal lens fragments in one case (Table 10.1).

Endoscopy allowed successful completion of surgery in 37 of the 39 cases (95%) by permitting observation of microscopically inaccessible areas (25 cases) and/or facilitating the use of additional surgical maneuvers (12 cases) (Table 10.1). All surgical maneuvers were single handed (Table 10.2). In two cases, endoscopic visualization was insufficient to continue surgery. Both cases required extensive membranectomy for retinal detachments caused by proliferative retinopathy. The lack of stereopsis and the need for bimanual dissection made endoscopic completion of these cases difficult.

Table 10.2 Endoscope-controlled surgical maneuvers

Surgical maneuver	*No. of cases*
Vitrectomy	16
Endocautery	1
Endolaser	9
Air–fluid exchange	4
Placement and removal of perfluorocarbon liquid	1
Membrane removal (limited)	1
Total	32

DISCUSSION

Endoscopy expands visual control for vitreoretinal surgery when ocular media opacification produces microscopic imaging limitation or obstruction. In this consecutive series of vitreoretinal procedures, endoscopy was used for observation and successful completion in a variety of surgical manipulations, obviating the need for additional surgery usually required to regain microscopic control. The majority of cases (64%) involved imaging within the retroiridal area, where microscopic viewing was difficult or impossible. Most of these cases were predictable from preoperative examination. Quite interestingly, however, was the usefulness of endoscopy for cases in which operating room microscopic visualization was predicted to be adequate based upon preoperative examination but unexpectedly became limited or obstructed by media opacification during surgery. Endoscopy provided a rapid means of regaining visual control, permitting continuation and completion of surgery in almost all cases.

Limited surgical dissection of membranes from a detached retina was possible in one case; however, endoscopic membranectomy in general remains limited and difficult even with experience. The lack of stereopsis, resolution limitations, and inability to perform bimanual manipulations are the major obstacles.

Endoscopic imaging and operative techniques are most quickly and safely acquired in laboratory practice by utilizing model eyes. Image orientation, limited fields of view and two-dimensional monitor viewing comprise the greatest challenges; however, most surgeons rapidly adapt. The technique of ophthalmic endoscopy expands and extends visual control during vitreoretinal surgery when microscopic imaging is limited or obstructed, often providing restoration of visualization in order to continue or complete necessary surgical maneuvers.

REFERENCES

1. Thorpe HE. Ocular endoscopy: an instrument for the removal of intravitreous non-magnetic foreign bodies, *Trans Am Acad Ophthalmol* (1934) **39**:422–4.
2. Butterworth RF, Bignell JL. A new type of eye endoscope, *Br J Ophthalmol* (1952) **36**:217–20.
3. Neubauer H. The removal of non-magnetic foreign bodies in the vitreous by aspiration, *Trans Ophthalmol Soc UK* (1963) **83**:143–52.
4. Norris JL, Cleasby GW. An endoscope for ophthalmology, *Am J Ophthalmol* (1978) **85**:420–2.
5. Norris JL. Orbital endoscopy, *Trans Pac Coast Ophthalmol Soc* (1978) **59**:145–8.
6. Norris JL, Cleasby GW. Endoscopic orbital surgery, *Am J Ophthalmol* (1981) **91**:249–52.
7. Norris JL, Cleasby GW, Nakanishi AS, Martin LJ. Intraocular endoscopic surgery, *Am J Ophthalmol* (1981) **91**:603–6.
8. Funk R, Rohen JW. Intraocular microendoscopy of the ciliary-process: Vasculature in albino rabbits: effects of vasoactive agents, *Exp Eye Res* (1987) **45**:597–606.
9. Funk R, Rohen JW. Microendoscopy of the anterior segment vasculature in the rabbit eye, *Ophthalmic Res* (1989) **21**:8–17.
10. Eguchi S, Araie M. A new ophthalmic electronic videoendoscope system for intraocular surgery, *Arch Ophthalmol* (1990) **108**:1778–81.
11. Volkov VV, Danilov AV, Vassin LN, Frolov YA. Flexible endoscopes, *Arch Ophthalmol* (1990) **108**:956–7.
12. Koch F, Spitznas M. Videoendoskopie in der Glaskorperchirurgie, *Oftalmochirurgie* (1990) **2**:70–8.
13. Leon CS, Leon JA. Microendoscopic ocular surgery: a new intraoperative, diagnostic and therapeutic strategy. Part I: Endoscopic equipment/methodology applied to cataract surgery with intraocular implantation, *J Cataract Refract Surg* (1991) **17**:568–72.
14. Leon CS, Leon JA. Microendoscopic ocular surgery: a new intraoperative, diagnostic and therapeutic strategy. Part II: Preliminary results from the study of glaucomatous eyes, *J Cataract Refract Surg* (1991) **17**:573–6.
15. Koch F, Spitznas M. The videoendoscope as a useful adjunct to vitreous surgery. In: Stirpe M, ed, *Advances in Vitreoretinal Surgery*, Acta of the 3rd International Congress of Vitreoretinal Surgery, (Rome, 1991) (New York, Ophthalmic Communications Society, 1992): 5–7.
16. Uram M. Ophthalmic laser microendoscope endophotocoagulation, *Ophthalmology* (1992) **99**:1829–32.
17. Althaus C, Sundmacher R. Intraoperative intraocular endoscopy in transscleral suture fixation of posterior chamber lenses: consequences for suture technique, implantation procedure, and choice of PCL design, *Refractive Corneal Surg* (1993) **9**:333–9.
18. Fisher YL, Slakter JS. A disposable ophthalmic endoscopic system, *Arch Ophthalmol* (1994) **112**:984–6.

Chapter 11 Mechanical dilation of the pupil

Dwain Fuller

INTRODUCTION

Excellent visualization of the peripheral retina and vitreous base is critical for many complex vitreoretinal cases. Despite multiple preoperative dilating drops, topical flurbiprofen and possible epinephrine in the infusion fluid, intraoperative pupillary constriction is common. Lengthy procedures, mechanical irritation of the iris, introduction of gas into the eye and episodes of hypotony can, singly or in concert, induce miosis. A number of intraoperative techniques have been described to obtain wide pupillary dilation for vitreoretinal surgery.

HISTORY

The simplest gambit for attempting to enhance pupillary dilation for vitreous surgery is the standard injection of 0.3 ml of 1:10 000 epinephrine (preservative free) into the anterior chamber. Sometimes intracameral epinephrine works brilliantly, but in elderly or diabetic patients the pupil often shows meager or no response to this pharmacologic endeavor. When epinephrine fails, mechanical pupillary dilation must be employed if a larger pupil is necessary to complete the surgery effectively.

Time-honored cataract surgical techniques for pupillary enlargement have been abandoned by most modern vitreoretinal surgeons. Among the cataract surgery techniques are a limbal scissors sphincterotomy or a superior sector iridectomy with subsequent iris suture closure. If a permanently enlarged pupil is acceptable, vitreous surgeons may 'nibble' the iris margin with a vitreous cutter, either via the pars plana or through the limbus. Diathermy can be used to smooth the cut edges and achieve a round pupil, although it will remain enlarged forever.

Eckardt was the first to describe the use of iris sutures for temporary pupillary dilation during vitreous surgery.[1] The concept of a translimbal approach to mechanical pupillary dilation was a definite advancement, but the suture technique proved cumbersome and has become obsolete. Fuller conceptualized the idea of using translimbal iris hooks with fixation slides for pupillary dilation, and Wilson built the first prototype.[2] The initial commercial iris hooks were single-use only. Iris hooks are now available that are reusable. Translimbal iris hooks are used frequently, not only by vitreoretinal surgeons but also by glaucoma specialists. The hooks are often employed at the outset of surgery for pupils that cannot be dilated pharmacologically as a result of the chronic use of miotics or posterior synechiae. Translimbal iris hooks have solved the problem of inadequate pupils for vitreoretinal surgery for pseudophakic and aphakic eyes. Iris hooks generally are not used in phakic eyes unless removal of the crystalline lens is planned.

TECHNIQUES

INJECTION OF INTRACAMERAL EPINEPHRINE

In phakic or posterior-chamber pseudophakic eyes, injecting 1:10 000 epinephrine via the limbus with a 30-gauge needle often will deepen the anterior chamber, thus forcing the lens–iris diaphragm posteriorly to give temporary mechanical dilation of the pupil as well as potential drug mydriasis. In phakic or posterior-chamber pseudophakic eyes, it is important to avoid injecting trapped air bubbles from the tip of the needle into the anterior chamber, which may compromise visibility by causing a clustering of small bubbles centrally against the endothelium. Such inadvertent air injection is easily avoided by gentle depression of the syringe plunger while approaching the limbus, so that fluid is flowing marginally from the needle as the corneal limbus is perforated.

IRIS HOOKS

Translimbal mechanical pupillary dilation is achieved quite simply by inserting flexible hooks through 27-gauge needle perforations. Each hook engages the iris margin in one quadrant. The shaft of each hook then is pulled slowly out of the eye until the pupil is as dilated as the surgeon wishes (Figs 11.1 and 11.2). Fixation slides are pushed down the shaft of each hook toward the limbus to maintain iris traction. At the conclusion of the case, it is easy to grasp the distal end of the iris hooks with forceps and then to slide the fixation device away from the limbus. The iris edge is released by pushing the hook toward the center of the eye, rotating the shaft of the hook 90° and then pulling the hook from the eye. The limbal entrance sites generally do not require sutures.

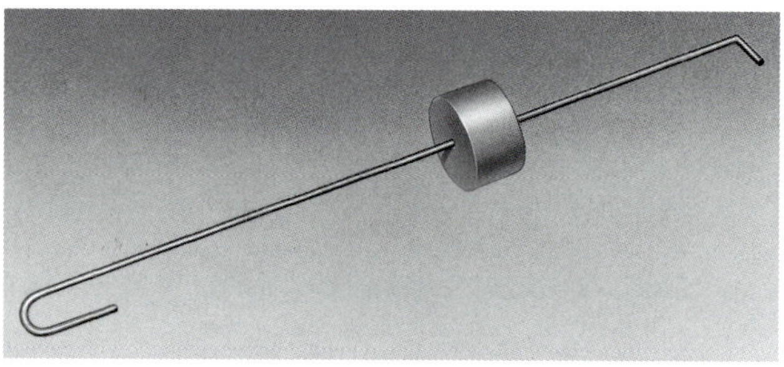

Figure 11.1 *Magnified view of a single translimbal iris hook. (Courtesy of Synergetics, Inc.)*

OTHER APPROACHES

Cataract surgeons continue to employ their own evolving means of mechanical pupillary dilation. Some of their techniques may be applicable to vitreoretinal surgery. Beehler has developed a three-point mechanical dilator that is inserted through a 2.5-mm limbal incision[3] (Fig. 11.3). The pupil is stretched, and then the dilating prongs are withdrawn into the shaft of the instrument for translimbal removal. Beehler cautions that adequate preoperative cycloplegia is essential for maintaining a 6–7 mm pupil after the stretching procedure.

Nirenberg and Nirenberg (personal communication) have described a 'twin pupil' stretching technique that uses Kuglen hooks through horizontal meridian limbal stab wounds followed by vertical stretching of the pupil via the cataract section. Viscoelastic is then used to maintain a deep anterior chamber in order to maintain an enlarged pupil for lens extraction and pseudophakos placement.

Pupillary rings have been suggested as a potentially less traumatic means of temporary pupillary enlargement. Arpa[4] described a technique for pupillary dilation that allows observation of the vitreous cavity

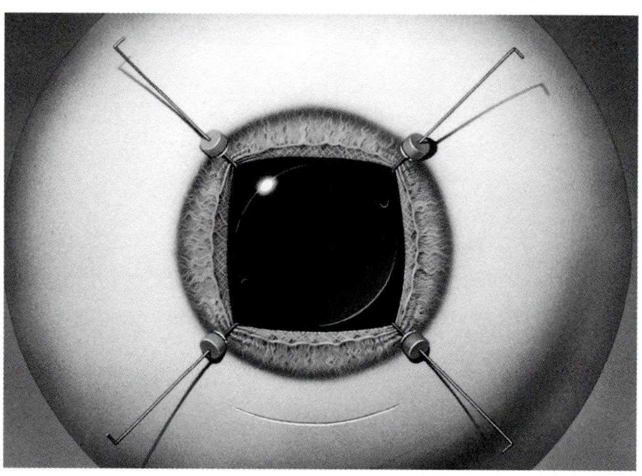

Figure 11.2 *Four translimbal iris hooks in place in a pseudophakic eye. (Courtesy of Synergetics, Inc.)*

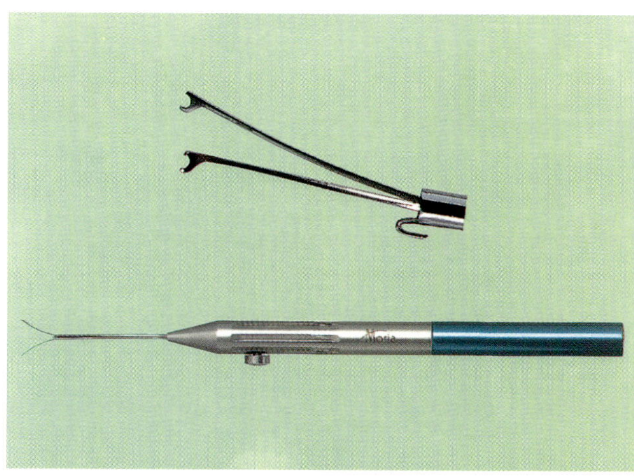

Figure 11.3 *The three-point Beehler pupil dilator. (Courtesy of Dr Cecil Beehler and Microtech, Inc.)*

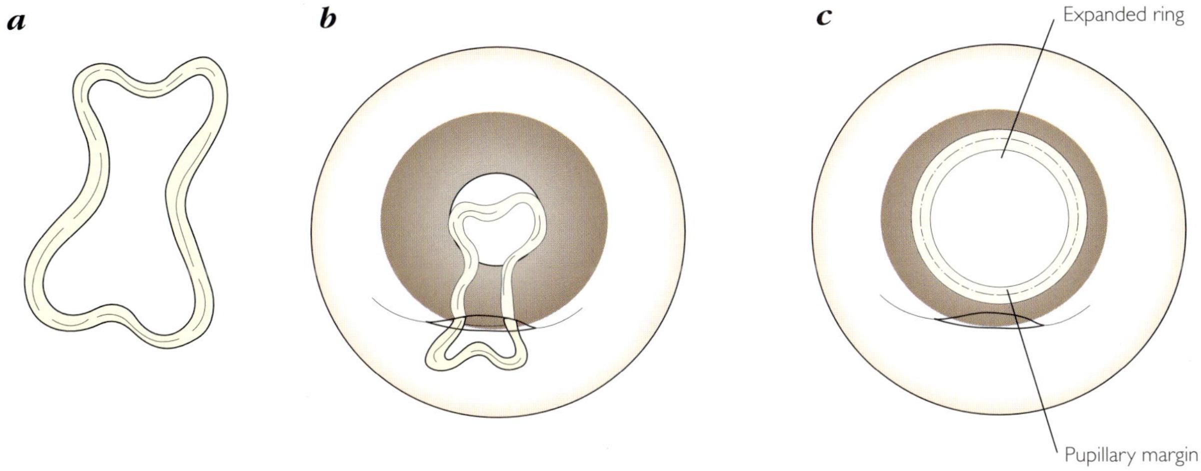

Figure 11.4 *Artist's sketches of the hydrogel iris ring: (a) desiccated hydrogel ring; (b) introduction of the ring into the anterior chamber via a cataract section; (c) fully hydrated hydrogel ring in position, maintaining iris dilation.*

during surgery in both phakic and aphakic patients. A silicone elastomer (Silastic, Dow Corning, Midland, MI) ring with a C-shaped groove on the outer edge is inserted into the eye through an opening in the limbus. When positioned properly, the external groove of the ring engages the pupillary rim. This technique has been used successfully to treat 12 patients (three phakic and nine aphakic) without any apparent damage to the iris. Difficulty with inserting the device was encountered because of the lubricating effect of silicone oil in two patients whose eyes had received this substance as a tamponading agent in a previous surgery. Siepser,[5] Federman and Cook have invented a desiccated hydrogel ring that expands inside the eye during a 30–60-second hydration period, thereby slowly enlarging the pupil to 7 mm (Fig. 11.4). The desiccated ring requires a 3.5-mm limbal incision for insertion, which will likely limit its use to anterior segment surgeons.

Wide-angle viewing systems for vitreous surgery may obviate the necessity of a large pupil in some simple cases, but when proliferative vitreoretinopathy (PVR) demands a meticulous, two-handed vitreous base dissection, there is no substitute for the 9-mm pupil that can be achieved routinely with iris hooks. Wide pupillary dilation and scleral depression permit excellent vitreous base and ciliary body exposure without the need for a surgical contact lens.

One potential problem of all forms of mechanical pupillary dilation is a permanently enlarged pupil. Sphincter tears can occur with overly aggressive dilation, particularly with irides that are fibrotic. In cases of severe PVR, the surgeon and the patient may consider a pupil that remains moderately dilated a small price to pay for a reattached retina. Iridoplasty may be possible as a subsequent procedure, if the enlarged pupil causes photophobia or if it is of cosmetic concern.

CONCLUSION

Mechanical dilation of pupils is now much more sophisticated than it was in the early days of vitreous surgery, when the vitreous cutter frequently was used aggressively to remove substantial amounts of central iris tissue. Translimbal iris hooks have become the primary weapon in the vitreoretinal surgeon's armamentarium for dealing with inadequate pupils in the operating room.

REFERENCES

1. Eckardt C. Pupillary stretching: a new procedure in vitreous surgery, *Retina* (1985) **5**:235–8.
2. Fuller DG, Wilson DL. Translimbal iris hook for pupillary dilation during vitreous surgery (letter), *Am J Ophthalmol* (1990) **110**:577.
3. Beehler CC. Personal communication: www.microtech.com.
4. Arpa P. A new device for pupillary dilatation in vitreous surgery, *Retina* (1992) **12** (Suppl 3):S87–S89.
5. Siepser SB. Personal communication: www.clear-sight.com.

Chapter 12 Use of the temporary keratoprosthesis in ocular trauma repair

Maurice B Landers III and Steven M Williams

INTRODUCTION

Massive ocular trauma that causes both anterior and posterior segment injury presents a difficult surgical challenge. Visualization of posterior structures is necessary to repair a detached retina, remove an intraocular foreign body or relieve abnormal vitreoretinal traction. However, the view is often limited by damage to anterior ocular structures. Corneal clouding caused by edema, blood staining, recently repaired wounds, scar formation and corneal vascularization is common following anterior segment trauma (Fig. 12.1). Treatment options for posterior segment repair in the setting of such corneal opacities previously have been limited to open-sky vitrectomy, penetrating keratoplasty followed by pars plana vitrectomy and a corneal graft followed by vitreous surgery after the graft had cleared. In some cases, no intervention at all was carried out.

The development of the temporary keratoprosthesis has permitted timely surgical repair of the injured posterior segment in the presence of a damaged opaque cornea.[1] The original temporary keratoprosthesis was a polymethylmethacrylate (PMMA) threaded biconcave optical cylinder 5.0 mm in length and 7.2 mm in diameter (Fig. 12.2). Subsequent modification by Eckardt produced a silicone rubber temporary keratoprosthesis that is 10 mm in diameter on the outer convex surface, 7 mm in diameter in the inner cylinder and 2.8 mm in length (Fig. 12.2).[2] The Eckardt temporary keratoprosthesis facilitated the view of the peripheral retina and is compatible with phakic and pseudophakic eyes.[3] The Eckardt temporary keratoprosthesis was originally designed to be disposable and it was found that the silicone became damaged by multiple suture tracks that occurred with repeated use (Fig. 12.2).

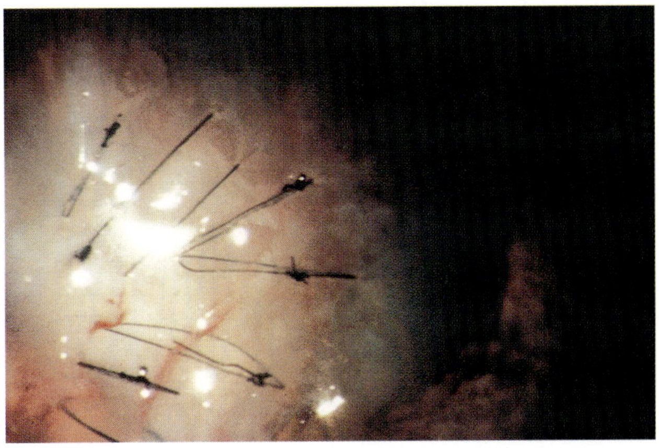

Figure 12.1 *Severe corneal opacification after repair of corneal injury.*

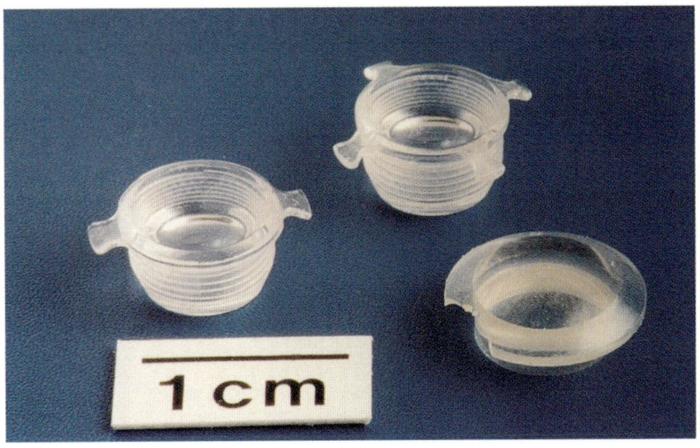

Figure 12.2 *(Left and center) Temporary keratoprosthesis with polymethylmethacrylate threaded biconcave optical cylinder 5.0 mm in length and 7.2 mm in diameter. (Right) Eckardt silicone rubber temporary keratoprosthesis 10 mm in diameter on outer convex surface, 7 mm in diameter of inner cylinder and 2.8 mm in length.*

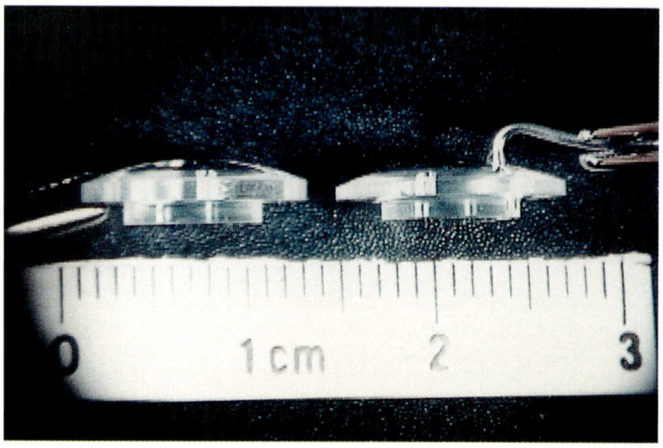

Figure 12.3 *(Left) Landers wide-field temporary keratoprosthesis with hard plastic polymethylmethacrylate device with 1-mm central cylinder protruding into anterior chamber, choice of diameters of 6.2, 7.2 or 8.2 mm, topped by a large, mushroom-shaped corneal surface with anterior radius of curvature of 15.5 mm. (Right) Device modified to include 20-gauge stainless steel infusion cannula.*

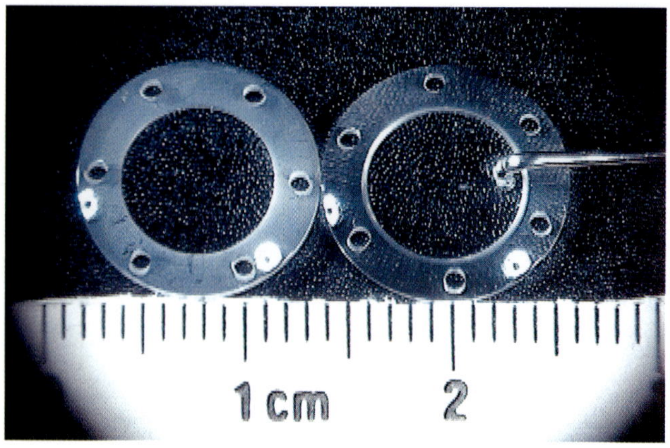

Figure 12.4 *(Left) Landers wide-field temporary keratoprosthesis peripheral flange has six marginal suture holes. (Right) Flange modified to include 20-gauge stainless-steel infusion cannula.*

The further development of the Landers wide-field temporary keratoprosthesis[4] included a hard plastic PMMA device with a 1-mm central cylinder protruding into the anterior chamber, with the choice of diameter of 6.2, 7.2 or 8.2 mm, topped by a large, mushroom-shaped corneal surface with an anterior radius of curvature of 15.5 mm and with six marginal suture holes in the peripheral flange (Figs 12.3 and 12.4). This wide-field temporary keratoprosthesis is reusable, can be sutured firmly to the globe and gives a view of both the posterior pole and the periphery without the use of ancillary lenses.[4] Recently, the wide-field temporary keratoprosthesis has been modified to include a 20-gauge stainless-steel cannula to allow standard infusion into the vitreous through the temporary keratoprosthesis when media opacity precludes safe placement of a pars plana cannula (Figs 12.3 and 12.4).[5]

In the surgical procedure, the keratoprosthesis is positioned after the removal of the central host cornea (Fig. 12.5). The clear wide-field temporary keratoprosthesis is placed in the corneal opening and sutured firmly in place. A pars plana vitrectomy and subsequent penetrating keratoplasty are carried out during one operative procedure. This technology allows surgical repair of eyes that otherwise might be irreparably damaged by combined anterior and posterior segment trauma.

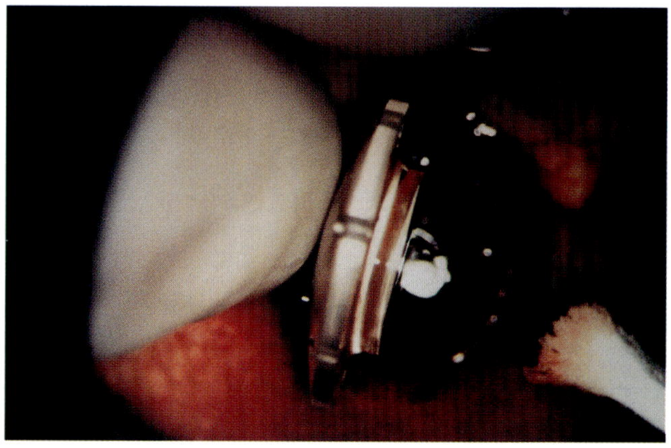

Figure 12.5 *Keratoprosthesis is positioned after removal of central host cornea.*

SURGICAL TECHNIQUE

General anesthesia is recommended when there is a question of globe integrity. The corneal wound, if not previously repaired, is sutured closed. A 360° conjunctival peritomy may be performed at the limbus. The four rectus muscles may be isolated for stabilization of the eye. A Flieringa ring can be sutured to the sclera to prevent collapse of the globe, particularly in children. A 4-mm infusion cannula is inserted through a pars plana sclerotomy placed

a

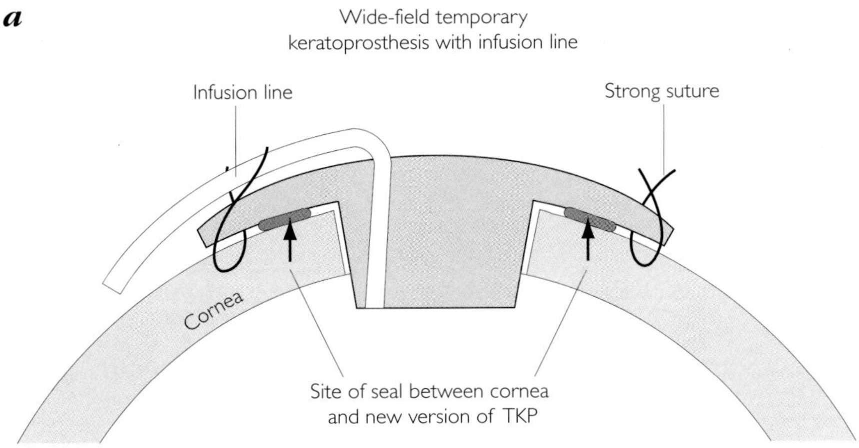

b

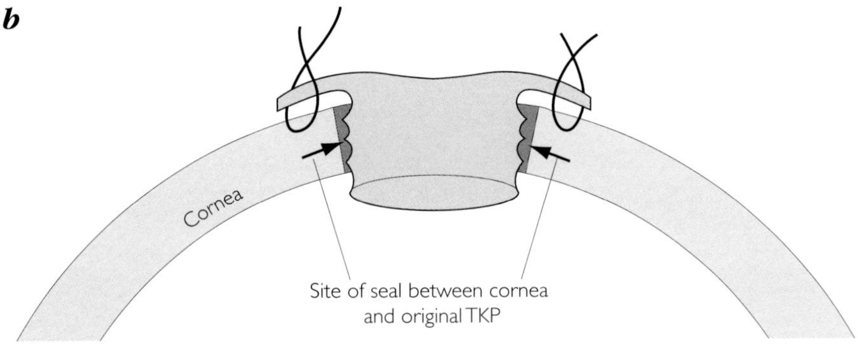

Figure 12.6 *Schematic drawing of wide-field temporary keratoprosthesis with infusion line. (a) Site of seal between cornea and new version of temporary keratoprosthesis (TKP). (b) Site of seal between cornea and original TKP.*

3–4 mm posterior to the limbus; it is held in place with one suture. Infusion permits control of the intraocular pressure throughout the procedure. If it appears impossible to place an infusion cannula safely through the pars plana directly into the vitreous cavity, the use of an infusion temporary keratoprosthesis can be considered.[5]

Typically, a trephine 0.25 mm smaller than the diameter of the central peg of the temporary keratoprosthesis is used. However, with the new wide-angle PMMA temporary keratoprosthesis, it is no longer mandatory that a water-tight fit be obtained between the central peg of the keratoprosthesis and the corneal stroma. The actual seal between the intraocular contents and the atmosphere is located between the undersurface of the keratoprosthesis flange and the anterior surface of the host cornea. This is particularly true when strong fixation sutures are used, such as 5-0 Mersiline (Fig. 12.6).

The trephine is centered on the cornea whenever possible; this location is preferred even in the setting of a freshly closed corneal wound. Partial trephinization of the corneal button is performed with a hand-held trephine. The corneal button then can be excised with a diamond knife and microcorneal scissors.

The disorganized anterior segment now can be repaired directly. Blood clots, portions of disrupted iris, pupillary membranes and lens remnants may be removed under direct visualization. The tip of the infusion cannula and the potential sclerotomy sites can be inspected for overlying tissue or local retinal detachments.

The wide-field temporary keratoprosthesis is placed in the corneal bed (Fig. 12.5) and sutured to the limbus with six interrupted sutures. Strong sutures, such as 5-0 Mersilene, work well and can be used to seal the underside of the wide-field

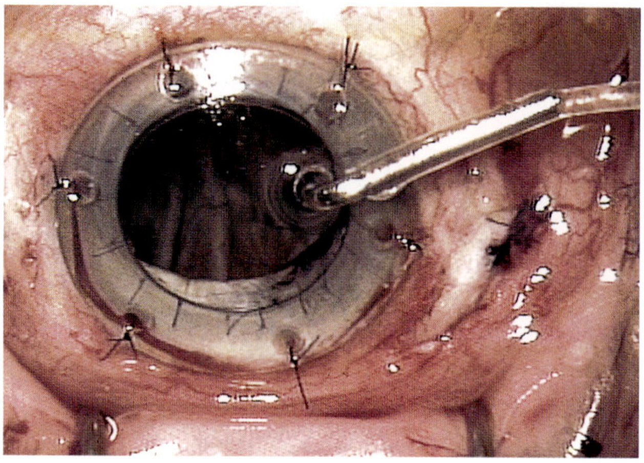

Figure 12.7 *Infusion temporary keratoprosthesis in place.*

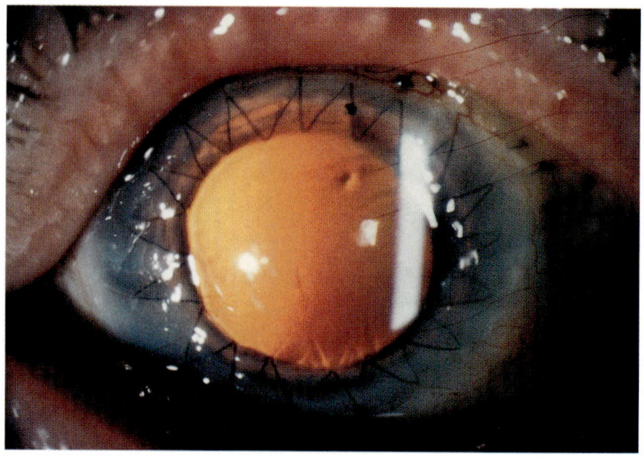

Figure 12.8 *Donor cornea button is sutured in place after removal of wide-angle temporary keratoprosthesis, using interrupted and running 10-0 nylon sutures.*

temporary keratoprosthesis firmly to the anterior surface of the cornea. The scleral bites can be made either parallel or perpendicular to the limbus (Fig. 12.7).[5]

After placement of the temporary keratoprosthesis and visualization of the infusion cannula, the globe is pressurized by opening the infusion line. Additional sclerotomies for the insertion of the fiberoptic light pipe and vitrectomy probe are created. A closed-system pars plana vitrectomy can be performed.

Occasionally, it is desirable to enhance the peripheral view with ancillary lenses such as prism lenses or wide-field viewing lenses. A wide-angle indirect viewing system also can be used. It is possible also to get an excellent view of the peripheral retina when using the wide-field temporary keratoprosthesis through the use of scleral depression. The tight seal between the wide-field temporary keratoprosthesis and the cornea permits extensive scleral depression without loss of intraocular fluid through the corneal opening.

If water droplets develop on the internal surface of the wide-field temporary keratoprosthesis during fluid–gas exchange, these droplets may be wiped away with the side of a silicone extrusion cannula. Scleral buckling can be performed with the temporary keratoprosthesis in place. When a large, retained intraocular foreign body is present, the wide-field temporary keratoprosthesis can be removed temporarily to facilitate removal of the foreign body through the trephine opening in the cornea.

Following completion of the vitrectomy, scleral plugs are placed in the pars plana incisions and a donor cornea is prepared; this is usually made 0.2 mm larger than the recipient bed using an endothelial punch technique. The infusion pressure is lowered slowly before removal of the wide-field temporary keratoprosthesis in order to avoid sudden intraocular pressure changes. The donor cornea button is sutured in place after removal of the wide-field temporary keratoprosthesis, using interrupted and running 10-0 nylon sutures (Fig. 12.8). Running sutures may become loosened in cases in which hypotony or phthisis bulbi occurs.[3] Sterile gas or silicone oil can be placed in the vitreous cavity through a sclerotomy site when indicated. The view remains good through the wide-field temporary keratoprosthesis, even in the air-filled eye. While in place, the wide-field temporary keratoprosthesis generally provides an air-tight vitreous cavity into which fluid–gas exchange can be carried out.

The sclerotomies are closed with 7-0 Vicryl suture. If necessary, balanced salt solution is injected through the pars plana into the vitreous cavity to return the eye to normal pressure. The conjunctival peritomy is sutured and ocular medications are administered.

OUTCOMES

The visual outcome for eyes experiencing both anterior and posterior segment trauma is frequently poor; this is most often a reflection of the initial trauma. Reported visual acuities following the use of the temporary keratoprosthesis in trauma cases ranged widely from 20/20 to no light perception. The majority of patients achieved vision of 5/200 or less. The percentage of eyes with clear corneas ranged from 40% to 80% in case series including four or more eyes with a minimum follow up of six months. The retinal reattachment rate varied from 27% to 100%.[1,6–9] There is no evidence that corneal graft survival is impaired by the use of the temporary keratoprosthesis. Problems with corneal grafts are generally caused by hypotony, phthisis or glaucoma.

The visual recovery in cases involving severe anterior and posterior trauma will likely remain poor. However, the use of a temporary keratoprosthesis offers these eyes a chance to achieve useful vision. The visual recovery in these patients will likely improve as experience with the newer versions of the temporary keratoprosthesis, including the wide-field temporary keratoprosthesis and the infusion temporary keratoprosthesis, increases.

CONCLUSIONS

The development of the temporary keratoprosthesis has allowed the surgical repair of eyes that have experienced anterior and posterior segment trauma. Improvements in the keratoprosthesis design now permit the use of strong anchoring sutures, which offers fluid- and air-tight seals between the cornea and the wide-field temporary keratoprosthesis in nearly all cases. This allows the use of fluid–gas exchange, dissection of the peripheral vitreous, infusion through an infusion temporary keratoprosthesis, when indicated, and the use of silicone oil and perfluorocarbon liquids in the initial management of severe trauma cases. Modifications of the anterior radius of curvature and the central optical peg permit easy viewing of both the posterior pole and the peripheral retina. The temporary keratoprosthesis provides the opportunity for vitreoretinal and anterior segment surgeons to combine their expertise in an attempt to salvage those eyes with injuries requiring both penetrating keratoplasty and pars plana vitrectomy.

REFERENCES

1. Landers MB III, Foulks GN, Landers DM, Hickingbotham D, Hamilton RC. Temporary keratoprosthesis for use during pars plana vitrectomy, *Am J Ophthalmol* (1981) **91**:615–19.
2. Eckardt C. A new temporary keratoprosthesis for pars plana vitrectomy, *Retina* (1987) **7**:34–7.
3. Gallemore RP, Bokosky JE. Penetrating keratoplasty with vitreoretinal surgery using the Eckardt temporary keratoprosthesis: modified technique allowing use of larger corneal grafts, *Cornea* (1995) **14**:33–8.
4. Toth CA, Landers MB III. A new wide-field temporary keratoprosthesis (letter), *Retina* (1993) **13**:353–5.
5. Benner JD, Landers MB III. An infusion temporary keratoprosthesis for pars plana vitrectomy, *Am J Ophthalmol* (1996) **122**:579–80.
6. Koenig SB, McDonald HR, Williams GA, Abrams GW. Penetrating keratoplasty after placement of a temporary keratoprosthesis during pars plana vitrectomy, *Am J Ophthalmol* (1986) **102**:45–9.
7. Gelender H, Vaiser A, Snyder WB, Fuller DG, Hutton WL. Temporary keratoprosthesis for combined penetrating keratoplasty, pars plana vitrectomy, and repair of retinal detachment, *Ophthalmology* (1988) **95**:897–901.
8. Gross JG, Feldman S, Freeman WR. Combined penetrating keratoplasty and vitreoretinal surgery with the Eckardt temporary keratoprosthesis, *Ophthalmic Surg* (1990) **21**:67–71.
9. Soheilian M, Ahmadieh H, Sajjadi H, et al. Temporary keratoprosthesis for surgical management of complicated combined anterior and posterior segment injuries to the eye: combat- versus noncombat-injury cases, *Ophthalmic Surg* (1994) **25**:452–7.

Part III Techniques of Pars Plana Vitrectomy

Chapter 13 Simple vitrectomy

Alan J Ruby and George A Williams

INTRODUCTION

No advance in the treatment of vitreoretinal diseases has been as significant as the introduction of pars plana vitrectomy by Machemer in 1971.[1] With the advent of closed system vitrectomy, vitreoretinal surgeons were able to remove media opacities and repair complicated retinal detachments that had not been amenable to treatment. Over the years, many advances have been made in the equipment and technique of pars plana vitrectomy. This chapter will provide an introduction to basic pars plana vitrectomy, including the equipment used for the procedure, the basic set-up for vitrectomy, core vitrectomy, peripheral vitrectomy, as well as removal of the posterior hyaloid during pars plana vitrectomy.

EQUIPMENT

The basic equipment required for pars plana vitrectomy includes a vitrectomy machine, a light source, an air pump, a lens viewing system and an operating microscope. Each piece of equipment will be discussed in detail, with consideration given to their set-up as well as their use in vitrectomy surgery.

VITRECTOMY MACHINE

Various models of vitrectomy machines are available for vitreoretinal surgery (Fig. 13.1). However, all of them share some basic components. Each machine is equipped with an infusion system that allows control of intraocular pressure (IOP) during surgery. Infusion systems may use gas-forced infusion in which a bottle of balanced salt solution (BSS) is attached to an air pump that regulates the pressure that forces the BSS into the eye through infusion tubing. Other systems rely on gravity, specifically the height of the bottle above the patient's eye, in order to maintain the IOP. Both systems allow the surgeon to raise the IOP by either increasing the gas pressure forcing the fluid into the eye or by raising the bottle height.

For those systems using bottle elevation and the effect of gravity to maintain the IOP, the bottle is usually positioned approximately 18 inches above the eye level to maintain a normal IOP. For those systems that employ gas-forced infusion, the air pump is usually set at a pressure of 20–30 mmHg during normal operations. An air pump is built into most vitrectomy machines; a separate air pump is available when not included in the vitrectomy machine.

The infusion bottle is connected to the eye by an infusion line. This infusion line may also include multiple three-way stopcocks, which allow the surgeon to control the infusion going into the eye, whether fluid or air (Fig. 13.2). The infusion line is connected to an infusion cannula that is sewn into the sclera for control of the IOP (Fig. 13.3).

VITREOUS CUTTER

The primary instrument used during pars plana vitrectomy is a vitreous cutter, which allows high-speed cutting of formed vitreous and controlled removal of the vitreous gel with low suction. There are various types of vitreous cutters, each consisting of a handpiece connected to a metal cutter with a side port positioned a variable distance from the tip of the shaft (Fig. 13.4). The cutter employs a guillotine-type mechanism, which is pneumatically driven by the vitrectomy machine. Most currently available vitreous cutters feature a side-cutting port with the guillotine action in the vertical plane. Some of the newer vitreous cutters have a side-cutting port closer to the tip

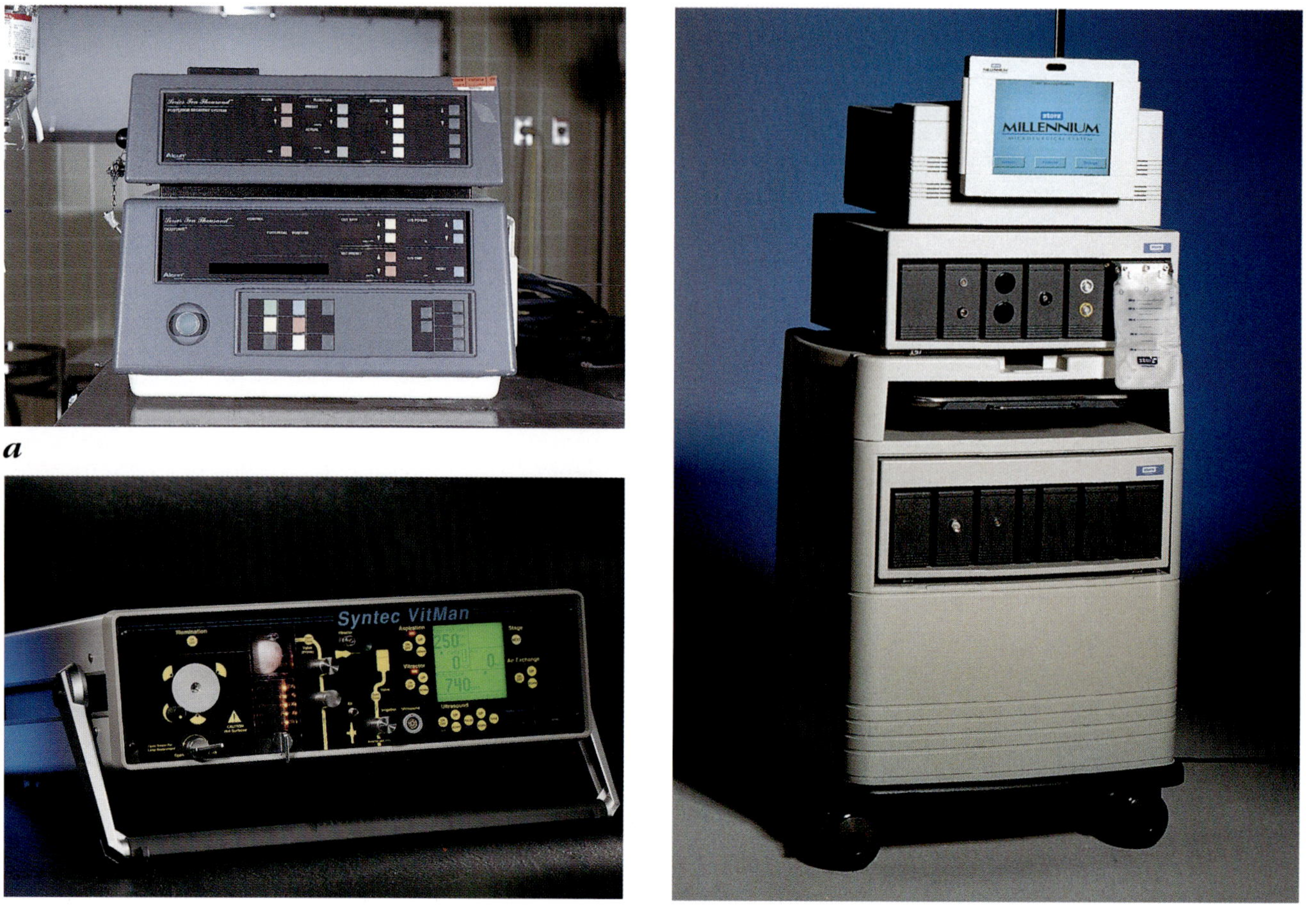

Figure 13.1 *(a) Vitrectomy machine made by Alcon with internal illumination source and air pump. A bottle of balanced salt solution is hung on an intravenous pole and connected to an infusion cannula to maintain normal intraocular pressure during surgery. The intraocular pressure is controlled by the height of the bottle above the patient's eye. (b) Bausch & Lomb vitrectomy machine. (c) Portable vitrectomy unit from Syntec, Inc., which works similarly to the Alcon unit.*

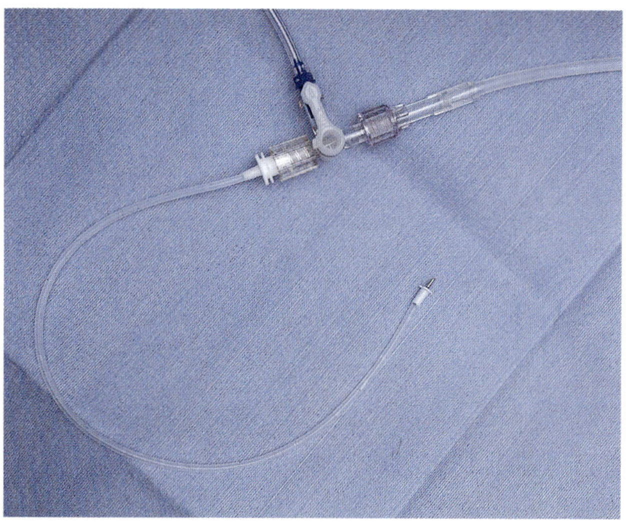

Figure 13.2 *An infusion cannula is attached with tubing to a three-way stopcock that allows control of the infusion into the eye. Tubing from the balanced salt solution is attached to one end of the three-way stopcock. A separate tube is attached to the other stopcock and is connected to the air pump on the vitrectomy machine. The infusion is controlled by the position of the three-way stopcock.*

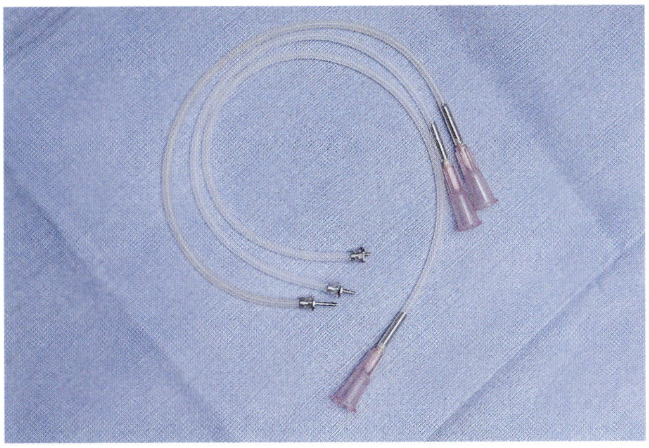

Figure 13.3 *A 2-mm, 4-mm or 6-mm infusion cannula is connected by tubing to the infusion solution for maintenance of intraocular pressure during surgery.*

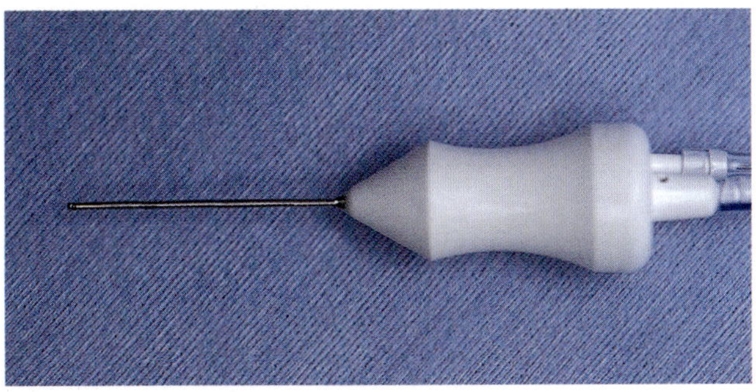

a

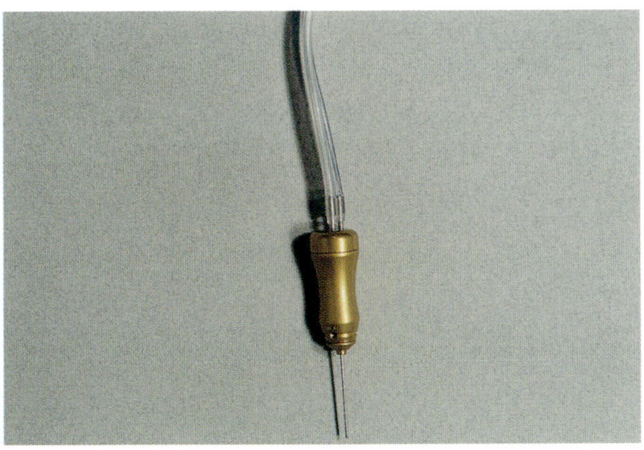

b

Figure 13.4 *(a) A pneumatically driven vitrectomy handpiece with a side-cutting port near its tip. Two separate tubes connect the handpiece to the cutting drive on the vitrectomy machine as well as to the vacuum to allow suction during surgery. (b) Vitrectomy handpiece from Syntec.*

of the steel shaft and may actually use a horizontal cutting mechanism. However, regardless of the design of the vitreous cutter, the principles involved in removal of the vitreous gel remain the same (a cutting rate sufficient to prevent traction and a suction rate that allows removal of the vitreous without exerting undue traction on underlying surfaces).

A suction line connects the cutter to the vitrectomy machine. Typical settings for suction range from 100 to 150 mmHg but can be increased to a maximum of 400 mmHg on most machines. For most vitrectomies, the cutting rate is set at 600 cuts per minute (cpm); some machines have cutting rates up to 1200 cpm.

The vitreous cutter is connected to the vitrectomy machine through two lines. The first line goes from the cutter to the cutting drive on the machine (Fig. 13.4). This line usually will plug into the vitrectomy machine at the port labeled 'cutter'. The second line is the aspiration line from the vitreous cutter to the vitrectomy machine. In most machines, this line will plug into a cartridge that is placed in the vitrectomy machine. Many machines have a priming mode that allows the vitreous cutter to be primed before its use in the eye. The machine is primed by placing the vitreous cutter tip into a solution of fluid and pressing the priming command on the vitrectomy machine. If no priming mode is available, fluid can be aspirated through the vitreous cutter by use of a foot pedal, by either the surgeon or by the scrub technician.

FOOT PEDAL

Control of the vitreous cutter is by way of a foot pedal placed on the floor next to the surgeon's right or left foot (Fig. 13.5). The foot pedal allows the surgeon to control the vitrector, deploying suction only or cutting and suction together. The surgeon selects a predetermined aspiration setting that will be reached as the foot pedal is maximally depressed. The majority of systems feature linear control of suction by the surgeon, as determined by the extent the foot pedal is depressed toward the floor. The surgeon can switch between modes via a control on the foot pedal, which may vary according to the vitrectomy machine. Some machines allow the surgeon to click the foot pedal either to the right or left to switch between the modes, whereas other machines have separate buttons that must be

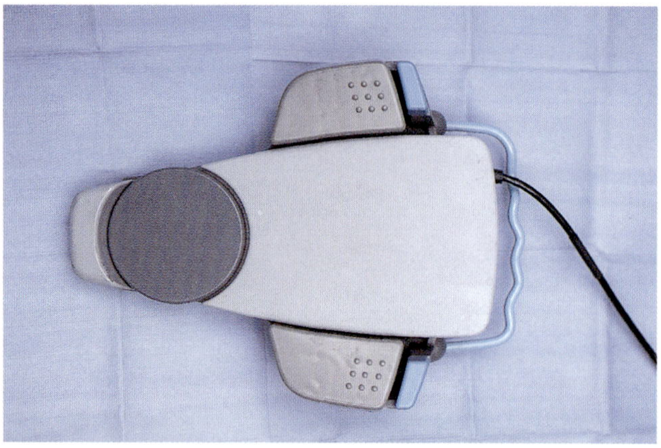

a

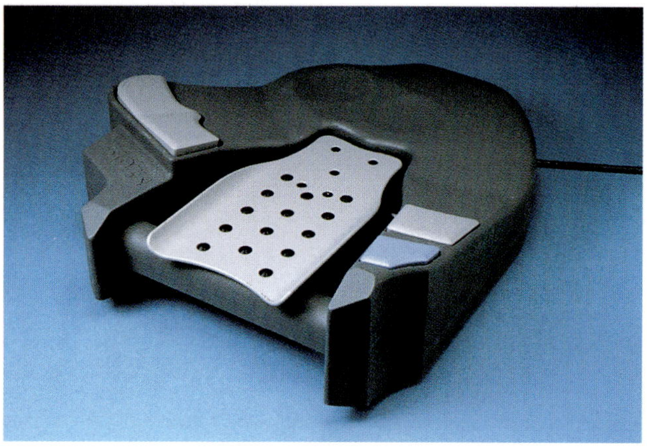

b

Figure 13.5 *(a) A foot pedal for control of the Alcon vitrectomy machine. The surgeon controls the cutting and aspiration modes by clicking the pedal to the right to switch between modes. Cautery may also be controlled by depressing the gray knob to the left of the foot pedal. (b) Foot pedal of Bausch & Lomb unit with various control mechanisms.*

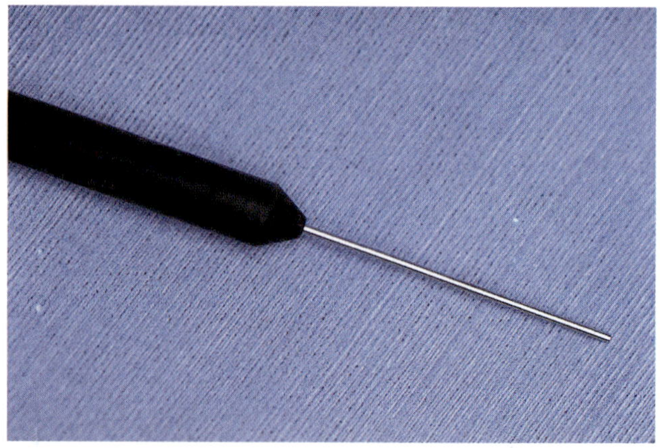

a

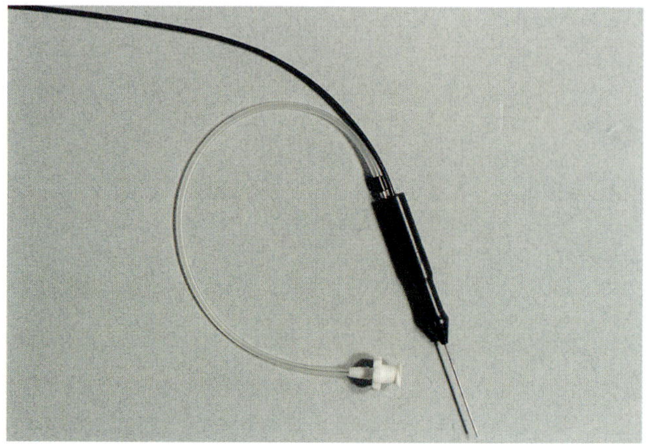

b

Figure 13.6 *(a) A standard light probe. A metal shaft is connected to a plastic handpiece with a fiberoptic cable running from the light source to the tip of the metal shaft. (b) Infusion light pipe for Syntec vitrectomy unit is connected to the light source and an infusion bottle.*

engaged in order for the cutting and aspiration modes to be interchanged.

ILLUMINATION SOURCE

A light source is required during vitrectomy surgery to illuminate the material being removed. Most vitrectomy machines are equipped with a built-in light source, usually employing yellow light. Some of the newer systems may use white light. A separate light source is also available. A light pipe that employs a fiberoptic cable encased in a plastic handpiece is connected to the vitrectomy machine's light source and infusion attachment. The light pipe is available in various shapes and sizes (Fig. 13.6).

The intensity of the light used during vitreous surgery should be set at the minimum that allows visualization of the area of interest, to minimize the risk of phototoxicity. Additionally, the light pipe should be positioned as far from the retina as possible in order to reduce the intensity of the light at the retinal surface. A corneal cover may be utilized during the vitrectomy set-up and for closure of the ports and conjunctiva at the conclusion of surgery in order to minimize the risk of phototoxicity.

VIEWING SYSTEM

The unique structure of the eyeball with multiple refractive surfaces, including the lens and the cornea, prevents clear viewing of the retina without a neutralizing lens. Various viewing systems are available to facilitate visualization of the retina as well as the vitreous cavity. The most commonly used systems for viewing the posterior segment of the eye include hand-held contact lenses, which are attached to an irrigating handpiece and held on the cornea by the surgical assistant (Fig. 13.7), and sew-on contact lenses (Fig. 13.8). A ring held in place by sutures sewn at the limbus holds the various contact lenses. A solution of BSS or viscoelastic couples the lenses to the cornea.

Lenses of various strengths and configurations allow viewing of the macula or, with the aid of prism lenses, the retinal periphery. High-minus lenses (biconcave) are used for air–fluid exchanges because of the change in the refractive status of the eye as the vitreous fluid is replaced with air. One disadvantage of the sew-on contact lens system is that any blood present in the operating field may migrate under the contact lens and reduce visualization. This problem is eliminated by constant infusion with the hand-held irrigating system.

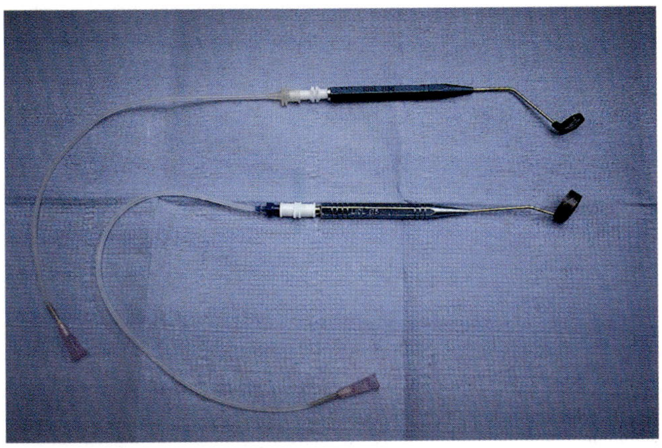

Figure 13.7 *Irrigating contact lenses for viewing during vitreous surgery. A flat lens is used for viewing in a fluid-filled eye. A high-minus biconcave lens is used in an air-filled eye.*

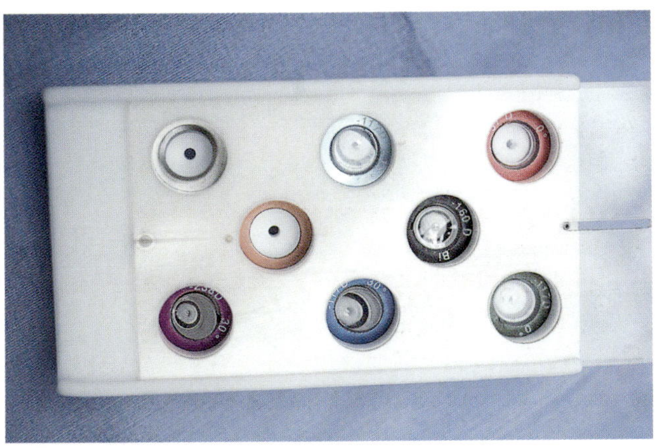

Figure 13.8 *Sew-on contact lens set made for various lenses used for viewing the posterior pole and peripheral retina. High-minus lenses are used for viewing during air–fluid exchange.*

OPERATING MICROSCOPE

An operating microscope is absolutely essential for pars plana vitrectomy. Although some components of the vitrectomy can be completed by utilizing the indirect ophthalmoscope for visualization, the majority of surgery is done with the aid of an operating microscope (Fig. 13.9).

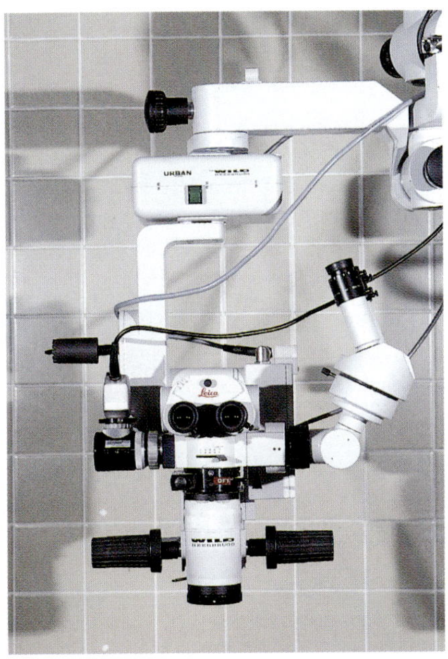

Figure 13.9 *A Wild operating microscope with a video monitor hook-up, as well as a teaching assistant's scope.*

The primary objective of the operating microscope is to allow clear visualization of the structures being manipulated, with a preferential importance placed on depth of field. The greater the depth of field available on the microscope, the greater is the ability of the surgeon to focus finely.

The operating microscope should be equipped with an assistant's scope. Optional equipment may include a video camera to allow monitoring of the surgery on a video screen.

Some vitreoretinal surgeons prefer a microscope cover while performing vitreous surgery. This microscope drape allows the surgeon to move the microscope freely without concern for a break in sterile technique. No studies have demonstrated any association between the use of a microscope drape and the development of endophthalmitis.

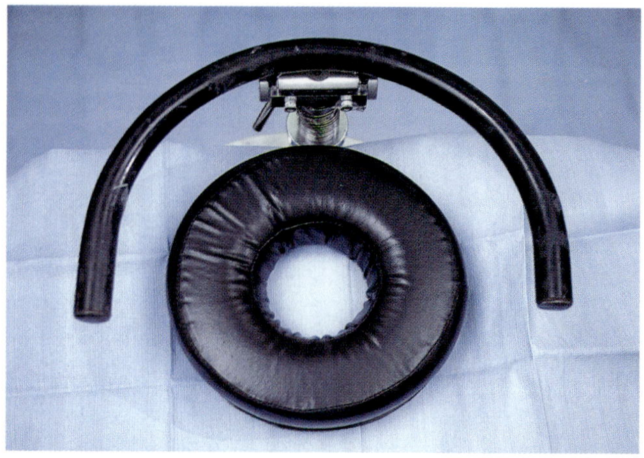

Figure 13.10 *A donut-shaped head support with a wrist rest.*

SET-UP

Once the surgeon is familiar with the basic equipment necessary for a pars plana vitrectomy, the set-up of the patient and the equipment becomes a primary concern. In this section, we will discuss the set-up of the patient as well as the equipment immediately before surgery.

POSITIONING OF PATIENT

The positioning of the patient is the first critical stage in the performance of any surgical procedure. It is imperative that the patient be positioned so that the surgical eye is in the primary position. In many cases, a small shoulder roll under the patient will facilitate a slight extension of the patient's neck and place the eye in primary position. The surgery becomes increasingly difficult when the position of the eye is altered from primary because the surgeon's ability to visualize the peripheral retina will be severely compromised.

The patient should be positioned so that he or she is comfortable lying on the table. A pillow or rolled towel under the patient's knees may reduce the stress on the lower back and prevent discomfort during the procedure if performed under local anesthetic. The patient's head is usually positioned on a donut-shaped head support device, which will prevent the head from rolling. A wrist rest is usually employed around the patient's head (Fig. 13.10).

The patient should be draped in a sterile fashion for eye surgery. This procedure usually entails the use of a head drape placed across the patient's forehead and a body drape that covers all but the operated eye. A 1060 Steri-Drape or comparable drape can be used to cover the operative site and allow placement of a lid speculum. The microscope then should be positioned over the surgical eye so that the eye is in primary position. Once the patient and microscope are in position, attention then can be directed toward the set-up of the infusion, vitrectomy cutter, light pipe and air pump.

VITRECTOR SET-UP

The vitrectomy machine is usually placed toward the foot of the bed to allow easy access for the surgical scrub. The light pipe is usually placed on one side of the eye and the vitreous cutter on the other side of the eye, to reduce the risk of the lines becoming entangled during the surgery, because most of the procedure is performed in the dark.

SURGICAL PREPARATION OF THE EYE

The eye should be prepped and draped in a sterile fashion as for other eye surgery. Cleansing of the operative site with povidone–iodine 5% has been shown to reduce the incidence of postoperative endophthalmitis.[2]

A conjunctival incision is performed at the limbus, both nasally and temporally, to facilitate placement of the vitrectomy ports. The nasal incision usually extends from the horizontal approximately 1.5–2 clock-hours superiorly. The temporal incision usually extends for

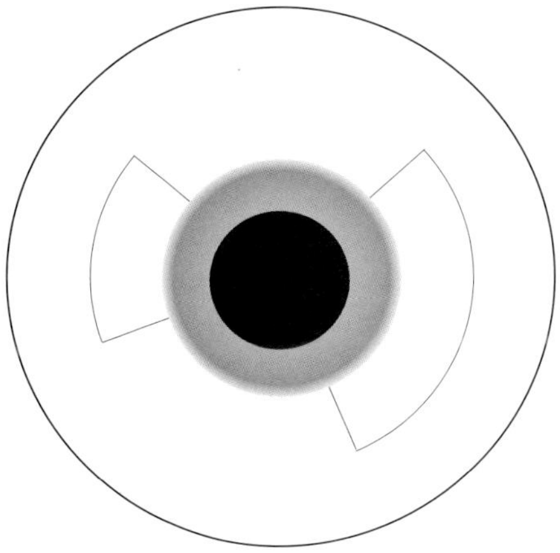

Figure 13.11 *A conjunctival peritomy, left eye. Relaxing incisions are seen at 10:30, 1:30 and 4:30 positions to minimize the risk of conjunctival tearing during the procedure.*

the 4 clock-hours. Relaxing incisions should be made to prevent ripping of the conjunctiva during the remainder of the procedure (Fig. 13.11).

If a sew-in contact lens system is to be used, a suture is placed at the 3 and 9 o'clock positions at the limbus to facilitate placement of the lens ring. A 4-0 silk suture on a spatulated needle or 4-0 Mersilene on a spatulated needle is used. A spatulated needle reduces the risk of perforation into the globe. Wet-field cautery is performed throughout the area of exposed sclera in order to reduce subsequent bleeding and oozing during the procedure.

A site is picked inferotemporally for placement of the infusion. An infusion cannula is used to deliver the BSS into the vitreous cavity. The infusion cannulas usually measure 2, 4 or 6 mm in length (Fig. 13.3). During a standard pars plana vitrectomy, most surgeons will employ a 4-mm infusion cannula. The length of the infusion cannula should be adequate to deliver solution into the vitreous cavity while minimizing the risk of hitting the lens or the retina during manipulation. A longer infusion cannula may be employed with aphakic or pseudophakic patients or in patients with high myopia or peripheral retinal elevations (such as choroidal detachments) in order to reduce the risk of the cannula entering the subretinal space. A 2-mm cannula is employed by some surgeons to reduce the risk of lens damage.

Typically the infusion cannula is placed through a sclerotomy inferotemporally made approximately 3.5–4 mm posterior to the limbus in phakic eyes and 3–3.5 mm posterior to the limbus in aphakic or pseudophakic eyes (Fig. 13.12). The sclerotomy should perforate the pars plana without causing damage to the retina or lens. A caliper is set at the desired distance and a mark made on the external sclera. A microvitreoretinal (MVR) blade is used to create a sclerotomy. The MVR blade is kept perpendicular to the sclera and aimed toward the midvitreous cavity to reduce the risk of hitting the lens or damaging the retina (Fig. 13.13). If possible, the MVR blade

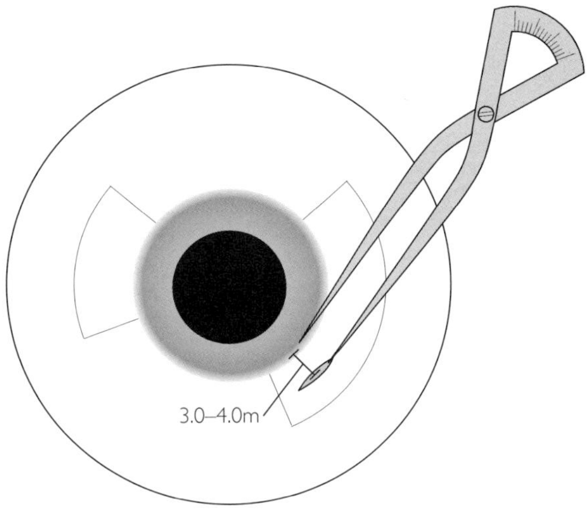

Figure 13.12 *A sclerotomy site is marked on the external sclera 3.0–3.5 mm posterior to the limbus in an aphakic or pseudophakic eye or 3.5–4.0 mm posterior to the limbus in a phakic eye. A caliper placed on the sclera can be used to mark the proposed sclerotomy site.*

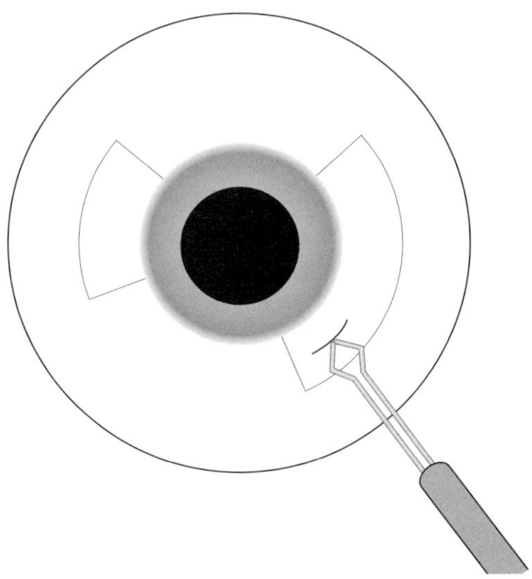

Figure 13.13 *A microvitreoretinal blade held perpendicular to the sclera is used to create the sclerotomy.*

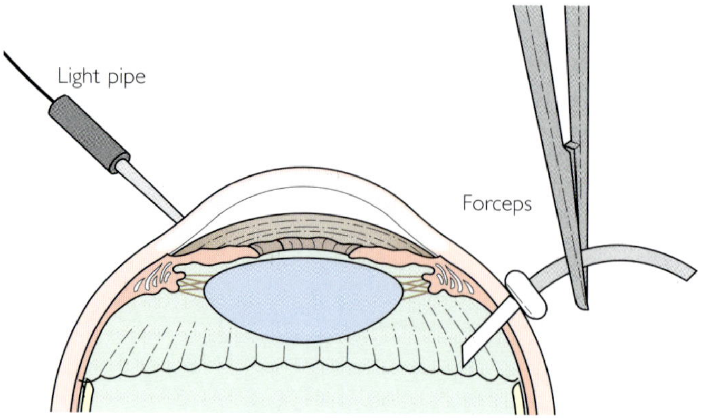

Figure 13.14 *The infusion cannula is grasped with a smooth forceps and rotated away from the surgeon. A light pipe held at the limbus is used to illuminate the cannula, which is visualized through the dilated pupil.*

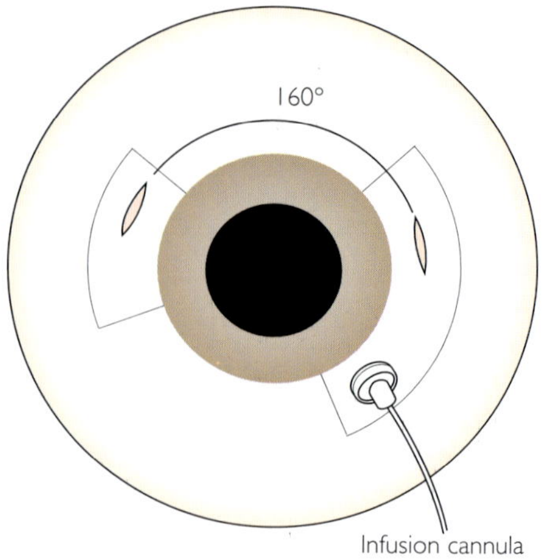

Figure 13.15 *Sclerotomies are placed superonasally and superotemporally approximately 160° apart. The temporal sclerotomy is placed as low to the horizontal as possible, to facilitate inferior rotation of the eye. The infusion cannula is shown sewn into the sclera inferotemporally.*

is visualized directly in the vitreous cavity as it passes through the pars plana.

The infusion cannula is held in place with a 6-0 Vicryl suture on a spatulated needle. A vertical mattress suture is placed before or after the creation of the sclerotomy. The 6-0 Vicryl suture can be left in place following removal of the infusion cannula at the conclusion of surgery. Some surgeons prefer to use a 6-0 nylon or Mersilene suture, which is cut at the conclusion of the surgical case and then replaced with a 6-0 Vicryl suture following removal of the infusion cannula. If a 6-0 Vicryl suture is used to anchor the cannula, a slip knot can be used so that the knot can be loosened and the infusion cannula removed at the conclusion of the procedure without replacing the suture. The ends of the suture are left approximately 0.5–1 inch long to facilitate grasping at the conclusion of the procedure.

After the cannula is sewn into the sclerotomy, it is critical that the surgeon directly visualizes the position of the cannula in the vitreous cavity before turning on the infusion. This is done by grasping the infusion cannula with a smooth forceps and gently pushing the cannula toward the central vitreous cavity while tilting the eye toward the cannula itself. The illuminating light pipe is then used to facilitate visualization of the infusion tip (Fig. 13.14). If the tip is not visualized using this technique, the indirect ophthalmoscope can be tried. Once the position of the cannula is confirmed in the vitreous cavity, the infusion is turned on to maintain normal IOP.

Similar sclerotomy sites are made superotemporally and superonasally, 3.5–4 mm posterior to the limbus in a phakic eye and 3–3.5 mm posterior to the limbus in an aphakic or pseudophakic eye. The sclerotomies should ideally be approximately 160° apart to facilitate manipulation in the vitreous cavity (Fig. 13.15). Twenty-gauge scleral plugs fill the sclerotomies in order to maintain normal IOP, prevent egress of formed vitreous and prevent incarceration of detached retina in the sclerotomy. At this time, the sew-on ring is tied in place on the cornea using the preplaced limbal sutures.

CORE VITRECTOMY

The vitreous cavity usually consists of formed and liquefied vitreous and has a volume of 3–4 ml. The vitreous is strongly adherent to the retina at the vitreous base, which extends approximately 2 mm anterior to the ora serrata and 2–3 mm posterior to the ora serrata. This portion of the vitreous is not removed during a pars plana vitrectomy. The posterior hyaloid is also strongly adherent to the optic nerve and variably attached to the retinal blood vessels, over the macula and to any retinal scars. The goal of the vitrectomy is to remove the centrally formed vitreous first and then to move the vitrectomy gradually toward the retinal periphery so that a complete vitrectomy may be performed.

Incision of the central vitreous gel is performed initially. A light pipe is introduced through one of the sclerotomies after the scleral plug has been removed by the assistant. The vitreous cutter is introduced through the other sclerotomy. If a hand-held contact lens system is being deployed, the surgical assistant then places the flat planoconcave lens onto the cornea and the irrigating fluid to the handpiece is turned on. If a sew-on contact lens system is being deployed, a planoconcave flat lens is placed onto the corneal surface using either BSS or a viscoelastic substance as a coupler.

Positioning of the light pipe and vitrector in the midvitreous cavity (Fig. 13.16) can be simplified by keeping the instruments perpendicular to the external surface of the sclera and advancing the instruments toward the central cavity until they can be visualized through the operating microscope. The light pipe should be positioned a few millimeters away from the vitreous cutter so that the tip of the cutter is illuminated by the fiberoptic light. The further away from the vitreous cutter the light pipe is positioned, the greater the field of view that will be illuminated.

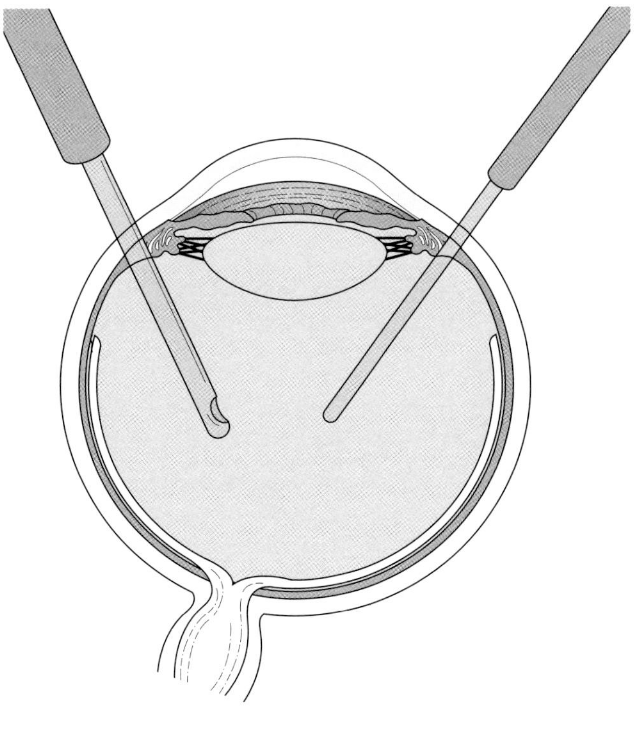

Figure 13.16 *The vitreous cutter and the light pipe positioned in the midvitreous cavity.*

Once the instruments are positioned in the midvitreous cavity, the surgeon depresses the foot pedal to begin aspiration and cutting. The cutting port on the vitreous cutter should face the vitreous to be cut, so that the surgeon can visualize the cutting port at all times. The vitreous will appear to gravitate toward the vitreous port and be aspirated through the opening in the tip. Any reflection of the light off the cutter can be minimized by changing the angle of illumination from the fiberoptic source.

The instruments are held steady in the central vitreous cavity so that the vitreous is allowed to come to the vitreous cutter. Any excessive waving of the vitreous cutter or the light pipe can lead to peripheral retinal traction and peripheral retinal tears.

When the vitreous appears to stop its migration toward the vitreous cutter, the cutter is advanced further posteriorly in the central vitreous cavity to engage any remaining posterior vitreous. Usually the posterior vitreous face will be visualized as the vitrectomy progresses, if the posterior vitreous is detached. Once the posterior vitreous has been excised, the vitrectomy is continued toward the retinal periphery. The vitreous cutter should be positioned with the port facing the vitreous to be removed and the light pipe illuminating the vitreous immediately in front of the cutter. The peripheral retina is visualized with the aid of a hand-held contact lens.

Scleral depression by the assistant with a cotton-tipped applicator permits trimming of the vitreous toward the peripheral vitreous base (Fig. 13.17). When scleral depression is being used, it is important for the assistant to reduce the amount of depression as the suction increases because of the propensity for the peripheral retina to collapse toward the vitreous cutter as the eye becomes soft. If a sew-in lens set is being used, angled lenses of 30° or 50° may be used to aid in visualization of the peripheral retina anterior to the equator.

Scleral depression may be employed to facilitate viewing of the vitreous base and ora serrata. Wide-angle viewing (see Chapter 9) also facilitates peripheral visualization.

The vitreous is shaved toward the vitreous base, taking care to reduce any unnecessary traction on the retina. Certain newer vitrectomy machines have cutting rates of 800–1200 cpm, which may be beneficial in trimming the peripheral vitreous. This procedure is carried out for 360° until a total pars plana vitrectomy is completed.

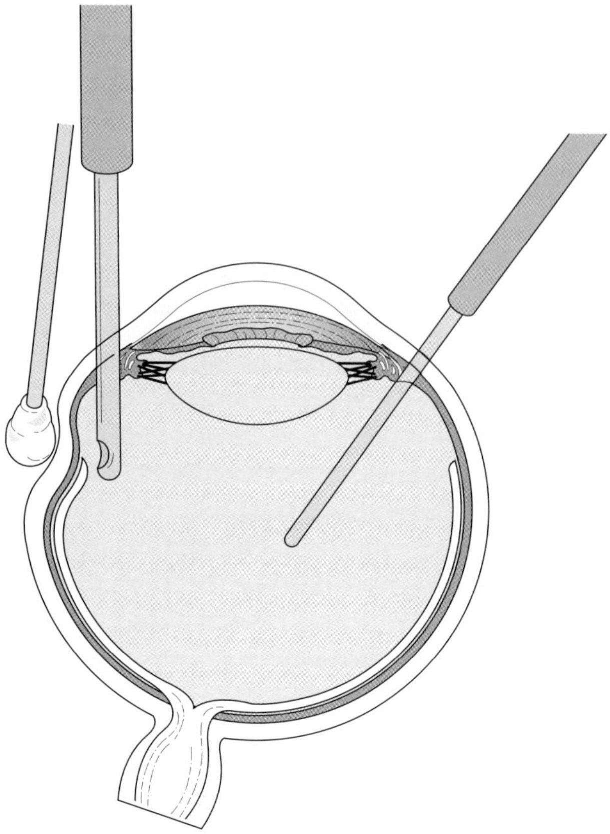

Figure 13.17 *A cotton-tipped applicator is used to perform scleral depression to facilitate removal of the peripheral vitreous.*

REMOVAL OF THE POSTERIOR HYALOID

The vitreous cavity consists of core vitreous gel and a posterior vitreous face, which represents the posterior hyaloid. In a patient without a posterior vitreous separation, the posterior hyaloid is attached to the optic nerve, the retinal vessels, over the macula, and to areas of old retinal scarring. The spectrum of diseases that involve abnormal attachments of the posterior hyaloid has expanded significantly over the last decade, increasing the indications for removal of the posterior hyaloid.

Extreme caution is necessary when removing the posterior hyaloid. Any undue traction on the hyaloid will be transmitted to the vitreous base and can result in retinal tears or detachment. The posterior hyaloid is typically engaged in the peripapillary region, where the potential for damage to the retina is the lowest.[3] Various instruments can be used to engage the posterior hyaloid. A soft-tipped extrusion cannula with active suction may facilitate removal of the posterior hyaloid. A silicone-tipped cannula cut to approximately 3 mm is attached to suction through the aspiration line of the vitrectomy machine and is brought to the peripapillary region with a suction setting of approximately 100 mmHg.

Engagement of the posterior hyaloid can be recognized in numerous ways. First, the infusion line will stop dripping. Once the tip of the cannula is blocked by the engaged posterior hyaloid, no fluid will be seen to enter the eye and the BSS bottle will not drip. Additionally, the 'fish-strike sign' may be seen (Fig. 13.18). This is evidenced by a bending of the soft-tipped cannula as it is moved to and fro over the retinal surface. Any one of these signs is helpful in confirming engagement of the posterior hyaloid when using a soft-tipped infusion cannula.

The surgeon may also employ the vitreous cutter on low aspiration to engage the posterior hyaloid. A barbed MVR blade or other pick may also be used. The posterior hyaloid, once engaged either with a soft-tipped cannula or with the Microvit, is gently pulled toward the central vitreous cavity. When the posterior hyaloid is completely detached, it will be seen to pop off the optic nerve and a Weiss ring will be present in the central vitreous cavity.

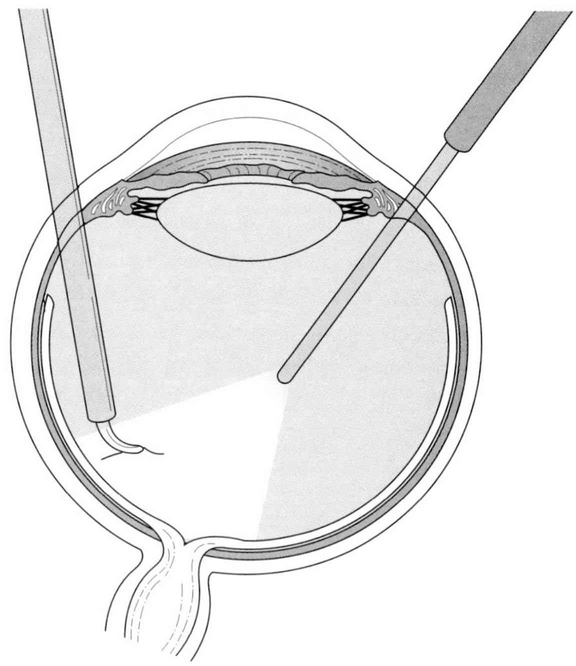

Figure 13.18 *A soft-tipped extrusion cannula is used to engage the posterior hyaloid in the peripapillary region. A 'fish-strike sign' can be seen as the hyaloid is engaged and elevated.*

One must take care not to exert undue traction to the elevated hyaloid because this may increase the risk of peripheral retinal tears. After the Weiss ring is lifted off the optic nerve and the hyaloid is lifted off the macula, removal of the posterior hyaloid is complete.

The posterior hyaloid should be removed from posterior to anterior using the Microvit. The peripheral vitrectomy should proceed toward the vitreous base, either with or without scleral depression, depending on the underlying pathologic condition.

Removal of the posterior hyaloid can be confirmed using a soft-tipped extrusion cannula, which is introduced into the eye in the peripapillary region. Aspiration is then performed. If, upon moving the tip around the peripapillary region, no fish-strike sign is seen and the infusion is observed to flow freely into the eye, one can conclude that the posterior hyaloid has been removed successfully. This process also can be performed around the macular region in a careful fashion to confirm the absence of the posterior hyaloid over any macular structures.

INSPECTION OF THE PERIPHERAL RETINA

A careful inspection of the peripheral retina should be performed after vitrectomy with indirect ophthalmoscopy and scleral depression, to ascertain that no retinal tears occurred as a result of the surgery. Special attention should be directed to the region of the retina directly posterior to each of the sclerotomies. Any retinal tears should be treated with either retinal cryopexy or laser photocoagulation.

CLOSURE FOLLOWING VITRECTOMY

After completion of the surgical procedure, the sclerotomy ports, as well as the conjunctiva, are closed in an orderly fashion. If a sew-on contact lens system was used during the procedure, the sutures at the limbal region are cut and removed before closure of the sclerotomies. The superonasal and superotemporal sclerotomies are usually closed first using a 7-0 Vicryl suture. Some surgeons prefer a permanent closure with a nylon or Mersilene suture. Any vitreous that is protruding from the sclerotomy may be trimmed with a Weck-cel sponge and Westcott scissors before placement of the suture.

The infusion should be clamped temporarily while the sclerotomies are being sutured closed in order to ensure a water-tight seal. The infusion cannula is then removed from its sclerotomy and the preplaced 6-0 Vicryl suture is pulled up and tied down tight. If a temporary suture was not used, the infusion cannula should be removed and a suture placed in the sclerotomy to ensure permanent closure.

The IOP is measured at this time either by tactile touch or by the use of a Schiötz tonometer. If the pressure is normal, the conjunctiva is closed nasally and temporally using interrupted 6-0 plain gut sutures. Subconjunctival injections of antibiotic or steroid can be used at the discretion of the surgeon, as well as atropine drops to ensure adequate postoperative cycloplegia and dilation.

CONCLUSION

Pars plana vitrectomy has greatly expanded the scope of diseases that are amenable to surgical intervention by the vitreoretinal surgeon. This chapter should provide a basic knowledge of the equipment, set-up and surgical technique necessary to perform a core vitrectomy and remove the posterior hyaloid. More complex surgical procedures will be discussed in later chapters.

REFERENCES

1. Machemer R, Buettner H, Norton EW, Parel JM. Vitrectomy: a pars plana approach, *Trans Am Acad Ophthalmol Otolaryngol* (1971) **75**:813–20.
2. Speaker MG, Menikoff JA. Prophylaxis of endophthalmitis with topical povidone–iodine, *Ophthalmology* (1991) **98**:1769–75.
3. Kelly NE, Wendel RT. Vitreous surgery for idiopathic macular holes: Results of a pilot study, *Arch Ophthalmol* (1991) **109**:654–9.

Chapter 14 Pars plana lensectomy

Andrew W Eller and Brian B Berger

INTRODUCTION

The removal of a lens or cataract via the pars plana was introduced coincidentally with vitrectomy by the same approach. Initially, lenses were removed with the vitreous cutting instrument alone.[1,2] This was a rather tedious process, because pieces of lens had to be retrieved from the surface of the retina and fed manually into the cutting port. With the introduction of the ultrasonic fragmentation needle, the lens or cataract could be removed with increased ease and efficiency.[3–8] The ultrasonic fragmentation tip now serves as the standard instrument for pars plana lensectomy.

When cataract surgery is performed by intra- or extracapsular techniques, the creation of a large limbal wound is necessary. These large wounds are not conducive to the placement of scleral buckles or gas–fluid exchanges during vitrectomy. Therefore, the removal of the lens through a small pars plana incision offers many advantages. Phacoemulsification also allows the removal of a lens through a small wound, but in selected cases there is a benefit to the pars plana lensectomy technique.

INDICATIONS

There are several indications for removal of the crystalline lens by the pars plana technique. The lens should be removed whenever opacification prevents sufficient visualization of the retina and vitreous gel to complete the surgical objectives. In some cases, a clear lens may be removed to permit adequate access to anterior locations within the vitreous cavity, as in proliferative vitreoretinopathy (PVR) and trauma. Although this technique is not advocated for routine cataract extraction, concomitant pars plana vitrectomy and lensectomy in patients with uveitis have been shown to be very successful.[9–13] Pars plana lensectomy is also useful in managing patients with subluxation of the lens and vitreous prolapse into the anterior chamber.[14–19]

PREOPERATIVE EVALUATION

The anterior segment should be examined carefully. If corneal guttata are present, a viscoelastic may be used to protect the corneal endothelium. The iris is inspected for its ability to dilate, because iris retractors may be necessary. The presence of posterior and peripheral anterior synechiae and iris neovascularization should be determined. The lens should be assessed for hardness which will determine how much energy will be required. In general, it is best to use the minimal amount of power that is necessary for removal of the lens.

If there is a possibility of placing an intraocular lens (IOL) implant on the anterior capsule (with the haptics in the ciliary sulcus), then a preoperative A-scan should be performed. In cases in which silicone oil injection is anticipated, it is useful to obtain an A-scan measurement if the macula is attached. This determination is important because it can be difficult to measure the axial length of the eye that is filled with silicone oil.

In addition to the standard preoperative eye drops for dilation, one may consider the use of a nonsteroidal anti-inflammatory agent to help maintain dilation during the procedure.

SURGICAL TECHNIQUE

The eye is prepared for a standard three-port vitrectomy. A 4-mm infusion cannula is placed through a sclerotomy that is located 3.5 mm behind the limbus.

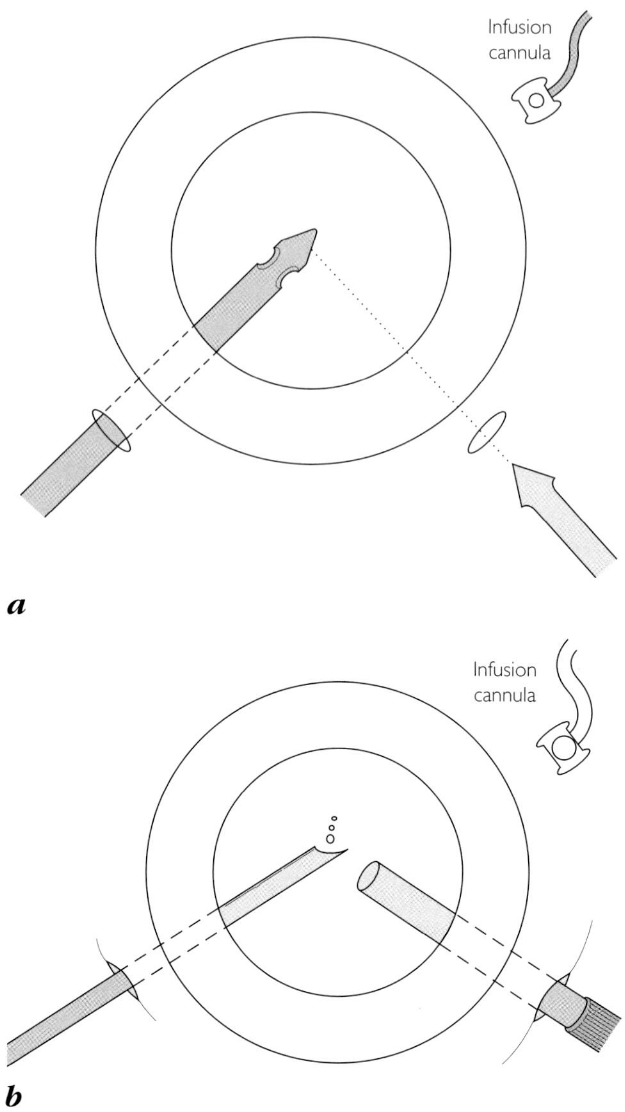

Figure 14.1 *(a) From each of the two superior sclerotomies, the microvitreoretinal blade is directed into the nucleus through the equator of the lens. (b) If the tip of the infusion cannula cannot be identified in the vitreous cavity, then a 20-gauge infusion needle should be placed directly into the lens.*

It is important to visualize the tip of the cannula in the vitreous cavity before turning on the infusion. Once the infusion has been started, then a microvitreoretinal (MVR) blade is used to make two additional sclerotomies, also 3.5 mm behind the limbus, superiorly at the 2:30 and 9:30 clock positions. From each of these sclerotomies, the MVR blade is directed into the nucleus through the equator of the lens (Fig. 14.1a). If the lens is fairly clear, it is useful to remove at least the anterior one-third of the vitreous with a vitrectomy instrument. This will prevent inadvertent aspiration of the vitreous in the event that the posterior lens capsule is damaged during fragmentation.

If the tip of the infusion cannula cannot be identified in the vitreous cavity, then a 20-gauge infusion needle should be placed directly into the lens (Fig. 14.1b). When the infusion cannula is finally visualized, it is turned on as the needle is withdrawn from the eye.

Hydrodissection has become an important part of modern cataract surgery because it separates the nucleus from the lens capsule and allows it to be mobilized.[20] This is a useful technique because the nucleus can be manipulated without putting stress on the lens capsule or zonules, thereby reducing the risk of a rupture. Preservation of the posterior capsule eliminates the potential problem of lens fragments drifting to the posterior pole.

The technique of hydrodissection can be applied easily to pars plana lensectomy. Using either a 20-gauge irrigation cannula or a specialized hydrodissection needle, a stream of balanced saline solution is forced between the lens capsule and the epinucleus (Fig. 14.2). It is important to avoid injecting air into the lens. The tip of the cannula should be placed as close to the inner surface of the anterior lens

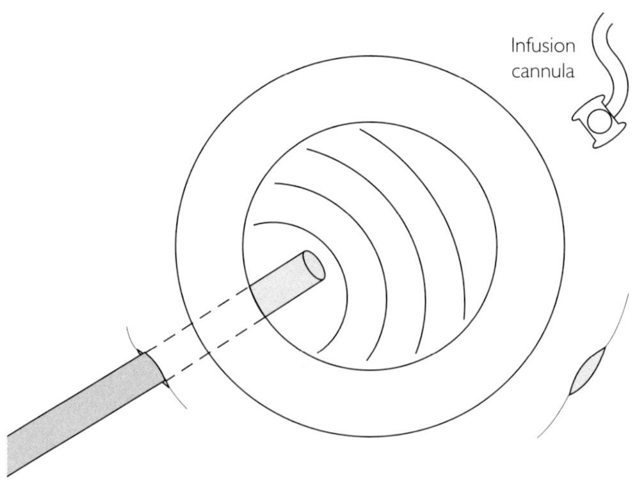

Figure 14.2 *In hydrodissection, the tip of the cannula should be placed as close to the inner surface of the anterior lens capsule as possible. This maneuver is complete after a fluid wave has been observed passing inside both the anterior and posterior capsules.*

capsule as possible. This maneuver is complete after a fluid wave has been observed passing inside the anterior and posterior capsules.

The fragmentation needle is passed through the nucleus from each of the two superior sclerotomies. The power of the fragmentation needle is set at the minimal energy necessary to bore through the lens. Often, a power setting of 10% is sufficient. The aspiration pressure is usually set at 150 mmHg. This technique creates two tunnels that cross in an 'x' configuration (Fig. 14.3).

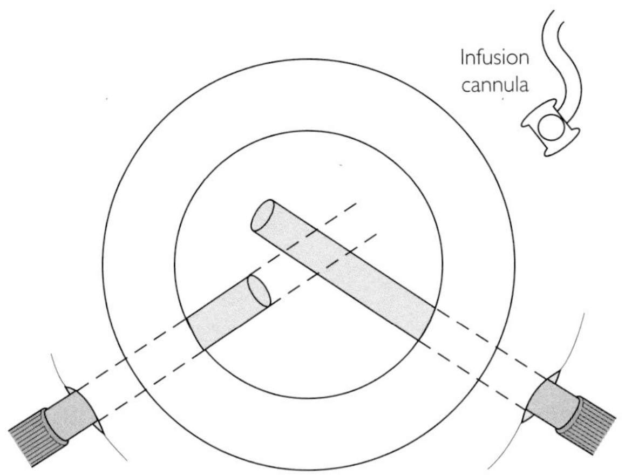

Figure 14.3 *The ultrasonic fragmentation needle is passed through the nucleus from each of the two superior sclerotomies. This technique creates two tunnels that cross in an 'x' configuration.*

A variety of techniques introduced for anterior segment phacoemulsification surgery has provided a major advance in cataract surgery. One of the most important is the 'divide-and-conquer' technique of nuclear disassembly.[21,22] This technique reduces surgical time and lessens stress on the zonules. One of the greatest benefits of nuclear disassembly is that it allows the surgeon to visualize the entire depth or thickness of the lens. When the posterior extent of the nucleus can be seen, damage or rupture of the posterior lens capsule can be avoided. We have found that the divide-and-conquer technique can be applied to pars plana lensectomy, and offers similar advantages. The Barraquer iris sweep and the fragmentation needle are placed in the two tunnels and the nucleus is 'cracked' into two or four sections (Fig. 14.4).

The quarters of the nucleus are rotated with the iris sweep and fragmentation tip, and each one is removed separately. The iris sweep is used to manipulate the nucleus and can be placed under or over the nuclear fragments to protect the lens capsule from the fragmentation needle. Preservation of the anterior lens capsule protects the corneal endothelium, and can be used for placement of a posterior chamber IOL. Maintenance of the posterior lens capsule prevents lens fragments from falling onto the retina (Fig. 14.5).

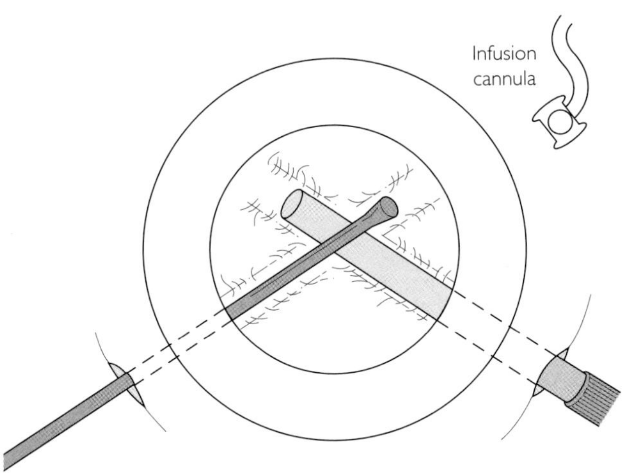

Figure 14.4 *The 'divide-and-conquer' technique can be applied to pars plana lensectomy. The Barraquer iris sweep and the fragmentation needle are placed in the two tunnels and the nucleus is 'cracked' into two or four sections.*

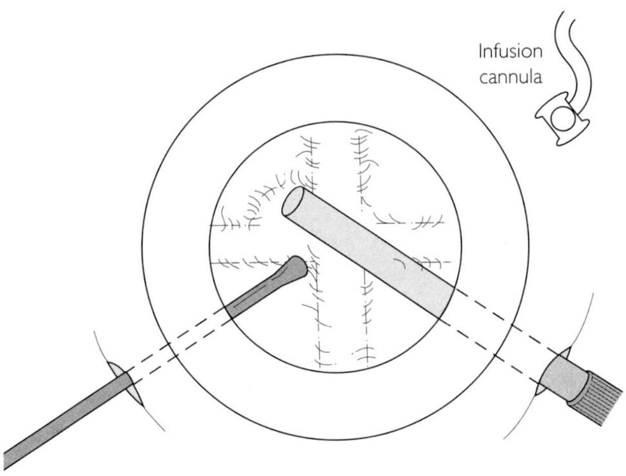

Figure 14.5 *The quarters of the nucleus are rotated with the iris sweep and fragmentation tip, and each one is removed separately. Maintenance of the posterior lens capsule prevents lens fragments from falling onto the retina.*

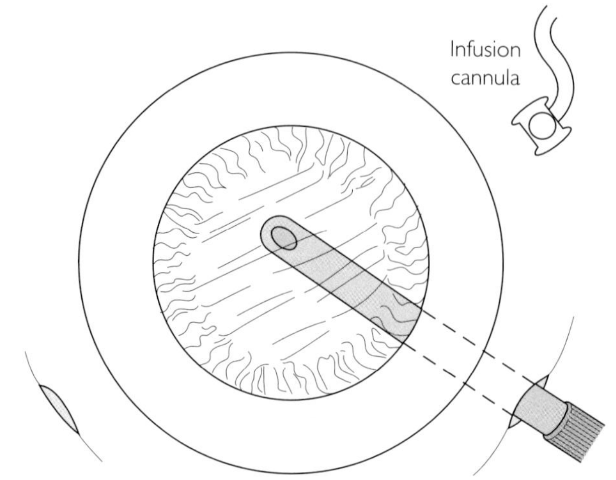

Figure 14.6 *Using a gentle teasing motion, the lens cortex is stripped from the capsular bag and aspirated with the vitreous cutter.*

After the nucleus has been removed, the vitreous cutter is used to aspirate the cortex (Fig. 14.6). If the posterior capsule is intact, the vitrectomy instrument is placed into the lens. Using a gentle teasing motion, the cortex is stripped from the capsular bag and aspirated (Fig. 14.7). One must exert care to avoid aspiration of the lens capsule. A teasing motion is used with minimum aspiration pressure until the tip is completely occluded by the cortex. If the posterior capsule has been ruptured, the central portion may be removed, along with the remaining anterior vitreous.

It is important to remove as much anterior vitreous gel as possible before aspiration of the lens cortex. Inadvertent traction on the vitreous can lead to a retinal detachment. Then the vitreous cutting tip is used to strip away the cortex as described previously (Figs 14.6 and 14.7). If the tip becomes obstructed, briefly switch the setting to the cutting mode to clear the port, or increase the aspiration pressure. It is important to check beneath the entire area of the iris to remove as much cortex as

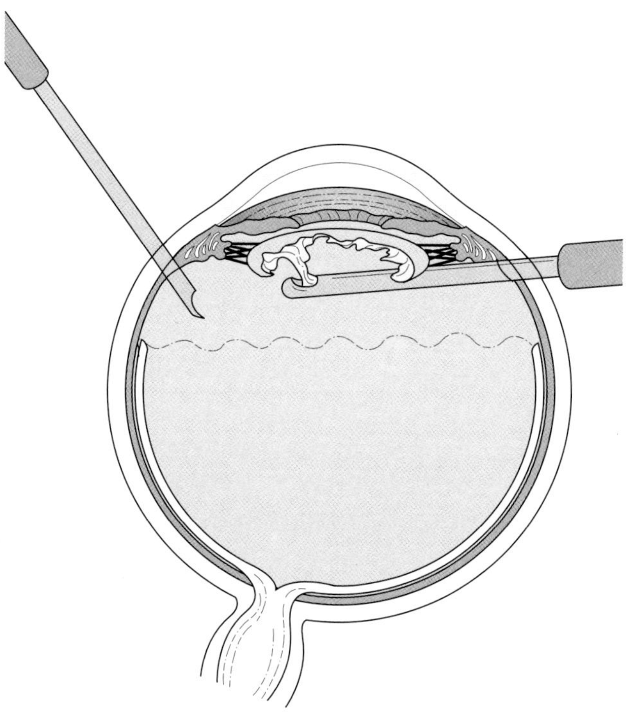

Figure 14.7 *If the posterior capsule has been ruptured, the central portion may be removed, along with the remaining anterior vitreous. It is important to remove as much anterior vitreous gel as possible before aspiration of the lens cortex. Inadvertent traction on the vitreous can lead to a retinal detachment.*

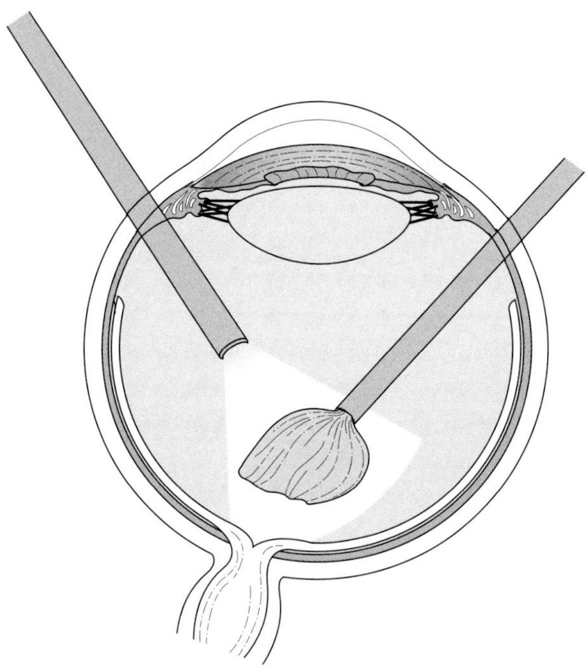

Figure 14.8 *The fragmentation tip is introduced into the vitreous cavity along with the endoilluminator. Using aspiration alone, each fragment is elevated into the midvitreous cavity and then ultrasound power is added to remove the fragment. With a low power level of 5%, the lens fragment will remain close to the fragmentation tip, and can be cartwheeled with the assistance of the endoilluminator until it has been removed completely.*

possible. If necessary, scleral indentation can be performed to help visualize the area under the iris.

If nuclear fragments fall onto the retina, the cortex should first be removed to facilitate visualization of the posterior pole. This is followed by removal of as much of the vitreous gel as possible. The posterior hyaloid should also be separated from the retina and removed, unless there has been a pre-existing posterior vitreous detachment. The fragmentation tip is introduced into the vitreous cavity again, along with the endoilluminator. The power setting is placed at 5% unless the fragments are particularly hard. Using aspiration alone, each fragment is elevated into the midvitreous cavity and then ultrasound power is added to remove the fragment (Fig. 14.8). With a low level of power, the lens fragment will remain close to the fragmentation tip, and can be cartwheeled with the assistance of the endoilluminator until it has been removed. If the power of the ultrasound is too high, the fragment will be propelled forcefully onto the retina. As in all vitrectomies, it is important to inspect the peripheral retina with the indirect ophthalmoscope and with scleral depression for any possible retinal breaks.

MANAGEMENT OF THE ANTERIOR CAPSULE

After the vitrectomy has been completed, a decision must be made about the anterior lens capsule. At one time, it was popular to remove the entire lens capsule, often with the assistance of alpha-chymotrypsin.[23] This procedure was done to prevent adhesions between the iris, lens capsule and the anterior vitreous, and was felt to be particularly important in patients with penetrating trauma and PVR. We feel that the anterior capsule can be preserved safely if the vitreous is 'shaved' carefully from the area of the vitreous base. This allows concurrent or future placement of a posterior chamber IOL, with haptic fixation in the ciliary sulcus. In uncomplicated cases, it has become routine to use the lens capsule and ciliary sulcus for support of a posterior chamber IOL.[24–29]

Our preferred IOL is made entirely of polymethylmethacrylate, with an optic diameter of 6.5 mm and an overall diameter of 13.5 mm. A sulcus-fixated IOL should have a lens power that is 0.5 diopters less than that calculated for an IOL placed in the capsular bag. A small, central opening can be made in the lens capsule with the vitreous cutter during surgery, or an opening can be made postoperatively with an Nd–YAG laser in the event of opacification.

In summary, the crystalline lens can be removed safely and efficiently via the pars plana using a standard 20-gauge fragmentation instrument in combination with a vitrectomy. This is particularly useful for patients with subluxation of the lens, trauma and in uveitis. In most cases, the anterior capsule can be preserved for the placement of a posterior chamber IOL.

REFERENCES

1. Machemer R. *Vitrectomy: a Pars Plana Approach* (Grune & Stratton: New York, 1975).
2. Peyman GA, Dodich NA. Experimental vitrectomy: instrumentation and surgical technique, *Arch Ophthalmol* (1971) **86**:548–51.
3. Girard LJ. Pars plana lensectomy by ultrasonic fragmentation. I. Versatile and simple technique for cataract removal, *Surv Ophthalmol* (1982) **27**:96–101.
4. Girard LJ. Pars plana lensectomy by ultrasonic fragmentation: 1984. Part I: Updated surgical technique, *Ophthalmic Surg* (1984) **15**:212–16.
5. Girard LJ. Pars plana lensectomy by ultrasonic fragmentation: 1984. Part II: Operative and postoperative complications—avoidance or management, *Ophthalmic Surg* (1984) **15**:217–20.
6. Eide N, Vatne HO, Syrdalen P. Pars plana lensectomy, *Acta Ophthalmol* (1985) **63**:250–3.
7. Girard LJ, Monasterio R, Rodriguez J, Mailman ML, Romano TJ. Pars plana lensectomy and vitrectomy by ultrasonic fragmentation. Part III: Results in eyes without other ocular pathology or an implant, *Ophthalmic Surg* (1985) **16**:765–8.
8. Charles S. *Vitreous Microsurgery*, 2nd edn (Williams and Wilkins: Baltimore, 1987).
9. Flynn HW Jr, Davis JL, Culbertson WW. Pars plana lensectomy and vitrectomy for complicated cataracts in juvenile rheumatoid arthritis, *Ophthalmology* (1988) **95**:1114–19.
10. Fox GM, Flynn HW Jr, Davis JL, Culbertson W. Causes of reduced visual acuity on long-term follow-up after cataract extraction in patients with uveitis and juvenile rheumatoid arthritis, *Am J Ophthalmol* (1992) **114**:708–14.
11. Girard LJ, Rodriguez J, Mailman ML, Romano TJ. Cataract and uveitis management by pars plana lensectomy and vitrectomy by ultrasonic fragmentation, *Retina* (1985) **5**:107–14.
12. Petrilli AM, Belfort R Jr, Abreu MT, et al. Ultrasonic fragmentation of cataract in uveitis, *Retina* (1986) **6**:61–5.

13. Verbraeken H. Pars plana lensectomy in cases of cataract with juvenile chronic uveitis, *Graefes Arch Clin Exp Ophthalmol* (1996) **234**:618–22.
14. Girard LJ, Canizales R, Esnaola N, Rand WJ. Subluxated (ectopic) lenses in adults: long-term results of pars plana lensectomy–vitrectomy by ultrasonic fragmentation with and without a phacoprosthesis, *Ophthalmology* (1990) **97**:462–5.
15. Girard LJ. Pars plana lensectomy for subluxated and dislocated lenses, *Ophthalmic Surg* (1981) **12**:491–5.
16. Hakin KN, Jacobs M, Rosen P, Taylor D, Cooling RJ. Management of the subluxed crystalline lens, *Ophthalmology* (1992) **99**:542–5.
17. Halpert M, BenEzra D. Surgery of the hereditary subluxated lens in children, *Ophthalmology* (1996) **103**:681–6.
18. Koenig SB, Mieler WF. Management of ectopia lentis in a family with Marfan syndrome, *Arch Ophthalmol* (1996) **114**:1058–61.
19. Soheilian M, Ahmadieh H, Afghan MH, et al. Posterior segment triple surgery after traumatic eye injuries, *Ophthalmic Surg* (1995) **26**:338–42.
20. Fine IH. Cortical cleaving hydrodissection, *J Cataract Refract Surg* (1992) **18**:508–12.
21. Gimbel HV. Divide and conquer nucleofractis phacoemulsification: development and variations, *J Cataract Refract Surg* (1991) **17**:281–91.
22. Masket S. 'Phaco-chop' or 'divide and conquer'. *Oper Techn Cataract Refract Surg* (1998) **1**:47–50.
23. Lewis H, Aaberg TM, Abrams GW, Han DP, Kreiger AE. Management of the lens capsule during pars plana lensectomy, *Am J Ophthalmol* (1987) **103**:109–10.
24. Blankenship GW, Flynn HW Jr, Kokame GT. Posterior chamber intraocular lens insertion during pars plana lensectomy and vitrectomy for complications of proliferative diabetic retinopathy, *Am J Ophthalmol* (1989) **108**:1–5.
25. Blankenship GW. Posterior chamber intraocular lens implantation during pars plana lensectomy and vitrectomy for diabetic complications, *Graefes Arch Clin Exp Ophthalmol* (1989) **227**:136–8.
26. Kokame GT, Flynn HW Jr, Blankenship GW. Posterior chamber intraocular lens implantation during diabetic pars plana vitrectomy, *Ophthalmology* (1989) **96**:603–10.
27. Pang MP, Peyman GA, Minatoya HK. Posterior chamber lens implantation following pars plana lensectomy and vitrectomy in severe proliferative diabetic retinopathy, *Can J Ophthalmol* (1989) **24**:175–8.
28. Slusher MM, Greven CM, Yu DD. Posterior chamber intraocular lens implantation combined with lensectomy–vitrectomy and intraretinal foreign-body removal, *Arch Ophthalmol* (1992) **110**:127–9.
29. Uchida H, Ogino N. Pars plana lensectomy preserving a clear anterior capsule in vitreous surgery, *Nippon Ganka Gakkai Zasshi* (1991) **95**:1117–23.

Chapter 15 Endocyclophotocoagulation

Jennifer I Lim

INTRODUCTION

Endocyclophotocoagulation is a useful treatment alternative to filtration surgery for selected patients with uncontrolled glaucoma. The goal is to achieve sufficient destruction of the ciliary body to lower the intraocular pressure (IOP) but to spare enough ciliary body to avoid hypotony. The idea of selective destruction of the ciliary body via laser was first reported by Lee in 1979.[1] Shields then showed that destruction of the anterior ciliary body could be achieved while sparing the posterior ciliary body.[2] However, transpupillary destruction required a clear media with a widely dilated pupil to allow visualization of the ciliary processes.

With the advent of vitrectomy surgery, a direct approach was possible. Charles reported direct photocoagulation of the ciliary body in the manuscript describing the initial applications of his xenon endolaser probe in 1981.[3] Patel et al showed that this could be achieved successfully in 14/18 treated eyes.[4] Later, Lim et al combined endocyclophotocoagulation with vitrectomy techniques to treat vitreoretinal diseases with concomitant glaucoma.[5] Haller reported a variety of eyes that underwent endocyclophotocoagulation, including eyes that failed prior conventional glaucoma surgery, those with combined vitreoretinal disease and uncontrolled glaucoma, those with anterior-segment scarring precluding filtration surgery and eyes with corneal scars and penetrating keratoplasty.[6] The argon laser was used in these series. Recent work by Immonen et al in rabbits demonstrated that the diode laser can also achieve destructive lesions in the ciliary body.[7]

INDICATIONS

Indications for the use of endocyclophotocoagulation include:

- Prior failed filtration surgeries.
- Conjunctival scarring and uncontrolled glaucoma.
- Neovascular glaucoma with no view posteriorly.
- Penetrating keratoplasty and glaucoma.
- Vitreoretinal diseases requiring vitrectomy and uncontrolled glaucoma.

For eyes with glaucoma alone, this procedure is reserved as an alternative cyclodestructive procedure when filtration surgery has failed. When filtration surgery cannot be performed readily because of severe conjunctival scarring, endocyclophotocoagulation is a good procedure. For eyes with both uncontrolled glaucoma and vitreoretinal disease requiring pars plana vitrectomy, ciliary body ablation is a good alternative to conventional filtration surgery with or without a seton procedure. Children and adults with uncontrolled glaucoma despite prior surgical procedures may benefit from this procedure.

METHODS

A pars plana vitrectomy is performed and any vitreoretinal pathology is addressed before attention is turned to the ciliary body. In aphakic or pseudophakic patients, direct visualization of the entire length of the ciliary processes is achieved through the pupillary space by using scleral depression.

When visualizing the processes through the pupillary space, tangential illumination from the operating microscope is best. A scleral plug is placed into one sclerotomy site and the endolaser probe is placed through the other sclerotomy site. The IOP is lowered to the 8–12 mmHg range to soften the eye and allow firm scleral depression and rotation of the ciliary processes into view. The surgeon uses one hand to depress the ciliary body into view and the other hand to apply the laser treatment (Fig. 15.1).

The peripheral retina is brought into view by using a cotton-tipped applicator held slightly horizontally to the sclera, corresponding to the ora serrata. The cotton-tipped applicator is then rolled anteriorly (twirled between the thumb and forefinger) until the ciliary processes are seen through the pupillary space. The globe will be significantly distorted at this point.

The laser is set to a continuous mode of energy delivery. The area opposite the probe entry site is treated first (Fig. 15.2). The argon laser energy is increased or decreased at 50-mW increments from 300 mW until a white spot is created on the ciliary process, without excessive energy delivery. Excessive

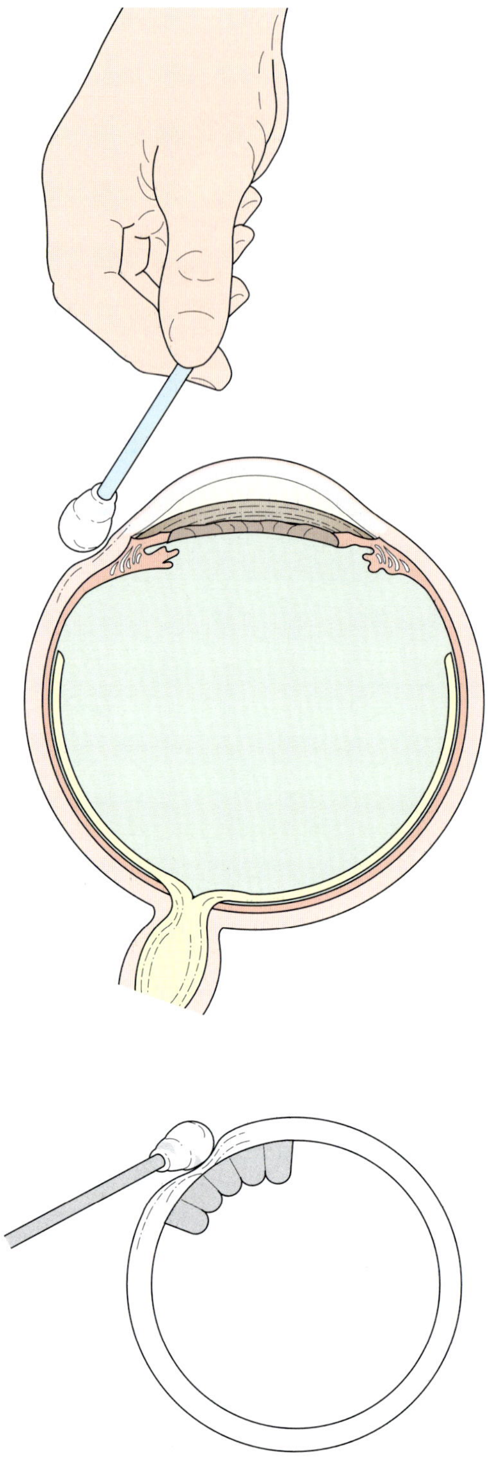

Figure 15.1 *Scleral depression with a cotton-tipped applicator brings the processes into view through the dilated pupil in aphakic or pseudophakic patients. Surgeon's hand in area to be treated depresses ciliary body into view; other hand uses endolaser to treat processes. (a) Scleral depression. (b) Processes seen through the pupil.*

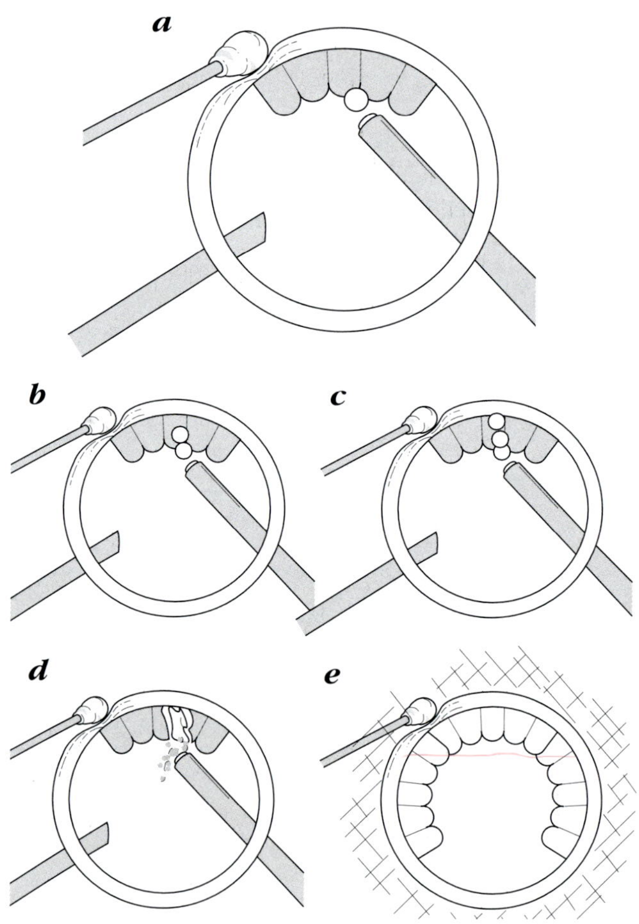

Figure 15.2 *(a) Begin laser treatment to the processes at anterior-most tip. (b,c) Proceed down length of process. (d) Excessive energy results in liberated pigment cloud. (e) Treat the inferior 270°.*

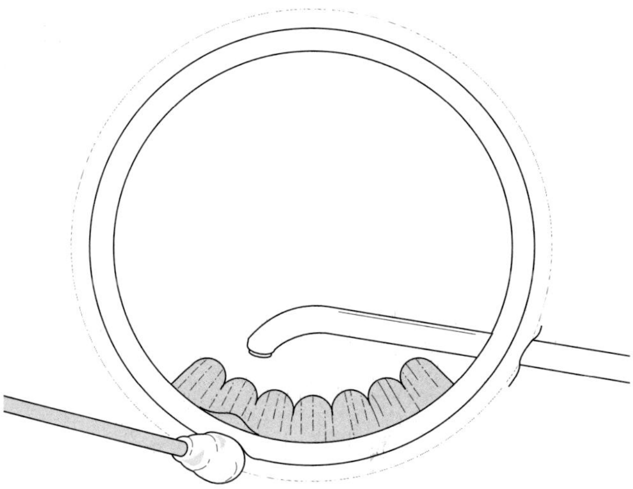

Figure 15.3 *In patients who require additional treatment, the curved laser probe is useful for treating the superior clock-hours.*

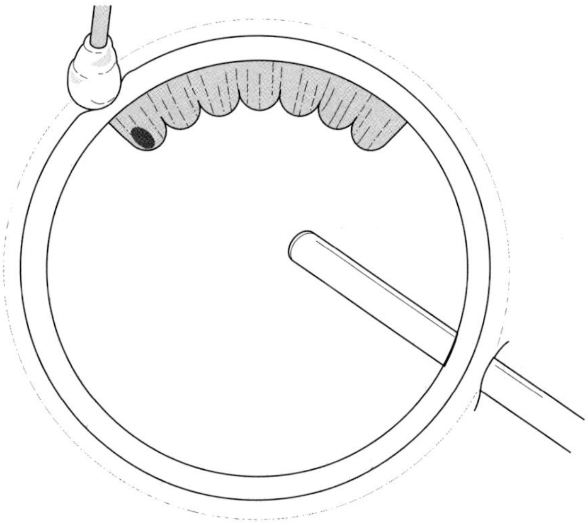

Figure 15.5 *Illuminated laser probe allows use of a contact lens system.*

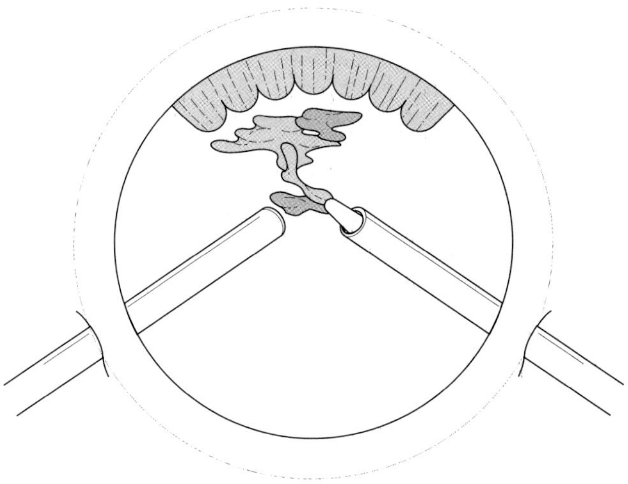

Figure 15.4 *Aspirating silicone-tipped instrument removes the liberated pigment debris.*

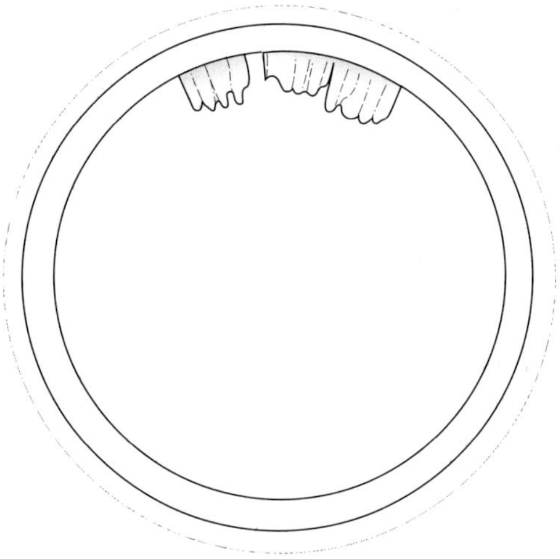

Figure 15.6 *The treated ciliary processes should appear gray-white and shrunken.*

energy may result in an audible 'popping' sound, a visible bubble and liberated pigment intraocularly. This situation should be avoided while still achieving whitening and shrinkage of the ciliary body processes.

The inferior 240–270° of the ciliary body are the easiest to treat. Treatment should proceed from one sclerotomy site toward the 6 o'clock meridian, at which point treatment sites are switched and the laser probe is inserted into the other sclerotomy site. The remaining clock-hours from 6 o'clock to the other sclerotomy site are then treated. When it is necessary to treat more superior areas of the ciliary body, the curved laser probe is useful (Fig. 15.3).

After completion of the laser treatment, any liberated pigment or ciliary body debris is aspirated using the silicone-tipped cannula (Fig. 15.4). If an illuminated laser probe is used, a contact lens system may be employed through the cornea (Fig. 15.5). After completion of laser treatment, the ciliary processes should appear gray-white and shrunken (Fig. 15.6). Topical prednisolone sulfate 1% is given every 4–6

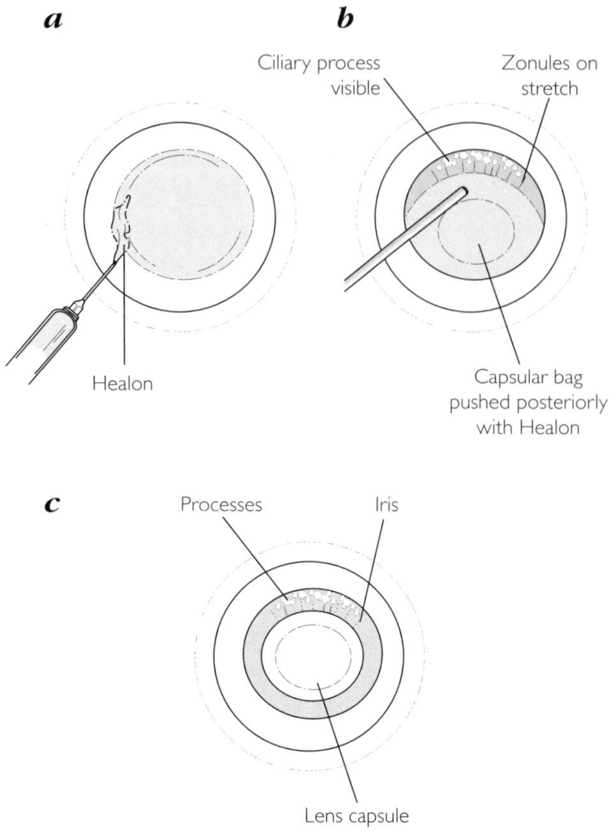

Figure 15.7 *(a) In pseudophakic patients, deepen the retropupillary space and anterior chamber with Healon. (b) Insert endoscopic laser probe held 2–3 mm from ciliary processes to treat the processes. (c) The entire length of the processes is then whitened.*

hours postoperatively, along with atropine 1%. If the IOP is elevated, topical glaucoma medications may be added. The medications will require titration as the laser effect becomes manifest over the next 4–6 weeks.

Scleral depression is not required for visualization if an endoscopic delivery system is available (see Chapter 16). In that case, a 20-gauge endoscopic diode laser probe is directed toward the ciliary processes and visualization is via a monitor. Endoscopic visualization of the ciliary processes enables direct visualization during delivery of endolaser photocoagulation to the ciliary processes.[8]

Uram described endoscopic laser delivery to the ciliary processes combined with phacoemulsification and intraocular lens implantation.[9] The anterior chamber is entered and a viscoelastic substance is injected to deepen the chamber (Fig. 15.7) and to displace the bag posteriorly. The endolaser probe tip is inserted through a limbal incision, posterior to the iris but 'over the bag' and posterior to the area of ciliary body to be treated. The viscoelastic substance keeps the lens capsular bag away from the iris and allows visualization of the processes to be treated. This method can be used in pseudophakes.

The entire length of the ciliary process is then whitened and shrunken using the endolaser endoscopic probe with direct visualization. The diode laser is set to 200 mW initially and the energy is increased in 50-mW increments to achieve the desired results. The duration is set for 2–3 seconds.

RESULTS

Patel et al reported transient vitreous hemorrhage in 2/18 eyes, transient choroidal detachment in 2/18 eyes and hypotony in one eye.[4] Lim et al described 24 eyes of patients with concomitant retinal conditions and uncontrolled glaucoma treated by pars plana vitrectomy and endolaser to the ciliary body.[5] Control of the IOP was achieved in 86%. Visual acuity fell in 47%; most of these were eyes with severe proliferative diabetic retinopathy and neovascular glaucoma. In the series by Lim et al,[5] 19% of eyes developed hypotony. Complications other than those related to hypotony were not seen in this series.

In the series by Haller et al, IOP control was achieved in 87% of patients 1 year postoperatively and in 68% at the last follow-up.[6] The complication rate was 12% and included hypotony, choroidal detachments (spontaneously resolved), uveitis with fibrin and graft failure. Sixteen percent required reoperation to control the IOP. Visual acuity increased in 32%, decreased in 27% and remained unchanged in 41%. The eyes with the best IOP response were eyes with glaucoma and prior or simultaneous penetrating keratoplasty. The IOP was controlled successfully in 91% of the penetrating keratoplasty eyes and in 87% at 1 year overall (68% of final follow-up). In eyes with significant conjunctival scarring, this approach may be a useful alternative.

Uram noted a mean decrease of 65% in the IOP in eyes with intractable neovascular glaucoma following microendoscopic laser ablation of the ciliary processes.[9] In eyes with intraocular lenses, the mean

IOP decrease was 57%; visual acuity improved in all patients postoperatively and there were no significant complications. The IOP decreased from a mean of 31.4 to 13.5 mmHg. Good IOP control without any topical medication was achieved in half of the patients. Visual acuity improved. Only one eye developed a transient vitreous hemorrhage postoperatively.

POSTOPERATIVE MANAGEMENT

Topical prednisolone forte 1% and atropine sulfate 1% are used to control inflammation after surgery. Any topical glaucoma medication is tapered over the ensuing 4–6 weeks. The best IOP is not achieved until that time postoperatively.

Indications for reoperation include both uncontrolled glaucoma after waiting at least 2 months postoperatively and any retinal condition that requires intervention.

Ciliary body ablation is an alternative treatment to conventional filtration surgery or to filtration surgery with setons for eyes with uncontrolled glaucoma. In patients with conjunctival scarring or extensive vitreoretinal conditions, endocyclophotocoagulation is a good choice. Treatment of more than 270° may lead to hypotony postoperatively and should be avoided. The full effect of the endolaser treatment requires several weeks to become manifest.

REFERENCES

1. Lee PF. Argon laser photocoagulation of the ciliary processes in cases of aphakic glaucoma, *Arch Ophthalmol* (1979) **97**:2135–8.
2. Shields MB, Chandler DB, Hickingbotham D, Klintworth GK. Intraocular cyclophotocoagulation: histopathologic evaluation in primates, *Arch Ophthalmol* (1985) **103**:1731–5.
3. Charles S. Endophotocoagulation, *Retina* (1981) **1**:117–20.
4. Patel A, Thompson JT, Michels RG, Quigley HA. Endolaser treatment of the ciliary body for uncontrolled glaucoma, *Ophthalmology* (1986) **93**:825–30.
5. Lim JI, Lynn M, Capone A Jr, et al. Ciliary body endophotocoagulation during pars plana vitrectomy in eyes with vitreoretinal disorders and concomitant uncontrolled glaucoma, *Ophthalmology* (1996) **103**:1041–6.
6. Haller JA. Transvitreal endocyclophotocoagulation, *Trans Am Ophthalmol Soc* (1996) **94**:589–676.
7. Immonen I, Viherkoski E, Peyman GA. Experimental retinal and ciliary body photocoagulation using a new 670-nm diode laser, *Am J Ophthalmol* (1996) **122**:870–4.
8. Uram M. Ophthalmic laser microendoscope endophotocoagulation, *Ophthalmology* (1992) **99**:1829–32.
9. Uram M. Combined phacoemulsification, endoscopic ciliary process photocoagulation, and intraocular lens implantation in glaucoma management, *Ophthalmic Surg* (1995) **26**:346–52.

Chapter 16 Endolaser

Jennifer I Lim

INTRODUCTION

The development of endophotocoagulation significantly advanced the scope of vitreoretinal surgery. The argon green and diode lasers are most frequently used for vitreoretinal surgery. The erbium–YAG laser has been evaluated recently for use in vitreoretinal surgery; however, this chapter will focus upon vitreoretinal surgical applications of the argon green and diode lasers.

The first photocoagulation probe for vitreoretinal surgery was developed by Charles in 1979[1,2] using a portable xenon arc coagulator. He reported his experience with the initial 169 eyes in which the endophotocoagulator was used to stop bleeding, treat retinal tears, apply scatter photocoagulation, coagulate ciliary processes and enlarge the pupil in eyes with miotic pupils and iris neovascularization. The indications described by Charles are applicable to the lasers in use today.

The xenon arc light, however, was not ideal for vitreoretinal surgery. The xenon arc light's angle of divergence required a short working distance and the xenon arc generated heat that prohibited rapid firing applications. Peyman and associates developed an endolaser probe for the argon laser and reported its use for panretinal photocoagulation and laser wall-off around posterior retinal breaks during vitrectomy surgery.[3–8]

The advantages of the argon laser over the xenon light are its smaller angle of divergence, which facilitates a more comfortable and safe working distance, a finer spot size and a reproducible endpoint. In addition, the argon endoprobe tip withstands rapid laser applications and may be fired through air or gas.

Proper endolaser filter positioning is important to protect the operating surgeon from the laser flash; the filter was developed initially by Carroll and Peyman.[9] Currently used lasers are not functional unless the filter is connected properly to the operating microscope. However, it is possible that the filter may be connected above the observer scope and that the assistant may not be protected from the laser light. Thus, one should check that the filter connection is positioned to protect both the surgeon and the assistant (Fig. 16.1).

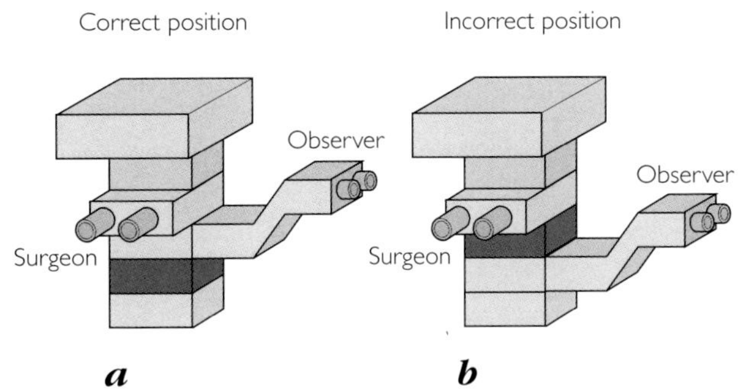

Figure 16.1 *Laser filter (shaded area) should be connected to the microscope to protect both the surgeon and assistant. (a) Correct placement. (b) Incorrect placement.*

The intensity of the laser burn depends upon the duration and power settings of the laser, the degree of underlying pigmentation, the working distance of the endolaser tip from the retinal surface and the angulation of the endolaser tip relative to the retinal surface. Longer duration, higher power settings, more pigmentation of tissues and decreased working distance of the endolaser probe tip to the retinal surface result in more intense laser uptake (Table 16.1). Blood on the retinal surface, which will absorb the laser energy and could result in inadvertent retinal scarring, should be avoided.

During vitrectomy procedures, the endolaser is used most commonly to create a laser barricade around retinal holes, surround retinectomy edges or giant retinal tear margins and deliver scatter laser photocoagulation. Less common applications include

Table 16.1 Treatment parameters that vary the laser energy output

	Increased coagulation response	*Decreased coagulation response*
Duration	Longer	Shorter
Power	Higher	Lower
Underlying pigment	More	Less
Working distance	Shorter	Longer
Angulation of tip	Less	More

endolaser to ciliary processes and to choroidal neovascular membranes.

INSTRUMENTATION

The 20-gauge endolaser probe is available in various styles: straight versus curved,[6] blunt versus tapered tip and simple versus aspirating[7] or illuminating (Fig. 16.2).[8,10] The straight blunt or tapered tip is the most commonly used style. The tapered tip facilitates insertion into the sclerotomy site.

The curved tip[6] is used to apply laser photocoagulation around curves, in the superior clock-hours and in the more anterior peripheral retina. This tip is most useful for applying laser treatment on the anterior superior ridge of retina supported on a scleral buckle and on the peripheral retina near the surgeon's dominant hand (Fig. 16.3).

Modifications of the basic endolaser probe include illumination, aspiration or a combination of these functions.[7,8,10] The aspirating tip is useful for applying endolaser around retinal holes (Fig. 16.4). The passive aspiration system removes accumulated subretinal fluid or blood from the edges of retinal holes. The illuminated endolaser probe frees the surgeon's other hand, which then can be used for bimanual surgical techniques within the eye or scleral

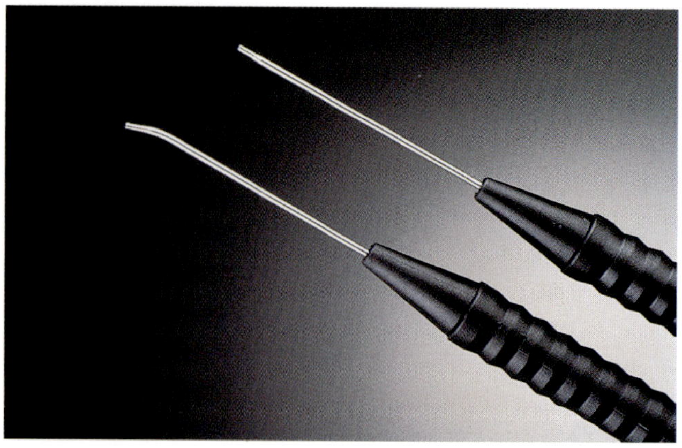

a

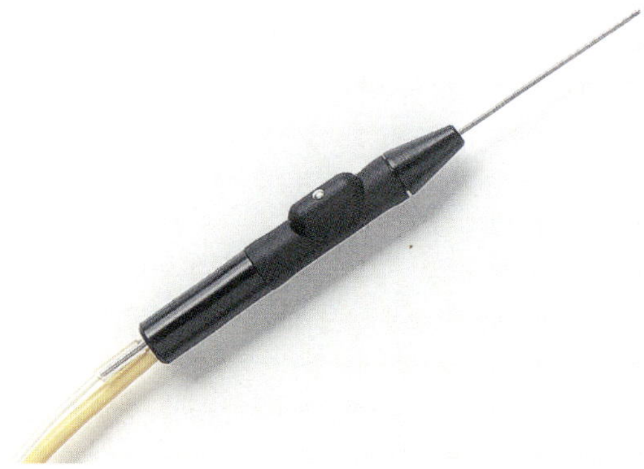

b

Figure 16.2 *Endolaser probe styles. (a) Left: Occulite curved, tapered tip. Right: Occulite straight tapered tip, courtesy of Coherent Co. (b) Aspirating probe, courtesy of Iris Medical Company.*

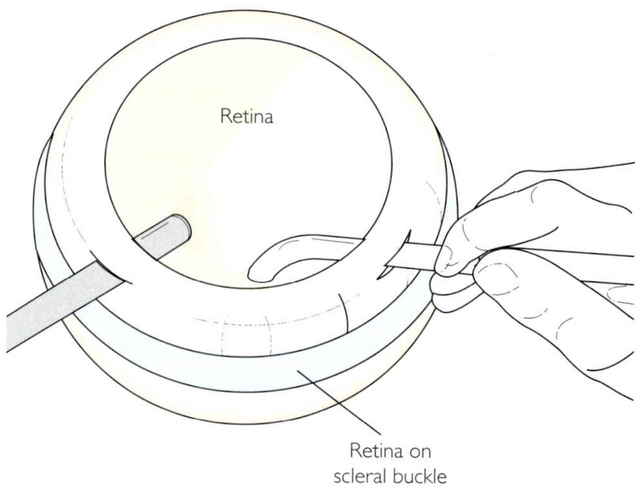

Figure 16.3 *Curved tip is useful for applying endolaser around curved surfaces. Note the utility of the curved tip in applying laser onto the anterior retina supported on the scleral buckle and onto the retina adjacent to the surgeon's operating hand.*

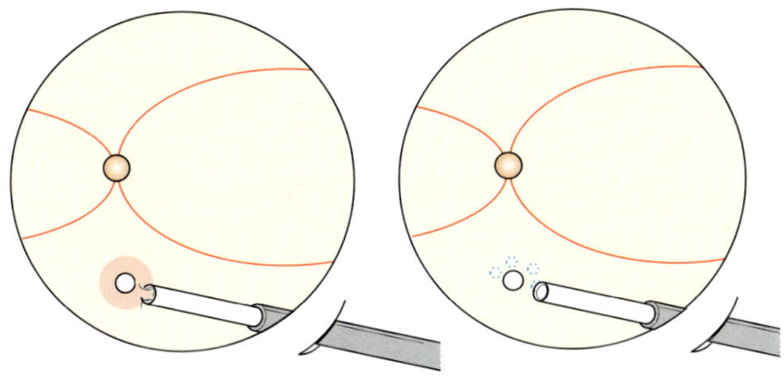

Figure 16.4 *Aspirating laser probe is useful for removing subretinal fluid from around the edges of retinal holes.*

depression to aid visualization of peripheral retina while applying laser internally. Awh et al described a probe in which illumination and laser emission are fused.[10]

Another mode of endolaser delivery is the ophthalmic laser endoscopic system.[11] This system consists of a 20-gauge probe that permits endoscopic visualization of internal ocular structures, delivers diode laser spots and illuminates the retina. The view is via a television monitor. It is useful when there are anterior segment or other anatomic factors that are impediments to a clear posterior view.

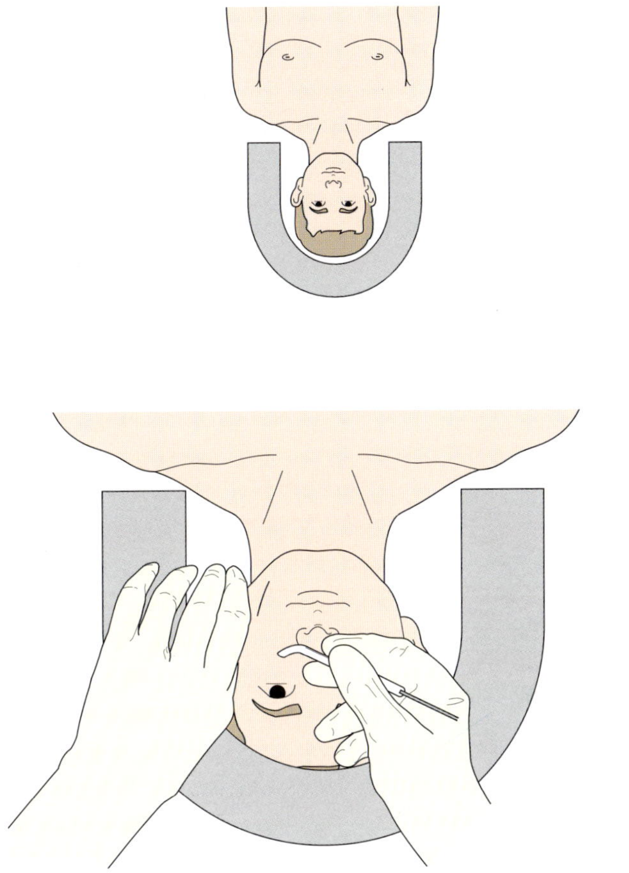

Figure 16.5 *The surgeon's hand should be supported on wrist rests. The endolaser probe should be held as a writing instrument.*

SURGICAL TECHNIQUE

The surgeon's hand should be supported firmly on wrist rests and the instrument held as a writing instrument (Fig. 16.5). The endolaser tip should be perpendicular to a tangent along the retinal surface to be treated. This will ensure that the aiming beam casts a round spot onto the retina and that a uniform laser burn is achieved. Oblique positioning of the probe at the retinal surface results in an irregular and elliptical laser spot and non-uniform laser burns (Fig. 16.6).

The initial settings of the argon laser should be for a duration of 0.1–0.2 seconds and a power of 200 mW. The initial diode laser settings should be 0.2–0.3 seconds with 300 mW. The power should be adjusted incrementally (30–50-mW steps) until a light gray-white spot is achieved. Increasing the duration to the next level to gain the desired effect at lower energy settings than otherwise required may be advisable. A continuous setting is sometimes useful for

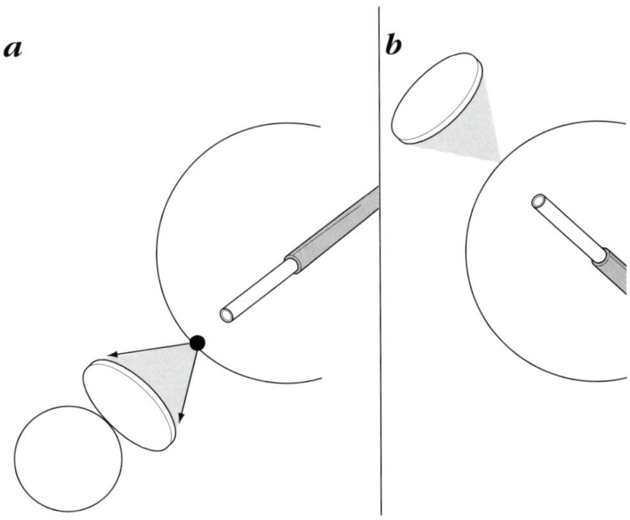

Figure 16.6 *The position of the endolaser probe relative to the retinal surface varies the effect achieved. (a) Probe perpendicular: round, even spot. (b) Probe oblique: oblong, non-uniform spot.*

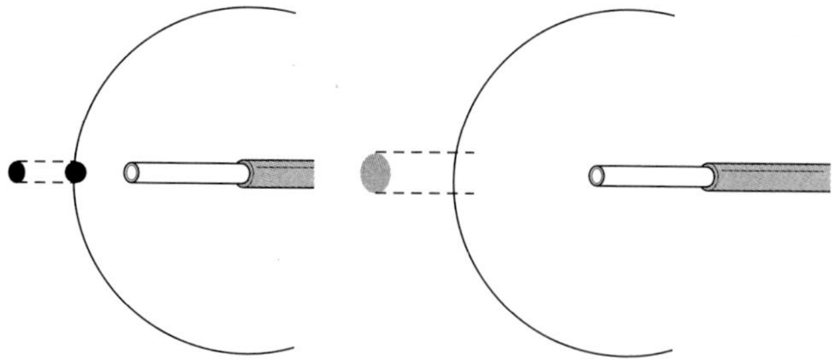

Figure 16.7 *Working distance and effect on laser output. Increasing the working distance with the same laser energy results in less uptake.*

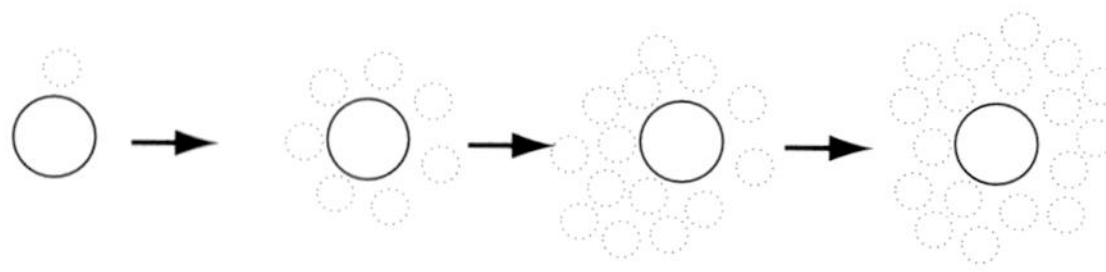

Figure 16.8 *Laser treatment around the retinal hole. Individual spots to surround the hole.*

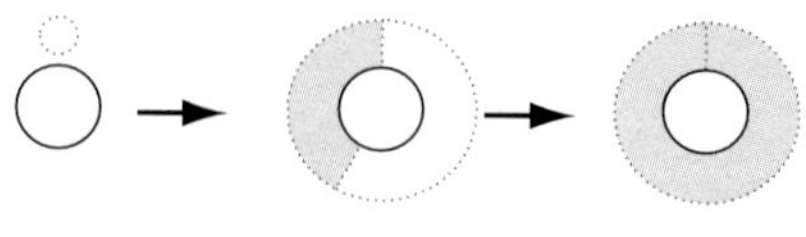

Figure 16.9 *Continuous laser band around the hole.*

treating retinotomies and for achieving hemostasis in areas of active hemorrhage.

The diode laser[7,12,13] has been proven safe, reliable and as effective as the argon laser. One must wait a few seconds for the laser treatment spot to become visible in order to achieve maximum intensity when using the diode. Thus, adjustments of laser power or other parameters should be staged to allow laser spot maturation.

If the laser burn spot size is too small, the working distance should be increased and the power setting adjusted. As the laser spot size increases, the intensity of the laser burn decreases (if no adjustment of laser power is made). Thus, the laser power must be increased to achieve the same burn intensity (Fig. 16.7).

INDICATIONS

RETINAL HOLE

The goal of laser treatment is to surround the retinal hole with two to three rows of laser photocoagulation. In order to achieve a laser burn, there must be no surrounding subretinal fluid. The presence of subretinal fluid around the hole insulates the retinal pigment epithelium from the laser. Subretinal fluid can be removed from the edges of the hole using a passive aspirating fluted needle, preferably silicone tipped. The endolaser probe with a surrounding aspiration tube is useful for removing subretinal fluid or hemorrhage from the area to be treated, obviating the need to switch instruments within the eye; the laser is applied before more fluid accumulates.

Multiple individual laser spots may be applied to surround the hole (Fig. 16.8). Alternatively, one continuous band of laser may be placed around the hole. The endolaser probe may be used to 'paint' the area around the hole with a continuous ring of laser treatment (Fig. 16.9).

RETINECTOMIES AND GIANT RETINAL TEARS

When retinal photocoagulation is placed around large areas of detached retina, a perfluorocarbon liquid may be used to hold the retina in position and the laser is applied through the perfluorocarbon liquid, which is then exchanged with air. This sequence maximizes the opportunity for laser placement when the visibility is at its best, before the air–fluid exchange.

Rows of peripheral laser treatment are sometimes applied to 'wall-off' the area of prior detachment in eyes with reattached retinas in the setting of proliferative vitreoretinopathy and cytomegalovirus retinitis. The reattached retina is frequently lasered on the scleral buckle. Scleral depression can facilitate visualization of the peripheral retina to be treated (Fig. 16.10). If a wide-angle viewing system is available, scleral depression may not be necessary (Fig. 16.11).

PANRETINAL LASER PHOTOCOAGULATION

For panretinal laser treatment, the goal is to achieve a laser pattern similar to that obtained using the slit-lamp or indirect laser delivery systems. With the endolaser, however, the more peripheral areas of retina are accessible (Fig. 16.12). The lens must be

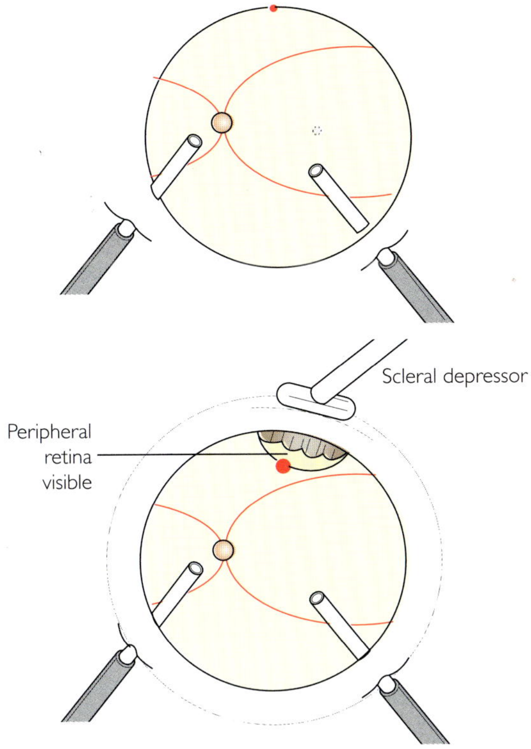

Figure 16.10 *Scleral depression of the peripheral retina enables visualization of the peripheral retina and allows laser application.*

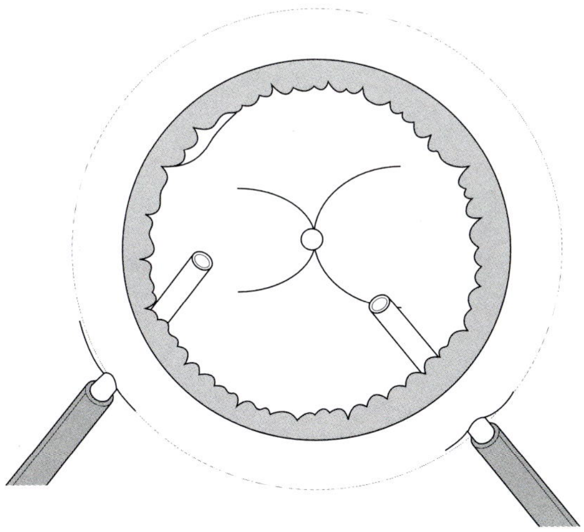

Figure 16.11 *Wide-angle viewing system affords a view of the peripheral retina without scleral depression.*

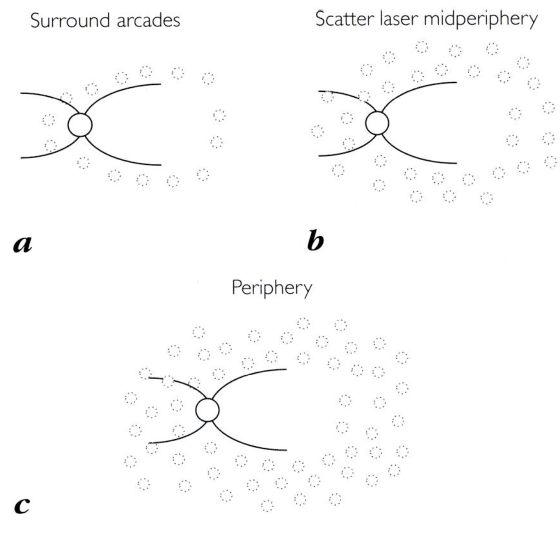

Figure 16.12 *Laser scatter pattern in eyes with proliferative retinopathy: (a) surround arcades, (b) scatter laser midperiphery, (c) periphery.*

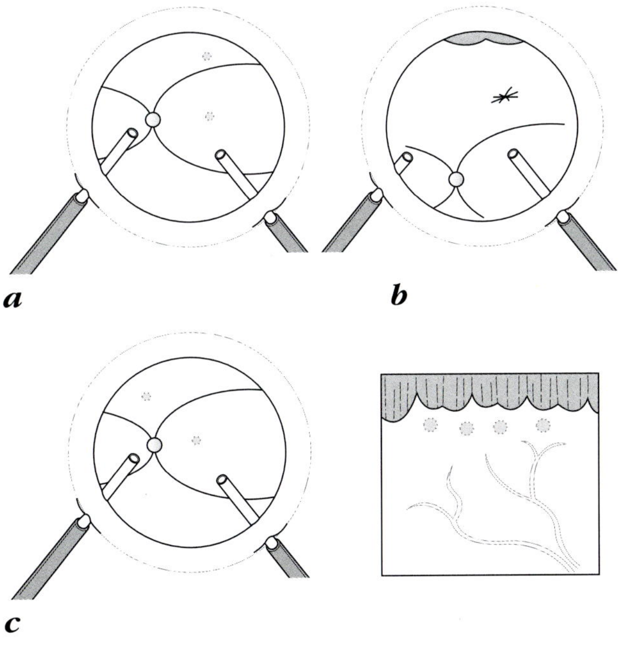

Figure 16.13 *Other methods to visualize the peripheral retina: (a) normal position; (b) tilted eyeball position; (c) endoscopic delivery of endolaser.*

avoided during the procedure by careful attention to the location of the instruments when crossing the lens equator. One can also tilt the eyeball in the direction of retinal photocoagulation, use a prism or wide-angle viewing contact lens system or use an endoscopic delivery system to view the periphery (Fig. 16.13).

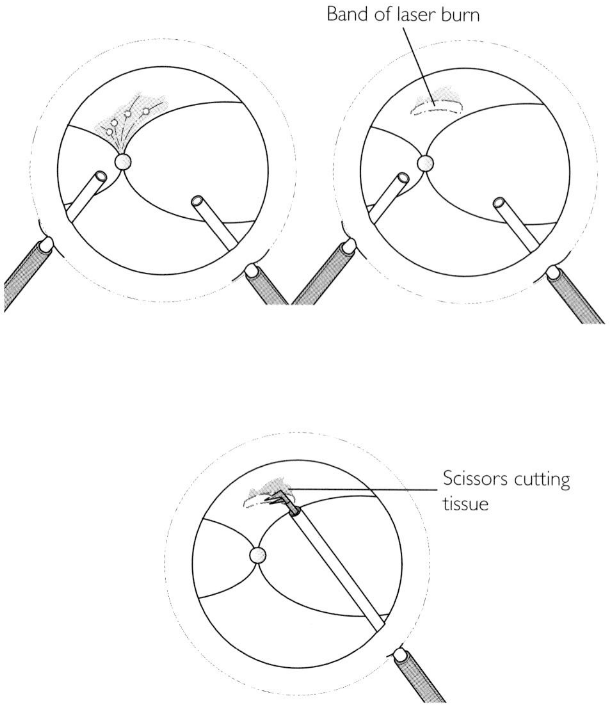

Figure 16.14 *Apply laser to neovascularized tissue prior to transecting membranes.*

RETINAL VESSEL PHOTOCOAGULATION

Application of laser photocoagulation to tissues before cutting neovascular tissues or performing retinectomies may minimize bleeding (Fig. 16.14). An argon green laser is the laser of choice because it is best absorbed by blood. Caution is necessary in applying this laser to areas of vascularized retina in order to prevent inadvertent vascular occlusions.

Diathermy remains another useful alternative for elevated areas of neovascularization. Subretinal vessel photocoagulation has been described in combination with subretinal surgery for choroidal neovascularization.[14]

COMPLICATIONS

Retinal complications of endolaser, including retinal necrosis, choroidal neovascularization and tears, result from laser treatment that is too intense or from direct impact onto the retinal surface. Choroidal neovascularization is a known complication of intense laser applications. A retinal hemorrhage with breaks in Bruch's membrane may result in an audible 'popping' sound. This break in Bruch's membrane may serve as the site of ingrowth of the choroidal neovascularization.

Laser energy that is too intense may cause retinal necrosis, which may be avoided by titrating the energy from barely visible levels to the desired light gray to light yellow-white spot. Areas covered with retinal hemorrhage, which absorb the laser energy, should be avoided. When approaching areas of heavier pigmentation than the preceding area of treatment, one should titrate the power to a lower setting in order to avoid excessive delivery of laser to that region.

Positioning the probe tip too close to the retina may result in inadvertent retinal adhesion to the tip. Contusions from the probe tip may lead to retinal holes, subretinal hemorrhage and possible choroidal neovascularization or scar formation in the future.[15]

Endolaser is an extremely useful and sometimes indispensable component of vitreoretinal surgery. With the proper laser energy settings and careful application of the endolaser probe, the benefits of endolaser far exceed the potential complications.

REFERENCES

1. Charles S. Endophotocoagulation, *Ophthalmol Times* (1979) **4**:68–9.
2. Charles S, Endophotocoagulation, *Retina* (1981) **1**:117–20.
3. Peyman GA, Grisolano JM, Palacio MN. Intraocular photocoagulation with the argon-krypton laser, *Arch Ophthalmol* (1980) **98**:2062–64.
4. Peyman GA, Salzano TC, Green JL Jr. Argon endolaser, *Arch Ophthalmol* (1981) **99**:2037–8.
5. Peyman GA, Conway MD, Ganti SD, Durant W, Viherkoski E. Argon, krypton, and neodymium–YAG–endolasers, *Doc Ophthalmol Proc Ser* (1984) **36**:277–87.
6. Peyman GA. A bent-tipped endolaser probe, *Ophthalmic Surg* (1987) **18**:185–6.
7. Peyman GA, D'Amico DJ, Alturki WA. An endolaser probe with aspiration capability, *Arch Ophthalmol* (1992) **110**:718.
8. Peyman GA, Lee KJ. Multifunction endolaser probe (letter), *Am J Ophthalmol* (1992) **114**:103–4.

9. Carroll CP, Peyman GA. A microscope filter for endophotocoagulation, *Arch Ophthalmol* (1981) **99**:327.
10. Awh CC, Schallen EH, de Juan E Jr. An illuminating laser probe for vitreoretinal surgery, *Arch Ophthalmol* (1994) **112**:553–4.
11. Uram M. Ophthalmic laser microendoscope endophotocoagulation, *Ophthalmology* (1992) **99**:1829–32.
12. Smiddy WE. Diode endolaser photocoagulation, *Arch Ophthalmol* (1992) **110**:1172–4.
13. Sasoh M, Smiddy WE. Diode laser endophotocoagulation, *Retina* (1995) **15**:388–93.
14. Thomas MA, Ibanez HE. Subretinal endophotocoagulation in the treatment of choroidal neovascularization, *Am J Ophthalmol* (1993) **116**:279–85.
15. Escoffery RF. Subretinal neovascularization following endophotocoagulation, *Retina* (1981) **1**:211–15.

Chapter 17 Intraocular gases and techniques for air–fluid exchange

John T Thompson

INTRODUCTION

Intraocular gas bubbles are important tools in vitreoretinal surgery, used primarily for their ability to provide an internal tamponade for retinal breaks. The high surface tension between gas and saline prevents vitreous fluid from entering a retinal break as long as the gas bubble covers the retinal break. This allows the retinal pigment epithelium (RPE) to absorb any remaining subretinal fluid, permitting the retina to reattach.

Intraocular gas bubbles are used less commonly as a temporary vitreous replacement in conjunction with removal of vitreous hemorrhage following vitrectomy to decrease the total amount of blood that must be absorbed. Intraocular gas bubbles are used occasionally for their flotation force, for example, unrolling the edges of a giant retinal tear.

Intraocular gas bubbles are injected into the eye using two basic techniques. The first technique exchanges the vitreous fluid with a gas bubble, where most or all of the vitreous fluid is replaced by gas. This allows placement of a large gas bubble that will tamponade a large area of retina. The second technique involves the injection of a small intraocular gas bubble in an eye without prior vitrectomy, to provide a focal tamponade for a retinal break. This is typically done in an office setting, such as the treatment of rhegmatogenous retinal detachment using pneumatic retinopexy.

INTRAOCULAR GASES AND KINETICS

There are four different intraocular gases that are commonly used in vitreoretinal surgery: air, sulfur hexafluoride (SF_6), perfluoroethane (C_2F_6) and perfluoropropane (C_3F_8). All of these gases are inert in the vitreous cavity. Air does not expand if injected into the vitreous cavity, but pure SF_6, C_2F_6 and C_3F_8 will expand in the vitreous cavity as dissolved air from the bloodstream enters the gas bubble to equilibrate with the intraocular gas bubble. Each of the gases is ultimately absorbed into the bloodstream.

The physical properties of each gas help to determine the indications for usage in vitreoretinal surgery. Each of these gases has different absorption rates in the vitreous cavity, which can allow the surgeon to choose the gas that provides the appropriate tamponade duration based on the characteristics of the retinal pathology, such as the number and location of retinal breaks.

There are two variables concerning the intraocular gas bubble that can be controlled by the surgeon: the size of the intraocular gas bubble and the duration of the gas bubble. In some eyes, it is desirable to have a large, short-acting intraocular gas bubble, such as for treating an inferior tear without vitreoretinal traction in an eye with vitrectomy for a vitreous hemorrhage. A small, short-acting gas bubble may be used for closure of a retinotomy site, such as following removal of submacular choroidal neovascular membrane. A small, long-acting expansile intraocular gas bubble is required in pneumatic retinopexy to tamponade a superior retinal break. A large, long-acting intraocular gas bubble is useful in eyes with multiple retinal breaks in association with proliferative vitreoretinopathy (PVR) or giant retinal tears. Knowledge of the kinetics of intraocular gas mixtures helps the surgeon to choose the most appropriate intraocular bubble size and duration based on the etiology and location of the retinal breaks.

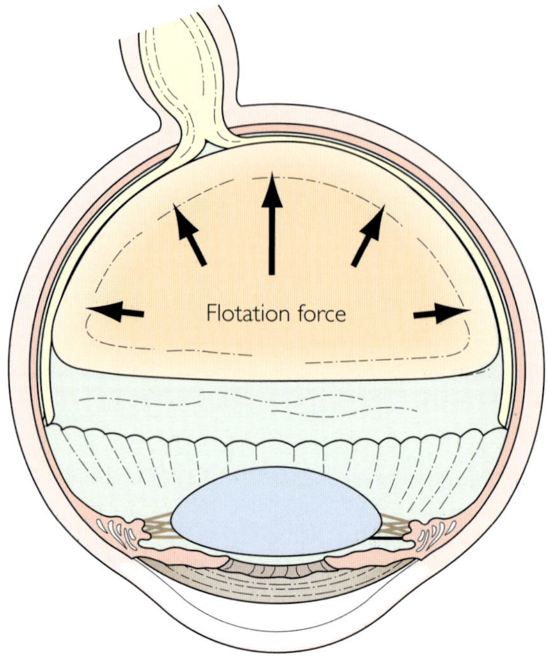

Figure 17.1 *The flotation force of an intraocular gas bubble is maximal at the apex of the bubble. The flotation force and extent of retinal tamponade are also greater for a large intraocular gas bubble compared to a small intraocular gas bubble.*

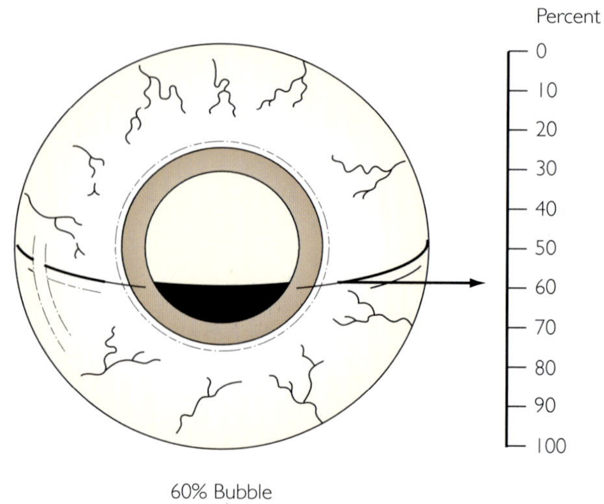

Figure 17.2 *Intraocular gas bubbles are measured in a clinical setting by estimating the percentage of the vertical height of the bubble in the vitreous cavity. A bubble that fills 6/10 of the vitreous cavity is a 60% gas bubble. The superior limbus corresponds to a 25% bubble and the inferior limbus to a 75% gas bubble. It is important to have the patient and examiner level, so that the visual axis is parallel to the floor, to avoid estimation errors induced by parallax.*

The volume of an intraocular gas bubble determines the buoyancy of the intraocular gas bubble. The flotation force is maximal at the apex of the gas bubble, which explains why it is desirable to position patients with the retinal break in the most superior position (Fig. 17.1). The surface tension between the gas bubble and the vitreous fluid is very high, so even a relatively small, perfectly positioned bubble will result in absorption of subretinal fluid in an eye with a retinal detachment. It is usually desirable to use a larger intraocular gas bubble than is needed, because positioning of the patient may not be optimal and nonexpansile bubbles decrease in size as the gas is absorbed from the vitreous. The vitreous cavity volume determines the extent of retinal coverage by a given intraocular gas bubble volume.

Intraocular gas bubbles are normally measured as the vertical meniscus height of the intraocular gas bubble in the eye. This is commonly expressed as a percentage. A 60% gas bubble has the meniscus sixty percent of the way inferior to the superior pole of the eye with the patient upright (Fig. 17.2). It is important when measuring intraocular gas bubbles to have the patient and examiner at the same height, with the patient looking directly ahead, in order to minimize parallax errors, which can be substantial.

The volume of an intraocular gas bubble can be estimated if the bubble meniscus height is known based on geometric models of the average human eye. The relationship between meniscus height and intraocular bubble volume is shown by Eqn. (1) (Fig. 17.3).

$$\int_{-r}^{r-h} \int_{y_0}^{r} \sqrt{r^2 - x^2 - y^2}\, \mathrm{d}y\mathrm{d}x \qquad (1)$$

Table 17.1 gives the approximate volume of the gas bubble with different meniscus heights for phakic, aphakic and pseudophakic eyes.[1,2]

The arc of coverage of the retina by a particular size of intraocular gas bubble can also be estimated based on the volume of the intraocular gas bubble.

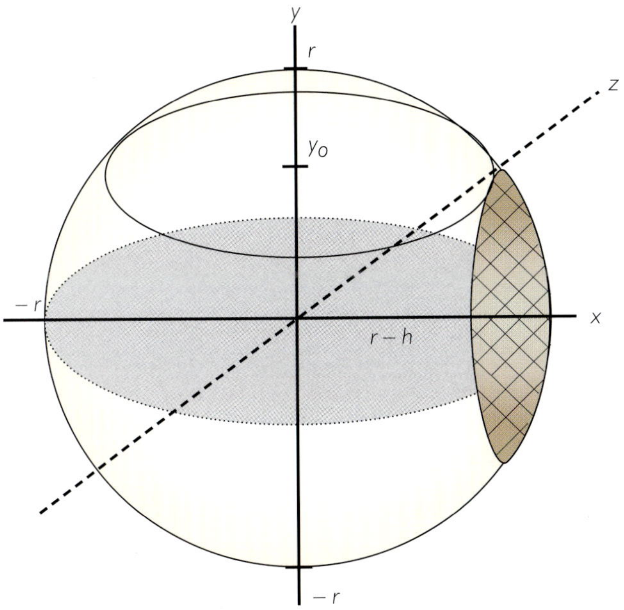

Figure 17.3 *Equation (1). (Reproduced with permission from Thompson JT. Kinetics of intraocular gases: disappearance of air, sulfur hexafluoride, and perfluoropropane after pars plana vitrectomy,* Arch Ophthalmol *(1989)* ***107****:687–91.*[2] *Copyright © 1989, American Medical Association.)*

The extent of coverage is predicted by Eqn. (2):[3,4]

$$\text{Arc of contact} = 2\cos^{-1}[1-(h/r)] = 2\cos^{-1}(1-2p) \quad (2)$$

where h is the height of the gas bubble, r is the radius of the vitreous cavity and p is the percentage of gas fill, expressed as a decimal. In general, an intraocular gas bubble greater than 50% can provide a tamponade for inferior tears with the patient prone because the arc of contact is 180°. An intraocular gas bubble of greater than 20% will provide a tamponade for superior tears with the patient upright or for a macular hole with the patient prone because the arc of contact is about 106°.

The goal of selecting the intraocular gas bubble composition and size is to provide tamponade of sufficient duration to allow a stable chorioretinal adhesion to form around the retinal break (s). A corollary goal is to have an intraocular gas bubble absorb rapidly once the stable chorioretinal adhesion has formed. A small round hole without vitreous traction may only require a few days of tamponade, whereas larger retinal breaks with residual vitreous traction, such as a giant retinal tear with PVR, may warrant several weeks of gas tamponade.

When pure SF_6 or C_3F_8 is placed in an eye, the gas bubble does most of its expansion in 8 hours but may expand slowly up to 96 hours after injection, depending on multiple factors such as the concentration of gas, volume of gas and how rapidly it mixes in the vitreous fluid. The bubble expansion occurs as air (80% nitrogen/20% oxygen) enters the intraocular gas bubble to achieve an equilibrium between the composition of the gas bubble and the bloodstream. The SF_6 or C_3F_8 is relatively insoluble in the bloodstream, so nitrogen and oxygen dissolved in blood initially enter the vitreous cavity gas bubble much faster than SF_6 or C_3F_8 can be absorbed into the circulation. The net effect of air

Table 17.1 Conversion of intraocular bubble size to volume

Bubble meniscus size	*Bubble volume in aphakic eye (ml)*	*Bubble volume in pseudophakic eye (ml)*	*Bubble volume in phakic eye (ml)*
0%	0.0	0.0	0.0
10%	0.15	0.15	0.13
20%	0.54	0.53	0.45
30%	1.12	1.06	0.88
40%	1.83	1.69	1.40
50%	2.60	2.37	1.95
60%	3.37	3.04	2.51
70%	4.08	3.67	3.02
80%	4.66	4.20	3.46
90%	5.06	4.58	3.78
100%	5.20	4.73	3.91

entering the bubble is to increase the volume of the intraocular gas bubble.

The sclera is relatively inelastic compared to a balloon, therefore the intraocular pressure (IOP) may increase because the sclera cannot expand to accommodate the increased gas volume. Aqueous outflow increases to compensate for the increased volume of the gas bubble as it slowly expands, which re-equilibrates the IOP in most eyes with a normal outflow facility. Because it is undesirable to face potentially large increases in IOP in the peri-operative period, most vitreoretinal surgeons use gas mixtures with minimal or no expansion during vitrectomy. A small, pure expansile gas is used in an eye without vitrectomy for pneumatic retinopexy if the goal is a moderate-size gas bubble in the vitreous cavity because it cannot accommodate a large initial bubble volume. The maximum nonexpansile concentration of SF_6 is 20% SF_6/80% air;[5] the maximum nonexpansile concentration of C_3F_8 is 12% C_3F_8/88% air.[6]

The concentration of the intraocular gas is chosen to achieve the desired duration of tamponade based on the number and location of the tears. The absorption of intraocular gas bubbles is described reasonably accurately by a first-order kinetic equation, similar to the decay of a radioisotope. First-order kinetics predict that a constant percentage of the volume of the intraocular gas bubble absorbs over a given unit of time (Eqn. (3)):

$$V = V_0 e^{-kt} \qquad (3)$$
$$T_{1/2} = 0.693/k$$

where V is the volume of the gas bubble, V_0 is the initial volume of the gas bubble, k is the decay constant for the particular gas, t is the time and $T_{1/2}$ is the half-life.

The time required for a 50% reduction in volume is called the half-life. This is the time that it takes a 4-ml intraocular gas bubble to decrease to 2 ml, for example. It will take the same amount of time for the 2-ml gas bubble to be absorbed to a 1-ml gas bubble (Fig. 17.4). The absorption of an intraocular gas bubble is not predicted precisely by a first-order kinetic equation because this would predict that the gas bubble would *never* be completely absorbed from the eye. Figure 17.4 shows that the predicted gas bubble volume approaches zero asymptotically, but never equals zero.

It is important to distinguish between the meniscus height and intraocular bubble volume because the absorption of an intraocular gas bubble is dependent on the volume of the gas bubble and not the meniscus height (although the two can be interconverted using Eqn. (1)). The half-lives of some commonly used mixtures of intraocular gases are given in Table 17.2.

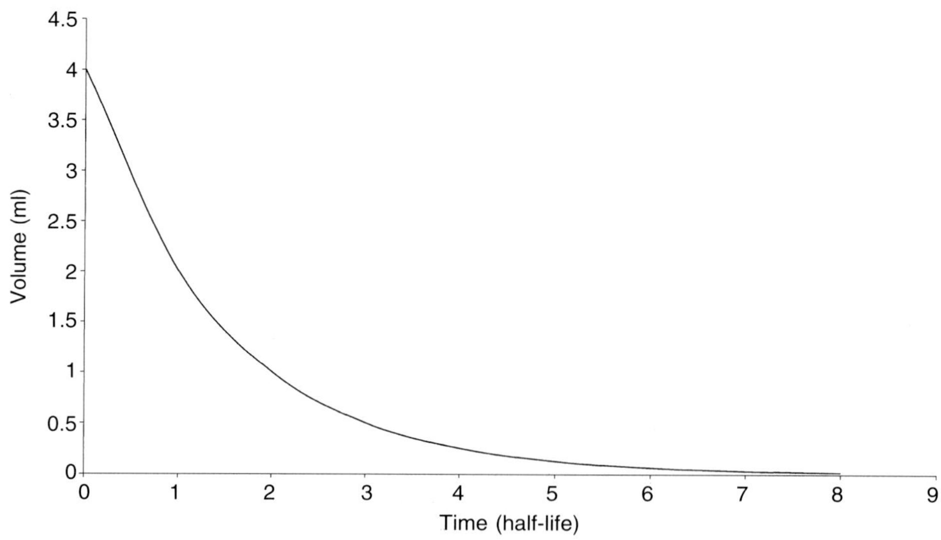

Figure 17.4 *Absorption of an intraocular gas bubble in the vitreous cavity approximates to a first-order exponential decay equation. The bubble volume (y-axis) decreases by 50% for each half-life (x-axis). A 4-ml gas bubble will decrease to 0.5 ml in three half-lives.*

Table 17.2 Kinetics of intravitreal gas absorption in the vitreous

Gas mixture	*Half-life (days)*	*Maximum effective duration of tamponade[a] (days)*
Air	1.3	4
20% SF_6	2.6	8
5% C_3F_8	4.2	13
10% C_3F_8	6.5	20
15% C_3F_8	8.0	24
20% C_3F_8	12.5	38

[a]The maximum effective duration of tamponade is approximately equal to three half-lives.
Adapted with permission from Thompson JT. The absorption of mixtures of air and perfluoropropane after pars plana vitrectomy, *Arch Ophthalmol* (1992) **110**:1594–7.[1] Copyright © 1992, American Medical Association; and Thompson JT. Kinetics of intraocular gases: disappearance of air, sulfur hexafluoride, and perfluoropropane after pars plana vitrectomy, *Arch Ophthalmol* (1989) **107**:687–91.[2] Copyright © 1989, American Medical Association.

TECHNIQUES OF FLUID–GAS EXCHANGE AND INTRAOCULAR GAS INJECTION

Intraocular gases are usually injected via the pars plana infusion line during vitrectomy. Intraocular gas bubbles are injected via the limbus in aphakic eyes or via the pars plana in phakic or pseudophakic eyes in an office setting. Small intraocular gas bubbles (>0.2 ml) may be injected into the vitreous cavity without removal of vitreous or aqueous, but larger injection volumes must be accompanied by removal of an approximately equal volume of vitreous or aqueous. Several techniques have evolved to remove vitreous or aqueous to accommodate injection of an intravitreal gas bubble. These can be subdivided into procedures performed in the operating room or the office.

OPERATING ROOM: FLUID–AIR EXCHANGE DURING VITRECTOMY

The standard way to inject an intraocular gas bubble in the operating room during a vitrectomy is to switch the vitreous cavity infusion from balanced saline to a continuous air pump. The intravitreal infusion cannula is attached via intravenous tubing to a three-way stopcock with inflow that can be selected for balanced saline or the air pump. The outflow stopcock is attached to the infusion cannula in the vitreous cavity. The vitreous infusate may be changed rapidly from balanced saline to air by rotating the three-way stopcock. The air pump has a feedback control designed to maintain a constant air pressure in the vitreous cavity, which can be preset according to the surgeon's preference. The vitreous fluid is aspirated via the pars plana using a vacuum-cleaner needle (passive aspiration) vented to the atmosphere (Fig. 17.5) or using active aspiration into the vitrectomy cassette.

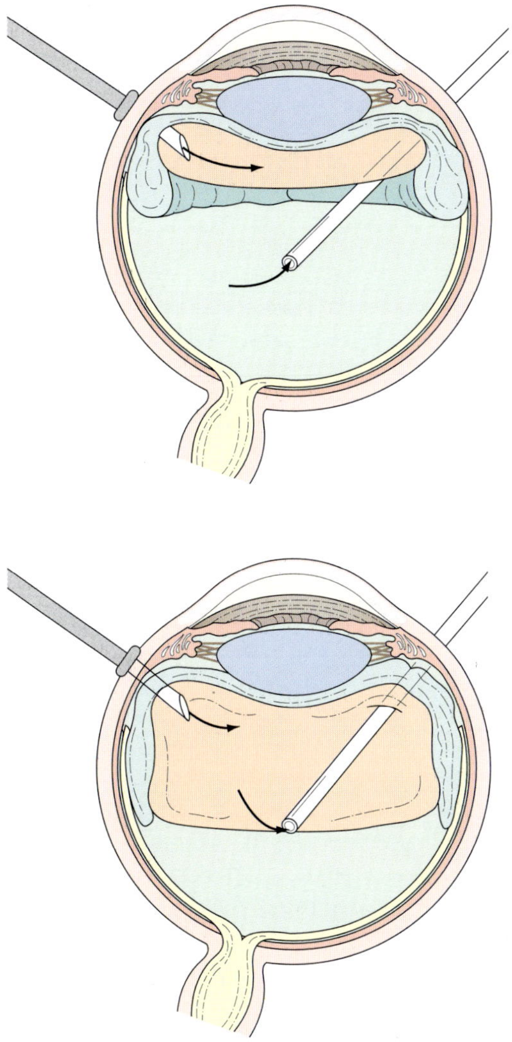

Figure 17.5 *Vitreous fluid may be removed and exchanged with air using a passive-aspiration vacuum-cleaner needle. The force of air entering through the vitreous infusion cannula causes the vitreous fluid to egress through the vacuum-cleaner needle, which is vented to the atmosphere. If the air enters the vitreous at a pressure of 35 mmHg, then the suction pressure at the vacuum-cleaner needle tip is 35 mmHg.*

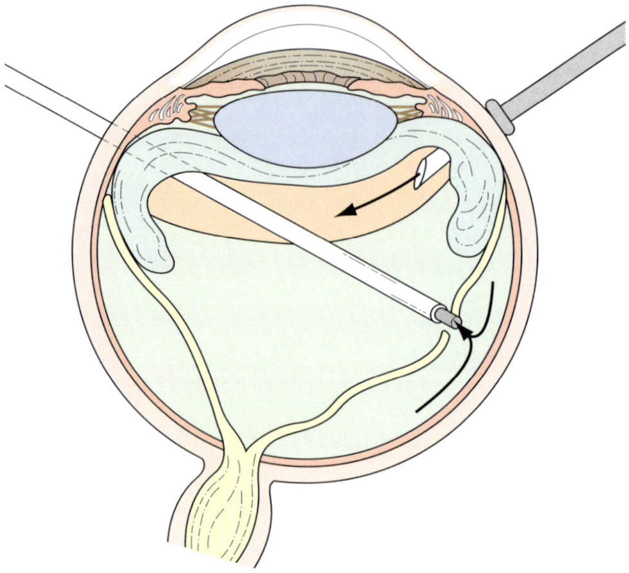

Figure 17.6 *Subretinal fluid is removed by passive aspiration by placing the tip of the aspiration cannula through the retinal break. The subretinal fluid is removed preferentially as air fills the vitreous cavity. Then the vacuum-cleaner needle is withdrawn just anterior to the retinal surface once the retina is flat, to remove the intravitreal fluid until the vitreous cavity is filled with air.*

With passive aspiration, the pressure driving the removal of vitreous fluid is equal to the height of the infusion bottle minus the height of the vacuum-cleaner outflow port for fluid exchange or equal to the air infusion pressure for an air–fluid exchange. This results in a reasonably rapid fluid–gas exchange while avoiding a negative pressure of 150 mmHg or more, from active aspiration into the vitrectomy cassette. The fluid–gas exchange with active aspiration is more rapid but hypotony sometimes results if the aspiration of vitreous fluid is faster than the response of the air pump to increase inflow of gas when the IOP decreases below the preset gas pressure. Overall, control is better with passive aspiration and the author prefers this technique for fluid–air exchange.

Subretinal fluid in eyes with a retinal detachment is usually removed during surgery via the retinal break or a drainage retinotomy (Fig. 17.6). Removal of the subretinal fluid is advantageous to allow a larger gas bubble to be injected and to allow intraoperative laser photocoagulation around the retinal breaks, which is possible when all of the subretinal fluid has been removed.

OPERATING ROOM: EXCHANGING AIR WITH LONGER ACTING INTRAOCULAR GAS BUBBLE

Often, it is desirable to exchange the intravitreal air with a longer acting intraocular gas such as C_3F_8 or SF_6 before closing the sclerotomy sites. A specific percentage of inert gas is exchanged for the vitreous cavity air by the following technique. A 60-ml syringe is flushed to remove any air in the syringe and pure C_3F_8 or SF_6 is infused via the gas tank into the 60-ml syringe through an air filter. Typically 10–15 ml of pure gas is placed in the 60-ml syringe after flushing the dead space of the tank and connecting the filter. The filter is removed and the syringe tip is quickly covered with a finger. Some of the pure gas is expelled while partially covering the syringe tip so that the remaining volume will result in the correct concentration of gas when air is added to the pure gas (Fig. 17.7). For example, if a 10% C_3F_8 intraocular gas bubble is needed, then the excess pure C_3F_8 is expelled until 6 ml of pure gas remains. Then the air filter is attached to the syringe and 54 ml of filtered (sterile) air is withdrawn into the syringe over approximately 30 seconds, so the syringe is now filled with 60 ml of 10% C_3F_8/90% air. The superonasal sclerotomy site is closed and the second sclerotomy site is sutured but left open without tying the knot. Then the syringe is attached quickly to the infusion cannula via the three-way stopcock and about 50 ml of gas is lavaged through the eye. The air in the vitreous cavity is expelled through the open sclerotomy as the 50 ml of gas is injected. Sometimes the gas does not exit the sclerotomy because of vitreous plugging the sclerotomy. A tapered tip vacuum needle can be placed into the sclerotomy to allow the gas to escape the vitreous as the 10% C_3F_8 is injected. Then the suture is tied permanently to close the supertemporal sclerotomy site, the infusion cannula is removed and a suture is used to close the final sclerotomy site.

A variation of this technique is to close the second sclerotomy site and lavage the 10% C_3F_8 via the infusion cannula and allow gas to be expelled using a 25-gauge needle inserted through the pars plana, which is attached to the vacuum-cleaner handle. A 30-gauge needle is attached to the 60-ml syringe or the gas is transferred to a smaller 3-ml syringe and additional gas may be injected via the pars plana if the eye became hypotonus during closure of the third sclerotomy site.

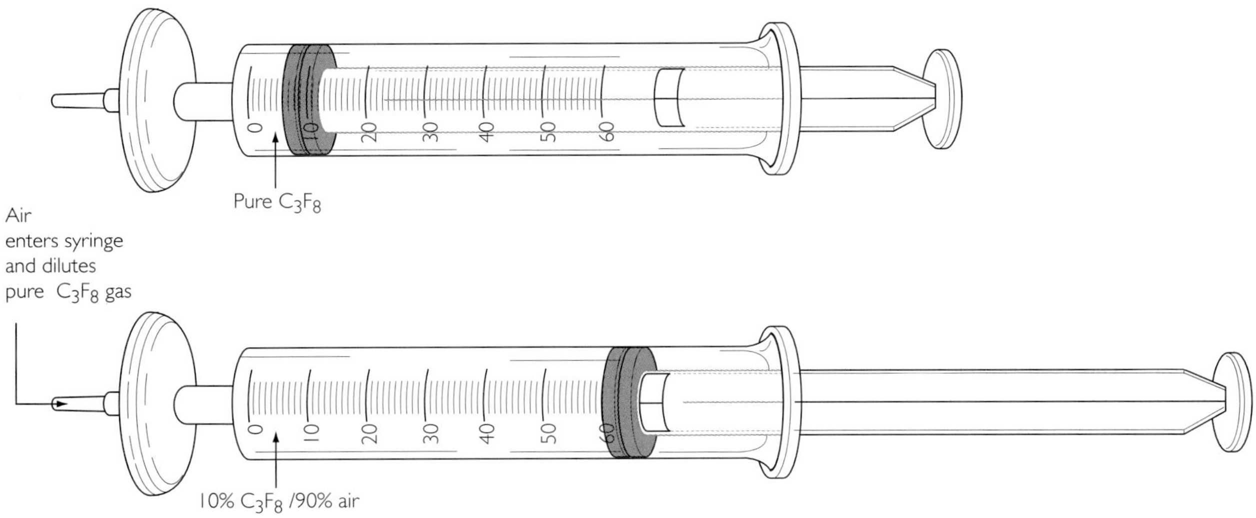

Figure 17.7 *A long-acting intraocular gas bubble mixture is prepared by taking a syringe partially filled with a pure gas such as C_3F_8 or SF_6 and diluting the gas with sterile (filtered) air until the desired concentration is achieved. The gas mixture contained in a 60-ml syringe is then exchanged continuously with the air in the vitreous cavity so that the vitreous is filled with the premixed gas concentration.*

OPERATING ROOM: INJECTION OF GAS IN EYE WITHOUT VITRECTOMY

In some eyes, it is desirable to inject an intraocular gas bubble as part of the repair of a rhegmatogenous retinal detachment using a scleral buckle when there is still substantial subretinal fluid around the retinal break(s). The gas may be injected from a 3-ml syringe with a 30-gauge needle if the eye is hypotonus. If the eye is not already hypotonus from drainage of subretinal fluid, vitreous or aqueous fluid must be removed to allow injection of more than 0.2 ml of gas, which is approximately the maximum volume of gas that can be injected in a normotensive eye.

There are two techniques to remove aqueous or vitreous fluid, depending on the volume of fluid to be removed. The first technique injects gas using a 3-ml syringe filled with gas via the pars plana and then aqueous paracentesis is performed to normalize the IOP. A repeat paracentesis after 5–10 minutes may normalize the pressure if it remains elevated. A gas volume of 0.2–0.6 ml usually can be injected using this technique. An expansile gas such as pure C_3F_8 is usually injected. Pure C_3F_8 expands to four times the initial volume, so a gas bubble of up to 2.4 ml can be created when the bubble expands.

The second method aspirates vitreous fluid to allow injection of the intraocular gas bubble. A 22- to 25-gauge 1.5-inch needle attached to a 1- or 3-ml syringe is placed via the pars plana to aspirate liquid vitreous. The position of the needle tip is monitored with indirect ophthalmoscopy as it is advanced deeper in the vitreous cavity, and a pocket of fluid vitreous can be aspirated anterior or lateral to the optic nerve in eyes with a posterior vitreous detachment (Fig. 17.8). The needle must pierce the posterior hyaloid to position the tip in the liquid vitreous in the posterior vitreous cavity. It may be difficult to find a pocket of liquid vitreous in some eyes but, if successful, often 0.5–1.0 ml of fluid may be withdrawn. Intraocular gas then is injected immediately via the pars plana using a 30-gauge needle to replace the vitreous fluid withdrawn; it is best to have the premixed gas ready in the syringe before the vitreous fluid is aspirated, to minimize the duration of hypotony.

If the liquid vitreous pocket cannot be aspirated, then an external drainage site may be made in the sclera to remove subretinal fluid. The drainage site and choroidal perforation should be performed before the gas is injected, to avoid puncturing the choroid when the IOP is high. The amount of subretinal fluid must be monitored and drainage stopped before the retina completely settles, to avoid retinal incarceration in the drainage site. The drainage site is closed and the gas then is injected slowly using a finger to monitor the IOP to avoid raising the IOP above 20 mmHg.

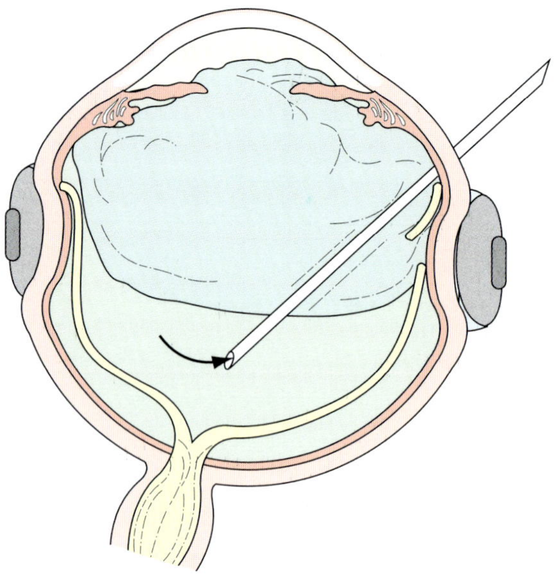

Figure 17.8 *Liquid vitreous may be removed to lower the intraocular pressure and allow a large scleral buckle to be tightened to indent the eye wall. Liquid vitreous is aspirated posterior to the formed vitreous gel. A 22- to 25-gauge, 1-inch needle is inserted into the pars plana through the posterior hyaloid, slightly lateral to the optic nerve. The liquid vitreous is aspirated until sufficient vitreous fluid volume has been removed to accommodate the volume displacement required to elevate the scleral buckle.*

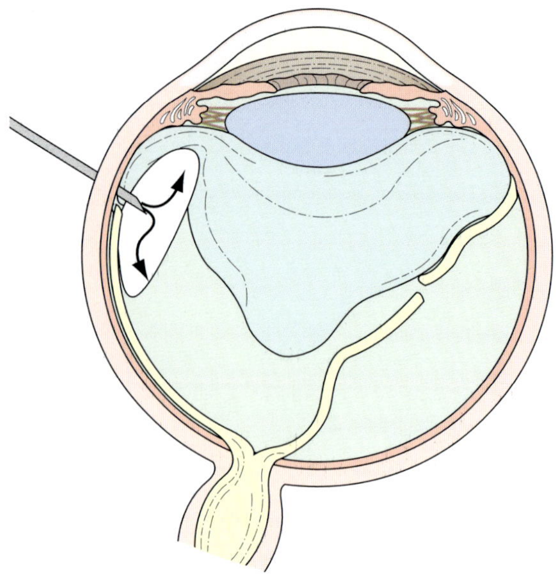

Figure 17.9 *Pure expansile gases such as SF_6 or C_3F_8 are injected into the anterior vitreous in a phakic or pseudophakic eye. The gas bubble expands, creating a larger intraocular gas bubble, and the patient is positioned so that the gas bubble covers the retinal break, allowing subretinal fluid to absorb.*

The second technique of vitreous fluid aspiration allows a larger volume of gas to be injected than the first technique of paracentesis. The second technique often allows the surgeon to inject a larger volume of air or a nonexpansile mixture of intraocular gas, which will be absorbed more rapidly than the smaller volume of long-acting pure gas injected using the paracentesis technique. A short-duration gas bubble is usually all that is needed, because the goal is to encourage the remaining subretinal fluid to absorb by using internal tamponade of the retinal tear(s). Once the retina is flat on the buckle within the first 24 hours after surgery, the gas bubble is no longer needed.

OFFICE: INJECTION OF A SMALL-VOLUME EXPANSILE INTRAOCULAR GAS BUBBLE IN PHAKIC OR PSEUDOPHAKIC EYES

Injection of a gas bubble in phakic or pseudophakic eyes is done through the pars plana. This technique is most commonly performed as part of a pneumatic retinopexy[7] or to encourage absorption of persisting subretinal fluid after a scleral buckling procedure. The eye is prepped with an iodine solution and a lid speculum is placed in the eye. A 1-ml or 3-ml syringe filled with pure SF_6 or C_3F_8 is attached to a half-inch 30-gauge needle and injected through the pars plana 4 mm behind the limbus in the temporal sclera, with the needle directed toward the center of the vitreous cavity (Fig. 17.9). The patient may be seated at the slit lamp for the injection or placed supine, tilting the head slightly so that the injection site is superior. The desired volume of gas (generally 0.3 ml) is injected rapidly to try to minimize the formation of small 'fish-egg' gas bubbles. The needle is then withdrawn; a cotton-tipped applicator is placed immediately over the puncture site as the needle is withdrawn in order to try to prevent gas from escaping through the needle puncture site.

The IOP is usually very high (40–60 mmHg) immediately after injection and a limbal paracentesis using a Ziegler knife (Grieshaber 681.05, Kennesaw, GA) is often necessary at the slit lamp to drain a small volume of aqueous in order to normalize the IOP. The chamber will become shallow as the aqueous drains through the paracentesis site and it is desirable to remove the paracentesis knife to stop drainage before the anterior chamber becomes flat. The IOP is then checked to be certain that the paracentesis was adequate to lower the IOP.

The anterior chamber usually reforms partially within several minutes as aqueous from the posterior chamber shifts forward. A topical antibiotic and a topical steroid are usually used for several days after the procedure.

OFFICE: FLUID–GAS EXCHANGE IN PHAKIC OR PSEUDOPHAKIC EYES WITH PRIOR VITRECTOMY

Several techniques have been described in the literature,[8,11] most of which require injection of gas with simultaneous or sequential removal of excess vitreous fluid. The patient is placed in a sideways position after sterilizing the eye with iodine. A wire lid speculum is used to hold the eye open. It is best to give retrobulbar or peribulbar anesthesia so that the patient does not feel the pain from changes in IOP during the procedure. The aspiration site is placed in a dependent position, rotating the patient's head toward the aspiration site. Then, a 25- or 27-gauge needle attached to a three-way stopcock is inserted into the vitreous cavity 4 mm behind the limbus. The needle is aimed into the midvitreous. The three-way stopcock is attached to a 3- or 5-ml syringe filled with a desired concentration of intraocular gas and an empty 3- or 5-ml syringe is attached to the other arm of the three-way stopcock (Fig. 17.10). The stopcock is turned initially to allow aspiration of vitreous fluid into the empty syringe. A second pair of hands is necessary for this procedure to help turn the stopcock when switching from fluid aspiration to gas injection. About 0.5–1 ml of vitreous fluid is withdrawn slowly. When the eye begins to soften and collapse, aspiration is stopped and the stopcock is

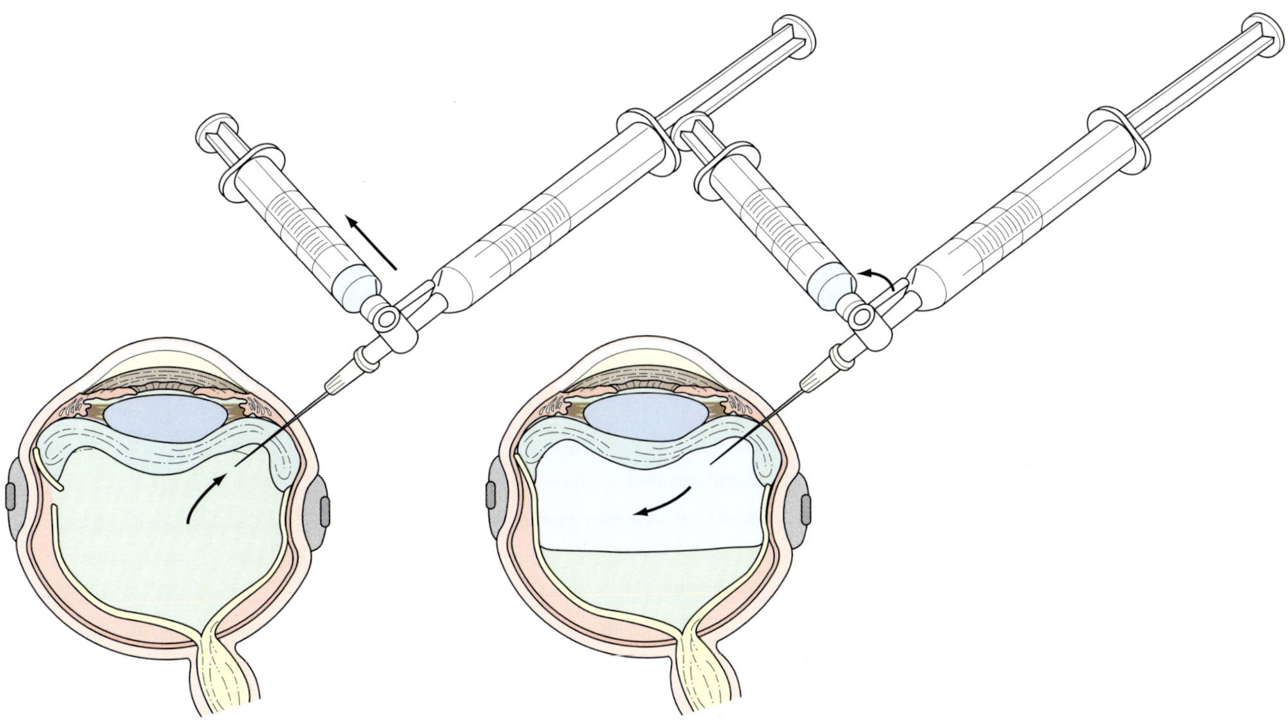

Figure 17.10 *A sequential fluid–gas exchange in a phakic or pseudophakic eye with a prior vitrectomy allows a moderate volume of gas to be injected. Vitreous fluid is removed as the first step and then the stopcock is rotated to allow injection of gas to normalize the intraocular pressure. This may be repeated as the needle is advanced into the vitreous below the meniscus level of the vitreous fluid.*

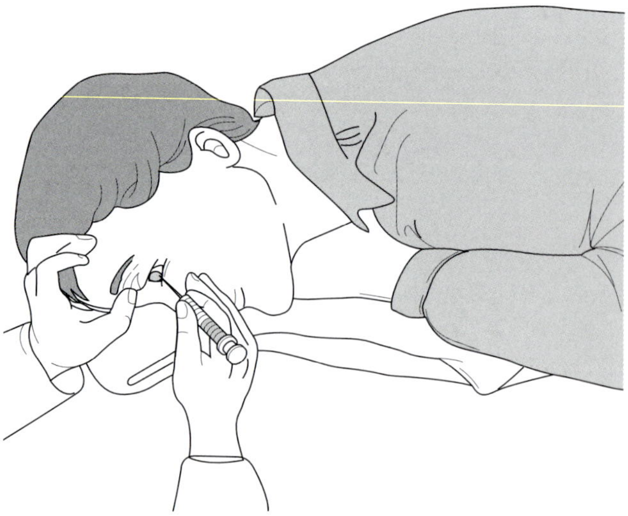

Figure 17.11 *A second technique for fluid–air exchange in a phakic or pseudophakic eye with prior vitrectomy uses a single syringe. The vitreous fluid is aspirated via a 22- to 25-gauge needle into the syringe, with the patient in a dependent position. The vitreous fluid, which is heavier than gas, dribbles to the most dependent portion of the syringe against the plunger. The gas in the syringe is then injected into the hypotonus eye until normal pressure is re-established. Then, more vitreous fluid may be aspirated, followed by additional gas injection.*

turned to allow injection of some gas. The gas is injected until the eye is again firm. The needle may then be placed in a more dependent position in the vitreous cavity below the air bubble, repeating the same sequence of fluid aspiration followed by gas injection.

A second variation of this technique for fluid–gas exchange in phakic and pseudophakic eyes can be done by one person. The patient is placed in a prone position and the surgeon takes a 5-ml syringe filled with approximately 3 ml of premixed gas. The syringe, which is attached to a 25-gauge needle, is placed through the pars plana with the syringe facing upwards (Fig. 17.11). Some vitreous fluid is aspirated into the syringe. The fluid collects in the dependent position against the plunger and then the gas in the syringe is injected into the vitreous. Some additional vitreous fluid is aspirated and more gas is injected. This technique is repeated until no more vitreous fluid can be withdrawn. The technique has the advantage that it requires only one person, but the disadvantage is that vitreous fluid in the needle and syringe tip is reinjected with the gas and gas is often withdrawn into the syringe during aspiration. It is possible to replace about 40–60% of the vitreous cavity using either technique in phakic eyes.

OFFICE: FLUID–GAS EXCHANGE IN APHAKIC EYES WITH PRIOR VITRECTOMY

This technique can be performed by one person at the slit lamp. The eye is prepped with iodine and a wire lid speculum is placed in the eye after retrobulbar or peribulbar anesthesia. A Ziegler knife (Grieshaber 681.05, Kennesaw, GA) is used to make an oblique paracentesis tract into the temporal inferior limbus in the 7 o'clock meridian in a right eye or the 5 o'clock meridian in a left eye. Then a 30-gauge needle attached to a 5 ml syringe filled with the desired gas mixture is inserted into the paracentesis tract. The gas then is injected slowly. If the IOP becomes elevated, the needle can be rotated obliquely within the paracentesis tract to allow some additional aqueous to escape around the needle. The gas is injected sequentially as aqueous drains around the needle, to keep the IOP approximately normal (Fig. 17.12). Gas injection will

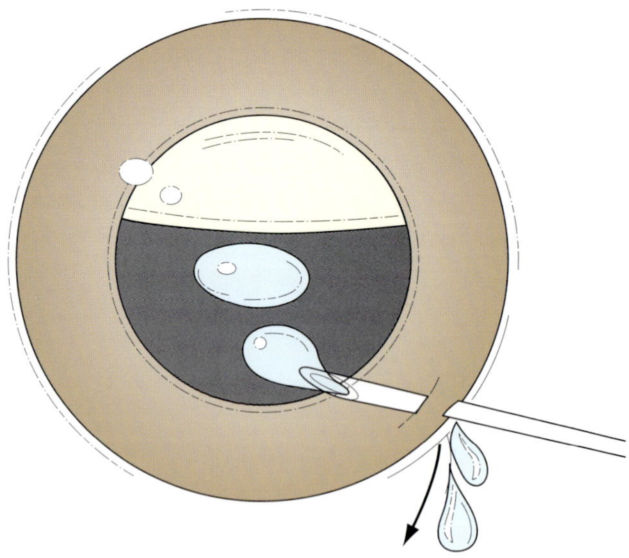

Figure 17.12 *Fluid–gas exchange in an aphakic eye is performed at the slit lamp. A 30-gauge needle is passed obliquely through a paracentesis tract and the gas is injected. The needle is rotated about 15° to allow aqueous fluid to escape around the needle so that aqueous drains continuously as the gas is slowly injected.*

usually result in multiple fish-egg bubbles but these coalesce into one or several bubbles as the gas fill increases.

Sometimes vitreous fluid unavoidably is trapped in the inferior vitreous cavity posterior to the inferior iris. The vitreous fluid can be made accessible to removal by asking the patient to assume a prone position for 10–15 seconds after withdrawing the needle from the limbus. The prone positioning also causes most of the remaining fish-egg bubbles to coalesce. Then the needle is again placed in the anterior chamber and more gas is injected. This process is repeated two or three times until no more vitreous fluid moves into the anterior chamber when the patient is prone. It is possible to replace as much as 90% of the vitreous fluid using this technique in aphakic eyes.

USE OF INTRAOCULAR GAS BUBBLE TO REMOVE VITREOUS HEMORRHAGE

The technique is identical to a fluid–gas exchange in a phakic, pseudophakic or aphakic eye as described above. The goal is to remove as much bloody vitreous fluid as can be done safely and to replace this with air. As aqueous fluid forms and replaces the air, the remaining blood is diluted and exits the eye via the aqueous outflow. This technique is most successful if at least 50% and preferably 80% or more of the bloody vitreous fluid can be removed.

USE OF INTRAOCULAR GAS BUBBLE TO UNROLL EDGES OF A GIANT RETINAL TEAR

An intraocular gas bubble may be used to help unroll the edge of a giant retinal tear, although this technique increasingly is being supplanted by the use of perfluorocarbon liquids. The patient can be turned to a prone position in the operating room and the fluid–gas exchange performed by infusing gas while removing fluid from the anterior chamber or vitreous (upside down fluid–gas exchange). The gas rises over the optic nerve, which is in the most superior position during the prone fluid–gas exchange. The expanding bubble will push the retina against the RPE, unrolling the edges of the giant retinal tear (Fig. 17.13). Vitreous fluid drains through a vacuum-cleaner needle held in the sclerotomy site, which is in a dependent position.

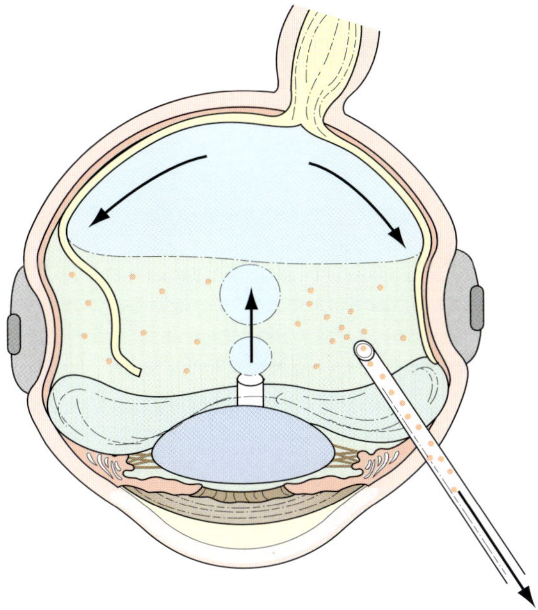

Figure 17.13 *A giant retinal tear may be unrolled using an intraocular gas bubble by placing the patient in a prone position and injecting air via the infusion cannula as the vacuum-cleaner needle is used to remove fluid that accumulates in the anterior vitreous cavity. The retina is pushed against the eye wall as the bubble expands in the vitreous cavity and the subretinal fluid moves to the anterior vitreous cavity. The patient is then returned to a supine position. There will be no slippage of the edge of the giant retinal tear as long as the subretinal fluid has been removed completely, because capillary attraction between the retina and the retinal pigment epithelium will hold the retina in the correct anatomic position. The patient must remain prone postoperatively to keep the fluid from dissecting under the edge of the giant retinal tear.*

Slippage of the giant retinal tear edge in the first 12 hours following surgery can be minimized by asking the patient to do slow forward somersaults if the giant retinal tear is inferior and backward somersaults if the giant retinal tear is superior but this procedure may be difficult for some patients. The intraocular gas bubble displaces the remaining subretinal fluid into the vitreous cavity, unrolling the edges of the giant retinal tear. This technique is also useful in eyes where slippage of the edge of the giant retinal tear is noted within the first 24 hours following surgery, to try to avoid returning to the operating room.

POSTOPERATIVE POSITIONING AND DURATION OF POSITIONING

The appropriate position of the patient postoperatively is dictated by the size of the intraocular gas bubble, the location of the retinal tear and whether the crystalline lens is present or not. The patient's position must keep the intraocular gas bubble away from the crystalline lens if the patient is phakic, because posterior capsular changes, termed 'lens feathering', will develop. Lens feathering is a branching pattern of posterior subcapsular lens changes that develops from gas contact with the lens. Feathering will develop within hours of continuous contact of the gas bubble with the posterior lens capsule, but is reversible if the patient improves compliance with prone positioning.

The presence of posterior capsular feathering on the first postoperative day strongly suggests that the patient has not been sufficiently compliant with prone positioning. The physician must emphasize the importance of prone positioning to the patient and demonstrate the correct position to the patient. Improved compliance with prone positioning will generally cause reversal of the posterior subcapsular lens feathering within 24 hours.

Prolonged contact of the intravitreal gas bubble with the lens will result in permanent posterior subcapsular vacuoles or opacification. The intraocular gas bubble-induced cataracts generally involve most or all of the posterior capsule and hence differ from typical idiopathic posterior subcapsular cataracts, which are usually predominantly central. These gas-induced cataracts are usually visually significant and may result in poor visualization of the retina by the surgeon during the critical first few weeks following surgery.

Pseudophakic patients and aphakic patients with intraocular gas bubbles may avoid prolonged prone positioning if the retinal break is in the superior periphery because the gas bubble will provide good tamponade for a superior break with the patient upright. For aphakic eyes that are to be managed with upright positioning, the use of postoperative mydriasis should be avoided because a small pupil will keep the intraocular gas bubble in the vitreous cavity, thus preventing prolonged gas contact with the corneal endothelium.

The duration of prone positioning is determined by the location of the retinal break and the absorption rate of the intraocular gas bubble. Most phakic patients should remain prone until the gas bubble decreases to about 20% of the vitreous cavity, to avoid gas contact with the crystalline lens when the patient resumes an upright position. The particular gas concentration is chosen to provide a sufficient duration of tamponade for the location and etiology of the retinal break(s). The absorption of the gas bubble is monitored and the prone positioning is discontinued when appropriate.

In general, superior retinal breaks do not require prolonged prone positioning; a short-acting gas mixture is usually sufficient. Superior retinal breaks without retinal detachment can be treated with air, and superior retinal breaks associated with retinal detachment are treated with 5% C_3F_8 or 20% SF_6.

Inferior retinal breaks associated with retinal detachment may be treated with 10% C_3F_8, so the gas bubble will remain large enough for the first 10 days to provide adequate tamponade for the inferior retina. Prolonged tamponade for complex retinal detachments with PVR or giant retinal tears usually requires a 10–15% C_3F_8 gas mixture. Macular holes are usually treated with a 15% C_3F_8 gas bubble because a long-duration tamponade appears helpful to achieve higher macular hole closure rates.[12,13]

CONTRAINDICATIONS FOR INTRAOCULAR GAS

The use of an intraocular gas bubble is inadvisable in the eyes of patients who must travel by air or ascend a mountain when the gas bubble is still large. Decreased atmospheric pressure under these conditions leads to enlargement of the intraocular gas bubble and increases in the IOP. The author recommends that air travel be avoided until the gas bubble is less than 5%.

Nitrous oxide anesthesia must be avoided during retinal surgery when an intraocular gas bubble is placed in the eye. If nitrous oxide anesthesia is used, it should be discontinued about half an hour before the gas is instilled into the eye. Dissolved nitrous oxide in the blood is very soluble in the vitreous cavity and begins to enter the intraocular gas bubble as soon as it is injected in the eye. Nitrous oxide anesthesia leads to large increases in the IOP within 10–15 minutes of sclerotomy closure in a gas-filled eye as nitrous oxide in the bloodstream enters the intraocular gas bubble. Later, the nitrous oxide in the gas bubble returns to the bloodstream, causing the bubble to decrease in volume, thus leading to hypotony.

COMPLICATIONS

ELEVATED IOP

Elevated IOP is one of the more common complications in eyes with an intraocular gas bubble but usually is not caused directly by the intraocular gas bubble when nonexpansile mixtures of gases are used. The inflammation from surgery, presence of intravitreal blood and placement of encircling scleral buckles, all of which may cause a transient reduction in aqueous outflow, are usually the major factors that contribute to elevated IOP.

The incidence of an IOP of 30 mmHg or greater was 35.6% in one study of 222 eyes treated with vitrectomy and an intraocular gas bubble.[14] The IOP increased to greater than 25 mmHg in 43% of 171 eyes in another study of vitrectomy with an intraocular gas bubble.[15]

The elevation in IOP is transient in the vast majority of eyes and usually can be managed with topical or systemic aqueous suppressants. It is rarely necessary to remove a portion of the intraocular gas bubble to manage elevated IOP if the appropriate gas is chosen during surgery.

The mechanism for elevated IOP must be evaluated and angle-closure glaucoma should be considered in eyes with a shallow or flat anterior chamber. Gonioscopy is essential to make this diagnosis accurately. The intraocular gas bubble may cause the lens–iris diaphragm to shift forward, leading to an iatrogenic angle-closure glaucoma, which can be treated by reformation of the anterior chamber with a viscoelastic to reverse the angle closure.

Eyes with narrow angles after absorption of the intraocular gas bubble should be evaluated for laser iridectomy because such eyes appear to be predisposed toward this complication. Aphakic eyes appear to be more prone to angle closure with instillation of a very large intraocular gas bubble because the bubble easily can push the iris forward, closing the angle whenever the patient is supine. It is helpful to place a thin layer of viscoelastic substance between the anterior iris and cornea at completion of surgery in aphakic eyes in order to prevent apposition of the iris and posterior corneal surface in the first 24 hours.

Some angle-closure episodes can be treated by keeping the patient prone, because poor compliance with prone positioning probably precipitates this complication. A laser iridectomy may help to avoid repeat angle closure but laser iridectomy is usually not sufficient to break the angle closure if the gas bubble is pushing the iris forward.

Reformation of the anterior chamber may be performed at a slit lamp in most eyes, although occasional patients may require a procedure in the operating room to allow greater sedation. A paracentesis tract is made with a Ziegler knife, which usually releases some aqueous or a portion of the gas bubble. The viscoelastic substance is injected between the iris and cornea. The goal is to inject enough viscoelastic substance to open at least two-thirds of the peripheral angle. Sometimes, a second paracentesis tract is made to allow injection of the viscoelastic substance over another area of the iris. The injection of the viscoelastic substance alone is successful in reforming the flat anterior chamber in most eyes and breaking the angle-closure episode. The viscoelastic substance itself may lead to moderately elevated IOP for 1–2 days after injection, but this is generally transient.

If viscoelastic injection is successful, then subsequent evaluation of the formed anterior chamber angle by gonioscopy will help to determine whether a laser peripheral iridectomy is indicated. Careful evaluation of the angle of the fellow eye may help to determine whether the operative eye had a narrow angle preoperatively that was predisposed to angle closure.

Removal of a portion of the intraocular gas bubble should be considered if the IOP remains elevated in an eye with an open angle where maximal aqueous-suppressant antiglaucoma therapy fails to control the IOP. Most eyes with elevated IOP respond to beta-blockers, apraclonidine, latanoprost or carbonic anhydrase inhibitors, but a few eyes fail to respond adequately to any antiglaucoma therapy. If the pressure remains substantially elevated despite maximal aqueous suppression, then removal of a portion of the intraocular gas bubble should be considered. The amount of gas to be removed is determined by the IOP. A sufficient amount of gas should be removed to lower the IOP to about 5–10 mmHg and antiglaucoma therapy should be continued for at least one to two more days until it is certain that the IOP has normalized. Decreased aqueous outflow with placement of a high encircling scleral buckle and severe postoperative inflammation or vitreous hemorrhage are the most frequent causes of this problem. Mixing errors in the intraocular gas bubble, where the surgeon injects pure rather than diluted C_3F_8, is a less common cause of uncontrollable elevated IOP in the early postoperative period. A portion of the gas bubble should be removed if a gas mixing error is certain or strongly suspected.

The presence of an intraocular gas bubble results in errors in IOP measurement, so this must be considered when evaluating the IOP in a gas-filled eye postoperatively. The intraocular gas bubble causes a change in scleral rigidity, which in turn alters the accuracy of IOP determination. Previous studies have shown that the Goldmann tonometer gives accurate IOP measurements in gas-filled eyes. The Tonopen® underestimates the IOP by about 10 mmHg or more when the IOP is 30 mmHg or more.[16] The Schiotz tonometer also substantially underestimates the true IOP when the pressure is elevated in a gas-filled eye.[17]

INADEQUATE GAS BUBBLE SIZE

Some eyes have an intraocular gas bubble following vitreous surgery that is too small to adequately tamponade retinal breaks. First, inadequate gas fill may result if the surgery is completed with a smaller-than-desired intraocular gas bubble. The volume of intraocular gas bubble in the vitreous may be too small when insufficient vitreous or subretinal fluid is removed and exchanged with gas. Second, intraocular gas may escape through the sclerotomy in the perioperative period, leading to loss of intravitreal gas and transient hypotony. Loss of gas through the sclerotomy most often results from poor surgical technique for sclerotomy closure, or from an increased IOP, such as a spontaneous choroidal detachment, which pushes gas out of an otherwise adequately closed sclerotomy. The third cause of inadequate gas fill is premature absorption of the intraocular gas bubble. Rapid absorption of the intraocular gas bubble is usually a sign of a mixing error in the concentration of long-acting intraocular gas, where too much air was added at the time of surgery.

MIGRATION OF THE INTRAOCULAR GAS BUBBLE

The intraocular gas bubble may migrate into the subretinal space on rare occasions. Migration of intravitreal gas into the subretinal space during fluid–gas exchange only occurs when there is unrelieved traction on the retina or where the gas is injected accidentally into the subretinal space. A subretinal intraocular gas bubble will be absorbed much as an intravitreal gas bubble, but the subretinal gas bubble obviously will not properly tamponade the retinal break(s). Migration of the intraocular gas bubble into the anterior chamber is rarely a problem as long as the patient remains prone so that the endothelium is still bathed by aqueous. Small gas bubbles in the anterior chamber of phakic eyes usually do not produce cataracts from contact with the anterior lens capsule. Long-term contact of the corneal endothelium with the intraocular gas bubble will lead to endothelial cell damage.[18–20]

AIR TRAVEL AND ELEVATED IOP

Air travel is contraindicated in eyes with an intraocular gas bubble unless the gas bubble is small. Most commercial jet airliners are pressurized between 5000 and 8000 feet at their cruising altitude. This is equivalent to going from a pressure of 760 mmHg at sea level to an atmospheric pressure of 564 mmHg at 8100 feet.[21] The pressure (P) is inversely related to the volume (V) by Boyle's Law:

$$PV_{\text{sea level}} = nRT = PV_{\text{8100 feet}}$$

because the nRT portion of the equation remains essentially constant at sea level and 8100 feet. A 1-ml intraocular gas bubble at sea level expands to become 1.35 ml at 8100 feet.

Lincoff et al have suggested that air travel is safe if the intraocular gas bubble is 10% or less, because the eye usually can compensate for the increased volume of the intraocular gas bubble.[22,23] This is a useful guideline but the author has allowed patients to fly with a 10% intraocular gas bubble and a few have reported severe ocular pain during ascent, sometimes requiring modification of the aviation flight plan. The high IOP and severe pain usually can be relieved by asking the pilot to decrease the airplane altitude by several thousand feet. Dieckert et al have observed elevated IOP to 42 mmHg with a gas volume as small as 0.25 ml in rhesus monkeys in a simulated altitude of 8100 feet.[21] Kokame and Ing have reported toleration of low-altitude air travel in a patient with a 65% intraocular gas bubble, although the IOP did increase to 49 mmHg during the flight.[24]

There are a number of factors, such as the baseline IOP at sea level, aqueous outflow, rapidity of ascent, forward shift of the lens–iris diaphragm and other factors, that may alter the response of an individual eye to decreased atmospheric pressure. Hence, the author recommends against flying with an intraocular gas bubble of 5% or greater. The same problem of increased IOP from an expanding intraocular gas bubble may occur when ascending a mountain range by automobile or rail, although the rate of ascent is generally slower, which gives the eye more time to compensate for the increased bubble size.

Most of the published literature about intraocular gas bubbles and air travel is related to intravitreal gas bubbles, but the presence of a gas bubble in the anterior chamber of a pseudophakic or phakic eye may create more significant problems. Some eyes with zonular dehiscence or large posterior capsulotomies may have migration of the gas bubble into the anterior chamber when the patient lies supine. If the patient then travels on an airplane, a posterior chamber intraocular lens may become dislocated as the gas bubble expands in the anterior chamber.

HYPERBARIC CONDITIONS AND INTRAOCULAR GAS BUBBLES

Hyperbaric conditions may lead to problems in eyes with an intraocular gas bubble. Hyperbaric pressure occurs with SCUBA diving and with hyperbaric oxygen therapy used for the treatment of burns. The intraocular gas bubble decreases in size when atmospheric pressure increases, leading to hypotony under hyperbaric conditions. The most serious problems occur as the eye goes from hyperbaric pressure to normal atmospheric pressure, particularly as the patient just reaches the surface atmospheric pressure. The eye continues to make aqueous humor during the dive and tends to compensate for the hypotony, but return from hyperbaric conditions to normal sea-level atmospheric pressure leads to re-expansion of the intraocular gas bubble and large increases in IOP. Diving to depths of 33 feet or equivalent decreases the IOP to 0 mmHg, and the IOP increases to 50 mmHg or greater upon reascent to the surface in eyes with a gas bubble filling about 50% of the vitreous cavity.[25] Similar problems develop in gas-filled eyes during treatment with hyperbaric oxygen.

VISUAL FIELD LOSS AND INTRAOCULAR GAS BUBBLES

Intraocular gas bubbles may cause visual field defects; this has been reported primarily in eyes with macular hole surgery.[26–30] There are a number of theories about the pathogenesis of the visual field loss, but dehydration of the retina from air infusion during vitrectomy and prolonged contact of the intraocular gas bubble with the nerve-fiber layer could potentially cause damage to the nerve-fiber layer.[31,32] Visual field defects have been noted primarily in eyes with long-duration gas tamponade, although some eyes with short-duration tamponade may be at risk.[33] The possible damage to the nerve-fiber layer by an intraocular gas bubble is another reason to avoid long-acting intraocular gas bubbles, unless they are necessary to treat the retinal pathology.

CATARACTS

Cataracts in the posterior lens capsule will develop from excessive contact of the intraocular gas bubble with the posterior lens capsule. The mechanism is unknown, but posterior subcapsular feathering develops when the intraocular gas bubble contacts the posterior capsule in patients who are poorly compliant with prone positioning. The posterior subcapsular feathering may be reversed by diligent prone positioning. The posterior subcapsular feathering usually develops in the first postoperative day in patients who do not understand or comply with prone positioning. Proper instructions on the first postoperative day will generally reverse the lens changes. If the patient remains poorly compliant with prone positioning for a week or more, the posterior subcapsular lens opacities become permanent as the posterior subcapsular feathering evolves into posterior lens vacuoles or a diffuse posterior subcapsular cataract.

Vitrectomy alone leads to progressive nuclear sclerotic cataracts and it is not known if the addition of an intraocular gas bubble accelerates the progression of the nuclear sclerosis, although one study found similar nuclear sclerosis progression in eyes with macular holes treated with air versus long-acting 16% C_3F_8.[34]

SUMMARY AND CONCLUSIONS

The intraocular gas bubble is one of the vitreous surgeon's most useful ancillary tools in treating retinal breaks. The high surface tension between gas and fluid allows gas bubbles effectively to close retinal tears internally. The gas bubble disappears after it has provided the internal tamponade that closes the retinal break. A thorough understanding of the appropriate uses and limitations of an intraocular gas bubble gives the vitreous surgeon a powerful tool to treat retinal detachments and retinal breaks.

REFERENCES

1. Thompson JT. The absorption of mixtures of air and perfluoropropane after pars plana vitrectomy, *Arch Ophthalmol* (1992) **110:**1594–7.
2. Thompson JT. Kinetics of intraocular gases: disappearance of air, sulfur hexafluoride, and perfluoropropane after pars plana vitrectomy, *Arch Ophthalmol* (1989) **107:**687–91.
3. Parver LM, Lincoff H. Mechanics of intraocular gas, *Invest Ophthalmol Vis Sci* (1978) **17:**77–9.
4. Wilkinson CP, Rice TA. *Michels Retinal Detachment* (Mosby: St Louis, 1997): 468–70.
5. Abrams GW, Edelhauser HF, Aaberg TM, Hamilton LH. Dynamics of intravitreal sulfur hexafluoride gas, *Invest Ophthalmol* (1974) **13:**863–8.
6. Peters MA, Abrams GW, Hamilton LH, Burke JM, Schrieber TM. The nonexpansile, equilibrated concentration of perfluoropropane gas in the eye, *Am J Ophthalmol* (1985) **100:**831–9.
7. Hilton GF, Grizzard WS. Pneumatic retinopexy: a two-step outpatient operation without conjunctival incision, *Ophthalmology* (1986) **93:**626–41.
8. Landers MB III, Robinson D, Olsen KR, Rinkoff J. Slit-lamp fluid–gas exchange and other office procedures following vitreoretinal surgery, *Arch Ophthalmol* (1985) **103:**967–72.
9. Stern WH, Blumenkranz MS. Fluid–gas exchange after vitrectomy (letter). *Am J Ophthalmol* (1983) **96:**400–2.
10. Devenyi RG. Outpatient postvitrectomy fluid–gas exchange using long-acting gases, *Can J Ophthalmol* (1995) **30:**148.
11. Lambrou FH, Devenyi RG, Han DP. Fluid–gas exchange after vitrectomy using long-acting gases in an outpatient setting (letter), *Arch Ophthalmol* (1988) **106:**1344.
12. Thompson JT, Smiddy WE, Glaser BM, Sjaarda RN, Flynn HW Jr. Intraocular tamponade duration and success of macular hole surgery, *Retina* (1996) **16:**373–82.
13. Thompson JT, Glaser BM, Sjaarda RN, Murphy RP, Hanham A. Effects of intraocular bubble duration in the treatment of macular holes by vitrectomy and transforming growth factor-beta 2, *Ophthalmology* (1994) **101:**1195–200.
14. Han DP, Lewis H, Lambrou FH Jr, Mieler WF, Hartz A. Mechanisms of intraocular pressure elevation after pars plana vitrectomy, *Ophthalmology* (1989) **96:**1357–62.
15. Chen PP, Thompson JT. Risk factors for elevated intraocular pressure after the use of intraocular gases in vitreoretinal surgery, *Ophthalmic Surg Lasers* (1997) **28:**37–42.
16. Lim JI, Blair NP, Higginbotham EJ, et al. Assessment of intraocular pressure in vitrectomized gas-containing eyes. A clinical and manometric comparison of the Tono-Pen to the pneumotonometer, *Arch Ophthalmol* (1990) **108:**684–8.
17. Del Priore LV, Michels RG, Nunez MA, et al. Intraocular pressure measurement after pars plana vitrectomy, *Ophthalmology* (1989) **96:**1353–6.
18. Matsuda M, Tano Y, Inaba M, Manabe R. Corneal endothelial cell damage associated with intraocular gas tamponade during pars plana vitrectomy, *Jpn J Ophthalmol* (1986) **30:**324–9.
19. Van Horn DL, Edelhauser HF, Aaberg TM, Pederson HJ. In vivo effects of air and sulfur hexafluoride gas on rabbit corneal endothelium, *Invest Ophthalmol* (1972) **11:**1028–36.
20. Green K, Cheeks L, Stewart DA, Norman BC. Intraocular gas effects on corneal endothelial permeability, *Lens Eye Toxic Res* (1992) **9:**85–91.
21. Dieckert JP, O'Connor PS, Schacklett DE, et al. Air travel and intraocular gas, *Ophthalmology* (1986) **93:**642–5.
22. Lincoff H, Weinberger D, Reppucci V, Lincoff A. Air travel with intraocular gas. I. The mechanisms for compensation, *Arch Ophthalmol* (1989) **107:**902–6.
23. Lincoff H, Weinberger D, Stergiu P. Air travel with intraocular gas. II. Clinical considerations, *Arch Ophthalmol* (1989) **107:**907–10.
24. Kokame GT, Ing MR. Intraocular gas and low-altitude air flight, *Retina* (1994) **14:**356–8.
25. Jackman SV, Thompson JT. Effects of hyperbaric exposure on eyes with intraocular gas bubbles, *Retina* (1995) **15:**160–6.
26. Hutton WL, Fuller DG, Snyder WB, Feffman RL, Swanson WH. Visual field defects after macular hole surgery: a new finding, *Ophthalmology* (1996) **103:**2152–9.
27. Boldt HC, Munden PM, Folk JC, Mehaffey MG. Visual field defects after macular hole surgery, *Am J Ophthalmol* (1996) **122:**371–81.
28. Ezra E, Arden GB, Riordan-Eva P, Aylward GW, Gregor ZJ. Visual field loss following vitrectomy for stage 2 and 3 macular holes, *Br J Ophthalmol* (1996) **80:**519–25.
29. Pendergast SD, McCuen BW II. Visual field loss after macular hole surgery, *Ophthalmology* (1996) **103:**1069–77.
30. Kerrison JB, Haller JA, Elman M, Miller NR. Visual field loss following vitreous surgery, *Arch Ophthalmol* (1996) **114:**564–9.
31. Welch JC. Dehydration injury as a possible cause of visual field defect after pars plana vitrectomy for macular hole, *Am J Ophthalmol* (1997) **124:**698–9.
32. Thompson JT. Reply to Letter to Editor by Brucker AJ and Berger, *Retina* (1998) **18:**87–8.
33. Melberg NS, Thomas MA. Visual field loss after pars plana vitrectomy with air/fluid exchange, *Am J Ophthalmol* (1995) **120:**386–8.
34. Kaplan JA, Thompson JT, Glaser BM. Intraocular gas tamponade duration and progression of cataracts after macular hole surgery, *Ophthalmology* (1996) **103S**(9A):160.

Chapter 18 Use of perfluorocarbon liquids

Kevin J Blinder

INTRODUCTION

Investigation of the vitreous substitutes was first begun by Cibis et al over a quarter of a century ago.[1] Originally, both lighter-than-water silicone oil and heavier-than-water vitreous substitutes were studied, with the former demonstrating good clinical application.[2] The first heavier-than-water vitreous substitute, fluorosilicone oil, also proved effective intraoperatively and postoperatively but its poor ocular tolerance and high viscosity limited its usefulness.[3]

The perfluorocarbon liquids (PFCLs), originally introduced by Clark and Gollan as high-oxygen-content blood substitutes, constitute the second category of heavier-than-water vitreous substitutes.[4] The PFCLs have had numerous applications in medicine as blood substitutes, as diagnostic imaging aids and in organ transplant preservation. Haidt et al[5] were the first to inject PFCL experimentally into the vitreous cavity of animals, noting that its unique physical properties were desirable for vitreoretinal surgery. Other investigations soon followed, searching for the least toxic substance for intraocular surgery.[6–10]

The PFCLs are fluorinated, synthetic liquids containing carbon–fluorine bonds. Toxicity is usually due to small amounts of unsaturated hydrogen-containing compounds. Impurities found in PFCLs include compounds with nitrogen–fluoride bonds, as well as hydrogen–fluoride bonds. Purification can be accomplished through the removal of these compounds.[11]

The physical properties of the PFCLs are uniquely suitable for vitreoretinal surgery (Table 18.1). With specific gravities ranging between 1.7 and 2.03, the PFCLs are denser than water, allowing hydrokinetic manipulation of the retina. With the assistance of gravity, the heavy liquid fills the eye in a posterior-to-anterior fashion, hydrokinetically tamponading the retina against the underlying retinal pigment epithelium

Table 18.1 Perfluorocarbon characteristics

Perfluorocarbon	*Chemical formula*	*Specific gravity*	*Viscosity (cSt at 25°C)*	*Refractive index*	*Vapor pressure (mmHg at 37°C)*	*Surface tension (dyne/cm at 25°C)*
Perfluorotributylamine	$C_{12}F_{27}N$	1.89	2.6	1.29	1.14	16
Perfluorodecalin	$C_{10}F_{18}$	1.94	2.7	1.31	13.5	16
Perfluorooctane	C_8F_{18}	1.76	0.8	1.27	50	14
Perfluorooctylbromide	$C_8F_{17}Br$	1.93	2.3	1.30	1.1	18.2
Perfluoroethylcyclohexane	C_2F_6	1.83	0.94	1.29	55	
Perfluoroperhydrophenanthrene	$C_{14}F_{24}$	2.03	8.03	1.33	<1	21.6

(RPE). Subretinal fluid is 'steamrolled' out through an anterior retinal defect into the vitreous cavity. The intravitreal fluid then egresses through the sclerotomies as the PFCL level rises.

The PFCLs are optically clear, immiscible with water and have an index of refraction close to that of water. Visualization during surgery is not hindered when PFCLs are employed. Unlike silicone oil, the PFCLs have a low viscosity, allowing injection and removal through small-gauge needles or cannulas.

The high surface tension of PFCLs in water both creates an effective internal tamponading effect and prevents the substance from passing through a retinal tear into the subretinal space. Silicone oil and the PFCLs have similar surface tension properties, but PFCLs exert a greater tamponading force than silicone oil;[12] a 1.0-ml silicone oil bubble produces a buoyant force of 0.06 g, whereas a 0.3-ml PFCL bubble produces a transretinal force of 0.25 g. This might be even more important than the surface tension characteristics in determining the ability of an intraocular tamponading agent to resist the development of a traction retinal detachment.[13]

INDICATIONS AND TECHNIQUES

The clinical indications for the PFCLs have grown rapidly over the past decade. This chapter describes the basic technique for the use of PFCLs, and the most common indications. A brief mention of a wide variety of other, less-common indications will conclude the discussion.

Whatever the case scenario, the surgeon begins with the standard three-port pars plana vitrectomy, consisting of an infusion cannula (infusing the normal vitrectomy fluid of balanced salt solution plus (BSS Plus) and/or enriched with customized ingredients) and two other ports to accommodate the vitrectomy probe and endoilluminator. A standard core vitrectomy is followed by identification of the posterior hyaloid face. If no pre-existent posterior vitreous detachment is present, the posterior hyaloid is engaged and detached with the vitrectomy probe, a flexible silicone-tipped cannula, or a hyaloid lifter (designed by Matthew A. Thomas, MD, personal communication). The vitrectomy is extended peripherally along the edge of the posterior hyaloid face. The vitreous base may need to be trimmed at this time, with or without the assistance of scleral depression. A wide-angle viewing system may assist in performing this maneuver.

Approximately 5 ml of the PFCL is drawn up by the scrub technician in a sterile fashion with a 20- to 27-gauge needle attached to a luer-lock syringe to prevent loosening of the needle or cannula and inadvertently injecting it into the eye. The PFCL injection process requires a 20- to 30-gauge cannula (Fig. 18.1a). If the retina is detached, a partial air–fluid exchange should be performed (Fig. 18.1b) to prevent the subretinal fluid from being displaced anteriorly and bypassing the retinal defect (Fig. 18.1c).[10] This will result in a small air bubble tamponading the anterior peripheral retina, forcing the subretinal fluid to exit through the peripheral retinal defect. The injection phase is completed once the PFCL reaches the level of the sclerotomies.

At this point, the surgeon may perform endolaser photocoagulation, membranectomy, retinal cryopexy, scleral buckling procedure or whatever other surgical manipulation is required for that particular case. All of these maneuvers can be performed easily under PFCL.

The visibility of the PFCL bubble varies, depending on which specific PFCL is utilized. The difference between the index of refraction of water (1.33) and that of the PFCL is the main factor that determines the visibility of the PFCL in a saline solution. Perfluoroperhydrophenanthrene has an index of refraction equal to that of water, making the bubble more difficult to visualize in BSS than the other PFCLs, which have a lower index of refraction. The interface is easier to see when blood or debris is on the surface of the bubble, with other visual clues evident with experience. Under air, of course, visibility of the bubble is not a problem.

The PFCL can be removed with active aspiration via an extrusion needle (20-gauge blunt cannula, with or without a tapered end) or with passive aspiration via a silicone-tipped flute needle (Fig. 18.1d,e). During removal of the PFCL, air is infused through the infusion cannula, creating an air–PFCL exchange. If complete removal of the PFCL is unclear, instill a few drops of BSS Plus after the air–fluid exchange, wait a few minutes and then remove the remaining fluid (Fig. 18.1f).

Although one may perform a PFCL–silicone oil exchange directly, this may hinder the complete removal of the PFCL bubble. To address this, Peyman and Mehta developed an instrument for simultaneous removal of PFCL and injection of silicone oil.[14] Most surgeons, however, prefer to inject silicone oil under air.

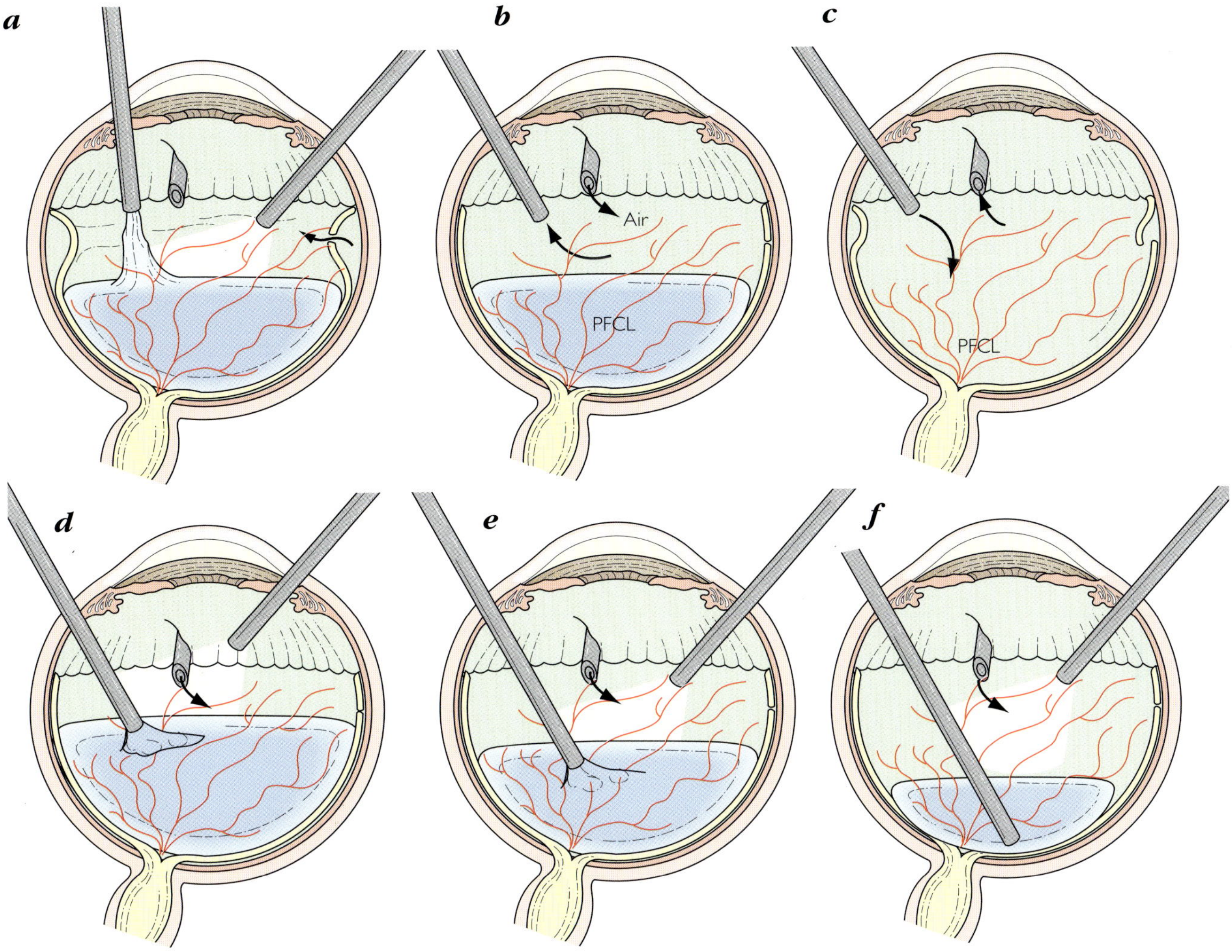

Figure 18.1 *Schematic representation of the injection and removal phases of perfluorocarbon liquids (PFCLs). (a) Injection of the liquid with a 20- to 30-gauge cannula. (b) A partial air–fluid exchange is performed, during the injection phase, in the presence of a retinal detachment. (c) This is performed to prevent the subretinal fluid from being displaced anteriorly and bypassing the retinal defect, resulting in an anteriorly displaced ring of subretinal fluid. (d, e) The PFCL is removed with an extrusion needle or flute needle, while infusing air through the infusion cannula. (f) To ensure complete removal of the PFCL, a few drops of BSS Plus are reinjected into the eye, and slowly removed again. This step may be repeated if necessary.*

GIANT RETINAL TEARS

Repair of the giant retinal tear (GRT) with retinal detachment remains one of the great surgical challenges for even the more experienced vitreoretinal surgeon. GRTs are breaks that are greater than or equal to 90° of the retinal circumference.[15] Treatment modalities have varied over the past three to four decades, beginning with the prone positioning technique of Schepens et al, to unfold the inverted retinal flap.[16] Peyman later modified this technique with the introduction of a new rotating table.[17] Norton was the first to advocate air injection to tamponade the posterior retinal flap.[18]

With the advent of vitrectomy and air–fluid exchange, other more innovative ideas evolved. Suturing the retina both transsclerally[19] and transvitreally[20–22] were other techniques attempted over the years. Peyman et al suggested microincarceration of the retina via a penetrating diathermy needle to fixate the retinal flap.[23] Retinal tacks were also attempted, with varying success rates and the added difficulties of introducing a foreign body into the eye.[24–29] Most of these techniques also involved manipulation of the inverted retinal flap with vitreoretinal microinstrumentation, creating the possibility of surgical trauma and damage during retinal repair.

With the introduction of the PFCLs, repair of a GRT with retinal detachment has been greatly simplified.[30,31] This complicated retinal detachment remains the best clinical indication for PFCL use. A core vitrectomy is performed and during peripheral vitrectomy great care is taken to trim the vitreous base, especially along the tear edges. To accomplish this, the surgeon or assistant performs scleral depression under the operating microscope (Fig. 18.2). A wide-angle viewing system may suffice, but scleral depression may be required.

The PFCL is injected over the posterior pole, filling the eye in a posterior-to-anterior direction. With an extremely inverted retinal flap, the PFCL initially is directed beneath the flap, with unfolding of the retina as the PFCL bubble enlarges (Fig. 18.3a). The subretinal fluid is forced anteriorly as the retina is

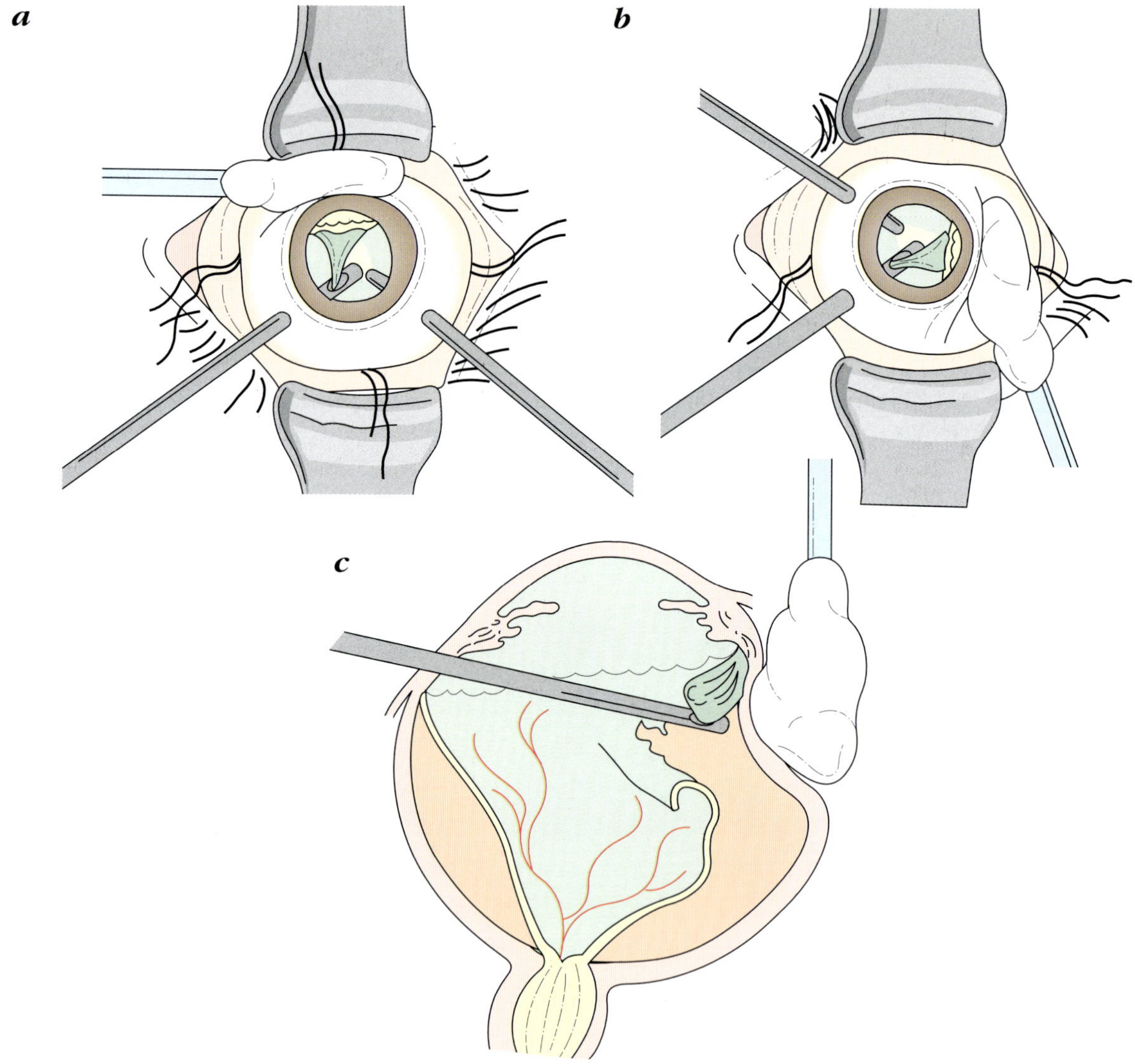

Figure 18.2 *Scleral depression under the operating microscope. (a) The surgical assistant may depress, while the surgeon holds the vitrector and light pipe. (b) The surgeon can perform his own depression, with the assistant holding the light pipe over the cornea or over the contact lens. (c) Another view of the scleral depression and trimming of the vitreous base.*

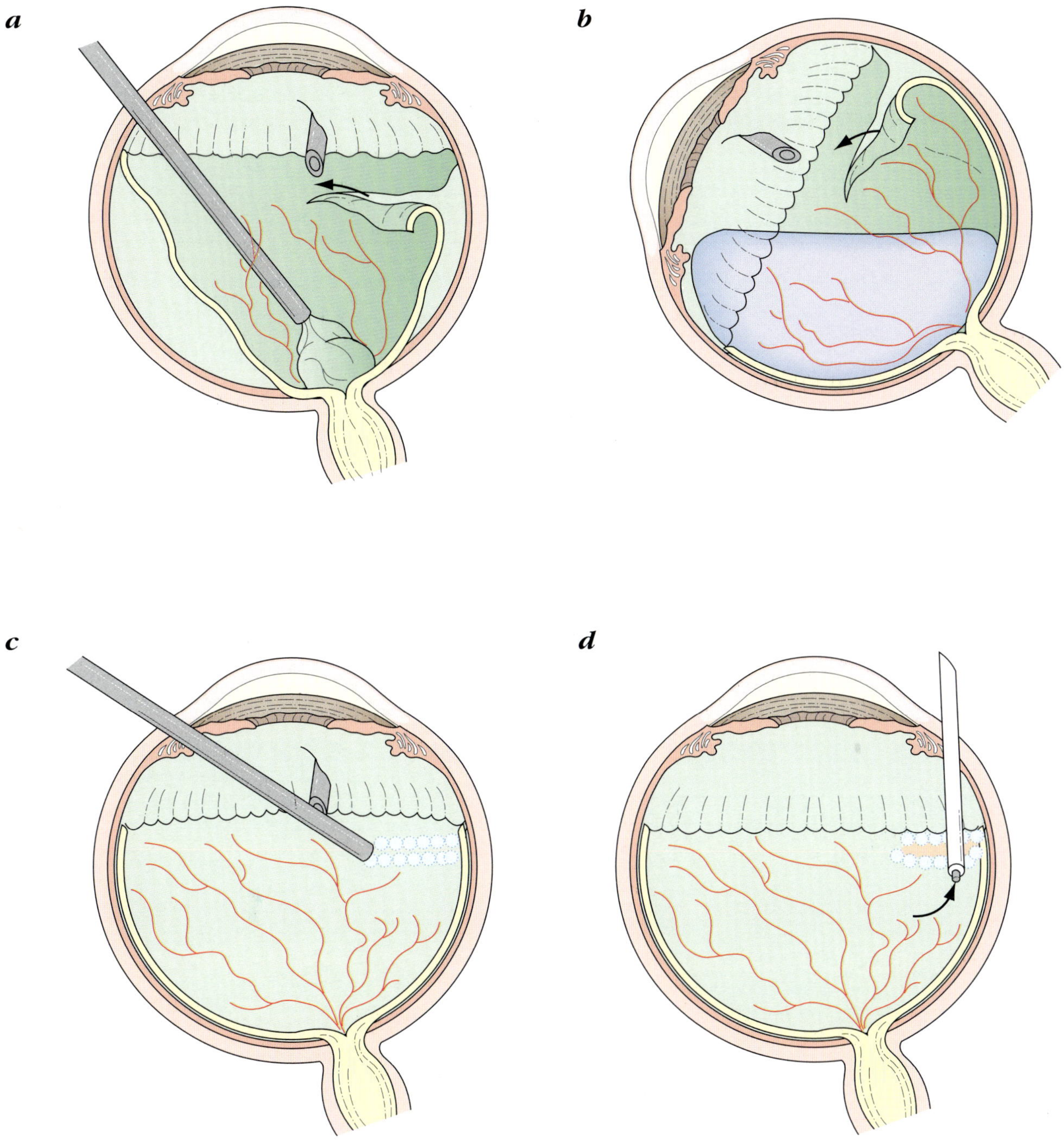

Figure 18.3 *Repair of giant retinal tear with retinal detachment. (a) The perfluorocarbon liquid (PFCL) is injected over the posterior pole, under the inverted retinal flap. (b) The subretinal fluid is 'steam-rolled' anteriorly, through the giant retinal tear and out of the sclerotomies. (c) Once the retina is flat, with the PFCL in place, endolaser photocoagulation (or cryopexy) is performed to the edge of the tear. (d) An air–PFCL exchange is performed, drying the edge of the tear to prevent any fluid from re-entering the subretinal space.*

hydrokinetically repositioned against the RPE (Fig. 18.3b). This obviates the need for direct physical manipulation of the retina, thus reducing the possibility of surgical trauma to the retina. No posterior retinotomy is necessary, eliminating another source of potential complications, such as bleeding or membrane formation.[32] The force of the PFCL tamponade is great enough to prevent slippage of the retina.

The injection phase of the PFCL is complete once the bubble level reaches the edge of the tear. Endolaser photocoagulation, cryotherapy or both are then applied to the edges of the tear (Fig. 18.3c). An encircling element may be placed around the eye at this point in the procedure. The need for a buckle is somewhat debatable. If the surgeon decides against this step, then *extra* care must be taken to closely trim the vitreous base along the tear edges with the assistance of scleral depression.

The need for performing a lensectomy is also somewhat controversial. Some surgeons remove the lens in order to accomplish more complete vitreous base trimming.

Removal of the PFCL is initiated in a slow, cautious fashion with an air–fluid exchange. The eye is rotated toward the tear and aspiration is performed along the tear edge. This dries the edge of the tear and prevents fluid from re-entering the subretinal space (Fig. 18.3d). To ensure complete PFCL removal, a partial fluid–PFCL exchange (wherein a small amount of BSS Plus is injected into the eye and removed), may be performed. The surgeon then chooses a long-acting postoperative tamponading agent: perfluoropropane gas (C_3F_8, 10–15%) or silicone oil.

The repair of a GRT with retinal detachment and proliferative vitreoretinopathy (PVR) is somewhat more complex. After the vitrectomy is performed, the preretinal membrane is removed as completely as possible. A small amount of PFCL may be injected to provide countertraction and stabilization of the retina, thus facilitating membrane dissection (Fig. 18.4).

The PFCL bubble also can determine if all of the traction has been relieved and if the retina can be flattened. If the retina does not flatten with the PFCL bubble in place, then residual traction exists, necessitating further membranectomy with possible relaxing retinotomy.[33,34] The surgeon may elect to place an encircling element in the presence of severe PVR to relieve traction on the peripheral retina.

Kreiger and Lewis reported a series of 11 patients with GRTs without PVR treated with perfluorooctane.[35] They performed careful vitreous base trimming without scleral buckling. One eye required further surgery for redetachment secondary to PVR. Eight additional major procedures were necessary in seven eyes, with all retinas remaining reattached with a visual acuity of 5/200 or better in nine eyes.

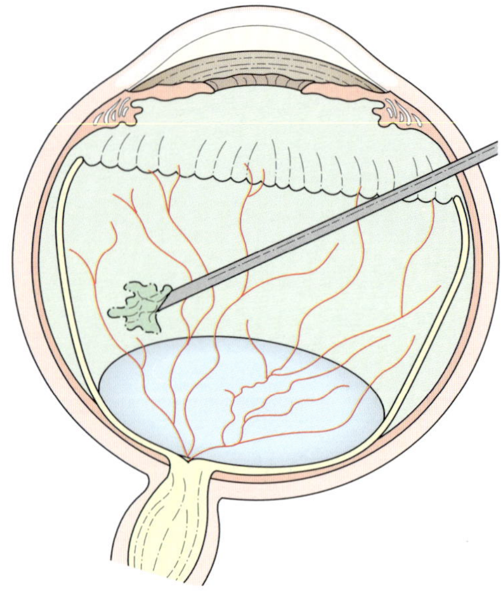

Figure 18.4 *Perfluorocarbon liquid injection in the presence of proliferative vitreoretinopathy. This allows better visualization of the membrane formation and provides countertraction and stabilization of the retina, facilitating the membrane dissection.*

Freeman and associates reported on the intraoperative use of perfluorooctane to manage atraumatic GRTs.[36] Twenty-five clinical sites enrolled 214 patients. PVR was present preoperatively in 57 eyes (26.7%). The retina was reattached at 6-month follow-up in 179 eyes (83.7%), with a visual acuity of 20/400 or better in 69 eyes (32.3%). Intraoperative retinal slippage occurred in 33 eyes (15.5%), with subretinal PFCL in 11 eyes (5.2%).

Kertes et al reported the Vitreon Collaborative Study Group's results for the management of GRTs using perfluoroperhydrophenanthrene.[37] Twenty-three study centers enrolled 162 consecutive eyes with GRTs 90° or greater in circumferential extent. One hundred and fifty-eight eyes (97.5%) were reattached intraoperatively and 147 eyes (90.7%) remained attached at their most recent follow-up. Ninety-five eyes (58.6%) required at least a second procedure, ranging from scatter laser photocoagulation to complex retinal detachment–PVR surgery.

Data analysis showed that neither a scleral buckling procedure nor a lensectomy had any effect on the postoperative visual or anatomic outcome. The preoperative factors associated with a poor visual outcome included macular detachment, hypotony, pseudophakia or aphakia, poor preoperative visual acuity, higher grade PVR and GRTs greater than 180° in extent. The intraoperative factors associated with a poor visual outcome included the need for a relaxing retinotomy and a silicone oil tamponade. Patients with postoperative hypotony or persistent retinal detachments were more likely to have a poor visual result.

A patient presenting with a GRT in one eye should have a careful examination of the fellow eye with indirect ophthalmoscopy and scleral depression. One should consider prophylactic treatment of fellow eyes at risk for development of GRTs. These would include high myopes, eyes with areas of white without pressure and eyes that show increasing condensation of the vitreous base.[38]

PROLIFERATIVE VITREORETINOPATHY

Utilization of PFCLs has altered the surgeon's approach to complicated retinal detachments with PVR. The traditional strategy has been to address the anterior PVR first, followed by dissection of the

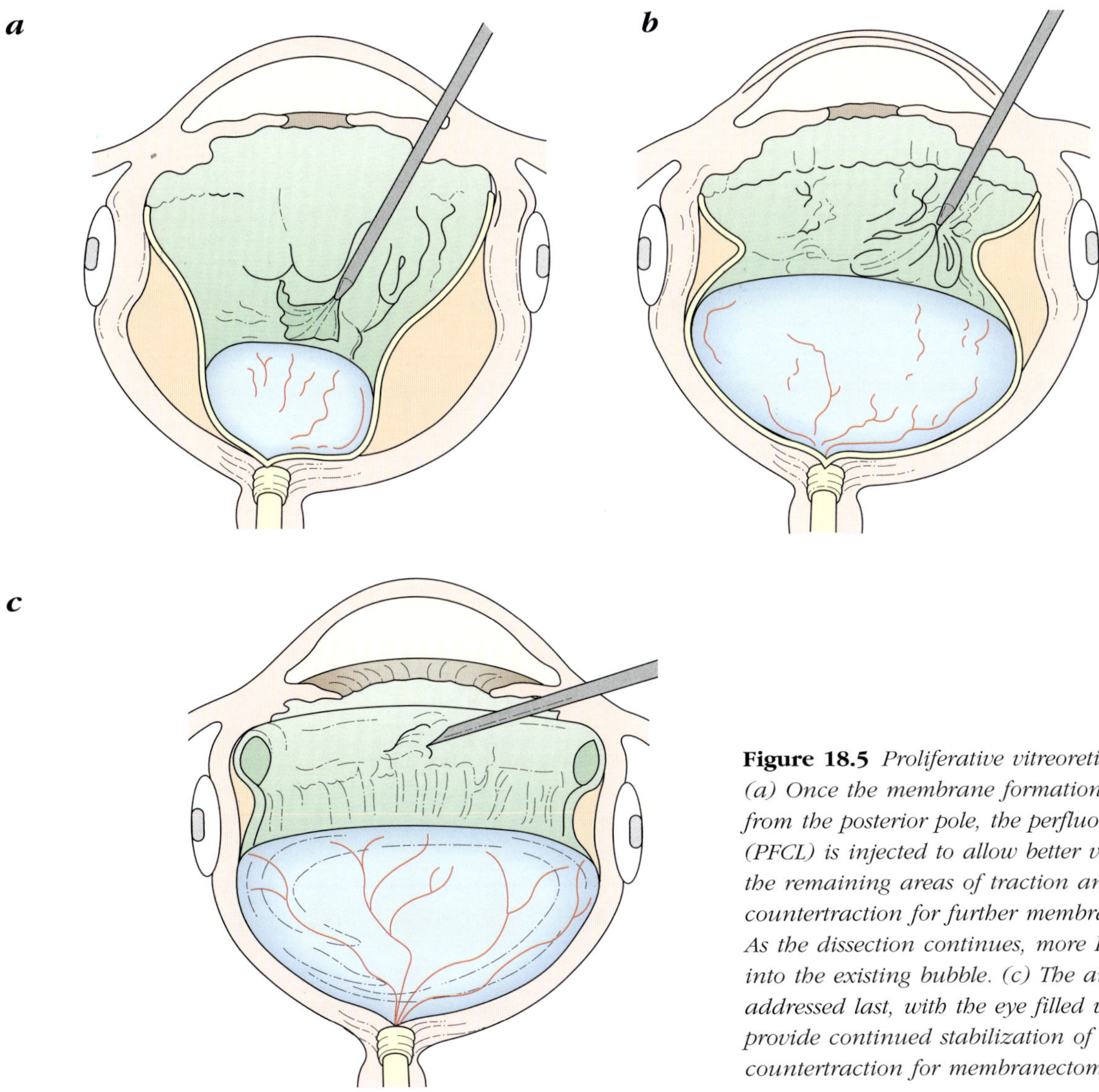

Figure 18.5 *Proliferative vitreoretinopathy (PVR). (a) Once the membrane formation is removed from the posterior pole, the perfluorocarbon liquid (PFCL) is injected to allow better visualization of the remaining areas of traction and to provide countertraction for further membranectomy. (b) As the dissection continues, more PFCL is injected into the existing bubble. (c) The anterior PVR is addressed last, with the eye filled with the PFCL to provide continued stabilization of the eye and countertraction for membranectomy.*

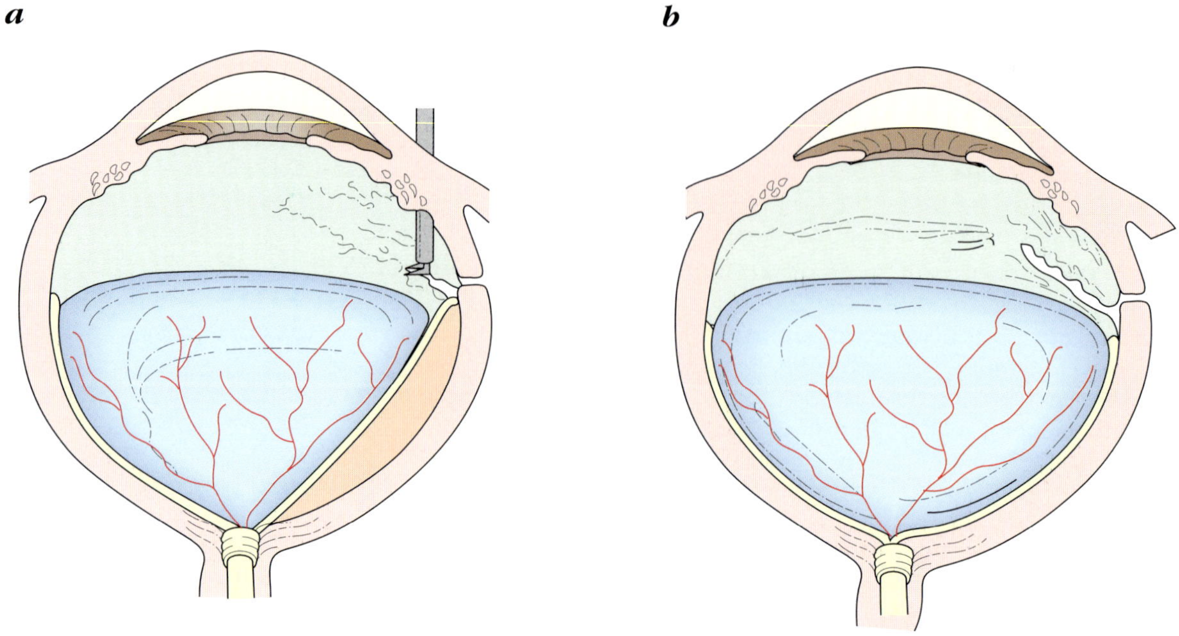

Figure 18.6 *A relaxing retinotomy may be necessary and can be performed under perfluorocarbon liquid (PFCL). (a) The PFCL stabilizes the globe and assists the surgeon in determining how much is enough. (b) The end point is reached once the traction is relieved and the retina flattens. This can be visualized as the retinotomy is performed.*

posterior PVR. Use of PFCLs has reversed this strategy to a posterior-to-anterior approach in a very systematic, controlled fashion.

The surgeon begins with the standard three-port pars plana vitrectomy. The preretinal membrane formation is then addressed by developing an edge of the membrane located close to the optic nerve. The membrane dissection is then begun posteriorly with a pick, a bent microvitreoretinal (MVR) blade or a pair of vitreoretinal forceps and is extended in an anterior direction.

After the initial dissection, a small amount of PFCL is injected over the optic nerve and posterior pole, below the level of the membrane formation. This flattens the posterior retina and provides better visualization of the areas of remaining traction and membrane formation, thus allowing more complete removal of the membrane formation (Fig. 18.5a).[39,40] The PFCL also helps to open tight funnel formations in severe PVR, and provides countertraction for further membrane dissection. As the dissection continues anteriorly, more PFCL is added to the bubble posteriorly to provide continued stabilization of the posterior retina (Fig. 18.5b). The PFCL bubble also acts as a barrier, protecting the posterior retina from cells and (possibly) biochemically active substances that may contribute to reproliferation.[41] The anterior PVR formation is then addressed with the assistance of scleral depression under the microscope (Fig. 18.5c). In severe anterior PVR cases, the lens is often removed to provide adequate visualization for the anterior dissection. The subretinal fluid is displaced anteriorly and drained through a peripheral retinal defect, thus avoiding the necessity for a posterior retinotomy.

After the preretinal membrane dissection is complete and the eye is filled with PFCL, a persistent retinal detachment becomes an ominous sign, indicating the presence of significant subretinal band formation or foreshortening of the retina. The subretinal bands may produce sufficient traction to require the creation of a small retinotomy and band removal. In the case of persistent traction and retinal detachment, a relaxing retinotomy would be the next logical step,[33,34,42] which may be performed under the PFCL in a controlled manner (Fig. 18.6).[43,44] Intraocular diathermy is applied in a circumferential fashion, peripheral to the area of retina exhibiting the most traction, with a sharp 23-gauge Mentor diathermy tip that can cut while cauterizing. Grieshaber intraocular scissors may be used, if necessary, to complete the retinotomy. With the PFCL in place, the retina will flatten when sufficient traction has been relieved. With persistent elevation, the retinotomy should be extended until the retina flattens. Endolaser photocoagulation is then applied to the retinotomy edges. The PFCL is removed in a similar manner as described for the GRTs. At this point, the surgeon must decide which postoperative tamponading agent to use: C_3F_8 or silicone oil.[45]

Carroll et al reported a series of 140 patients with retinal detachments and PVR grades C_2–D_3 repaired with the assistance of perfluoroperhydrophenanthrene.[46] In seven patients, the PFCL was left in the eye as a postoperative tamponading agent. Intraoperative reattachment was achieved in 98% of patients. At final follow-up (mean of 7.5 months), 84% of retinas remained attached and 92% of patients had stable or improved visual acuity.

Coll et al reported a series of 223 patients who underwent surgery for retinal detachment with PVR grades C_1–D_3 with the assistance of perfluorooctane.[47] Seventy-eight percent of the retinas were reattached posterior to the scleral buckle after a single vitreoretinal surgery, with 96% reattached after multiple surgeries (mean follow-up of 13 months). Visual acuity was 20/400 or better in 74% of eyes and 20/80 or better in 30% of eyes. Retained perfluorooctane was noted postoperatively in the vitreous cavity in 1.3% and in the subretinal space in 0.9%.

DISLOCATED CRYSTALLINE AND INTRAOCULAR LENSES

Both crystalline and intraocular lenses are lighter than the PFCLs and thus float on the surface of a PFCL bubble.[48] Use of the PFCLs has facilitated the safe removal of posteriorly dislocated crystalline lenses,[49] lenticular fragments[50] and intraocular lenses (IOLs).[51] The technique is similar for all cases but the actual physical removal may be different.

A dislocated crystalline lens or lenticular fragments may be secondary to spontaneous dislocation, trauma or complicated cataract surgery. A three-port pars plana vitrectomy is performed to release and remove any vitreous adhesions and inflammatory debris (Fig. 18.7a). The PFCL is then injected into the vitreous cavity, allowing the lens or lenticular material to float on the surface of the PFCL bubble (Fig. 18.7b). Hard lenticular material can be elevated into the anterior chamber and removed through a corneoscleral limbal wound, as in the case of dense nuclear sclerosis (Fig. 18.7c). More commonly, the lens material is removed with the phacofragmatome or vitrector on the surface of the PFCL bubble (Fig. 18.7d).[52] The lens material will break into smaller pieces which remain on the surface of the bubble above the retina. This allows safer lens removal, avoiding damage to the retina from dropping particles and eliminating high aspiration close to the surface of the retina. Care must be taken not to overfill the eye with PFCL, maintaining the PFCL interface near the equator for adequate visualization of the lens particles. With too high a PFCL level, the lens particles may disappear behind the iris root and/or become entrapped in the vitreous base.

The technique is similar for posteriorly dislocated IOLs, with the IOL floating on the surface of the PFCL bubble and eliminating direct manipulation of the IOL posteriorly (Fig. 18.8a,b). This avoids potential retinal complications of contusion, break formation, detachment and hemorrhage. The IOL may be floated up to the level of the ciliary sulcus, where it can be fixated by transscleral suturing. Fanous and Friedman described a technique for scleral fixation utilizing perfluoroperhydrophenanthrene (Fig. 18.8c).[53] One haptic is held with intraocular forceps and the other is lassoed in a 10-0 polypropylene loop that has been threaded through a standard 25-gauge needle and inserted into the eye at the level of the ciliary sulcus (1 mm posterior to the surgical limbus). The needle is withdrawn and the loop remains around the haptic. The second haptic is similarly fixated and the sutures are tied in the scleral bed, covered with a flap of sclera and then conjunctiva.

Another technique for posteriorly dislocated IOLs is removal from the eye through a corneoscleral limbal wound (Fig. 18.8d). The PFCL is very helpful when converting from a closed three-port system to an open wound by providing internal eye-wall support and preventing collapse of the globe. An IOL exchange can be performed, suturing in an IOL specifically designed for sulcus fixation (Fig. 18.8e) or simply implanting an anterior chamber IOL.

Greve et al reported the Vitreon Collaborative Study Group's experience with the management of posteriorly dislocated crystalline and intraocular lenses.[54] Their series consisted of 28 patients with dislocated lenses managed with the assistance of perfluoroperhydrophenanthrene. Postoperative visual acuity improved in 73% of patients, remained the same in 15% and worsened in 12%.

Anterior segment surgeons have questioned their own possible use of PFCL to retrieve a dislocated

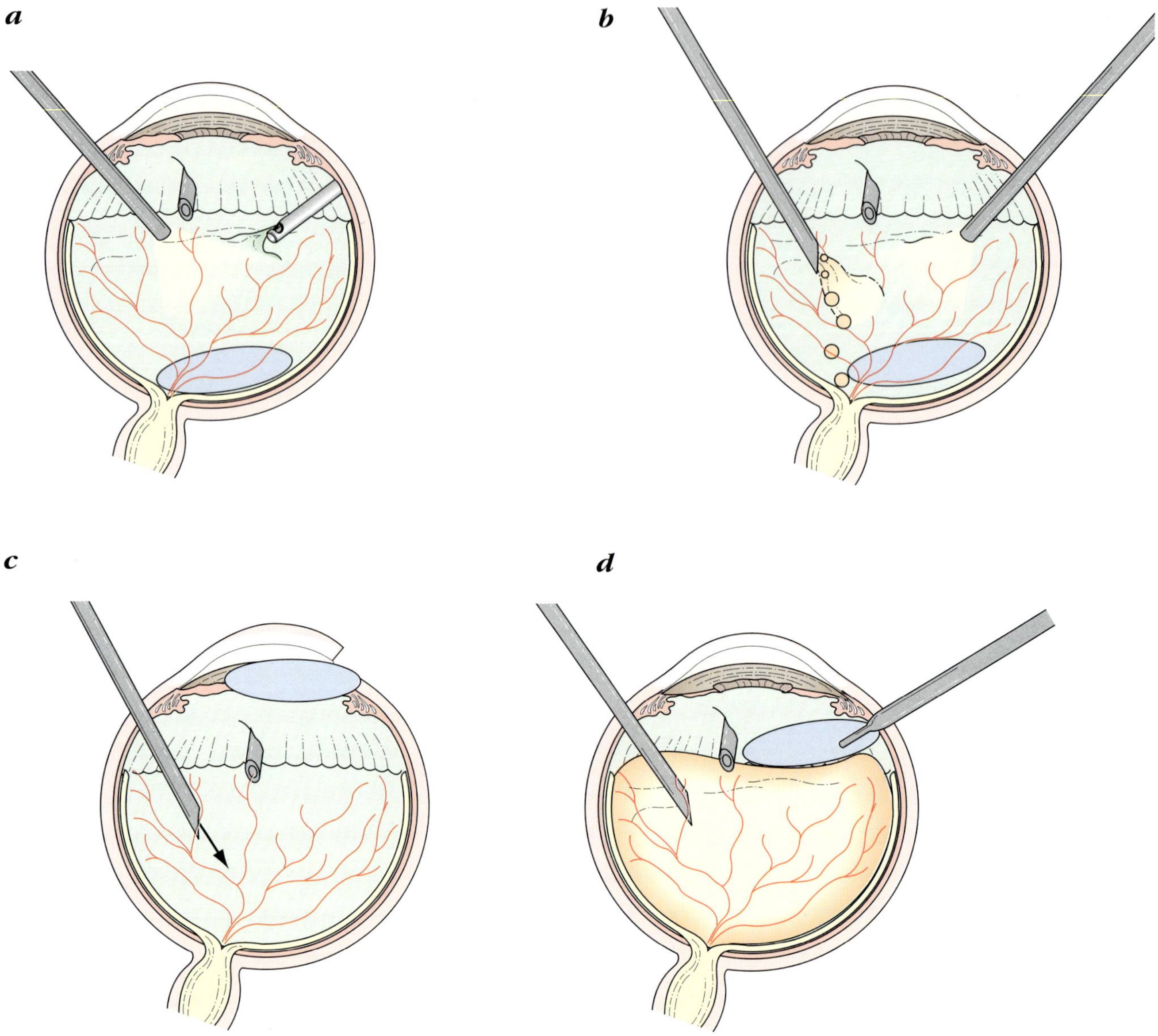

Figure 18.7 *Perfluorocarbon liquid (PFCL) use in the removal of dislocated crystalline lenses or lenticular fragments. (a) Standard three-port pars plana vitrectomy with release of any vitreous strands or adhesions to the lens. (b) Injection of PFCL is begun, resulting in the lens material floating on the surface of the PFCL bubble. (c) With dense nuclear sclerosis, the lens can be floated into the anterior chamber and removed through a corneoscleral wound. (d) The more common option is to remove the lens with a phacofragmatome or vitrector on the surface of the PFCL bubble. As the lens material breaks up into smaller pieces, the pieces will remain on the surface of the PFCL bubble, minimizing the risk of retinal damage.*

lenticular fragment or IOL during the original surgery. This would necessitate an anterior PFCL injection through the disrupted posterior capsule. This technique would most likely allow removal of the lens in question, but then the anterior segment surgeon must remove the PFCL. Without a three-port pars plana set-up, the PFCL cannot be removed by irrigation alone because of its high specific gravity. Therefore, it is recommended that PFCL only be used by experienced vitreoretinal surgeons.[55,56]

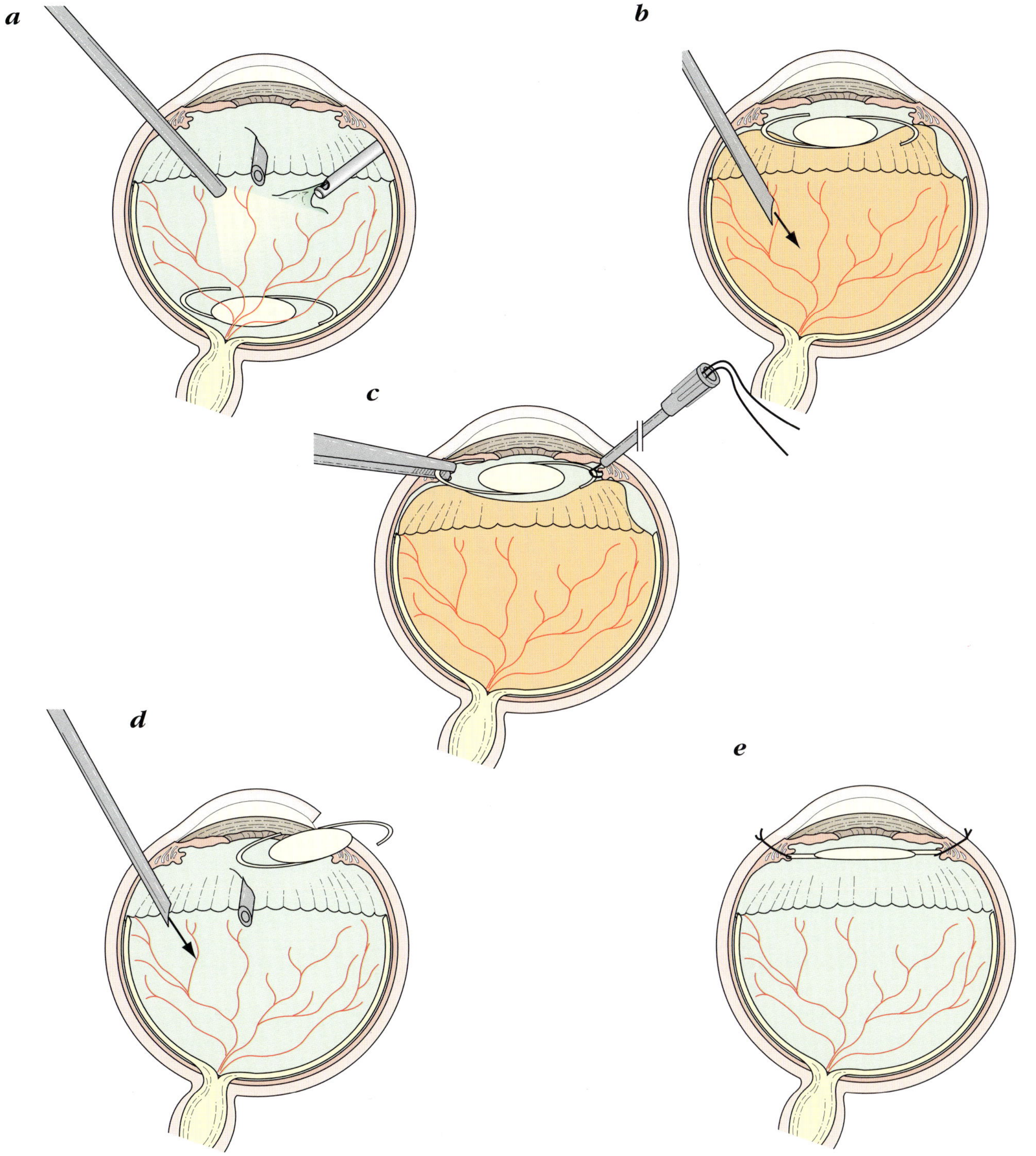

Figure 18.8 *Perfluorocarbon liquid (PFCL) use in the removal of a dislocated intraocular lens (IOL). (a) Standard three-port pars plana vitrectomy with release of any vitreous strands or adhesions to the IOL. (b) Injection of PFCL is begun, resulting in the IOL floating on the surface of the PFCL bubble. (c) The IOL can be fixated by transscleral suturing. One haptic is held with intraocular forceps and the other is caught in a 10-0 polypropylene loop that has been threaded through a standard 25-gauge hypodermic needle. This is repeated for the other haptic, and sutures are tied in the scleral bed. (d) The IOL can be removed from the eye through a corneoscleral limbal wound. (e) An IOL designed for sulcus fixation can then be implanted.*

The combination of a dislocated IOL or crystalline lens and a rhegmatogenous retinal detachment presents an even more difficult management problem to the vitreoretinal surgeon. Use of PFCLs has greatly simplified this once-very-complex surgical procedure.[48,57] The PFCL hydrokinetically flattens the retina, displacing the subretinal fluid through an anteriorly located retinal tear, while elevating the IOL or crystalline lens on the surface of the bubble. With the retina flat, the lens then can be managed as described above. Retinopexy is applied to the retinal tear, and an encircling element can be placed, if desired. The PFCL is then removed, as described previously.

Lewis and associates reported a series of four patients with dislocated crystalline lenses and retinal detachments treated with the assistance of PFCLs.[58] The lenses were removed and the retinas successfully reattached in each eye without complications. The visual acuity improved and the retinas remained reattached in all four eyes, with a follow-up of 6–9 months.

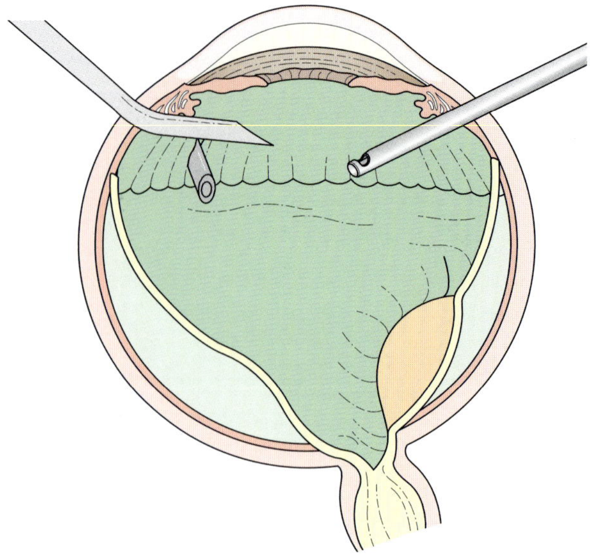

Figure 18.9 *A two-port system is utilized when the infusion cannula cannot be confirmed visually. A bent 20-gauge needle for infusion is held in one hand and the vitrector in the other hand, until the infusion cannula can be visualized.*

OCULAR TRAUMA

The PFCLs in ocular trauma, whether it is a vitreous hemorrhage with retinal detachment, intraocular foreign body, or retinal incarceration, have again proven to be very useful surgical adjuncts. Treatment of penetrating trauma with vitreous hemorrhage and retinal detachment repair are often technically difficult with limited visibility intraoperatively. The timing of the secondary repair (after primary wound closure) is somewhat controversial.[59] Many surgeons wait 7–14 days after the primary wound closure to allow resolution of choroidal congestion, decreased intraocular inflammation and partial or total posterior vitreous detachment.[60–62] Investigators have shown better surgical results with decreased complications with total vitrectomy, including removal of the posterior hyaloid membrane, in traumatized eyes.[63,64] However, secondary complications, including preretinal and subretinal membrane formation, may begin as early as 4 days post-trauma, thus favoring earlier vitrectomy.[65]

Regardless of the timing of the repair, the eye is prepared for a standard three-port pars plana vitrectomy. The infusion cannula is not utilized until its placement can be confirmed visually. It is best to begin with a two-port system, infusing BSS Plus with a bent 20-gauge needle or infusion light pipe visualized in the pupillary space in one hand, and the vitrector in the other (Fig. 18.9). The lens frequently has been expelled during the trauma, or is cataractous and therefore must be removed. A core vitrectomy is then performed until a hole in the posterior hyaloid is created (Fig. 18.10a). The PFCL is injected into the retrohyaloid space with a 25- to 27-gauge cannula, forcing the retina posteriorly and simultaneously dissecting the posterior hyaloid face and creating a complete posterior vitreous detachment (Fig. 18.10b). The vitrector may then be positioned anteriorly to safely remove the remaining vitreous hemorrhage and peripheral vitreous with minimal chance of inadvertent retinal damage (Fig. 18.10c).

Vitrectomy in traumatized eyes frequently is complicated by active bleeding into the vitreous cavity, but the PFCL will confine and control the bleeding due to its immiscibility with blood. More PFCL can be injected at this point to flatten the peripheral retina. Often schlieren is seen as the thick subretinal fluid exits from the retinal hole toward the vitreous cavity, indicating the site of the retinal defect. The remainder of the procedure is completed as described previously (Fig. 18.10d).

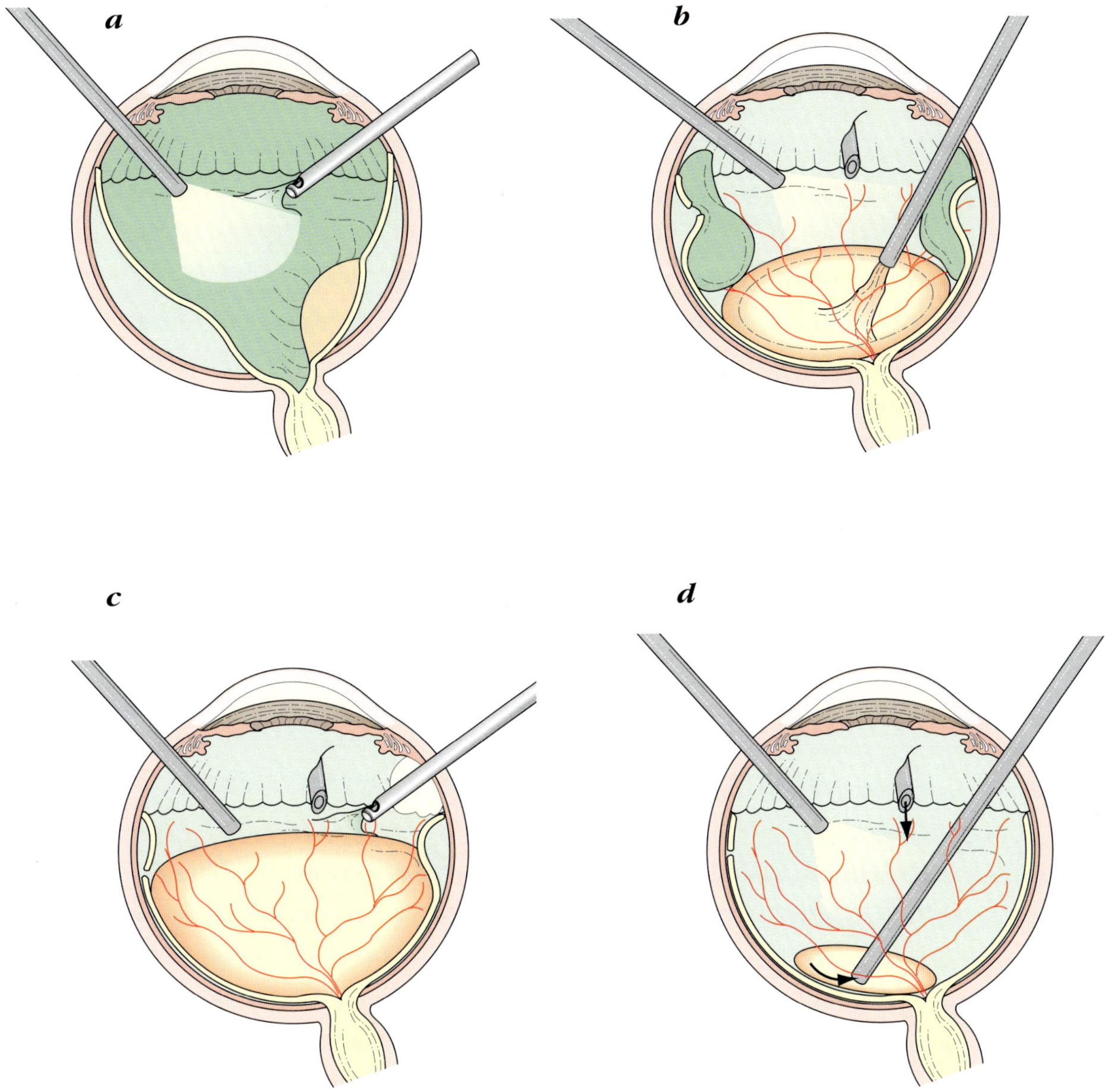

Figure 18.10 *Traumatic retinal detachment with vitreous hemorrhage. (a) A normal three-port pars plana vitrectomy is begun, locating or creating a hole in the posterior hyaloid face. (b) The perfluorocarbon liquid (PFCL) is then injected into the retrohyaloid space, hydrokinetically forcing the retina posteriorly, while dissecting the posterior hyaloid face and forming a complete posterior vitreous detachment. (c) The vitrector may now be positioned anteriorly to remove the vitreous hemorrhage and remaining vitreous body. (d) The retinopexy step is then performed, with a possible scleral buckling procedure if necessary. The PFCL is then removed as described previously.*

Desai et al presented three cases of penetrating ocular trauma with vitreous hemorrhage and associated retinal detachment.[66] The authors utilized the PFCL to separate the partially detached posterior hyaloid face, flatten the retina and simplify removal of the vitreous hemorrhage. In all cases, the retina was reattached successfully and documented as stable for a minimum of 8 months' follow-up.

Chang et al used PFCL in the management of 14 traumatic retinal detachments.[67] The PFCL flattened the retina intraoperatively in all eyes, avoiding the need for a posterior retinotomy. With a minimum follow-up of six months, eight of 11 eyes were anatomically reattached, with six gaining visual acuity of 20/400 or better.

Traumatic retinal incarceration can be a very difficult surgical challenge.[68] Depending on the extent of incarceration, a retinotomy may be required to relieve the tractional forces and flatten the retina. The PFCL can be utilized in this scenario (as with PVR), to provide countertraction and assist with deciding how much retinotomy is necessary.

The Vitreon Collaborative Study Group presented its results of 111 patients with a history of trauma (109 had retinal deatchment, 50 had PVR) repaired with perfluoroperhydrophenanthrene.[69] At the last follow-up, 75.6% remained reattached with 49.5% achieving a visual acuity of greater than or equal to 5/200 and 30.6% attaining a visual acuity of greater than or equal to 20/200. Factors predictive of a poor visual outcome were the type of trauma, the presence of GRT and poor preoperative visual acuity.

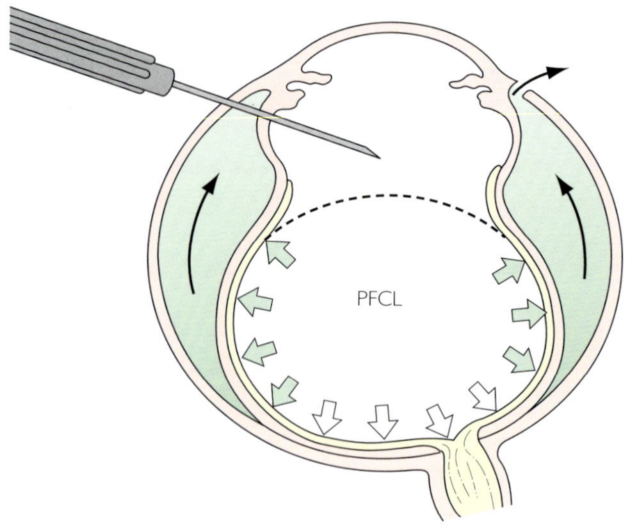

Figure 18.11 *Perfluorocarbon liquid (PFCL) in the treatment of massive suprachoroidal hemorrhage. The PFCL evacuates the suprachoroidal space in a posterior-to-anterior fashion, with the blood exiting through the anteriorly placed sclerotomies.*

MASSIVE SUPRACHOROIDAL HEMORRHAGE

Massive suprachoroidal hemorrhage (discussed in detail in Chapter 42) is one of the complications most feared by the ophthalmic surgeon, whether occurring intraoperatively or postoperatively, in an expulsive or nonexpulsive form.[70,71]

Desai et al described the surgical management of suprachoroidal hemorrhages utilizing PFCLs in three patients.[72] The sclerotomies were placed anteriorly only 4 mm posterior to the limbus in a circumferential fashion. The PFCL was injected with a 30-gauge needle at the limbus in aphakes, or at the pars plana in pseudophakic and phakic patients. The PFCL evacuated the suprachoroidal space in a posterior-to-anterior fashion, similar to subretinal fluid drainage, allowing the blood to exit through the anteriorly placed sclerotomies (Fig. 18.11). The PFCL also provided stabilization of the globe during pars plana vitrectomy, with less chance of intraoperative hypotony and exacerbation or recurrence of the suprachoroidal hemorrhage. The PFCL then was removed, with air, gas or silicone oil left in postoperatively. All three patients had complete resolution of the suprachoroidal blood, with retinas attached at the 5-month follow-up visit and improved visual acuity.

RETINAL DETACHMENT ASSOCIATED WITH CHOROIDAL COLOBOMA

Dysembryogenesis of the fetal fissure may result in a choroidal coloboma, consisting of hypoplastic retina overlying an area devoid of RPE and choroid.[73] About 40% of eyes with choroidal colobomas will develop an associated retinal detachment.[74] Surgical repair of these eyes has had poor anatomic success rates in the past.[75] With the advent of vitrectomy, the results have improved yet still are somewhat disappointing. Retinopexy alone is impossible in the area of the coloboma because of the absence of choroid and RPE. Treatment, whether laser or cryotherapy, must be directed to the healthy tissue beyond the edges of the coloboma. Colobomas are most often located inferiorly, which complicates the surgical repair of coloboma-related retinal detachments due to strict postoperative positioning requirements.

Lee and associates described a case of recurrent retinal detachment associated with coloboma after pars plana vitrectomy and sulfur hexafluoride injection.[76] The patient was examined 2 days postoperatively and noted to have recurrent subretinal fluid inferonasally, adjacent to a probable retinal defect in the coloboma. Two milliliters of perfluoroperhydrophenanthrene were injected at the pars plana into the vitreous cavity, with an equal amount of gas removed in an outpatient setting. No special positioning requirements were necessary owing to the inferior location of the retinal defect and the physical properties of the PFCL. Several days after the injection, when the subretinal fluid had reabsorbed, argon laser photocoagulation was performed around the coloboma and over the buckle. The PFCL was removed 4 weeks later, as described previously with multiple air–fluid exchanges. The patient's postoperative vision of counting fingers at 5 feet was attributed to cystoid macular edema and past corneal graft.

Perfluoroperhydrophenanthrene has been shown to be well tolerated in the eye postoperatively[9,77] and, under certain special circumstances, perfluoroperhydrophenanthrene has been left in the eye to ease postoperative positioning restrictions to provide a short-term tamponading effect.[78] However, the current Food and Drug Administration (FDA) recommendations are for use as an intraoperative tool.

OTHER LESS COMMON USES OF THE PFCLs

RETINAL DETACHMENT FOLLOWING PROSTHOKERATOPLASTY

Prosthokeratoplasty is a procedure to permanently replace the cornea with an artificial keratoprosthesis, reserved for patients in whom penetrating keratoplasty is likely to fail.[79] With the procedure, excellent initial results have been tempered by numerous long-term complications, including a retinal detachment rate of approximately 20%.[80,81] Traditional retinal detachment repair in these patients is difficult, with a high failure rate.

Paris and associates successfully repaired a retinal detachment in an eye with a Cardona keratoprosthesis by utilizing PFCL[82] (Fig. 18.12). Porting was done directly through the lids and the vitrectomy had to be performed with the indirect ophthalmoscope and an endoilluminator serving as the sole light source. The PFCL was injected after a partial air–fluid exchange, as described previously. Usually the retinal hole cannot be located owing to limited visibility, thus necessitating 360° of peripheral retinal cryopexy and an encircling element. The PFCL in Paris's case was removed 3 weeks later and the retina remained attached.

RETINOPATHY OF PREMATURITY

Management of advanced retinopathy of prematurity (ROP) presents a surgical challenge to the vitreoretinal specialist. Millsap and associates used PFCL to assist in the surgical repair of an infant with bilateral ROP[83] (Fig. 18.13). They recommended a two-port vitrectomy with the sclerotomy sites immediately posterior to the iris root. With the infusion light pipe and vitrectomy instrument, the lens is aspirated (for advanced cases) with removal of the posterior capsule and anterior vitreous condensation. Intraocular scissors may be necessary for more difficult posterior capsules. Following establishment of a pathway posteriorly, 2 ml of PFCL can be injected toward the posterior pole. The posterior retina may flatten at this time, while the anterior retina may remain detached and adherent to the fibrous tissue composed of vitreous base and lens capsule. The PFCL provides countertraction and improves the visibility of the membranes. If sharp dissection with intraocular scissors is required, the retina and neovascular tissue must be avoided. More PFCL may be injected to displace the subretinal fluid anteriorly. A drainage sclerotomy can be fashioned 6 mm posterior to the limbus, to allow external drainage of the subretinal fluid. Because of its density, the PFCL helps to maintain the shape of the eye, even if the infusion light pipe is removed. After the dissection is complete, the PFCL is removed and exchanged with some other vitreous substitute, if needed. An encircling no. 40 band may then be placed.

OTHER INDICATIONS

Investigators have reported numerous other uses of the PFCLs. Lambert et al described the use of PFCLs to control hemorrhagic complications during excision of choroidal neovascular membranes.[84] Forlini and associates reported the use of PFCLs during vitrectomy for endophthalmitis to assist in visualization.[85] Other authors have described the use of PFCLs in vitrectomy for complications of diabetic retinopathy.[86–88]

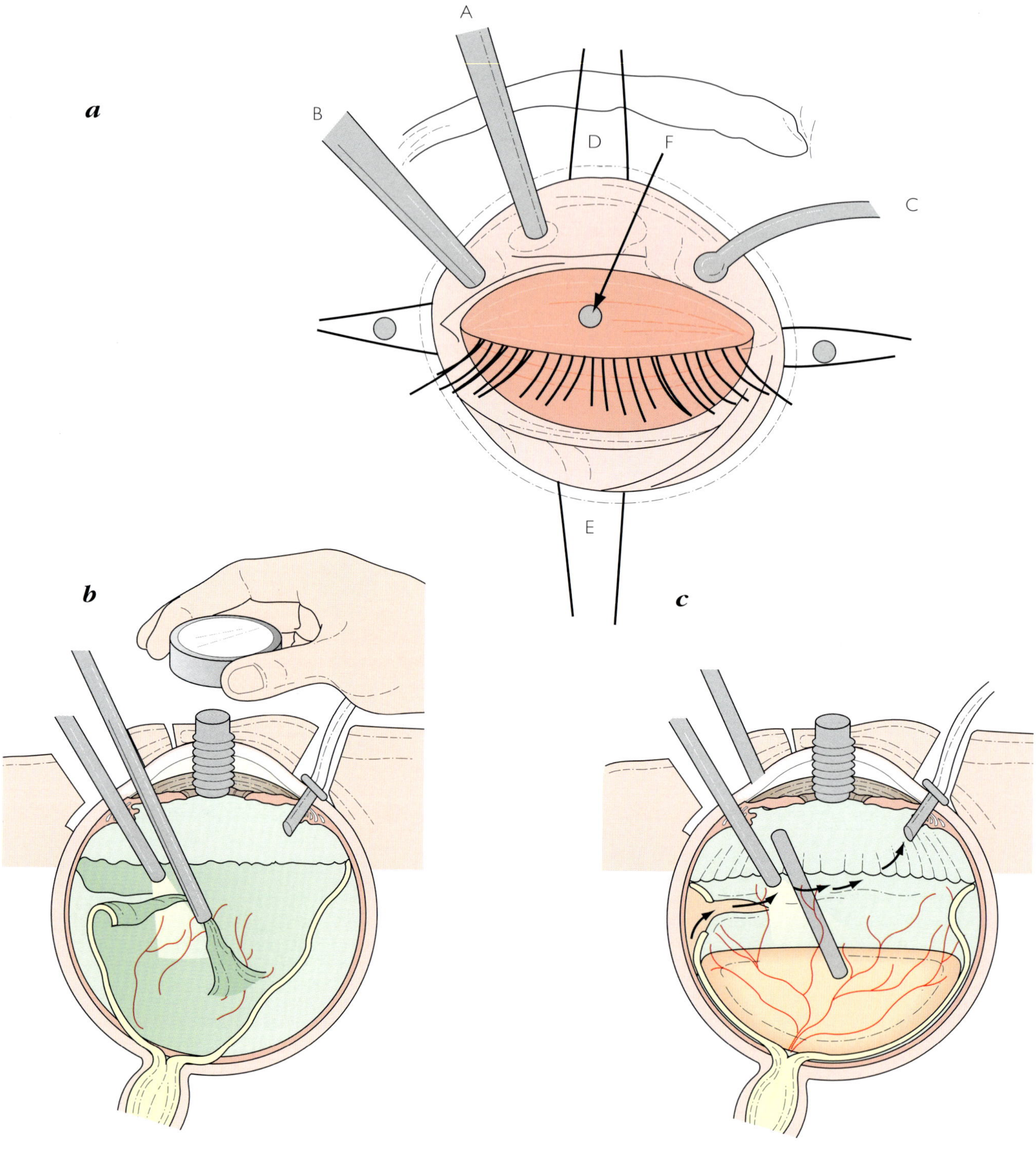

Figure 18.12 *Perfluorocarbon liquid (PFCL) in the repair of a retinal detachment in an eye with a Cardona keratoprosthesis. (a) Porting is done directly through the lids: (A) endoilluminator; (B) vitrector; (C) infusion cannula; (D, E) isolated recti muscles; (F) prosthetic device. (b) Vitrectomy is performed with the indirect ophthalmoscope, with the scope's light source turned off. (c) The PFCL injection phase after a partial air–fluid exchange, followed by 360° of retinal cryopexy.*

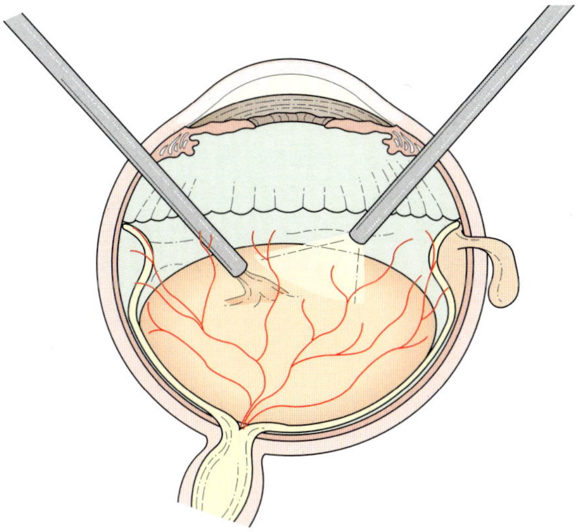

Figure 18.13 *Perfluorocarbon liquid (PFCL) in the surgical management of retinopathy of prematurity. More PFCL may be injected, displacing the subretinal fluid anteriorly and out through an anteriorly placed sclerotomy.*

Especially when there is a rhegmatogenous component to the detachment, the PFCL can greatly assist in the surgery and possibly help control bleeding during the vitrectomy.[89] The PFCL may sequester the clot at the site of bleeding, controlling the intraocular hemorrhage. Additional indications for the use of the PFCLs include: treatment of a rhegmatogenous retinal detachment when no retinal break can be found;[90] repair of a retinal detachment secondary to a macular hole after a vitrectomy;[90] removal of submacular hemorrhage with tissue plasminogen activator;[91] and removal of subretinal gas.[92]

CONCLUSION

The PFCLs have been a welcome addition to the limited arsenal of the vitreoretinal surgeon against the wide variety of vitreoretinal pathology. The primary indication for its use is surgical repair of GRTs. In this chapter, there are examples of many other indications for the PFCLs where their use (although not mandatory for the success of the case) may greatly simplify or shorten the surgical procedure. Whatever the vitreoretinal pathology may be, the surgeon must use his or her best judgment to determine if the use of a PFCL is indicated.

REFERENCES

1. Cibis PA, Becker B, Okun E, Canaan S. The use of liquid silicone in retinal detachment surgery, *Arch Ophthalmol* (1962) **68:**590–9.
2. Okun E. Intravitreal surgery utilizing liquid silicone: a long-term follow-up, *Trans Pac Coast Ophthalmol Soc* (1968) **49:**141–59.
3. Gremillion CM Jr, Peyman GA, Liu KR, Naguib KS. Fluorosilicone oil in the treatment of retinal detachment, *Br J Ophthalmol* (1990) **74:**643–6.
4. Clark LC Jr, Gollan F. Survival of mammals breathing organic liquids equilibrated with oxygen at atmospheric pressure (letter), *Science* (1966) **152:**1755–6.
5. Haidt SJ, Clark LC, Ginsberg J. Liquid perfluorocarbon replacement of the eye, *ARVO Supplement to Invest Ophthalmol Vis Sci* (JB Lippincott: Philadelphia, 1982): 233 (abst).
6. Zimmerman NJ, Faris D. The use of *N*-perfluorocarbon amines in complicated retinal detachments, *Invest Ophthalmol Vis Sci* (1984) **25** (Suppl):258 (abst).
7. Miyamoto K, Refojo MF, Tolentino FI, et al. Perfluoroether liquid as a long-term vitreous substitute: an experimental study, *Retina* (1984) **4:**264–8.
8. Chang S, Zimmerman NJ, Iwamoto T, et al. Experimental vitreous replacement with perfluorotributylamine, *Am J Ophthalmol* (1987) **103:**29–37.
9. Nabih M, Peyman GA, Clark LC Jr, et al. Experimental evaluation of perfluorophenanthrene as a high specific gravity vitreous substitute: a preliminary report, *Ophthalmic Surg* (1989) **20:**286–93.
10. Blinder KJ, Peyman GA, Paris CL, et al. Vitreon®, a new perfluorocarbon, *Br J Ophthalmol* (1991) **75:**240–4.
11. Clark LC Jr. Methods of treating disorders of an eye with liquid perfluorocarbons. US Patent No. 4,490,351, Dec. 25, 1984.
12. Chang S. Low viscosity liquid fluorochemicals in vitreous surgery, *Am J Ophthalmol* (1987) **103:**38–43.
13. Sparrow JR, Jayakumar A, Berrocal M, et al. Experimental studies of the combined use of vitreous substitutes of high and low specific gravity, *Retina* (1992) **12:**134–40.
14. Peyman GA, Mehta NJ. Intravitreal infusion–aspiration instrument for silicone oil–perfluorocarbon liquid exchange (letter), *Retina* (1993) **13:**177–8.
15. Freeman HM, Castillejos ME. Current management of giant retinal breaks: results with vitrectomy and total air fluid exchange in 95 cases, *Trans Am Ophthalmol Soc* (1981) **79:**89–102.
16. Schepens CL, Freeman HM, Thompson RF. A power-driven multipositional operating table, *Arch Ophthalmol* (1965) **73:**671–3.
17. Peyman GA. A new operating table for the management of giant retinal breaks, *Arch Ophthalmol* (1981) **99:**498–9.
18. Norton EWD, Aaberg T, Fung W, Curtin VT. Giant retinal tears, I: Clinical management with intravitreal air, *Am J Ophthalmol* (1969) **68:**1011–21.

19. Heimann K. Behandlung kimplizieter Riesenrisse der Netzhaut, *Klin Monatsbl Augenheilkd* (1980) **176:**491.
20. Federman JL, Shakin JL, Lanning RC. The microsurgical management of giant retinal tears with trans-scleral retinal sutures, *Ophthalmology* (1982) **89:**832–9.
21. Scott JD. A new approach to the vitreous base, *Mod Probl Ophthalmol* (1974) **12:**407–10.
22. Rappazzo JA, Michels RG. A new system of intraocular instruments. II. Intraocular needleholder, *Retina* (1983) **3:**239–40.
23. Peyman GA, Rednam KRV, Seetner AA. Retinal micro-incarceration with penetrating diathermy in the management of giant retinal tears, *Arch Ophthalmol* (1984) **102:**562–5.
24. Ando F, Kondo J. A plastic tack for the treatment of retinal detachment with giant tear (letter), *Am J Ophthalmol* (1983) **95:**260–1.
25. De Juan E Jr, Hickingbotham D, Machemer R. Retinal tacks, *Am J Ophthalmol* (1985) **99:**272–4.
26. Ando F, Kondo J. Surgical techniques for giant retinal tears with retinal tacks, *Ophthalmic Surg* (1986) **17:**408–11.
27. Abrams GW, Williams GA, Neuwirth J, McDonald HR. Clinical results of titanium retinal tacks with pneumatic insertion, *Am J Ophthalmol* (1986) **102:**13–19.
28. De Juan E Jr, McCuen BW II, Machemer R. The use of retinal tacks in the repair of complicated retinal detachments, *Am J Ophthalmol* (1986) **102:**20–4.
29. O'Grady GE, Parel JM, Lee W, et al. Hypodermic stainless steel tacks and companion inserter designed for peripheral fixation of retina, *Arch Ophthalmol* (1988) **106:**271–5.
30. Chang S, Lincoff H, Zimmerman NJ, Fuchs W. Giant retinal tears: surgical techniques and results using perfluorocarbon liquids, *Arch Ophthalmol* (1989) **107:**761–6.
31. Millsap CM, Peyman GA, Mehta NJ, et al. Perfluoroperhydrophenanthrene (Vitreon) in the management of giant retinal tears: results of a collaborative study, *Ophthalmic Surg* (1993) **24:**759–63.
32. McDonald HR, Lewis H, Aaberg TM, Abrams GW. Complications of endodrainage retinotomies created during vitreous surgery for complicated retinal detachment, *Ophthalmology* (1989) **96:**358–63.
33. Haut J, Larricart P, van Effenterre G. Localized retinectomy indications in the treatment and prevention of retinal detachment, *Ophthalmologica* (1984) **188:**212–15.
34. Machemer R. Retinotomy, *Am J Ophthalmol* (1981) **92:**768–74.
35. Kreiger AE, Lewis H. Management of giant retinal tears without scleral buckling: use of radical dissection of the vitreous base and perfluoro-octane and intraocular tamponade, *Ophthalmology* (1992) **99:**491–7.
36. Freeman HM, Chang S, Mosher C. Perfluoro-*n*-octane in the management of giant retinal tears, Annual Meeting of American Academy of Ophthalmology, San Francisco (1997): 147.
37. Kertes PJ, Wafapoor H, Peyman GA, et al. Vitreon Collaborative Study Group. The management of giant retinal tears using perfluoroperhydrophenanthrene: a multicenter case series, *Ophthalmology* (1997) **104:**1159–65.
38. Freeman HM. Current management of giant retinal breaks and fellow eyes. In: Ryan SJ, ed, *Retina*, 2nd edn (Mosby: St Louis, 1994): 2313–28.
39. Chang S, Ozmert E, Zimmerman NJ. Intraoperative perfluorocarbon liquids in the management of proliferative vitreoretinopathy, *Am J Ophthalmol* (1988) **106:**668–74.
40. Glaser BM, Carter JB, Kuppermann BD, Michels RG. Perfluoro-octane in the treatment of giant retinal tears with proliferative vitreoretinopathy, *Ophthalmology* (1991) **98:**1613–21.
41. Forlini C. Centrifugal surgical strategy with early introduction of PFCL in the management of retinal tractional detachment: effect on reproliferation, *J Vitreo Retina* (1992) **1:**44–51.
42. Morse LS, McCuen BW II, Machemer R. Relaxing retinotomies: analysis of anatomic and visual results, *Ophthalmology* (1990) **97:**642–8.
43. Han DP, Rychwalski PJ, Mieler WF, Abrams GW. Management of complex retinal detachment with combined relaxing retinotomy and intravitreal perfluoro-*n*-octane injection, *Am J Ophthalmol* (1994) **118:**24–32.
44. Greve MDJ, Peyman GA, Millsap CM. Relaxing retinotomy under perfluorocarbon liquid, *Ophthalmic Surg Lasers* (1996) **27:**154–5.
45. Silicone Study Group. Vitrectomy with silicone oil or perfluoropropane gas in eyes with severe proliferative vitreoretinopathy: results of a randomized clinical trial. Silicone study group report 2, *Arch Ophthalmol* (1992) **110:**780–92.
46. Carroll BF, Peyman GA, Mehta NJ, et al. Repair of retinal detachment associated with proliferative vitreoretinopathy using perfluoroperhydrophenanthrene (Vitreon®), *Can J Ophthalmol* (1994) **29:**66–9.
47. Coll GE, Chang S, Sun J, et al. Perfluorocarbon liquid in the management of retinal detachment with proliferative vitreoretinopathy, *Ophthalmology* (1995) **102:**630–9.
48. Liu KR, Peyman GA, Chen MS, Chang KB. Use of high-density vitreous substitutes in the removal of posteriorly dislocated lenses or intraocular lenses, *Ophthalmic Surg* (1991) **22:**503–7.
49. Shapiro MJ, Resnick KI, Kim SH, Weinberg A. Management of the dislocated crystalline lens with a perfluorocarbon liquid, *Am J Ophthalmol* (1991) **112:**401–5.
50. Wallace RT, McNamara JA, Brown G, et al. The use of perfluorophenanthrene in the removal of intravitreal lens fragments, *Am J Ophthalmol* (1993) **116:**196–200.
51. Lewis H, Sanchez G. The use of perfluorocarbon liquids in the repositioning of posteriorly dislocated lenses, *Ophthalmology* (1993) **100:**1055–9.
52. Alfaro DV, Liggett PE. Indications and management of pars plana vitrectomy for retained lens fragments following cataract surgery, *Vitreoretinal Surg Technol* (1993) **15:**3–4.
53. Fanous MM, Friedman SM. Ciliary sulcus fixation of a dislocated posterior chamber intraocular lens using liquid perfluorophenanthrene, *Ophthalmic Surg* (1992) **23:**551–2.
54. Greve MDJ, Peyman GA, Mehta NJ, Millsap CM. Use of perfluoroperhydrophenanthrene in the management of posteriorly dislocated crystalline and intraocular lenses, *Ophthalmic Surg* (1993) **24:**593–7.
55. Foster RE, Smiddy WS, Alfonso EC, Parrish RK II. Secondary glaucoma associated with retained perfluorophenanthrene (letter), *Am J Ophthalmol* (1994) **118:**253–5.
56. Peyman GA, Schulman JA, Sullivan B. Perfluorocarbon liquids in ophthalmology, *Surv Ophthalmol* (1995) **39:**375–95.
57. Brod RD, Flynn HW Jr, Clarkson JG, Blankenship GW. Management options for retinal detachment in the presence of a posteriorly dislocated intraocular lens, *Retina* (1990) **10:**50–6.

58. Lewis H, Blumenkranz MS, Chang S. Treatment of dislocated crystalline lens and retinal detachment with perfluorocarbon liquids, *Retina* (1992) **12:**299–304.
59. Mieler WF. The role and timing of pars plana vitrectomy in penetrating ocular trauma, *Arch Ophthalmol* (1997) **115:**1191–2.
60. Abrams GW, Topping TM, Machemer R. Vitrectomy for injury: the effect on intraocular proliferation following perforation of the posterior segment of the rabbit eye, *Arch Ophthalmol* (1977) **97:**743–8.
61. Coleman DJ. Early vitrectomy in the management of the severely traumatized eye, *Am J Ophthalmol* (1982) **93:**543–51.
62. Ryan SJ. Guidelines in the management of penetrating ocular trauma with emphasis on the role and timing of pars plana vitrectomy, *Int Ophthalmol* (1979) **1:**105–8.
63. Gregor Z, Ryan SJ. Complete and core vitrectomies in the treatment of experimental posterior penetrating eye injury in the rhesus monkey. I. Clinical features, *Arch Ophthalmol* (1983) **101:**441–5.
64. Gregor Z, Ryan SJ. Complete and core vitrectomies in the treatment of experimental posterior penetrating eye injury in the rhesus monkey. II. Histologic features, *Arch Ophthalmol* (1983) **101:**446–50.
65. Cleary PE, Ryan SJ. Histology of wound, vitreous, and retina in experimental posterior penetrating eye injury in the rhesus monkey, *Am J Ophthalmol* (1979) **88:**221–31.
66. Desai UR, Peyman GA, Harper CA III. Perfluorocarbon liquid in traumatic vitreous hemorrhage and retinal detachment, *Ophthalmic Surg* (1993) **24:**537–41.
67. Chang S, Reppucci V, Zimmerman NJ, et al. Perfluorocarbon liquids in the management of traumatic retinal detachments, *Ophthalmology* (1989) **96:**785–92.
68. Han DP, Mieler WF, Abrams GW, Williams GA. Vitrectomy for traumatic retinal incarceration, *Arch Ophthalmol* (1988) **106:**640–5.
69. Soheilian M, Peyman GA, Wafapoor H, et al. The Vitreon Collaborative Study Group. Surgical management of traumatic retinal detachment with perfluorocarbon liquid, *Int Ophthalmol* (1996) **20:**241–9.
70. Welch JC, Spaeth GL, Benson WE. Massive suprachoroidal hemorrhage: follow-up and outcome of 30 cases, *Ophthalmology* (1988) **95:**1202–6.
71. Reynolds MG, Haimovici R, Flynn HW Jr, et al. Suprachoroidal hemorrhage: clinical features and results of secondary surgical management, *Ophthalmology* (1993) **100:**460–5.
72. Desai UR, Peyman GA, Chen CJ, et al. Use of perfluoroperhydrophenanthrene in the management of suprachoroidal hemorrhages, *Ophthalmology* (1992) **99:**1542–7.
73. Spencer WH. *Ophthalmic Pathology: an Atlas and Textbook*, 3rd edn, Vol. 3 (WB Saunders: Philadelphia, 1986): 1415–24.
74. Gopal L, Kini MM, Badrinath SS, Sharma T. Management of retinal detachment with choroidal coloboma, *Ophthalmology* (1991) **98:**1622–7.
75. Wang K, Hilton GF. Retinal detachment associated with coloboma of the choroid, *Trans Am Ophthalmol Soc* (1985) **83:**49–62.
76. Lee KJ, Peyman GA, Paris CL, et al. Management of retinal detachment associated with choroidal coloboma using perfluoroperhydrophenanthrene (Vitreon®), *Ophthalmic Surg* (1992) **23:**553–4.
77. Blinder KJ, Peyman GA, Desai UR, et al. Vitreon, a short-term vitreoretinal tamponade, *Br J Ophthalmol* (1992) **76:**525–8.
78. Peyman GA, Conway MD, Soike KF, Clark LC Jr. Long-term vitreous replacement in primates with intravitreal Vitreon® or Vitreon® plus silicone, *Ophthalmic Surg* (1991) **22:**657–64.
79. Cardona H. Prosthokeratoplasty, *Cornea* (1983) **2:**179–83.
80. Girard LJ. Keratoprosthesis, *Cornea* (1983) **2:**207–24.
81. Rao GN, Blatt HL, Aquavella JV. Results of keratoprosthesis, *Am J Ophthalmol* (1979) **88:**190–204.
82. Paris CL, Peyman GA, Blinder KJ, et al. Surgical technique for managing rhegmatogenous retinal detachment after prosthokeratoplasty, *Retina* (1991) **11:**301–4.
83. Millsap CM, Peyman GA, Ma PE, Greve MDJ. The surgical management of retinopathy of prematurity using a perfluorocarbon liquid, *Int Ophthalmol* (1994) **18:**97–100.
84. Lambert HM, Capone A Jr, Aaberg TM, et al. Surgical excision of subfoveal neovascular membranes in age-related macular degeneration, *Am J Ophthalmol* (1992) **113:**257–62.
85. Forlini C, Dal Fiume E, Cicognani A, D'Eliseo D. Use of PFCL in the surgical management of endophthalmitis: new indication, *J Vitreo Retina* (1992) **1:**55–63.
86. Corcostegui B. Use of perfluorocarbon liquid in vitrectomy for diabetic rhegmatogenous retinal detachment, *J Vitreo Retina* (1992) **1:**30–4.
87. Mathis A. The use of perfluorodecalin in diabetic vitrectomy, *J Vitreo Retina* (1992) **1:**28–9.
88. Mathis A, Pagot V, David JL. The use of perfluorodecalin in diabetic vitrectomy, *Fortschr Ophthalmol* (1991) **88:**148–50.
89. Skolik SA, Moreira CA, Freeman WR, et al. Liquid perfluorocarbons for control of bleeding during pars plana vitrectomy: an animal model and human clinical correlation, *Invest Ophthalmol Vis Sci* (1994) **35** (Suppl):1618 (abst).
90. Berrocal MH, Chang S. Perfluorocarbon liquids in vitreous surgery, *Ophthalmol Clin North Am* (1994) **7:**67–76.
91. Kamei M, Tano Y, Maeno T, et al. Surgical removal of submacular hemorrhage using tissue plasminogen activator and perfluorocarbon liquid, *Am J Ophthalmol* (1996) **121:**267–75.
92. Brown AD, Kirkby GR. Removal of subretinal gas using perfluorocarbon liquid, *Retina* (1997) **17:**70–1.

Chapter 19 Use of silicone oil in vitreous surgery

Peter J Kertes and Gholam A Peyman

INTRODUCTION

Silicone oil is the term used to designate a group of clear inert hydrophobic polymer compounds based on siloxane chemistry of varying viscosities. The length of the polymer determines the viscosity, and the silicone oils in usage today range from 1000 to 12 500 cSt in viscosity. Silicone oil has a refractive index of 1.4035, which is slightly higher than that of the vitreous (1.33).[1,2]

Its use as a vitreous substitute was first described by Stone in 1958.[3] Unlike other vitreous substitutes, silicone oil may remain in the eye almost permanently. It has a density of 0.975 – less than water – and thus floats on water in the vitreous. It is always found at the top of the vitreous cavity, so superior tears are easily and nearly always closed by silicone oil. Because it is impossible to fill the vitreous cavity completely with silicone oil, inferior tears frequently require a scleral buckle to achieve permanent closure (Fig.19.1).

The interfacial tension of silicone oil is high (40 dyne/cm^2), but less than the gas–water interface (70 dyne/cm^2).[4] For this reason, air often is used first to flatten the retina; then the air is replaced with silicone oil to provide a long-term internal tamponade (Fig. 19.2).[5]

INDICATIONS

There are few hard-and-fast rules about the indications for the use of silicone oil. These will vary from patient to patient and from surgeon to surgeon. There are some important principles, however, that may help to guide its use.[6]

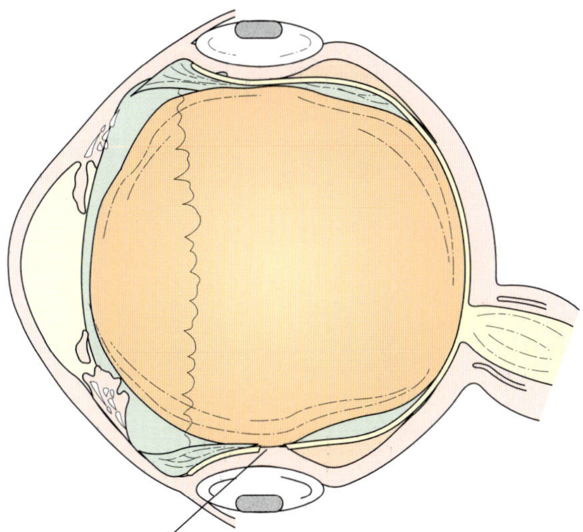

Figure 19.1 *The use of a scleral buckle with a silicone oil tamponade can help to achieve closure of inferior retinal breaks.*

PROLONGED TAMPONADE

Chief among these principles is the length of the internal tamponade provided by silicone oil. This is important when an initially closed break may be expected to reopen, such as occurs in cases complicated by significant proliferative vitreoretinopathy (PVR), or in eyes at high risk for the development of PVR.

POSTOPERATIVE POSITIONING

In addition to a tamponade of longer duration, silicone provides a more complete and consistent fill *a*

b

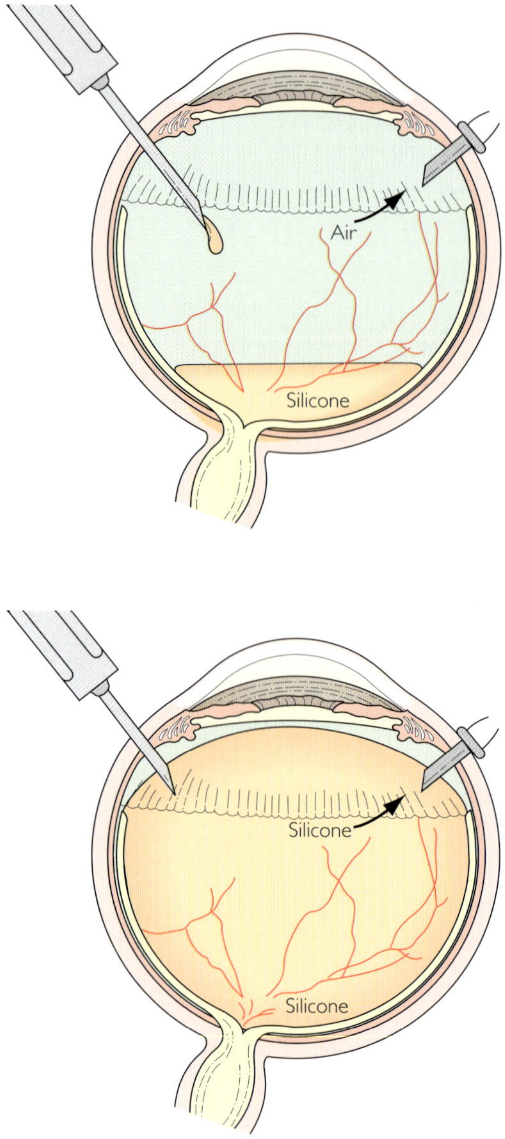

Figure 19.2 *Silicone–air exchange. (a) Silicone oil is injected into the eye through a 16-gauge cannula as the air infusion pressure is lowered. (b) Silicone–air exchange continues until the silicone reaches the posterior surface of the lens or the iris diaphragm and oil can be seen to reflux into the air infusion cannula.*

so that issues of positioning become less critical. Silicone oil can be considered for patients with orthopedic problems, for children or for any patient who, for whatever reason, cannot maintain the position required for effective intraocular gas tamponade.

VITREOUS HEMORRHAGE

Vitreous surgery is commonly complicated by postoperative vitreous hemorrhage. This is particularly true of diabetic vitrectomies, but can occur whenever extensive membrane dissection or retinotomy is required. Such postoperative hemorrhage is limited with the use of silicone oil,[7] which has the effect of concentrating and compartmentalizing clotting factors at the site of hemorrhage and thereby limits the amount and extent of the bleeding. Moreover, this effect combined with the immiscibility of silicone and blood also serves to maintain media clarity, which, in the event of a postoperative vitreous hemorrhage, can be a significant problem in air- or fluid-filled eyes.[8]

PRACTICAL CONSIDERATIONS

There are several practical patient issues that might sway a surgeon to use silicone oil over a long-acting gas. If a patient is monocular or has relatively high or immediate visual demands, silicone oil offers faster and earlier visual rehabilitation. If a patient needs to travel by air or to a higher elevation in the early postoperative period, then clearly silicone is a safer and more sensible choice.

PROLIFERATIVE VITREORETINOPATHY

Several factors have improved the success of retinal detachment and PVR surgery. Eyes previously considered unsalvageable because of significant PVR now enjoy a relatively good prognosis for the recovery of functional vision. There is no question that our ability to provide prolonged intraocular tamponade, such as with silicone oil, has contributed importantly to this success. In one series of 500 cases with 2 years of follow-up, anatomic success was achieved in 70% of cases and functional success in 60%.[9] Yeo et al reported similar findings in 1987.[10]

The Silicone Study Group conducted a multicenter, randomized, clinical trial involving 101 eyes with rhegmatogenous retinal detachment and severe PVR (grade C_3 or worse) to compare the effectiveness of silicone oil to sulfur hexafluoride (SF_6). The study demonstrated the superiority of silicone oil to SF_6 in achieving a visual acuity of 5/200 or better (50–60% vs 30–40%) and macular attachment (80% vs 60%).[11]

The Silicone Study Group went on to compare the efficacy of silicone oil to perfluoropropane (C_3F_8) gas in 265 eyes with rhegmatogenous retinal detachment and severe PVR (grade C_3 or worse). The investigators found no significant difference between silicone oil and C_3F_8 in their achievement of retinal reattachment or visual acuity (≥ 5/200). Hypotony was twice as prevalent in eyes that received C_3F_8 and occurred more often in eyes that had undergone previous vitrectomy and were tamponaded with C_3F_8.[12–14] Of note, the Silicone Study Group found silicone oil and C_3F_8 to be equally effective tamponading agents, even when a retinotomy was required.[15]

DIABETIC VITRECTOMY

No firm rules exist for the use of silicone oil in proliferative diabetic retinopathy as an adjunct to diabetic vitrectomy. There are, however, situations where its use can be rationalized easily and encouraged. These indications might include: eyes with severe tractional retinal detachment; eyes with combined tractional/rhegmatogenous retinal detachment with or without some component of PVR; recurrent nonclearing vitreous hemorrhage where injection of silicone oil can be expected to keep the vitreous cavity relatively clear by preventing and limiting the dispersion of postoperative vitreous hemorrhage; and rubeosis iridis in the setting of proliferative diabetic retinopathy.[16]

Diabetic retinopathy is a major cause of anterior segment neovascularization and neovascular glaucoma.[17] The incidence of rubeosis after vitrectomy and lensectomy has been reported to be in the range of 30–50%.[18–20] When only vitrectomy is performed, the incidence is in the range of 10–15%.[21] Some investigators have postulated that silicone oil may somehow prevent or arrest the progress of rubeosis.[16,17] This effect has been attributed to a barrier effect created by silicone that, in some way, prevents the diffusion of the angiogenic substance(s) elaborated by the ischemic and/or detached retina from reaching the anterior segment. This is supported by evidence from animal experiments that demonstrates a higher anterior chamber oxygen concentration in aphakic vitrectomized eyes filled with silicone oil than in similar eyes not filled with silicone.[20] This salutary effect is far from universal and has been disputed by several authors.[22–25]

The prolonged and stable internal tamponade provided by silicone may be desirable in cases with pre-existing (especially posterior) retinal breaks or in cases where extensive membrane dissection has led to the creation of iatrogenic retinal tears. The optical clarity afforded by silicone facilitates the intra- and postoperative laser photocoagulation that may be necessary in these silicone-filled diabetic eyes.[9,23] Similarly, if pre- or subretinal hemorrhage prevents the placement of adequate laser retinopexy at the time of surgery at the site of a retinal break or relaxing retinotomy, the permanent and stable tamponade of silicone oil, in contrast to gas, allows the surgeon to wait for clearing and resorption of the hemorrhage before applying the necessary retinopexy.

Silicone essentially prevents the recurrent vitreous hemorrhage that so often complicates diabetic vitrectomy, particularly in eyes where extensive dissection of neovascular tissue or a large retinotomy has been performed.[26] Silicone concentrates and compartmentalizes clotting factors at the site of bleeding, thus preventing its extension. The immiscibility of silicone and blood further prevents diffusion of the blood, keeping the media relatively clear and the retinal details visible.

The confinement of the hemorrhage to the preretinal space, however, may delay its clearance and contribute to the formation of fibrosis and epiretinal membranes. This can be avoided by the injection of intravitreal tissue plasminogen activator (tPA) in the early postoperative period.[8] This technique is reserved for silicone-filled eyes with significant posterior preretinal hemorrhage on the first postoperative day. Typically, 12.5–25 µg of tPA in a volume of 0.05–0.1 ml of balanced salt solution (BSS) is injected through the pars plana into the midvitreous cavity under topical anesthesia. The patient is positioned supine for the first 12–24 hours to allow the tPA to mix with the premacular hemorrhage, and subsequently upright to allow the newly liquefied hemorrhage to be displaced inferiorly.

Interestingly, the 12% incidence of retinal redetachment after silicone oil removal in diabetics is lower than that reported for nondiabetics.[27–29] This likely relates to differences in pathophysiology and natural history, the more typically posterior location of retinal breaks in proliferative diabetic retinopathy, and the near-universal presence of scatter laser photocoagulation in the setting of diabetic vitrectomy.

INFECTIOUS RETINITIS

Viral retinitis is a relatively frequent finding in patients with acquired immunodeficiency syndrome (AIDS) or other causes of immunosuppression. Cytomegalovirus (CMV) is the most common infectious agent, although herpes zoster and herpes simplex infection also occur. Such retinitis is the single greatest risk factor for the development of a retinal detachment, occurring in probably 40% of cases. The incidence of bilaterality is also very high, in the range 17–67%.[30–32]

CMV retinitis-related detachments differ from rhegmatogenous detachments seen in immunocompetent patients in several important ways. These detachments are often associated with multiple tiny retinal breaks and areas of thinned, atrophic and gliotic retina. These patients are generally young and the vitreous may be well formed and often not detached at the time of surgery. Interestingly, PVR is an infrequent complication of CMV retinitis-related detachments, occurring less than 20% of the time.[30,33,34]

Conventional techniques of retinal detachment repair, such as scleral buckling and pneumatic retinopexy, have been disappointing. Silicone oil has the advantage of a more rapid recovery of vision and offers a permanent tamponade of multiple retinal breaks. Vitrectomy, combined with endolaser photocoagulation and silicone oil tamponade, is the favored management for the repair of such retinitis-associated retinal detachments, particularly when the detachment is extensive.[35–37] García and coworkers found that the addition of a scleral buckle adds little to the success of vitrectomy, laser or silicone oil surgery alone. They reported a total retinal reattachment rate of 84% and a macular reattachment rate of 91%.[38] These principles and indications for the use of silicone oil can be extrapolated to retinal detachments that occur in the setting of progressive outer retinal necrosis,[39,40] acute retinal necrosis,[41,42] and other necrotizing retinitides, although the prognosis following surgery is somewhat more guarded.

INTRAVITREAL DRUG DELIVERY

Silicone oil has been suggested and tested as a repository for lipophilic antiproliferative agents. Retinoic acid,[43] retinol,[44] and carmustine[45] dissolved in silicone oil were shown to be effective in the treatment of PVR in a rabbit model. The future may indeed see silicone used as an intravitreal drug delivery vehicle in eyes with PVR, for example, when silicone is used as an internal tamponading agent.

CAVEATS

The complications of silicone oil use relate largely to its migration into the anterior chamber. While aphakia is not a contraindication to its use, the absence of an intact iris diaphragm likely is. If the anterior displacement of silicone oil cannot be prevented, then keratopathy will certainly ensue and, as such, favor the use of a long-acting gas.[8,46]

Silicone provides a long-term and stable intraocular tamponade and may remain in place for as long as several years, but it is not permanent. Its removal or replacement requires a second operative procedure, usually 3–6 months following its instillation.[28,47] If the patient or surgeon expects to have limited access to an appropriate surgical facility, or if the patient's ill health makes him or her a poor repeat surgical candidate, then the use of gas may be preferred.

PREOPERATIVE EVALUATION

The decision to use silicone oil is often made at the time of surgery, but its likelihood can usually be ascertained during the preoperative evaluation. There are both important ophthalmologic and nonophthalmologic considerations that enter into the decision on whether or not to use silicone oil as a long-term intraocular tamponade. The decision to use silicone is generally one that is made over a long-acting gas, so the merits of each must be weighed in any given situation.

With respect to nonophthalmologic considerations, the surgeon has to judge whether the patient has the intellectual and physical ability to comply with any postoperative positioning that may be required, should the surgeon choose a gas tamponade. With the more complete and prolonged fill afforded by silicone oil, issues of postoperative positioning become less critical.[5,48] Certainly, in patients with orthopedic problems that prevent them from assuming the required position, in young children or in mentally disabled adults, silicone oil should be strongly considered when a prolonged postoperative tamponade is required. Other issues might include a patient who will travel by air or to a higher altitude soon after surgery. Silicone oil also leads to faster visual rehabilitation than a gas-filled eye, so a one-eyed patient and a binocular patient with higher visual demands might be candidates for the use of silicone oil.

The ophthalmologic indications for the use of silicone oil are enumerated above and need to be determined; the patient also needs to be evaluated carefully in the clinic preoperatively. Eyes with retinal detachments and PVR should be examined, with special attention paid to the configuration of the PVR, the state of the iris diaphragm and the presence and likelihood of future hypotony. In eyes with proliferative diabetic retinopathy, attention should be paid to the presence of rubeosis iridis, the presence of a tractional retinal detachment and the balance between neovascularization and fibrosis in the preretinal membranes that are present. With an ischemic retina and the requirement for extensive membrane dissection, the creation of iatrogenic retinal holes becomes quite likely, and this may sway the surgeon toward the use of a silicone oil tamponade.

OPERATIVE EVALUATION

The decision to use silicone oil is often made at the time of surgery. Important considerations that may favor the use of silicone oil may include: the number, extent and configuration of retinal breaks present at the end of surgery; the amount and nature of intraocular hemorrhage that was encountered during surgery; the need for a relaxing retinotomy or retinectomy; the status of the ciliary body; the integrity of the iris diaphragm; and the likelihood for laser treatment being required postoperatively.

INTRAOCULAR INJECTION OF SILICONE

Silicone oil can be injected intraocularly either by a direct fluid–silicone exchange (Fig. 19.3) or as a two-step procedure with an air–fluid exchange followed by an air–silicone exchange (see Fig. 19.2). The advantages of the former are improved visualization and more easily detected residual traction, because the retina flattens slowly. The advantages of a two-step procedure include better control of intraocular pressure (IOP) during the exchange and the reduced danger of silicone oil entering the subretinal space through a retinal hole.[6]

The two-stage procedure for silicone injection involves a modification of techniques used for gas–fluid exchange. Following a complete vitrectomy and relief of all the traction, the infusion cannula is connected to an air pump system, and an active or

a

b

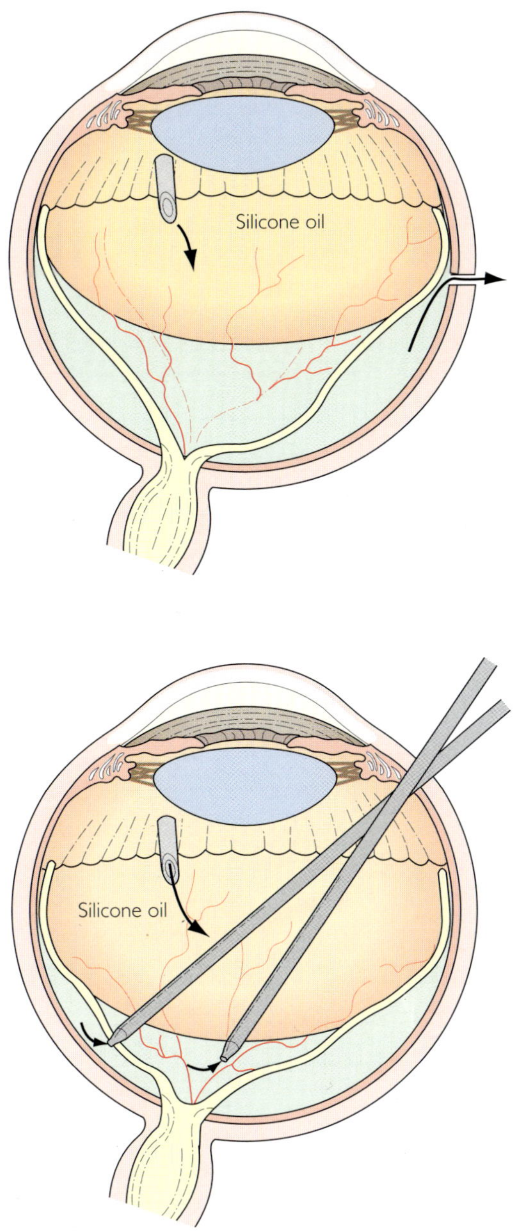

Figure 19.3 *Techniques of silicone–fluid exchange: (a) subretinal fluid is drained through a sclerotomy as silicone oil is injected; (b) alternatively, silicone is delivered through the infusion cannula as subretinal fluid is drained through an extrusion needle.*

passive extrusion needle is introduced to perform a complete air–fluid exchange. Any remaining subretinal fluid should be drained internally at this time and laser photocoagulation performed as necessary. The fiberoptic light pipe then is removed and the sclerotomy is closed securely with the appropriate suture

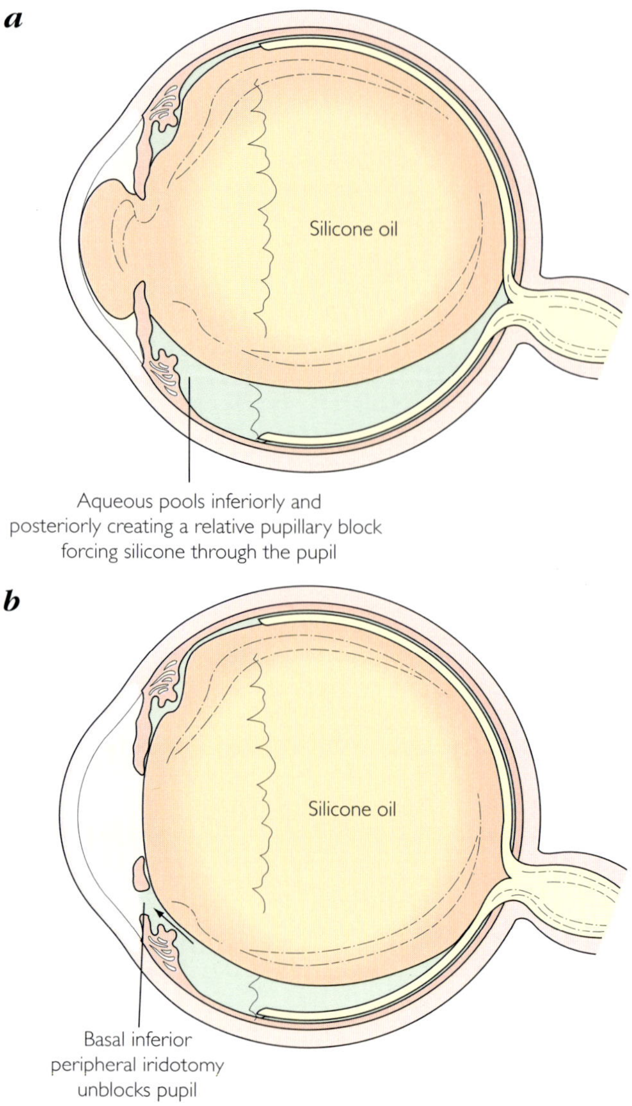

Figure 19.4 *(a) Pupillary block caused by silicone. (b) Pupillary block relieved by an inferior peripheral iridotomy.*

material. The other sclerotomy then is closed temporarily. When indicated, a scleral buckle is placed at this juncture.

The force required to inject silicone oil varies with the viscosity. Silicone oil of viscosity 1000 cSt probably can be injected through the infusion line of a short 20-gauge cannula, but for silicone of greater viscosity a short 16-gauge needle should be used.[49] Viscous fluid injectors controlled by the surgeon with a foot pedal have been recommended for intravitreal silicone injection. They give the surgeon more control over the amount of silicone injected intravitreally and prevent undesirable variations in IOP during injection, which can cause complications. Because pressures are greatest near the silicone container, and to prevent the tubing from becoming disconnected from the syringe, the injectors should have a locking syringe assembly.[50,51] Injection is facilitated by enlarging the 20-gauge sclerotomy site with the microvitreoretinal blade to accommodate the 5- to 6-mm beveled, blunt-tipped 16-gauge needles.

For manual injection of silicone, a 5- to 6-mm, bevel-tipped, 16-gauge needle connected to a 10-ml syringe containing at least 6 ml of silicone oil is similarly used, and is introduced through the previously enlarged sclerotomy site. To keep the eye expanded by air, for both the automated and manual delivery systems, the air infusion pressure is gradually lowered to approximately 10 mmHg as the injection of silicone proceeds.[50,52] In such a silicone–air exchange, the silicone oil fills the eye in a posterior-to-anterior direction. After the vitreous cavity is filled with silicone oil, the needle used to inject the silicone is removed and the sclerotomy is securely closed. The authors favor the use of a preplaced 6-0 Vicryl (polyglactin) suture in a figure-of-eight configuration. The air infusion cannula is then loosened, clamped and removed and the sclerotomy similarly is securely closed with a preplaced 6-0 Vicryl suture in a figure-of-eight configuration.

When the lens is removed at the time of vitrectomy, the anterior or posterior capsule should be preserved, depending on the surgical technique. An intact lens capsule largely prevents the anterior displacement of the silicone oil from the vitreous cavity to the anterior chamber, and the attendant complications of glaucoma and keratopathy, such as can occur in aphakic patients who have received intravitreal silicone oil.[52,53]

In aphakic eyes, an inferior peripheral iridectomy is performed to decrease the possibility of pupillary block glaucoma and to help keep the silicone oil in the posterior segment (Fig. 19.4).[8,52,54] Because silicone floats in an aqueous medium, a superior iridectomy can become blocked by the oil. In one series of 88 aphakic eyes that underwent vitrectomy with silicone oil fill, anterior segment complications were diminished in those aphakic eyes that had an inferior rather than a superior iridectomy. After 6 months of follow-up in eyes with a patent inferior iridectomy, silicone was not found in the anterior chamber but was seen in 50% of eyes with a superior iridectomy.[55]

The aphakic eye is filled nearly to the level of the iris diaphragm. Care must be taken not to fill the anterior chamber with silicone oil.[56] In phakic and pseudophakic eyes, the silicone bubble is allowed to touch the posterior lens surface.[10]

The other method of silicone injection is that of a silicone–fluid exchange. In this technique, after vitrectomy and membranectomy, silicone is injected through the infusion line as a fluted needle, or the tip of an extrusion handpiece is used to drain subretinal fluid through a posterior hole or drainage retinotomy. Residual traction detected during silicone injection can be relieved by a variey of vitreoretinal surgical techniques.[50,57] The silicone–fluid exchange continues until all detectable fluid is removed from the vitreous cavity and subretinal space and the eye is filled with silicone oil (see Fig. 19.3).

Fluid–silicone exchange is preferred by some surgeons for the following situations: suspected or 'lost' retinal breaks obscured by preretinal hemorrhage; posterior retinal breaks, especially if not treated with intraoperative photocoagulation or cryopexy; persistent tangential traction associated with retinal breaks; multiple retinal breaks, particularly when widely separated; and eyes requiring permanent intraocular tamponade because of tightly adherent and permanently contracted epiretinal membranes that require retinal resection to relieve traction.[58]

a

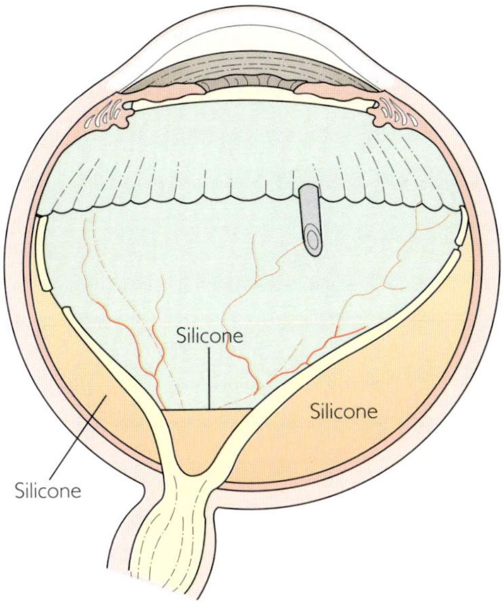

b

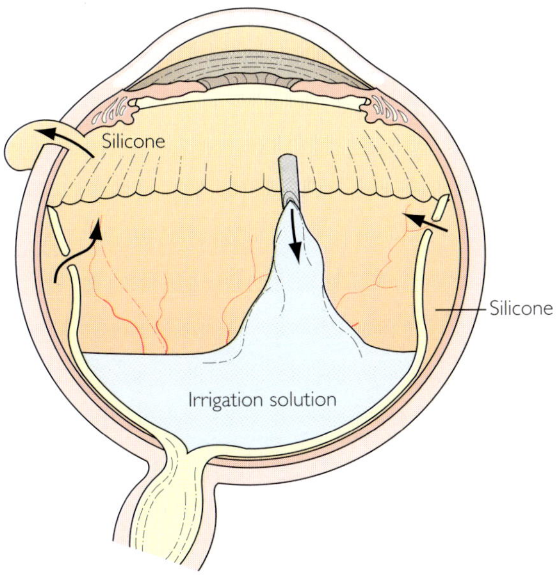

Figure 19.5 *Management of subretinal silicone oil: (a) a peripheral retinotomy is created; (b) irrigating solution is injected into the vitreous cavity, pushing the subretinal silicone anteriorly and out of the retinotomy and subretinal space.*

POSTOPERATIVE CONSIDERATIONS

POSITIONING

Not unlike air or gas, silicone oil has a lower specific gravity than water, and this property can be an advantage in the early postoperative period. The patient may be positioned in such a way that the buoyant force of the silicone oil may help to achieve or maintain retinal attachment. Nonetheless, the more complete and more permanent tamponade that is achieved by silicone oil makes the issues of postoperative positioning less critical than they would be in a comparable gas-filled eye.

RECURRENT RETINAL DETACHMENT

Repair of recurrent inferior retinal detachments under silicone oil may be achieved with prone positioning and later, when and if the retina flattens, with supplemental laser photocoagulation. This face-down position may allow the silicone to tamponade the inferior retina and the responsible retinal hole to achieve retinal reattachment.[59] If this fails or if a significant tractional component remains, repeat surgery may be necessary. Additional membrane dissection and relaxing retinotomy as necessary generally can be done under silicone oil. The drainage of subretinal fluid can be achieved with the infusion of air or silicone oil and either passive or active fluid extrusion. The silicone oil-fill has to be supplemented before the conclusion of surgery to make up for the silicone that may have been lost from the sclerotomy sites and to achieve a more complete tamponade.[60] In general, additional surgery is reserved for cases with posterior or progressive retinal detachments.

COMPLICATIONS OF SILICONE OIL USE

INTRAOPERATIVE

The main intraoperative complication that occurs with silicone oil instillation is that of overfill. Silicone oil is viscous and has to be injected under considerable pressure. If the IOP is not controlled during silicone injection, and an attempt is made to overfill the eye with silicone oil, then zonular rupture generally ensues and silicone oil gains access to the anterior chamber.[61] This is a problem that is more easily prevented than managed. Care should be taken to lower the air infusion pressure to a low level as silicone injection begins and to stop injecting once silicone can be seen touching the posterior lens surface or refluxing back up the air infusion line. Silicone should be injected until the IOP is normalized but not exceeded.

Another problem that arises with silicone injection occurs when silicone gains access to the subretinal space through a pre-existing retinal tear or hole.[62] This complication may be avoided by removing the traction around retinal tears before intravitreal injections, by prior drainage of subretinal fluid and by performing an air–fluid exchange initially. If silicone gains access to the subretinal space, air should be replaced with fluid and the silicone aspirated through an anterior hole or retinotomy (Fig. 19.5).[6]

REFRACTIVE CHANGES

Because the refractive index of silicone oil is higher than that of aqueous or lens cortex, the change in refractive error is determined by the shape of the anterior refractive surface of the silicone bubble. A negative lens effect occurs in phakic eyes in which the oil surface is concave because of the effect of the posterior lens surface. Consequently, phakic eyes become more hyperopic when filled with silicone oil. Aphakic eyes experience a myopic shift because of the convex anterior surface of silicone oil.[63]

Positioning also affects refraction. In the supine position, the silicone oil, which floats on water, moves forward and separates from the retina. This produces a positive posterior oil surface that contributes towards a myopic shift. In aphakic eyes, the oil can move forward through the pupil to increase the anterior convexity of the surface. This results in more of a myopic shift in aphakic than in phakic patients.[63,64]

INTRAOCULAR LENSES

With respect to intraocular lenses (IOLs), two issues deserve particular attention in the context of silicone oil: the potential interaction of silicone oil with an IOL that is in place at the time of silicone instillation;[65–69] and the choice of IOL type when cataract surgery is performed on a silicone oil-filled eye.[70–72]

Foldable posterior chamber IOLs of various materials have become quite popular and are encountered increasingly in patients undergoing pars plana vitrectomy for vitreoretinal disease. When silicone oil comes into contact with a silicone IOL, the silicone oil irreversibly coats the lens and obscures both the view in and the view out. The silicone coating is manifest as a thick coating with droplet formation on the lens surface that is tenaciously adherent and cannot be dislodged by instruments or viscoelastics. Although other lens biomaterials are not immune to this complication, adherence is maximal with the silicone IOLs.[65–69] When the use of silicone oil is contemplated in an eye with a foldable silicone IOL in place and an opening in the posterior capsule, consideration should be given to either removing the lens or using a long-acting gas instead.

The second important issue has to do with the choice of lens material, design and power when cataract surgery with IOL implantation is to be done on a silicone oil-filled eye. This is perhaps most often a concern after retinal detachment repair with silicone oil in patients with AIDS. The comparatively high refractive index of silicone oil significantly alters the power of the eye. If standard formulae are used to determine lens power, major refractive errors result with most IOL styles. A number of various modifications to the standard formulae have been put forward, and a few general principles should be kept in mind. The meniscus-style IOL followed by the convexoplano lens yields the smallest difference between predicted and actual postoperative refraction. These lens styles also minimize the change in refractive error that accompanies subsequent alterations in the content of the vitreous cavity, including the removal of silicone oil and replacement with a BSS.[70–72] The speed of sound is different in silicone oil than it is in normal vitreous. This different sound velocity has to be used in axial length determinations. Silicone IOLs should be avoided in all cases. While heparin-surface-modified lenses appear to have the least coverage by silicone oil, other lens materials probably also are acceptable.[68]

ANTERIOR SEGMENT COMPLICATIONS

Early complications of silicone oil injection are primarily confined to the anterior segment and can be limited by preventing the anterior migration of silicone. When such anterior migration is not prevented, irreversible silicone keratopathy occurs as often as 50% of the time in eyes followed for an average of 8.5 months. Corneal changes frequently present as bullous keratopathy in older patients and as band keratopathy in younger patients (Fig. 19.6).[28]

This high rate of corneal decompensation emphasizes the importance of frequent ocular examinations and prompt removal of any silicone oil discovered in the anterior chamber. Surgical methods that minimize prolapse of silicone oil into the anterior chamber include the avoidance of silicone oil overfill, maintaining a normal IOP at the conclusion of surgery and filling the anterior chamber with air in aphakic eyes before silicone oil injection.[73]

Silicone-induced corneal damage may be reduced by creating and ensuring the patency of an inferior peripheral iridotomy in aphakic eyes.[8,74] This prevents pupillary block and the attendant prolapse of silicone into the anterior chamber (see Fig. 19.5). Additionally, prompt repair of recurrent retinal detachment is required because this condition, by shrinking the intravitreal volume, can lead to the migration of silicone oil into the anterior chamber.

When the lens is left in place, 60–100% of eyes will demonstrate some degree of cataract formation.[61,75–78] The basis for this is felt to be mechanical rather than toxic, with the silicone oil bubble preventing the diffusion of nutrients for lens function.[79] The rapidity of cataract formation is proportional to the duration of silicone oil contact with the lens, although prompt removal of the silicone oil may delay but not prevent cataract formation.[80]

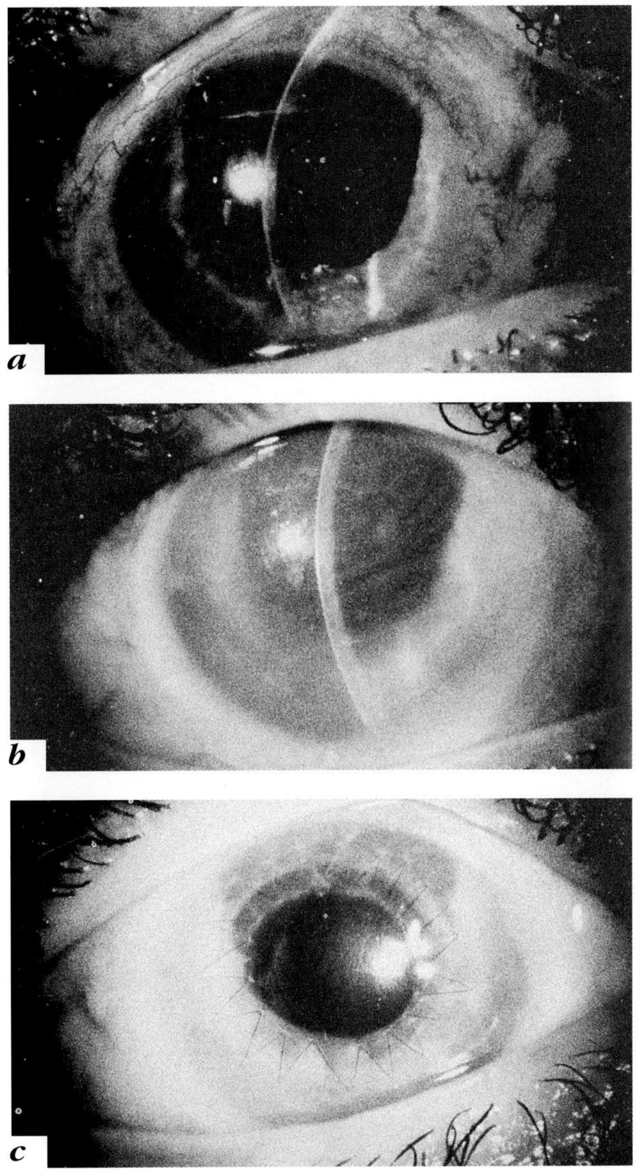

Figure 19.6 *Silicone keratopathy. (a) Anterior segment 3 weeks after silicone oil injection for proliferative vitreoretinopathy. Silicone fills the anterior chamber. (b) Silicone keratopathy 4 months after silicone oil injection. (c) Appearance of the anterior segment 6 months after removal of silicone oil and penetrating keratoplasty. (Reproduced with permission from McCuen BW II, de Juan E Jr, Landers MB III, Machemer R. Silicone oil in vitreoretinal surgery: II. Results and complications,* Retina *(1985)* **5***:198–205.[28])*

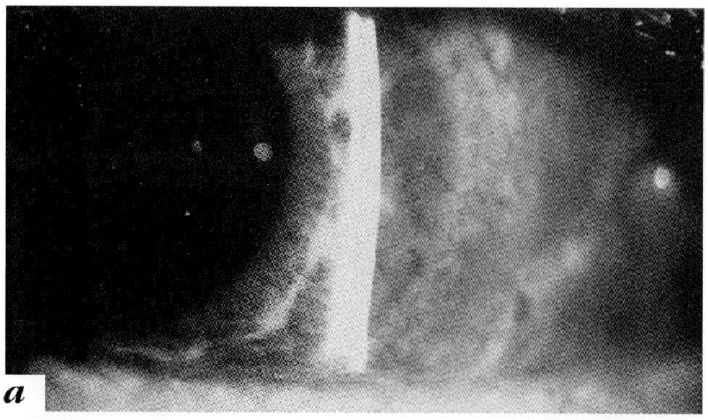

a

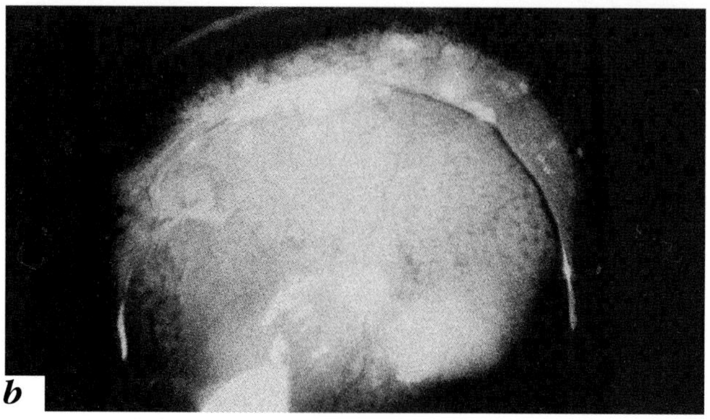

b

Figure 19.7 *Glaucoma after silicone oil injection: (a) acute angle-closure glaucoma 1 day after silicone oil injection caused by silicone-induced pupillary block; (b) emulsification of silicone oil with tiny silicone bubbles present superiorly just posterior to the scleral buckle. (Reproduced with permission from McCuen BW II, de Juan E Jr, Landers MB III, Machemer R. Silicone oil in vitreoretinal surgery: II. Results and complications,* Retina *(1985)* ***5****:198–205.*[28]*)*

INTRAOCULAR PRESSURE

After cataract, postoperative glaucoma is the second most common complication of intravitreal silicone oil (Fig. 19.7a).[53,81–83] The Silicone Study noted a 5% incidence of chronically elevated IOP in eyes with severe PVR. Eyes randomized to silicone oil had a higher incidence of glaucoma than eyes in the C_3F_8 group (8% vs 2%).[84] This occurs in both phakic and aphakic eyes. Pupillary block and angle closure that occur in aphakic eyes filled with silicone oil can be prevented largely with a patent inferior iridotomy. Emulsified silicone oil droplets can block the trabecular meshwork and can cause glaucoma refractory to conventional medical management or even removal of the emulsified silicone oil.[85,86] One should bear in mind that eyes undergoing vitrectomy and silicone oil injection may have other contributors to their elevated IOP, such as rubeosis iridis, hemolytic or erythroclastic causes, phakolytic causes, inflammation and steroid response.[87] Any or all of these factors should be considered and managed when approaching a patient with elevated IOP and silicone oil.

The results of the Silicone Study suggest that hypotony is a more important clinical problem than elevated IOP. Hypotony was present in 24% of eyes in the Silicone Study compared to 5% of eyes with chronically elevated IOP, and hypotony was nearly twice as prevalent in eyes randomized to C_3F_8 gas as those randomized to silicone oil (31% vs 18%).[84]

EMULSIFICATION

Emulsification is a major complication of intravitreal silicone oil use. Generally, when silicone oil is in contact with fluid, interfacial tension keeps both liquids immiscible and the silicone bubble whole. Emulsification describes the formation of silicone oil droplets on the surface of ocular tissues or at the interface between silicone oil and intraocular fluids (Fig. 19.7b).[1,88–90]

Emulsification facilitates migration of silicone oil into the anterior chamber, where mechanical contact with the cornea may result in keratopathy and obstruction of the trabecular meshwork, causing glaucoma.[90,91] The longer silicone oil is present, the more likely some degree of emulsification is to have taken place, so that after 12 months nearly 100% of eyes will demonstrate some emulsified silicone.[61]

Fibrin and serum are strong biologically active emulsifiers.[85] In addition, the lower the viscosity of silicone, the greater its tendency to emulsify. This difference is particularly marked among silicone oils with viscosities varying from 1000 to 5000 cSt.[85]

LATE COMPLICATIONS

Late complications attributed to silicone oil injection include cataract, glaucoma, keratopathy, iritis, endophthalmitis and recurrent retinal detachment.[61,62,77] Inflammatory membranes have been found to occur at the silicone–fluid interface as both an early and late complication of intravitreal silicone oil injection and may contribute to recurrent tractional retinal detachment (Fig. 19.8).[61,77,92–94]

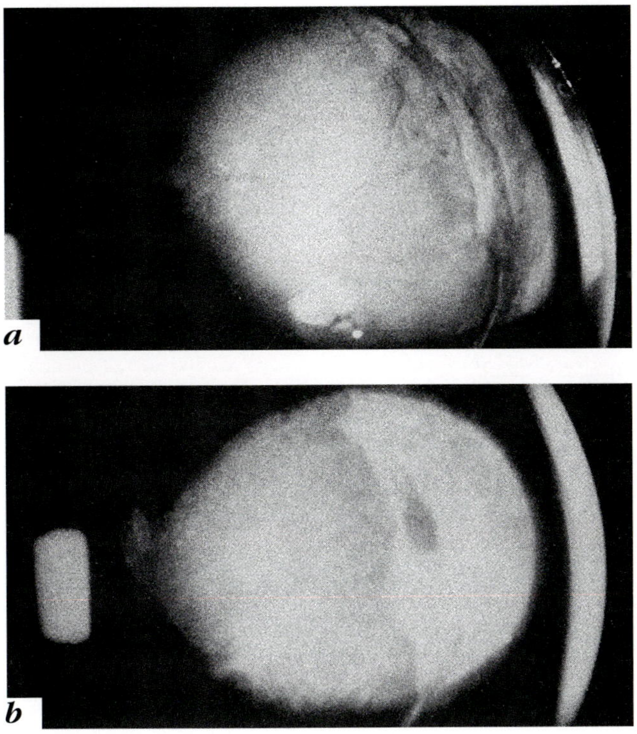

Figure 19.8 *Recurrent retinal detachment with reproliferation after silicone oil injection: (a) fundus appearance 6 weeks after silicone oil injection for proliferative vitreoretinopathy; (b) fundus of same eye 4 months after silicone oil injection with the development of reproliferation and tractional retinal redetachment nasally. (Reproduced with permission from McCuen BW II, de Juan E Jr, Landers MB III, Machemer R. Silicone oil in vitreoretinal surgery: II. Results and complications,* Retina *(1985)* **5***:198–205.[28])*

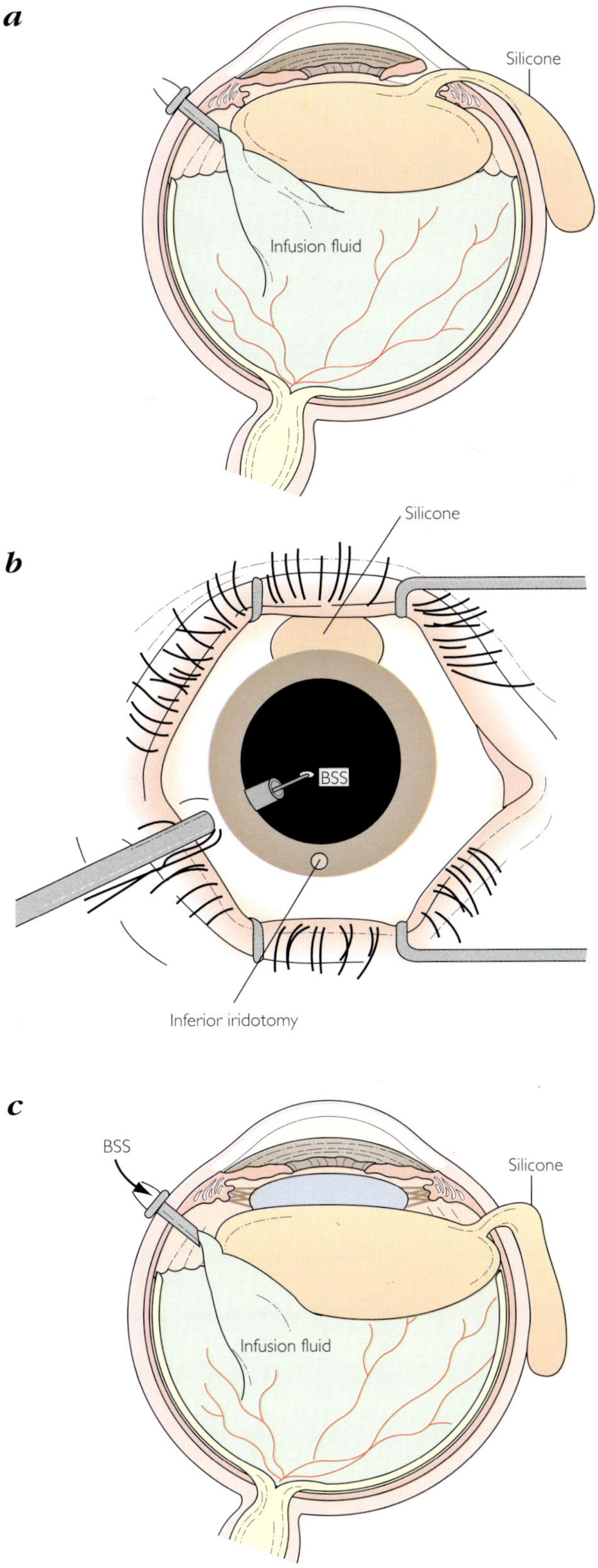

Figure 19.9 *Techniques of silicone oil removal: (a) in an aphakic eye; (b) front view; (c) in a phakic eye.*

SILICONE OIL REMOVAL

INDICATIONS

To avoid complications related to intraocular silicone oil, silicone usually is removed from the eye when the retina is attached, when chorioretinal scars are formed and when there is no significant traction on the retina. McCuen et al[28] suggested removal 3–6 months after intravitreal injection. Others have suggested intervals ranging from 6 weeks to as long as 30 months.[9,57,61,95,96] Vision-threatening complications attributable to intraocular silicone include cataract formation, elevated IOP, corneal clouding and diplopic symptoms related to the silicone–aqueous interface.[91,97] When such complications are present, silicone removal may be therapeutic.

A number of techniques have been described for the removal of intraocular silicone.[28,57,98,99] A 21-gauge butterfly needle or an infusion cannula can be connected to the infusion fluid and secured through the inferotemporal pars plana into the vitreous cavity. A small superior limbal incision can then be made in aphakic eyes. In phakic or pseudophakic eyes a superior or superotemporal pars plana sclerotomy is created and held open with Calibri forceps or an iris spatula. Silicone oil floats on water so that as the infusion begins silicone is pushed through the limbal opening or sclerotomy, particularly when the eye is rotated in a dependent inferior or nasal direction. The infusion continues until the infusion fluid flows freely from the limbal incision or sclerotomy (Fig. 19.9).[28,57,98] Alternatively, silicone oil can be aspirated actively using a three-port pars plana technique and a short blunt 16-gauge needle.

REDETACHMENT

In a series involving silicone oil removal from 120 consecutive eyes after a mean of 30 weeks, postoperative retinal detachment occurred in 19% of eyes.[80] Other series report rates of retinal redetachment ranging from 8% to 25%.[28,95,100,101] Visual acuity otherwise generally improved in most eyes after silicone oil removal. Factors contributing to visual improvement included the removal of emulsified silicone oil, cataract extraction and the absence of optical effects caused by the silicone oil bubble. Although nearly all eyes eventually developed cataracts, the rate of progression was slowed when silicone oil was removed.[80] Interestingly, the 12% incidence of retinal redetachment after silicone oil removal in diabetics is lower than that reported for nondiabetics.[27–29] This most likely relates to differences in pathophysiology and natural history, the more typically posterior location of retinal breaks in proliferative diabetic retinopathy and the nearly universal presence of scatter laser photocoagulation in the setting of diabetic vitrectomy.

REFERENCES

1. Crisp A, de Juan E Jr, Tiedeman J. Effect of silicone oil viscosity on emulsification, *Arch Ophthalmol* (1987) **105:**546–50.
2. Gabel VP, Kampik A, Burkhardt J. Analysis of intraocularly applied silicone oils of various origins, *Graefes Arch Clin Exp Ophthalmol* (1987) **225:**160–2.
3. Stone W Jr. Alloplasty in surgery of the eye, *N Engl J Med* (1958) **258:**486–90.
4. De Juan E Jr, McCuen B, Tiedeman J. Intraocular tamponade and surface tension, *Surv Ophthalmol* (1985) **30:**47–51.
5. Kreiner CF. Chemical and physical aspects of clinically applied silicones, *Dev Ophthalmol* (1987) **14:**11–19.
6. Peyman GA, Schulman JA. *Vitreous Substitutes* (Appleton & Lange: Norwalk, CT 1995): 1–52.
7. Peyman GA, Kao GW, de Corral LR. Randomized clinical trial of intraocular silicone vs gas in the management of complicated retinal detachment and vitreous hemorrhage, *Int Ophthalmol* (1987) **10:**221–34.
8. Kertes PJ, Peyman GA, Chou F, et al. The use of tissue plasminogen activator in silicone oil-filled eyes, *Can J Ophthalmol* (1998) **33:**28–9.
9. Lucke KH, Foerster MH, Laqua H. Long-term results of vitrectomy and silicone oil in 500 cases of complicated retinal detachments, *Am J Ophthalmol* (1987) **104:**624–33.
10. Yeo JH, Glaser BM, Michels RG. Silicone oil in the treatment of complicated retinal detachments, *Ophthalmology* (1987) **94:**1109–13.
11. The Silicone Study Group. Vitrectomy with silicone oil or sulfur hexafluoride gas in eyes with severe proliferative vitreoretinopathy: results of a randomized clinical trial. Silicone Study Report 1, *Arch Ophthalmol* (1992) **110:**770–9.
12. The Silicone Study Group. Vitrectomy with silicone oil or perfluoropropane gas in eyes with severe proliferative vitreoretinopathy: results of a randomized clinical trial. Silicone Study Report 2, *Arch Ophthalmol* (1992) **110:**780–92.
13. McCuen BW, Azen SP, Stern W, et al. Vitrectomy with silicone oil or perfluoropropane gas in eyes with severe proliferative vitreoretinopathy. Silicone Study Report 3, *Retina* (1993) **13:**279–84.
14. Abrams GW, Azen SP, McCuen BW II, et al. Vitrectomy with silicone oil or long-acting gas in eyes with severe proliferative vitreoretinopathy: results of additional and long-term follow-up. Silicone Study Report 11, *Arch Ophthalmol* (1997) **115:**335–44.
15. Blumenkranz MS, Azen SP, Aaberg TM, et al. Relaxing retinotomy with silicone oil or long-acting gas in eyes with severe proliferative vitreoretinopathy. Silicone Study Report 5, *Am J Ophthalmol* (1993) **116:**557–64.
16. Heimann K, Dhal B, Dimopoulos S, Lemmen KD. Pars plana vitrectomy and silicone oil injection in proliferative diabetic retinopathy, *Graefes Arch Clin Exp Ophthalmol* (1989) **227:**152–6.
17. De Corral LR, Peyman GA. Pars plana vitrectomy and intravitreal silicone oil injection in eyes with rubeosis iridis, *Can J Ophthalmol* (1986) **21:**10–12.
18. Blankenship GW. The lens influence on diabetic vitrectomy results: report of a prospective randomized study, *Arch Ophthalmol* (1980) **98:**2196–8.
19. Aiello LM, Wand M, Liang G. Anterior and posterior segment neovascularization following cataract extraction in patients with diabetes mellitus, *Ophthalmology* (1982) **89**(Suppl):115 (abst).
20. Rice TA, Michels RG, Maguire MG, Rice EF. The effect of lensectomy on the incidence of iris neovascularization and neovascular glaucoma after vitrectomy for diabetic retinopathy, *Am J Ophthalmol* (1983) **95:**1–11.
21. Schachat AP, Oyakawa RT, Michels RG, Rice TA.

Complications of vitreous surgery for diabetic retinopathy, *Ophthalmology* (1983) **90:**522–9.
22. Rinkoff JS, de Juan E Jr, McCuen BW II. Silicone oil for retinal detachment with advanced proliferative vitreoretinopathy following failed vitrectomy for proliferative diabetic retinopathy, *Am J Ophthalmol* (1986) **101:**181–6.
23. Brourman ND, Blumenkranz MS, Cox MS, Trese MT. Silicone oil for the treatment of severe proliferative diabetic retinopathy, *Ophthalmology* (1989) **96:**759–64.
24. Azzolini C, Brancato R, Camesasca FI, Codenotti M. Influence of silicone oil on iris microangiopathy in diabetic vitrectomized eyes, *Ophthalmology* (1993) **100:**1152–9.
25. McCuen BW II, Rinkoff JS. Silicone oil for progressive anterior ocular neovascularization after failed diabetic vitrectomy, *Arch Ophthalmol* (1989) **107:**677–82.
26. Blankenship GW. Management of vitreous cavity hemorrhage following pars plana vitrectomy for diabetic retinopathy, *Ophthalmology* (1986) **93:**39–44.
27. Sternberg P Jr, Hatchell DL, Foulks GN, Landers MB III. The effect of silicone oil on the cornea, *Arch Ophthalmol* (1985) **103:**90–4.
28. McCuen BW II, de Juan E Jr, Landers MB III, Machemer R. Silicone oil in vitreoretinal surgery: II. Results and complications, *Retina* (1985) **5:**198–205.
29. Pearson RV, McLeod D, Gregor ZJ. Removal of silicone oil following diabetic vitrectomy, *Br J Ophthalmol* (1993) **77:**204–7.
30. Jabs DA, Enger C, Haller J, de Bustros S. Retinal detachments in patients with cytomegalovirus retinitis, *Arch Ophthalmol* (1991) **109:**794–9.
31. Freeman WR, Quiceno JI, Crapotta JA, et al. Surgical repair of rhegmatogenous retinal detachment in immunosuppressed patients with cytomegalovirus retinitis, *Ophthalmology* (1992) **99:**466–74.
32. Sidikaro Y, Silver L, Holland GN, Kreiger AE. Rhegmatogenous retinal detachments in patients with AIDS and necrotizing retinal infections, *Ophthalmology* (1991) **98:**129–35.
33. Regillo CD, Vander JF, Duker JS, et al. Repair of retinitis-related retinal detachments with silicone oil in patients with acquired immunodeficiency syndrome, *Am J Ophthalmol* (1992) **113:**21–7.
34. Irvine AR. Treatment of retinal detachment due to cytomegalovirus retinitis in patients with AIDS, *Trans Am Ophthalmol Soc* (1991) **89:**349–67.
35. Lim JI, Enger C, Haller JA, et al. Improved visual results after surgical repair of cytomegalovirus-related retinal detachments, *Ophthalmology* (1994) **101:**264–9.
36. Nasemann JE, Mutsch A, Wiltfang R, Klauss V. Early pars plana vitrectomy without buckling procedure in cytomegalovirus retinitis-induced retinal detachment, *Retina* (1995) **15:**111–16.
37. Davis JL, Serfass MS, Lai MY, et al. Silicone oil in repair of retinal detachments caused by necrotizing retinitis in HIV infection, *Arch Ophthalmol* (1995) **113:**1401–9.
38. García RF, Flores-Aguilar M, Quiceno JI, et al. Results of rhegmatogenous retinal detachment repair in cytomegalovirus retinitis with and without scleral buckling, *Ophthalmology* (1995) **102:**236–45.
39. Irvine AR, Lonn L, Schwartz D, et al. Retinal detachment in AIDS: long-term results after repair with silicone oil, *Br J Ophthalmol* (1997) **81:**180–3.
40. Spaide RF, Martin DF, Teich SA, et al. Successful treatment of progressive outer retinal necrosis syndrome, *Retina* (1996) **16:**479–87.
41. Saari KM, Boke W, Manthey KF, et al. Bilateral acute retinal necrosis, *Am J Ophthalmol* (1982) **93:**403–11.
42. Gerling J, Neumann-Haefelin D, Seuffert HM, et al. Diagnosis and management of the acute retinal necrosis syndrome, *Ger J Ophthalmol* (1992) **1:**388–93.
43. Araiz JJ, Refojo MF, Arroyo MH, et al. Antiproliferative effect of retinoic acid in intravitreous silicone oil in an animal model of proliferative vitreoretinopathy, *Invest Ophthalmol Vis Sci* (1993) **34:**522–30.
44. Manzanas L, Marin J, Refojo MF. Retinol in silicone oil for treating proliferative vitreoretinopathy, *Invest Ophthalmol Vis Sci* (1990) **31** (Suppl):24 (abst).
45. Arroyo MH, Refojo MF, Araiz JJ, et al. Silicone oil as a delivery vehicle for BCNU in rabbit proliferative vitreoretinopathy, *Retina* (1993) **13:**245–50.
46. Abrams GW, Azen SP, Barr CC, et al. The incidence of corneal abnormalities in the Silicone Study. Silicone Study Report 7, *Arch Ophthalmol* (1995) **113:**764–9.
47. Hutton WL, Azen SP, Blumenkranz MS, et al. The effects of silicone oil removal. Silicone Study Report 6, *Arch Ophthalmol* (1994) **112:**778–85.
48. Petersen J. The physical and surgical aspects of silicone oil in the vitreous cavity, *Graefes Arch Clin Exp Ophthalmol* (1987) **225:**452–6.
49. Grisolano J, Peyman GA. Special short needles to inject and aspirate high-viscosity silicone oil, *Arch Ophthalmol* (1986) **104:**608.
50. McCuen BW II, de Juan E, Machemer R. Silicone oil in vitreoretinal surgery: I. Surgical technologies, *Retina* (1985) **5:**189–97.
51. Zivojnovic R. *Silicone Oil In Vitreoretinal Surgery* (Martinus Nijhoff/Dr W Junk Publishers: Dordrecht, The Netherlands, 1987): 25–8.
52. Peyman GA, de Corral LR. One-step extracapsular cataract extraction and silicone oil-injection in the management of proliferative vitreoretinopathy, *Br J Ophthalmol* (1986) **70:**382–6.
53. Alexandridis E, Daniel H. Results of silicone oil injection into the vitreous, *Dev Ophthalmol* (1981) **2:**24–7.
54. Ando F. Intraocular hypertension resulting from pupillary block by silicone oil, *Am J Ophthalmol* (1985) **99:**87–8.
55. Laganowski HC, Leaver PK. Silicone oil in the aphakic eye: the influence of a six o'clock peripheral iridectomy, *Eye* (1989) **3:**338–48.
56. De Corral LR, Peyman GA. Silicone oil injection in aphakic eyes: a modified technique, *Ophthalmic Surg* (1985) **16:**774–5.
57. Gonvers M. Temporary silicone oil tamponade in the management of retinal detachment with proliferative vitreoretinopathy, *Am J Ophthalmol* (1985) **100:**239–45.
58. McLeod D. Silicone-oil injection during closed microsurgery for diabetic retinal detachment, *Graefes Arch Clin Exp Ophthalmol* (1986) **224:**55–9.
59. Sternberg P Jr, Meredith T. Management of recurrent retinal detachment after silicone oil injection. Case report, *Arch Ophthalmol* (1987) **105:**27–8.
60. Kertes PJ, Peyman GA. Drainage of subretinal fluid under silicone oil, *Can J Ophthalmol* (1997) **32:**445–6.
61. Federman JL, Schubert HD. Complications associated with the use of silicone oil in 150 eyes after retina-vitreous surgery, *Ophthalmology* (1988) **95:**870–6.

62. Kanski JJ, Daniel R. Intravitreal silicone injection in retinal detachment, *Br J Ophthalmol* (1973) **57:**542–5.
63. Smith RC, Smith GT, Wong D. Refractive changes in silicone filled eyes, *Eye* (1990) **4:**230–4.
64. Dick HB, Schwenn O, Pavlovic S, et al. Effect of head position on refraction in aphakic and phakic silicone-filled eyes, *Retina* (1997) **17:**397–402.
65. Kusaka S, Kodama T, Ohashi Y. Condensation of silicone oil on the posterior surface of a silicone intraocular lens during vitrectomy, *Am J Ophthalmol* (1996) **121:**574–5.
66. Apple DJ, Federman JL, Krolicki TJ, et al. Irreversible silicone oil adhesion to silicone intraocular lenses. A clinicopathologic analysis, *Ophthalmology* (1996) **103:**1555–62.
67. Horgan SE, Cooling RJ. Irreversible silicone oil adhesion (letter), *Ophthalmology* (1997) **104:**898–900.
68. Apple DJ, Isaacs RT, Kent DG, et al. Silicone oil adhesion to intraocular lenses: an experimental study comparing various biomaterials, *J Cataract Refract Surg* (1997) **23:**536–44.
69. Senn P, Schmid MK, Schipper I, Hendrickson P. Interaction between silicone oil and silicone oil intraocular lenses: an in vitro study, *Ophthalmic Surg Lasers* (1997) **28:**776–9.
70. McCartney DL, Miller KM, Stark WJ, et al. Intraocular lens style and refraction in eyes treated with silicone oil, *Arch Ophthalmol* (1987) **105:**1385–7.
71. Grinbaum A, Treister G, Moisseiev J. Predicted and actual refraction after intraocular lens implantation in eyes with silicone oil, *J Cataract Refract Surg* (1996) **22:**726–9.
72. Meldrum ML, Aaberg TM, Patel A, Davis J. Cataract extraction after silicone oil repair of retinal detachments due to necrotizing retinitis, *Arch Ophthalmol* (1996) **114:**885–92.
73. Gao R, Neubauer L, Tang S, Kampik A. Silicone oil in the anterior chamber, *Graefes Arch Clin Exp Ophthalmol* (1989) **227:**106–9.
74. Madreperla SA, McCuen BW. Rate of closure of surgical inferior peripheral iridectomy and effect on silicone oil position in eyes treated with silicone oil extended tamponade, *Invest Ophthalmol Vis Sci* (1994) **35** (Suppl):2071 (abst).
75. Cockerham W, Schepens CL, Freeman HM. Silicone injection in retinal detachment, *Bibl Ophthalmol* (1969) **79:**525–40.
76. Pang MP, Peyman GA, Kao G. Early anterior segment complications after silicone oil injection, *Can J Ophthalmol* (1986) **21:**271–5.
77. Leaver PK. Silicone-oil injection in the treatment of massive preretinal retraction. In: McPherson A, ed, *New and Controversial Aspects of Vitreoretinal Surgery* (CV Mosby: St Louis, 1977): 397–401
78. Moisseiev J, Bartov E, Cahane M, et al. Cataract extraction in eyes filled with silicone oil, *Arch Ophthalmol* (1992) **110:**1649–51.
79. Lucke K, Laqua H. *Silicone Oil in the Treatment of Complicated Retinal Detachments: Techniques, Results and Complications* (Springer-Verlag: New York, 1990): 21–4.
80. Franks WA, Leaver PK. Removal of silicone oil: rewards and penalties, *Eye* (1991) **5:**333–7.
81. Grey RH, Leaver PK. Results of silicone oil injection in massive preretinal retraction, *Trans Ophthalmol Soc UK* (1977) **97:**238–41.
82. Ni C, Wang WJ, Albert DM, Schepens CL. Intravitreous silicone injection: histopathologic findings in a human eye after 12 years, *Arch Ophthalmol* (1983) **101:**1399–401.
83. Leaver PK, Grey RH, Garner A. Complications following silicone-oil injection, *Mod Probl Ophthalmol* (1979) **20:**290–4.
84. Barr CC, Lai MY, Lean JS, et al. Postoperative intraocular pressure abnormalities in the Silicone Study. Silicone Study Report 4, *Ophthalmology* (1993) **100:**1629–35.
85. Heidenkummer HP, Kampik A, Thierfelder S. Emulsification of silicone oils with specific physicochemical characteristics, *Graefes Arch Clin Exp Ophthalmol* (1991) **229:**88–94.
86. Moisseiev J, Barak A, Manaim T, Treister G. Removal of silicone oil in the management of glaucoma in eyes with emulsified silicone, *Retina* (1993) **13:**290–5.
87. Weinberg RS, Peyman GA, Huamonte FU. Elevation of intraocular pressure after pars plana vitrectomy, *Graefes Arch Clin Exp Ophthalmol* (1976) **200:**157–61.
88. Pon DM. Chemical characteristics of perfluorocarbon liquids and silicone oil for complex retinal detachments, *Vitreoretinal Surg Technol* (1990) **2:**6.
89. Zivojnovic R, *Silicone Oil in Vitreoretinal Surgery* (Martinus Nijhoff/Dr W Junk Publishers: Dordrecht, The Netherlands, 1987): 40–4.
90. Nakamura K, Refojo MF, Crabtree DV. Factors contributing to the emulsification of intraocular silicone and fluorosilicone oils, *Invest Ophthalmol Vis Sci* (1990) **31:**647–56.
91. Haut J, Ullern M, Chermet M, van Effenterre G. Complications of intraocular injections of silicone combined with vitrectomy. *Ophthalmologica* (1980) **180:**29–35.
92. Scott JD. A rationale for the use of liquid silicone in retinal detachment surgery. In: Shimizu K, Oosterhuis JA, eds, *Acta XXIII Consilium Ophthalmologicum, Kyoto, 1978* (Excerpta Medica: Amsterdam, 1979): 433–7.
93. Lewis H, Burke JM, Abrams GW, Aaberg TM. Perisilicone proliferation after vitrectomy for proliferative vitreoretinopathy, *Ophthalmology* (1988) **95:**583–91.
94. Charles S. *Vitreous Microsurgery*, 2nd edn (Williams & Wilkins: Baltimore, 1987): 146–7.
95. Casswell AG, Gregor ZJ. Silicone oil removal: II. Operative and postoperative complications, *Br J Ophthalmol* (1987) **71:**898–902.
96. Sell CH, McCuen BW II, Landers MB III, Machemer R. Long-term results of successful vitrectomy with silicone oil for advanced proliferative vitreoretinopathy, *Am J Ophthalmol* (1987) **103:**24–8.
97. Leaver PK, Grey RHB, Garner A. Silicone oil injection in the treatment of massive preretinal retraction: II. Late complications in 93 eyes, *Br J Ophthalmol* (1979) **63:**361–7.
98. Leaver PK, Lean JS. Management of giant retinal tears using vitrectomy and silicone oil/fluid exchange: a preliminary report, *Trans Ophthalmol Soc UK* (1981) **101:**189–91.
99. Fletcher ME, Peyman GA. A simplified technique for the removal of liquid silicone from vitrectomized eyes, *Retina* (1987) **5:**168–71.
100. Casswell AG, Gregor ZJ. Silicone oil removal: I. The effect on the complications of silicone oil, *Br J Ophthalmol* (1987) **71:**893–7.
101. Van Meurs JC, Mertens DAE, Peperkamp E, Post J. Five-year results of vitrectomy and silicone oil in patients with proliferative vitreoretinopathy, *Retina* (1993) **13:**285–9.

Chapter 20 Removal of silicone oil from the anterior chamber

Marta A Recasens

INTRODUCTION

The Silicone Study Group reported the incidence of complications of silicone oil use in the management of complex retinal detachments and proliferative vitreoretinopathy (PVR). Intra- and postoperative complications associated with the presence of silicone oil in the anterior chamber included:

- Secondary glaucoma
- Decreased visual acuity
- Corneal decompensation
- Chronic iritis
- Intraoperative appearance of silicone oil in the anterior chamber.

Although the removal of silicone oil from the anterior chamber in these instances may improve or reverse these conditions, intraocular pressure normalization may not occur.

INDICATIONS

The presence of secondary glaucoma caused by emulsified silicone in the anterior chamber may be an indication for removal of silicone oil. Valone and McCarthy[1] found emulsified oil in 56% of postoperative retinal detachment repairs with silicone oil; only 10% of the eyes developed new glaucoma within their 2-year follow-up. The removal of silicone oil may not reverse the glaucoma, as demonstrated by one series in which silicone oil removal controlled the glaucoma in only one of 11 eyes.[2]

The optical effects of the presence of silicone oil in the anterior chamber may further compromise visual acuity. Silicone oil removal from the anterior chamber reverses the optical and refractive changes caused by its presence in the anterior chamber.

Corneal complications occurred in 27% of eyes followed for 24 months in the Silicone Study.[3] Corneal decompensation as manifested by corneal haze and edema caused by silicone oil–corneal contact can progress to band keratopathy.[1] Silicone oil removal from the anterior chamber may arrest the progression of the corneal decompensation and the development of band keratopathy.

Chronic iritis with pain, photophobia and biomicroscopic cell and flare may be relieved with the removal of the silicone oil.

The intraoperative appearance of silicone oil in the anterior chamber can immediately obscure the surgeon's visualization of the posterior structures. Kirkby and Gregor[4] described the mechanism of passage of silicone oil in phakic eyes into the subretinal space and eventually into the anterior chamber. In pseudophakic or aphakic eyes, the passage of silicone oil from the posterior chamber to the anterior chamber is through direct communication between the two compartments.

Although there are preventive and nonsurgical methods of ridding the anterior chamber of the presence of silicone oil, prompt surgical removal of the silicone oil from the anterior chamber remains the preferred intervention.

PREVENTIVE MEASURES TO AVOID SILICONE OIL FROM FILLING THE ANTERIOR CHAMBER

Avoid an overfill of the vitreous cavity with silicone oil. Overfilling of aphakic eyes without intact capsules is more common because of the lack of barrier. When performing a lensectomy, all attempts should be made to maintain an intact anterior capsule.[5] Phakic eyes should not be filled with more than 3–3.5 ml of silicone oil. The amount of silicone

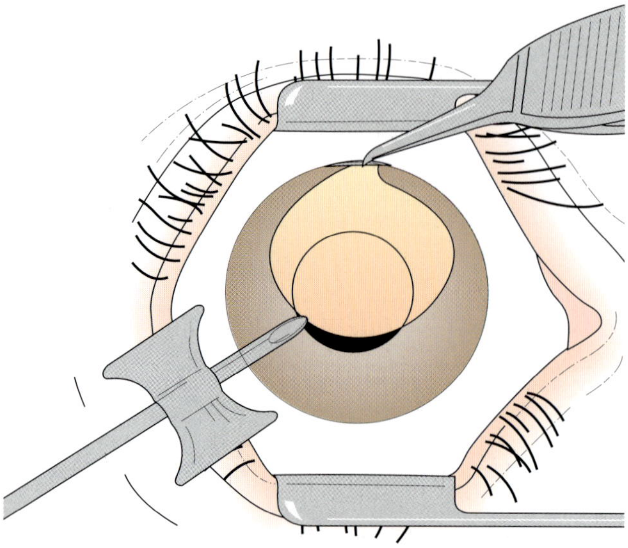

Figure 20.1 *Anterior chamber paracentesis technique for removal of silicone oil from the anterior chamber.*

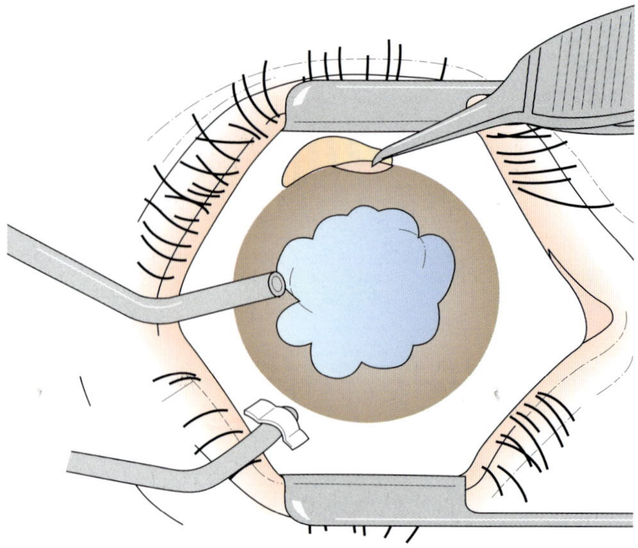

Figure 20.2 *Use of sodium hyaluronate for the removal of silicone oil from the anterior chamber.*

oil injected in pseudophakic or aphakic eyes should range from 3.0–4.0 ml; with volumes of less than 3 ml postoperative retinal detachments occur, whereas higher volumes produce increased intraocular pressure and anterior segment complications.[6]

An inferior peripheral iridectomy at the time of vitrectomy prior to silicone oil in the pseudophakic or aphakic eyes can prevent postoperative migration of the silicone oil into the anterior chamber and its associated complications.[7]

Patients should be instructed to avoid postoperative supine positioning, which facilitates forward displacement of the silicone oil from the posterior chamber.

NONSURGICAL MANAGEMENT TO PREVENT MIGRATION OF SILICONE OIL IN THE ANTERIOR CHAMBER

The patency of the inferior peripheral iridectomy must be maintained. Intracameral tissue plasminogen activator has been demonstrated to lyse early fibrin deposits that occlude inferior peripheral iridectomies after silicone oil implantation.[8] An Nd:YAG laser inferior peripheral iridectomy may enlarge and reopen previous iridotomy and permit the aqueous to move toward the anterior chamber.[7]

Topical miotics will reduce the size of the pupil and maintain the potency of the peripheral iridectomy patency.

SURGICAL REMOVAL OF SILICONE OIL FROM THE ANTERIOR CHAMBER

REMOVAL OF SILICONE OIL FROM THE ANTERIOR CHAMBER WITH AN ANTERIOR CHAMBER PARACENTESIS TECHNIQUE

A 25-gauge butterfly needle connected to a bottle of balanced salt solution (BSS) is inserted into the anterior chamber at the inferior temporal limbus while the infusion line is clamped. A 12 o'clock limbal stab incision is made with a Superblade (Alcon Surgical, Fort Worth, TX). The infusion line is unclamped and the anterior chamber fills with the BSS, forcing the silicone oil superiorly toward the 12 o'clock incision. The eye is rotated inferiorly, to force the silicone oil to exit superiorly from the wound. A 0.12-mm microsurgical forceps is used to spread the two lips of the wound as silicone oil exits the anterior chamber. By applying pressure to the lip of the wound, the remaining oil can emerge through this opening (Fig. 20.1). Once all of the silicone oil is

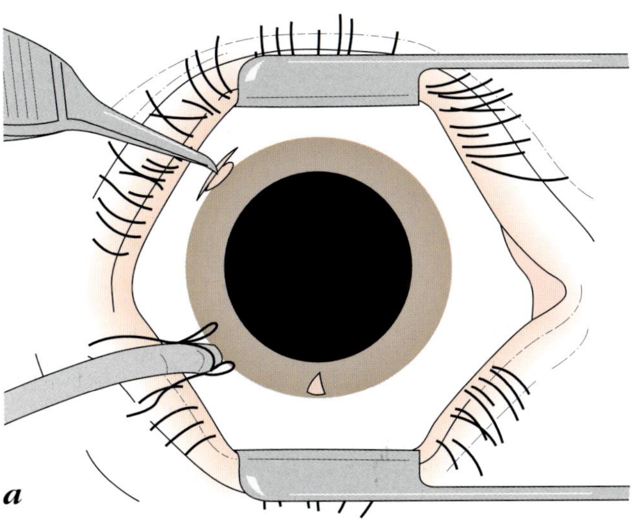

a

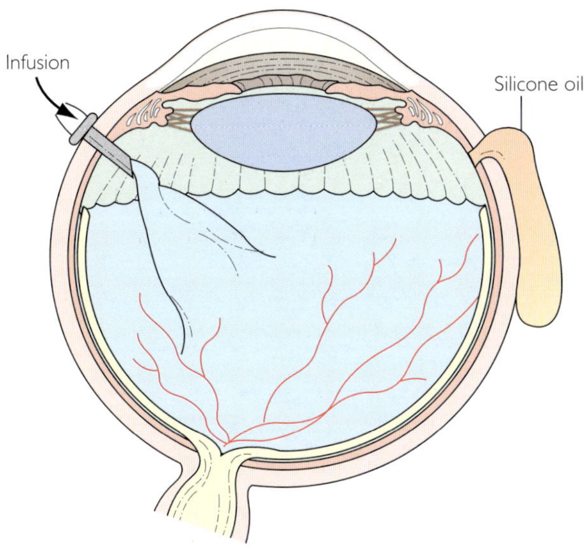

b

Figure 20.3 *Removal of silicone oil through a posterior sclerotomy: (a) top view; (b) cross-section.*

removed, the superior paracentesis site is closed with a single 10-0 nylon suture, embedding the knot in the corneal stroma. The infusion needle is then removed and subconjunctival antibiotic and steroid injections can be given inferotemporally.

Rarely, the appearance of silicone oil in the anterior chamber can occur during vitrectomy procedures. This can be managed by injecting sodium hyaluronate through a blunt-tipped cannula after an inferior temporal limbal stab incision is made with a Superblade. The sodium hyaluronate fills the anterior chamber, coats the corneal endothelium, and forces the silicone oil out of the superior wound incision and back toward the posterior chamber (Fig. 20.2). At the conclusion of the vitreous surgery, removal of the sodium hyaluronate is achieved by replacing it with BSS.

REMOVAL OF SILICONE OIL THROUGH A POSTERIOR SCLEROTOMY IN CASES OF SUSPECTED POSTERIOR CHAMBER OVERFILL

When an overfill of silicone oil in the vitreous cavity forces the silicone oil into the anterior chamber, a posterior sclerotomy may be necessary to remove part of the silicone oil and ameliorate the condition. With a phakic eye, a 4-mm infusion cannula is connected to an infusion of BSS through an inferotemporal sclerotomy 4 mm from the limbus. Another pars plana incision is prepared for removal of silicone oil, through which it exits passively (Fig. 20.3).

In pseudophakic eyes, we use a 6-mm infusion cannula placed 3.5 mm from the limbus. In aphakic eyes, the silicone oil overfill can be relieved using the anterior chamber infusion technique described previously. A superotemporal sclerotomy can be made with a 19-gauge microvitreoretinal blade and the incision is expanded slightly further. The sclerotomy is kept opened by expanding the lips of the wound with a 0.12-mm microsurgical forceps, which results in passive extrusion of silicone oil. At the end of the procedure, the sclerotomies are closed with 6-0 Vicryl sutures and the conjunctiva reapproximated with 7-0 Vicryl sutures.[8]

REFERENCES

1. Valone J Jr, McCarthy M. Emulsified anterior chamber silicone oil and glaucoma, *Ophthalmology* (1994) **101**:1908–12.
2. Moisseiev J, Barak A, Manaim T, Treister G. Removal of silicone oil in the management of glaucoma in eyes with emulsified silicone, *Retina* (1993) **13**:290–5.
3. Abrams GW, Azen SP, Barr CC, et al. Incidence of corneal abnormalities in the Silicone Study: Silicone Study Report 7, *Arch Ophthalmol* (1995) **113**:764–9.
4. Kirkby GR, Gregor ZJ. The removal of silicone oil from the anterior chamber in phakic eyes. *Arch Ophthalmol* (1987) **105**:1592.

5. Pang MP, Peyman GA, Kao GW. Early anterior segment complications after silicone oil injection, *Can J Ophthalmol* (1986) **21**:271–5.
6. Peyman GA, Kao GW, Corral LR. Randomized clinical trial of intraocular silicone vs. gas in the management of complicated retinal detachment and vitreous hemorrhage, *Int Ophthalmol* (1987) **10**:221–34.
7. Peyman GA, Schulman JA. *Intravitreal Surgery: Principles and Practice* (Appleton & Lange: Norwalk, CT, 1994): 616.
8. MacCumber MW, McCuen BW II, Toth CA, et al. Tissue plasminogen activator for preserving inferior peripheral iridectomy patency in eyes with silicone oil, *Ophthalmology* (1996) **103**:269–73.
9. Peyman GA, Schulman JA. *Intravitreal Surgery: Principles and Practice* (Appleton & Lange: Norwalk, CT, 1994) 334.

Chapter 21 Control of intraocular hemorrhage during vitrectomy

Famin Chou and Peter J Kertes

INTRODUCTION

Intraocular hemorrhage is a common problem during vitreoretinal surgery. Fortunately, severe bleeding is a rare occurrence. In a series of 400 consecutive vitrectomies, Peyman and associates[1] reported a 19% rate of intraoperative hemorrhage. Seventy-five percent of these were controlled with simple measures and the remaining 25% required cautery or diathermy to achieve hemostasis.

PREOPERATIVE EVALUATION

Any eye for which a pars plana vitrectomy is planned needs a careful and complete preoperative evaluation to devise a surgical plan and anticipate common sources of intraocular hemorrhage. These include areas of fibrovascular proliferation, vascularized preretinal membranes and neovascular iris vessels; normal vessels may be engorged and bleed in cases of hypotony. Attention should be directed to these anatomic structures to identify and prevent potential complicating factors. Other sources of intraoperative hemorrhage may be iatrogenic retinal tears or avulsed retinal vessels. Careful and meticulous attention to surgical technique, particularly during membrane dissection, avoids these sources of intraocular hemorrhage.

Intraoperative hemorrhage can accumulate in the vitreous cavity or in the subretinal space (from choroidal hemorrhage). Piper and associates reported 13 cases of choroidal hemorrhage at the time of vitrectomy in 683 consecutive vitreoretinal procedures. Risk factors that they identified for choroidal hemorrhage during pars plana vitrectomy included: older age, elevated preoperative intraocular pressure (IOP), retinal detachment, an aphakic or pseudophakic status and an accompanying scleral buckling procedure.[2] It is not feasible to eliminate all risk factors but careful preoperative planning, control of the IOP and careful scleral buckling techniques may help to decrease intra- or perioperative choroidal hemorrhage.

INSTRUMENTATION AND SURGICAL TECHNIQUE

INCREASING THE IOP

A simple and common technique for controlling intraocular hemorrhage is raising the IOP. This maneuver serves to compress the bleeding vessels and initiate the normal clotting process. As blood flows rapidly through a damaged vessel, thrombosis with hemostasis occurs with difficulty, particularly in a fluid-filled medium. The IOP is elevated by raising the height of the infusion bottle or by increasing the air pressure in the infusion. Some vitrectomy systems can regulate the IOP by infusing air into the space above the fluid in the infusion bottle.

The infusion pressure created by the fluid's gravitational force or the air pressure force in a nonexpandable sphere can be calculated theoretically, but the actual IOP is difficult to determine because different variables are involved.[3] The infusion bottle is lifted as high as the pole permits for the duration of 3 minutes. Then the bottle is lowered slowly 1 foot at a time every minute. At times oozing of blood will persist but at a slower rate. Raising the infusion pressure only increases the IOP if the system remains closed. Thus, the sclerotomies need to be plugged and the outflow stopped.

Increasing the IOP to achieve hemostasis may damage intraocular structures that are sensitive to ischemia, particularly in eyes with diabetic retinopathy

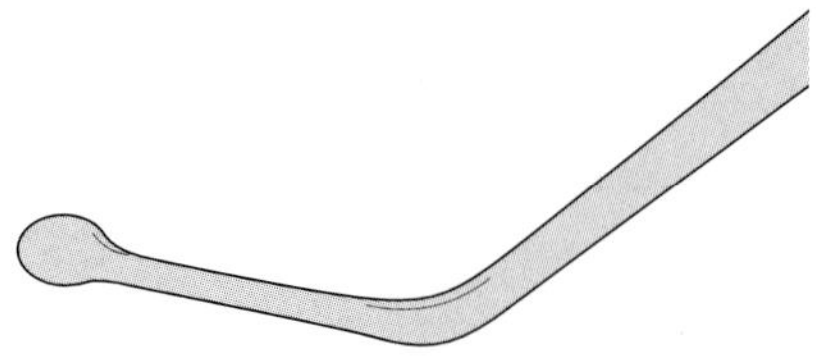

Figure 21.1 *The Eckardt Hem-Stopper. (Courtesy of Dutch Ophthalmic USA, Kingston, NH.)*

or glaucoma. Elevating the IOP may inadvertently produce retinal incarceration in the sclerotomy sites, especially when the retina is detached, when the infusion pressure remains high and when instruments are removed from the eye. Therefore, before the removal of instruments from the eye, the IOP should be lowered to normal.

A number of devices have been introduced over the last three decades to control intravitreal hemorrhage.[4–8]

THE HEM STOPPER

The Hem-Stopper (Dutch Ophthalmic USA, Kingston, NH) (Fig. 21.1) is a blunt-tipped intraocular device designed for the direct application of pressure to a bleeding site. It is held in place until blood flow through the affected vessel is stopped and a thrombus forms. This technique circumvents the unwanted effects of raised IOP.

INTERNAL DIATHERMY

Diathermy utilizes the tissue's resistance to the passage of high-frequency electromagnetic radiation or electric current. It induces protein denaturation and hemostasis. Cauterization differs because it uses an electric current, or heats up the tip of the probe to create tissue coagulation. Because no direct tissue contact is required, only close approximation between the tissue and diathermy tip is sufficient to produce the desired effect. The setting for the cautery or diathermy should be titrated gradually to produce prompt coagulation without excessive heat production, tissue damage or hemorrhage.

A useful approach is to pretreat fibrovascular membranes and vascularized preretinal membranes with internal diathermy before membrane dissection

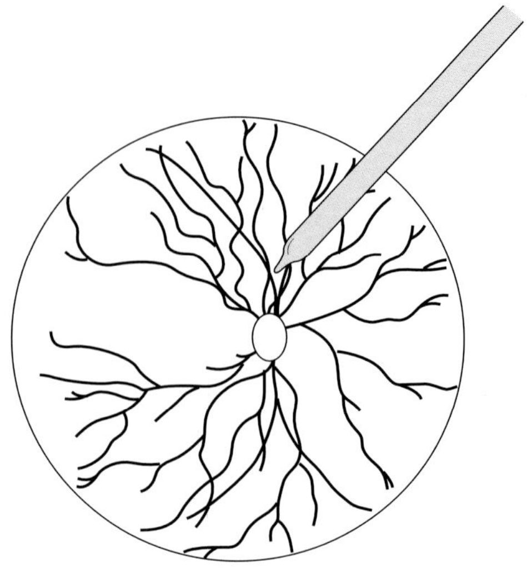

Figure 21.2 *Using diathermy or cautery to pretreat or treat vascularized fibrovascular membrane.*

(Fig. 21.2). In cases where a retinal vessel is inadvertently avulsed or in the setting of an iatrogenic retinal tear, internal diathermy may have to be used in conjunction with other methods to control intraocular hemorrhage and re-establish visualization. These include increasing the IOP, air–fluid exchange or the injection of perfluorocarbon liquids.

We prefer a unimanual coaxial bipolar diathermy probe over bimanual bipolar or unipolar probes. Because a bipolar electrode has a shorter ground path than a unipolar electrode, electrical current can be concentrated at the tip of the device, a more precise coagulation can be performed and excessive damage to surrounding tissue is avoided.

LASER PHOTOCOAGULATION

The absorption of laser energy by intraocular pigment produces a thermal effect that induces protein denaturation and subsequent hemostasis. Its effect is similar to that of intraocular cautery or diathermy. Laser delivery systems can be applied to flat areas of retinal bleeding without direct contact with the tissue. Aspirating laser probes[9,10] may be especially useful in cases of active bleeding. The aspiration of blood that prevents visualization can be accomplished without having to exchange instruments to achieve coagulation.

AIR–FLUID EXCHANGE

Intraocular air and gas have many applications in vitreoretinal surgery. Because gases are lighter than water, the gas bubble exerts a buoyant force that pushes on the retina and provides an intraocular tamponade. Because the gas bubble surface tension is higher than that exerted by fluid, an intraocular gas bubble slows the blood flow from an injured blood vessel and facilitates the coagulation process. Additionally, the IOP can be raised by increasing the air/gas pump pressure to slow the blood flow through the injured vessels and hasten thrombosis.

From a pure visualization standpoint, an air– or gas–fluid exchange removes the blood-filled infusion fluid in the vitreous cavity and allows better visualization of the retina and the bleeding site. Oozing of blood from a damaged vessel or neovascular frond can be identified and accessed to achieve hemostasis by a number of methods. We use an automatic air pump connected to the infusion cannula via a three-way stopcock to perform air–fluid exchange. The air pump pressure is set at 30–45 mmHg and a reflux soft-tipped extrusion needle is positioned at the nasal peripapillary area to perform a passive air–fluid exchange. An active air–fluid exchange is performed with a Grizzard cannula (VISITEC Co., Sarasota, FL) on tubing connected to the vitrector. Aspiration is controlled by the vitrectomy foot pedal. When the goal of thrombosis and hemostasis has been achieved, the three-way stopcock can be switched easily to resume infusion of fluid and to complete the surgery.

PERFLUOROCARBON LIQUIDS

The chemical stability, optical clarity, heavier-than-water specific gravity and high surface tension have made the perfluorocarbon liquids useful surgical adjuncts in the management of complicated vitreoretinal conditions. Their immiscibility with blood and water have made them particularly useful when intraocular hemorrhage occurs. This immiscibility combined with their optical clarity allows excellent visualization of the bleeding site and facilitates its cauterization.

These agents are typically injected through a small-gauge blunt-tipped needle over the optic nerve head. To prevent dispersion, the tip of the needle should be kept within the enlarging perfluorocarbon liquid bubble. The heavier-than-water liquid should be injected to a level above the bleeding site. The site can be identified and diathermized through the perfluorocarbon liquid.

SILICONE OIL

Silicone oil is frequently used in complex retinal detachments to provide a stable, long-term intraocular tamponade. It is immiscible with blood and concentrates clotting factors at the bleeding site, encouraging hemostasis. Silicone oil is typically injected at the end of surgery to stabilize the retina but has the added advantage of limiting postoperative vitreous hemorrhage. This is useful in some cases of severe trauma or proliferative diabetic retinopathy (PDR).

Some reports indicate that with severe trauma or PDR, minor postoperative vitreous hemorrhage can occur in up to 60% of cases.[11–14] In most situations, only observation is required. Outpatient air–fluid exchange has been advocated to improve the view to either allow additional retinopexy and/or to extend the duration of the intraocular tamponade. In a silicone oil-filled eye, postoperative hemorrhage can be managed with intravitreal tissue plasminogen activator injection, which will be discussed further in Chapter 32.

VISCOELASTICS

Viscoelastic agents effectively control hemorrhage in the anterior chamber by forming a physical barrier that slows the dispersion of blood and thus concentrates coagulation factors at the site of bleeding to achieve hemostasis. In the anterior chamber, the injection of viscoelastics also increases the IOP and stops bleeding from rubeotic vessels or bleeding iris vessels. Its utility in the posterior segment is not clear and it is usually not very effective.

THROMBIN

Thrombin is a coagulation protein that plays a pivotal role in the coagulation cascade. It is a potent agent in the induction of the platelet release reaction and also converts soluble plasma fibrinogen into fibrin. Fibrin plays a crucial role in the final formation of the hemostatic plug. The use of thrombin to control anterior chamber hemorrhage was described initially by Savory[15] and Hughes.[16] Subsequently, its use in the control of intraocular hemorrhage during vitreous surgery has been widely reported.[17,18] It has been particularly useful in cases of stage V retinopathy of prematurity,[19] severe PDR[20] and proliferative vitreoretinopathy.[21]

Bovine thrombin, a commercially available lyophilized powder, is diluted with balanced salt solution to a concentration of 100 U/ml. For vitrectomy, two infusion bottles are used in the set-up: one with a thrombin mixture (100 U/ml bottle) and the other with regular infusion fluid. They are connected to the infusion cannula through a three-way stopcock. The thrombin mixture can be accessed quickly in situations that require better hemostatic control. When intraocular hemostasis is achieved, the intraocular thrombin is washed out with regular infusion fluid to decrease the risk of postoperative inflammation and unwanted clot formation. The potential toxicity of thrombin limits the usefulness of this hemostatic agent and it should only be used if necessary to complete the surgical procedure.

SUMMARY

Intraoperative hemorrhage is a common intraoperative problem encountered during vitreous surgery. It impairs visualization intraoperatively and, postoperatively, residual hemorrhage may contribute to the development of proliferative vitreoretinopathy. With careful preoperative assessment and surgical planning, combined with the ability to perform a number of coagulation techniques, significant intraocular hemorrhage can be avoided or managed successfully.

REFERENCES

1. Peyman GA, Huamonte FU, Goldberg MF, et al. Four hundred consecutive pars plana vitrectomies with the vitrophage, *Arch Ophthalmol* (1978) **96**:45–50.
2. Piper JG, Han DP, Abrams GW, Mieler WF. Perioperative choroidal hemorrhage at pars plana vitrectomy: a case-control study, *Ophthalmology* (1993) **100**:699–704.
3. Parel JM, Parrish RK II, Nose I. An intraoperative intraocular pressure monitor, *Ophthalmic Surg* (1987) **18**:371–4.
4. McPherson SD Jr, Bipolar coagulation in ophthalmic operations. *Am J Ophthalmol* (1972) **73**:790–1.
5. Tate GW Jr, Hutton WL, Vaiser A, Snyder WB. A coaxial electrode for intraocular diathermy, *Am J Ophthalmol* (1975) **79**:691–3.
6. Charles S, White J, Dennison C, Eichenbaum D. Bimanual, bipolar intraocular diathermy, *Am J Ophthalmol* (1976) **81**:101–2.
7. Machemer R. Transvitreal radiofrequency diathermy (letter), *Am J Ophthalmol* (1977) **83**:282.
8. McCuen BW II, Hickingbotham D. A fiberoptic diathermy tissue manipulator for use in vitreous surgery (letter), *Am J Ophthalmol* (1984) **98**:803–4.
9. Peyman GA, D'Amico DJ, Alturki WA. An endolaser probe with aspiration capability, *Arch Ophthalmol* (1992) **110**:718.
10. Peyman GA, Lee KJ. Multifunction endolaser probe (letter), *Am J Ophthalmol* (1992) **114**:103–4.
11. Blankenship GW. Management of vitreous cavity hemorrhage following pars plana vitrectomy for diabetic retinopathy, *Ophthalmology* (1986) **93**:39–44.
12. De Bustros S, Glaser BM, Michels RG, Auer C. Effect of epsilon-aminocaproic acid on postvitrectomy hemorrhage, *Arch Ophthalmol* (1985) **103**:219–21.
13. Liggett PE, Lean JS, Barlow WE, Ryan SJ. Intraoperative argon endophotocoagulation for recurrent vitreous hemorrhage after vitrectomy for diabetic retinopathy, *Am J Ophthalmol* (1987) **103**:146–9.
14. Novak MA, Rice TA, Michels RG, Auer C. Vitreous hemorrhage after vitrectomy for diabetic retinopathy, *Ophthalmology* (1984) **91**:1485–9.
15. Savory M. Some uses of thrombin and fibrinogen in ophthalmic surgery, *Trans Ophthalmol Soc UK* (1947) **67**:323.
16. Hughes WL. Use of thrombin in the anterior chamber to control haemorrhage, *Acta Conc Ophthalmol (Britannia)* (1950) **XVI**:1299–1305.
17. De Bustros S, Glaser BM, Johnson MA. Thrombin infusion for the control of intraocular bleeding during vitreous surgery, *Arch Ophthalmol* (1985) **103**:837–9.
18. De Bustros S. Intraoperative control of hemorrhage in penetrating ocular injuries, *Retina* (1990) **10**(Suppl):S55–8.
19. Blacharski PA, Charles ST. Thrombin infusion to control bleeding during vitrectomy for stage V retinopathy of prematurity, *Arch Ophthalmol* (1987) **105**:203–5.
20. Verdoorn C, Hendrikse F. Intraocular human thrombin infusion in diabetic vitrectomies, *Ophthalmic Surg* (1989) **20**:278–9.
21. Glaser BM. The use of intravitreal thrombin to control hemorrhage during retinectomy, *Retina* (1988) **8**:1–2.

Part IV Surgical Techniques for the Management of Complications of Cataract Surgery

Chapter 22 Anterior vitrectomy

Brian B Berger

INTRODUCTION

Anterior vitrectomy is the removal of vitreous from the anterior chamber and the anterior one-third to one-half of the vitreous cavity. Both anterior and posterior approaches are possible. Entry sites may include clear cornea, limbus, pars plicata and pars plana in any meridian. The location of entry sites should be selected according to the goals of surgery and are only limited by the surgeon's imagination.

INDICATIONS

Indications for anterior vitrectomy include removal of vitreous from anterior segment structures, such as iris, lens, cornea or wounds in order to prevent or treat complications from anterior segment vitreous adhesions. Anterior vitrectomy for these purposes is either done at the time of cataract surgery or primary repair of anterior segment trauma, or as a subsequent procedure in conjunction with anterior segment reconstruction following cataract surgery or trauma. Specific situations include vitreous loss or prolapse through a ruptured posterior capsule during phacoemulsification, removal of retained lens fragments from anterior vitreous, removal of pupillary membranes or secondary cataracts, removal of adherent leukoma and vitreocorneal touch syndrome.

Other indications include the removal of vitreous from its normal location because it is inflamed or infected, such as chronic posterior uveitis or endophthalmitis, or because it is associated with other pathology, such as malignant glaucoma or persistent fetal vasculature.

PREOPERATIVE EVALUATION

Patients undergoing planned anterior vitrectomy should have a preoperative evaluation with special attention directed toward the cornea and retina. If the eye has undergone previous surgery or trauma, then it may be prudent to evaluate the cornea with pachymetry or endothelial microscopy. If there is evidence of corneal compromise, then this would favor a pars plana approach for both infusion and suction cutter in order to lessen corneal trauma. Visual potential is dependent upon the status of the retina. If the retina cannot be visualized preoperatively, then ultrasonography is indicated. This may reveal retinal detachment, vitreous hemorrhage, intraocular foreign body, or in persistent fetal vasculature, an abnormal anterior retinal insertion or persistent hyaloid vessels.

If the retina can be visualized and there is any suspicion of cystoid macular edema, then retinal angiography should be performed. If cystoid macular edema is confirmed, then the surgeon should plan to administer subTenon's steroid before the conclusion of surgery.

The location and extent of abnormal vitreous adhesions and other structures should be noted carefully and documented with photography. This will influence the surgical approach, such as the location of the ocular incisions.

INSTRUMENTATION

The basic instruments for anterior vitrectomy include a microvitreoretinal (MVR) knife, suction cutter and

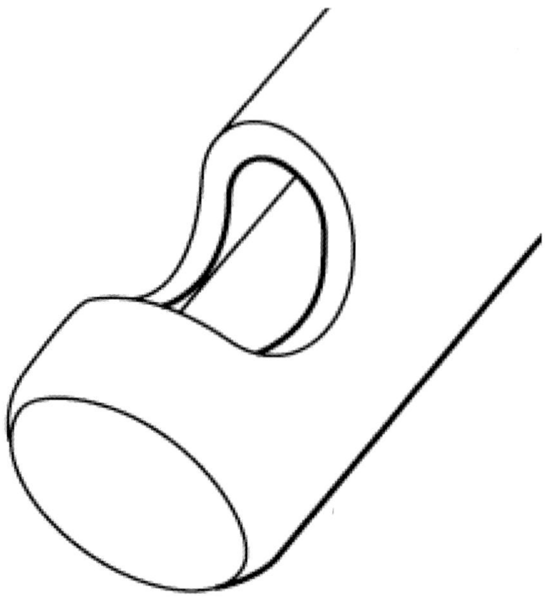

Figure 22.1 *Variable port suction cutter. The inner blade always stops in the open position so that the size of the port can be observed as it is adjusted. Alcon ATOP® probe.*

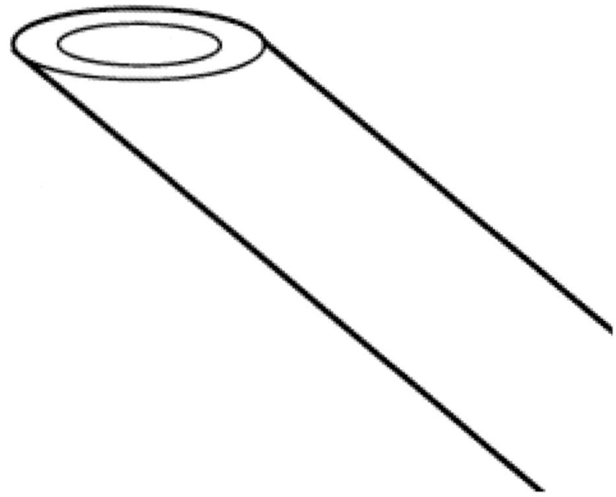

Figure 22.2 *Alcon reusable anterior segment infusion needle. Note the beveled blunt tip to allow easy entry into the eye and minimize trauma to intraocular structures.*

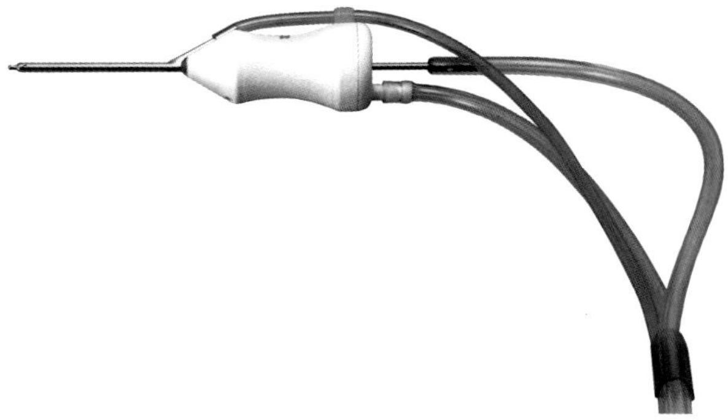

Figure 22.3 *Storz suction cutter with integrated infusion sleeve. Note that the infusion stream is directed perpendicular to the shaft of the suction cutter to minimize interference with the engagement of tissue.*

infusion device. The MVR knives are double-edged symmetrical knives that make full-thickness cuts through the eye and are available in 19- and 20-gauge sizes. A 20-gauge instrument is 0.89 mm in diameter. A 20-gauge MVR knife will make an incision that is longer than 0.89 mm in order to accommodate a 20-gauge instrument. The standard suction cutter is a 20-gauge instrument. A complete set of 23-gauge instruments is available from the Dutch Ophthalmic Research Center (DORC). Although modern posterior segment suction cutters generally have small fixed ports, it is helpful to have a variable size port for anterior vitrectomy work (Fig. 22.1).

Infusion devices include a reusable anterior segment infusion needle (Fig. 22.2), a disposable 21-gauge butterfly or Angiocath, self-retaining anterior chamber maintainer cannulas (Visitec 5061), a sutured anterior chamber cannula (Visitec 5196), a posterior segment infusion cannula, a suction cutter infusion sleeve (Fig. 22.3) or irrigating endoilluminator (Fig. 22.4). An infusion device is usually the first instrument placed in the eye for closed system vitrectomy.

Accessory instruments for bimanual surgery include 20-gauge scissors (Fig. 22.5), endoilluminators with or without picks, iris retractor or infusion, bipolar cauteries and forceps (Fig. 22.6). Iris retractors are useful to expose retroiridal pathology when the iris fails to dilate. Bipolar cauteries are available for external use (no. 22-1250) and 20-gauge with (no. 22-1202) or without (no. 22-1260) aspiration/infusion or 23-gauge sharp (no. 22-1265) and blunt (no. 22-1266) tapered are available for intraocular use (Mentor O&O, Inc., Santa Barbara, CA).

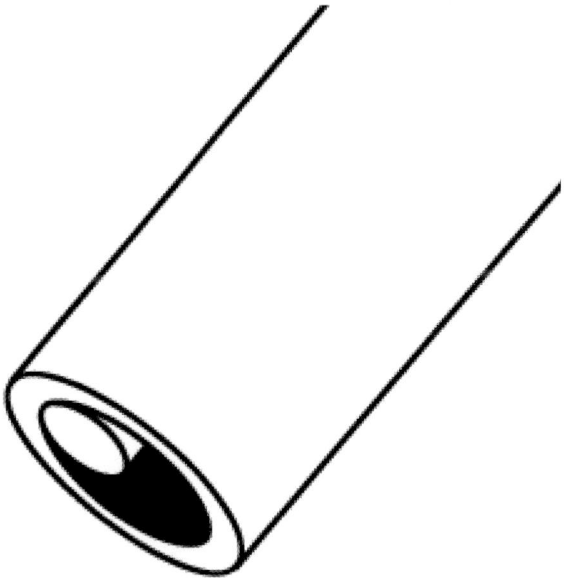

Figure 22.4 *20-Gauge irrigating endoilluminator.*

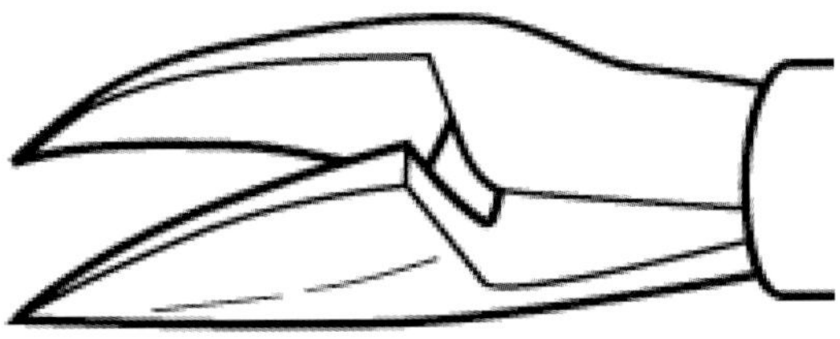

Figure 22.5 *Straight-end cutting 20-gauge scissors.*

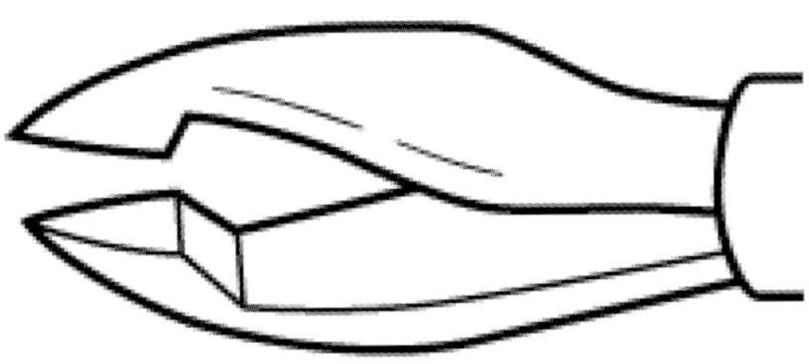

Figure 22.6 *Straight-end grasping 20-gauge forceps.*

Viscoelastic materials, such as chondroiton sulfate (Viscoat), can be helpful for anterior vitrectomy and should be available. A 27-gauge cannula or 30-gauge 5/8-inch needle should be available to inject a balanced salt solution (BSS Plus) in order to restore normal intraocular pressure (IOP) after wound closure.

Cellulose spears are used to clean the sclerotomy sites of prolapsed vitreous. Cotton-tipped applicators are useful for scleral depression to expose the pars plicata.

VITRECTOMY SETTINGS

The surgeon can control several parameters intraoperatively, including infusion pressure, cutting rate, suction pressure and suction cutter port size. These parameters are varied according to the tissue being cut and other factors.[1] The parameters are adjusted to maximize control and cutting efficiency. For example, in an open-sky vitrectomy when there is no infusion pressure to help guide tissue into the cutting port, suction pressure must be much higher. When cutting stiffer tissues, such as lens capsule or lens fragments, it is necessary to use low-to-moderate suction pressures to engage these tissues but higher suction pressures to maintain engagement and to cut the tissues. Obviously, surgeon-operated foot control of suction pressure is very helpful. A slower cutting rate, such as 300 cuts per minute (cpm), allows more time for stiffer tissues to mold into the cutting port. When cutting vitreous, high cutting rates of 600 cpm are desirable. In cutting the vitreous base or near the retina, even higher cutting rates, such as 1000 cpm, are desirable and now attainable. Recently, a surgeon-controlled cutting rate has become available (Storz Millennium). A smaller cutting port is also helpful to engage lens capsule and other membranes.

With higher suction pressures, it is relatively easy for suction to get ahead of infusion if the cutting port suddenly is no longer engaging the tissue. This can lead to collapse of the anterior chamber. To avoid this, higher infusion pressures are necessary and can be achieved by bottle placement 20–30 cm above the eye. In the situation of a ruptured posterior capsule with vitreous prolapse, the goal is to minimize further vitreous prolapse. This is achieved by using gentle cutting and aspiration with a suction pressure of 100 mmHg and an infusion bottle height of 10 cm above the eye to avoid hydration and expansion of the vitreous.

SUTURES

Twenty-gauge corneal incisions are closed with 10-0 nylon sutures, although these beveled incisions are frequently self-sealing. Twenty-gauge scleral incisions are usually closed with modified figure-of-eight 9-0 nylon except for the infusion cannula, which is closed with a 7-0 Vicryl mattress suture. Sclerotomy sites are cleaned with cellulose sponges before closure. Conjunctiva is closed with 6-0 plain gut suture as needed.

PHARMACEUTICALS

BSS Plus is the preferred infusion fluid. If cystoid macular edema was diagnosed preoperatively, then I prefer to irrigate 1 ml of triamcinolone diacetate into the posterior subTenon's space. This is performed by using a curved 19-gauge retrobulbar anesthesia cannula on a 1-cc tuberculin syringe. The cannula is placed in the superotemporal quadrant and the infusion is given slowly to avoid reflux. The objective is to place the steroid against the sclera over the macula.

Prophylactic antibiotics generally include a subconjunctival injection of a combination of an aminoglycoside and a cephalosporin and a subconjunctival injection of a steroid if there has been chronic inflammation or significant surgical trauma. Therapeutic antibiotics in cases of suspected endophthalmitis would include intraocular injections of antibiotics and steroids as appropriate. Topical agents may include a miotic such as Miochol (acetylcholine chloride) if there has been vitreous adherent to the iris, or a medium-to-long acting cycloplegic in other cases, and a combination antibiotic–steroid ointment.

POSTOPERATIVE CARE

If general or retrobulbar anesthesia is used, then the eye is patched the first day and night after surgery. If there has been no retinal involvement or intraoperative hemorrhage, then activities are not restricted. The head is kept elevated if intraoperative hemorrhage has occurred.

SURGICAL RESULTS

In cases of abnormal vitreous adhesions, anatomical improvement should be achieved in virtually every case. It is generally agreed that vitreous adhesions to the anterior segment are associated with an increased rate of long-term complications and that these complications can be reduced by correcting the anterior segment anatomy.[2] A number of published series of consecutive patients have shown that with modern anterior vitrectomy techniques and phacoemulsification cataract surgery, the visual results and postoperative complications in eyes with ruptured posterior capsules and/or vitreous loss are comparable to those in patients with uncomplicated cataract surgery.[3–6] Other series have shown that the delayed removal of retained lens material by an experienced retinal surgeon results in satisfactory vision with minimal long-term complications in most cases.[7,8] Controlled studies have shown that aphakic and pseudophakic eyes with cystoid macular edema associated with vitreous adhesions to the anterior segment have a reduction of macular edema and improved acuity following anterior vitrectomy.[9,10]

Several series have reported that malignant glaucoma can be cured by anterior vitrectomy alone in 50–100% of cases.[11,12] The majority of eyes with persistent fetal vasculature can achieve growth and avoid phthisis with anterior vitrectomy techniques, although only 20% or less will achieve 20/200 or better acuity.[13–15]

In the following techniques and illustrations, the orientation of the eye is irrelevant. For example, whether vitreous loss occurs using a temporal cataract incision or a traditional superior incision, the technique is the same. It is the relative relationship of the instruments that is important.

PHACOEMULSIFICATION WITH RUPTURED POSTERIOR CAPSULE

Phacoemulsification with a ruptured posterior capsule is the most common indication for an anterior vitrectomy that a general ophthalmologist will encounter. The anterior vitrectomy technique is determined by the point during cataract surgery when vitreous loss is noted and by the extent of vitreous loss. Vitreous loss is the movement of vitreous outside the globe through the surgical wound. Vitreous prolapse is the movement of vitreous into the anterior chamber through the anterior capsulorhexis resulting from a rupture in the posterior capsule. In general, the sooner the surgeon notices vitreous prolapse, the smaller the anterior vitrectomy that will be required to treat it.

SURGICAL TECHNIQUE FOR VITREOUS PROLAPSE DURING PHACOEMULSIFICATION OF NUCLEUS OR FOLLOWING PLANNED EXTRACAPSULAR CATARACT EXTRACTION

OPERATIVE PROCEDURE

When vitreous presents during phacoemulsification of the lens nucleus, the first priority is to prevent dislocation of the nucleus through the break in the posterior capsule into the vitreous cavity. As soon as the phacoemulsification tip encounters vitreous, phacoemulsification is stopped. The anterior chamber is filled with viscoelastic through the side port incision before removing the phaco tip. The incision is extended to convert the procedure to an extracapsular cataract extraction. The incision is enlarged only to the extent necessary to remove the nuclear fragment. The nucleus is removed with a pick or forceps following the instillation of a viscoelastic.[16] The incision is closed temporarily with an 8-0 mattress suture of either polyglycolic acid or silk.

A 23-gauge infusion cannula is placed into the anterior chamber through a corneal stab incision with the nondominant hand. The infusion stream should be directed towards the angle of the eye, avoiding both the vitreous cavity and the corneal endothelium. The infusion bottle should be placed 15 cm above the eye.

The suction cutter is placed through the incision with the dominant hand. The cutting port should be set to its maximum opening, if it is adjustable, and oriented towards the cornea. Using a suction pressure of 50–100 mmHg, any mobile-retained lens fragments are removed using aspiration only. The suction cutter is then directed through the rent in the posterior capsule and held just behind it. Using a cutting rate of 500–600 cpm, a vitrectomy is performed (Fig. 22.7a). Within minutes, the posterior chamber should be free of vitreous. Retained lens cortex is removed with the suction cutter using the aspiration-only mode of the vitrectomy instrument (Fig. 22.7b). The cutting port is partially closed, if possible. If additional vitreous presents during the aspiration of lens cortex, the cutting mode should be activated immediately and the vitreous removed before proceeding with cortical aspiration. During cortical aspiration, the suction pressure is varied from 50 mmHg for engagement to higher pressures in order to mold the material into the port. Once the port is free, suction must be lowered immediately to prevent collapse of the anterior chamber.

If vitreous adhesions are noted to the iris or wound, then the suction cutter can be withdrawn to the anterior chamber to remove these adhesions. Frequently, vitreous is adherent to the underside of the iris at the incision site. It can be difficult to access this area from the entrance site. A nylon iris retractor can be used to expose this area (Fig. 22.7c). Other ways to retract the iris include an irrigating iris retractor (Visitec, Sarasota, FL; no. 5091, 23-gauge) and an illuminated iris retractor (Escalon, Skillman, NJ; no. TR 9809, 23-gauge).

Both sides of the iris at the entrance site area should be swept with the irrigation cannula to be sure that it is free of vitreous. Following the anterior vitrectomy, either a posterior chamber lens in front of the anterior capsule in the ciliary sulcus or an anterior chamber lens can be placed. The infusion cannula is removed and the stab incision checked for leaks. Miochol is instilled into the anterior chamber to ensure that the pupil is round. The cataract incision and conjunctiva are closed.

This basic approach may be used also when vitreous presents during a lens exchange.

SURGICAL TECHNIQUE FOR VITREOUS PROLAPSE DURING ASPIRATION OF LENS CORTEX

OPERATIVE PROCEDURE

The suction cutter is placed with the dominant hand through the phacoemulsification incision and through the break in the posterior capsule and held with the port facing anteriorly 1–2 mm below the posterior capsule (Fig. 22.7a). The cataract incision does not have to be extended. The vitrectomy is begun using the settings described in the preceding section. A few seconds later, a 23-gauge cannula is placed into the anterior chamber through a temporal stab incision.[17] The infusion bottle is at a height of 15 cm. In this position, the suction cutter should be held perfectly still. After several minutes, an adequate anterior vitrectomy will have been achieved. The procedure is completed according to the steps in the preceding section.

SURGICAL TECHNIQUE FOR VITREOUS PROLAPSE DURING PHACOEMULSIFICATION WITH DISLOCATED LENS FRAGMENTS

In general, the dislocation of lens fragments into the anterior vitreous is accompanied by a large break in

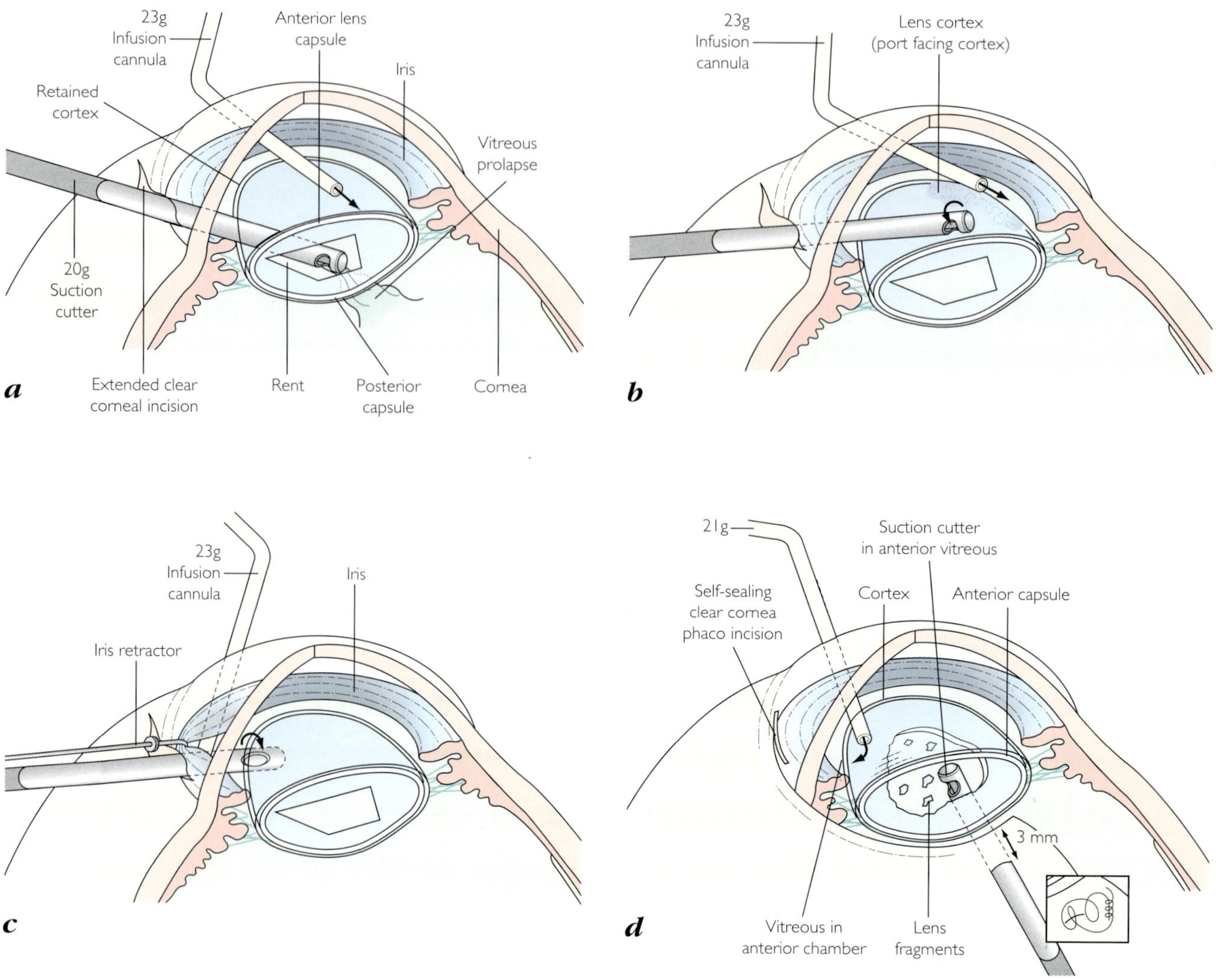

Figure 22.7 *(a) Clear cornea approach bimanual anterior vitrectomy with the suction cutter placed through a rupture in the posterior capsule. Note that the infusion stream is directed away from the rent. (b) Following removal of prolapsed vitreous, retained lens cortex is aspirated. Note that the cutting port is oriented toward the cortex and away from the iris. (c) Sweep the entrance site area to be sure the iris is free of vitreous adhesions. Note the nylon iris retractor, and the cutting port oriented posteriorly. (d) Pars plana approach with the suction cutter passed into the anterior vitreous to remove retained lens fragments and infusion cannula in anterior chamber. Insert: modified figure-of-eight sclerotomy closure.*

the posterior lens capsule and a significant prolapse of vitreous. Chasing after posteriorly dislocated lens fragments with a suction cutter entails a significant risk for retinal damage, including giant retinal tears.[18] Lens loops, forceps, cryoprobes and phacoemulsification tips should not be used in the vitreous. In this situation, a pars plana approach maximizes the opportunity to remove the dislocated lens fragments and relieve any vitreous incarceration in the wound.[1,19] The following procedure uses a combined anterior and posterior approach.

OPERATIVE PROCEDURE

If the phacoemulsification incision is not self-sealing, it should be closed temporarily. Because vitreous hydration is not a concern, a 21-gauge infusion cannula is placed through a corneal stab incision and a bottle height of 20 cm is used. A 20-gauge MVR knife is placed through the sclera 3 mm posterior to the limbus in the inferotemporal quadrant into the vitreous cavity. A suction cutter with the port fully opened is placed through the sclerotomy into the vitreous cavity. Using a cutting rate of 500–600 cpm and a suction pressure of 150 mmHg, a vitrectomy is performed (Fig. 22.7d). Through this entrance site, the suction cutter can be maneuvered into any position behind the posterior capsule to remove dislocated lens fragments. If there is a large rupture in the posterior capsule, the probe also can be angulated into the anterior chamber to remove any vitreous adhesions. If this maneuver does not remove all vitreous in the anterior segment, then the suction cutter can be removed and placed into the anterior chamber through the phacoemulsification incision (Fig. 22.7a). The sclerotomy site is closed. Miochol should be instilled to ensure that the pupil is round. The infusion cannula is removed and an anterior chamber lens can be placed with the use of a viscoelastic.

SURGICAL TECHNIQUE FOR REMOVAL OF ADHERENT LEUKOMA

Following primary repair of a penetrating injury, there may be a mixture of lens material, vitreous and iris adherent to the wound, which can lead to an adherent leukoma. Frequently, there is retained lens material, iridocapsular adhesions and vitreous prolapse into the anterior chamber. The following procedure uses a bimanual clear cornea approach.

OPERATIVE PROCEDURE

Corneal incisions are made with an MVR knife 120° to either side of the adherent leukoma. A 20-gauge blunt-tipped needle is placed into the anterior chamber with the nondominant hand. The infusion bottle is positioned 20 cm or higher above the eye. If the adherent tissue is vascularized, it may have to be treated with 23-gauge tapered, bipolar cautery (Fig. 22.8a). Through one of the incisions, the adherent material is incised with either an MVR knife or end-cutting scissors (Fig. 22.8b). With the suction cutter in the dominant hand, the adhesion is excised, as well as the prolapsed vitreous and any retained lens material. The cutting rate is 200–300 cpm and suction is 200 mmHg. Iridocapsular and iridovitreal adhesions are incised with either an MVR knife or scissors (Fig. 22.8c). Excision of the tissue may be difficult because of an inability to engage the tissue in the cutting port. Engagement of the tissue may be facilitated by raising the infusion bottle height, increasing suction pressure and reducing the cutting rate. An anterior vitrectomy is performed using a cutting rate of 500–600 cpm, 150 mmHg of suction and an infusion bottle height of 25 cm. This is done to prevent any recurrence of anterior segment vitreous adhesions. The instruments are removed from the eye. The wounds are checked for leaks and, if necessary, closed with a single suture.

SURGICAL TECHNIQUE FOR EXCISION OF DENSE PUPILLARY MEMBRANE

Occasionally, a dense pupillary membrane is encountered in an eye after distant surgery or trauma. The following procedure uses a combined anterior and posterior approach and can be used in an aphakic eye or in the presence of an anterior chamber lens but not a posterior chamber lens. This so-called chopping block technique is useful for very dense membranes.

OPERATIVE PROCEDURE

The conjunctiva is incised in a temporal quadrant at the limbus and reflected posteriorly. A sclerotomy is marked 3 mm posterior to the limbus. A 21-gauge infusion needle is placed through the cornea and the tip placed in the inferior angle. Alternatively, an anterior chamber maintainer or sutured anterior-chamber cannula can be used. The disadvantage of these fixed infusion devices is that they cannot be used as a second instrument.

The sclerotomy is made with the MVR knife and an attempt may be made to pierce the pupillary membrane during its passage into the vitreous cavity. The suction cutter is then placed with the dominant hand through the sclerotomy into the middle of the pupil just posterior to the membrane but is not activated. Next, the MVR knife is passed with the nondominant hand 90° away from the suction cutter through clear cornea into the anterior chamber and positioned over the suction cutter. The MVR knife is then used to cut down on the pupillary membrane,

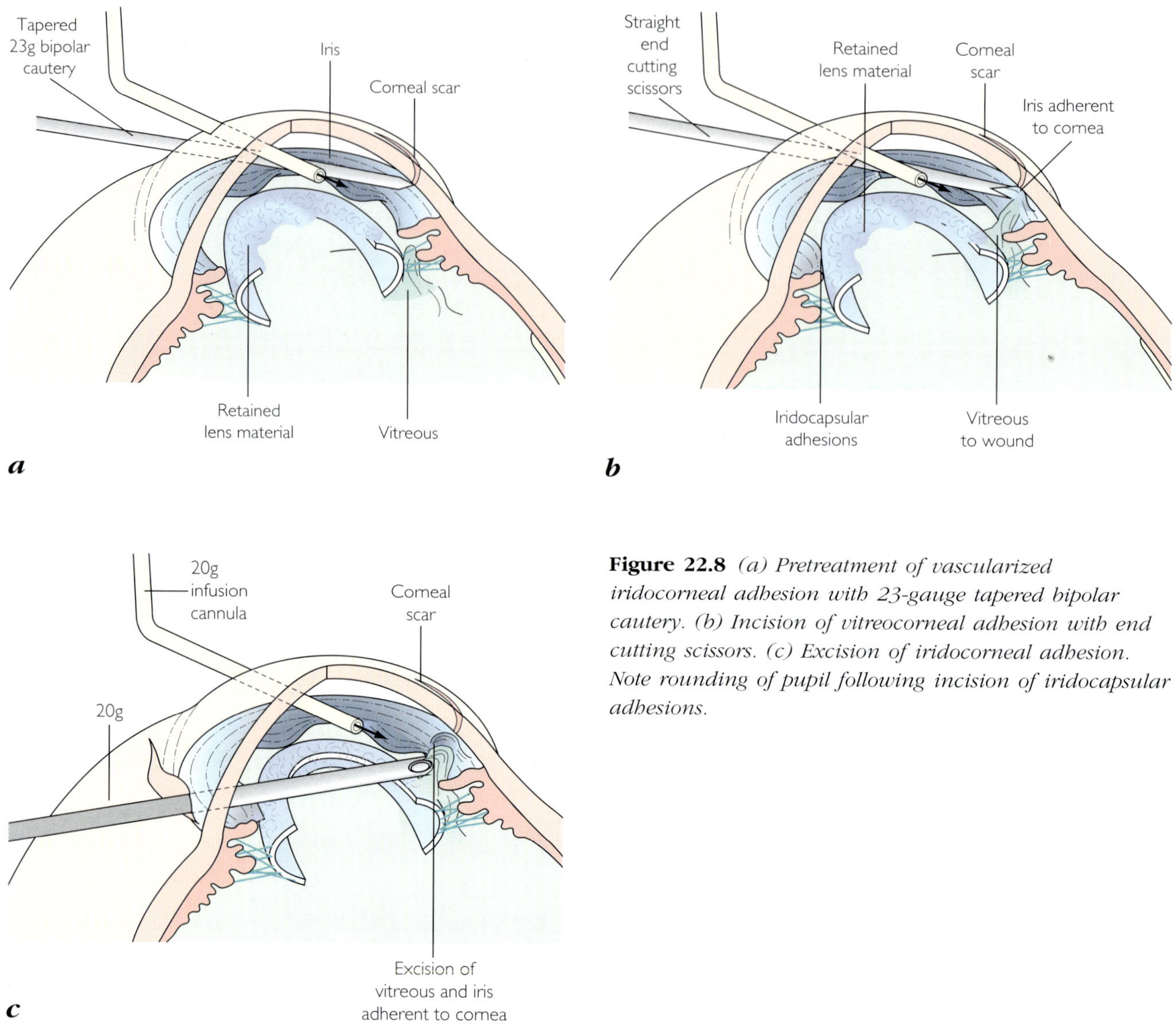

Figure 22.8 *(a) Pretreatment of vascularized iridocorneal adhesion with 23-gauge tapered bipolar cautery. (b) Incision of vitreocorneal adhesion with end cutting scissors. (c) Excision of iridocorneal adhesion. Note rounding of pupil following incision of iridocapsular adhesions.*

which is supported underneath by the suction cutter. Supporting the pupillary membrane in this manner allows the incision of even the toughest membranes while minimizing traction on the ciliary body. The membrane is incised repeatedly to create free edges in order to permit excision of the membrane by the suction cutter (Fig. 22.9a). Once the membrane has been incised adequately, the MVR knife can be removed. Scissors also can be used to fenestrate the membrane.

The cutting port should be opened fully. The cutting rate is only 100–200 cpm and the suction pressure is 200–300 mmHg. The infusion bottle should be 60–70 cm above the eye in order to increase tissue engagement. The membrane is excised. With the free nondominant hand, a cotton-tipped applicator can be used to indent the pars plicata in order to improve visualization of the retroiridal membrane. In this manner, the ciliary processes can be cleaned of all tissue (Fig. 22.9b). All iridovitreal and iridocapsular adhesions should be incised using the suction cutter at low suction, the infusion needle, the MVR knife or the scissors. The instrument settings are then changed to appropriate vitrectomy parameters and an anterior vitrectomy is performed to prevent any prolapse of vitreous into

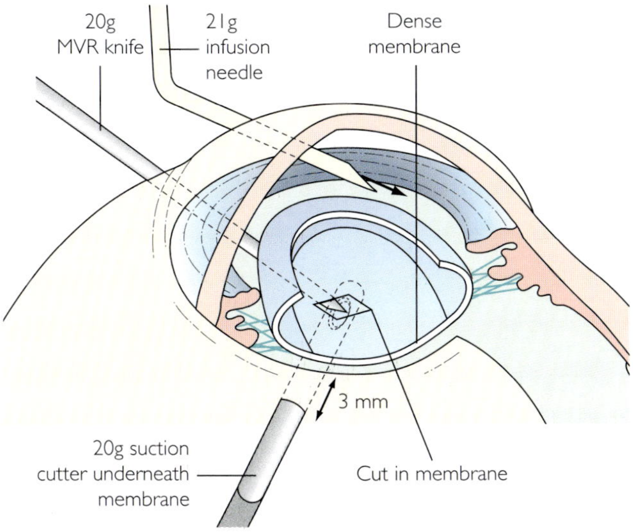

a

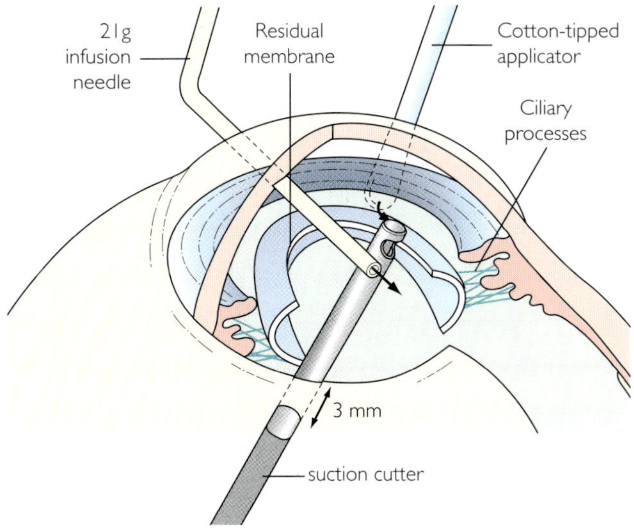

b

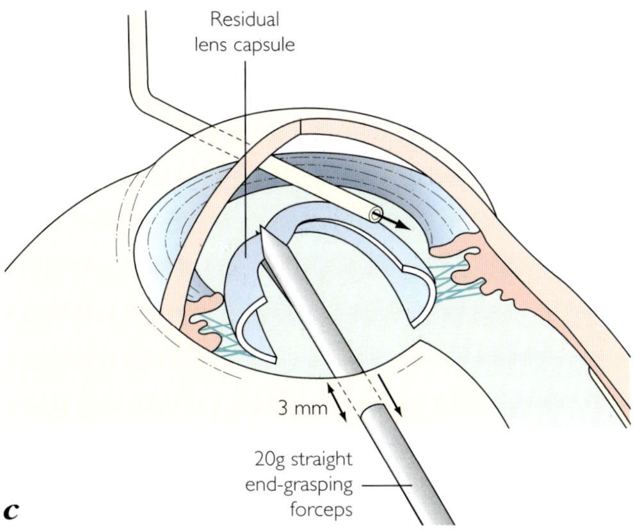

c

Figure 22.9 *(a) Anterior–posterior bimanual chopping block technique for cutting dense pupillary membrane. (b) Depression of the pars plicata for removal of retroiridal membranes. Note rounding of pupil following incision of iridocapsular adhesions. (c) Total capsulectomy through the pars plana using 20-gauge end-opening forceps.*

the anterior chamber. The suction cutter is then removed and the sclerotomy site cleaned and closed. The infusion needle is removed, and the corneal incision is checked for leaks.

Sometimes it is desirable to remove the entire lens capsule. This can be accomplished by instilling alpha-chymotrypsin over the zonules. Infusion is stopped. After waiting a few minutes, an edge of the posterior capsule is grasped with a 20-gauge forceps. With gentle traction, the zonules can be broken and frequently the entire capsular bag is removed in one piece (Fig. 22.9c).[20] An anterior vitrectomy is then performed as described above.

SURGICAL TECHNIQUE FOR MALIGNANT GLAUCOMA, PUPILLARY BLOCK GLAUCOMA AND VITREOUS BIOPSY

In malignant glaucoma there is a misdirection of aqueous humor into the vitreous cavity, which expands the vitreous, forces the lens–iris diaphragm forward and raises the intraocular pressure (IOP). A patent iridectomy to exclude pupillary block must be present to make the diagnosis. In phakic eyes, it is thought that there is an abnormal interface between the anterior vitreous face and the ciliary body and zonules. In the aphakic or pseudophakic eye, it is thought that there is an abnormal interface between the vitreous and iris or lens capsule. Anterior vitrectomy can be curative.

The objective in the phakic eye is to remove the anterior hyaloid in order to restore normal anterior aqueous flow. In phakic eyes, a combined vitrectomy–lensectomy should be considered when there is marked corneal edema, a cataractous lens or failure of the anterior chamber to deepen during vitrectomy. Incomplete pupillary dilation should be overcome with iris retractors if necessary (see Fig. 22.7c). Locating the sclerotomy at the meridian of the iridectomy allows improved access and visualization of the anterior hyaloid and zonules.

The objective in the aphakic or pseudophakic eye is to remove iridovitreal or vitreocapsular adhesions in order to re-establish normal anterior aqueous flow. Pupillary block can occur in aphakic eyes when vitreous occludes the pupil and iridectomy. This results in aqueous humor expanding the vitreous and forcing the iris forward. Because aqueous cannot reach the anterior chamber, it expands the vitreous, forcing the iris forward and making the anterior chamber shallower. This closes the angle, raises the pressure and causes pain. If a laser iridotomy is not successful in relieving the block, then anterior vitrectomy is indicated.

Vitreous biopsy is most commonly used in the diagnosis of endophthalmitis but is also helpful in posterior uveitis to identify malignant cells or infectious agents through immunoassays such as deoxyribonucleic acid polymerase chain reaction (DNA-PCR) or standard cultures. In these situations, an anterior vitrectomy can be performed through a single posterior sclerotomy with the use of an infusion sleeve.

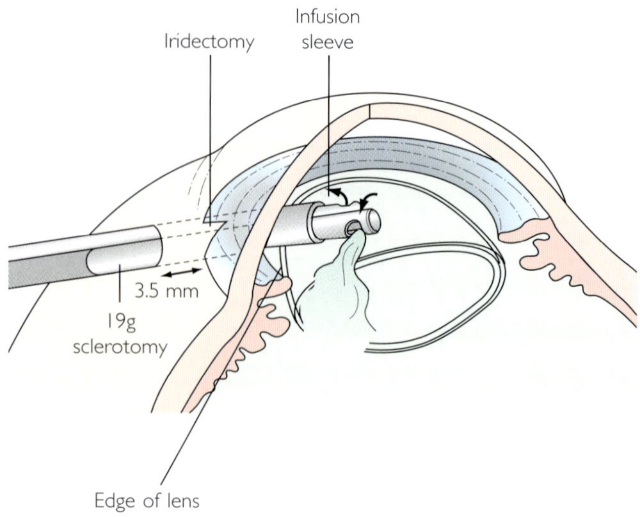

Figure 22.10 *Aqueous block. A single sclerotomy pars plana anterior vitrectomy using an infusion sleeve.*

OPERATIVE PROCEDURE

An L-shaped conjunctival peritomy is performed in the quadrant of the iridectomy. A sclerotomy is marked 3 mm posterior to the limbus in an aphakic or pseudophakic eye and 3.5 mm posterior to the limbus in a phakic eye; it is made in the same meridian as the iridectomy. The vitreous cavity is entered with a 19-gauge MVR knife. Using a suction cutter with an open port, 150 mmHg of suction pressure and a cutting rate of 600 cpm, the vitrectomy probe is placed into the midvitreous cavity with an attached infusion sleeve (Fig. 22.10). The infusion sleeve is attached to an infusion bottle 50 cm above the eye. The high infusion pressure helps the suction cutter to engage the anterior hyaloid. An anterior vitrectomy is performed, keeping the cutting port directed anteriorly and visualized at all times. Using suction alone, the suction is increased until the anterior hyaloid is engaged; cutting is then activated. An endoilluminator may be necessary for adequate visualization (Fig. 22.4).

In aphakic or pseudophakic eyes, the iridectomy site is cleared of anterior hyaloid, lens zonules, lens capsule and debris to ensure a permanent pathway for anterior aqueous flow. At least the anterior one-third of the vitreous should be removed, because following hydration of the remaining vitreous, there will be expansion of the vitreous anteriorly. The vitrectomy must be continued until the anterior chamber deepens, which indicates that the aqueous block is broken.

When a vitreous biopsy is performed, a pure specimen can be obtained by removing approximately 0.5 ml of vitreous before activating the infusion of fluid. After completion of the vitrectomy, the suction cutter is removed and the sclerotomy is cleaned and sutured closed. The globe is reformed by injecting BSS Plus solution with a half-inch 30-gauge needle through the pars plana or limbus. The conjunctiva is closed.

An alternative procedure for vitreous biopsy is possible with a specially designed 23-gauge vitrector. Because the knife is integral to the tip of the suction cutter, it can be passed transconjunctivally through

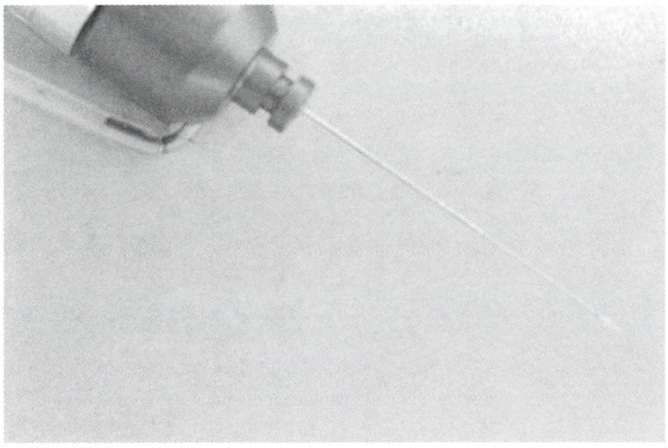

Figure 22.11 *23-Gauge suction cutter with integral knife. (Photograph courtesy of Robert G Josephberg MD.)*

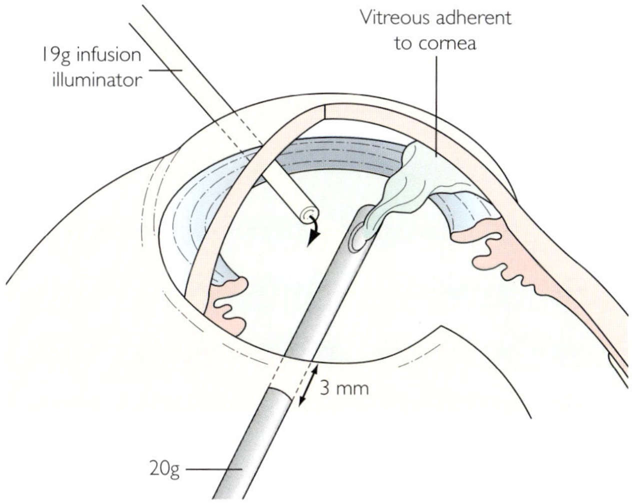

Figure 22.12 *Vitreocorneal touch. Bimanual pars plana vitrectomy with infusion endoilluminator and suction cutter.*

the sclera without the need for a sclerotomy, and obviates the need for infusion or wound closure (Fig. 22.11). Therefore, it can be performed in the office but can only obtain a small specimen.

SURGICAL TECHNIQUE FOR VITREOCORNEAL TOUCH

Occasionally, vitreous can prolapse into the anterior chamber and adhere to the cornea, resulting in corneal decompensation. This situation was uncommon even with intracapsular cataract surgery, but in the modern era of phacoemulsification it is even more rare. Nevertheless, it is an important condition to recognize and is very amenable to a two-instrument pars plana approach utilizing an infusion endoilluminator.

OPERATIVE PROCEDURE

The conjunctiva is incised at the limbus superotemporally and superonasally and reflected posteriorly. Sclerotomy sites are marked on the sclera 3 mm posterior to the limbus in these two quadrants. After creating a 20-gauge sclerotomy, a 20-gauge infusion endoilluminator is placed into the vitreous cavity and held with the nondominant hand. A sclerotomy is made with the dominant hand and a suction cutter is placed into the vitreous cavity behind the pupil. The cutting port is fully open and directed anteriorly (Fig. 22.12). The cutting rate is 500–600 cpm and the suction pressure is 100 mmHg. The infusion bottle is 40 cm above the eye because of the restricted flow of the infusion system. The endoilluminator is used to visualize the vitreous. The vitreous in the anterior chamber is excised as well as the anterior one-third of the vitreous in the vitreous cavity. Surgery should be minimized to reduce the risk of irrigation damage to the cornea. The instruments are removed from the eye and the sclerotomies and conjunctiva are sutured closed. Normal IOP is established by injecting BSS Plus solution with a half-inch 30-gauge needle through the pars plana or limbus.

SURGICAL TECHNIQUE FOR PERSISTENT HYPERPLASTIC PRIMARY VITREOUS (PERSISTENT FETAL VASCULATURE)

In this rare condition, recently termed persistent fetal vasculature,[21] the goals of surgery are to restore a visual pathway and relieve all traction on the ciliary processes. This is achieved by first performing a pars

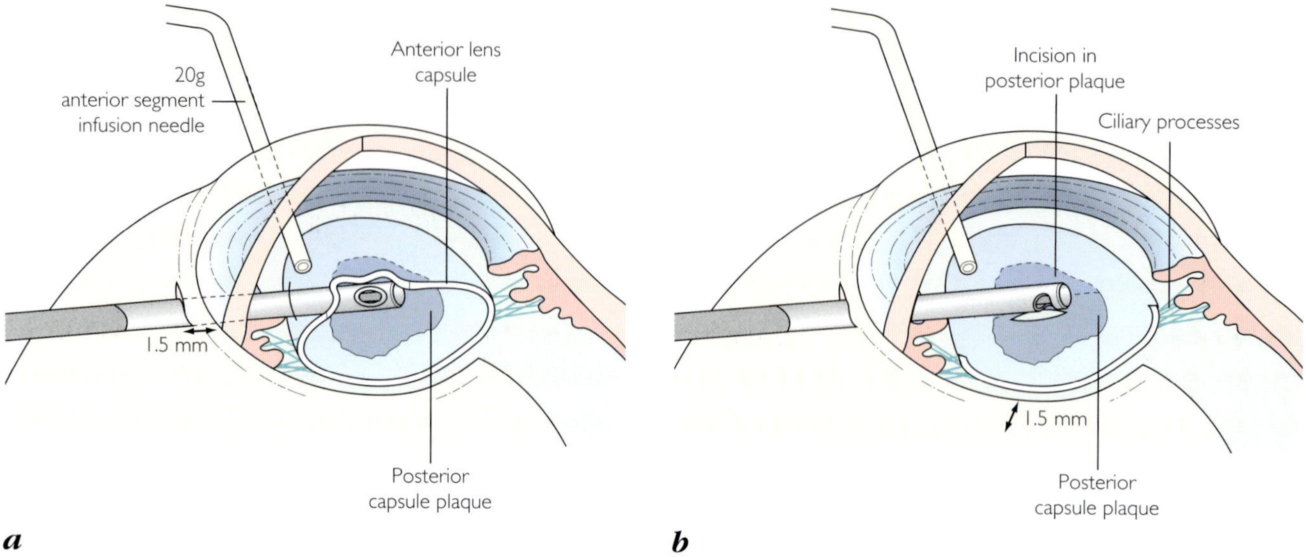

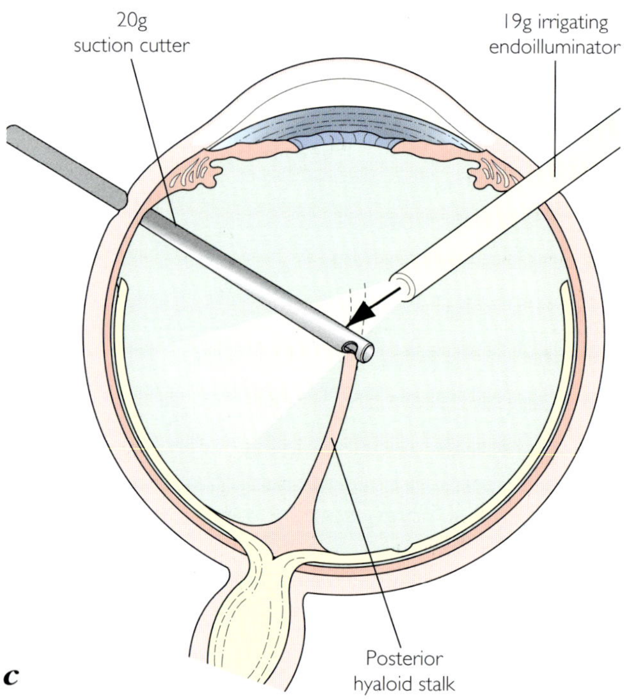

Figure 22.13 *(a) Persistent fetal vasculature. Removal of anterior lens capsule with suction cutter. (b) Excision of central posterior capsule and attached remnants of posterior hyaloid artery with suction cutter. (c) Bimanual pars plicata anterior vitrectomy.*

plicata lensectomy followed by removal of the retrolental fibrovascular membrane. Finally, the hyaloid artery is incised and cauterized. Because this surgery is usually performed in infants within the first few months of life and the eyes are usually microphthalmic, an anterior limbal approach has been advocated.[15] However, unless echography demonstrates a retinal detachment, the pars plicata is a safe and more effective approach. Also, 23-gauge pediatric vitrectomy instruments (DORC) are now available, which should further reduce the risk of retinal dialysis and retinal detachment. Because an IOL is not recommended in these cases, a total lensectomy is performed.

OPERATIVE PROCEDURE

The conjunctiva is incised at the limbus superotemporally and superonasally and reflected posteriorly. In an infant, the sclerotomy sites are usually marked 1.5 mm posterior to the limbus at the 10 and 2 o'clock positions. Transillumination may help to identify the pars plicata and influence the location of the sclerotomies.

Sclerotomies are made with an appropriate gauge MVR knife. An anterior segment infusion needle (Alcon 800-22) is placed into the lens first and then, using the suction cutter with the port fully opened, the lens is aspirated. This technique reduces the risk of anterior chamber collapse and posterior dislocation of lens fragments.

Because of the low blood pressure in an infant, the infusion bottle is kept at a height of only 30 cm. The anterior lens capsule is excised by placing the cutter between the iris and the anterior lens capsule, with the cutting port facing posteriorly (Fig. 22.13a). The cutting rate is 300 cpm but the suction is varied as high as 300 mmHg as necessary.

The posterior lens capsule is intimately involved with the retrolental fibrovascular membrane. Hemostasis of the abnormal persistent fetal vessels is obtained with a 23-gauge tapered bipolar endocautery or raising the IOP or both. The plaque is incised in its center with the MVR knife. The more fenestrations that are made in the posterior capsule, the easier it is to excise with the suction cutter. After the initial incision is made, additional incisions may be made less traumatically by using scissors (Fig. 22.5). The cutting port is directed posteriorly and an opening is made in the plaque (Fig. 22.13b).

Traction on the ciliary processes should be avoided. Care is taken to identify the ciliary processes and avoid incising them. The opening in the plaque is gradually enlarged, relieving traction on the ciliary body. All material adherent to the ciliary processes is excised.

A total capsulectomy may be performed (Fig. 22.9c). A central core vitrectomy is performed in order to excise the hyaloid artery so that it extends no more than half the distance from the plane of the optic nerve to the iris. If necessary to aid in visualization, an infusion endoilluminator can be used for this portion of the procedure (Fig. 22.13c).

The instruments are then removed from the eye and the sclerotomy sites are cleaned and sutured closed, as well as the conjunctiva. Usually it is necessary to inject BSS Plus solution with a half-inch 30-gauge needle through the limbus or pars plicata to restore normal IOP.

REFERENCES

1. Stern WH, Diddie KR, Smith RE. *Vitrectomy Techniques for the Anterior Segment Surgeon* (Grune & Stratton: New York, 1983).
2. Berger BB. Vitreous loss managed by anterior vitrectomy, *Arch Ophthalmol* (1980) **98**:1245–7.
3. Spigelman AV, Lindstrom RL, Nichols B, Lindquist TD. Visual results following vitreous loss and primary lens implantation, *J Cataract Refract Surg* (1989) **15**:201–4.
4. Osher RH, Cionni RJ. The torn posterior capsule: its intraoperative behavior, surgical management and long term consequences, *J Cataract Refract Surg* (1990) **16**:490–4.
5. Cruz OA, Wallace GW, Gay CA, Matoba AY, Koch DD. Visual results and complications of phacoemulsification with intraocular lens implantation performed by residents, *Ophthalmology* (1992) **99**:448–52.
6. Koch PS. Anterior vitrectomy. In: Nordan LT, Maxwell WA, Davison JA, eds, *The Surgical Rehabilitation of Vision: An integrated approach to anterior segment surgery* (Gower Medical Publishing: London, 1994): *17.1–17.7.*
7. Kim JE, Flynn HW, Smiddy WE. Retained lens fragments after phacoemulsification, *Ophthalmology* (1994) **101**:1827–32.
8. Margherio RR, Margherio AR, Pendergast SD, et al. Vitrectomy for retained lens fragments after phacoemulsification, *Ophthalmology* (1997) **104**:1426–32.
9. Harbour JW, Smiddy WE, Rubsamen PE, et al. Pars plana vitrectomy for chronic pseudophakic cystoid macular edema, *Am J Ophthalmol* (1995) **120**:302–7.
10. Fung WE. Vitrectomy for chronic aphakic cystoid macular edema: results of a national collaborative prospective randomized investigation, *Ophthalmology* (1985) **92**:1102–11.
11. Byrnes GA, Leen MM, Wong TP, Benson WE. Vitrectomy for ciliary block (malignant) glaucoma, *Ophthalmology* (1995) **102**:1308–11.
12. Harbour WJ, Rubsamen PE, Palmberg P. Pars plana vitrectomy in the management of phakic and pseudophakic malignant glaucoma, *Arch Ophthalmol* (1996) **114**:1073–8.
13. Karr DJ, Scott WE. Visual acuity results following treatment of persistent hyperplastic primary vitreous, *Arch Ophthalmol* (1986) **104**:662–7.
14. Federman JL, Shields JA, Altman B, Koller H. The surgical and nonsurgical management of persistent hyperplastic primary vitreous, *Ophthalmology* (1982) **89**:20–4.
15. Stark WJ, Lindsey PS, Fagadau WR, Michels RG. Persistent hyperplastic primary vitreous, surgical treatment, *Ophthalmology* (1983) **90**:452–7.
16. Koch PS. Managing the torn posterior capsule and vitreous loss, *Int Ophthalmol Clin* (1994) **34**:113–30.
17. Kusaka S, Tsjioka M, Mano T, Tsuboi S, Ohashi Y. Two-

port vitrectomy for vitreous loss during sutureless cataract surgery (letter), *Am J Ophthalmol* (1994) **117**:533–4.

18. Aaberg TM Jr, Rubsamen PE, Flynn HW Jr, et al. Giant retinal tear as a complication of attempted removal of intravitreal lens fragments during cataract surgery, *Am J Ophthalmol* (1997) **124**:222–6.
19. Eller AW, Barad RF. Miyake analysis of anterior vitrectomy techniques, *J Cataract Refract Surg* (1996) **22**:213–7.
20. Berger BB. Total capsulectomy through the pars plana, *Ocutome Newsletter* (1982) **7**:1.
21. Goldberg MF. Persistent fetal vasculature (PFV): an integrated interpretation of signs and symptoms associated with persistent hyperplastic primary vitreous (PHPV), LIV Edward Jackson Memorial Lecture, *Am J Ophthalmol* (1997) **124**:587–626.

Chapter 23 Removal of retained lens fragments

Harry W Flynn Jr and William E Smiddy

INTRODUCTION

Retained lens fragments, including both nuclear and cortical remnants, occur more often following phacoemulsification compared to other strategies for cataract surgery.[1,2] The exact incidence of posteriorly displaced lens fragments after phacoemulsification is unknown. In a survey of the membership of the American Society of Cataract and Refractive Surgery, the incidence of retained lens fragments was reported as being 0.3%.[1] In a similar survey from the UK, the incidence was 1.1%.[2] Because approximately 1.3 million operations are performed each year in the USA,[3] this complication following phacoemulsification is not rare in clinical practice.

This chapter will review the surgical strategies for managing this condition, as well as follow-up outcomes based on studies in the literature. The issues of timing of surgery, placement of intraocular lenses (IOLs) and occurrence of chronic glaucoma will be addressed, based on published studies from the Bascom Palmer Eye Institute.

CAUSES OF RETAINED LENS FRAGMENTS FOLLOWING PHACOEMULSIFICATION

The exact causes of posteriorly displaced lens fragments are often difficult to determine but this complication occurs more commonly in the elderly patient with a very hard nucleus. Pseudoexfoliation of the lens capsule is also associated with unplanned rupture of the posterior capsule. Loose zonules may cause the entire capsular bag and its contents to be dislocated during phacoemulsification.

Previous vitreous surgery for macular epiretinal membrane or macular hole also may be associated with a greater risk of posterior capsular rupture and subsequent displacement of lens material into the vitreous cavity. Phacoemulsification through clear cornea produces a more vertical angle of approach to the lens, which at times can force the nucleus into the vitreous cavity. The learning curve for this procedure may be associated with a greater initial frequency of rupture of the posterior capsule, causing retained lens fragments.

PREOPERATIVE EVALUATION

The preoperative examination includes a standard ophthalmological work-up including slit-lamp biomicroscopy of the anterior segment and examination of the posterior segment with the indirect ophthalmoscope. Some eyes with retained lens fragments present with marked intraocular inflammation and secondary glaucoma.[4–6] When a hypopyon occurs within 1 week of cataract surgery, there should be a strong clinical suspicion for endophthalmitis.[4,5] In eyes with endophthalmitis and no view of fundus details, echography generally is recommended to rule out the presence of a retained lens fragment as part of the inflammatory process. In this setting of retained lens fragments and endophthalmitis, a needle tap and injection of antibiotics alone will not resolve the intraocular inflammation. A pars plana vitrectomy with removal of retained lens fragments is necessary in the initial treatment of endophthalmitis in these eyes.

In eyes with both retained lens fragments and a dislocated IOL, standard A-scan measurements should be determined in order (possibly) to remove or exchange the dislocated IOL for the appropriate IOL during the vitrectomy procedure.

INDICATIONS FOR SURGERY

Large pieces of retained nuclear or epinuclear fragments are not well tolerated and should be removed at a convenient operating time after the initial cataract surgery.[6–11] However, very small lens fragments (less than 25% or less than 2 mm in size) may be tolerated in the vitreous cavity and surgical intervention can be delayed while evaluating the clinical course. Also, residual lens cortex may become flocculent but will be reabsorbed in many cases. If secondary glaucoma occurs as a result of retained lens fragments, surgery is almost always required.[6–11]

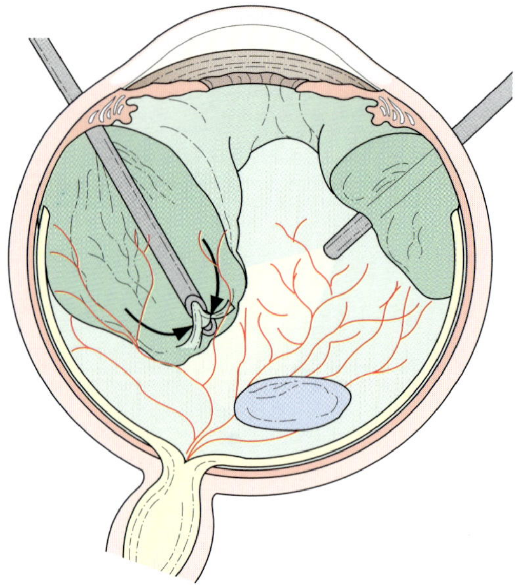

Figure 23.1 *A standard three-port pars plana vitrectomy is performed initially to remove the formed vitreous gel and smaller fragments of lens material suspended in the vitreous. Harder fragments consisting of epinucleus or nucleus are not easily removed with the vitrectomy instrument.*

INSTRUMENTATION

The specific instruments are those required for a standard three-port pars plana vitrectomy approach. The vitrectomy settings are similar to those of standard vitreous surgery. A fragmatome is also necessary for removing harder pieces of lens nucleus in the posterior segment. Sclerotomy sites are closed with 7-0 Dexon sutures. We do not use intravitreal antibiotics either in an injection form or in the infusion fluid. However, standard postoperative subconjunctival antibiotics and steroids are utilized at the end of the surgical procedure.

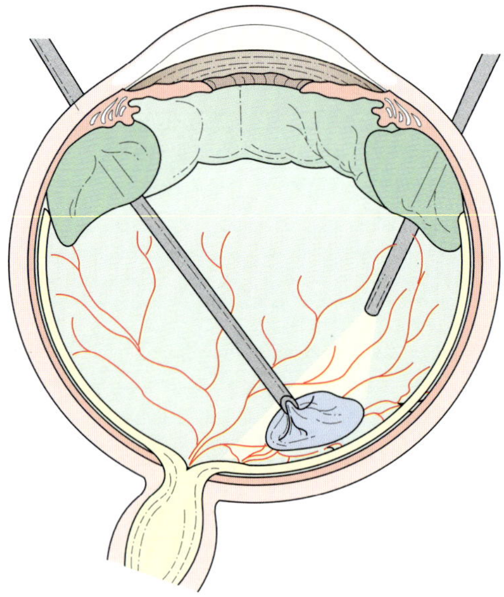

Figure 23.2 *The fragmatome is used to aspirate and lift nuclear fragments from the surface of the retina. Using a power setting of 5–10% and aspiration in the range 150–200 mmHg, the fragment can be slowly fragmented and aspirated into the fragmatome tip. This procedure is performed more safely in the midvitreous cavity, away from the surface of the retina.*

SURGICAL TECHNIQUES

A standard three-port pars plana vitrectomy is performed initially to remove the formed vitreous gel and smaller fragments of lens material suspended in the vitreous (Fig. 23.1). It is not necessary to perform scleral depression to remove formed vitreous overlying the vitreous base region unless the lens nucleus has become adherent to the ora serrata region. In most cases, the lens nucleus will remain mobile and will migrate into the posterior pole after removal of the central vitreous gel.

Residual lens cortex covering the nucleus can be removed with the vitrectomy handpiece. Then the fragmatome can be used to fragment and aspirate the harder nuclear fragments using a power setting of 5–10% with aspiration at 150–200 mmHg (Fig. 23.2).

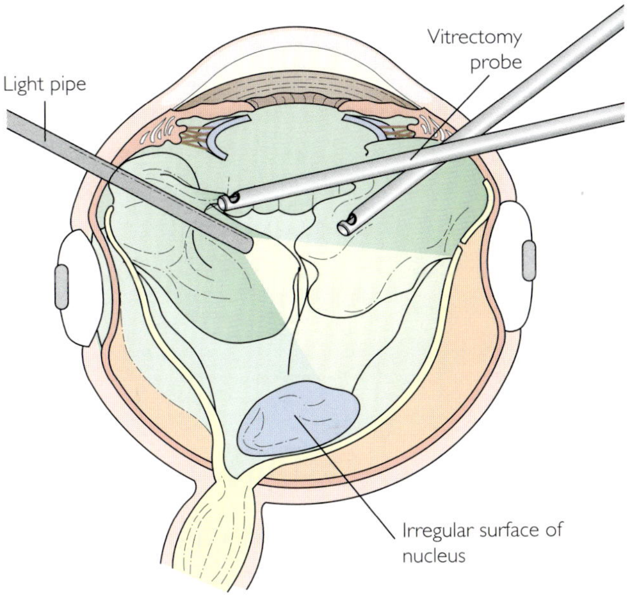

Figure 23.3 *If a coexisting retinal detachment and a retained nuclear fragment are present, an encircling scleral buckle generally is recommended. After placement of the encircling scleral buckle, a standard three-port pars plana vitrectomy is performed to remove the vitreous gel and smaller lens fragments.*

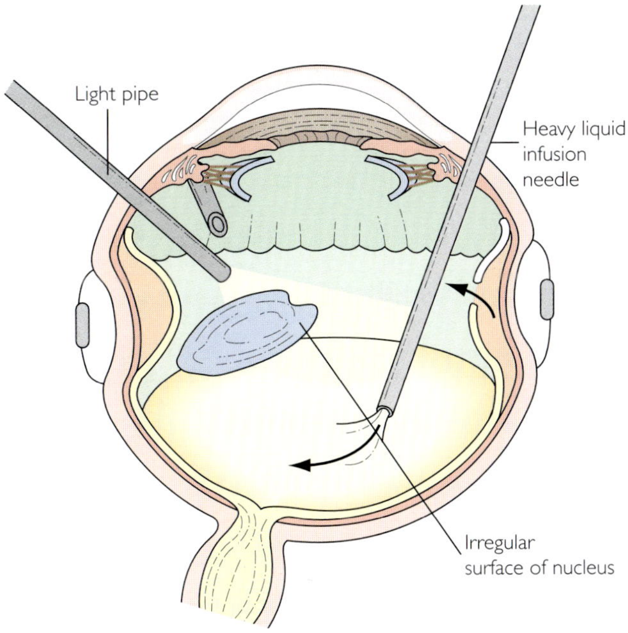

Figure 23.4 *Perfluorocarbon liquids are used to achieve retinal reattachment while simultaneously floating the lens nucleus anteriorly.*

The actual fragmentation of the nucleus should not be performed on or near the retinal surface but should be in the midvitreous cavity. This avoids unplanned contact with the retina or propelling hard nuclear fragments into the macular region.

If no IOL is present, consideration for placement of an IOL should be made at the time of the vitrectomy. After placement of scleral plugs into the sclerotomy sites, the retinal periphery should be inspected to rule out retinal breaks or retinal detachment.

If coexisting retinal detachment and a retained nuclear fragment are present, an encircling scleral buckle generally is recommended (Fig. 23.3). After placement of the buckle, a standard three-port pars plana vitrectomy is performed. The vitreous gel is removed in order to gain access to the lens nucleus. Perfluorocarbon liquids[12–14] may be used to achieve retinal reattachment while simultaneously floating the lens nucleus forward for phacofragmentation (Fig. 23.4).

The majority of the lens nucleus is removed by phacofragmentation. A cyclodialysis spatula can be used to move the nucleus near the tip of the instrument (Fig. 23.5). Small residual fragments are aspirated

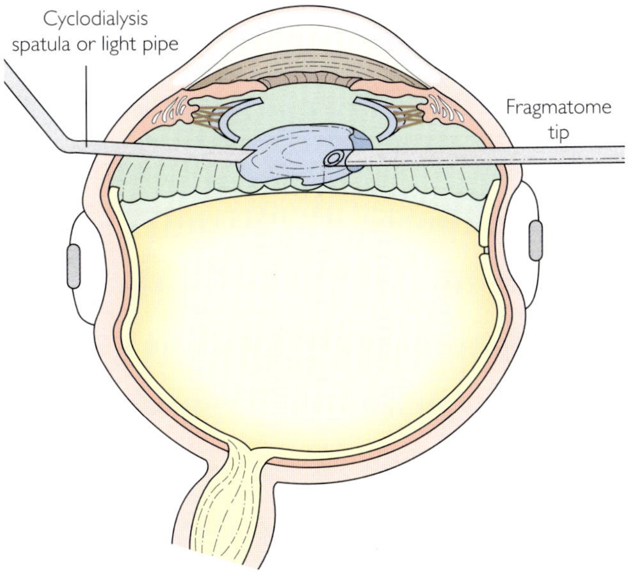

Figure 23.5 *The majority of the lens nucleus is removed by phacofragmentation. A cyclodialysis spatula can by used to move the nucleus near the tip of the instrument.*

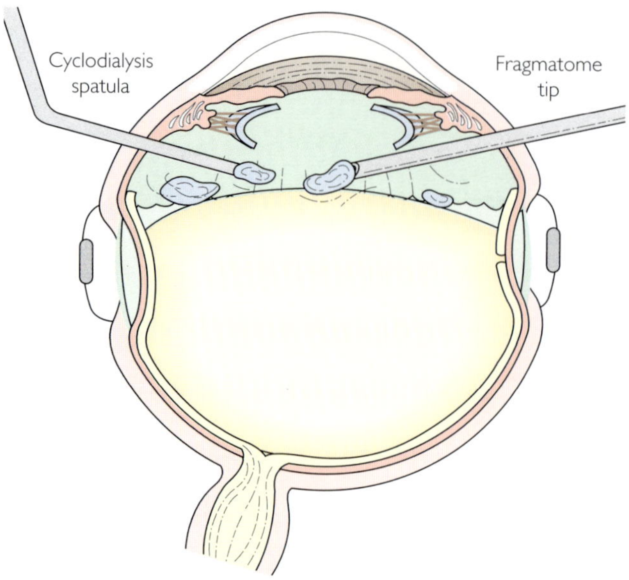

Figure 23.6 *The small fragments can be pushed toward the tip of the instrument for aspiration.*

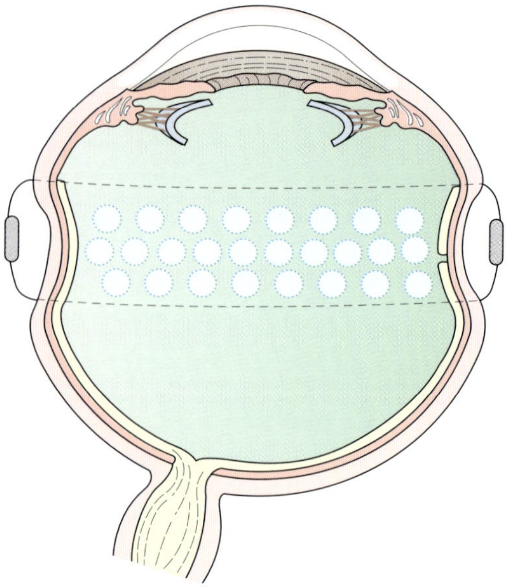

Figure 23.7 *When the lens removal has been completed, endolaser treatment is applied around retinal breaks and on the scleral buckle for 360°. Laser treatment can be performed either before or after a fluid–air exchange. Finally, the use of a long-acting gas tamponade is recommended to increase the chance of long-term retinal reattachment.*

into the fragmatome tip (Fig. 23.6). When lens removal is completed, endolaser treatment is applied around retinal breaks and on the scleral buckle for 360° (Fig. 23.7). The perfluorocarbon liquid is then removed and replaced with a long-acting gas tamponade.

If no IOL was inserted during the initial surgery, it is generally preferable to delay IOL implantation until stable retinal reattachment has been accomplished.

POSTOPERATIVE FOLLOW-UP

The patient is usually examined on the first postoperative day. Often the corneal edema worsens on the first postvitrectomy day, but it should clear within the first few weeks following surgery. Similarly, intraocular pressure (IOP) elevated after cataract surgery may remain elevated following vitrectomy but is usually lower than before vitrectomy.

There are no special requirements for postoperative positioning in these patients, except in cases treated for coexisting retinal detachment. Standard topical antibiotics and steroids are used postoperatively and the patient is examined again approximately 1 week after vitrectomy. Topical glaucoma medications may be necessary if the IOP remains high during the early postoperative course.

The indications for reoperation are few; these would include a very large piece of lens nucleus that was missed during the first vitrectomy. Also, a newly diagnosed retinal detachment would certainly constitute an indication for reoperation. Rarely, secondary glaucoma does not respond to removal of retained lens fragments and standard glaucoma surgery may become necessary in this uncommon situation.

SURGICAL RESULTS: VISUAL ACUITY AND GLAUCOMA OUTCOMES IN PATIENTS WITH RETAINED LENS FRAGMENTS

The visual outcomes in reported series are variable.[6–11] More than 50% of patients achieve 20/40 or better

Table 23.1 Retained lens fragments: visual acuity and glaucoma outcomes

Series	*Year*	*No. of patients*	*Visual acuity ≥ 20/40 (%)*	*IOP ≥ 30 mmHg*	
				Before PPV[a] (%)	*After PPV[a] (%)*
Gilliland[7]	1979–1991	56	50	52	25
Borne[8]	1991–1994	121	68	32	11
Margherio[9] [b]	1986–1996	126	44	52	25
Bascom Palmer Eye Inst.[10,11]	1990–1995	188	62	40	6

[a] PPV, pars plana vitrectomy

[b] Margherio et al reported intraocular pressure (IOP) >25 mmHg before and after vitrectomy

visual acuity unless retinal detachment, corneal edema or cystoid edema is present (Table 23.1). In reported series, coexisting diseases such as macular degeneration, glaucoma and diabetic retinopathy are other causes of poor visual acuity outcomes in these patients.

COMPLICATIONS IN EYES WITH RETAINED LENS FRAGMENTS

Retinal detachment occurs in a high percentage of these patients with retained lens fragments before and after vitrectomy (Table 23.2).[6–11] The causes of retinal detachment are complex and include various factors associated with previous cataract surgery as well as factors associated with the vitrectomy.

During cataract surgery, aggressive attempts to retrieve the posteriorly displaced nucleus may create retinal detachment or a giant retinal tear.[15] Risk factors for retinal detachment during or after cataract surgery include the use of the phacoemulsification probe in formed vitreous, copious vitreous cavity irrigation with balanced salt solution or deep posterior vitrectomy through a limbal incision.[16–18] During vitrectomy, retinal detachment may result from vitreous traction on the peripheral retina during fragmentation or vitrectomy.

RECOMMENDATIONS FOR MANAGEMENT

The anterior segment surgeon usually recognizes the futility of attempted retrieval through a limbal

Table 23.2 Distribution of retinal detachment in the four largest series before and after vitrectomy in eyes with retained lens fragments

Largest reported series	*Years*	*Before or during vitrectomy*	*After vitrectomy*	*Cumulative numbers*
Gilliland[7]	1979–1991	4/56	4/56	8/56
Borne[8]	1991–1994	8/121	11/121	19/121
Margherio[9]	1986–1996	7/126	13/126	20/126
Bascom Palmer Eye Inst.[10,11]	1990–1995	12/188	13/188	25/188
Totals		31/491 (6.3%)	41/491 (8.4%)	72/491 (14.7%)

Table 23.3 Recommendations for management by the anterior segment surgeon

- Attempt fragment retrieval only if readily accessible
- Perform anterior vitrectomy only as necessary, to avoid vitreous prolapse into the wound
- Insert intraocular lens if possible
- Close cataract wound with interrupted sutures
- Prescribe topical medications as needed
- Refer patient to vitreoretinal consultant

Table 23.4 Recommendations for management by the vitreoretinal surgeon

- Initial observation of eyes with minimal inflammation and/or a small nuclear fragment
- Continue topical medications as needed
- Schedule vitrectomy:
  - if inflammation or intraocular pressure is not controlled
  - if fragment is >25% of the nucleus (>2 mm in size)
- Delay vitrectomy, if necessary, to allow clearing of corneal edema or reduction of conjunctival congestion
- Perform adequate core vitrectomy before phacofragmentation
- Start with low fragmentation power (5–10%) for safe, efficient removal of the nucleus
- Prepare for secondary intraocular lens insertion if necessary
- Examine the retinal periphery for retinal tears or retinal detachment

approach. If a posterior segment colleague is readily available in the same hospital or surgical center, an immediate consultation in the same operating room for retrieval of the lens nucleus can be made. The theoretical advantages of this approach are to save the patient another operation at a later time (a second operative procedure, a second anesthesia administration and a second postoperative recovery time).

In these cases with a large posteriorly displaced nuclear fragment, the anterior segment surgeon should perform an anterior vitrectomy, leave as much posterior capsule as possible, insert a sulcus-fixated IOL and close the wound in a standard manner with sutures (Table 23.3).[14] The patient then can be referred to a posterior segment colleague to retrieve the retained lens fragments using a pars plana vitrectomy approach.

When patients are seen in consultation by the vitreoretinal surgeon regarding retained lens fragments, some eyes can be observed when there is minimal inflammation or a very small (less than 2 mm) nuclear fragment (Table 23.4).[14] Topical medications can be continued while observing the clinical features during the follow-up course. If marked intraocular inflammation occurs or the IOP is not controlled, vitrectomy is usually recommended. If the fragment is large (even with minimal inflammation and normal IOP), vitrectomy should be considered.

A delay in vitrectomy may be considered in order to allow clearing of corneal edema and improvement in conjunctival congestion before a second surgical procedure is done. The surgeon should be prepared with IOL calculations if an IOL was not placed initially or if IOL exchange appears to be a possibility.

The vitreoretinal surgeon should always examine the peripheral retina for retinal tears or retinal detachment in these eyes. Small pieces of nucleus may migrate into the inferior part of the anterior chamber, causing marked inflammation and corneal edema.[19] These fragments should be removed at the time of the posterior vitrectomy.

CONCLUSIONS

The incidence of retained lens fragments following phacoemulsification ranges between 0.3% and 1.1% in reported surveys. Because phacoemulsification is the method of choice today for many cataract surgeons and because approximately 1.3 million cataract operations are performed in the USA each year, a large number of patients will require vitrectomy for retained lens fragments. The timing of vitrectomy can be delayed in order to allow clearing of corneal edema and conjunctival congestion. Placement of a posterior chamber IOL at the initial cataract surgery does not adversely influence the final visual results. Retinal detachment is frequent in these eyes and occurred in about 15% of eyes in the four largest reported series. Causes of poor visual acuity outcomes include postoperative retinal detachment, corneal edema and cystoid macular edema, but pre-existing diseases (macular degeneration, diabetic retinopathy and glaucoma) also contribute to poor outcomes in reported series. Vitrectomy and removal of retained lens fragments reduce secondary glaucoma and restore good visual acuity for most patients.

REFERENCES

1. Leaming DV. Practice styles and preferences of ASCRS members – 1994 survey, *J Cataract Refract Surg* (1995) **21:**378–85.
2. Pande M, Dabbs TR. Incidence of lens matter dislocation during phacoemulsification, *J Cataract Refract Surg* (1996) **22:**737–42.
3. Prevent Blindness America. Vision problems in the US. In: *Prevent Blindness America* (Prevent Blindness America: New York, 1994): 8–10.
4. Irvine WD, Flynn HW Jr, Murray TC, Rubsamen PC. Retained lens fragments after phacoemulsification manifesting as marked intraocular inflammation and hypopyon. *Am J Ophthalmol* (1992) **114:**610–14.
5. Kim JE, Flynn HW Jr, Rubsamen PE, et al. Endophthalmitis in eyes with retained lens fragments, *Ophthalmology* (1996) **103:**575–8.
6. Blodi BA, Flynn HW Jr, Blodi CF, et al. Retained nuclei after cataract surgery, *Ophthalmology* (1992) **99:**41–4.
7. Gilliland GD, Hutton WL, Fuller DG. Retained intravitreal lens fragments after cataract surgery, *Ophthalmology* (1992) **99:**1263–9.
8. Borne MJ, Tasman W, Regillo C, et al. Outcomes of vitrectomy for retained lens fragments, *Ophthalmology* (1996) **103:**971–6.
9. Margherio RR, Margherio AR, Pendergast SD, et al. Vitrectomy for retained lens fragments after phacoemulsification, *Ophthalmology* (1997) **104:**1426–32.
10. Kim JE, Flynn HW Jr, Smiddy WE, et al. Retained lens fragments after phacoemulsification, *Ophthalmology* (1994) **101:**1827–32.
11. Vilar NF, Flynn HW Jr, Smiddy WE, et al. Removal of retained lens fragments after phacoemulsification reverses secondary glaucoma and restores visual acuity, *Ophthalmology* (1997) **104:**787–92.
12. Abrams GW, Arrindell EL, Wolf MD, et al. Advances in vitreous surgery: perfluorocarbon liquids. In: Franklin RM, ed, *Retina and Vitreous* (Kugler Publications: New York, 1993): 237–47.
13. Lewis H, Blumenkranz MS, Chang S. Treatment of dislocated crystalline lens and retinal detachment with perfluorocarbon liquids, *Retina* (1992) **12:**299–304.
14. Smiddy WE, Flynn HW Jr. Managing retained lens fragments and dislocated posterior chamber IOLs after cataract surgery. Focal points (modules), American Academy of Ophthalmology, San Francisco, CA, publication (1996) **14:**1–14.
15. Aaberg TM Jr, Rubsamen PE, Flynn HW Jr, et al. Giant retinal tears as a complication of attempted removal of intravitreal lens fragments during cataract surgery, *Am J Ophthalmol* (1997) **124:**222–6.
16. Schecter RJ. Glass-slide vitrectomy for use by the cataract surgeon, *Am J Ophthalmol* (1991) **112:**100.
17. Truhlsen SM. Approaching nuclear slippage, *Arch Ophthalmol* (1991) **109:**627.
18. Weinstein GW, Charlton JF, Esmer E. The 'lost lens': a new surgical technique using the Machemer lens, *Ophthalmic Surg* (1995) **26:**156–9.
19. Bohighian GM, Wexler SA. Complications of retained nuclear fragments in the anterior chamber after phacoemulsification with posterior chamber lens implant, *Am J Ophthalmol* (1997) **123:**546–7.

Chapter 24 Surgical techniques for the management of dislocated posterior chamber intraocular lens

William E Smiddy and Harry W Flynn Jr

INTRODUCTION

A posterior chamber intraocular lens (PC-IOL) may become dislocated when there is suboptimal posterior capsule support following posterior capsular rupture during cataract extraction. Because it has become widely recognized that PC-IOLs may be implanted even after the posterior capsule is ruptured, this problem has become somewhat more common.

The early postoperative dislocation frequently is caused by unknowingly placing part or all of the IOL through a posterior capsular defect onto the anterior hyaloid, or misjudging haptic placement or capsular support. When dislocation occurs more than a few days or weeks after surgery, it may be the result of spontaneous IOL haptic rotation away from the meridians of posterior capsule remnants or zonular dehiscence. Dislocation months or years after placement is even less common and may be due to traumatic[1] or spontaneous loss of zonular support, particularly in eyes with pseudoexfoliation syndrome.

PREOPERATIVE EVALUATION

Completely dislocated PC-IOLs (into the vitreous cavity) are observed typically within the first week following surgery (26/32 cases in one series).[2] The presenting symptoms of patients with dislocated IOLs depend mostly upon the degree of lens decentration.[3] Decentration usually refers to mild malposition with the optic still covering more than half of the pupillary space. In many cases of decentration, one haptic is in the ciliary sulcus and the other is in the capsular bag. Decentration may increase with progressive capsular fibrosis and subsequent capsular contraction.

Patients at the milder end of the decentration spectrum usually present several weeks following cataract extraction with good visual acuity, normal intraocular pressure and without inflammation. Visual symptoms usually are mild and may be related to glare from the edge of the optic. Patients with subluxated PC-IOLs are usually more symptomatic because of the decentered or variable position of the optic in the visual axis. The presenting visual acuity with aphakic correction may be very good, but is frequently unacceptable despite best spectacle correction. A mobile, luxated PC-IOL may generate unique floater-like symptoms, or even induce pupillary block glaucoma.

In addition to the routine ocular examination, preoperative evaluation should include checking the aphakic refracted visual acuity, assessing the mobility or fixation points of the IOL and evaluating the status of residual lens capsular components (Fig. 24.1). Specifically, a judgment should be made as to whether there is sufficient capsular support to allow IOL repositioning into the sulcus or whether suture fixation or IOL removal techniques should be planned. Generally, at least 6 clock-hours of peripheral capsule, at least half of which is in the inferior quadrants, is necessary for satisfactory PC-IOL support.

INDICATIONS FOR SURGERY

There are four general classes of management options for dislocated IOLs: observation, IOL removal, IOL exchange and IOL repositioning.[4–9] The management plan and timing are formulated based on clinical factors such as the type of IOL and any observed secondary complications.

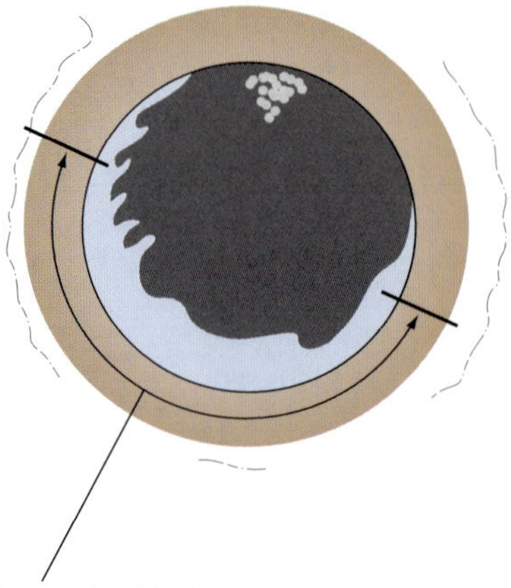

Figure 24.1 *Assessment of degree of residual posterior capsular support. At least 6 clock-hours of well-defined peripheral capsule, much of which must be located inferiorly, is necessary for reliable support without sutures.*

IOLs with simple decentration are usually managed satisfactorily by observation or the use of topical miotics. Surgery also may be deferred, even for luxated PC-IOLs, if phakic contact lens correction is visually satisfactory and convenient to the patient, if other superseding medical or ocular problems prohibit further surgery or if the patient simply elects not to pursue further surgery. A mobile PC-IOL may be associated with, or even induce, other complications. In a series of 15 patients where a dislocated anterior chamber or iris plane IOL was observed, a visual acuity of 20/40 or better was reported in 60%, but retinal detachment occurred in two patients.[4]

Substantial intraocular inflammation, retinal detachment or cystoid macular edema (CME) (especially when associated with vitreous in the cataract wound) constitute relative indication for surgery. Although a completely dislocated PC-IOL may be well tolerated in many eyes, the difficulties in visual rehabilitation necessitate surgical intervention in most of them. For symptomatically subluxated PC-IOLs, surgery may be performed via a limbal or a pars plana approach. Eyes with less extensive IOL subluxation may be managed via a limbal incision with minimal or no anterior vitrectomy if the posterior capsule is largely intact. However, if there is a large posterior capsular rent, vitrectomy using a pars plana approach may offer optimal control to achieve the goals of surgery.

IOL exchange may be performed if the PC-IOL has been damaged during surgical manipulation (e.g. broken haptic), if instrument availability or familiarity with repositioning techniques is lacking, or if PC-IOL design features (e.g. highly flexible haptics or short, C-loop haptics) make it unsuitable for sulcus or suture fixation.

SILICONE IOL REPOSITIONING

A recently encountered circumstance in which IOL exchange may be considered is in certain cases with silicone IOLs.[10] Silicone IOLs are slippery and more difficult to grasp than polymethylmethacrylate IOLs, but usually can be engaged and elevated from the retinal surface with a vitreoretinal pick or a lighted pick. A serrated or diamond-dusted forceps may be necessary to gain a firm purchase, but care should be exercised to avoid scratching the center of the optic if the IOL is to be repositioned. Although silicone-plate haptic IOLs are extremely floppy and difficult to manipulate, and the dimension of the IOL is designed for capsular fixation, usually it can be repositioned onto the anterior capsular remnants satisfactorily (Figs 24.2 and 24.3).[11]

IOL PLACEMENT

Following the removal of a dislocated IOL, the placement of an anterior chamber (AC)-IOL or a scleral suture-fixated PC-IOL may be performed. Exchange for a suture-fixated PC-IOL has been simplified by IOL designs with holes in the haptics. However, explanting and reimplanting an IOL may risk more corneal endothelial cell trauma compared to repositioning techniques. Exchange for an AC-IOL may be less traumatic to the corneal endothelium and may be easier and faster to accomplish, especially in selected circumstances such as with an elderly patient at risk for choroidal hemorrhage.

The mechanical side-effects of earlier AC-IOL designs reportedly have been lessened by newer AC-IOL designs.[12,13] In general, scleral suture fixation with a PC-IOL is preferred by the authors over AC-IOL implantation. The possibility of either PC-IOL or AC-IOL implantation should be anticipated by obtaining IOL power calculations before vitreous surgery.

Another undesirable option is retention of the dislocated PC-IOL in the vitreous and implantation of a secondary (usually AC) IOL.[14–16] Some have advocated this option as a last resort; however, this

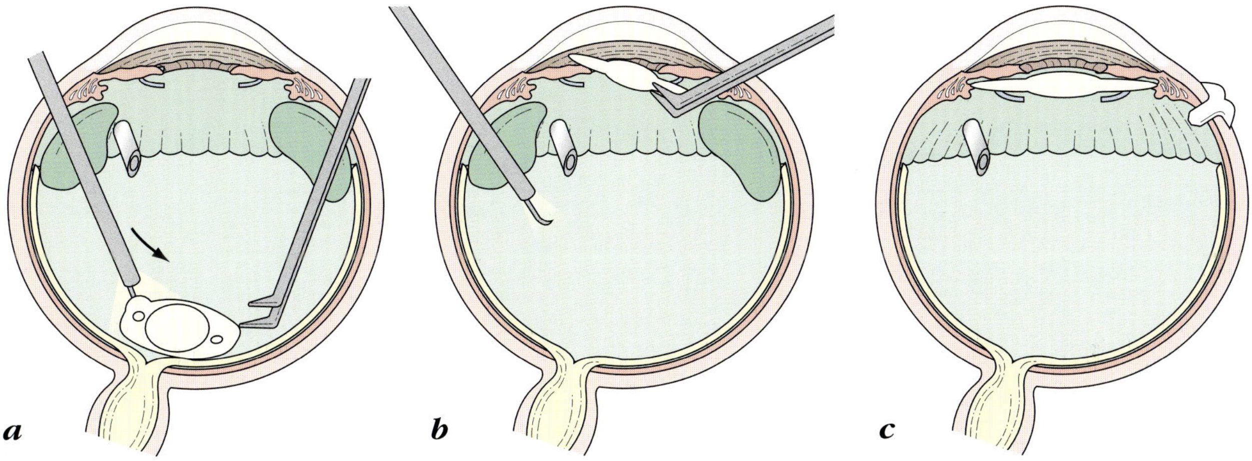

Figure 24.2 *Retrieval and repositioning of silicone-plate intraocular lens (IOL). (a) After core vitrectomy, the IOL edge is lifted with a lighted pick and grasped firmly using serrated or diamond-dusted forceps. (b) The IOL is brought anteriorly through the posterior capsule defect and into the anterior chamber. (c) The haptics then are directed sequentially into the sulcus using a vitreoretinal pick to decenter the haptic central to the pupil and then allowing it to go over the residual anterior capsule.*

can be considered in circumstances, when the patient or the eye cannot tolerate prolonged surgery.

PC-IOL repositioning completes the initial surgical objectives of the cataract surgery and is the most commonly elected surgical approach. There are three basic approaches to IOL repositioning:

- PC-IOL repositioning without sutures using residual peripheral anterior or posterior capsular remnants.
- Iris suture fixation.
- Scleral suture fixation.

Recognizing and using adequate capsular support is as important for successful IOL repositioning as it is for primary placement. Repositioning by sulcus fixation in front of residual capsular support is the most common management technique (in reported series[2,4–9]) and is the authors' first choice when technically possible. Generally, the IOL remains well supported if at least 180° of peripheral capsular

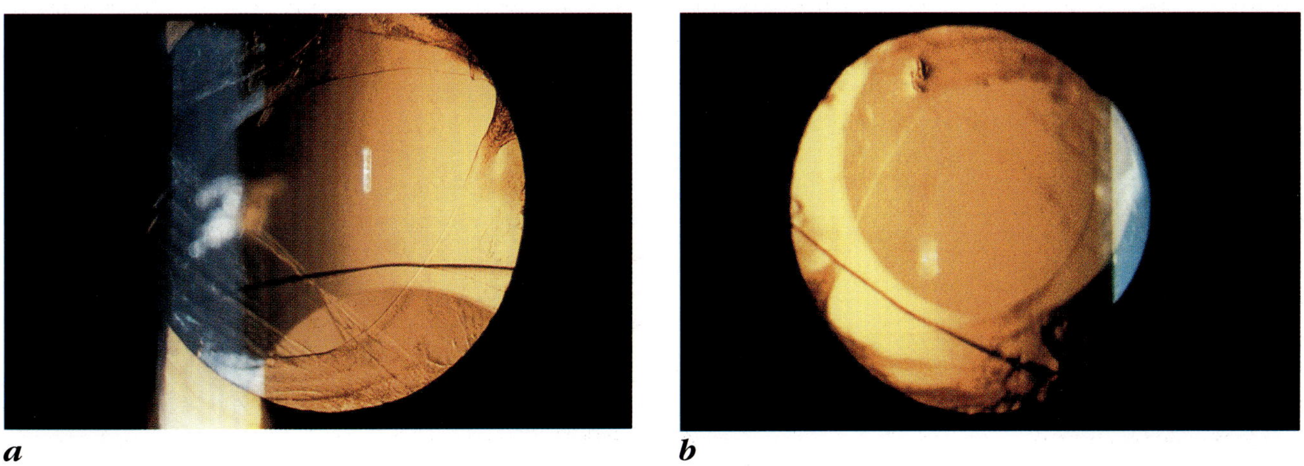

Figure 24.3 *(a) Preoperative and (b) postoperative clinical appearance of an eye in which a silicone-plate haptic posterior chamber intraocular lens was repositioned anterior to capsular remnants.*

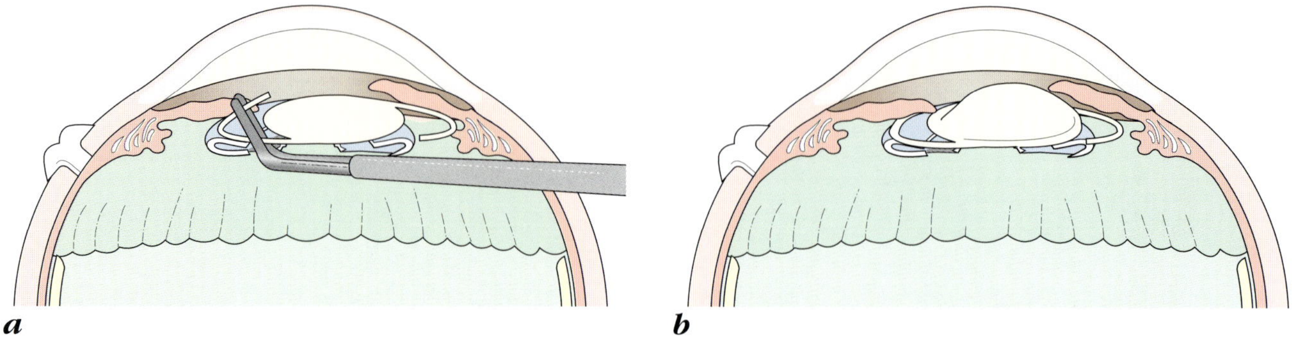

Figure 24.4 *(a) When repositioning a posterior chamber intraocular lens (PC-IOL) into the sulcus in an eye with adequate capsular support, it is convenient to bring at least one of the haptics anterior to the iris, capturing the IOL anteriorly. The first haptic usually can be placed into the sulcus during this maneuver while still grasping the optic with forceps. The second haptic can then be placed using the forceps from either a limbal paracentesis or the sclerotomy. (b) The IOL should be rotated strategically before placing the second haptic, to minimize the need for subsequent manipulation of the IOL, which avoids risking rotating the IOL out of a stable position.*

material is intact. More extensive support is necessary, however, when the inferior capsule is absent or if the margin of the residual capsule is of questionable integrity to support the PC-IOL haptics.

Surgical success depends on accurate placement of the haptics into the ciliary sulcus. Adequate visualization of the residual capsule[17,18] is helpful to accomplish this and iris hooks are useful in selected cases. Sometimes it is easier to use strategic local iris retraction with a hooked instrument to gain adequate visualization. A useful maneuver in a pars plana approach is to bring one PC-IOL haptic into the anterior chamber while placing the opposite haptic into the sulcus over the residual capsule (Fig. 24.4). The second haptic can be guided between the residual capsule and posterior iris surface either by rotating the lens or by grasping the haptic with intraocular forceps via a pars plana or limbal incision. Most cataract surgeons perform a capsulorrhexis. Thus, the remaining anterior capsule is usually intact and provides a shelf on which the IOL can be placed.

Repositioning a PC-IOL permanently into the anterior chamber also has been reported (and used satisfactorily by the authors on two occasions),[19] but should be reserved for only selected cases because chronic chafing of the iris by the PC-IOL (which is usually vaulted posteriorly) may induce chronic inflammation. An additional consideration is that positioning a PC-IOL that originally was intended for capsular fixation into the sulcus usually makes the eye about 1 diopter myopic. This should also be considered when implanting a PC-IOL during IOL exchange.

Iris fixation sutures initially were described for use with dislocated AC-IOLs.[20] However, their use has been modified for posterior chamber implant fixation using a limbal or a pars plana approach.[17,21] This technique requires that a suture pass through the cornea, iris, around the PC-IOL haptic and back out through the iris and cornea. Because accurate placement of the needle is difficult, it is challenging to optimize PC-IOL centration. Also, concern regarding iris-mediated chronic inflammation and the technical difficulty encountered during suture placement has led to the development of other techniques.[22]

Scleral fixation sutures were introduced for implantation of secondary IOLs and for primary IOL placement in the absence of satisfactory peripheral capsular support from the limbal or pars plana approach.[23–34] Early reports[35–37] described externalizing the haptic through a sclerotomy, looping it with a suture and then repositioning the haptic into the eye and suturing it to the internal lip of the sclerotomy. Subsequently, IOL repositioning using transscleral fixation sutures via a pars plana approach (mimicking the techniques of secondary IOL fixation) was described,[38] meaning that the haptic was looped intraocularly and sutures were brought out of the eye. Numerous innovative modifications have made IOL fixation technically easier and safer and these will be reviewed below.

Components common to all scleral suture fixation techniques include:

- Retrieving the IOL.
- Introducing a suture loop through the ciliary sulcus region into the vitreous cavity.

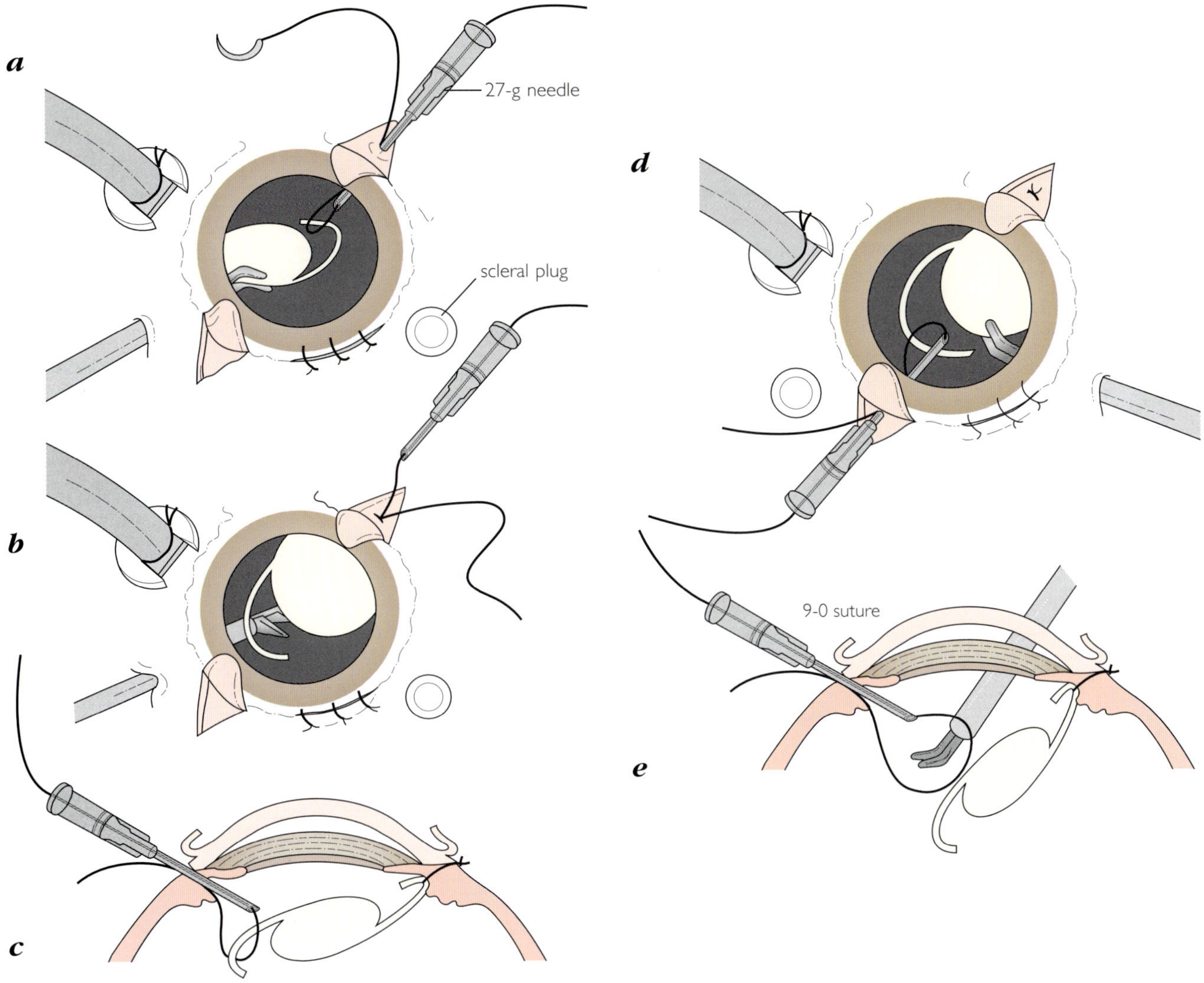

Figure 24.5 *(a) A 9-0 suture (with needle) threaded through a 27-gauge straight needle is introduced into the vitreous cavity 1.0 mm posterior to the limbus through the bed of a partial-thickness scleral flap. Under direct visualization, the haptic is threaded through the loop of the suture. A scleral plug is placed in the unused open sclerotomy. (b) The 27-gauge needle is withdrawn and the suture is tied under the scleral flap in the usual fashion. (c and d) A similar procedure is performed for the other haptic, unless the second haptic can be secured by capsular fixation; c shows side view. (e) Depending upon factors such as pupillary dilation, capture of the second haptic may be facilitated by using intraocular forceps to pull or guide it through the loop.*

- Passing the suture loop around the IOL haptic.
- Securing the suture to the sclera.
- Covering or burying the scleral suture knot.

A variety of techniques have been described to achieve these goals.

Most proposed techniques modify how the suture loop is introduced and attached to the IOL haptic. Such techniques have included imbricating the IOL haptic into the sutures used to close the sclerotomy,[39] externalizing the haptics to attach a suture,[40] using a needle guide to thread the suture around the haptic,[41] introducing and reversing a small suture needle intraocularly to capture the haptic,[38] suturing through IOL optic positioning holes,[42,43] backing a large needle into the eye to introduce a suture loop,[44] grasping a loop with intraocular forceps[45,46] and suturing techniques involving or introducing the suture from a third sclerotomy.[47] Other proposed technique variations include achieving three- or four-point fixation to lessen lens torsion,[48] using specially designed, small-gauge forceps to aid in maneuvering the loop around the haptic,[49] and using perfluorocarbon liquids to place the implant in an accessible position for suturing.[5,50–53] Most posterior segment surgeons find the use of perfluorocarbon liquids unnecessary for routine cases.

TECHNIQUE FOR FIXATION OF DISLOCATED PC-IOL

The current technique preferred by the authors for fixation of a dislocated PC-IOL is described (Fig. 24.5).[54] A standard three-port pars plana vitrectomy is performed to remove the vitreous around the IOL and to mobilize it. Partial-thickness, limbal-based scleral flaps are prepared, most conveniently in the 1 and 7 o'clock meridians to avoid the previous cataract wound and yet be accessible for scleral suture placement. A disposable 27-gauge needle with or without a hole located in the bevel[55] is pre-threaded with 9-0 polypropylene (Prolene®) suture and introduced into the eye 1 mm posterior to the limbus in the bed of the partial-thickness scleral flap. Slack is created in the suture along the shaft of the needle by withdrawing it slightly. The IOL haptic is guided through this loop using the intraocular forceps to grasp the optic. The haptic is captured in the loop as the needle is withdrawn. A partial-thickness scleral needle pass in the bed of the scleral flap allows fixation of the scleral suture. A similar procedure is repeated for the other haptic, unless capsular fixation is possible for the opposite haptic. Occasionally it is necessary to guide the haptic through the loop by using intraocular forceps. The scleral flap is then closed with an absorbable suture and, if necessary, the vitrectomy is completed through the original sclerotomies.

Histopathological and ultrasound biomicroscopic studies have shown that little or no fibrosis occurs around sutured PC-IOL haptics,[56] but one study has shown cicatrization around the haptics.[57] Either way, it is vital to use a nondissolving suture material because it may provide the sole means of support at the ciliary sulcus. Indeed, the authors have observed redislocation after cutting an exposed scleral suture knot.

IOL torsion and decentration can be avoided by accurate ciliary sulcus placement and by adequate excision of bulky capsular and cortical remnants. Anatomic studies have located the sulcus approximately 1 mm posterior to the limbus.[58] Consequently, suture placement more posteriorly may cause IOL optic torsion by forcing the circumferentially oriented haptic over radially oriented ciliary processes. Identification of the location of the ciliary sulcus can be facilitated by transillumination techniques[59] or via a specially designed intraocular mirror.[60] The sutures must be placed diametrically apart for proper centration. Also, the IOL must be rotated minimally and cautiously to the center at the end of the case. It may be necessary to exchange some IOLs that are too short from haptic to haptic for sulcus fixation, because tension on the haptics will cause optic torsion.

OUTCOMES AND COMPLICATIONS

The final visual acuity probably depends not only on preoperative macular function but also on complications from the original cataract surgery, such as CME and retinal detachment. Still, recent series report a final visual acuity of at least 20/40 in more than 90% of eyes (Table 24.1).[2,4,6,9,40,41,61] However, surgical series are difficult to compare accurately because of a nonhomogeneous study population and the variety of surgical techniques.

Managing a dislocated PC-IOL in the presence of a retinal detachment typically involves standard vitreoretinal surgical techniques,[62] but perfluorocarbon liquids may be useful in selected cases to manipulate the IOL better while avoiding retinal trauma (Fig. 24.6). Postoperative complications are difficult to separate from those associated with complicated cataract surgery. Both CME and retinal detachment have been described after IOL repositioning surgery.[63] Retinal

Table 24.1 Results of pars plana vitrectomy for dislocated intraocular lens

Series	*No. of patients*	*Visual acuity ≥ 20/40 (%)*
Campo[41] (1989)	17	59
Flynn[4] (1990)	25	68
Smiddy[2] (1991)	32	69
Chan[40] (1992)	12	92
Panton[6] (1993)	31	94
Smiddy[9] (1995)	46	50
Mello[61] (2000)	110	57

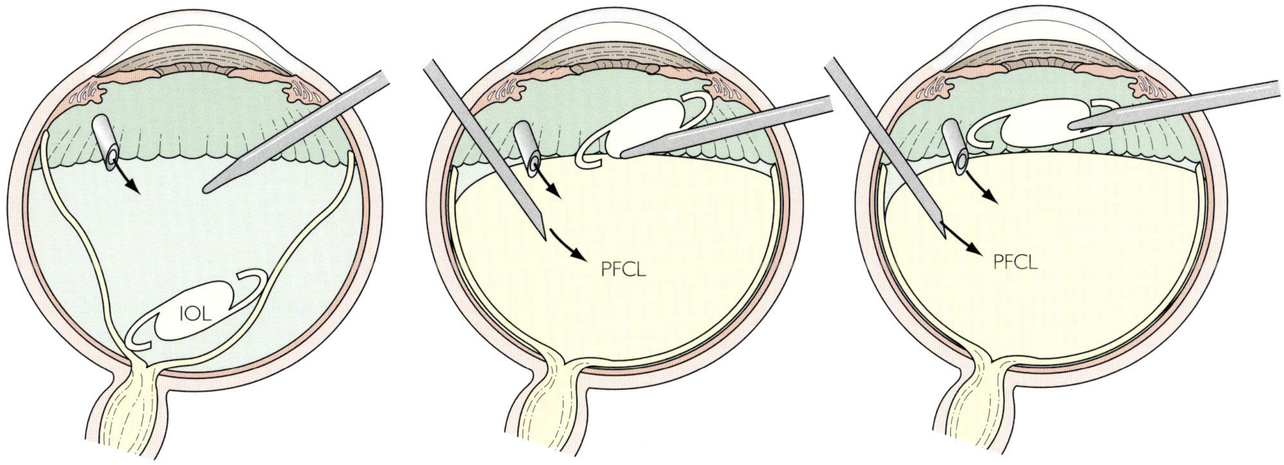

Figure 24.6 *Perfluorocarbon liquids (PFCL) may facilitate intraocular lens (IOL) repositioning in the presence of retinal detachment by floating the IOL anteriorly while keeping the retina posteriorly.*

detachment occurs in about 2% of cases (Table 24.2), but may be less frequent than with retained lens fragments.[63] Retinal detachment may be more common and more difficult to repair when scleral suture fixation has been performed,[64,65] but this may reflect more the complexities of eyes requiring scleral sutures rather than the technique itself.

There are a few considerations in complications that are specific to scleral suture fixation techniques. An intraoperative or postoperative vitreous hemorrhage commonly occurs because sutures are placed through the vascular ciliary body, but the hemorrhage is almost always self-limited, of little clinical significance and resolves spontaneously. Bacterial migration along the transscleral suture tract has been described as a possible route for infection in cases of delayed-onset endophthalmitis.[4,66] The use of a partial-thickness scleral flap to cover the scleral suture knot should reduce the risk of this complication, but the suture knot may erode through the flap.

SUMMARY AND RECOMMENDATIONS FOR MANAGEMENT

For the anterior segment surgeon, avoiding PC-IOL dislocation depends upon accurate assessment of posterior capsular status intraoperatively. With the

Table 24.2 Incidence of retinal detachment occurring before and after vitrectomy for dislocated posterior chamber intraocular lens

Series	*Initial co-existing retinal detachment*	*Retinal detachment after vitrectomy*	*Combined rates*
Flynn[4] (1990)[a]	1/20 (5%)	0/20 (0%)	1/20 (5%)
Smiddy[2] (1991)[a]	1/32 (3%)	1/32 (3%)	2/32 (6%)
Chan[40] (1992)	0/12 (0%)	0/12 (0%)	0/12 (0%)
Panton[6] (1993)	0/31 (0%)	0/31 (0%)	0/31 (0%)
Smiddy[9] (1995)[a]	0/59 (0%)	0/59 (0%)	0/59 (0%)
Total	2/154 (1.3%)	1/154 (0.6%)	3/154 (1.9%)

[a] These three series are from the same institution but data are abstracted and are listed here as consecutive series without overlap of cases.

increased use of phacoemulsification, capsular ruptures are now more commonly central, rather than peripheral, as was usually created by extracapsular techniques. However, the anterior segment surgeon must be suspicious enough to evaluate the integrity of the peripheral capsule carefully before implanting a PC-IOL in the presence of a posterior capsular rupture. Generally, at least 6 clock-hours of peripheral capsule (including the inferior meridians) are necessary to maintain PC-IOL support. Once it is deemed safe to proceed with PC-IOL placement, it is vital that the haptics are placed precisely. Viscoelastic substances and iris retraction may facilitate this evaluation and placement.

Recommendations to the anterior segment surgeon encountering PC-IOL dislocation intraoperatively include performing an anterior vitrectomy to avoid vitreous incarceration in the wound. Postoperatively, frequent topical corticosteroids and, as clinically indicated, intraocular pressure-reducing agents should be prescribed. For most cases, vitreoretinal referral for definitive management is advisable, but some eyes may be observed or may be amenable to management with limbal incisions. Careful attention is necessary to detect other complications such as retinal detachment.

Recommendations to the vitreoretinal surgeon include:

- Careful assessment of existing capsular anatomy.
- Detection of coexisting complications to formulate a treatment plan in terms of timing and technique options.
- Generally allowing a week or more for treatment and resolution of acute postoperative inflammation.
- IOL power calculations if an IOL exchange is a possibility.

There are many management options available for dislocated PC-IOLs; the optimal approach must be determined individually for each eye and based upon many aspects of existing ocular anatomy and the surgeon's experience. Although postoperative visual results are good, it will depend on pre-existing, intraoperative or postoperative complications.

REFERENCES

1. Murphy GE. Traumatic dislocation of a shearing lens 31 months after implantation, *Ophthalmic Surg* (1983) **14:**53–4.
2. Smiddy WE, Flynn HW Jr. Management of dislocated posterior chamber intraocular lenses, *Ophthalmology* (1991) **98:**889–94.
3. Smith SG, Lindstrom RL. Malpositioned posterior chamber lenses: etiology, prevention, and management, *J Am Intraocular Implant Soc* (1985) **11:**584–91.
4. Flynn HW Jr, Buus D, Culbertson WW. Management of subluxated and posteriorly dislocated intraocular lenses using pars plana vitrectomy instrumentation, *J Cataract Refract Surg* (1990) **16:**51–6.
5. Capone A Jr, Mandell BA, Aaberg TM Sr, et al. Contemporary vitreoretinal surgical management of posteriorly dislocated intraocular lenses, *Proceedings of the Symposium on Retina and Vitreous* (New Orleans Academy of Ophthalmology: New Orleans, 1993): 271–81.
6. Panton RW, Sulewski ME, Parker JS, et al. Surgical management of subluxed posterior-chamber intraocular lenses, *Arch Ophthalmol* (1993) **111:**919–26.
7. Smiddy WE, Flynn HW Jr. Management options for posteriorly dislocated intraocular lenses, *Ophthalmic Practice* (1994) **12:**72–7.
8. Shakin EP, Carty JB Jr. Clinical management of posterior chamber intraocular lens implants dislocated in the vitreous cavity, *Ophthalmic Surg Lasers* (1995) **26:**529–34.
9. Smiddy WE, Ibanez GV, Alfonso E, Flynn HW Jr. Surgical management of dislocated intraocular lenses, *J Cataract Refract Surg* (1995) **21:**64–9.
10. Batlan SJ, Dodick JM. Explanation of a foldable silicone intraocular lens, *Am J Ophthalmol* (1996) **122:**270–2.
11. Schneiderman TE, Johnson MW, Smiddy WE, et al. Surgical management of posteriorly dislocated silicone plate haptic intraocular lenses, *Am J Ophthalmol* (1997) **123:**629–35.
12. Ellerton CR, Rattigan SM, Chapman FM, et al. Secondary implantation of open-loop, flexible, anterior chamber intraocular lenses, *J Cataract Refract Surg* (1996) **22:**951–4.
13. Schein OD, Kenyon KR, Steinert RF, et al. A randomized trial of intraocular lens fixation techniques with penetrating keratoplasty, *Ophthalmology* (1993) **100:**1437–43.
14. Jacobi KW, Krey H. Surgical management of intraocular lens dislocation into the vitreous: case report, *J Am Intraocular Implant Soc* (1983) **9:**58–9.
15. Brockman EB, Franklin RM, Kaufman HE. Visual disability resulting from a dislocated intraocular lens, *J Cataract Refract Surg* (1993) **19:**312–13.
16. Sinskey RM. Posterior chamber implant removal with or without replacement, *Cataract* (1983) **1:**8–10.
17. Stark WJ, Bruner WE, Martin NF. Management of subluxed posterior-chamber intraocular lenses, *Ophthalmic Surg* (1982) **13:**130–3.
18. Eifrig DE. Two principles for repositioning intraocular lenses, *Ophthalmic Surg* (1986) **17:**486–9.
19. Allara RD, Weinstein GW. A new surgical technique for managing sunset syndrome, *Ophthalmic Surg* (1987) **18:**811–14.
20. McCannel MA. A retrievable suture idea for anterior uveal problems, *Ophthalmic Surg* (1976) **7:**98–103.
21. Sternberg P Jr, Michels RG. Treatment of dislocated posterior chamber intraocular lenses, *Arch Ophthalmol* (1986) **104:**1391–3.
22. Busin M, Brauweiler P, Boker T, Spitznas M. Complications of sulcus-supported intraocular lenses with iris sutures, implanted during penetrating keratoplasty after intracapsular cataract extraction, *Ophthalmology* (1990) **97:**401–6.

23. Malbran ES, Malbran E Jr, Negri I. Lens guide suture for transport and fixation in secondary IOL implantation after intracapsular extraction, *Int Ophthalmol* (1986) **9:**151–60.
24. Lindquist TD, Agapitos PJ, Lindstrom RL, et al. Transscleral fixation of posterior chamber intraocular lenses in the absence of capsular support, *Ophthalmic Surg* (1989) **20:**769–75.
25. Smiddy WE, Sawusch MR, O'Brien TP, et al. Implantation of scleral-fixated posterior chamber intraocular lenses, *J Cataract Refract Surg* (1990) **16:**691–6.
26. Grehn F, Sundmacher R. Fixation of posterior chamber lenses by transscleral sutures: techniques and preliminary results (letter), *Arch Ophthalmol* (1989) **107:**954–5.
27. Lewis JS. Sulcus fixation without flaps, *Ophthalmology* (1993) **100:**1346–50.
28. McCluskey P, Harrisberg B. Long-term results using scleral-fixated posterior chamber intraocular lenses, *J Cataract Refract Surg* (1994) **20:**34–9.
29. Teichmann KD. Pars plana fixation of posterior chamber intraocular lenses, *Ophthalmic Surg* (1994) **25:**549–53.
30. Tomikawa S, Hara A. Simple approach to secondary posterior chamber intraocular lens implantation in patients without a complete posterior lens capsule support, *Ophthalmic Surg* (1995) **26:**160–3.
31. Vajpayee RB, Angra SK, Sandramouli S, Rewari R. Direct scleral fixation of posterior chamber intraocular lenses using a special needle-holder, *Ophthalmic Surg* (1992) **23:**383–7.
32. Mittelviefhaus H, Wiek J. A refined technique of transscleral suture fixation of posterior chamber lenses developed for cases of complicated cataract surgery with vitreous loss, *Ophthalmic Surg* (1993) **24:**698–701.
33. Lyle WA, Jin JC. Secondary intraocular lens implantation: anterior chamber vs posterior chamber lenses, *Ophthalmic Surg* (1993) **24:**375–81.
34. Regillo CD, Tidwell J. A small-incision technique for suturing a posterior chamber intraocular lens, *Ophthalmic Surg Lasers* (1996) **27:**473–5.
35. Lyons CJ, Steele AD. Report of a repositioned posteriorly dislocated intraocular lens via pars plicata sclerotomy. *J Cataract Refract Surg* (1990) **16:**509–11.
36. Moretsky SL. Suture fixation technique for subluxated posterior chamber IOL through stab wound incision, *J Am Intra-Ocular Implant Soc* (1984) **10:**477–80.
37. Insler MS, Mani H, Peyman GA. A new surgical technique for dislocated posterior chamber intraocular lenses, *Ophthalmic Surg* (1988) **19:**480–1.
38. Smiddy WE. Dislocated posterior chamber intraocular lens: a new technique of management, *Arch Ophthalmol* (1989) **107:**1678–80.
39. Girard LJ, Nino N, Wesson M, Maghraby A. Scleral fixation of a subluxated posterior chamber intraocular lens, *J Cataract Refract Surg* (1988) **14:**326–7.
40. Chan CK. An improved technique for management of dislocated posterior chamber implants, *Ophthalmology* (1992) **99:**51–7.
41. Campo RV, Chung KD, Oyakawa RT. Pars plana vitrectomy in the management of dislocated posterior chamber lenses, *Am J Ophthalmol* (1989) **108:**529–34.
42. Koch DD. New optic hole configuration for iris fixation of posterior chamber lenses (letter), *Arch Ophthalmol* (1988) **106:**163–4.
43. Nabors G, Varley MP, Charles S. Ciliary sulcus suturing of a posterior chamber intraocular lens, *Ophthalmic Surg* (1990) **21:**263–5.
44. Friedberg MA, Pilkerton AR. A new technique for repositioning and fixating a dislocated intraocular lens, *Arch Ophthalmol* (1992) **110:**413–15.
45. Maguire AM, Blumenkranz MS, Ward TG, Winkelman JZ. Scleral loop fixation for posteriorly dislocated intraocular lenses, *Arch Ophthalmol* (1991) **109:**1754–8.
46. Lawrence FC II, Hubbard WA. 'Lens lasso' repositioning of dislocated posterior chamber intraocular lenses, *Retina* (1994) **14:**47–50.
47. Bloom SM, Wyszynski RE, Brucker AJ. Scleral fixation suture for dislocated posterior chamber intraocular lens, *Ophthalmic Surg* (1990) **21:**851–4.
48. Anand R, Bowman RW. Simplified technique for suturing dislocated posterior chamber intraocular lens to the ciliary sulcus (letter), *Arch Ophthalmol* (1990) **108:**1205–6.
49. Chang S, Coll GE. Surgical techniques for repositioning a dislocated intraocular lens, repair of iridodialysis, and secondary intraocular lens implantation using innovative 25-gauge forceps, *Am J Ophthalmol* (1995) **119:**165–74.
50. Lewis H, Sanchez G. The use of perfluorocarbon liquids in the repositioning of posteriorly dislocated intraocular lenses, *Ophthalmology* (1993) **100:**1055–9.
51. Fanous MM, Friedman SM. Ciliary sulcus fixation of a dislocated posterior chamber intraocular lens using liquid perfluorophenanthrene, *Ophthalmic Surg* (1992) **23:**551–2.
52. Liu KR, Peyman GA, Chen MS, Chang KB. Use of high-density vitreous substitutes in the removal of posteriorly dislocated lenses or intraocular lenses, *Ophthalmic Surg* (1991) **22:**503–7.
53. Greve MDJ, Peyman GA, Mehta NJ, Millsap CM. Use of perfluoroperhydrophenanthrene in the management of posteriorly dislocated crystalline and intraocular lenses, *Ophthalmic Surg* (1993) **24:**593–7.
54. Smiddy WE, Flynn HW Jr. Needle-assisted scleral fixation suture technique for relocating posteriorly dislocated IOLs (letter), *Arch Ophthalmol* (1993) **111:**161–2.
55. Murray TG, Abrams GW. Pars plana vitrectomy in the management of dislocated posterior chamber lenses (letter), *Am J Ophthalmol* (1990) **109:**362.
56. Pavlin CJ, Rootman D, Arshinoff S, et al. Determination of haptic position of transsclerally fixated posterior chamber intraocular lenses by ultrasound biomicroscopy, *J Cataract Refract Surg* (1993) **19:**573–7.
57. McDermott ML, Puklin JE. Pars plana cicatrization of sewn-in posterior chamber intraocular lens haptics, *Ophthalmic Surg Lasers* (1997) **28:**239–40.
58. Duffey RJ, Holland EJ, Agapitos PJ, Lindstrom RL. Anatomic study of transsclerally sutured intraocular lens implantation, *Am J Ophthalmol* (1989) **108:**300–9.
59. Horiguchi M, Hirose H, Koura T, Satou M. Identifying the ciliary sulcus for suturing a posterior chamber intraocular lens by transillumination, *Arch Ophthalmol* (1993) **111:**1693–5.
60. Tsai JC, Rowsey JJ, Fouraker BD, et al. Use of a mirror needle holder with transsclerally sutured posterior chamber intraocular lenses, *Ophthalmic Surg Lasers* (1996) **27:**720–4.
61. Scott MD Jr, Scott IU, Smiddy WE, et al. Surgical management and outcomes of dislocated intraocular lenses, *Ophthalmology* (2000) **107:**62–7.
62. Brod RD, Flynn HW Jr, Clarkson JC, Blankenship GW. Management options for retinal detachment in the presence of a posteriorly dislocated intraocular lens, *Retina* (1990) **10:**50–6.

63. Smiddy WE, Flynn HW Jr, Kim JE. Retinal detachment in patients with retained lens fragments or dislocated posterior chamber intraocular lenses, *Ophthalmic Surg Lasers* (1996) **27:**856–61.
64. Sheu SJ, Wu TD. Is a transsclerally sutured intraocular lens a poor prognostic factor for the management of rhegmatogenous retinal detachment? *Ann Ophthalmol* (1996) **28:**244–9.
65. Bourke RD, Gray PJ, Rosen PH, Cooling RJ. Retinal detachment complicating scleral-sutured posterior chamber intraocular lens surgery, *Eye* (1996) **10** (4):501–8.
66. Epstein E. Suture problems (letter), *J Cataract Refract Surg* (1989) **15:**116.

Part V Surgical Techniques in Diabetic Retinopathy

Chapter 25 Membrane dissection in proliferative diabetic retinopathy

Michael S Lee and Gary W Abrams

INTRODUCTION

The development of closed vitrectomy techniques has allowed the surgical management of a variety of disease processes. One such entity falls under the category of proliferative vascular retinopathy. These disease processes, such as diabetic retinopathy, Eales' disease, branch retinal vein occlusion, central retinal vein occlusion and sickle cell retinopathy, may develop proliferative vascular membranes due to retinal ischemia. The most common cause of proliferative vascular retinopathy is diabetes mellitus, which will be the focus of this chapter. However, the techniques described may be applied to the surgical treatment of any of these diseases.

The past 25 years have led to a marked change in surgical intervention for proliferative diabetic retinopathy (PDR). In 1970, pars plana vitrectomy was developed by Machemer et al, in order to treat nonclearing vitreous hemorrhages from PDR, as well as reattach the retina by removing vitreous traction.[1] An early series of vitrectomy cases demonstrated that surgery was often limited to less severe complications related to diabetic retinopathy. Surgical intervention was undertaken 70% of the time for longstanding, nonclearing vitreous hemorrhages but only 30% of the time for retinal detachments.[2] Since then there has been a dramatic alteration in the indications for diabetic vitrectomy, whereby 75% of the time the main indication for surgical intervention is a retinal detachment.[3] This change may be related to a variety of factors.

Significant advances in technique, in instrumentation and in knowledge of the disease process have allowed the repair of more complex diabetic ocular complications and, consequently, have expanded the vitrectomy indications for intervention in PDR. In addition, the development and utilization of laser treatment has altered the natural course and history of PDR.[4] Clinical observations have not only led to a better understanding of the surgical anatomy in PDR but also have spurred the development of new surgical approaches and techniques. Clinical trials have better defined the indications and timing of vitrectomy for nonclearing vitreous hemorrhage and for severe fibrovascular proliferation. These factors have led to the evolution of vitrectomy for PDR.

PATHOPHYSIOLOGY AND PATHOANATOMY

A firm grasp of the underlying pathophysiology and pathoanatomy of PDR is crucial in understanding the surgical approach for diabetic vitrectomy. The initial insult appears to be ischemia, which results in the production of an angiogenic factor.[5] The growth factors that are thought to play a role in retinal neovascularization are insulin-like growth factor I (IGF-I), basic fibroblast growth factor (bFGF) and vascular endothelial growth factor (VEGF).[6–9] This signal then leads to the development of neovascular buds or 'vascular epicenters' from retinal blood vessels. The fibrovascular tissue proliferates in the potential space between the vitreous and retina. Eventually, the continued growth leads to invasion of the posterior lamellae of the cortical vitreous, producing a very firm adhesion.[10,11]

The vessels continue to proliferate in size and extent, with the subsequent development of a more fibrous component. This fibrous element of the neovascularization may contract, causing the vitreous to exert traction on the friable vascular tissue. This could potentially result in a vitreous hemorrhage, which may then stimulate further fibrosis and vitreous contraction, and eventually lead to a tractional retinal detachment. If there is significant tractional force exerted on the neovascularization from

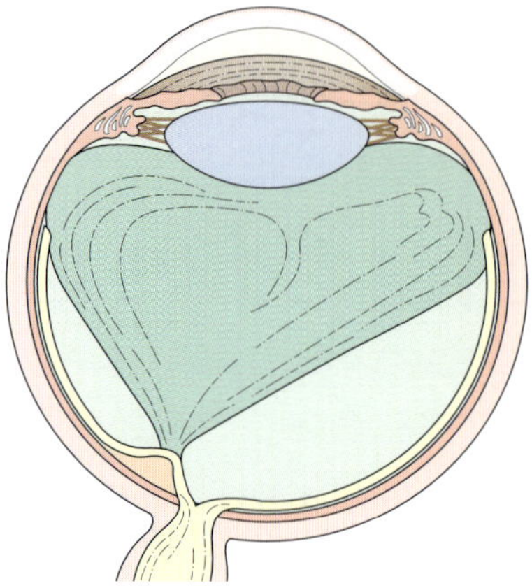

Figure 25.1 *In a focal vitreoretinal adhesion there is a point-like attachment of the vitreous to a vascular epicenter.*

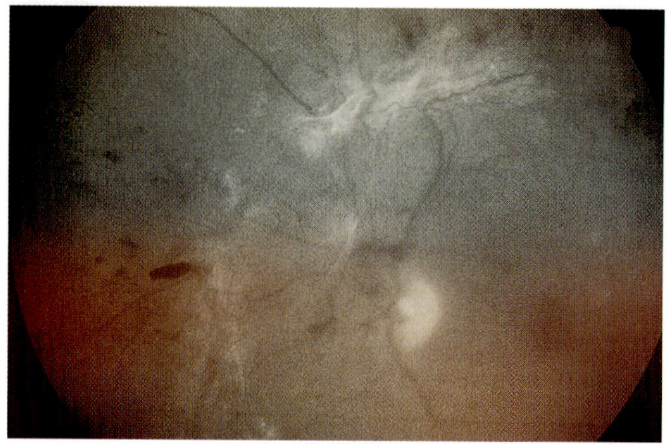

Figure 25.2 *Multiple focal vitreoretinal adhesions nasal and superior to the optic nerve. The posterior hyaloid is separated from the retina temporally, but not nasally.*

adhesions at the vitreoretinal junction, a retinal break may form. Therefore, in a combined rhegmatogenous–traction retinal detachment, the retinal break is often located near fibrovascular proliferative epicenters.

Because the basic pathophysiology involves vitreoretinal adhesions via vascular epicenters, vitrectomy for PDR demands an assessment of posterior vitreous separation, which can have several configurations. There may be minimal or no posterior vitreous detachment. In diabetic retinopathy, this may manifest as a preretinal hemorrhage, a dragged macula or tractional diabetic macular edema.[12] There may also be a partial vitreous separation, which remains attached at the posterior pole and at the midperipheral retina. On the other hand, the vitreous may be detached at the midperiphery, but remain attached at the posterior pole. Rarely, patients with PDR will have a complete posterior vitreous detachment. The only indication for vitrectomy in these patients is a longstanding, nonclearing vitreous hemorrhage.

In addition to the degree of posterior vitreous separation, the type of vitreoretinal adhesion also has a strong influence on the approach to vitrectomy for diabetic retinopathy. There are two basic types of adhesions, focal and broad, that develop from vascular epicenters. The simpler type is a focal vitreoretinal adhesion, which is essentially a point-like attachment (Fig. 25.1). Although occasionally there may be a single adhesion, it is more common to have multiple focal adhesions (Fig. 25.2). The degree of vitreous separation between the focal adhesions varies from no separation to partial separation. There may be epiretinal membranes on the retina surrounding the adhesion, even when the vitreous is separated (Fig. 25.3). These adhesions can, potentially, cause a purely tractional or a combined rhegmatogenous and tractional retinal detachment.

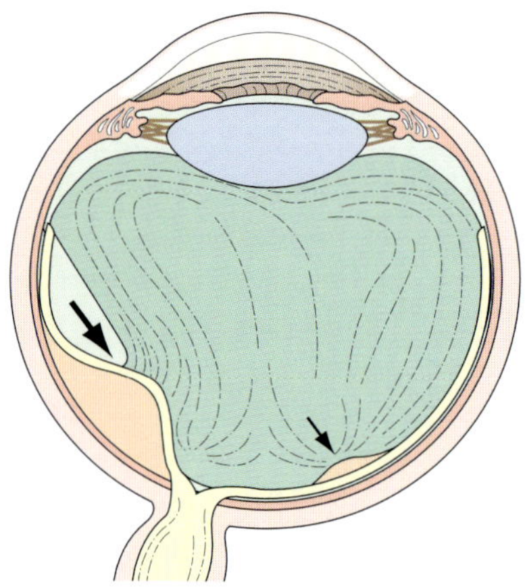

Figure 25.3 *Epiretinal membranes may be associated with focal vitreoretinal adhesions, producing a broader vitreous attachment. The vitreous may be partially separated from the retina (large arrow) or there may be no posterior vitreous separation (small arrow).*

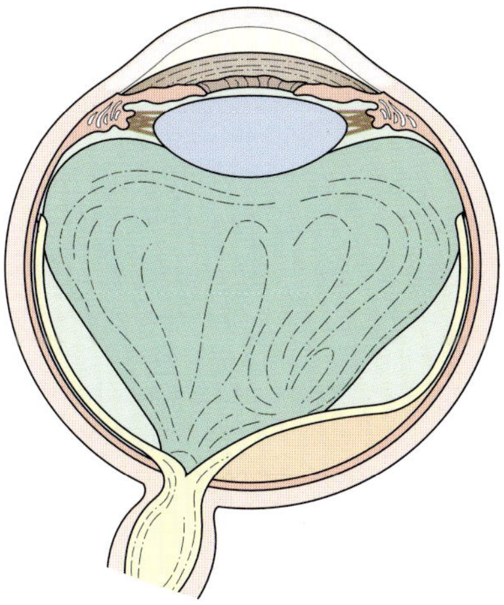

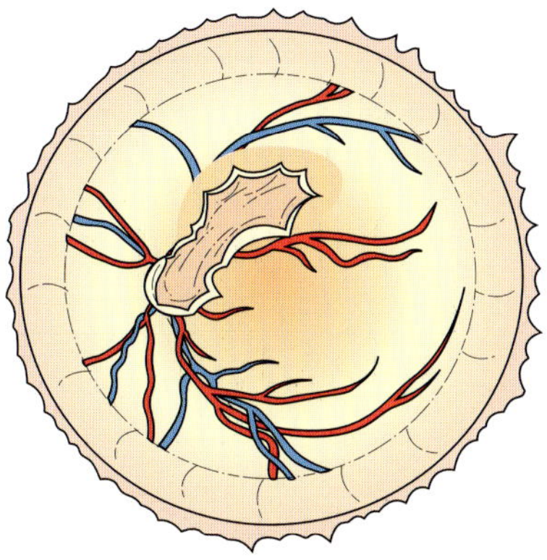

Figure 25.4 *Plaque-like broad vitreoretinal adhesion without underlying retinal folds.*

True broad vitreoretinal adhesions can be separated into two subtype categories: those associated and those not associated with folding of the underlying retina (Figs 25.4 and 25.5). The latter is the least common type of vitreoretinal adhesion and probably is created by a large segment of retinal neovascularization. Although there may only be a single, focal vascular adhesion underneath the large flat plaque, there are usually multiple epicenters of attachments between the vitreous and retina. Clinically, this type of vitreoretinal adhesion appears gray with variable vascularization. It often has thickened margins, which are the result of an opacified, fibrotic posterior cortical vitreous. In addition, the vitreous around the lesion is often separated.

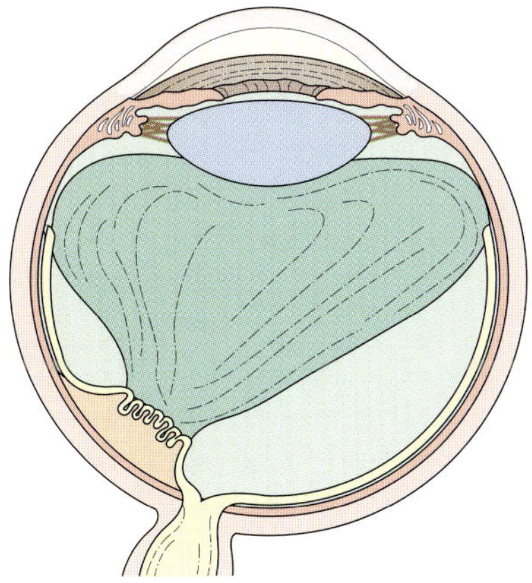

Figure 25.5 *The coalescence and contraction of multiple focal vitreoretinal adhesions lead to the formation of a plaque-like broad vitreoretinal adhesion with underlying retinal folds.*

The more common subtype of broad vitreoretinal adhesion, which is associated with underlying retinal folds, develops as a consequence of a fibrotic posterior hyaloid between multiple focal adhesions that coalesce and contract. Although this lesion may have a smooth plaque-like appearance, the underlying retina is often folded with a corrugated appearance (see Fig. 25.5). There may be an associated epiretinal membrane surrounding the adhesion, and there is usually at least a partial vitreous separation around the broad attachment. Although broad vitreoretinal adhesions with underlying retinal folds and those without underlying retinal folds may be associated with attached retina, the former type more often overlies areas of retinal detachment.

SURGICAL INDICATIONS

Currently, the most common indication for diabetic vitrectomy is a tractional retinal detachment. Although fibrosis of vascular epicenters commonly produces tractional detachments, the natural history of these detachments suggests that they often do not progress to cause severe visual loss. In a series of 99 eyes followed for 2 years, Charles and Flinn reported that only 21% of extramacular tractional retinal detachments extended into the macula without surgical intervention.[13] In addition, the Diabetic

Retinopathy Vitrectomy Study (DRVS) reported that 23% of eyes with tractional retinal detachments developed severe visual loss at 2 years.[14]

However, if the detachment does extend into the macula and leads to visual loss, this is an indication for surgical intervention. Numerous studies have documented the benefit of surgical treatment for diabetic tractional retinal detachments involving the macula. Investigators have found that 45–72% of eyes had visual improvement after vitrectomy.[15–19] Macular reattachment was achieved in 66–75% of eyes and a visual acuity of 5/200 or better was attained in 59–67% of eyes.[15,16,18] However, approximately 10–20% of diabetic vitrectomies resulted in vision of no light perception. Because of better surgical techniques and instrumentation, as well as a better understanding of the disease process, many surgeons have broadened the indication to include tractional detachments threatening the macula or causing macular distortion. Many of these patients will have visual loss, or visual symptoms such as metamorphopsia.

Further contraction of fibrovascular membranes may lead not only to worsening of a tractional retinal detachment but also to the creation of retinal breaks, producing a combined tractional–rhegmatogenous retinal detachment. This type of detachment often has a different configuration than that of the typical concave appearance of a tractional detachment. It usually has a convex appearance that may be bullous, and is more typical of rhegmatogenous retinal detachments. Because breaks in these detachments are produced by fibrous contraction, the holes are often found next to areas of traction. The retinal breaks may be difficult to identify, because they may be hidden underneath areas of vitreoretinal adhesions.

Combined tractional–rhegmatogenous retinal detachments more likely require vitrectomy regardless of the macular status. Surgical repair has led to a 48–53% improvement of visual acuity in these eyes.[20,21] Although there was a similar rate of eyes experiencing no light perception vision after vitrectomy compared with those with purely tractional retinal detachment, there was a lower rate of eyes achieving a visual acuity of 5/200 or better (45–56%).

Although a vitreous hemorrhage is a very common finding in PDR, the indication for vitrectomy had not been outlined clearly until the DRVS was undertaken. This was a multicenter, prospective, randomized clinical trial that was designed to evaluate the risks and benefits of performing early pars plana vitrectomy for advanced PDR. One arm of the study examined the outcomes of early and deferred vitrectomy (1 year) for severe vitreous hemorrhages, which was defined as hemorrhages reducing the visual acuity to 5/200 or less for at least 1 month.[22] There was no difference in either group in achieving a visual acuity of 10/100 or better, and both groups had a similar incidence of no light perception vision (approximately 20%). However, the study found that eyes of Type I diabetics had more severe proliferative retinopathy and vitreoretinal adhesions and were more likely to achieve a visual acuity of 10/20 or better with early vitrectomy when compared to eyes in which the vitrectomy was deferred (36% vs 12%, $P = 0.0001$). Early vitrectomy for eyes of Type II diabetic patients did not show a similar advantage of achieving 10/20 acuity or better when compared to the deferred group (18% vs 16%).

The DRVS also examined vitrectomy outcomes for eyes with advanced active PDR without opacified media or macular detachment.[23] Eyes that were eligible for the study had a visual acuity of 10/200 or better with extensive, active, neovascular or fibrovascular proliferation, which was defined by one of the following:

- Severe new vessels and severe fibrous proliferation.
- Severe new vessels and red vitreous hemorrhage.
- Moderate new vessels, severe fibrous proliferation and red vitreous hemorrhage.

Eyes were randomized to early vitrectomy or conventional management (observation, photocoagulation, or vitrectomy for other complications, such as vitreous hemorrhage obscuring the media or macular detachment).

At the 4-year follow-up, eyes that underwent early vitrectomy were more likely to attain 10/20 visual acuity than those that were managed conventionally (44% vs 28%), and the greatest advantage was demonstrated in eyes with the most severe proliferation.

There are other, less common indications for diabetic vitrectomy. Eyes with hemolytic glaucoma that have failed medical management may require a vitrectomy.[24] In addition, surgical intervention may be indicated for eyes with subhyaloid, premacular hemorrhages to prevent premacular fibrosis.[25,26] Vitrectomy may be considered in a specific subset of patients with diffuse macular edema who have not responded to photocoagulation. These patients have decreased vision with a thickened, taut and glistening posterior hyaloid, and on fluorescein angiography have diffuse leakage. One report of a small series of these eyes has demonstrated visual improvement with surgical intervention.[12]

PREOPERATIVE EVALUATION

Although there are some well-defined indications for surgical intervention, the decision to undertake surgical repair for complications related to PDR should be made with circumspection. Vitrectomy techniques have improved dramatically over the past 25 years, but there are still numerous complications that may develop, resulting in untoward outcomes. First, a careful, global assessment of the patient's general health status should be made because patients with PDR often have other concomitant illnesses, especially related to their diabetes. The patient's lifespan and anesthetic risks must be weighed against the potential outcome of a vitrectomy. Because diabetes is a systemic disease, and the extent of the PDR tends to be relatively symmetrical in both eyes, the condition of the fellow eye often does not contribute very much to the decision-making process. Occasionally, however, the status of the other eye is helpful, especially when a monocular patient has been incapacitated by a dense vitreous hemorrhage. In this situation, earlier intervention may be indicated.

Case selection also may be influenced by the status of the PDR and the estimated ease of dissection. In addition, vitrectomy undertaken for the immature stage of PDR has a better prognosis than the chronic fibrotic stage, which is often more difficult to dissect. Therefore, patients with PDR that has become fibrotic usually should not have a vitrectomy, unless there is an urgent indication for intervention, such as a macular detachment.

Another important aspect to consider is the degree of ischemia. Eyes that are highly ischemic are associated with poor outcomes. Manifestations of the ischemia may be poor initial visual acuity, rubeosis and neovascular glaucoma, all of which have been found to be poor prognostic factors.[15,20,21]

A complete and meticulous preoperative evaluation and examination are necessary before intervening for complications related to PDR. The visual acuity should be measured because more severe loss may be an indication for a vitrectomy. The iris should be examined carefully for rubeosis, which is prognostic of a poor outcome; the iris may stiffen, causing the pupil to dilate poorly. Preoperative knowledge of inadequate pupil dilation that requires mechanical stretching or breaking of synechiae will facilitate surgery. Gonioscopy, especially in eyes with rubeosis, should be performed to assess the presence and severity of angle neovascularization. Lens clarity also should be assessed, in order to determine the need for removal to achieve adequate visualization. Eyes requiring a lensectomy have a poorer outcome because they have a higher incidence of iris and angle neovascularization.[15,27–29]

In the posterior segment, vitreous separation and pathoanatomy should be examined and evaluated, as an aid in the surgical approach. In addition, the severity of PDR may prompt earlier intervention with a vitrectomy. Finally, an assessment of previous photocoagulation should be made. Eyes without preoperative photocoagulation are not only likely to have a poorer outcome but are more likely to develop a bullous retinal detachment from peripheral retinal breaks.[15,16]

A meticulous ophthalmologic examination often will be sufficient to make an adequate determination for surgical intervention, as well as the vitrectomy approach. In cases with opaque ocular media preventing visualization of the fundus, an ultrasound may be helpful to assess vitreoretinal adhesions and retinal detachment. If the patient has not had panretinal photocoagulation, laser treatment should be given preoperatively, if possible, to prevent intraoperative bullous retinal detachments, as well as to control the neovascular process.

SURGICAL PROCEDURE

The ultimate goal of surgery is to restore vision, which may be accomplished by clearing the media and/or reattaching the retina by separating membranes to relieve traction. The instrumentation that we prefer to manage PDR surgically includes a vitreous cutter, a tissue manipulator with diathermy, membrane peeler–cutter (MPC) scissors, an active suction soft-tipped cannula and a microvitreoretinal (MVR) blade. However, some instruments may be substituted if these are not available. An illuminated pick may be utilized for membrane or hyaloid elevation rather than a tissue manipulator, and horizontally cutting vitreoretinal scissors can be used.

The tissue manipulator is advantageous because it has multiple functions.[30] It can infuse fluid to displace hemorrhage from the retina, as well as aspirate to

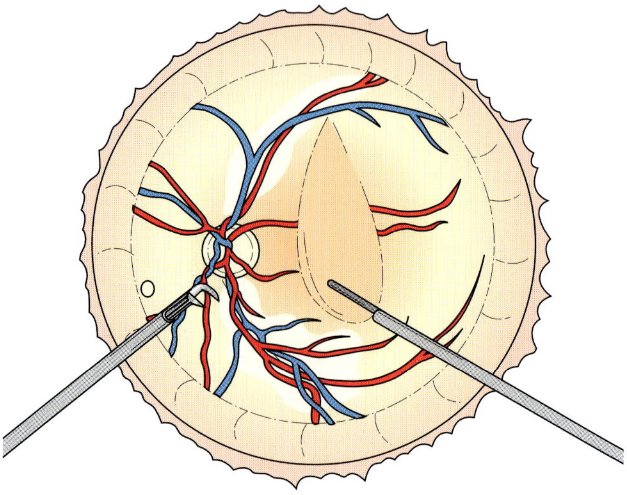

Figure 25.6 *A tissue manipulator and membrane peeler–cutter (MPC) scissors are the preferred instrumentation for membrane dissection in proliferative diabetic retinopathy. The tissue manipulator has multiple functions that include diathermy and endoillumination, as well as a manipulator with an aspiration system. The automated MPC scissors offer better control than manual scissors for cutting vitreoretinal adhesions.*

elevate membranes for dissection. In addition, it has a bipolar diathermy that allows rapid control of intraocular hemorrhage.

Horizontal scissors can be substituted for MPC scissors to cut vitreoretinal adhesions; however, automated scissors offer better control than manual scissors (Fig. 25.6). In addition, it is important to use glucose-fortified balanced salt solution (BSS Plus, 400 mg/dl) for the infusion fluid because the higher glucose concentration may prevent lenticular fluid fluxes from osmotic gradients, leading to intraoperative cataract formation.[31] This concentration is obtained by adding 3 ml of nonpreserved 50% dextrose to a 500 ml bottle of BSS Plus.

The surgical approach for diabetic vitrectomy is dictated largely by the pathoanatomy. In eyes with a posterior vitreous detachment, the only indication for surgical intervention is a nonclearing vitreous hemorrhage, and the objective is to clear the media. Although this is the simplest vitrectomy to perform on diabetics, severe complications may still occur, leading to poor outcomes, including no light perception vision.[15,16,18,20–22]

Initially, a core vitrectomy is performed to remove the central vitreous. Because there is a posterior vitreous separation, the vitreous cutter will easily incise the posterior hyaloid face. After an opening has been created, it should be enlarged to allow adequate posterior visualization. There is often hemorrhage layered over the posterior pole. Because the hemorrhage is unclotted blood, it generally can be aspirated easily with an active suction soft-tipped cannula. This will result in improved visualization of the vitreous and ocular structures by allowing more light from the endoilluminator to be reflected off the retina, thus improving the overall illumination.

At this point, a peripheral vitrectomy should be performed to remove as much of the vitreous as possible without damaging the lens. In uncomplicated cases, it is usually unnecessary to utilize scleral depression for more complete removal of the peripheral vitreous. If there is inadequate panretinal photocoagulation, laser endophotocoagulation should be applied.

All other diabetic vitrectomies have an incomplete separation of the posterior vitreous. In these cases, the posterior cortical vitreous must be separated from the retina, and vitreoretinal adhesions produced by vascular epicenters must be excised. Several factors contribute to the difficulty of dissection in these cases. Focal vitreoretinal adhesions are generally easier to remove than broad adhesions, especially those with underlying retinal folds. More difficult diabetic vitrectomies have little posterior vitreous separation, very fibrotic membranes and epiretinal membranes surrounding vitreoretinal adhesions. Associated retinal detachments, especially those that are chronic with atrophic, thinned retina and have retinal breaks, make the surgery more complicated.

Although a variety of techniques have been developed for diabetic vitrectomies, we primarily use the *en bloc* dissection technique.[32] With this approach, some of the posterior hyaloid is left attached to membranes, in order to maintain anterior–posterior traction and fixate membranes. After all of the vitreoretinal adhesions have been separated, the remaining posterior hyaloid can be removed, along with the membranes, as a single unit. However, the surgeon should be familiar with other approaches that may be preferred in selected cases.

Sectioning techniques involve relieving anterior–posterior traction and simply transecting membranes with scissors, leaving behind the vitreoretinal adhesions.[33,34] The delamination approach entails excising the vitreous around fibrovascular epicenters, releasing anterior–posterior traction and then amputating the vitreoretinal adhesions from the retina.[35] It is often necessary to use all three techniques in a

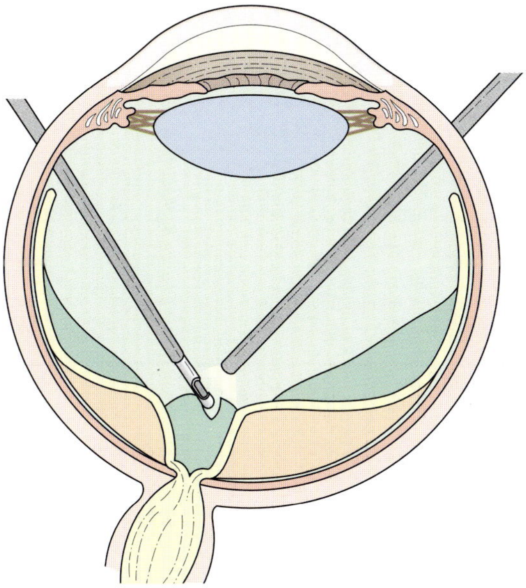

Figure 25.7 *A vitreous cutting instrument is used to create an opening in the posterior hyaloid between two vascular epicenters.*

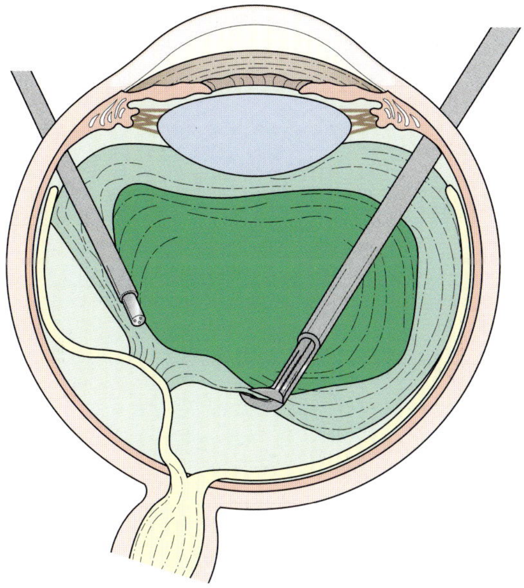

Figure 25.8 *Initially, the posterior hyaloid is usually separated from the retina around the optic nerve. A plane is developed between the posterior hyaloid and the retina, using blunt dissection with either the tips of scissors or a membrane pick. This technique will expose individual vascular epicenters.*

single case. Removing or sectioning the posterior hyaloid may facilitate access to membranes.

In the presence of a rhegmatogenous retinal detachment, maintaining the posterior hyaloid and anterior–posterior traction may cause the retina to become bullously detached. In that situation, it is preferable to excise the hyaloid and delaminate the membranes. Larger membranes are sometimes excised more easily after sectioning.

Regardless of the type of vitreoretinal adhesion present, the initial approach with the *en bloc* technique is the same. A core vitrectomy is performed to remove media opacities and to create an opening in the posterior hyaloid (Fig. 25.7). In eyes with minimal posterior vitreous separation, it may be difficult to incise the posterior hyaloid with the vitreous cutting instrument. In this situation, an MVR blade and a membrane pick may be necessary to induce a separation and produce an opening in the posterior hyaloid. The opening in the posterior hyaloid is enlarged widely and extended adjacent to vitreoretinal adhesions with the vitreous cutter, allowing access to the fibrovascular epicenters. Some of the posterior hyaloid attached to the vitreoretinal adhesions is not cut, thus maintaining some anterior–posterior traction. This will fixate, as well as sometimes elevate the edges of membranes, facilitating the dissection. Any posterior hyaloid that limits access to vitreoretinal adhesions should be excised with the vitreous cutter or sectioned with scissors.

Generally, the dissection is initiated posteriorly and then directed anteriorly. Usually a plane between the posterior hyaloid and the retina can be developed around the optic nerve, using either the tips of the scissors or a membrane pick, and any fibrovascular tissue from the disc should be removed (Fig. 25.8). Membranes tightly adherent to the optic disc should be sectioned adjacent to the nerve. The next step involves stripping the hyaloid from the retina and isolating individual areas of vitreoretinal adhesions. This can be accomplished by sliding an illuminated pick or the closed tips of the MPC or horizontal cutting scissors parallel to the surface of the retina, and then lifting the instrument, thus separating the hyaloid (Fig. 25.9).

Frequently, as the posterior cortical vitreous is stripped, adhesions between the vascular arcade vessels and the hyaloid are encountered. These points of attachment should not be stripped aggressively because this often leads to retinal break formation and hemorrhage. They should be isolated and

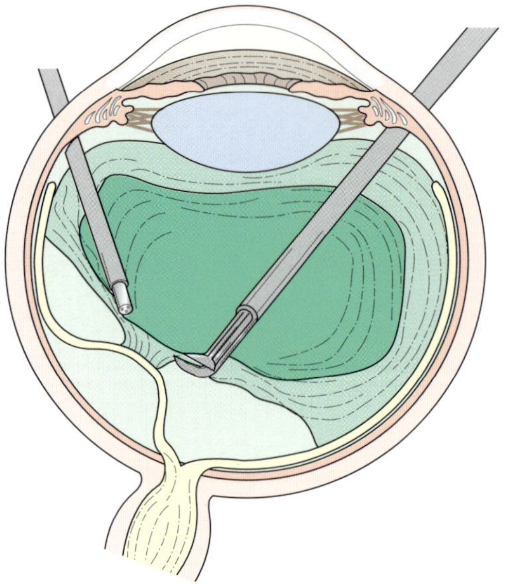

Figure 25.9 *The posterior hyaloid and any epiretinal membranes encountered are stripped toward vascular epicenters, isolating areas of vitreoretinal adhesions.*

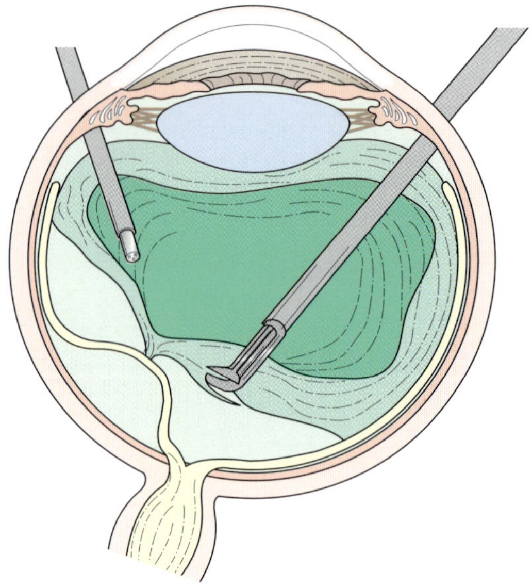

Figure 25.10 *After isolating areas of vitreoretinal adhesions, a tissue manipulator can be used to elevate the hyaloid for exposure and scissors are used to excise points of attachments parallel to the retinal surface.*

then excised parallel to the retinal surface, with either the horizontal cutting scissors or the MPC.

As the blunt dissection is carried out to isolate each vitreoretinal adhesion, associated epiretinal membranes may be found, which should also be stripped from the retina toward the vascular epicenter. After separating the hyaloid and epiretinal membranes, focal vitreoretinal adhesions can be excised easily from the surface of the retina by elevating them for exposure with either an illuminated pick or the tissue manipulator, and cutting them with the scissors parallel to the retinal surface (Fig. 25.10). As the posterior cortical vitreous is separated further, other vascular epicenters may be encountered, which should be removed in a similar fashion (Fig. 25.11 and 25.12). After all the vitreoretinal attachments have been excised, the posterior hyaloid and membranes are removed with a vitreous cutting instrument (Fig. 25.13).

Broad plaques without underlying retinal folds are somewhat more difficult to remove than focal adhesions and require a bimanual technique (Fig. 25.14). In this type of vitreoretinal adhesion there is often a central vascular epicenter surrounded by multiple, small, peg-like adhesions. To extirpate the broad plaque, the edge of the adhesion is elevated with an illuminated pick or a tissue manipulator and each individual adhesion is excised with the scissors. In order to gain further access to more centrally located attachments, it may be necessary to remove additional vitreous attached to the edges of the membrane and segment the membrane into smaller pieces. The dissection proceeds centrally until the entire plaque has been removed.

Broad plaque-like adhesions with underlying retinal folds are the result of multiple focal adhesions drawn together by contracted fibrous membranes and generally are the most difficult to excise. The retinal folds are hidden by the broad adhesions and often there are associated epiretinal membranes. The procedure described above should be performed, whereby the membranes and hyaloid are stripped to isolate the plaque and then each focal adhesion encountered is excised until the plaque has been removed.

When stripping the posterior cortical vitreous, the surgeon should be aware that there may be a 'split' in the posterior hyaloid, around the vitreoretinal adhesion (Fig. 25.15). Occasionally, a condensed vitreous strand inserts at a vascular epicenter and forms a bridge between the membrane and the vitreous base, creating the illusion of a partially separated posterior hyaloid.

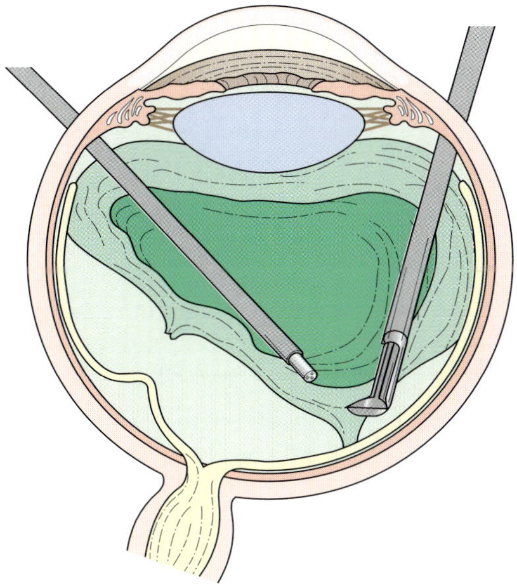

Figure 25.11 *After cutting a vitreoretinal adhesion, further blunt dissection with the tips of the scissors will often expose other areas of attachments.*

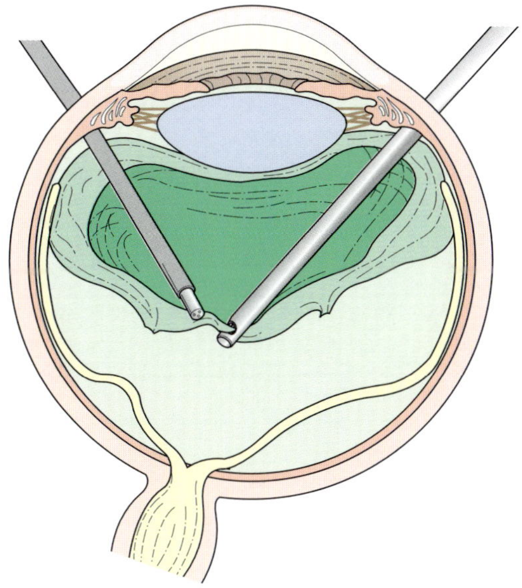

Figure 25.13 *After all the vitreoretinal adhesions have been excised from the retinal surface, the posterior hyaloid and the membranes are removed with a vitreous cutting instrument.*

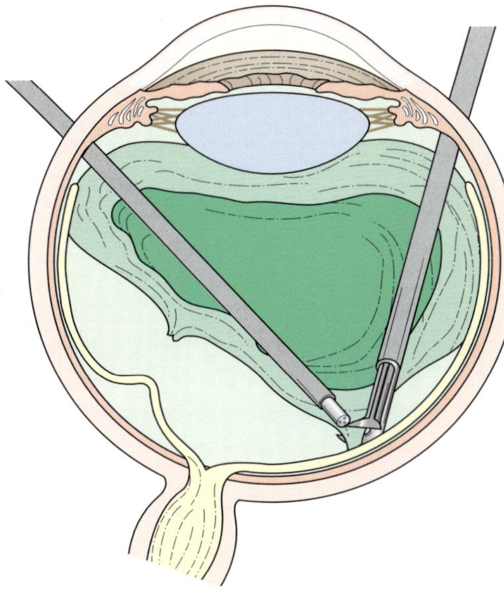

Figure 25.12 *Each vitreoretinal adhesion encountered should be treated in a similar manner. The hyaloid and epiretinal membranes are stripped toward the vitreoretinal adhesion. After isolating the point of attachment, it should be excised parallel to the retinal surface.*

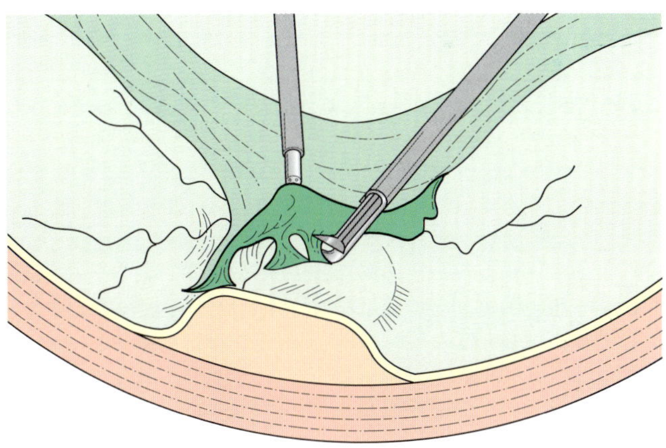

Figure 25.14 *Bimanual technique used for plaque-like broad vitreoretinal adhesions. A tissue manipulator is used to elevate the plaque while scissors are used to cut the vitreoretinal attachments, which are often multiple, fine, focal adhesions.*

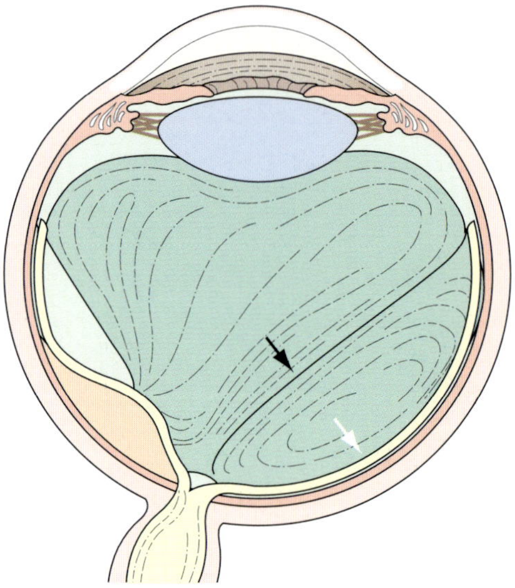

Figure 25.15 *Split hyaloid with partial vitreous separation. Although there is unseparated posterior hyaloid (white arrow), there is a pseudohyaloid membrane (dark arrow), giving the illusion of vitreous separation. The pseudohyaloidal membrane may be the result of condensed vitreous collagen that is often found after a hemorrhage in formed vitreous.*

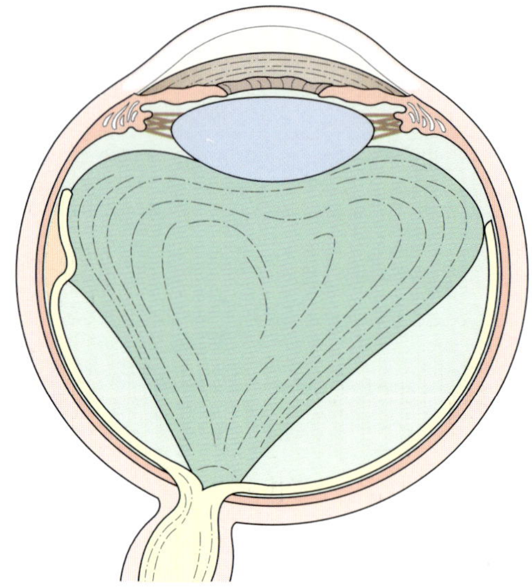

Figure 25.16 *Peripheral vascular epicenters leading to a tractional retinal detachment with partially separated posterior hyaloid.*

Although the etiology of a 'split' posterior cortical vitreous is unknown, it may be the result of hemorrhage into formed vitreous from the neovascularization at a vascular epicenter. The extent of the split is variable and may range from only a partial division, surrounding a single vascular epicenter, to a total division with no separation of the entire posterior hyaloid. If this phenomenon is unrecognized when excising a vitreoretinal adhesion, then only the condensed vitreous on the inner surface of the adhesion will be removed. Hence, the true posterior hyaloid will not be separated and the traction may be unrelieved. It is crucial for the ultimate success of a diabetic vitrectomy that the true posterior cortical vitreous be identified, separated and stripped toward the vascular epicenter, allowing complete excision of the adhesion.

After separation of all the posterior vitreoretinal adhesions and the posterior hyaloid, the dissection is continued anteriorly. If the midvitreous is still adherent to the retina, blunt dissection with either the illuminated pick or closed tips of scissors is utilized to achieve separation. Occasionally, midperipheral vitreoretinal adhesions at vascular epicenters will be encountered, requiring excision. They should be treated in the same manner as posterior attachments. However, excision of these membranes is not as crucial and sometimes they may be circumscribed simply using the vitreous cutter. It is important that all vitreous attachments to the membrane be completely excised, in order to relieve all traction.

Vitreoretinal adhesions located in the far periphery should be handled in a similar fashion to those in the midperiphery, but they are more difficult to manage for many reasons (Fig. 25.16): the anterior edge of the adhesion may be close to the vitreous base, making it difficult to separate and excise the vitreous around the attachment; and gaining access to the adhesions also can be problematic.

In phakic eyes, bimanual dissection is compromised, especially in the horizontal meridians where there is the greatest risk of lenticular damage from the instruments. It may be possible to gain access to the horizontal meridian by placing the sclerotomies in the vertical meridians and approaching the eye from the temporal side. This allows bimanual dissection in the horizontal meridians. An alternative is to perform a lensectomy to facilitate access to peripheral membranes. Finally, visualization of the membranes can be difficult; sometimes it can be enhanced by scleral depression.

Another means of circumventing the problem is to utilize indirect ophthalmoscopy, which provides excellent visualization of the periphery for unimanual dissection. However, the reversal of orientation by this approach can be problematic for surgeons unfamiliar with this technique, and may lead to inadvertent damage to the lens or retina. Newer wide-angle viewing systems can provide excellent peripheral visualization. The disadvantages with these systems include poor stereopsis and image minification. If peripheral traction cannot be relieved, an encircling scleral buckle should be placed.

The creation of retinal breaks is one of the major complications related to surgical intervention for PDR. A retinal dialysis may occur as a result of engaging vitreous with the tip of an instrument placed through the sclerotomy. Vitreous prolapse may lead to horseshoe tears at the posterior edge of the vitreous base, behind the sclerotomy sites. Stopping the infusion fluid while removing the instruments can minimize this problem.

As in any vitrectomy procedure, a careful and meticulous indirect ophthalmoscopic examination with scleral depression should be performed at the conclusion of the case prior to air insufflation in order to locate any retinal breaks. Small breaks without traction in the superior 200° of the retina often may be treated with cryotherapy or laser photocoagulation in conjunction with a gas bubble tamponade. An inferior retinal break or a break with persistent traction requires an encircling scleral buckle.

Posterior retinal breaks often are located near areas of vitreoretinal adhesions and usually occur when stripping the posterior hyaloid. They are less likely to occur in eyes with attached retinas. Eyes with tractional retinal detachments from chronic atrophic fibrovascular proliferation are especially prone to developing breaks. In cases of minimal tractional retinal detachment, membrane sectioning may be a preferable technique to avoid creating retinal breaks, provided that it will adequately relieve traction.

On the other hand, eyes with extensive retinal detachment and traction require separation of the posterior hyaloid and excision of the vitreoretinal adhesions. Although stripping of the hyaloid may create retinal breaks, this outcome is preferable to having an unseparated hyaloid with persistent traction. Occasionally, minimal extramacular traction may not extend and thus would not require membrane removal. However, if there is a retinal break, it is crucial that all the traction is released. Residual traction along a retinal break may prevent retinal reattachment and lead to recurrent retinal detachments. Retinal breaks can be managed adequately when all traction has been released.

Producing retinal breaks by separating the hyaloid can lead to a bullous retinal detachment, which is more difficult to manage. In this situation, there is no advantage to the *en bloc* technique because the countertraction force has been lost. Therefore, the peripheral vitreous should be excised and the delamination approach employed. Removing all of the associated vitreous, followed by segmentation between vitreoretinal adhesions, should isolate each individual vitreoretinal adhesion. A bimanual technique is utilized to remove the remaining membranes. A tissue manipulator or an illuminated pick is used to elevate the edge of the membrane while scissors are used to excise it.

After all traction has been relieved, the retinal break is marked with diathermy so that it can be visualized under air. The retina is reattached with a fluid–air exchange. The subretinal fluid is drained through the posterior break with a soft-tipped silicone cannula. In cases of posterior detachment with a peripheral retinal break, the subretinal fluid may be drained with a cannulated extrusion needle via the peripheral break, rather than creating a posterior drainage retinotomy.

Alternatively, perfluorocarbon liquid can be used to reattach the retina. It is initially injected over the optic disc and, as it fills the eye, it reattaches the retina from posteriorly to anteriorly. It is removed subsequently with a fluid–air exchange. Once the retina has been reattached, endolaser photocoagulation is applied around the retinal breaks. The retinal break then is usually tamponaded with a gas bubble.

Another serious complication of diabetic vitrectomy is an intraocular hemorrhage. Extensive hemorrhage may prevent the successful conclusion of surgery. In addition, clotted hemorrhage can be very tightly adherent to the retina. The removal of a hemorrhage not only may extend a pre-existing retinal break but also may create new retinal breaks, therefore hemorrhages should be avoided whenever possible. They should be anticipated, so that when they occur they can be controlled promptly. The *en bloc* technique is advantageous in minimizing hemorrhages because vascular epicenters are excised at their origin, so that only a single vessel will bleed rather than multiple small vessels in the fibrovascular membrane. In addition, when cut, the vessel at the base of a vascular epicenter will often stop bleeding spontaneously or will require only a short period of elevated intraocular pressure (IOP) to control the bleeding.

Generally, when a hemorrhage occurs, the infusion bottle should be raised promptly to increase the IOP, which is often sufficient to control the bleeding. Newer vitrectomy systems may employ pneumatic pressurization of the infusion system, which raises the IOP more rapidly. If the IOP is normalized and rebleeding occurs, then diathermy is used to cauterize the source vessel.

The tissue manipulator is advantageous in controlling any further hemorrhage. Infusion of a stream of BSS can displace any blood obscuring the focus of bleeding, and its bipolar diathermy function can then cauterize the source of hemorrhage. Any blood on the retina should be removed immediately before clotting occurs.

Clotted blood should be stripped away from the retina cautiously, because it may be tightly adherent to the retina, causing significant traction. The clot rarely may need to be excised from areas of adhesion with scissors. On rare occasions, it may be necessary to infuse thrombin to control extensive, widespread hemorrhaging.

POSTOPERATIVE MANAGEMENT

INTRAOCULAR PRESSURE ELEVATION

Postoperative complications are common after diabetic vitrectomies. However, with careful follow-up, the majority can be managed without serious consequences. During the immediate postoperative period, one of the most common problems is an elevated IOP. Han et al demonstrated that the incidence of postvitrectomy-elevated IOP of 30 mmHg or greater within 48 hours of surgery was approximately 35%.[36]

Risk factors for developing postoperative IOP elevations include eyes that have had extensive scatter photocoagulation, a scleral buckle placement, lensectomy and a gas tamponade. In addition, eyes with PDR may be at an increased risk for visual loss from increased IOP because they have relative ischemia. Therefore, it is important that the IOP is left in a normal range at the end of the case.

For eyes at high risk of pressure elevation, we typically give prophylactic topical medical treatment at the conclusion of surgery to prevent postoperative IOP elevations. In high-risk cases we may include a beta-blocker, an alpha-agonist, a carbonic anhydrase inhibitor and a prostaglandin analog. The IOP should be measured at 2 and 4 hours postoperatively, but more frequent checks may be necessary to ensure adequate IOP control. If the IOP cannot be controlled medically, then an anterior chamber or vitreous tap may be required. Watchful management of the IOP is crucial because significant elevations may lead to loss of light perception. However, with prompt IOP control, there may be significant return of vision.[37]

CORNEAL EROSION

Another common early postoperative complication is a corneal erosion. The reported incidence of postvitrectomy corneal problems in diabetics is 28–52%.[18,28] Corneal complications, especially persistent epithelial defects, may be very frequent because diabetic eyes have abnormal epithelial basement membranes and attachments.[38] Erosion often will heal when treated with emollients and patching. If the erosion is persistent, it should be treated with a bandage contact lens. Rarely, a tarsorrhaphy will be necessary to allow a chronic, nonhealing corneal erosion to re-epithelialize.

INTRAOCULAR FIBRIN DEPOSITION AND PUPILLARY BLOCK

Vitrectomy surgery may lead to breakdown of the blood–retinal barrier, which subsequently can result in intraocular fibrin deposition and pupillary block. Diabetics may be at higher risk for development of fibrin. Injections of subconjunctival dexamethasone at the conclusion of surgery, as well as frequent topical corticosteroid drops, are given as prophylaxis against postoperative fibrin and inflammatory response. However, when a significant fibrin response occurs, it should be treated with recombinant tissue plasminogen activator (tPA).[39,40] The tPA (as little as 3 μg) is injected intracamerally with a 30-gauge needle through the limbus. The tPA should not be administered in the immediate postoperative period because it can cause an intraocular hemorrhage.

CATARACT

A cataract may develop as a result of numerous insults. The lens may be damaged inadvertently by surgical instruments or from intraocular gas bubble contact. In addition, intraoperative fluid shifts caused by differences in glucose concentration between the infusion fluid and lens may lead to cataract formation. Vitrectomy procedures have been shown to cause progression of nuclear sclerotic cataracts.[41]

Although some lenticular opacities will clear spontaneously, others will result in visual impairment. Several studies have demonstrated that persistent visually significant cataracts may occur in 17–37% of diabetic eyes undergoing vitrectomy.[24,42,43] These eyes may be managed with cataract extraction and placement of an intraocular lens. It is recommended that the cataract extraction not be performed for at least 6 months after a successful vitrectomy procedure.[43] In addition, a silicone intraocular lens should not be placed because it may cause complications with other vitrectomies that may be required in the future. It has been shown that a silicone lens may develop condensation on its posterior surface during a fluid–air exchange and may bind irreversibly to silicone oil.[44,45]

RUBEOSIS IRIDIS AND NEOVASCULAR GLAUCOMA

Serious complications of diabetic vitrectomy are the development of postoperative rubeosis iridis and neovascular glaucoma. The incidence of iris neovascularization after vitrectomy is at least two to three times more common in aphakic diabetic eyes than in phakic diabetic eyes.[27–29] Many eyes with iris neovascularization will not progress to the more severe complication of neovascular glaucoma.

Neovascular glaucoma has been reported in 8–11% of diabetic eyes undergoing vitrectomy and seems to occur more frequently in aphakic than in phakic eyes.[16,20] Treatment with panretinal photocoagulation and reattachment of rhegmatogenous retinal detachments will reduce the frequency of postoperative rubeosis, as well as cause its regression.[16,20,28,29,46] Initially, these eyes should be managed conservatively with topical medications, but many eyes with neovascular glaucoma will require surgical intervention to control the IOP.

ANTERIOR HYALOIDAL FIBROVASCULAR PROLIFERATION

A severe postoperative complication after diabetic vitrectomy is anterior hyaloidal fibrovascular proliferation (AHFVP), which has been reported to occur in approximately 13% of the cases.[47] The patients who develop AHFVP are typically young phakic males who were recently diagnosed with diabetic retinopathy but may not have nephropathy or hypertension.[48] This retinopathy is highly ischemic, with neovascularization that responds poorly to panretinal photocoagulation. These patients may have had a scleral buckle, as well as a vitrectomy. This complication is often heralded by the onset of a hemorrhage into the vitreous cavity or the anterior vitreous 3–12 weeks following vitrectomy. This is the result of fibrovascular proliferation from the peripheral retina extending toward the equator of the lens and onto the lens capsule. A similar picture can result from fibrovascular proliferation from a sclerotomy site. As the fibrovascular tissue progresses, it may lead to a peripheral tractional detachment, anterior retinal displacement and ciliary body detachment. If untreated, these eyes have a poor prognosis because the condition often leads to hypotony and atrophic bulbi.

The best treatment for AHFVP depends upon high clinical suspicion and early detection. In the early phase, the media are clear and there is only fibrovascular proliferation without traction. At this stage, AHFVP may be amenable to extensive photocoagulation applied to the anterior retina and pars plana. However, if a significant vitreous hemorrhage or tractional detachment occurs, then surgical intervention may be necessary. A lensectomy with anterior membrane dissection is performed to release the traction and the eye is treated with extensive laser photocoagulation.

VITREOUS HEMORRHAGE

Although a vitreous hemorrhage may be the primary manifestation of AHFVP, most hemorrhages result from recurrent bleeding from cut vascular epicenters. These hemorrhages usually occur within 1 week of surgery. Postoperative vitreous hemorrhages may occur in 29–60% of eyes at some time during the postoperative period, but many of these will clear spontaneously without requiring another operation.[28,49,50]

If there is a significant vitreous hemorrhage, it may be cleared with a fluid–air or gas exchange.[51–53] In phakic or pseudophakic eyes, the exchange is performed through the pars plana. Five percent povidone–iodine solution is used to sterilize the lids and the conjunctiva. The patient is placed on his or her side with the affected eye in the dependent position and a 30-gauge needle, which is attached to an air pump, is inserted nasally into the vitreous cavity. A second 27-gauge needle connected to a syringe is placed in the dependent portion of the eye, which is temporal. As the air pump insufflates the eye at 30 mmHg, fluid is gently aspirated with the other syringe. The patient's head is rotated into a more prone position to achieve a more complete exchange. If an air pump is not accessible, then the exchange is performed in a stepwise fashion with two syringes by aspirating 0.5 ml of fluid and then filling the eye with 0.5 ml of air until the exchange has been completed. To prevent extreme fluctuations in IOP, it is important to exchange small and equal amounts of fluid and gas.

In aphakic eyes, the patient is placed in the prone position. A Ziegler-type blade is used to make an incision through the limbus. A 30-gauge needle attached to a syringe filled with air is inserted through the keratotomy. As the eye is filled with air, the fluid will egress from the eye through the incision around the needle shaft. The limbal incision is usually self-sealing, so after the fluid–air exchange has been completed the needle can simply be removed. Although this procedure is often successful in clearing recurrent vitreous hemorrhages, some hemorrhages will persist and may even recur. In these situations, and especially if AHFVP is suspected, another vitrectomy, with possible lensectomy, may be necessary.

MASSIVE FIBRIN FORMATION

Massive fibrin formation is another severe complication that may occur after a vitrectomy for PDR.[54] These eyes are typically very ischemic and have a poor visual prognosis. Postoperatively, the vitreous cavity is filled with massive fibrin deposits that may lead to the development of pupillary membranes, recurrent tractional retinal detachments and ciliary body detachments with resultant hypotony. If the retina is detached, fibrin may form in the subretinal space.

Dabbs et al investigated the use of tPA in eyes with a massive fibrin response after diabetic vitrectomy.[55] Although they found a rapid resolution of the fibrin with relief of tractional retinal detachments from fibrin membranes, all eyes developed intraocular hemorrhages and reaccumulation of the fibrin, as well as recurrence of tractional retinal detachments. Massive fibrin formation may be managed best with a repeat vitrectomy, removal of fibrin and injection of silicone oil.

REOPERATION PROGNOSIS

Many of the indications for reoperation, such as a nonclearing vitreous hemorrhage, recurrent tractional retinal detachment involving the macula, rhegmatogenous retinal detachment, combined tractional–rhegmatogenous retinal detachment, AHFVP, fibrinoid syndrome and retinal detachments associated with proliferative vitreoretinopathy, have been discussed above. Generally, the prognosis for diabetic eyes undergoing a second vitrectomy is not as good as those undergoing a primary vitrectomy. The second procedure is more likely to involve a relaxing retinotomy. In primary vitrectomies for complications related to PDR, the incidence of retinotomies was approximately 5%, whereas on repeat vitrectomies there was a much higher rate of 50%.[56] In addition, these cases may require the use of silicone oil as an intraocular tamponade.[57–59]

In a reported series of 37 eyes, 35% achieved anatomic success (defined as attachment posterior to the buckle, if present, or attachment of the retina posterior to the equator) and 24% of eyes had a visual acuity of 5/200 or better.[59]

SURGICAL RESULTS

The anticipated surgical outcomes have been discussed along with the indications. However, these results are reported regardless of the technique employed. The results of the primary approach described *en bloc* have been reported.[60] A case series of 69 eyes of 63 patients with tractional retinal detachments as a consequence of PDR were evaluated. All retinas were completely reattached at the conclusion of surgery. All eyes were followed for at least 6 months; 57 eyes (83%) were completely attached, whereas the macula was attached in 61 eyes (88%). The final visual acuity was 5/200 or better in 49 eyes (71%) and 20/100 or better in 30 eyes (43%). The most common intraoperative complication was the production of iatrogenic retinal tears in 24 eyes (35%), which was a poor prognostic factor with regard to final visual outcome and macular attachment.

REFERENCES

1. Machemer R, Buettner H, Norton EWD, Parel JM. Vitrectomy: a pars plana approach, *Trans Am Acad Ophthalmol Otolaryngol* (1971) **75:**813–20.
2. Aaberg TM. Vitrectomy for diabetic retinopathy. In: Freeman HM, Hirose T, Schepens CL, eds, *Vitreous Surgery and Advances in Fundus Diagnosis and Treatment* (Appleton-Century-Crofts: New York, 1977): 297–313.
3. Aaberg TM, Abrams GW. Changing indications and techniques for vitrectomy in management of complications of diabetic retinopathy, *Ophthalmology* (1987) **94:**775–9.
4. Diabetic Retinopathy Study Research Group. Preliminary report on the effects of photocoagulation therapy, *Am J Ophthalmol* (1976) **81:**383–96.
5. Henkind P. Ocular neovascularization: The Krill Memorial Lecture, *Am J Ophthalmol* (1978) **85:**287–301.
6. Meyer-Schwickerath R, Pfeiffer A, Blum WF, et al. Vitreous levels on the insulin-like growth factors I and II, and the insulin-like growth factor binding proteins 2 and 3, increase in neovascular eye disease: studies in nondiabetic and diabetic subjects, *J Clin Invest* (1993) **92:**2620–5.
7. Sivalingam A, Kenney J, Brown GC, et al. Basic fibroblast growth factor levels in the vitreous of patients with proliferative diabetic retinopathy, *Arch Ophthalmol* (1990) **108:**869–72.
8. Aiello LP, Avery RL, Arrigg PG, et al. Vascular endothelial growth factor in ocular fluid of patients with diabetic retinopathy and other retinal disorders, *N Engl J Med* (1994) **331:**1480–7.
9. Frank RN, Amin R, Kennedy A, Hohman TC. An aldose reductase inhibitor and aminoguanidine prevent vascular endothelial growth factor expression in rats with long-term galactosemia, *Arch Ophthalmol* (1997) **115:**1036–47.
10. Faulborn J, Bowald S. Microproliferations in proliferative diabetic retinopathy and their relationship to the vitreous: corresponding light and microscopic studies, *Graefes Arch Clin Exp Ophthalmol* (1985) **223:**130–8.
11. Davis MD. Vitreous contraction in proliferative diabetic retinopathy, *Arch Ophthalmol* (1965) **74:**741–51.
12. Lewis H, Abrams GW, Blumenkranz MS, Campo RV. Vitrectomy for diabetic macular traction and edema associated with posterior hyaloidal traction, *Ophthalmology* (1992) **99:**753–9.
13. Charles S, Flinn CE. The natural history of diabetic extramacular tractional retinal detachment, *Arch Ophthalmol* (1981) **99:**66–8.
14. Diabetic Retinopathy Vitrectomy Study Research Group. Two-year course of visual acuity in severe proliferative diabetic retinopathy with conventional management. Diabetic Retinopathy Vitrectomy Study (DRVS) Report 1, *Ophthalmology* (1985) **92:**492–502.
15. Thompson JT, de Bustros S, Michels RG, Rice TA. Results and prognostic factors in vitrectomy for diabetic traction retinal detachment of the macula, *Arch Ophthalmol* (1987) **105:**497–502.
16. Rice TA, Michels RG, Rice EF. Vitrectomy for diabetic traction retinal detachment involving the macula, *Am J Ophthalmol* (1983) **95:**22–33.
17. Peyman GA, Huamonte FU, Goldberg MF, et al. Four hundred consecutive pars plana vitrectomies with the vitrophage, *Arch Ophthalmol* (1978) **96:**45–50.
18. Tolentino FI, Freeman HM, Tolentino FL. Closed vitrectomy in the management of diabetic traction retinal detachment, *Ophthalmology* (1980) **87:**1078–89.
19. Aaberg TM. Pars plana vitrectomy for diabetic traction retinal detachment, *Ophthalmology* (1981) **88:**639–42.
20. Rice TA, Michels RG, Rice EF. Vitrectomy for diabetic rhegmatogenous retinal detachment, *Am J Ophthalmol* (1983) **95:**34–44.
21. Thompson JT, de Bustros S, Michels RG, Rice TA. Results and prognostic factors in vitrectomy for diabetic traction–rhegmatogenous retinal detachment, *Arch Ophthalmol* (1987) **105:**503–7.
22. Diabetic Retinopathy Vitrectomy Study Research Group. Early vitrectomy for severe vitreous hemorrhage in diabetic retinopathy: two-year results of a randomized trial. Diabetic Retinopathy Vitrectomy Study Report 2, *Arch Ophthalmol* (1985) **103:**1644–52.
23. Diabetic Retinopathy Vitrectomy Study Research Group. Early vitrectomy for severe proliferative diabetic retinopathy in eyes with useful vision: results of a randomized trial. Diabetic Retinopathy Vitrectomy Study Report 3, *Ophthalmology* (1988) **95:**1307–20.
24. Brucker AJ, Michels RG, Green WR. Pars plana vitrectomy in the management of blood-induced glaucoma with vitreous hemorrhage, *Ann Ophthalmol* (1978) **10:**1427–37.
25. Ramsay RC, Knobloch WH, Cantrill HL. Timing of vitrectomy for active proliferative diabetic retinopathy, *Ophthalmology* (1986) **93:**283–9.
26. O'Hanley GP, Canny CL. Diabetic dense premacular hemorrhage: a possible indication for prompt vitrectomy, *Ophthalmology* (1985) **92:**507–11.
27. Blankenship G, Cortez R, Machemer R. The lens and pars plana vitrectomy for diabetic retinopathy complications, *Arch Ophthalmol* (1979) **97:**1263–7.
28. Schachat AP, Oyakawa RT, Michels RG, Rice TA. Complications of vitreous surgery for diabetic retinopathy: II. Postoperative complications, *Ophthalmology* (1983) **90:**522–30.
29. Rice TA, Michels RG, Maguire MG, Rice EF. The effect of lensectomy on the incidence of iris neovascularization and neovascular glaucoma after vitrectomy for diabetic retinopathy, *Am J Ophthalmol* (1983) **95:**1–11.
30. McCuen BW II, Hickingbotham D. A fiberoptic diathermy tissue manipulator for use in vitreous surgery (letter), *Am J Ophthalmol* (1984) **98:**803–4.
31. Haimann MH, Abrams GW. Prevention of lens opacification during diabetic vitrectomy, *Ophthalmology* (1984) **91:**116–21.
32. Abrams GW, Williams GA. 'En bloc' excision of diabetic membranes, *Am J Ophthalmol* (1987) **103** (3 Pt 1): 302–8.
33. Meredith T, Kaplan HJ, Aaberg TM. Pars plana vitrectomy techniques for relief of epiretinal traction by membrane segmentation, *Am J Ophthalmol* (1980) **89:**408–13.
34. Michels RG. Proliferative diabetic retinopathy: pathophysiology of extraretinal complications and principles of vitreous surgery, *Retina* (1981) **1:**1–17.
35. Charles S. *Vitreous Microsurgery* (Williams & Wilkins: Baltimore, 1981): 115.
36. Han DP, Lewis HL, Lambrou FH Jr, et al. Mechanisms of intraocular pressure elevation after pars plana vitrectomy, *Ophthalmology* (1989) **96:**1357–62.
37. Kangas TA, Bennett SR, Flynn HW Jr, et al. Reversible loss of light perception after vitreoretinal surgery, *Am J Ophthalmol* (1995) **120:**751–6.

38. Azar DT, Spurr-Michaud SJ, Tisdale AS, Gipson IK. Decreased penetration of anchoring fibrils into the diabetic stroma: a morphometric analysis, *Arch Ophthalmol* (1989) **107:**1520–3.
39. Williams GA, Lambrou FH, Jaffe GA, et al. Treatment of postvitrectomy fibrin formation with intraocular tissue plasminogen activator, *Arch Ophthalmol* (1988) **106:**1055–8.
40. Jaffe GJ, Abrams GW, Williams GA, Han DP. Tissue plasminogen activator for postvitrectomy fibrin formation, *Ophthalmology* (1990) **97:**184–9.
41. Michels RG. Vitreous surgery for macular pucker, *Am J Ophthalmol* (1981) **92:**628–39.
42. Novak MA, Rice TA, Michels RG, Auer C. The crystalline lens after vitrectomy for diabetic retinopathy, *Ophthalmology* (1984) **91:**1480–4.
43. Hutton WL, Pesicka GA, Fuller DG. Cataract extraction in the diabetic eye after vitrectomy, *Am J Ophthalmol* (1987) **104:**1–4.
44. Eaton AM, Jaffe GJ, McCuen BW II, Mincey GJ. Condensation on the posterior surface of silicone intraocular lenses during fluid–air exchange, *Ophthalmology* (1995) **102:**733–6.
45. Apple DJ, Federman JL, Krolicki TJ, et al. Irreversible silicone oil adhesion to silicone intraocular lenses: a clinicopathological analysis, *Ophthalmology* (1996) **103:**1555–61.
46. Little HL, Rosenthal AR, Dellaporta A, Jacobson DR. The effect of pan-retinal photo-coagulation on rubeosis iridis, *Am J Ophthalmol* (1976) **81:**804–9.
47. Lewis H, Aaberg TM, Abrams GW, et al. Current causes of failure following diabetic vitrectomy, *Invest Ophthalmol Vis Sci* (1988) **29** (Suppl): 220 (abst).
48. Lewis H, Abrams GW, Williams GA. Anterior hyaloidal fibrovascular proliferation after diabetic vitrectomy, *Am J Ophthalmol* (1987) **104**:607–13.
49. Liggett PE, Lean JS, Barlow WE, Ryan SJ. Intraoperative argon endophotocoagulation for recurrent vitreous hemorrhage after vitrectomy for diabetic retinopathy, *Am J Ophthalmol* (1987) **103**:146–9.
50. Tolentino FI, Cajita VN, Gancayco T, Skates S. Vitreous hemorrhage after closed vitrectomy for proliferative diabetic retinopathy, *Ophthalmology* (1989) **96**:1495–500.
51. Blankenship GW. Management of vitreous cavity hemorrhage following pars plana vitrectomy for diabetic retinopathy, *Ophthalmology* (1986) **93**:39–44.
52. Blumenkranz M, Gardner T, Blankenship G. Fluid–gas exchange and photocoagulation after vitrectomy: indications, technique, and results, *Arch Ophthalmol* (1986) **104**:291–6.
53. Han DP, Murphy ML, Mieler WF, Abrams GW. Outpatient fluid–air exchange for severe postvitrectomy diabetic vitreous hemorrhage: long-term results and complications, *Retina* (1991) **11**:309–14.
54. Sebestyen JG. Fibrinoid syndrome: a severe complication of vitrectomy surgery in diabetics, *Ann Ophthalmol* (1982) **14**:853–6.
55. Dabbs CK, Aaberg TM, Aguilar HE, et al. Complications of tissue plasminogen activator therapy after vitrectomy for diabetics, *Am J Ophthalmol* (1990) **110**:354–60.
56. Eliott DE, Lewis JM, Townsend-Pico W, Abrams GW. Relaxing retinotomy performed during vitrectomy for proliferative diabetic retinopathy, *Invest Ophthalmol Vis Sci* (1997) **38** (Suppl): S483.
57. Yeo JH, Glaser BM, Michels RG. Silicone oil in the treatment of complicated retinal detachments, *Ophthalmology* (1987) **94**:1109–13.
58. Rinkoff JS, de Juan E Jr, McCuen BW II. Silicone oil for retinal detachment with advanced proliferative vitreoretinopathy following failed vitrectomy for proliferative diabetic retinopathy, *Am J Ophthalmol* (1986) **101**:181–6.
59. Brourman ND, Blumenkranz MS, Cox MS, Trese MT. Silicone oil for the treatment of severe proliferative diabetic retinopathy, *Ophthalmology* (1989) **96**:759–64.
60. Williams DF, Williams GA, Hartz A, et al. Results of vitrectomy for diabetic tractional retinal detachments using the *en bloc* excision technique, *Ophthalmology* (1989) **96**:752–8.

Chapter 26 Pars plana vitrectomy for diabetic macular edema associated with posterior hyaloidal traction

Peter K Kaiser and Hilel Lewis

INTRODUCTION

Diabetic macular edema is a significant source of visual deterioration in patients with diabetes mellitus. In the Wisconsin Epidemiologic Study of Diabetic Retinopathy, the incidence of diabetic macular edema over a 10-year period ranged from 13.9% in adult-onset patients not taking insulin, to 25.4% in adult-onset patients receiving insulin.[1]

The cause of diabetic macular edema is usually from leakage of intraretinal fluid from micro-aneurysms and abnormal retinal capillaries.[2] The pathogenesis of diabetic macular edema is likely multifactorial. Potential instigating factors include increased diastolic blood pressure, duration of diabetes, age at diagnosis, female gender, use of insulin, level of glycosylated hemoglobin, amount of proteinuria, cardiac decompensation, more severe diabetic retinopathy, and previous panretinal photo-coagulation.[1,3] A combination of these factors presumably leads to a breakdown in the blood–retinal barrier, causing macular edema.

The role of vitreous traction in producing macular edema has been demonstrated in cystoid macular edema resulting from peripheral uveitis, retinitis pigmentosa and aphakia.[4] Vitreous traction also has been shown to play a role in diabetic macular edema.[5,6] Diabetic eyes with macular edema have a significantly lower rate of posterior vitreous detachment than those without macular edema.[5,6] It is postulated that the attached posterior hyaloid causes tangential macular traction, leading to macular edema. This theory is supported by the fact that both spontaneous vitreous separation, as well as surgical vitreous detachment, can result in improvement of the diabetic macular edema.[5–9] In addition, it is also possible that the tangential traction exerted by the thickened, taut posterior hyaloid causes a very shallow macular detachment, further contributing to the decrease in vision.[9]

The Diabetes Control and Complications Trial (DCCT) reported a 23% reduction in the development of diabetic macular edema in patients receiving intensive insulin therapy compared with traditional therapy.[10] Once macular edema is present, laser photocoagulation may be advantageous. The Early Treatment Diabetic Retinopathy Study (ETDRS) established that focal macular photocoagulation is beneficial in the treatment of clinically significant diabetic macular edema.[11] In some cases of diffuse macular edema, laser photocoagulation is not beneficial. In these select cases, pars plana vitrectomy with separation and removal of the posterior hyaloid is effective at causing regression of the macular edema. This chapter will focus on the surgical management of diabetic macular edema associated with posterior hyaloidal traction.

INDICATIONS FOR SURGERY

Patients with clinically significant macular edema usually benefit from focal laser photocoagulation. However, we have observed and reported patients with diabetic retinopathy and diffuse diabetic macular edema who do not respond to laser treatment.[9] These patients have a thickened, taut, glistening premacular posterior hyaloid. This thickening is caused by abnormalities of the posterior vitreous surface and is not related to fibrovascular proliferation. When a thickened posterior cortical vitreous is present, pars plana vitrectomy and removal of the posterior hyaloid can result in resolution of the macular edema and improvement in visual acuity.[8,9]

PREOPERATIVE EVALUATION

It is essential to perform a complete preoperative ophthalmic examination to determine the appropriate surgical approach. Anterior segment examination is required to determine whether the view through anterior segment structures will be adequate to perform the precise surgical maneuvers that are required. If possible, preservation of the crystalline lens is advantageous to prevent anterior diffusion of vasoproliferative factors and to reduce the incidence of postoperative iris neovascularization. However, if significant lenticular opacities exist that would preclude adequate visualization of the fundus, we suggest cataract extraction either at the time of surgery or before surgery by an experienced cataract surgeon. In either situation, preservation of the posterior capsule and implantation of a posterior chamber intraocular lens are desirable.

The diagnosis of diabetic macular edema is made by careful ophthalmoscopy. Biomicroscopic examination of the posterior pole should be performed to verify the presence of the diabetic macular edema, to evaluate the vitreoretinal interface relationships and to check for any preretinal membranes. Evaluation for the presence of a posterior vitreous separation or a Weiss ring is necessary because surgical treatment of diabetic macular edema has been shown to be beneficial only in patients with an attached posterior hyaloid. In eyes in which the vitreous is already separated, other causes of macular edema should be entertained.

A careful fundus contact lens examination is imperative to differentiate the thickened, taut, glistening, premacular posterior hyaloid from fibrovascular proliferation or an epiretinal membrane. Epiretinal membranes usually cause straightening of nearby retinal vessels, retinal striae or shift the fovea from its original position. This is not the case with a thickened, opacified posterior hyaloid. In some instances, despite a careful contact lens examination, it may be difficult to assess how much the posterior cortical vitreous contributes to the macular edema.[8] Finally, examination of the retinal periphery with indirect ophthalmoscopy is suggested to determine the presence of preoperative retinal pathology that may require treatment before surgery.

Fluorescein angiography is a useful adjuvant to the clinical examination. Fluorescein angiography usually demonstrates a characteristic pattern of deep, diffuse, late retinal leakage in the central macula. This is in contrast to the traditional, multifocal vascular leakage seen in diabetic patients.[9] It is postulated that the tangential traction of the taut posterior cortical vitreous is more likely to produce diffuse leakage rather than the traditional discrete areas of leakage seen in diabetic macular edema. In some cases, late leakage in a petalloid pattern consistent with cystoid macular edema is also seen. Good capillary perfusion, especially of the fovea, is another important variable to consider on fluorescein angiography because patients with significant macular ischemia will likely not benefit from surgery.

SURGICAL TECHNIQUE

The choice of anesthesia for this surgery is based on several factors, including the patient's renal and cardiac status, the patient's preference and the anesthesiologist's skill. Although general anesthesia offers improved airway management, patient comfort and control of eye and head movements, we prefer performing this surgery under local anesthesia with monitored care by an anesthesiologist. The benefits of this approach are decreased cardiovascular morbidity, unaltered gas kinetics during gas tamponade, reduced recovery time and shorter operating times. Anesthesia and akinesia are obtained using retrobulbar injection of 150 units of hyaluronidase combined with a 50 : 50 mixture of 0.75% bupivacaine and 2% lidocaine without epinephrine. The addition of hyaluronidase allows quicker diffusion of the anesthesia mixture and a more comfortable block. In addition, given the fine surgical techniques that are required in this operation, we ask the anesthesiologist to keep the patient 'light'. This usually prevents the patient from awakening with a jolt, which is often seen with deeper forms of anesthesia.

The surgical technique begins with a limited, posterior vitrectomy using standard three-port pars plana vitrectomy techniques, including a separate infusion cannula, fiberoptic endoilluminator and automated vitrectomy probe (Fig. 26.1). Our usual vitrectomy settings are 600–800 cuts per minute (cpm) and suction levels of 150–200 mmHg.

In order to prevent opacification of the lens, it is important to add 3 ml of dextrose without preservatives

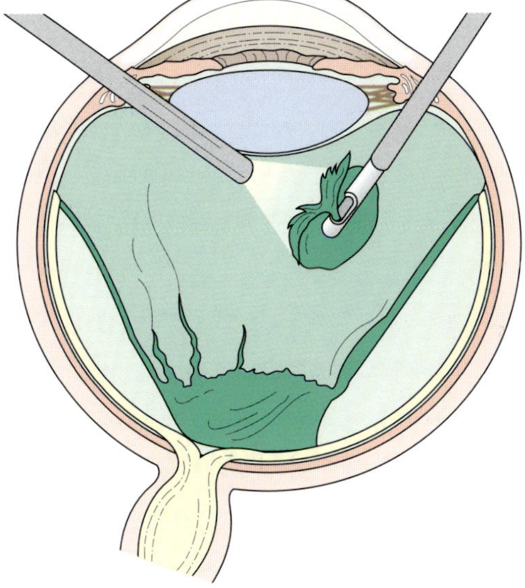

Figure 26.1 *A limited posterior core vitrectomy is performed using standard three-port pars plana vitrectomy techniques. As much as two-thirds of the vitreous gel is removed to relieve anterior–posterior traction. In aphakic and pseudophakic patients, the anterior vitreous is also removed. Notice the thickened premacular posterior hyaloid.*

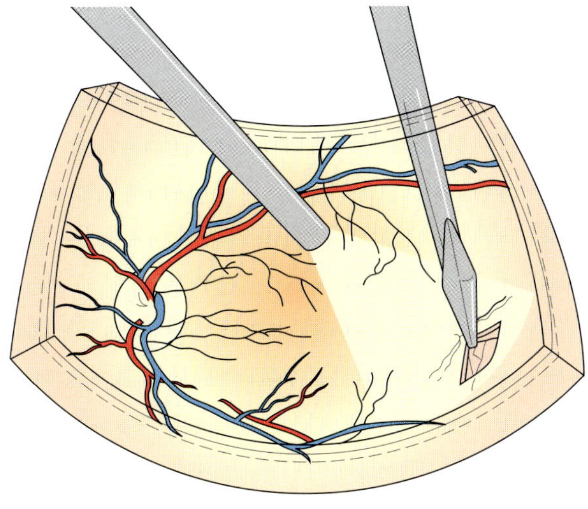

Figure 26.2 *A bent myringotomy blade is used to engage and make an opening into the posterior hyaloid at the thickest area. Holding the endoilluminator close to the retinal surface results in better visualization of the posterior hyaloid. The tip of the myringotomy blade should be directed toward the light source to avoid working in the shadow produced by the blade.*

or antioxidants to the 50-ml infusion bottle of balanced saline solution (BSS Plus) if the patient is phakic. We ordinarily use BSS Plus without any additional dextrose in aphakic and pseudophakic patients. Some authors have advocated adding epinephrine to the infusion solution to aid in pupillary dilation; however, we do not use epinephrine in diabetic patients because of the increased risk of vasoconstriction and decreased perfusion.

The posterior two-thirds of the vitreous gel is removed using the automated vitrector and endoilluminator in phakic patients. In aphakic and pseudophakic patients, the entire central vitreous gel, including the anterior vitreous, is removed.

After the core vitrectomy is completed, careful attention is paid to removing the posterior hyaloid. A bent myringotomy blade is used to engage and make an opening into the posterior hyaloid (Fig. 26.2). Ideally, the thickest area of the posterior hyaloid is chosen to engage with the myringotomy blade. Because the posterior vitreous surface is thickened and taut, this maneuver is accomplished relatively easily to form a nice dissection plane.

Once the edge is elevated, end-opening, diamond-dusted intraocular forceps are used to engage the posterior hyaloid and gently peel it off the retina (Fig. 26.3). By utilizing a circular motion, the entire thickened vitreous can be carefully elevated off the macula and peeled toward the periphery (Fig. 26.4).

We try to remove the posterior vitreous surface in one piece; however, the posterior hyaloid may fragment and require regrasping from other directions. In general, the thicker the posterior hyaloid, the easier it is to remove. During the peeling, very careful attention should be paid to the fovea in order to prevent any tearing. Rarely, we encounter a strong attachment at the optic nerve head. In these situations, diamond dusted forceps can be used to separate the hyaloid from the nerve. The automated vitrector is then used to trim the residual vitreous after it has been completely removed from the macula (Fig. 26.5).

After removing the remaining vitreous, indirect ophthalmoscopy and scleral depression should be performed on the fluid-filled eye to identify any iatrogenic breaks. If a retinal break is identified, it should

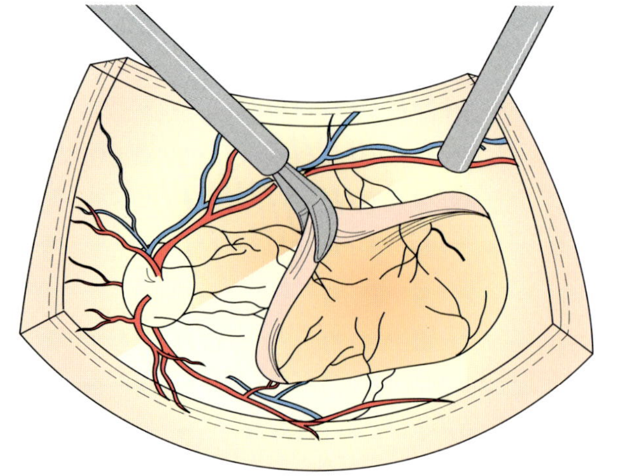

Figure 26.3 *Once an opening in the posterior hyaloid is made and the edge is elevated, intraocular forceps are used to engage the posterior hyaloid and gently peel it off the macula.*

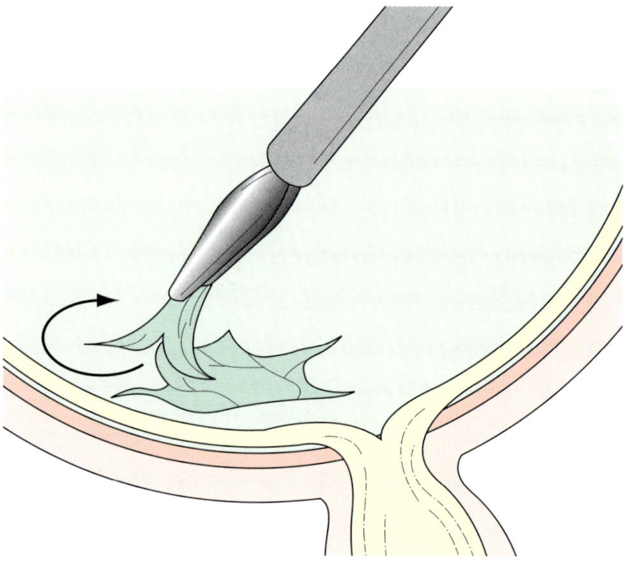

Figure 26.4 *The posterior hyaloid should be removed using a circular motion, pulling tangentially. During the peeling, careful attention should be paid to the fovea to prevent any tearing.*

be treated either with one application of cryotherapy or encircled with three rows of endolaser. A complete air–fluid exchange is then performed using the soft-tipped extrusion cannula and endoilluminator. This is

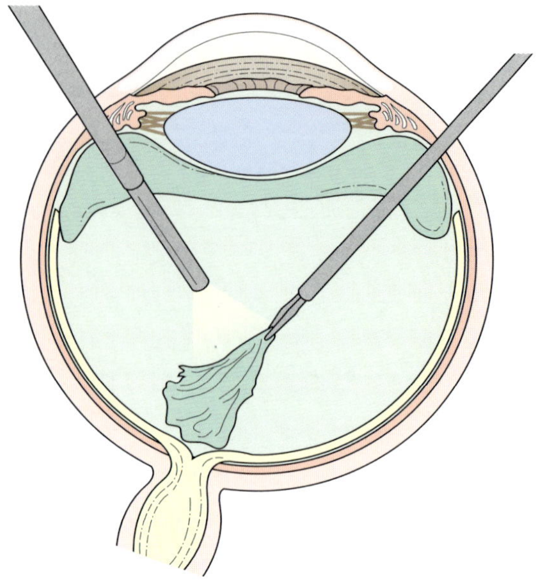

Figure 26.5 *The posterior hyaloid should be peeled entirely off the macula and toward the equatorial retina. Once the entire posterior cortical vitreous has been peeled off the macula, the automated vitrector can be used to remove it from the eye.*

followed by a gas–air exchange using a long-acting gas. We usually use nonexpansile concentrations of SF_6 produced by mixing the gas with filtered air. If no iatrogenic breaks are identified, an air–fluid exchange is not necessary.

We close the sclerotomy sites using 7-0 polyglactin suture in a figure-of-eight fashion with two or three bites. Next, the conjunctiva is reapproximated and closed with 6-0 plain gut suture in an interrupted fashion. Finally, subconjunctival injections of Ancef and Decadron are given.

COMPLICATIONS

Intraoperative complications occur with less frequency than postoperative complications. In phakic patients, the crystalline lens may be damaged, especially during maneuvers that cross the midline. Small amounts of bleeding may occur during the peeling of the posterior hyaloid, but these are usually minimal and stop spontaneously. The most important intraoperative complication is the formation of retinal breaks; therefore careful examination of the retinal periphery should be performed before finishing the case.

Postoperative complications include vitreous hemorrhage, rhegmatogenous retinal detachment, epiretinal membranes and cataracts. Retinal detachments should be treated immediately with traditional retinal detachment repair techniques. If a postoperative vitreous hemorrhage fails to clear after sufficient time, an outpatient air–fluid exchange can be performed. If epiretinal membranes or cataracts cause significant visual impairment, additional surgery can be considered to improve the visual outcome.

SURGICAL RESULTS

To date, no large-scale randomized trials have been performed to evaluate the effectiveness of vitreoretinal surgery in the treatment of diabetic macular edema associated with posterior hyaloidal traction. There have been several pilot studies. Results of our published pilot study showed that nine out of ten operated eyes had an improvement in visual acuity, with six achieving acuities of 20/60 or better after a mean follow-up of 16 months.[9] All eyes had a thickened posterior cortical vitreous preoperatively, 90% had focal laser photocoagulation preoperatively and none had epiretinal membranes identified intraoperatively. Eight out of ten patients had resolution of the macular edema and posterior hyaloidal traction, and the other two had an improvement in the macular edema postoperatively. Postoperative complications occurred in three eyes: one patient developed a vitreous hemorrhage 9 months after surgery; one patient suffered a rhegmatogenous retinal detachment 2 months after surgery; and another patient developed a visually significant epiretinal membrane with a pseudohole. The only patient who had a decrease in vision after surgery was the patient with the retinal detachment. Six patients had a worsening of their lenticular opacities; however, only one patient developed a dense cataract.

More recently, we studied 18 eyes of patients who underwent pars plana vitrectomy for diabetic macular edema associated with posterior hyaloidal traction. These patients were followed for a mean of 19 months (range 6–37 months). Preoperatively, all 18 eyes had diffuse macular thickening and 7/18 also had cystoid macular edema. The preoperative visual acuity ranged from 20/60 to 20/400. Intraoperatively, we found a thickened and taut posterior hyaloid attached over the macula in all patients, and there were no epiretinal membranes identified. Histopathologic findings in three eyes demonstrated vitreous condensation without any cellular elements or inner limiting lamina. At the end of follow-up, 14/18 eyes (78%) had complete resolution of the macular edema and 4/18 eyes (22%) had a decrease in macular edema. Of the 18 eyes: 13/18 (72%) had improvement in vision; only 1/18 eyes had worsening of the visual acuity; and 4/18 eyes (22%) were unchanged. Eight of the 18 eyes (44%) achieved a visual acuity of 20/50 or better and 11 of the 18 eyes (61%) had a visual acuity of 20/70 or better.

Another pilot study showed that five out of ten operated eyes had an improvement in visual acuity, with three patients improving by six lines of visual acuity.[8] The other five patients remained within one line of preoperative visual acuity. The authors found that a shorter interval between initial diagnosis and surgery was associated with better visual outcomes. Eyes with prolonged macular edema had poor outcomes. Postoperative diabetic macular edema improved in six eyes and persisted in four eyes. Interestingly, although all the patients were judged to have a thickened and taut posterior hyaloid preoperatively, two patients had a detached posterior vitreous and an epiretinal membrane intraoperatively. Both of these patients had an improvement in visual acuity after surgery. Postoperative complications occurred in four patients, including epiretinal membrane formation, transient vitreous hemorrhage, progressive macular ischemia and cataract.

Rather than having diabetic macular edema, we currently suspect that these patients probably have a shallow macular traction detachment caused by posterior hyaloidal traction. The late hyperfluorescence deep in the sensory retina seen on fluorescein angiography is consistent with pooling of dye into the subsensory space, which is seen in patients with a shallow neurosensory traction detachment. We were surprised by the improvement in visual acuity following vitrectomy in most of these patients.

The ETDRS showed that only 17% of patients had improvement in visual acuity within 5 years after focal laser photocoagulation for clinically significant diabetic macular edema.[11] Thus, the improvement in visual acuity following vitrectomy can be explained by the fact that, instead of diabetic macular edema, these patients had a shallow traction macular detachment secondary to posterior hyaloidal traction. Surgery allowed reattachment of the macula instead of reducing macular edema. This explains the significant improvement in vision.

REFERENCES

1. Klein R, Klein BE, Moss SE, Cruickshanks KJ. The Wisconsin Epidemiologic Study of Diabetic Retinopathy. XV. The long-term incidence of macular edema, *Ophthalmology* (1995) **102:**7–16.
2. Ferris FL, Patz A. Macular edema: a complication of diabetic retinopathy, *Surv Ophthalmol* (1984) **28** (Suppl):452–61.
3. McDonald HR, Schatz H. Macular edema following panretinal photocoagulation, *Retina* (1985) **5**:5–10.
4. Schepens CL, Avila MP, Jalkh AE, Trempe CL. Role of the vitreous in cystoid macular edema, *Surv Ophthalmol* (1984) **28** (Suppl):499–504.
5. Nasrallah FP, Jalkh AE, van Coppenolle F, et al. The role of the vitreous in diabetic macular edema, *Ophthalmology* (1988) **95**:1335–9.
6. Hikichi T, Fujio N, Akiba J, et al. Association between the short-term natural history of diabetic macular edema and the vitreomacular relationship in type II diabetes mellitus, *Ophthalmology* (1997) **104**:473–8.
7. Tachi N, Ogino N. Vitrectomy for diffuse macular edema in cases of diabetic retinopathy, *Am J Ophthalmol* (1996) **122**:258–60.
8. Harbour JW, Smiddy WE, Flynn HW Jr, Rubsamen PE. Vitrectomy for diabetic macular edema associated with a thickened and taut posterior hyaloid membrane, *Am J Ophthalmol* (1996) **121**:405–13.
9. Lewis H, Abrams GW, Blumenkranz MS, Campo RV. Vitrectomy for diabetic macular traction and edema associated with posterior hyaloidal traction, *Ophthalmology* (1992) **99**:753–9.
10. The Diabetes Control and Complications Trial Research Group. The effect of intensive treatment of diabetes on the development and progression of long-term complications in insulin-dependent diabetes mellitus, *N Engl J Med* (1993) **329**:977–86.
11. Early Treatment Diabetic Retinopathy Study Research Group. Photocoagulation for diabetic macular edema, ETDRS Report No. 1, *Arch Ophthalmol* (1985) **103**:1796–806.

Part VI Surgical Techniques in Proliferative Vitreoretinopathy and Macular Hole Surgery

Chapter 27 Membrane removal in proliferative vitreoretinopathy

Michael S Lee and Gary W Abrams

INTRODUCTION

Rhegmatogenous retinal detachment occurs in 1 per 10 000 persons annually.[1] Treatment consists of reattaching the retina to prevent severe visual loss. Although surgical repair of the retina is usually successful, the most common cause of failure of retinal reattachment surgery is proliferative vitreoretinopathy (PVR). PVR complicates approximately 5–10% of rhegmatogenous retinal detachment and typically occurs 6–8 weeks postoperatively.[2] It may occur following scleral buckling, pneumatic retinopexy or vitrectomy, but previous surgery is not a prerequisite for the development of PVR, because it may occur with longstanding retinal detachments. In order to develop a surgical approach to treat PVR, an understanding of both the pathophysiology and pathoanatomy of the disease is necessary.

Early investigators suggested that the cellular basis of PVR is the result of proliferating retinal pigment epithelial (RPE) cells, as well as retinal glial cells.[3–8] RPE cells have been identified by both light and electron microscopy on the retinal surface of longstanding detachments. Although the majority of the cells appeared to be normal RPE cells, some RPE cells had undergone metaplastic differentiation into macrophage-like cells with phagocytic activity and others had undergone a second transformation into fibrocyte-like cells with collagen-producing ability.[6] Retinal glial cells, which probably originate from Müller cells, can proliferate and break through the internal and external limiting membrane, forming epiretinal as well as subretinal membranes.[4,7]

In addition to RPE cells being identified on the inner retinal surface, they were also found in the vitreous. Proliferating RPE cells can transform into myofibroblast-like cells, which extend pseudopods to pull and contract a strand of collagen in a 'hand-over-hand' manner, resulting in retraction of the vitreous body. Because only a few cells are necessary to produce a great deal of vitreous contraction, this has been termed 'hypocellular gel contraction.'[9]

Another manifestation of PVR is retroretinal membranes. They are more likely to occur in the following: eyes with chronic retinal detachments, especially those caused by giant retinal tears; diabetic eyes with chronic subretinal hemorrhages or fibrin; eyes with retinal detachments following penetrating injuries; and eyes that have had multiple retinal reattachment surgeries.[10] Subretinal membranes develop in a process similar to epiretinal membranes. The RPE cells migrate underneath the retina and attach to the outer retinal surface as macrophage-like cells. These cells eventually transform into cells with fibroblast-like morphology, producing subretinal membranes.[8] Retinal glial cells also may proliferate and attach to the outer retinal surface, producing retroretinal membranes.[4] An early clinical sign of subretinal membranes may be the appearance of yellow spots, which, on pathological examination, represent a cluster of macrophages derived from pigment epithelial cells.[3] As these

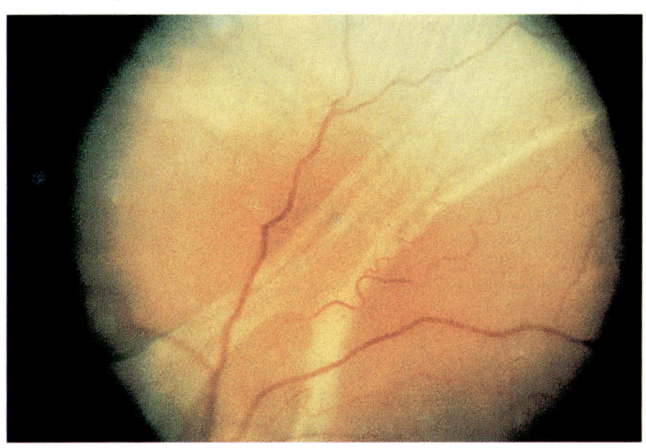

Figure 27.1 *Branching subretinal band.*

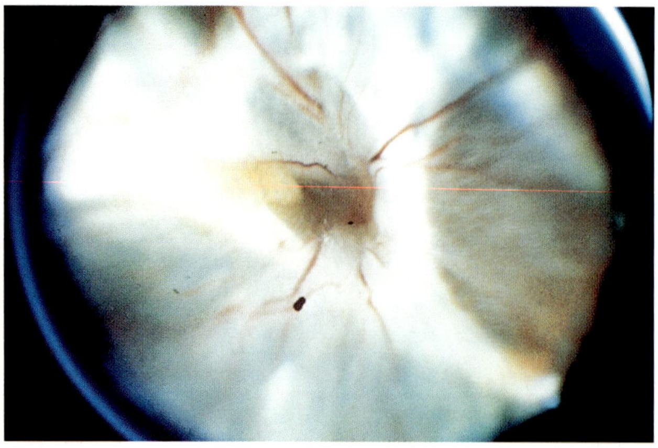

Figure 27.2 *Subretinal napkin-ring membrane.*

membranes enlarge, they begin to develop different configurations, which were described by Sternberg and Machemer.[11] The continued proliferation of pigment epithelial cells and the production of an acellular collagenous core lead to band formation (Fig. 27.1). Other cells that contribute to the formation of bands include glial cells, fibroblast-like cells and macrophages.[12–14] These cells can also form a ring or annular membrane around the posterior retina, encircling the retina anterior to the optic nerve (Fig. 27.2).[11] Another form of subretinal membrane is a sheet composed primarily of glial cells with little or no extracellular material (Fig. 27.3).[15,16]

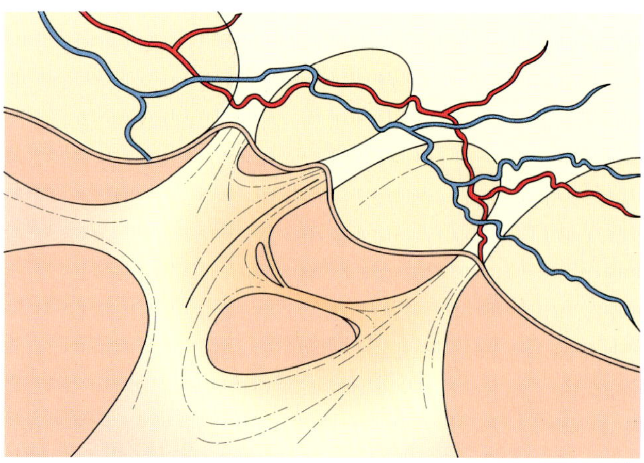

Figure 27.3 *Subretinal membrane sheet with moth-eaten appearance.*

CLASSIFICATION

The major clinical finding with PVR is fixed folds, which are classified by the extent of retinal folding. The Retina Society Classification, published in 1983, described PVR according to its severity.[17] It had four progressive grades, with grade A being the least severe and grade D being the most severe (Table 27.1).

In an attempt to eliminate the confusion caused by the various classification systems and to address observations by other investigators, the Retina Society published a revision of its classification system in 1991[18] (Tables 27.2 and 27.3). This new system retains the original grades of severity: grades A and B. Grade C has been modified and grade D has been eliminated. PVR is divided into posterior or anterior varieties, and clock-hours are now used instead of quadrants to describe the extent of involvement (Fig. 27.4).

Posterior PVR is characterized by three types of contraction. Type 1 or focal contraction consists of a single or multiple epicenters of PVR causing focal retinal contraction. The folds radiate away from each epicenter in a 'starfold' configuration, with the

Table 27.1 Original Retina Society Classification of proliferative vitreoretinopathy

Grade	*Name*	*Clinical signs*
A	Minimal	Vitreous haze Vitreous pigment clumps
B	Moderate	Wrinkling of the inner retinal surface Rolled edge of retinal breaks Retinal stiffness Vessel tortuosity
C	Marked	Full-thickness, fixed retinal folds
C_1		One quadrant
C_2		Two quadrants
C_3		Three quadrants
D	Massive	Fixed retinal folds in four quadrants
D_1		Wide funnel shape
D_2		Narrow funnel shape[a]
D_3		Closed funnel (optic nerve head not visible)

[a] Narrow funnel shape exists when the anterior end of the funnel can be seen by indirect ophthalmoscopy within the 45° field of a +20-D condensing lens (Nikon or equivalent). Adapted with permission from Retina Society Terminology Committee. The classification of retinal detachment with proliferative vitreoretinopathy, *Ophthalmology* (1989) **90**:121–5.[17] Copyright © 1989, Elsevier Science.

Table 27.2 Revised Retina Society Classification of proliferative vitreoretinopathy by grade

Grade	*Clinical features*
A	Vitreous haze Vitreous pigment clumps Pigment clusters on inferior retina
B	Wrinkling of the inner retinal surface Retinal stiffness Vessel tortuosity Rolled and irregular edges of retinal breaks Decreased mobility of vitreous
C_{P1}–C_{P12}	Posterior to equator Focal, diffuse or circumferential full-thickness folds[a] Subretinal strands[a]
C_{A1}–C_{A12}	Anterior to the equator Focal, diffuse or circumferential full-thickness folds[a] Subretinal strands[a] Condensed vitreous with strands

[a] Expressed by the number of clock-hours of involvement.
Adapted with permission from Machemer R, Aaberg TM, Freeman HM, et al. An updated classification of retinal detachment with proliferative vitreoretinopathy, *Am J Ophthalmol* (1991) **112**:159–65.[18] Copyright © 1991, Elsevier Science.

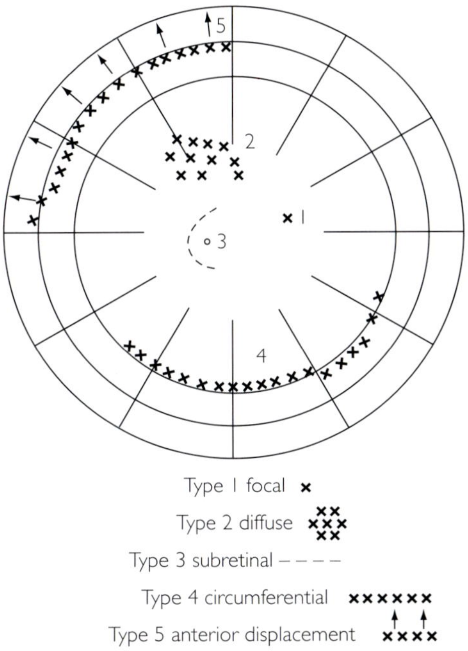

Figure 27.4 *Retinal diagram to depict the various types of full-thickness retinal folding. (Adapted with permission from Peyman GA, Schulman JA.* Intravitreal Surgery: Principles and Practice, *2nd edn (Appleton & Lange: Norwalk, CT, 1994): 595.[24])*

Table 27.3 Grade C proliferative vitreoretinopathy classification by type of contraction

Type	*Location*	*Clinical features*
1. Focal	Posterior	Starfold posterior to vitreous base
2. Diffuse	Posterior	Confluent starfolds posterior to vitreous base Optic disc may not be visible
3. Subretinal	Posterior/ anterior	Proliferation under the retina 'Napkin ring' around disc 'Clothes-line' Moth-eaten-appearing sheets
4. Circumferential	Anterior	Contraction along posterior vitreous base with central displacement of retina Peripheral retina stretched Posterior retina in radial folds
5. Anterior displacement	Anterior	Vitreous base pulled anteriorly by proliferative tissue Peripheral retinal trough Ciliary processes may be stretched or covered by membrane Iris may be retracted

Adapted with permission from Machemer R, Aaberg TM, Freeman HM, et al. An updated classification of retinal detachment with proliferative vitreoretinopathy, *Am J Ophthalmol* (1991) **112**:159–65.[18] Copyright © 1991, Elsevier Science.

resulting traction directed to a focal point rather than along an axis. Single focal contractions may have little effect on the overall configuration of the retinal detachment but multiple focal contractions can cause tight folds between the epicenters of contraction.

Diffuse posterior contraction (type 2) consists of confluent retinal folds in the posterior retina that cause a diffuse posterior retinal contraction (Fig. 27.5). A funneled configuration with folds radiating anteriorly toward the ora results from posterior circumferential traction. The normally bullous contours involving the more anterior retina are flattened when contraction occurs in an anterior–posterior direction.

Type 3 or subretinal contraction can be posteriorly or anteriorly located and is characterized by subretinal PVR and can take several forms.[19] An annular constriction caused by subretinal tissue constricting in a circumferential direction around the disc, also referred to as napkin-ring subretinal contraction,

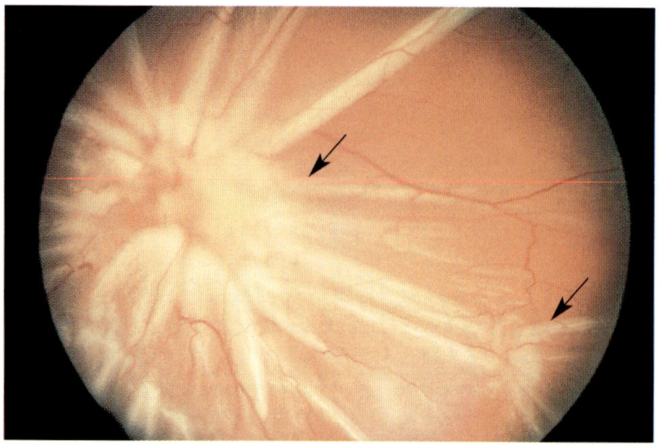

Figure 27.5 *Posterior proliferative vitreoretinopathy with focal or 'starfold' contraction (type 1, small arrow) and diffuse contraction (type 2, large arrow).*

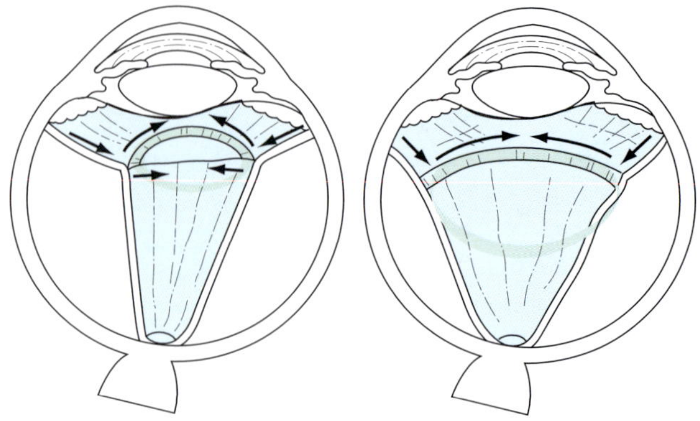

Figure 27.6 *Circumferential contraction (type 4, grade C proliferative vitreoretinopathy). The circumferential contraction is the result of proliferation immediately posterior to the insertion of the posterior hyaloid. The retina is pulled centrally, stretching the anterior retina and causing posterior retinal folds. Schematic drawing of nonvitrectomized eye (left) and vitrectomized eye (right), with arrows denoting direction of contractile forces.*

pulls the posterior retina together anterior to the disc while a series of radial folds involve the remainder of the retina. Another characteristic pattern caused by contraction of subretinal tissue is a linear fold, also referred to as a clothes-line configuration caused by a subretinal strand.[20,21] Sheets of subretinal membranes can elevate the retina without folds, preventing retinal reattachment. Frequently, the subretinal membranes seen in type 3 PVR are found intraoperatively but were not apparent before surgery.

Anterior PVR is also subdivided into three types (types 3–5), defined primarily on the basis of the primary vector forces produced by each type of anterior contraction. Additional vector forces besides the primary one may be created by a combination of forces. The combination of these vector forces produces characteristic patterns in each type of fixed retinal fold.[20,22]

Type 4 or circumferential contraction is caused by contraction of diffuse PVR located anterior to the equator (Fig. 27.6) and immediately posterior to the insertion of the posterior hyaloid, causing the retina to become circumferentially contracted to form a series of irregular folds. Posterior to the membrane, a series of radial retinal folds develop and extend toward the optic disc. In addition, a secondary traction vector extending toward the center of the vitreous cavity perpendicular to the retinal surfaces causes inward stretching of the anterior retina within the vitreous base (Fig. 27.7). With this type of PVR, the anterior retina will typically have a smooth appearance as it is stretched centrally, while retina posterior to the membrane will have radial folds. A form of type 4 contraction was described as 'perpendicular contraction' in the Silicone Study classification of PVR.[20] This manifested as a smooth circumferential fold of retina at the posterior border of the vitreous base caused by traction exerted by the contracted posterior hyaloid. Similar to other forms of type 4 PVR, the retina anterior to the fold was smooth while that posterior to the vitreous base had radial folds.

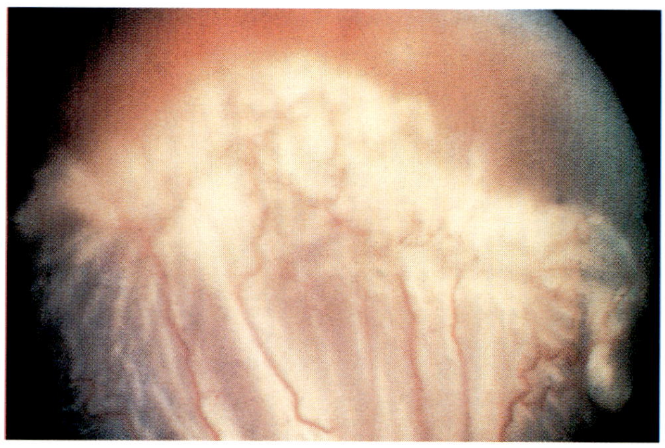

Figure 27.7 *Contraction along the posterior edge of the vitreous base pulling the retina centrally, producing posterior retinal folds and stretched anterior retina.*

This form of PVR can occur after vitrectomy owing to contraction of a ring of posterior hyaloid that was not removed during the procedure. This form of PVR was included with type 4 contraction in the revised Retina Society Classification (Table 27.3).

The posterior border of the vitreous base may be variable in location, which affects the prognosis in this type of anterior PVR. When the posterior hyaloid has an extremely posterior insertion in relation to the ora, these membranes can be difficult to remove surgically and tend to recur. Due to the posterior location, it may be difficult to support the traction on a scleral buckle.

The retina posterior to the vitreous base is displaced anteriorly and has developed abnormal attachments to other ocular structures, such as the pars plana, pars plicata, iris or lens capsule, producing a peripheral retinal trough (Fig. 27.8). In an eye that has not undergone vitrectomy, fibrous proliferation on the posterior hyaloid surface causes traction in the plane of the detached hyaloid across the vitreous cavity (Fig. 27.9).[20,22]

Anterior retinal displacement, or type 5 PVR, called anterior loop traction by Charles,[23] is observed most frequently following vitrectomy or penetrating trauma. It can sometimes be found in longstanding retinal detachments. Anterior retinal displacement is caused by contraction of the vitreous base, which is usually due to cellular proliferation and contraction on the surface of residual vitreous following vitrectomy. Cellular proliferation at the posterior aspect of the vitreous base can sometimes cause a similar picture in those eyes with trauma or longstanding retinal detachment that have not had a vitrectomy. This traction, in contrast to traction in type 4 PVR, which may also cause circumferential folds, is clinically apparent by the development of a trough at the vitreous base. This trough is caused by displacement of the posterior vitreous base toward its anterior

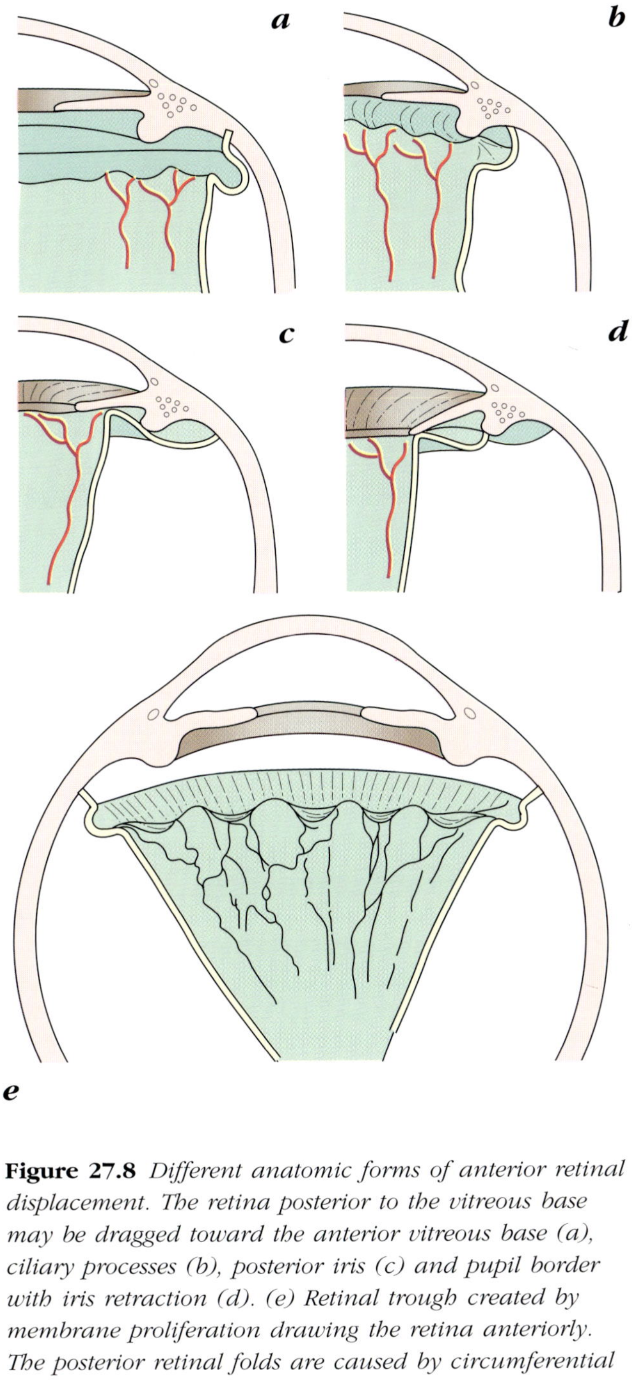

Figure 27.8 *Different anatomic forms of anterior retinal displacement. The retina posterior to the vitreous base may be dragged toward the anterior vitreous base (a), ciliary processes (b), posterior iris (c) and pupil border with iris retraction (d). (e) Retinal trough created by membrane proliferation drawing the retina anteriorly. The posterior retinal folds are caused by circumferential contraction.*

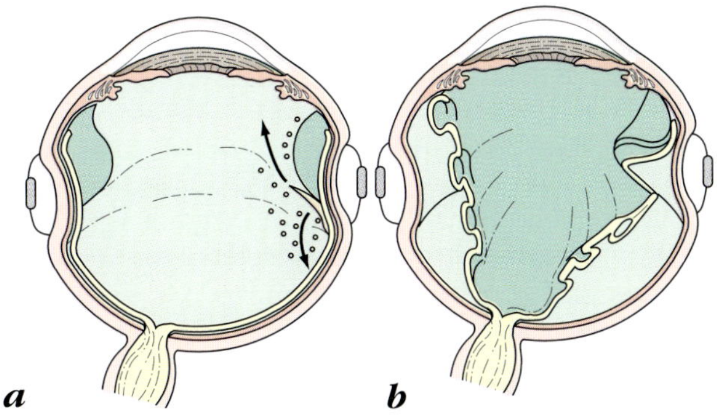

Figure 27.9 *Anterior retinal displacement (type 5, grade C proliferative vitreoretinopathy). (a) Proliferation of cells at the retina and vitreous base, following a vitrectomy and scleral buckle. (b) Resulting contraction of membranes, which drags the retina posterior to the vitreous base anteriorly.*

insertion, along with the detached anterior retina, which is also pulled forward. Hypotony may result when the proliferative tissue is adherent to the ciliary processes and causes this structure to stretch posteriorly. Posterior retraction of the iris may occur when abnormal adhesions also involve the posterior iris.[20,22]

A standard chart is available with a shaded and unshaded portion for recording the anterior and posterior forms of PVR, respectively. Different conventions are used to record the different types of contraction occurring in PVR. Grading is also done to indicate the number of clock-hours of anterior and posterior traction. The number of quadrants of posterior and anterior traction is reflected in the final PVR grade.[20,21,24]

SURGICAL INDICATIONS

We recommend that almost all eyes with retinal detachments with PVR undergo surgical repair. There has been a dramatic increase in the anatomic success rate of treatment of retinal detachments caused by PVR over the past two decades. With a better understanding of the pathophysiology and pathoanatomy of PVR, as well as improvements in surgical instruments and techniques, the retina may be reattached in up to 90% of cases of severe PVR.[25–28] Therefore, most eyes with recent retinal detachment and light perception vision or better should be offered an opportunity for surgical repair.

One factor that may influence the decision to intervene surgically is the chronicity of the detachment. With a longstanding retinal detachment, an estimate of visual potential should be made. The visual outcome is related to the status of the macula, as well as the length of time that the retina has been detached. The longer a macular detachment has existed, the less likely it is that the patient will have significant visual return. Retinal detachments of a year or longer have a poor visual prognosis, and we generally do not repair these cases. If the decision to repair a detachment has been made, we recommend that the surgery be performed as soon as possible. Some have recommended waiting for at least 6 weeks to allow membranes to mature, making their removal easier.[29] Because we have found it possible to remove immature membranes adequately, and we believe that delaying surgical intervention will likely result in a poorer visual outcome, we recommend that retinal detachment repair should not be postponed.

PREOPERATIVE EVALUATION

When evaluating a patient for surgery, the general health of the patient must be considered. A potentially long surgical case with a limited visual prognosis must be weighed against the patient's medical condition. In addition, the status of the fellow eye must be evaluated. Other ocular diseases, such as glaucoma or macular degeneration, or limited visual function in the fellow eye may influence the need for surgical intervention.

The surgical eye must be assessed carefully and undergo a complete examination. Although the cornea usually does not present a problem, it must be sufficiently clear to permit surgery. The iris should be evaluated for rubeosis, synechiae and pupillary dilation. Eyes with rubeosis have a poorer prognosis. Preoperative knowledge that the pupil does not dilate adequately, requiring pupil stretching or breaking of synechiae, will facilitate surgical planning. The eye should be evaluated for glaucoma and undergo gonioscopy. These eyes are more likely to develop postoperative intraocular pressure (IOP) problems, and they should be managed accordingly to minimize pressure elevation. If the eye is hypotonus, it should be examined carefully for anterior PVR and traction on the ciliary processes.

The lens status also should be noted. In most cases of severe PVR in phakic eyes, removal of the lens is necessary, regardless of lens clarity. The crystalline lens will prevent removal of the anterior vitreous and membranes, which is a critical aspect of surgical repair of PVR. In addition, removal of the crystalline lens will be helpful for postoperative management, such as performing a fluid–gas exchange or the placement of laser photocoagulation. These eyes will require prolonged internal tamponade, so they are likely to develop lenticular opacities.

If the patient has had a prior cataract extraction, the intraocular lens (IOL) must be evaluated carefully. If the lens is a stable, nonsilicone posterior chamber lens, it may be left in place. The IOL must be removed if it is unstable or if there are vitreous membranes adherent to it. If the lens is made of silicone and the posterior capsule is intact, it may be left in place. If the capsule has been violated, then a silicone IOL must be removed. During a fluid–air exchange, condensation may develop on a silicone lens without an intact capsule, which is difficult to remove and will limit the view of the retina.[30] In addition, silicone oil will adhere tightly to silicone IOLs.[31] The oil is irreversibly adherent to the lens and cannot be removed by any instrument or technique. Anterior chamber lenses are more likely to be displaced anteriorly by a gas bubble, resulting in lenticular corneal touch. Therefore, all unstable anterior chamber lenses should be removed.

Finally, every aspect of the posterior segment should be considered carefully. The vitreous should be examined for adherence to peripheral membranes posterior to the vitreous base. The extent of the retinal detachment, as well as membrane formation, should be evaluated. The development of anterior retinal displacement should be assessed as well, especially when the eye is hypotonus. Although subretinal membranes cannot always be identified preoperatively (especially when they are not pigmented), their presence should be noted. Subretinal membranes occasionally may prevent retinal reattachment, despite relief of all traction from epiretinal membranes.

After careful evaluation of the posterior segment has been completed, an estimate of prognosis of visual outcome can be made based on both the original Retina Society and Silicone Study classifications. The Silicone Study examined the reproducibility and prognostic utility of both classification schemes and found that preoperative visual estimations[32] could be made using the Silicone Study classification, which is similar to the revised Retina Society classification (Tables 27.2 and 27.3). Eyes with only posterior PVR had a better visual prognosis than those with anterior and posterior PVR and better than those with anterior and posterior PVR and subretinal membranes. Using the original Retina Society classification (Table 27.1), eyes had a progressively worse visual prognosis as the classification increased from C_3 (three quadrants of contraction) to D_3 (closed funnel obscuring a view of the optic disc). There was a strong concordance between preoperative and intraoperative assessment using the Silicone Study classification system, with respect to type of contraction (64%), number of involved clock-hours (77%), posterior PVR (67%), anterior and posterior PVR (88%) and anterior, posterior and subretinal PVR (94%). The reproducibility of the Retina Society classification was 99%. The Silicone Study classification scheme, using the location of PVR, predicted visual acuity and hypotony [hypotony more frequent with anterior and posterior PVR versus posterior (only) PVR], whereas the original Retina Society classification only predicted visual acuity outcomes by the severity of the PVR.

SURGICAL PROCEDURE

Because vitrectomies for PVR may be extremely complicated procedures, the surgeon ideally should have a full armamentarium of basic instruments at his/her disposal. The basic equipment needed includes a vitreous cutter, end-grabbing diamond-dusted forceps, an illuminated pick, membrane peeler–cutter (MPC) scissors, endodiathermy, endolaser and backflush brush. The surgeon also should be flexible enough to substitute other instruments when necessary. Perfluorocarbon liquid, perfluoropropane gas and silicone oil should be available as well.

In lesser grades of PVR (grades A and B), a scleral buckle can be used as the sole treatment for adequate relief of traction. However, most eyes with greater than 6 clock-hours of PVR, and many eyes with lesser grades, will require vitrectomy. If a vitrectomy is required to reattach a retina with PVR, and the eye does not have a scleral buckle, an encircling element should be placed to support the vitreous base. We most often use a no. 42 band, which is 4.0 mm wide. It should be placed just posterior to the vitreous base and tightened to achieve moderate height. We place the sutures before the vitrectomy because the eye is firmer, making it easier to pass the sutures. The buckling element is placed after the vitrectomy has been completed. If there is a pre-existing encircling element, generally we do not revise it. Occasionally it may be necessary to supplement a scleral buckle, especially in the inferior 180°, to provide further support. If there is only a radial element, it is usually removed and replaced with an encircling element.

For a vitrectomy, we use a three-port vitrectomy system. Sclerotomy sites are usually made 3 mm posterior to the limbus through the anterior pars plana. If the PVR displaces the retina anteriorly, the sclerotomies are made closer to the limbus through the ciliary processes. Eyes with retinal detachments and PVR often have had previous surgery; therefore, the sclera should be examined for previous sclerotomies. We prefer to make new sclerotomy sites, rather than reusing previous ones. Sometimes it is necessary to make a radial sclerotomy with a microvitreoretinal (MVR) blade (Alcon, Fort Worth, TX) to prevent the extension of sclerotomy sites into previous sclerotomies. We use a 4-mm infusion port and the tip is visualized before starting the infusion to ensure that the tip has penetrated the pigmented and nonpigmented epithelium of the pars plana. This

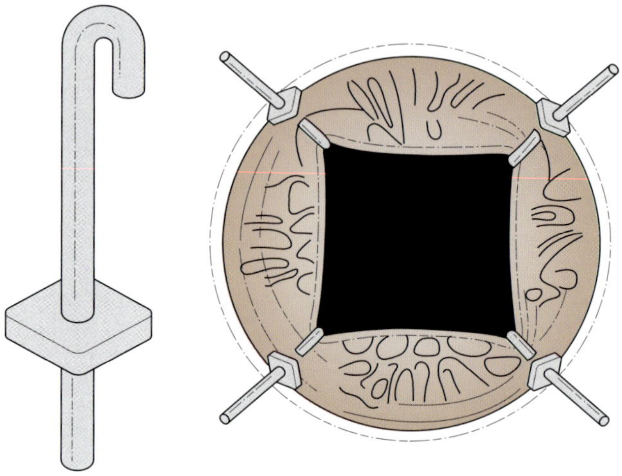

Figure 27.10 *Flexible iris retractors used for pupillary stretching.*

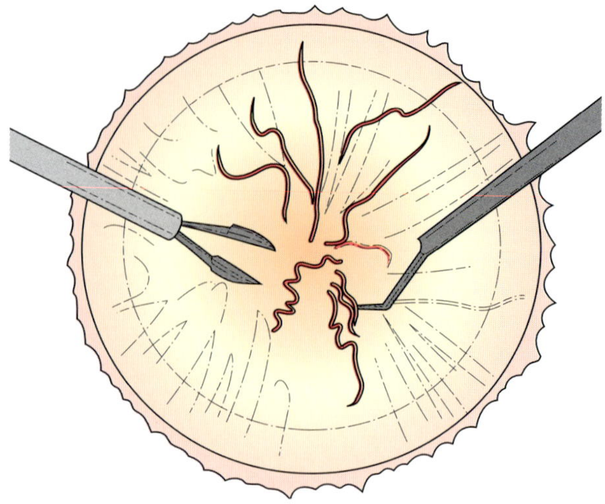

Figure 27.11 *The illuminated pick and the diamond-dusted forceps are the primary instruments used for membrane peeling in proliferative vitreoretinopathy.*

is done in order to prevent subretinal or choroidal infusion.

If the pupil dilates poorly, several procedures are undertaken to enlarge the pupil adequately. Initially, all synechiae are lysed and all residual capsular material is removed. Flexible iris retractors (Grieshaber, Inc., Kennesaw, GA), which are mechanical pupillary stretching devices, are utilized to dilate the pupil (Fig. 27.10).[33] A Ziegler-type blade is used to create four limbal incisions approximately 90° from each other. The openings are also made just parallel and anterior to the iris plane. After the hooks are placed appropriately, they are secured with an external locking device at the limbus.

Any manipulations of the lens may be performed at this point. If the nucleus is extremely hard or if an IOL must be removed, it is done through the limbus and the wound is sutured with closely placed 10-0 nylon sutures. Otherwise, the lens nucleus and cortex are removed with pars plana ultrasound fragmentation. Next, an opening is made through the anterior capsule with a vitreous cutter. The peripheral capsule then is grasped with the vitreous forceps, pulling the zonules centrally until they are visible through the pupil. The zonules then are cut with the MPC scissors (Alcon, Fort Worth, TX). Complete removal of the capsule will likely prevent the development of anterior PVR adhering to the lens capsule and also will prevent synechiae formation between the iris and lens capsule.[34]

We utilize a lens ring and a contact lens set to visualize the retina for a vitrectomy. The lens ring is sutured at the limbus, over the pupil-stretching devices, if they are present. Several different contact lenses may be necessary to visualize the retina. A planoconcave lens allows posterior visualization, while a prism lens provides views of the periphery.[35] In some situations, a wide-angle system with an image inverter is utilized, and is especially useful when there is a constricted view from an opacified capsule associated with a posterior chamber IOL.[36]

We perform a core vitrectomy and then remove the bulk of the peripheral vitreous with a vitreous cutting instrument. Membrane peeling is performed using a bimanual technique with an illuminated pick and diamond-dusted forceps (Fig. 27.11). The dissection is begun posteriorly. Membranes are elevated with the illuminated pick and then are grasped with the forceps, peeling the membranes anteriorly. If hemorrhage occurs, raising the infusion bottle usually provides adequate hemostasis. Occasionally, this maneuver will not control the bleeding and cautery with endodiathermy will be necessary.

Although membrane edges are usually visible, they may sometimes be difficult to identify. Subtle signs of the presence of membranes include obscuration of retinal vessels or a soft gray appearance of the retina. If a starfold is encountered, the illuminated pick is slipped into the fold and pulled centrally until the membrane is engaged (Fig. 27.12). After the edge has been elevated,

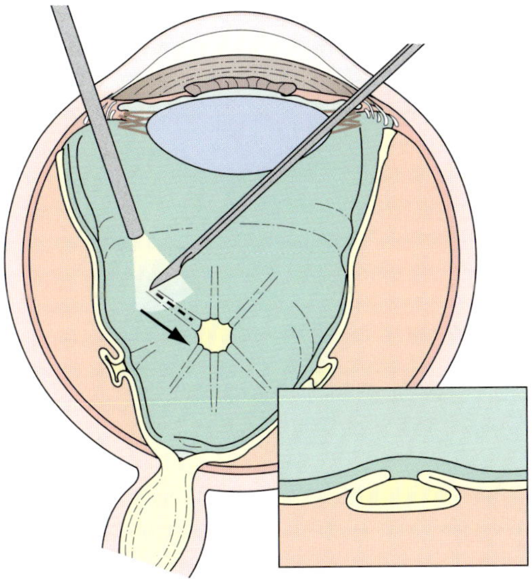

Figure 27.12 *Starfold membranes are engaged by stripping toward the center of the radiating folds. There is redundant retina obscured within the fold of retina, beneath the membrane.*

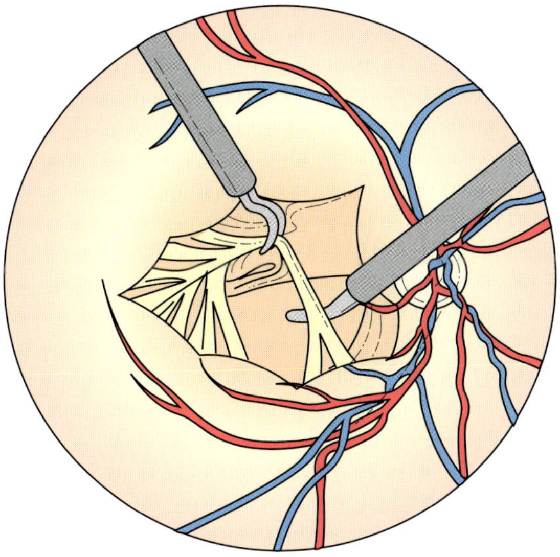

Figure 27.14 *Bimanual technique for membrane peeling. The retina is held back against the blunt edge of the pick as the membrane is stripped with the forceps.*

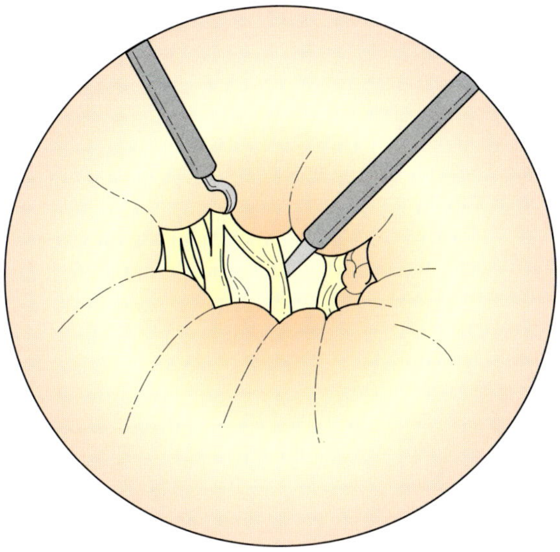

Figure 27.13 *Bimanual technique for membrane engagement. The membrane is engaged with the pick and then grasped with the forceps.*

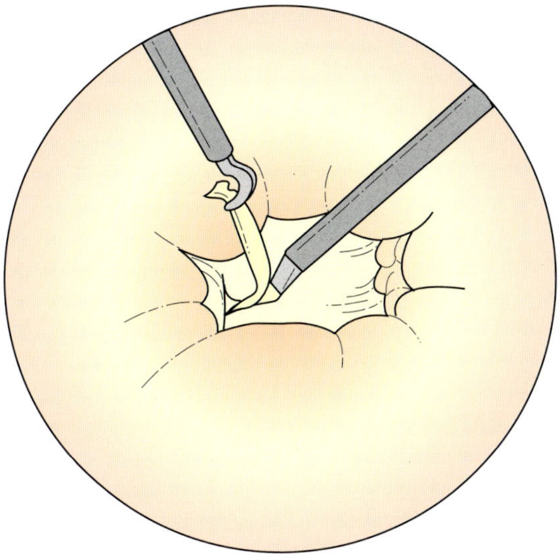

Figure 27.15 *Bimanual technique for membrane removal. The blunt portion of the membrane pick is held at the junction between the retina and membrane, creating a plane, as the retina is pulled centrally.*

the forceps are used to grasp the membrane (Fig. 27.13). Membrane stripping is achieved by placing the blunt portion of the pick against the retina for fixation, as the membrane is pulled centrally by the forceps (Fig. 27.14). This maneuver allows the instruments to develop a plane between the membrane and retina, thereby facilitating removal of the membrane from the surface of the retina (Fig. 27.15). This procedure should be repeated until all membranes have been separated meticulously from the retina.

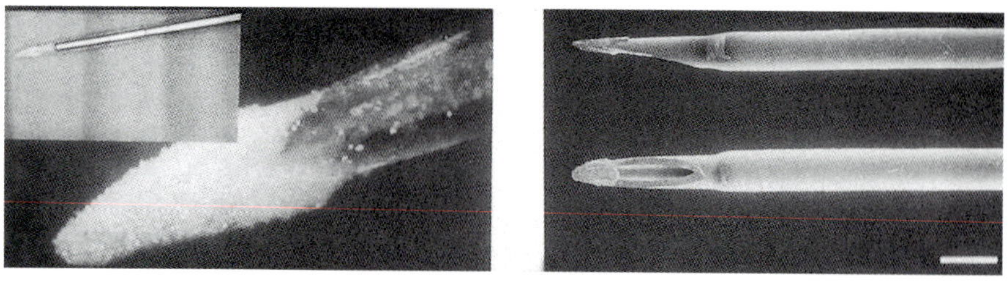

Figure 27.16 *Diamond-dusted silicone cannula used for immature membrane removal.*

Occasionally, it is necessary to use a sharp membrane pick. To engage tightly adherent membranes, we prefer to use a barbed MVR blade, which is created by pushing the blade tip against a flat metal surface of another instrument.

Immature membranes present special problems. They fragment easily during membrane stripping, requiring special attention to ensure that all the pieces have been removed. Sometimes they cannot be grasped adequately with the forceps. In this situation, the immature sheets of cells and fibrin are stroked with the silicone tip of a backflush brush to elevate them from the surface of the retina. The brush also can be used to remove pigmented cells from the retinal surface. Another instrument that is useful for separating immature membranes is the diamond-dusted silicone cannula (Fig. 27.16).[37]

As the membrane peeling is carried out progressively from posterior to anterior retina, one will often find the posterior hyaloid adherent to peripheral membranes posterior to horseshoe tears and the vitreous base. There may be membranes that result from RPE cell proliferation at the junction between the vitreous and peripheral retina. Progressive contraction of these membranes will drag the posterior hyaloid down against the retina, creating a firm attachment posterior to peripheral breaks and the vitreous base. It is important to recognize this phenomenon to ensure that the vitreous is stripped anteriorly to its base. This is accomplished with a bimanual technique, as described above, whereby forceps are used to pull the hyaloid centrally and the blunt edge of an illuminated pick is used to separate the vitreous from the retina. This technique also allows the surgeon to identify the posterior edge of the vitreous base. Once the vitreous has been stripped to its base, it should be trimmed with the vitreous cutter.

After the traction from posterior and peripheral membranes has been released, the retina becomes very mobile and bullous, making the peripheral vitrectomy more difficult and hazardous and increasing the risk of vitreous or retinal incarceration into the sclerotomy sites. This is especially true in the presence of an associated pars plana detachment. Perfluorocarbon liquid (PFCL) can be used to stabilize and fixate the posterior retina, allowing further peripheral vitreous and membrane removal, as well as preventing retinal incarceration at the sclerotomy sites (Fig. 27.17).[38] Before using the PFCL, it is very important to separate all of the posterior membranes. Excessive traction, even on a small retinal break, may allow PFCL to slip beneath the retina. Initially, a small volume of PFCL (approximately 1 ml) is injected over the optic nerve. The PFCL should not be injected directly over a retinal break because the stream produced may force it subretinally. Only enough PFCL is injected to flatten the retina posterior to the vitreous. Excessive PFCL will cover and compress the remaining vitreous and make

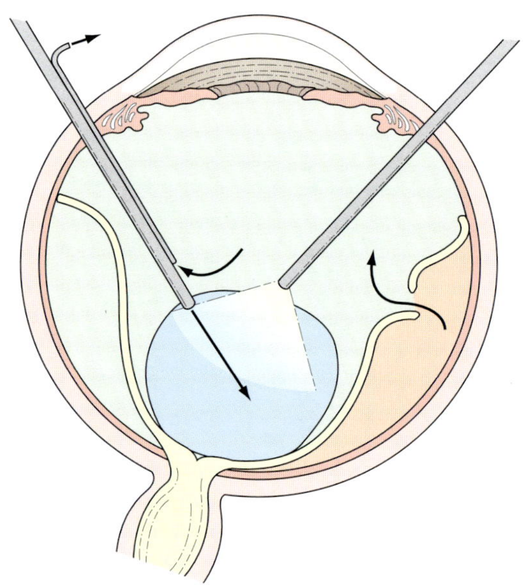

Figure 27.17 *Perfluorocarbon liquid bubble stabilizes the retina posteriorly, facilitating anterior membrane removal.*

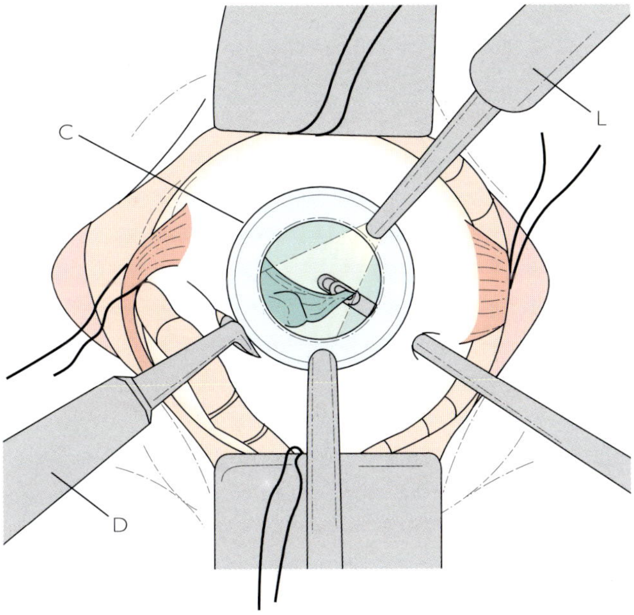

Figure 27.18 *Vitreous base shaving. A light pipe is held against the contact lens to provide illumination. As the vitreous base is pushed into view with the scleral depressor, the vitreous is trimmed carefully to its base with the vitreous cutter. C, contact lens; D, depressor; L, light pipe.*

removal difficult. As the dissection is carried out progressively toward the anterior retina, supplemental injections of PFCL can be given to provide further posterior stabilization of the retina.

After all membrane peeling has been completed, the vitreous base should be excised down to the retinal surface. During the vitreous base shaving, the PFCL will fixate the retina, preventing inadvertent aspiration of mobile retina into the vitreous cutter. Visualization for this step can be achieved using either a standard lens system (hand-held or sutured lens ring) with scleral depression or a wide-angle viewing system without depression. With the former method, the peripheral retina is depressed, bringing the vitreous base into view, and the vitreous is excised with the vitreous cutter. Visualization can be obtained with endoillumination or, alternatively, the fiberoptic light probe can be positioned against the contact lens outside the eye to illuminate the vitreous base (Fig. 27.18). The 125° wide-angle lens with an image inversion system and a 'bullet' light probe can be used to provide broad diffuse illumination to allow the vitreous base to be visualized directly without scleral depression. The wide-angle lens system does not afford good stereopsis and has low magnification, therefore it is not as useful in PVR cases as the standard lens system, which provides better visualization of the vitreous base and peripheral retina.

If anterior membranes are present, they must be dissected from the retinal surface.[22,39] Focal and diffuse anterior membranes are removed with a bimanual technique, similar to the approach used to peel posterior membranes. The most difficult type of anterior PVR to manage is anterior retinal displacement, which is the result of membranes extending from the peripheral retina (posterior to the vitreous base) to more anterior ocular structures, such as the pars plana, ciliary processes or iris. This produces both anterior–posterior and circumferential traction, resulting in the development of a circumferential 'trough' at the vitreous base between the anteriorly displaced retina and undisplaced anterior retina and pars plana (see Fig. 27.8). Usually, anteriorly displaced retina can be identified easily, but it can be very subtle and easily missed.

In some cases, the only sign of anterior displacement is a fibrous circumferential membrane adherent to the pars plana or ciliary processes. In order to release the anterior–posterior traction, the membrane producing the trough must be removed. An MVR blade may be necessary to create an opening in the membrane, which then is extended circumferentially with vertically cutting vitreoretinal scissors (Fig. 27.19). As the membrane is incised, the traction will relax and the anteriorly displaced retina should begin to settle posteriorly. The remaining membranes produce circumferential traction. They can be separated partially with a bimanual dissection, using the illuminated pick and forceps. Although the vitreous cannot be stripped from its base, the epiretinal membranes usually can be separated. The membranes and vitreous should be trimmed with a vitreous cutter to the vitreous base. If there is any remaining circumferential traction from incomplete removal of the membrane, vertically cutting scissors, such as the MPC, should be used to create multiple vertical sections through remnants of the membrane. During this dissection process, retinal breaks sometimes can occur. All breaks should be identified, and any remaining traction around them should be relieved.

After all the membranes have been removed, the retina is reattached with either an injection of PFCL or a fluid–air exchange. If the former technique is chosen, enough PFCL is introduced to reach the vitreous base. The PFCL level should not reach the infusion cannula tip because the fluid stream will

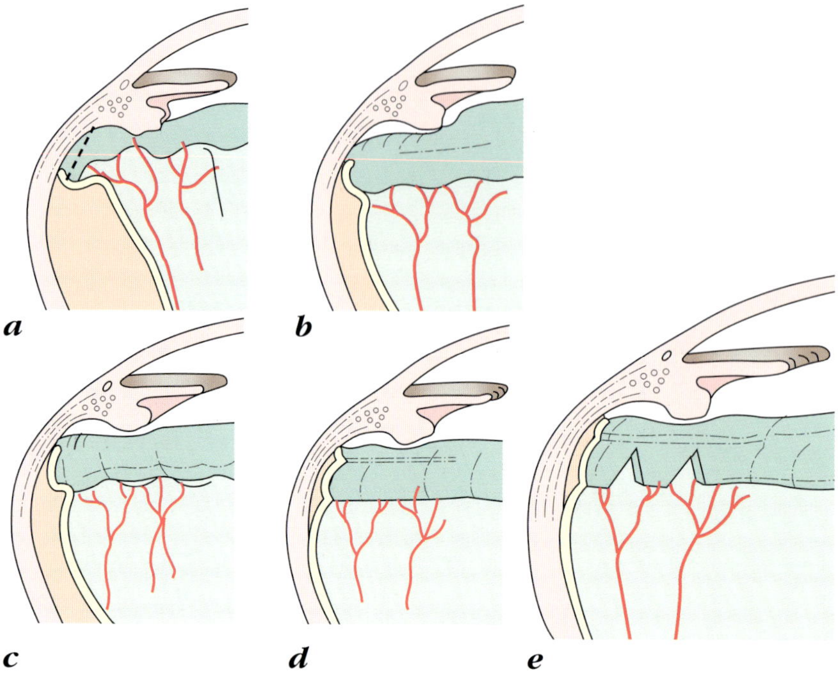

Figure 27.19 *(a) An incision (dotted line) with either a sharp blade or scissors, is made into the trough to release anterior–posterior traction. (b) Anterior–posterior contraction within the vitreous base has led to a reduction in the meridional distance between the anterior and posterior vitreous base insertions. (c) Traction from circumferentially contracted vitreous is relieved by making multiple vertical incisions (dotted line) with vertically cutting scissors. (d) Relief of circumferential traction after vertical incisions have been made, resulting in the disappearance of meridional pleat-like folds. (e) Circumferential vitreous base traction is eradicated by multiple wedge-like incisions of the posterior insertion without full-width radial transections of the vitreous base.*

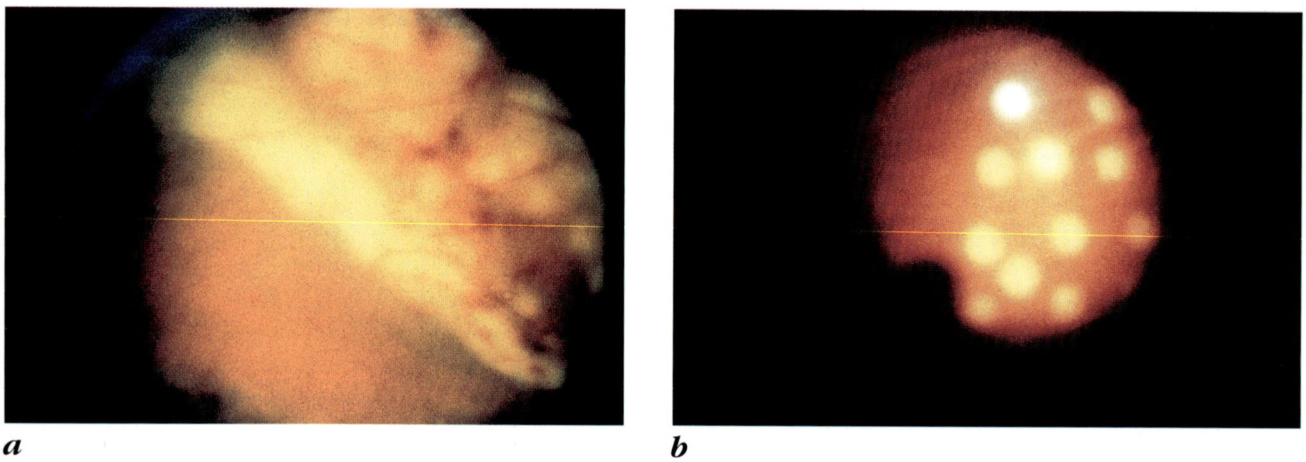

Figure 27.20 *(a) Excessive laser treatment to the peripheral retina on a scleral buckle. (b) Proper scatter laser treatment with each laser burn placed approximately one burn width apart.*

create multiple bubbles of PFCL. The small bubbles not only may compromise the view but also may enter the subretinal space through retinal breaks.

Laser photocoagulation is performed under PFCL.[40] The initial settings are usually at low power with 0.5-second duration. The power is increased until a moderately intense burn is achieved. Initially, the edges of the retinal breaks are treated with confluent laser burns, then 360° scatter photocoagulation in two to three rows is placed on the scleral buckle. For the scatter treatment, each laser burn should be placed one burn width apart (Fig. 27.20). Confluent treatment should be avoided on the scleral buckle because it may obstruct venous return from the ciliary body to the vortex veins, leading to postoperative increases in the IOP and possibly late hypotony.

The PFCL is removed during a fluid–air exchange. Before removing the PFCL, subretinal fluid anterior to

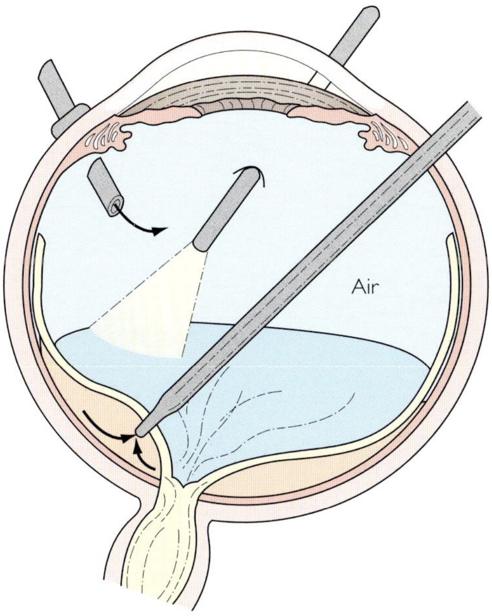

Figure 27.21 *Fluid–air exchange with posterior retinal break. Subretinal fluid is aspirated from a posterior retinal break as the eye is filled simultaneously with air.*

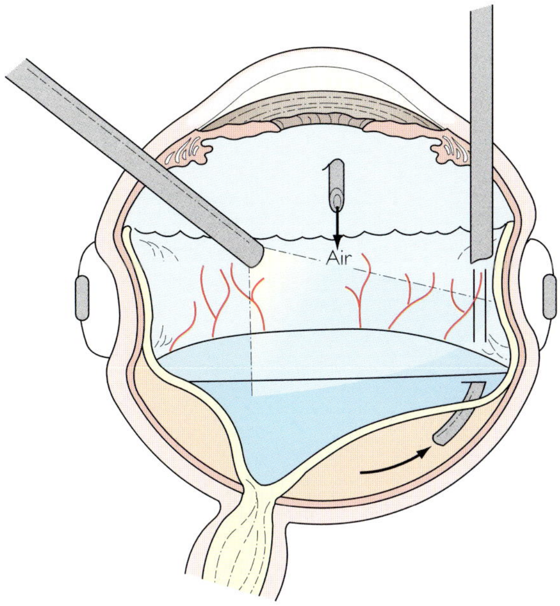

Figure 27.22 *Fluid–air exchange with peripheral retinal break. Drainage retinotomy is created anteriorly in an area supported by the scleral buckle. The extendable soft silicone tubing of a cannulated extrusion needle is passed through the retinotomy into the subretinal space.*

the PFCL is aspirated through anterior retinal breaks with a soft-tipped needle. A wide-angle system or indirect ophthalmoscopy will provide adequate visualization for this procedure. After all the subretinal fluid has been removed, the PFCL is aspirated. If perfluoro-*n*-octane is used, it can be identified easily and removed. Minuscule amounts on the retinal surface will evaporate at body temperature. Perfluorodecalin and perfluoroperhydrophenanthrene do not evaporate and are more difficult to identify. Therefore, a small aliquot of balanced saline is injected over the posterior pole to help detect any remaining PFCL, so that it can be removed.

Alternatively, a fluid–air exchange may be used to reattach the retina (Fig. 27.21). Initially, all retinal breaks should be marked with the endodiathermy. Either an active suction device, such as soft silicone-tipped needle, or an extrusion device, such as a backflush brush, is used to drain the subretinal fluid from a retinal break. It is generally easier to use a posterior retinal break, although it is also possible to drain through a peripheral break. In the latter case, an extendable cannulated extrusion needle can be placed in the break to provide access into the posterior subretinal space for fluid drainage (Fig. 27.22). However, in most cases, a nonextendable, soft-tipped cannula will be sufficient to remove the subretinal fluid. If a break is not present in an accessible area for drainage, then an endodiathermy probe is used to create a peripheral break in a location supported by the scleral buckle. After the retina has been reattached, laser is applied, as described above with the PFCL.

If the retina has not been mobilized enough to be reattached despite the removal of all epiretinal membranes, then further steps may be necessary. Persistent traction usually can be identified. However, in some cases it is discovered intraoperatively as air, PFCL or silicone oil migrates into the subretinal space. This may be the result of inadequate relief of anterior traction or the presence of subretinal membranes. Subretinal membranes often do not have to be removed because they usually do not prevent reattachment of the retina.[11,19] Because only 25% of subretinal membranes can be identified preoperatively, a careful intraoperative examination should be performed if unexplained traction is present.[19]

The surgical approach to subretinal membranes depends upon the type and location of the membrane. If there is an isolated band that has a

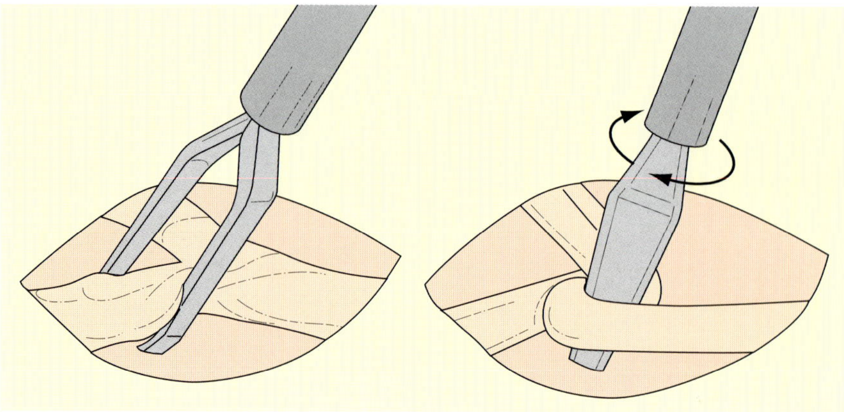

Figure 27.23 *Spaghetti-rolling technique for subretinal band removal. The membrane is grasped with the forceps and rolled in the hands of the surgeon.*

'clothes-line' appearance, a small retinotomy is created with endodiathermy. It is sometimes necessary to utilize a sharp instrument, such as a blade or scissors, to create an opening into the subretinal space. The retinotomy then can be extended, if necessary, with scissors. The retinotomy should be made adjacent to the membrane but as far as possible from the posterior pole. A superior retinotomy is preferable. Once the retinotomy has been created, forceps are used to grasp the membrane and gently pull to determine whether it will strip free. If the membrane is attached to the choroid and is pulled too aggressively, it may cause a choroidal hemorrhage. If the membrane can be stripped easily, it may be removed with a spaghetti-rolling technique (Fig. 27.23). While the membrane is grasped with the forceps, the instrument is rolled in the hands of the surgeon, wrapping the membrane around the forceps. If the membrane cannot be removed, it may be necessary to section it with scissors, which will sometimes cause the ends of the membranes to retract, relieving the traction (Fig. 27.24).

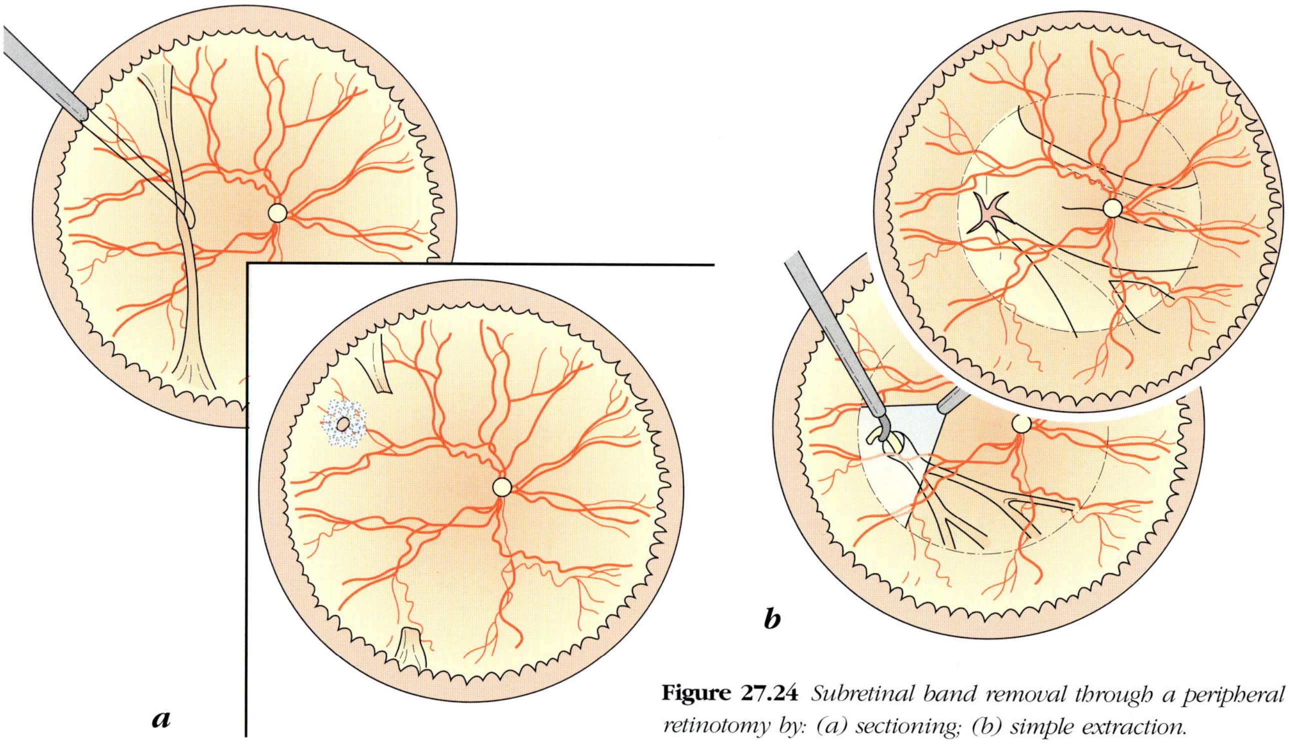

Figure 27.24 *Subretinal band removal through a peripheral retinotomy by: (a) sectioning; (b) simple extraction.*

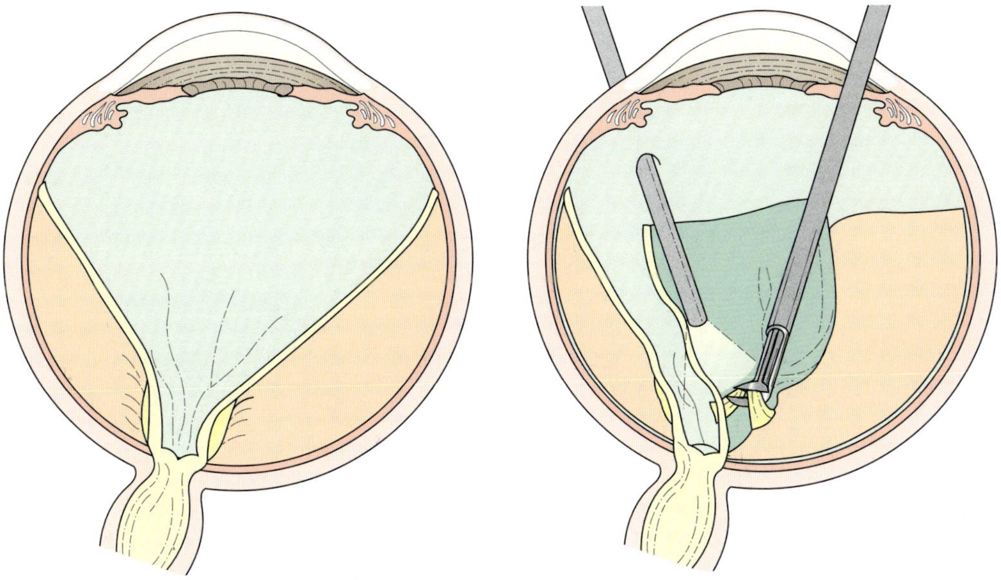

Figure 27.25 *(a) Subretinal napkin-ring removal. (b) Large peripheral retinotomy is created to allow adequate access, and the traction is relieved by membrane stripping.*

If the subretinal membrane has a sheet or latticework configuration, a larger peripheral retinotomy may be necessary. A posterior retinotomy should be avoided, because there is a risk of enlargement with resultant hemorrhage and visual field loss. A small peripheral retinotomy also may enlarge during stripping, so a retinotomy of adequate proportions should be made to remove the membrane. Occasionally, to allow adequate access for subretinal membrane removal, it is necessary to create a large enough peripheral retinotomy to allow the retina to be folded over. As the membrane is stripped, the retina should be observed carefully and excessive traction should be avoided.

The subretinal membranes that are most difficult to remove are those with a napkin-ring configuration, which is an annular membrane around the posterior retina. A peripheral retinotomy is created to allow access for membrane stripping (Fig. 27.25). Because these membranes are so difficult to remove, a very large retinotomy of 90° or even 180° will be necessary to provide direct visual exposure for membrane removal. If the subretinal membrane cannot be stripped from the undersurface of the retina, it may be necessary to section it in order to relieve traction adequately.

The other major indication for a relaxing retinotomy is unrelieved anterior traction, despite full membrane dissection. The retinotomy is made circumferentially and posterior to the scarred, organized retina. Initially, the area to be resected should be diathermized carefully to prevent hemorrhage, and then vertical cutting scissors are used to incise the retina. The retinotomy should continue into uninvolved retina on each side, extending beyond the area of contraction (Fig. 27.26). Each end should be angled anteriorly toward the ora serrata or, when

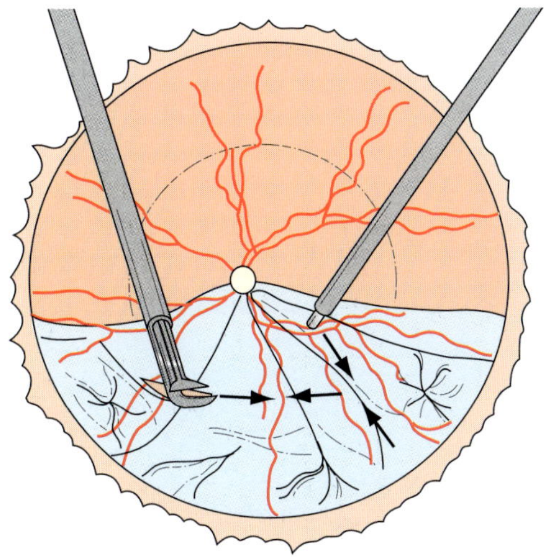

Figure 27.26 *Relaxing retinotomy technique: initially, the retina to be incised is diathermized; vertically cutting scissors are used to cut along the posterior edge of the contracted retina; the incision is extended into normal retina on each side.*

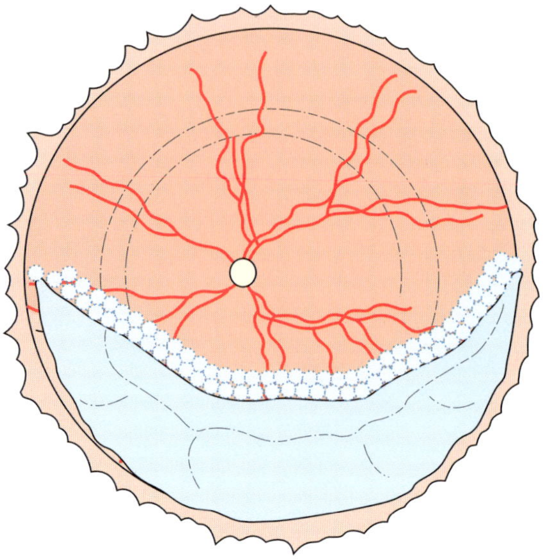

Figure 27.27 *Relaxing retinotomy: each end of the retinotomy is extended anteriorly to the ora serrata or the ciliary body (if pars plana involved); the retina anterior to the retinotomy is excised.*

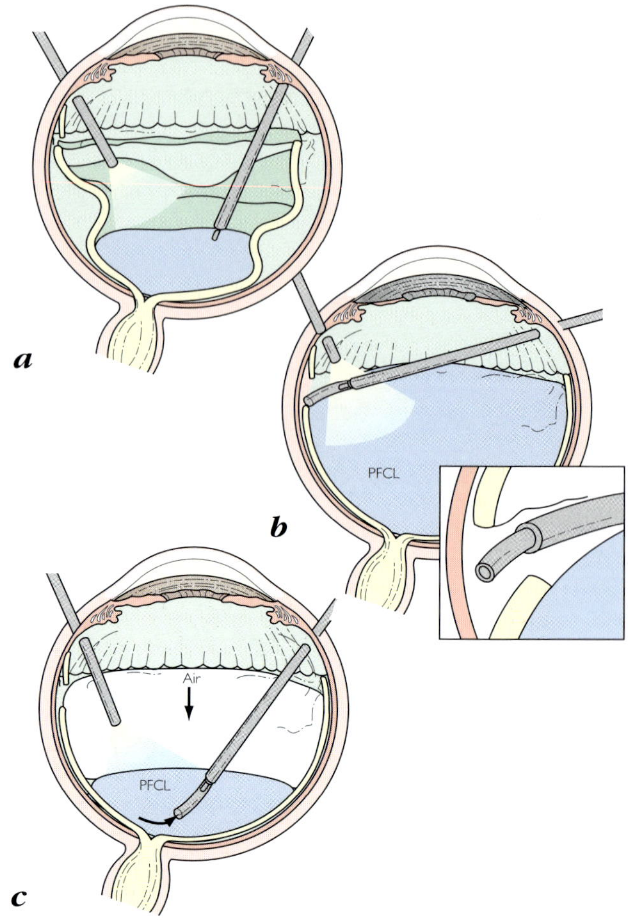

Figure 27.28 *Unfolding a large retinotomy with a perfluorocarbon liquid (PFCL). (a) The PFCL is injected over the posterior pole to unfold the flap of the giant retinal tear. After all the membranes have been removed, the PFCL can be injected anterior to the edge to reattach the retina completely. (b) Fluid–air exchange: the fluid anterior to the PFCL bubble is exchanged with air and then a soft-tipped needle is used to aspirate any remaining fluid behind the edge of the tear, to prevent slippage. (c) Perfluorocarbon liquid–air exchange: after the edge has been 'dried', the PFCL is removed with a soft-tipped needle and exchanged for air.*

the pars plana is detached, toward the posterior edge of the ciliary processes (Fig. 27.27). The remaining contracted and devitalized retina anterior to the retinotomy is excised with the vitreous cutter, because later it may contract circumferentially and exert traction on the ciliary body. Radial retinotomies are generally avoided because they often only inadequately relieve traction and may extend posteriorly, leading to poorer visual acuities.[41]

Making a retinotomy greater than 90° creates the problem of managing a giant retinal tear. The ideal method for reattaching the retina is to use PFCL, because it does not require manipulation of the flap under gas or air.[42] All of the traction must be relieved before using the PFCL. Unrelieved traction not only will prevent retinal reattachment but also may lead to subretinal migration of PFCL.

Initially, the PFCL is injected carefully over the posterior pole. As the bubble enlarges, it steamrolls the subretinal fluid anteriorly, flattening the retina. The PFCL should be infused until it flattens the edge of the giant tear. The PFCL level can extend anterior to the giant tear if all the traction has been relieved. The edge of the tear is treated with several rows of laser and the PFCL is exchanged for air, followed by gas or silicone oil. If the retinotomy is made 180° or more, there is a risk of retinal slippage during the air exchange. In order to prevent this complication, an air exchange is performed anterior to the flap and then fluid underneath the anterior edge of the retinotomy is aspirated with a soft silicone-tipped needle (Fig. 27.28). Visualization is achieved with either a wide-angle viewing system or an indirect ophthalmoscope. If the edge is not 'dried' before exchanging the PFCL for air, the fluid will be forced posteriorly, allowing posterior slippage of the edge of the tear.

INTRAOCULAR TAMPONADE FOR PROLIFERATIVE VITREORETINOPATHY

After the retina has been reattached under air, there are several choices for an intraocular tamponade. The Silicone Study concluded that silicone oil and perfluoropropane gas (C_3F_8) were equally efficacious in most respects for the management of PVR, and both modalities were superior to sulfur hexafluoride gas (SF_6).[27,43] Although the choice of tamponade is often made preoperatively by joint determination by the surgeon and the patient, intraoperative factors also may have significant influence on the decision. Perfluoropropane gas is preferred over silicone oil in some situations. C_3F_8 gas is preferred, if silicone oil is likely to herniate into the anterior chamber and contact the corneal endothelium.[44] Eyes at risk for this problem are those in which the iris diaphragm has been violated or those with an IOL without an intact iris–capsular–IOL diaphragm. Another indication for C_3F_8 is the presence of a large choroidal or subretinal hemorrhage, which precludes the possibility of an adequate silicone oil fill. If there is a retinal break at the base of a high scleral buckle, gas is preferred. Because silicone oil tends to retain a spherical configuration, it does not conform well to the shape of an excessively high scleral buckle and may not adequately tamponade the break.[45]

Silicone oil is preferred, however, for patients who cannot reliably maintain prone positioning (such as children or those who are mentally or physically impaired). Eyes at high risk for postoperative hypotony, such as those with preoperative hypotony, severe anterior PVR or giant retinotomies, should have a silicone oil tamponade.[46,47] Silicone oil also is used for patients who must travel by air or to higher elevations, or for patients who require a rapid visual recovery.[48,49]

If silicone oil is used, an inferior iridectomy is created in an aphakic eye to prevent herniation of the oil into the anterior chamber due to pupillary block. In pseudophakic eyes, an inferior iridectomy is unnecessary if the iris–capsular–IOL diaphragm is intact. If there is a posterior chamber lens with a violated diaphragm, an anterior chamber lens or the silicone oil herniates around the IOL into the anterior chamber, then an inferior iridectomy should be created in an attempt to keep the oil out of the anterior chamber (Fig. 27.29). If the silicone oil enters the anterior chamber in spite of an iridectomy, it may be the result of capsular or fibrous material obstructing the iridectomy, therefore it

a

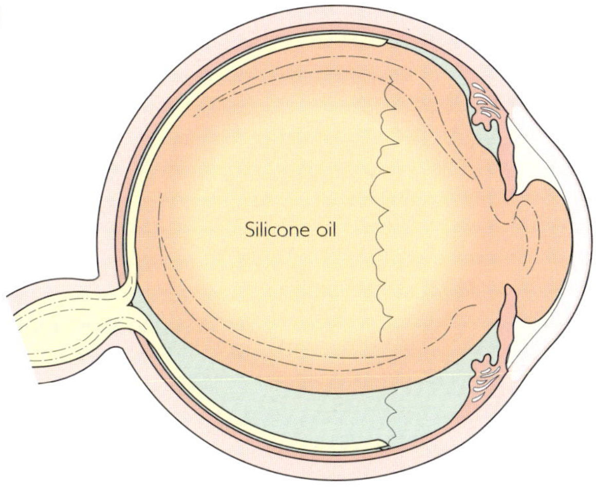

b

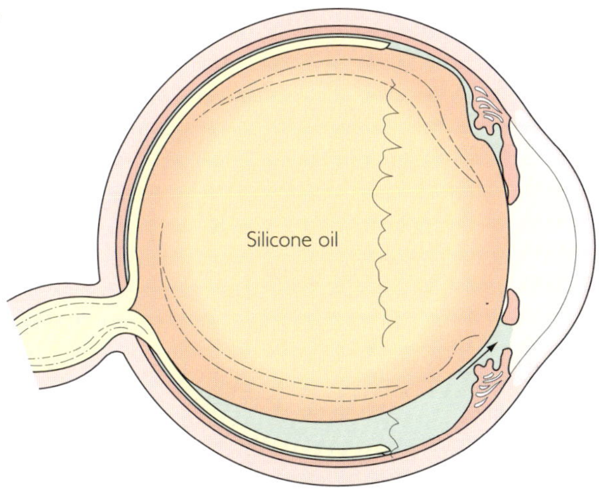

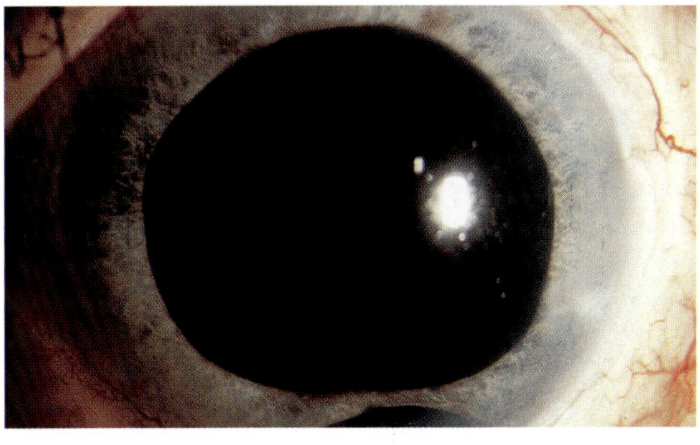

c

Figure 27.29 *Inferior iridectomy for silicone oil. (a) Without a patent inferior iridectomy, the silicone oil herniates into the anterior chamber secondary to a pupillary block mechanism. (b) An inferior iridectomy allows the aqueous to enter the anterior chamber, relieving the pupillary block. (c) Proper placement of an inferior iridectomy.*

is crucial that the patency be confirmed intraoperatively. Sometimes the silicone oil can be forced posteriorly by an injection of viscoelastic material into the anterior chamber.

Silicone oil can be infused into the eye in several different ways. The retina can be reattached by directly exchanging the fluid in the eye after vitrectomy for silicone oil (fluid–silicone oil exchange). Alternatively, the retina can be reattached with PFCL, which is then exchanged for silicone oil (PFCL–silicone exchange). However, in most cases, the eye is air-filled at the end of the case. In air-filled eyes, we usually infuse 5000-cSt silicone oil, which has high viscosity and requires high-pressure tubing if injected through the infusion port. Before infusing the silicone oil in phakic patients, we close one of the sclerotomy sites and leave the infusion port connected to the air pump. The silicone oil is placed in a syringe connected to an 18- or 20-gauge needle (Angiocath, Becton Dickinson Infusion Therapy Systems, Sandy, UT) that is trimmed at an angle to a length of approximately 10 mm. The air pump maintains a constant preset low pressure as the silicone oil is injected up to the level of the lens. In aphakic eyes, both sclerotomies are closed and the infusion port is removed. The air pump is connected to a 27-gauge needle, which is placed through the pars plana temporally and positioned at the plane of the pupil to maintain the intraocular pressure at a normal level. Silicone oil is injected through the previous infusion port site through an angiocath until it reaches the iris plane. The anterior chamber should maintain its normal depth. If it becomes shallow, then some of the oil should be removed and the anterior chamber should be reformed with an air injection at the limbus. The target IOP after the silicone oil injection should be at the low range of normal, to ensure that the eye has not been inadvertently overfilled or underfilled.

POSTOPERATIVE MANAGEMENT

Careful postoperative management is crucial to the ultimate success following PVR procedures. One of the most common complications is an elevated IOP. Han et al found that 36% of patients undergoing vitrectomy developed an IOP of 30 mmHg or greater.[50] Extreme rises in IOP can cause vascular occlusions and lead to visual loss. Some eyes undergoing vitrectomy may have a loss of light perception, resulting from high IOP. However, with prompt control of the IOP some will achieve significant recovery of vision,[51] therefore it is crucial to manage the IOP carefully. Eyes undergoing repair of PVR often are at higher risk because they have had very extensive previous procedures. A previous history of glaucoma, placement of a scleral buckle, a lensectomy, scatter photocoagulation, intraocular tamponade and the development of postoperative fibrin are all factors that place these eyes at particular risk.[50]

At the end of the operation, the IOP should be measured and left in the normal range. In addition, the patient is placed in a prone position and eyes at high risk are given prophylactic treatment with immediate postoperative topical medications, including a beta-blocker, an alpha-agonist, a carbonic anhydrase inhibitor and a prostaglandin analog. The IOP should be checked at a minimum approximately 2 and 4 hours after the procedure, but further IOP checks may be necessary. In most cases the IOP can be managed medically, but if the IOP remains elevated then a tap may be necessary. Usually an anterior chamber paracentesis will provide adequate control, and only rarely will it be necessary to tap for gas or silicone oil.

Increases in IOP may be related to pupillary block from postoperative fibrin formation. The fibrin also may interfere with postoperative management, such as a fluid–gas exchange. To control inflammation and fibrin formation, we give postoperative subconjunctival dexamethasone, as well as frequent postoperative topical corticosteroids. Significant fibrin formation is treated with an intraocular injection of tissue plasminogen activator (tPA).[52] The tPA (3 μg in 0.1 ml) is injected with a 30-gauge needle through the limbus. To prevent intraocular hemorrhage, we usually do not administer tPA before 48–72 hours after surgery.

Pupillary block from intraocular gas or silicone oil may lead to a flat anterior chamber by physically pushing the iris against the cornea. In silicone-filled eyes, this is more likely to occur if the peripheral iridectomy has closed. If the iridectomy is occluded with fibrin, tPA may be used to open it. Proper positioning, either on the side or in the prone position, will prevent this complication in gas-filled eyes. If iridocorneal adhesions occur, viscoelastic can be used to separate the adhesions and reform the anterior chamber.

Because eyes with PVR are likely to have undergone several surgical procedures, they are at high risk for postoperative corneal complications, including erosions, bullous keratopathy and filamentary keratitis. Corneal complications after vitrectomy may be as high as 27–43%.[44,53,54] Postoperative erosions usually will respond to patching and emollients.

A persistent erosion may heal with a bandage contact lens. Rarely, a temporary tarsorrhaphy is necessary to promote re-epithelialization of the cornea.

Gas- and silicone-filled eyes are managed differently during the postoperative period. An eye adequately filled with an intraocular tamponade is crucial for the ultimate success of the surgery, especially in the presence of inferior retinal breaks. In eyes with perfluorocarbon gas, we prefer to have at least an 80% fill. If there is an inadequate gas bubble, a postoperative fluid–gas exchange is performed to augment the bubble.[55–58] In phakic or pseudophakic eyes, the exchange is performed through the pars plana. Five percent povidone–iodine solution is used to sterilize the lids and the conjunctiva. The patient is placed on the side of the surgical eye, and a 30-gauge needle attached to a 10-cc syringe filled with perfluorocarbon gas (usually 14% C_3F_8) is inserted nasally into the vitreous cavity through the pars plana. A second 27-gauge needle attached to a 10-cc syringe is placed in the dependent portion of the eye, which is temporal. Fluid is aspirated from the dependent syringe as the eye is filled simultaneously with gas from the non-dependent syringe. The volume aspirated is equalized with the volume of gas injected. The exchange is performed in a stepwise fashion by aspirating 0.5 ml of fluid and then filling the eye with 0.5 ml of 14% C_3F_8, until the exchange has been completed. In order to prevent extreme fluctuations in IOP, it is important to exchange small and equal amounts of fluid and gas. The patient's head is rotated into a more prone position during the exchange in order to achieve a more complete gas fill.

In aphakic eyes, the patient is placed in the prone position, a Ziegler-type blade is used to make an incision through the limbus and a 30-gauge needle attached to a syringe filled with 14% C_3F_8 is inserted through the limbal opening. As the eye is filled with gas, the fluid will egress from the eye through the incision around the needle shaft. The limbal incision is usually self-sealing, so after the fluid–gas exchange has been completed the needle can simply be removed.

Gas-filled eyes also must be monitored carefully for recurrent retinal detachments. If this occurs, the cause must be identified. It is usually the result of untreated breaks and/or excessive residual traction. If the pathology in gas-filled eyes is related to the presence of posterior epiretinal membranes, producing posterior retinal folds, a reoperation usually is necessary. If a fluid–gas exchange is attempted, it may produce further tension on the posterior epiretinal membranes, and the retina may tear spontaneously in response to the excessive traction. More commonly, the detachment is secondary to residual anterior traction, which opens an anterior break. In this case, a fluid–gas exchange may safely and effectively flatten the retina.

After the retina has been reattached, several rows of laser treatment should be placed on, and sometimes posterior to, the scleral buckle for 360°.[56] In air- or gas-filled eyes, more effective laser treatment can be achieved by using a panfunduscopic contact lens in conjunction with a longer wavelength laser, such as a diode or krypton red laser, and long exposure times. Although residual fluid may remain anterior to the buckle, it often can be demarcated, allowing the posterior retina to stay attached. Residual anterior retinal detachment sometimes can be associated with postoperative hypotony.

Some postoperative complications related to silicone oil are unlike those of gas and thus require different management. As described previously, an eye filled with silicone oil requires an inferior peripheral iridectomy to prevent pupillary block, and closure of the iridectomy may lead to angle-closure glaucoma as well as corneal touch by the silicone oil. If the iridectomy is occluded by a postoperative fibrin response, tPA can be injected into the anterior chamber as described above. Fibrous proliferation sometimes will contract and close the iridectomy. In this case, the patency can be re-established only by mechanical means. A 25-gauge needle inserted through the limbus at the slit lamp may reopen the iridectomy. If this maneuver is unsuccessful, then the patient should be taken back to the operating room and the iridectomy should be reopened with the vitreous cutter.

Recurrent retinal detachments also must be managed differently in silicone oil-filled eyes than in gas-filled eyes. Because silicone oil is a nonabsorbing tamponade, recurrent peripheral detachments can be observed initially. Sometimes these will reattach without intervention. However, if there is a reproliferation of peripheral membranes, producing significant traction, or if the detachment is rhegmatogenous, then surgical intervention may be indicated. If a reoperation is necessary, the procedure may be performed without removing the silicone oil. The vitrectomy is set up in the normal fashion, except that high-pressure tubing attached to a pump filled with silicone oil is used, rather than the normal infusion tubing. Alternatively, a syringe filled with silicone oil can be used. The silicone oil should be of the same viscosity and made by the same manufacturer as that in the eye.

Peripheral membranes causing traction and retinal detachment usually can be removed under oil. If the detachment is caused by organization of the peripheral retina with foreshortening, a relaxing retinotomy may be necessary, which also can be performed under oil. The retinotomy should be performed as described above. Initially, diathermy should be placed posterior to the area of contraction to achieve hemostasis and the retinotomy is made with vertically cutting scissors. It is important that the retinotomy extends beyond the area of contraction on each side. In order to reattach the retina, the subretinal fluid is removed passively with a soft-tipped silicone cannula such as a backflush brush as silicone oil is injected into the eye. Afterwards, the edge of the retinotomy should be treated with several rows of laser. If there are extensive membranes, the silicone oil may have to be removed with an 18-gauge angiocatheter on a 10-ml syringe. The procedure is then performed in a fluid environment and, following retinal reattachment, the silicone oil can be reinfused.

The silicone oil usually remains in the eye for between 3 and 6 months, although complications may require earlier removal of the oil. The IOP may be increased by oil emulsification blocking the trabecular meshwork, or there may be corneal decompensation from silicone oil touching the endothelium. Macular pucker or recurrent tractional membranes often can be peeled at the time of silicone oil removal. Although it is usually safe to remove the oil, the Silicone Study demonstrated a redetachment rate of approximately 20% following removal of the silicone oil.[59] However, if the eye has a residual peripheral retinal detachment, but the macula remains attached, the oil sometimes is left in place. If the oil is to be removed in eyes with relatively small retinal detachments, the subretinal fluid can sometimes be demarcated with laser. However, in eyes with extensive detachments, it will be necessary to carry out surgical revision and repair at the time of silicone oil removal. The silicone oil should remain in eyes that are hypotonus, even if the retina is attached. Removal of the oil in these eyes often will lead to phthisis.

SURGICAL RESULTS

Two decades ago, surgical management of PVR with scleral buckling techniques led to a retinal reattachment rate of 35%; vitrectomy with membrane peeling was not much more successful, with a reattachment rate of 36–42%.[60–62] The most common cause of anatomic failure in the early repair of eyes with PVR was the development of tissue proliferation at the vitreous base. A better understanding of the pathophysiology of PVR, especially its anterior form, along with improved instrumentation and technique have led to marked advances in the management of PVR. Lewis et al demonstrated significant improvement of both anatomic and visual results in eyes undergoing vitrectomy for retinal detachments resulting from severe PVR.[26] Although the total retinal reattachment rate was 90%, 94% were attached posterior to the scleral buckle. Ambulatory vision, which was defined as a visual acuity of at least 5/200, was achieved in 85% of eyes with complete retinal reattachment. The surgical outcomes were not as favorable for recurrent PVR in eyes that had undergone a previous vitrectomy for PVR.[25] In those eyes, there was a 73% complete retinal reattachment rate and an 86% reattachment rate posterior to the scleral buckle. Ambulatory vision was attained in 67% of eyes with total retinal reattachment.

Eyes that require a relaxing retinotomy may have poor anatomic as well as visual outcome. Morse et al reported 100 eyes undergoing relaxing retinotomies.[41] In their series, 58 eyes were completely attached and eight had partial reattachment with the macula on. Only 43% of eyes with attached maculae had a visual acuity of 5/200 or better. Han et al demonstrated similar results with an anatomic success rate of 64% in eyes with a relaxing retinotomy, with 26% of all eyes attaining ambulatory vision.[63]

Subretinal membrane removal also is a poor prognostic factor when considering the results of surgical repair of PVR. In the largest series examining the prevalence of subretinal membranes and the anatomic as well as the visual outcomes of their removal, 153 consecutive cases of eyes undergoing vitrectomy for PVR were entered into the study.[19] Subretinal membranes were encountered in 72 eyes (47%), but only 20 (28%) of the membranes that prevented retinal reattachment required removal. Of the 20 eyes requiring subretinal membrane removal, 13 (65%) were attached and only four (20%) achieved a visual acuity of 5/200 or better. Of 52 eyes with subretinal membranes that did not require removal, 41 (79%) were attached and 31 (60%) attained ambulatory vision.

The Silicone Study – a multicenter, randomized, prospective clinical trial – compared the use of silicone oil and gases in the management of PVR and helped to define the expected outcome for vitrectomy in these eyes.[27,43] The eyes were stratified into two groups: group 1 consisted of eyes that had not undergone a previous vitrectomy and group 2 consisted of eyes that had undergone at least one previous unsuccessful vitrectomy with gas tamponade. The study was conducted in two parts: phase 1 compared SF_6 (20% mixture) with silicone oil (1000 cSt); and phase 2, the major portion of the study, compared C_3F_8 (14% mixture) with silicone oil. The primary outcomes were anatomic success (defined as macular attachment) and functional success (defined as a visual acuity of 5/200 or better).

In phase 1 of the study, silicone oil was found to be superior to SF_6 as an intraocular tamponade for severe PVR with respect to functional and anatomic success.[43] Phase 2 found that silicone oil and C_3F_8 were similar in most respects and superior to SF_6.[27] At 36 months, C_3F_8 had a higher rate of complete retinal attachment posterior to the scleral buckle compared to silicone oil in group 1 eyes (approximately 80% vs 60%). No such difference was noted in group 2 eyes. Between 55% and 65% of group 1 and 2 eyes with complete posterior attachment treated with C_3F_8 and silicone oil had a visual acuity of 5/200 or better. In eyes treated with either silicone oil or C_3F_8, there was no significant difference between groups 1 and 2 in achieving functional success.[64]

Complications related to retinal tamponade also were evaluated by the Silicone Study. Chronically elevated IOP (IOP greater than 25 mmHg) was more prevalent in eyes treated with silicone oil than with C_3F_8 (8% vs 2%, $P < 0.05$).[46] However, chronic hypotony (IOP less than or equal to 5 mmHg):

- Occurred more frequently in eyes treated with C_3F_8 than with silicone oil (31% vs 18%, $P < 0.05$).
- Was more prevalent in eyes with anatomic failure (48% vs 16%, $P < 0.01$).
- Was associated with poor postoperative visual acuity ($P < 0.001$) and retinal detachment ($P < 0.01$).

Diffuse contraction anterior to the equator was an independent prognostic factor of chronic hypotony.

The incidence of corneal abnormalities did not differ between eyes randomized to silicone oil and C_3F_8 (26% vs 28%).[44] Independent prognostic risk factors for corneal abnormalities include preoperative iris neovascularization, preoperative aphakia or pseudophakia, postoperative aqueous flare and reoperations. In addition, corneal abnormalities correlated with poor visual acuity and hypotony.

At the 6-month postoperative examination, the incidence of macular pucker was 15%.[65] There was no difference in the incidence of macular pucker between group 1 and 2 eyes, and nor was there a difference between eyes randomized to gas or silicone oil. Postoperative macular pucker was three times more likely to occur in eyes that were preoperatively aphakic or pseudophakic compared with eyes that were preoperatively phakic. Functional success was more likely to occur in eyes without macular pucker than in eyes with macular pucker (60% vs 28%, $P < 0.01$).

The Silicone Study evaluated the outcomes of surgical procedures used in vitrectomies for PVR. Relaxing retinotomies were performed more frequently in group 2 than group 1 eyes (42% vs 20%, $P < 0.001$).[47] Eyes undergoing retinotomy were more likely to have anterior contraction, anterior retinal displacement and subretinal membranes. Eyes without a relaxing retinotomy were more likely to have complete posterior attachment and functional visual acuity compared to eyes with relaxing retinotomies. For eyes undergoing retinotomy, the incidence of hypotony was less when silicone oil was used instead of gas in group 1 eyes but not in group 2 eyes.

The results of silicone oil removal also were examined in the study.[28,59] Oil-removed eyes had a better outcome than oil-retained or gas-treated eyes. However, the removal of oil was left to the surgeon's discretion. Eyes in which the silicone oil was removed were more likely to have an attached retina, functional visual acuity, fewer complications and fewer reoperations than eyes with retained oil; therefore surgeon bias makes it difficult to determine whether or not it is advantageous to remove or retain oil. To minimize this prejudice, a matched–paired analysis was performed on 222 eyes in which 45% had silicone oil removed.[59] Eyes that had the silicone oil removed were more likely to experience an improvement in visual acuity (three or more lines) but also were more likely to develop recurrent retinal detachment when compared to eyes with retained silicone oil.

As expected, anterior PVR was more common in group 2 eyes than in group 1 eyes (88% vs 73%, $P < 0.001$).[66] When compared to eyes with anterior PVR, eyes with only posterior PVR had better outcomes, with higher rates of complete retinal attachment, functional visual acuity and normal IOP. Predictors of poor visual outcomes (less than 5/200) in eyes with anterior PVR were the use of C_3F_8 gas and preoperative PVR grade of D_1 or worse.

In an extension of the Silicone Study, more eyes were followed up to 36 months and further follow-up demonstrated no significant change from the 24-month results in eyes randomized to C_3F_8 or silicone oil.[28] Eyes with attached maculae were followed for up to 72 months and the outcomes demonstrated little change compared to earlier reports. Independent analyses were made between gas-treated, oil-retained and oil-removed eyes and it was found that:

- Oil-removed eyes, compared to oil-retained eyes, had a higher rate of macular attachment, complete posterior attachment, functional success and less keratopathy.
- Oil-removed eyes, compared to C_3F_8 eyes, were more likely to have functional success at 60 months and less hypotony and lower incidence of keratopathy at 48 months, but there was no difference in complete posterior retinal attachment.
- Gas-treated eyes, compared to oil-retained eyes, had a higher rate of complete posterior attachment and a visual acuity of 5/200 or better. There was no difference in hypotony, but there was a trend toward more keratopathy in oil-retained eyes.

The Silicone Study has provided valuable information regarding the expected outcomes of vitrectomy using perfluorocarbon gas and silicone oil. Although the surgical results for PVR are excellent, they may improve further with recent technical improvements, such as PFCLs and wide-angle viewing systems – surgical adjuncts that were not available for the Silicone Study. Despite these advances, the most difficult problem – recurrent proliferation – remains. Investigations into the inhibition of cellular proliferation, especially in the area of pharmacologic therapy, may provide invaluable tools for the treatment of PVR.

REFERENCES

1. Michaelson IC, Stein R. A study in the prevention of retinal detachment, *Ann Ophthalmol* (1969) **1:**49.
2. Rachal WF, Burton TC. Changing concepts of failure after retinal detachment surgery, *Arch Ophthalmol* (1979) **97:**480–3.
3. Laqua H, Machemer R. Clinical–pathological correlation in massive periretinal proliferation, *Am J Ophthalmol* (1975) **80:**913–29.
4. Laqua H, Machemer R. Glial cell proliferation in retinal detachment (massive periretinal proliferation), *Am J Ophthalmol* (1975) **80:**602–18.
5. Machemer R, van Horn D, Aaberg TM. Pigment epithelial proliferation in human retinal detachment with massive periretinal proliferation, *Am J Ophthalmol* (1978) **85:**181–91.
6. Mueller-Jensen K, Machemer R, Azarnia R. Autotransplantation of retinal pigment epithelium in intravitreal diffusion chamber, *Am J Ophthalmol* (1975) **80:**530–7.
7. Van Horn DL, Aaberg TM, Machemer R. Glial cell proliferation in human retinal detachment with massive periretinal proliferation, *Am J Ophthalmol* (1977) **84:**383–93.
8. Machemer R, Laqua H. Pigment epithelium proliferation in retinal detachment (massive periretinal proliferation), *Am J Ophthalmol* (1975) **80:**1–23.
9. Glaser BM, Cardin A, Biscoe B. Proliferative vitreoretinopathy: the mechanism of development of vitreoretinal traction, *Ophthalmology* (1987) **94:**327–32.
10. Wallyn RH, Hilton GF. Subretinal fibrosis in retinal detachment, *Arch Ophthalmol* (1979) **97:**2128–9.
11. Sternberg P Jr, Machemer R. Subretinal proliferation, *Am J Ophthalmol* (1984) **98:**456–62.
12. Schwartz D, De La Cruz ZC, Green WR, Michels RG. Proliferative vitreoretinopathy: ultrastructural study of 20 retroretinal membranes removed by vitreous surgery, *Retina* (1988) **8:**275–81.
13. Federman JL, Folberg R, Ridley M, Arbizo VA. Subretinal cellular bands, *Trans Am Ophthalmol Soc* (1983) **81:**172–81.
14. Trese MT, Chandler DB, Machemer R. Subretinal strands: ultrastructural features, *Graefes Arch Clin Exp Ophthalmol* (1985) **223:**35–40.
15. Hiscott P, Greierson I. Subretinal membranes of proliferative vitreoretinopathy, *Br J Ophthalmol* (1991) **75:**53.
16. Hiscott P, Marino I, Alexander R, et al. Cellular components of subretinal membranes in proliferative vitreoretinopathy, *Eye* (1989) **3** (5):606–10.
17. Retina Society Terminology Committee. The classification of retinal detachment with proliferative vitreoretinopathy, *Ophthalmology* (1983) **90:**121–5.
18. Machemer R, Aaberg TM, Freeman HM, et al. An updated classification of retinal detachment with proliferative vitreoretinopathy, *Am J Ophthalmol* (1991) **112:**159–65.
19. Lewis H, Aaberg TM, Abrams GW, et al. Subretinal membranes in proliferative vitreoretinopathy, *Ophthalmology* (1989) **96:**1403–15.
20. Lean JS, Stern WH, Irvine AR, et al. Classification of proliferative vitreoretinopathy used in the Silicone Study, *Ophthalmology* (1989) **96:**765–71.
21. Azen SP, Irvine AR, Davis MD, et al. The validity and reliability of photographic documentation of proliferative vitreoretinopathy, *Ophthalmology* (1989) **96:**352–7.
22. Lewis H, Aaberg TM. Anterior proliferative vitreoretinopathy, *Am J Ophthalmol* (1988) **105:**277–84.
23. Charles S. *Vitreous Microsurgery.* (Williams & Wilkins: Baltimore, 1981): 124–5.
24. Peyman GA, Schulman JA. *Intravitreal Surgery: Principles and Practice,* 2nd edn (Appleton & Lange: Norwalk, CT, 1994): 595.
25. Lewis H, Aaberg TM. Causes of failure after repeat vitreoretinal surgery for recurrent proliferative vitreoretinopathy, *Am J Ophthalmol* (1991) **111:**15–19.
26. Lewis H, Aaberg TM, Abrams GW. Causes of failure after initial vitreoretinal surgery for severe proliferative vitreoretinopathy, *Am J Ophthalmol* (1991) **111:**8–14.
27. Silicone Study Group. Vitrectomy with silicone oil or perfluoropropane gas in eyes with severe proliferative vitreoretinopathy: results of a randomized clinical trial, Silicone Study Report 2, *Arch Ophthalmol* (1992) **11:**780–92.

28. Abrams GW, Azen SP, McCuen BW II, et al. Vitrectomy with silicone oil or long-acting gas in eyes with severe proliferative vitreoretinopathy: results of additional and long-term follow-up, Silicone Study Report 11, *Arch Ophthalmol* (1997) **115:**335–44.
29. Michels RG. Surgery of retinal detachment with proliferative vitreoretinopathy, *Retina* (1984) **4:**63–83.
30. Eaton AM, Jaffe GJ, McCuen BW II, Mincey GJ. Condensation on the posterior surface of silicone intraocular lenses during fluid–air exchange, *Ophthalmology* (1995) **102:**733–6.
31. Apple DJ, Federman JL, Krolicki TJ, et al. Irreversible silicone oil adhesion to silicone intraocular lenses: a clinicopathological analysis, *Ophthalmology* (1996) **103:**1555–61.
32. Lean J, Azen SP, Lopez PF, et al. The prognostic utility of the Silicone Study Classification System: Silicone Study Report 9, *Arch Ophthalmol* (1996) **114:**286–92.
33. De Juan E Jr, Hickingbotham D. Flexible iris retractor (letter), *Am J Ophthalmol* (1991) **111:**776–7.
34. Lewis H, Aaberg TM, Abrams GW, et al. Management of the lens capsule during pars plana lensectomy, *Am J Ophthalmol* (1987) **103:**109–10.
35. Landers MB III, Stefansson E, Wolbarsht ML. The optics of vitreous surgery, *Am J Ophthalmol* (1981) **91:**611–14.
36. Spitznas M, Reiner J. A stereoscopic diagonal inverter (SDI) for wide-angle vitreous surgery, *Graefes Arch Clin Exp Ophthalmol* (1987) **225:**9–12.
37. Lewis JM, Park I, Ohji M, et al. Diamond-dusted silicone cannula for epiretinal membrane separation during vitreous surgery, *Am J Ophthalmol* (1997) **124:**552–4.
38. Chang S, Ozmert E, Zimmerman NJ. Intraoperative perfluorocarbon liquids in the management of proliferative vitreoretinopathy, *Am J Ophthalmol* (1988) **106:**668–74.
39. Aaberg TM. Management of anterior and posterior proliferative vitreoretinopathy: XLV Edward Jackson Memorial Lecture, *Am J Ophthalmol* (1988) **106:**519–32.
40. Parke DW II, Aaberg TM. Intraocular argon laser photocoagulation in the management of severe proliferative vitreoretinopathy, *Am J Ophthalmol* (1984) **97:**434–43.
41. Morse LS, McCuen BW II, Machemer R. Relaxing retinotomies: analysis of anatomic and visual results, *Ophthalmology* (1990) **97:**642–8.
42. Chang S, Lincoff H, Zimmerman NJ, Fuchs W. Giant retinal tears: surgical techniques and results using perfluorocarbon liquids, *Arch Ophthalmol* (1989) **107:**761–6.
43. Silicone Study Group. Vitrectomy with silicone oil or sulfur hexfluoride gas in eyes with severe proliferative vitreoretinopathy: results of a randomized clinical trial, Silicone Study Report 1, *Arch Ophthalmol* (1992) **110:**770–9.
44. Abrams GW, Azen SP, Barr CC, et al. The incidence of corneal abnormalities in the Silicone Study: Silicone Study Report 7, *Arch Ophthalmol* (1995) **113:**764–9.
45. Lean JS. Use of silicone oil as an additional technique in vitreoretinal surgery. In: Ryan SJ, ed, *Retina*, 2nd edn (Mosby Year Book: St Louis, 1994): 2158–9.
46. Barr CC, Lai MY, Lean JS, et al. Postoperative intraocular pressure abnormalities in the Silicone Study: Silicone Study Report 4, *Ophthalmology* (1993) **100:**1629–35.
47. Blumenkranz MS, Azen SP, Aaberg TM, et al. Relaxing retinotomy with silicone oil or long-acting gas in eyes with severe proliferative vitreoretinopathy: Silicone Study Report 5, *Am J Ophthalmol* (1993) **116:**557–64.
48. Dieckert JP, O'Connor PS, Schacklett DE, et al. Air travel and intraocular gas, *Ophthalmology* (1986) **93:**642–5.
49. Hanscom TA, Diddie KR. Mountain travel and intraocular gas bubbles, *Am J Ophthalmol* (1987) **104:**546.
50. Han DP, Lewis H, Lambrou FH, et al. Mechanisms of intraocular pressure elevation after pars plana vitrectomy, *Ophthalmology* (1989) **96:**1357–62.
51. Kangas TA, Bennett SR, Flynn HW Jr, et al. Reversible loss of light perception after vitreoretinal surgery, *Am J Ophthalmol* (1995) **120:**751–6.
52. Jaffe GJ, Abrams GW, Williams GA, Han DP. Tissue plasminogen activator for postvitrectomy fibrin formation, *Ophthalmology* (1990) **97:**184–9.
53. Perry HD, Foulks GN, Thoft RA, Tolentino FI. Corneal complications after closed vitrectomy through the pars plana, *Arch Ophthalmol* (1978) **96:**1401–3.
54. Brightbill FS, Myers FL, Bresnick GH. Postvitrectomy keratopathy, *Am J Ophthalmol* (1978) **85** (5): 651–5.
55. Landers MB III, Robinson D, Olsen KR, Rinkoff J. Slit-lamp fluid–gas exchange and other office procedures following vitreoretinal surgery, *Arch Ophthalmol* (1985) **103:**967–72.
56. Blumenkranz M, Gardner T, Blankenship G. Fluid–gas exchange and photocoagulation after vitrectomy: indications, technique, and results, *Arch Ophthalmol* (1986) **104:**291–6.
57. Miller JA, Chandra SR, Stevens TS. A modified technique for performing outpatient fluid–air exchange following vitrectomy surgery, *Am J Ophthalmol* (1986) **101:**116–17.
58. Han DP, Murphy ML, Mieler WF, Abrams GW. Outpatient fluid–air exchange for severe postvitrectomy diabetic vitreous hemorrhage: long-term results and complications, *Retina* (1991) **11:**309–14.
59. Hutton WL, Azen SP, Blumenkranz MS, et al. The effects of silicone oil removal: Silicone Study Report 6, *Arch Ophthalmol* (1994) **112:**778–85.
60. Grizzard WS, Hilton GF. Scleral buckling techniques for retinal detachment complicated by periretinal proliferation, *Arch Ophthalmol* (1982) **100:**419–22.
61. Machemer R, Laqua H. A logical approach to the treatment of massive periretinal proliferation, *Ophthalmology* (1978) **85:**584–93.
62. Ratner CM, Michels RG, Auer C, Rice TA. Pars plana vitrectomy for complicated retinal detachments, *Ophthalmology* (1983) **90:**1323–7.
63. Han DP, Lewis MT, Kuhn EM, et al. Relaxing retinotomies and retinectomies: surgical results and predictors of visual outcome, *Arch Ophthalmol* (1990) **108:**694–7.
64. McCuen BW, Azen SP, Stern W, et al. Vitrectomy with silicone oil or perfluoropropane gas in eyes with severe proliferative vitreoretinopathy: Silicone Study Report 3, *Retina* (1993) **13:**279–84.
65. Cox MS, Azen SP, Barr CC, et al. Macular pucker after successful surgery for proliferative vitreoretinopathy: Silicone Study Report 8, *Ophthalmology* (1995) **102:**1884–91.
66. Diddie KR, Azen SP, Freeman HM, et al. Anterior proliferative vitreoretinopathy in the Silicone Study: Silicone Study Report 10, *Ophthalmology* (1996) **103:**1092–9.

Chapter 28 Anterior retinectomy

Michael D Bennett and Paul Sternberg Jr

INTRODUCTION

The term 'retinotomy' means to make a hole in the retina, in contradistinction to a 'retinectomy', which means to excise the retina. Anterior relaxing retinotomies and retinectomies are most commonly indicated when peripheral contraction cannot be relieved adequately by membrane dissection. They may vary from a small defect created in order to drain subretinal fluid, to a 360° excision of the peripheral retina. This chapter will discuss the indications, techniques, instrumentation and potential pitfalls for anterior retinectomy.

RELAXING RETINOTOMY AND RETINECTOMY

Relaxing retinotomies and retinectomies are performed when retinal reattachment cannot be achieved because of retinal incarceration or retinal contraction resulting from fibrous proliferation. The first description of a relaxing retinotomy during pars plana vitrectomy was in an eye with retina incarcerated in a traumatic scleral wound site.[1] Machemer and colleagues described indications, techniques, complications and results of retinotomies and retinectomies.[2] Zivojnovic et al[3,4] were the first to report the use of anterior retinectomy in the management of retinal detachment with severe traction not associated with trauma. Parke and Aaberg[5,6] described the use of retinotomies and retinectomies for the management of eyes with severe proliferative vitreoretinopathy (PVR). In all of these reports, the authors suggested the sacrifice of peripheral retina in order to preserve function of posterior, more visually significant retina.

INDICATIONS

Relaxing retinotomies and retinectomies should be performed only when other surgical techniques have failed or have little chance of success. Table 28.1 shows indications involving cases in which the retina is foreshortened because of fibroglial membranes as in PVR, vascular membranes or following a penetrating injury (trauma or surgical) with incarceration of retinal tissue at the wound site.

Table 28.1 Indications for anterior retinectomy

Proliferative vitreoretinopathy
Focal starfold
Diffuse contraction
Circumferential contraction
Intrinsic retinal contraction
Anterior retinal displacement
Fibrous periretinal proliferation
Giant retinal tear
Proliferative vascular retinopathy/proliferative diabetic retinopathy
Longstanding fibrovascular proliferation
Anterior hyaloidal fibrovascular proliferation
Fibrous proliferation at sclerotomy site
Retinal incarceration
Penetrating trauma
Surgical sclerotomy site

GENERAL SURGICAL PRINCIPLES AND TECHNIQUES

In order to determine the most appropriate surgical course, one must have a general understanding of the

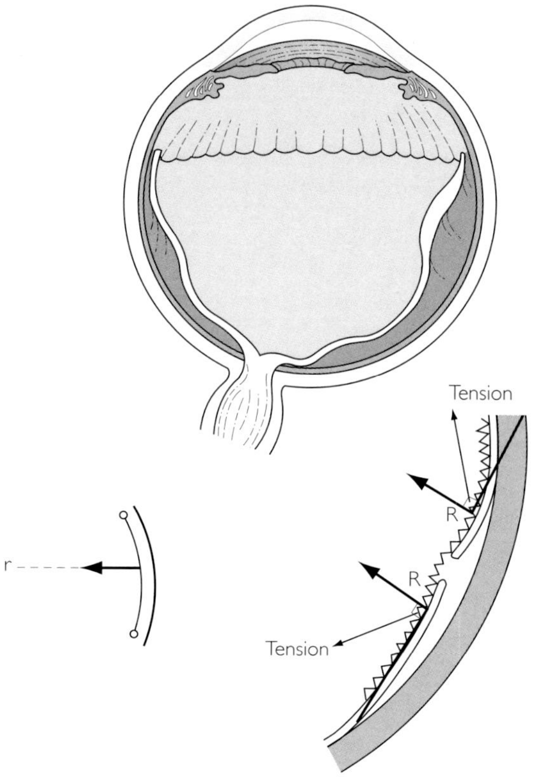

Figure 28.1 *Tension in an epiretinal membrane. The force exerted by an epiretinal membrane is ultimately directed toward the central vitreous cavity. The perpendicular vector force is especially important if a retinal break is present because it tends to pull the break away from the retinal pigment epithelium.*

pathophysiology leading to the retinal foreshortening. PVR is the leading cause of failure in retinal detachment surgery.

The pathogenesis of this proliferative tissue is believed to be derived from retinal pigment epithelial (RPE) cells that are liberated at the time of the original retinal detachment or its repair.[7,8] The RPE cells presumably undergo fibroblastic transformation with the ability to synthesize collagen and transform into macrophages. The fibroblasts arise from myofibroblasts; they contract and form mature fibrocytes, 'fixing' the tissue. These cells can cause retraction of the retina and vitreous body, leading to recurrent retinal detachment. The proliferative membranes, similar to those seen in proliferative vascular and diabetic retinopathy, can cause extensive contraction. Despite aggressive membrane dissection, the effective retinal foreshortening still may prevent reapproximation of the retina to the underlying RPE.

In contrast to retinal foreshortening that arises because of proliferative membranes, a true foreshortening can occur following penetrating or surgical trauma, with loss of retinal tissue.

When a retinectomy is considered, it is recommended that the eye be encircled with a scleral buckle. Supporting the vitreous base will relieve or reduce the tractional forces acting on the retinal surface. Michels et al[9] demonstrated that epiretinal membranes exert a perpendicular force on the retina that is directed toward the center of the vitreous cavity. This net vector force pulls the retina away from the underlying RPE (Fig. 28.1). Scleral buckle placement changes the eye wall from a concave surface at the vitreous base to a convex surface. This change reverses the vector force; the inherent elasticity of the retina, as well as any further epiretinal proliferation in this area, will pull the retina toward the underlying RPE (Fig. 28.2).

The decision whether to perform a retinectomy or to place or revise a scleral buckle is made at the time of surgery. Factors influencing the decision include the location and extent of the traction and the difficulty of revising or placing the buckle. Most traction can be relieved or minimized efficiently with a scleral buckle; membrane dissection should relieve the residual traction. Because posterior membranes are removed more easily, relaxing retinotomies or retinectomies are rarely indicated in these situations. Occasionally, despite encircling the eye and performing meticulous bimanual membrane dissection, significant traction remains, preventing retinal reattachment. Under these circumstances, anterior retinectomy is indicated.

Before tissue is incised, diathermy is applied to the retina surrounding the area to be excised, with particular attention paid to large-diameter retinal vessels. The retina then is elevated and cut with scissors or the vitrectomy instrument.

The general goal of a retinectomy is to excise surgically the entire remaining area of retinal contracture in order to optimize reapposition to the RPE. This excision is normally carried out into adjacent healthy retina. Failure to do so will likely leave residual proliferative tissue behind. For large areas of excision, the vitrectomy instrument is faster and more efficient; however, some fine control may be compromised.

The use of perfluorocarbon liquid (PFCL) may be helpful in determining the extent of the retinotomy

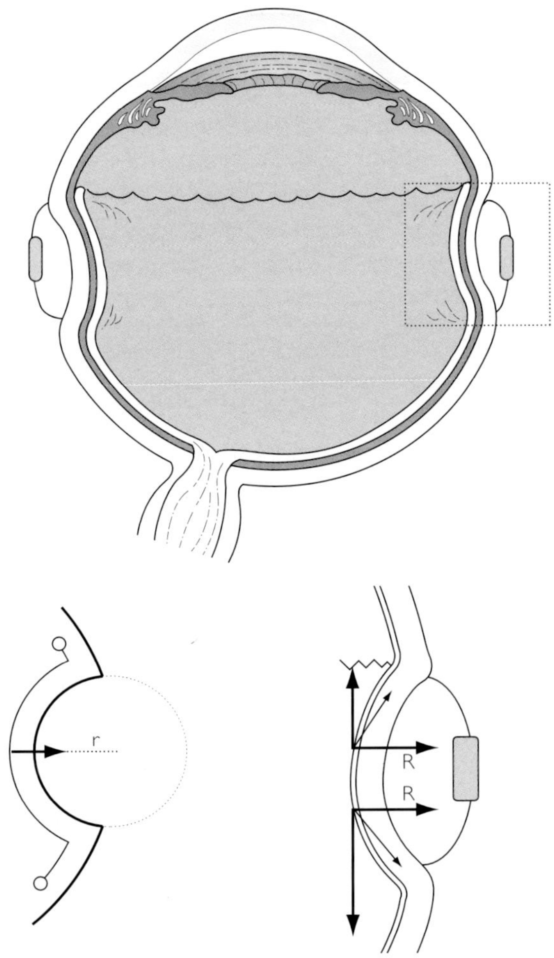

Figure 28.2 *Post-encircling element. When a scleral buckle is placed under an area of traction, the shape of the eye wall in that area is changed from concave to convex. This increases the magnitude and reverses the direction of the perpendicular vector force. The persistent traction then pulls the retina toward the pigment epithelium, rather than tending to cause the retina to detach.*

needed. The PFCL is injected centrally to stabilize the posterior retina. After the initial retinotomy, additional PFCL is injected; if the retina remains elevated or the PFCL moves subretinally, the retinotomy must be extended. The retinectomy is enlarged until the PFCL flattens the remaining retina. The retina should be reapposed with PFCL rather than air because the latter has a greater surface tension and can artifactually flatten residual tangential traction forces that will redetach the retina once the air or gas absorbs.

If the retina is successfully reapposed, photocoagulation is performed to stimulate retinal and RPE adherence. This adherence takes time to mature; therefore, some form of intraocular tamponade is usually indicated. Either a long-acting gas or silicone oil will help to facilitate the retinal reapposition process.

The size, location and configuration of the retinectomy will vary according to the indication. The following examples address specific scenarios in greater detail.

FOCAL STARFOLD/FOCAL INTRINSIC RETINAL CONTRACTION

A 360° application of diathermy is applied, surrounding the area of proliferation. On occasion, the larger diameter vessels may require sequential applications along their length. The treatment must be carried out into normal surrounding retina.

If a hole was not created with the diathermy, one may be created either with the scissors tip or with reapplication of diathermy. In areas where the retina is closely apposed to the RPE, there is a risk of choriocapillaris damage and significant bleeding if the underlying structures are engaged by the scissors. Following diathermy, an illuminated pick or scissors blade should enter the subretinal space in the area of the greatest elevation. The retina is subsequently elevated and lifted away from the RPE before cutting (Fig 28.3 and 28.4).

When cutting the retina, there may still be some areas that were not diathermized adequately. A two-function (illumination/coagulation) or three-function (illumination/coagulation/suction) instrument may be an efficient means to facilitate prompt hemostasis while cutting the retina.

Once the retinal contraction is relieved, the edges of the retinal defect are treated with endolaser and the eye is filled with a long-acting gas or silicone oil.

DIFFUSE CONTRACTION AND DIFFUSE FIBROUS PERIRETINAL PROLIFERATION (Fig. 28.5)

When diffuse areas of contracture are encountered, diathermy is used to surround the area of fibrous proliferation. If the area is large, laser endophotocoagulation can cover these larger areas efficiently. Usually two or three rows of treatment are used to surround the

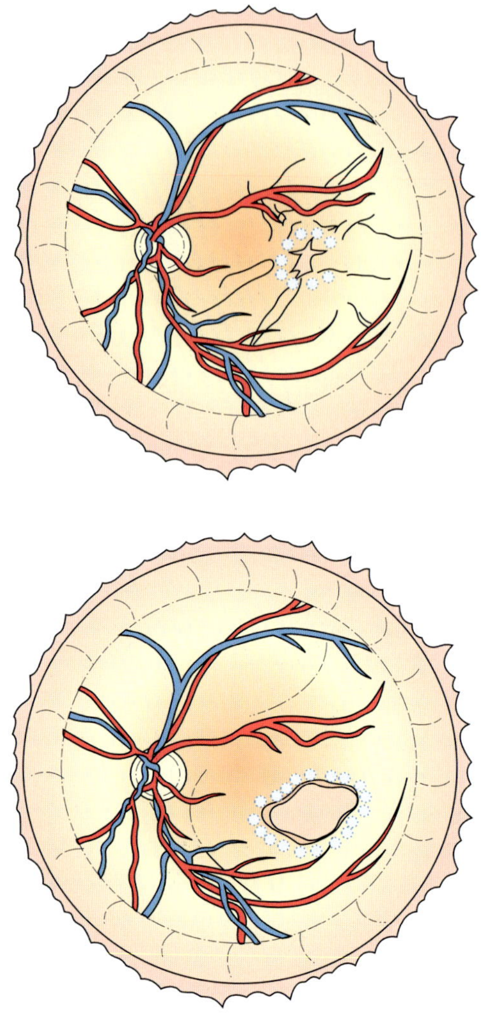

a

b

Figure 28.3 *(a) Focal contraction, starfold. Epicenter of proliferation surrounded by diathermy. (b) Focal contraction removed; surrounding retina attached. Photocoagulation applied.*

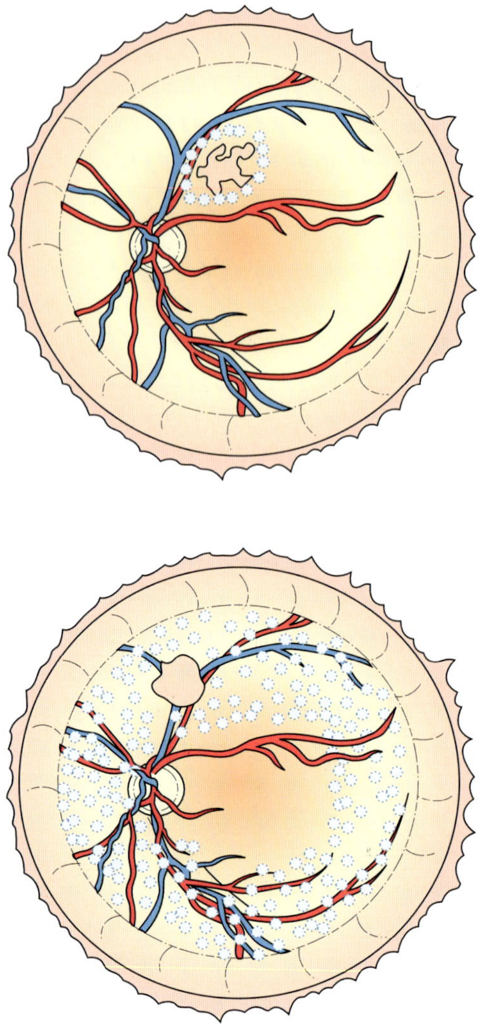

a

b

Figure 28.4 *(a) Diabetic eye with dense focal traction and macular detachment. (b) Frontal view of contracted membrane. Membrane removal unsuccessful with large break created.*

involved tissue. When the proliferation extends to the vitreous base, it is necessary to carry the coagulation out to the ora serrata in an oblique fashion. Usually larger areas of proliferation will necessitate extending the treatment further into normal surrounding retina.

The subretinal space may be entered in any area of elevation, taking care not to damage the underlying choriocapillaris. The retina then is elevated and the contracted area is excised. A two-function (illumination/coagulation) or three-function (illumination/coagulation/suction) instrument may be used to facilitate prompt hemostasis.

Once the retinal shortening is relieved, the edges of the retinal defect must be treated with laser. When the retinectomy approaches or extends into the vitreous base, thermal coagulation (endolaser or transscleral cryotherapy) should be carried across the ora serrata onto the pars plana so there is no 'gutter' accumulation of subretinal fluid later, resulting from contraction of the vitreous base.

The peripheral retina is an end artery system with minimal collateral circulation. Thus, when performing a large retinectomy, the remaining anterior retina is essentially nonviable and must be treated. Depending

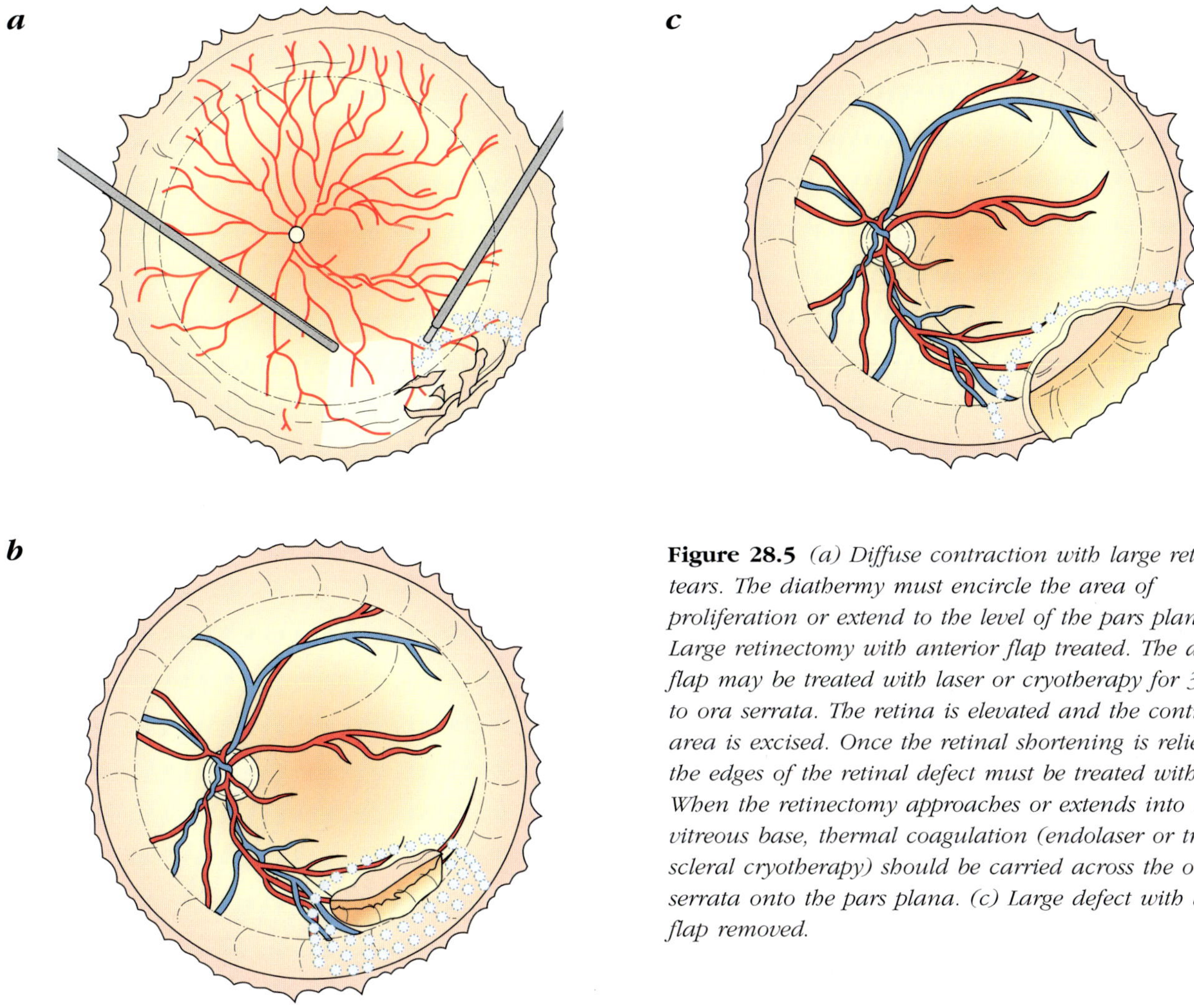

Figure 28.5 *(a) Diffuse contraction with large retinal tears. The diathermy must encircle the area of proliferation or extend to the level of the pars plana. (b) Large retinectomy with anterior flap treated. The anterior flap may be treated with laser or cryotherapy for 360° or to ora serrata. The retina is elevated and the contracted area is excised. Once the retinal shortening is relieved, the edges of the retinal defect must be treated with laser. When the retinectomy approaches or extends into the vitreous base, thermal coagulation (endolaser or transscleral cryotherapy) should be carried across the ora serrata onto the pars plana. (c) Large defect with anterior flap removed.*

on the individual circumstance, several options to treat anterior retina exist, including laser photocoagulation, cryoablation or extension of the retinectomy to the ora serrata. Following the retinectomy, the edges are photocoagulated and tamponaded further with a long-acting gas or silicone oil.

CIRCUMFERENTIAL CONTRACTION (Fig. 28.6)

Extensive circumferential contraction may occur because of marked contraction of membranes at the posterior aspect of the vitreous base. Circumferential contraction is a form of anterior–posterior contraction, in which the posterior hyaloid pulls the retina centrally into a funnel shape. This circumferential contraction creates tight retinal folds that radiate posteriorly (see Fig. 28.6b). Even with excision of the posterior hyaloid and sectioning of circumferential membranes, the retina may remain in a contracted state.

The first attempt to relieve the circumferential contraction is to place a broad, encircling scleral buckle and aggressively dissect all epiretinal membranes. If the contraction is not adequately relieved, then the vitreous should be trimmed to the retinal surface, starting at the posterior hyaloid and advancing anteriorly to the level of the vitreous base. The hyaloid is often adherent to the membranes just posterior to the vitreous base. The vitreous base should be shaved down to the level of the retina

a

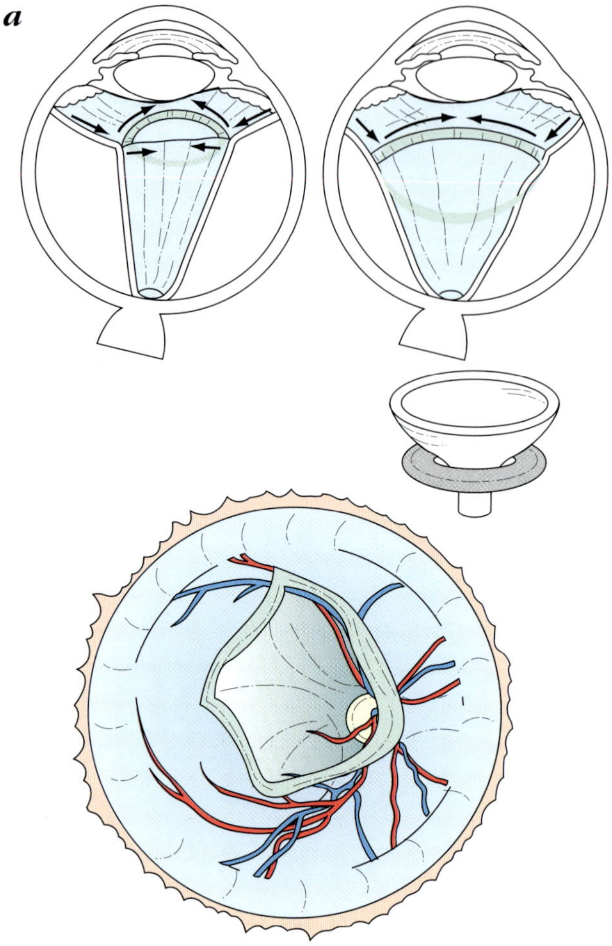

b

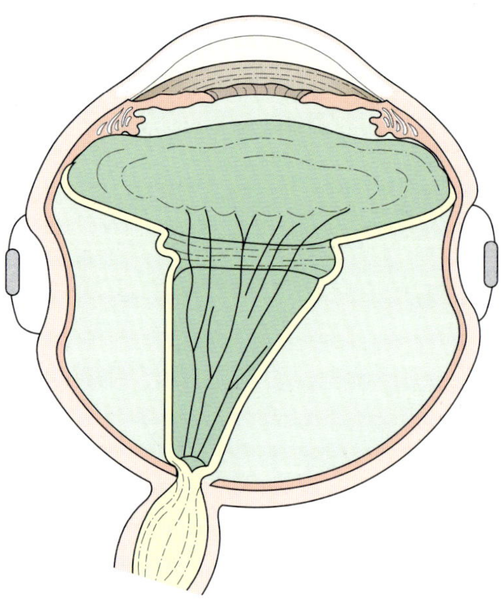

c

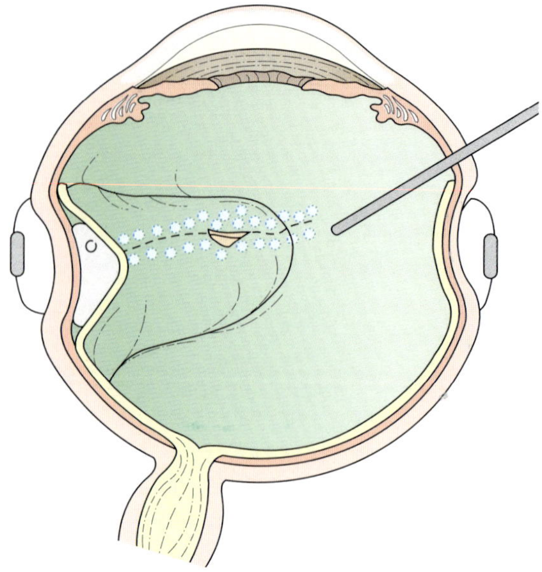

d

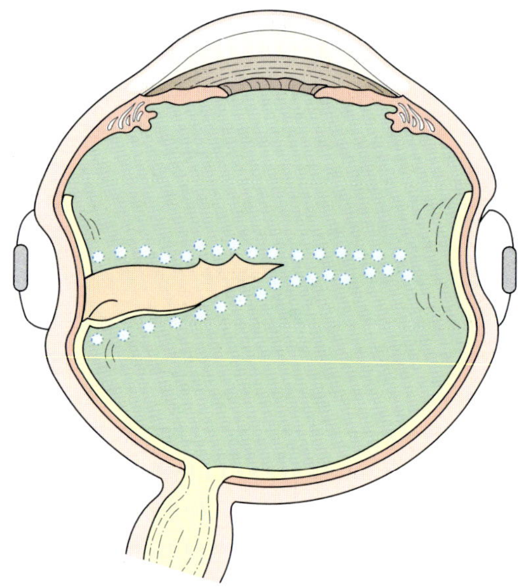

e

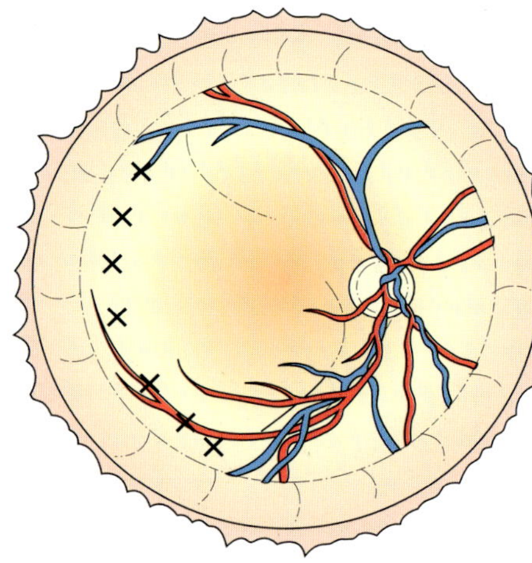

Figure 28.6 *(a) Circumferential traction with proliferation immediately behind insertion of the posterior hyaloid pulling the retina centrally, stretching the retina anterior to it and creating radial folds posteriorly. Schematic drawing of situation in nonvitrectomized eye* (left) *and vitrectomized eye* (right). *(b) Retina pulled into funnel configuration. Circumferential contraction of posterior vitreous base with radial folds. (c) After vitrectomy, membrane removal, scleral buckle and fluid–air exchange, air courses subretinally through retinal break. Dashed line indicates location of proposed retinotomy. (d) Circumferential retinotomy performed under air and retina flattens. Retinotomy is extended into attached retina on each end. (e) Following 360° anterior relaxing retinectomy, the retina is flat.*

either with scleral depression or with the use of a wide-angle viewing system.

A retinectomy is indicated if these measures have not adequately relieved the contraction. PFCL is injected, starting over the disc and filled toward the level of the residual contraction. The height of the scleral buckle can be raised at this time for a final attempt to diminish the tractional forces. If a retinectomy is indicated, it is carried out circumferentially and posteriorly into mobile, normal retina. Care must be taken at this point to excise well into normal retina because the tamponade of the air may flatten the retina in the presence of some remaining proliferative tissue. Anteriorly, the retinectomy is extended to the anterior-most level of traction, anywhere from the ora serrata to the ciliary body.

ANTERIOR RETINAL DISPLACEMENT (Fig. 28.7)

Anterior retinal displacement occurs mainly in eyes that have undergone prior pars plana vitrectomies[10–12] or some manipulation of the vitreous (i.e. trauma or pneumatic retinopexy). In these cases, fibrous proliferation and contraction at the level of the vitreous base pull the peripheral retina anteriorly toward the pars plana, ciliary body or even to the iris plane. This may lead to retinal detachment or ciliary body detachment with resultant hypotony.

In the presence of anterior retinal displacement, adequate dissection usually necessitates a lensectomy. When a pars plana lensectomy is indicated, care must be taken to remove the lens along with the entire capsular bag to limit any further contraction in this location. To eliminate the traction that has displaced the retina anteriorly, it is necessary to support the vitreous base with an encircling scleral buckle and to remove all associated membranes. The peripheral vitreous is removed and the vitreous base is shaved to the level of the retinal surface.

Limited dissection of the anterior membranes can be performed with the vitrectomy instrument. However, in most cases external depression and a bimanual technique using an illuminated pick or forceps and scissors are preferred.

Endoillumination may be inadequate in the presence of extremely anterior membranes. The coaxial light source from the operating microscope or external illumination may provide the best visualization. Use of a wide-angle viewing system may greatly facilitate the peripheral dissection.

If all of the anterior traction cannot be relieved following dissection and segmentation, a retinectomy should be performed to provide apposition of the retina to the underlying RPE. The retinectomy should be carried out well into normal surrounding retina in an attempt to limit any residual proliferative tissue.

Use of a wide-angle viewing system will assist in visualizing the overall status of the anterior retina, particularly in guiding the surgeon to determine the extent of the retinotomy needed.

GIANT RETINAL TEAR (Fig. 28.8)

In most giant retinal tears (GRT), the anterior edge will curl inward because of the intrinsic elastic properties of the retina and RPE cells growing over the edge of the GRT onto the internal limiting lamina. In the presence of PVR, this folded edge may become fixed. The resultant contraction occurs along the anteroposterior direction as well as circumferentially. If the retina does not settle following scleral buckling and aggressive membrane dissection, a retinectomy is indicated.

PFCL is injected over the posterior pole and filled to the posterior level of the GRT (Fig. 28.9). Diathermy is applied to the entire area to be excised, extending well into normal surrounding retina. The retinectomy can be performed segmentally in order to minimize tissue removal, taking care to remove all areas of residual contraction.

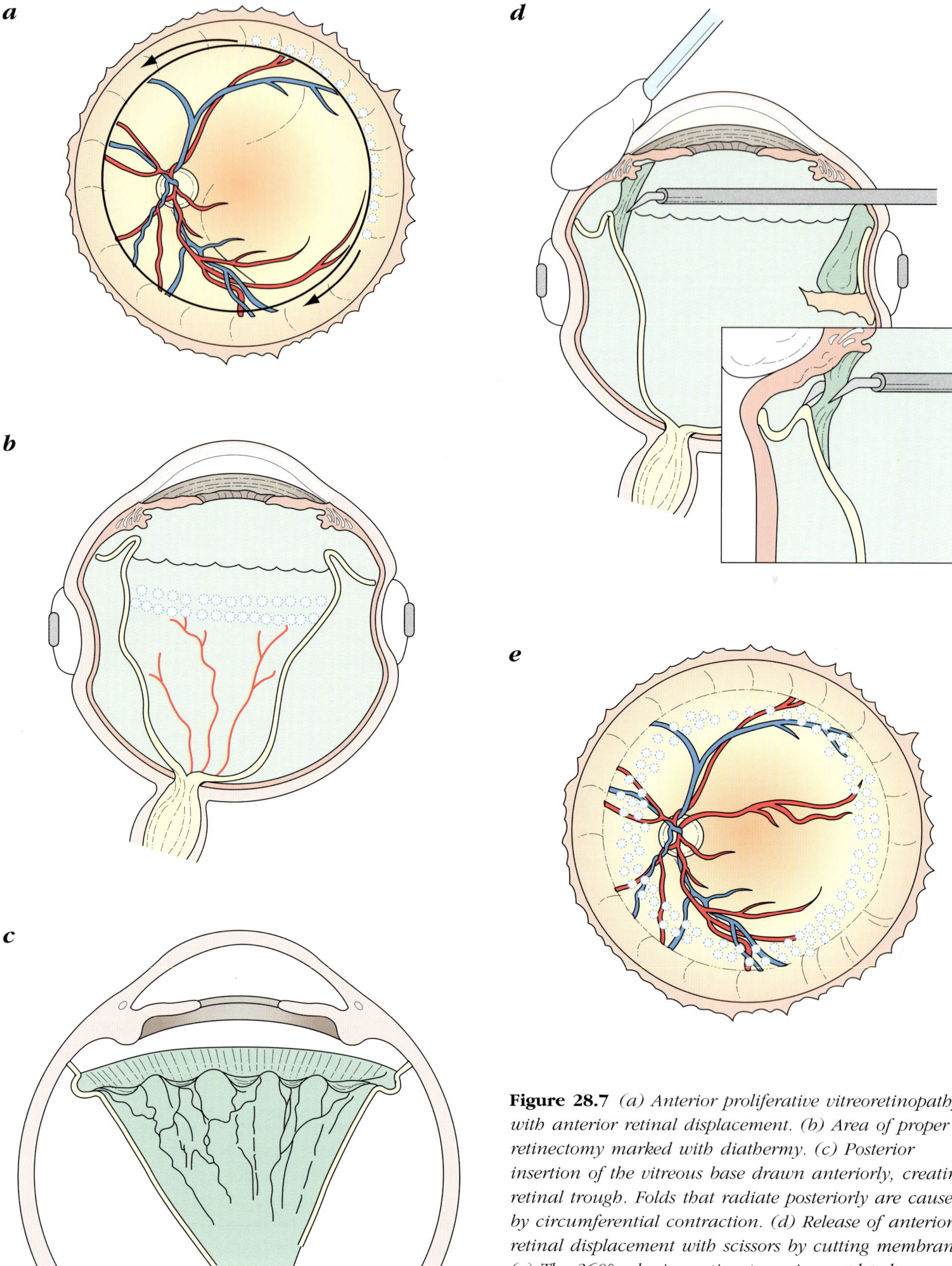

Figure 28.7 *(a) Anterior proliferative vitreoretinopathy with anterior retinal displacement. (b) Area of proper retinectomy marked with diathermy. (c) Posterior insertion of the vitreous base drawn anteriorly, creating a retinal trough. Folds that radiate posteriorly are caused by circumferential contraction. (d) Release of anterior retinal displacement with scissors by cutting membrane. (e) The 360° relaxing retinectomy is completed.*

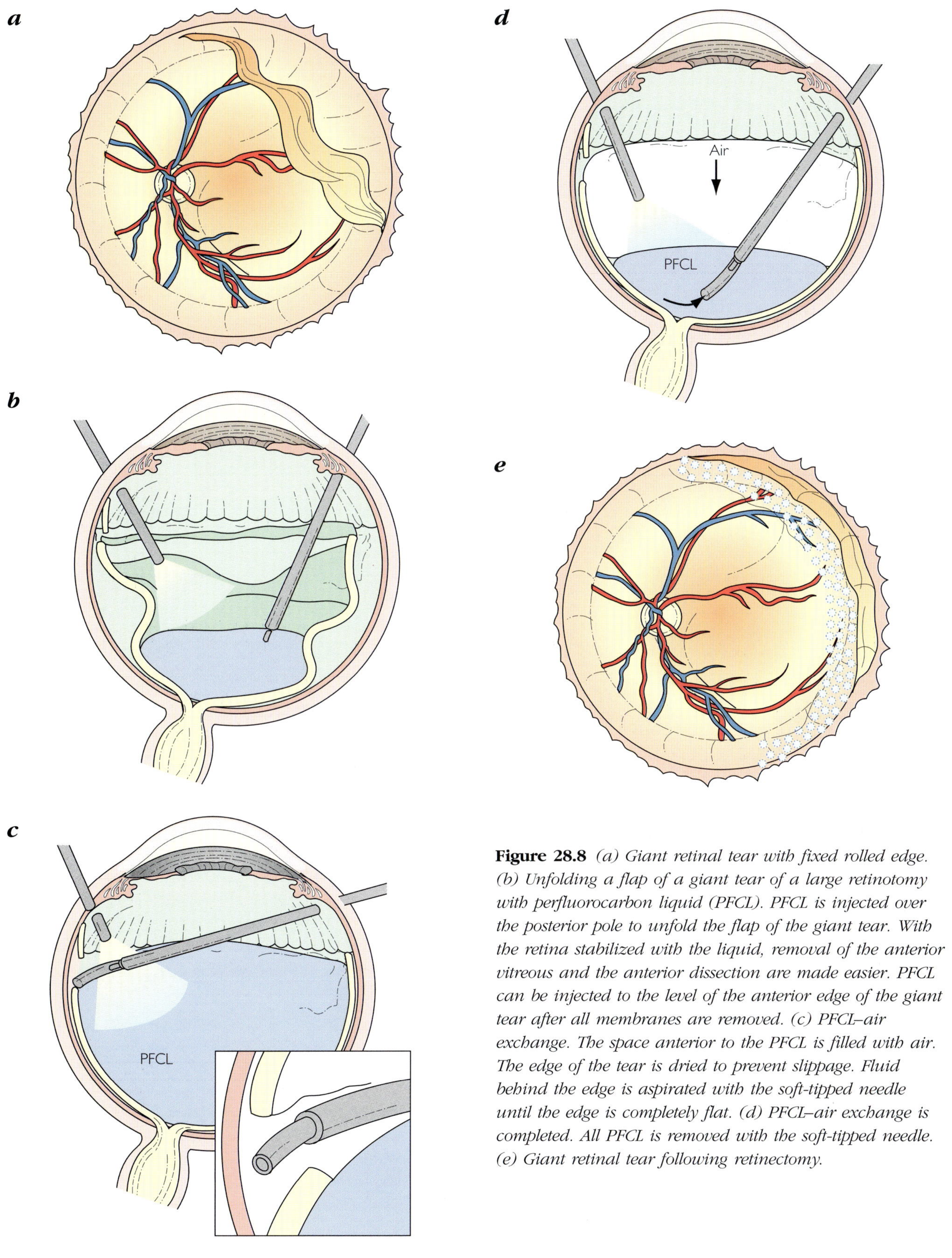

Figure 28.8 *(a) Giant retinal tear with fixed rolled edge. (b) Unfolding a flap of a giant tear of a large retinotomy with perfluorocarbon liquid (PFCL). PFCL is injected over the posterior pole to unfold the flap of the giant tear. With the retina stabilized with the liquid, removal of the anterior vitreous and the anterior dissection are made easier. PFCL can be injected to the level of the anterior edge of the giant tear after all membranes are removed. (c) PFCL–air exchange. The space anterior to the PFCL is filled with air. The edge of the tear is dried to prevent slippage. Fluid behind the edge is aspirated with the soft-tipped needle until the edge is completely flat. (d) PFCL–air exchange is completed. All PFCL is removed with the soft-tipped needle. (e) Giant retinal tear following retinectomy.*

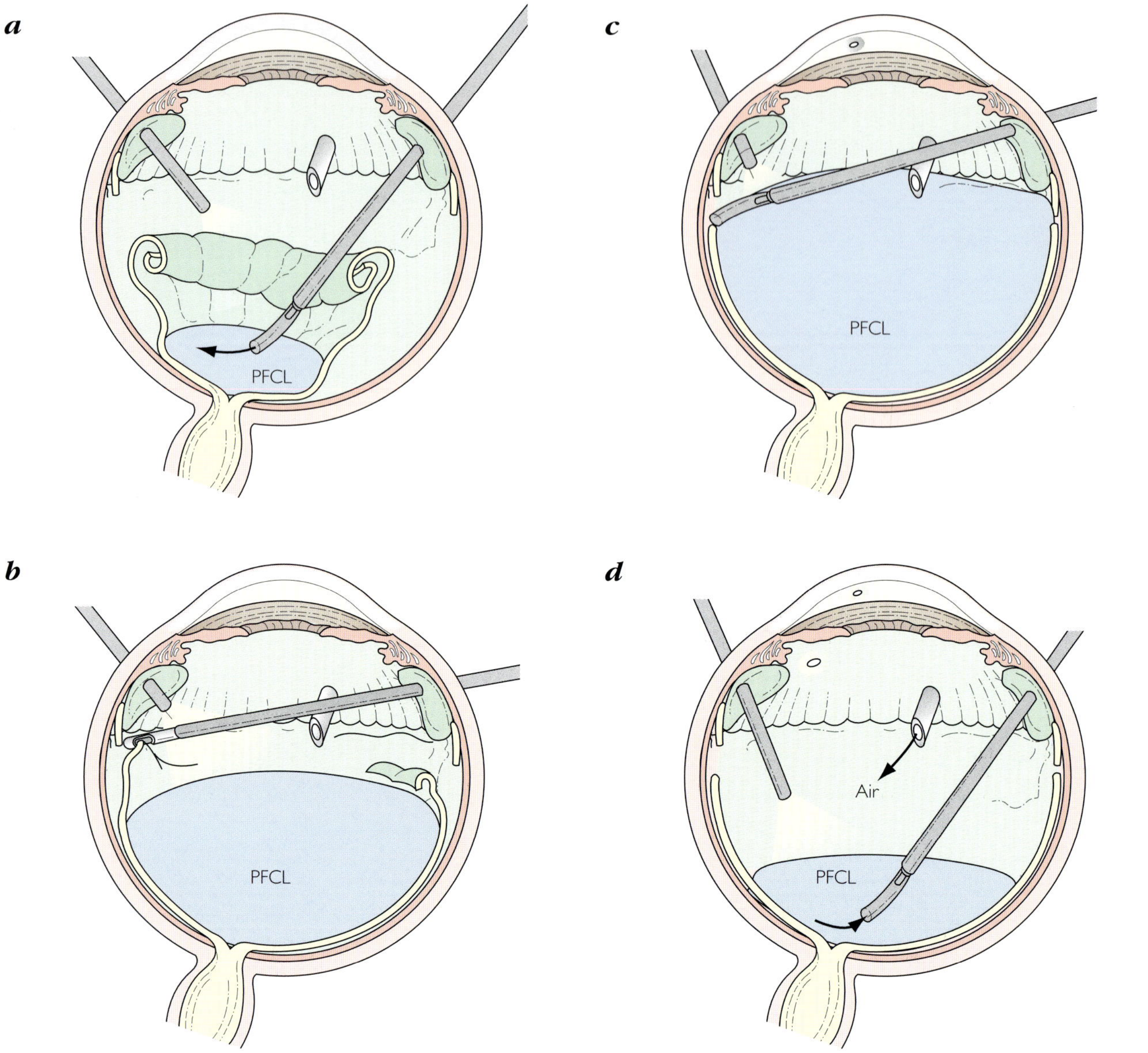

Figure 28.9 *Management of giant retinal tear or retinotomy with perfluorocarbon liquid (PFCL). (a) Folded-over giant tear with marked folding of the peripheral retina. PFCL injected over posterior pole after posterior epiretinal membrane removal. (b) Posterior retina reattached. Organized, folded edge of giant tear treated with diathermy and then excised with vitrectomy instrument. (c) Retina completely reattached with PFCL. 'Drying' anterior edge of giant tear during initial phase of fluid–air exchange by applying suction with soft-tipped needle beneath anterior edge of retina. (d) Continuing fluid–air exchange to remove residual PFCL. No retinal slippage has occurred.*

Occasionally following segmental trimming, a jagged edge will remain. At this point, it is best to freshen the edge in order to allow smooth apposition of the retina to the RPE. Theoretically, minimizing these jagged areas will reduce potential epicenters for further contraction in the future.

Endophotocoagulation is applied to the entire edge of the GRT and a fluid–air exchange is initiated. In order to minimize slippage of the retina, the eye can be rotated to orient the tear dependently. The anterior edge of the GRT must be dry during the initial phase of fluid–air exchange; this is accomplished by applying suction with a soft-tipped needle beneath the anterior edge of the retina. This maneuver will stabilize the retina in position until all of the subretinal fluid has been evacuated. The fluid–air exchange can be continued to remove residual PFCL.

PROLIFERATIVE VASCULAR RETINOPATHY/PROLIFERATIVE DIABETIC RETINOPATHY

Retinotomy or retinectomy is occasionally needed to repair longstanding tractional retinal detachments associated with diabetic retinopathy.[13] Traction outside of the posterior pole, away from the macula, may exist indefinitely without jeopardizing central acuity. However, if the traction extends to the macula, or if the macula is threatened, an attempt to restore the anatomic integrity of the retina is indicated.

With time, these ischemic areas become thin and atrophic. The retina tears with only mild manipulation during surgery; occasionally, large retinal breaks can develop. In the majority of cases, diabetic membranes can be segmented or delaminated in order to release residual traction. However, residual fibrovascular tissue may exert traction with associated posterior breaks, a combination that will preclude retinal reattachment. In these instances, the retina surrounding the areas of traction may have to be excised in order to reapproximate the retina.

LONGSTANDING FIBROVASCULAR PROLIFERATION

In the presence of proliferative vascular retinopathy, it is important to release all traction when retinal breaks are present. The same principles discussed for PVR apply here. The first steps in relieving traction require membrane dissection and the placement of a scleral buckle. The type of buckle (radial or encircling element) depends on the physical nature of the residual traction. Attempts are made to minimize the amount of retina that must be excised, ensuring that all of the traction is relieved. Diathermy is applied to the membrane and the surrounding retina that is to be excised.

The retinectomy is performed either with the vitrectomy instrument or the area is outlined with scissors and then excised with the vitrectomy instrument. Scissors allow better control and precision. Once the retinal contraction is relieved, the edges of the retinal defect are treated with endophotocoagulation and the vitreous cavity is filled with a long-acting gas or silicone oil.

ANTERIOR HYALOIDAL FIBROVASCULAR PROLIFERATION

Anterior hyaloidal fibrovascular proliferation (AHFVP) is associated with severe retinal ischemia and is usually found in diabetic patients with severe proliferative diabetic retinopathy after vitrectomy. The AHFVP is neovascularization and associated fibrovascular tissue proliferation that arises from the peripheral retina and extends to the anterior hyaloid and eventually along the posterior surface of the lens.[14,15]

With time, the fibrovascular tissue will contract to cause a peripheral traction retinal detachment in which the peripheral retina is pulled anteriorly and centrally toward the lens (Fig. 28.10). The retinal detachment that is observed is clinically very similar to the detachment seen in eyes with anterior retinal displacement. However, the fibrous tissue found in anterior retinal displacement is essentially avascular, whereas the proliferative tissue in AHFVP is highly vascular with a great propensity to bleed when engaged.

The surgical approach to AHFVP involves a pars plana vitrectomy and pars plana lensectomy. Usually these eyes have had prior panretinal photocoagulation and vitrectomy. The peripheral fibrous tissue is depressed into view following lens removal. Diathermy then is applied to the vessels and attempts are made to excise the fibrovascular tissue. In order to facilitate hemostasis, the height of the infusion bottle can be elevated to raise the intraocular pressure and a two-function (illumination/coagulation) or three-function (illumination/coagulation/suction) instrument can be used. The bottle height should be lowered as soon as possible in order to minimize the amount of limited perfusion in these highly ischemic eyes. If profound bleeding occurs, thrombin may be infused to aid hemostasis.[16]

If all of the traction cannot be relieved, a retinectomy is indicated. The size of the retinectomy is dictated by the extent of the disease, which may range from 1 clock-hour to a complete 360° excision. Then endophotocoagulation should be applied to the edges of the retinal defect and in a panretinal pattern. Silicone oil will aid in tamponading the retina and may reduce the risk of anterior segment neovascularization.

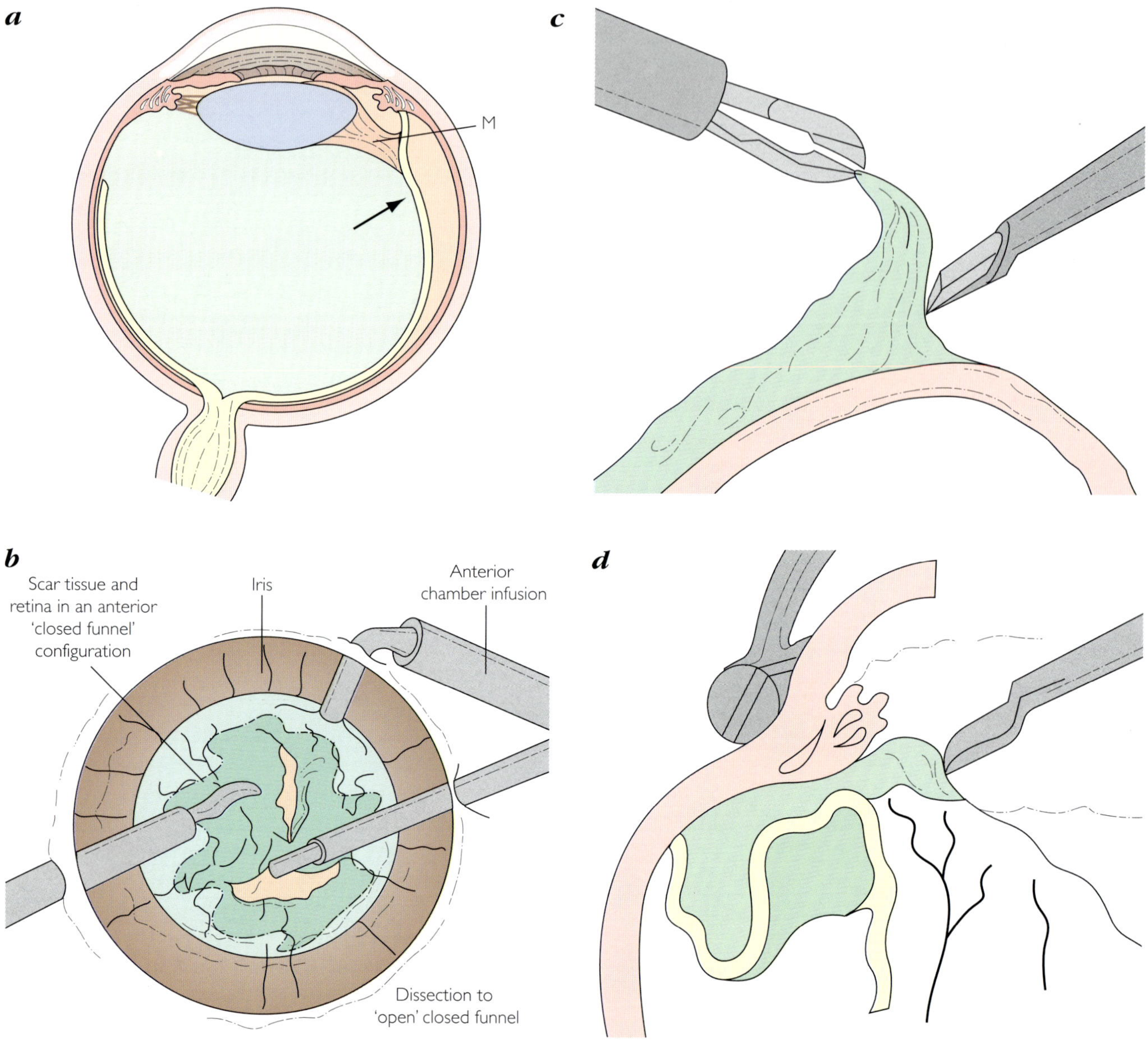

Figure 28.10 *(a) Advanced anterior hyaloidal fibrovascular proliferation. Fibrous proliferative membrane (M) and traction retinal detachment. (b) Once the lens has been removed, the bimanual technique is used to grasp the preretinal tissue and scissors are used to delineate the membranes from the retinal surface. (c) Artist's conception of bimanual surgery showing delamination of anterior membrane. (d) Drawing demonstrating peripheral scleral depression allowing access to the trough. (Note that the trough is filled with vitreous and fibrous tissues.)*

RETINAL INCARCERATION

Retinectomies are sometimes indicated to relieve traction resulting from perforating trauma. Retinal foreshortening can occur by a variety of mechanisms after a traumatic injury. The retina may be drawn into the wound site, resulting in true foreshortening with tissue loss. It may also shorten because of fibrous contraction associated with the healing process. Regardless of the mechanism, traumatic or surgical incarceration causes the surrounding retina to be pulled into folds. The degree of retinal shortening is

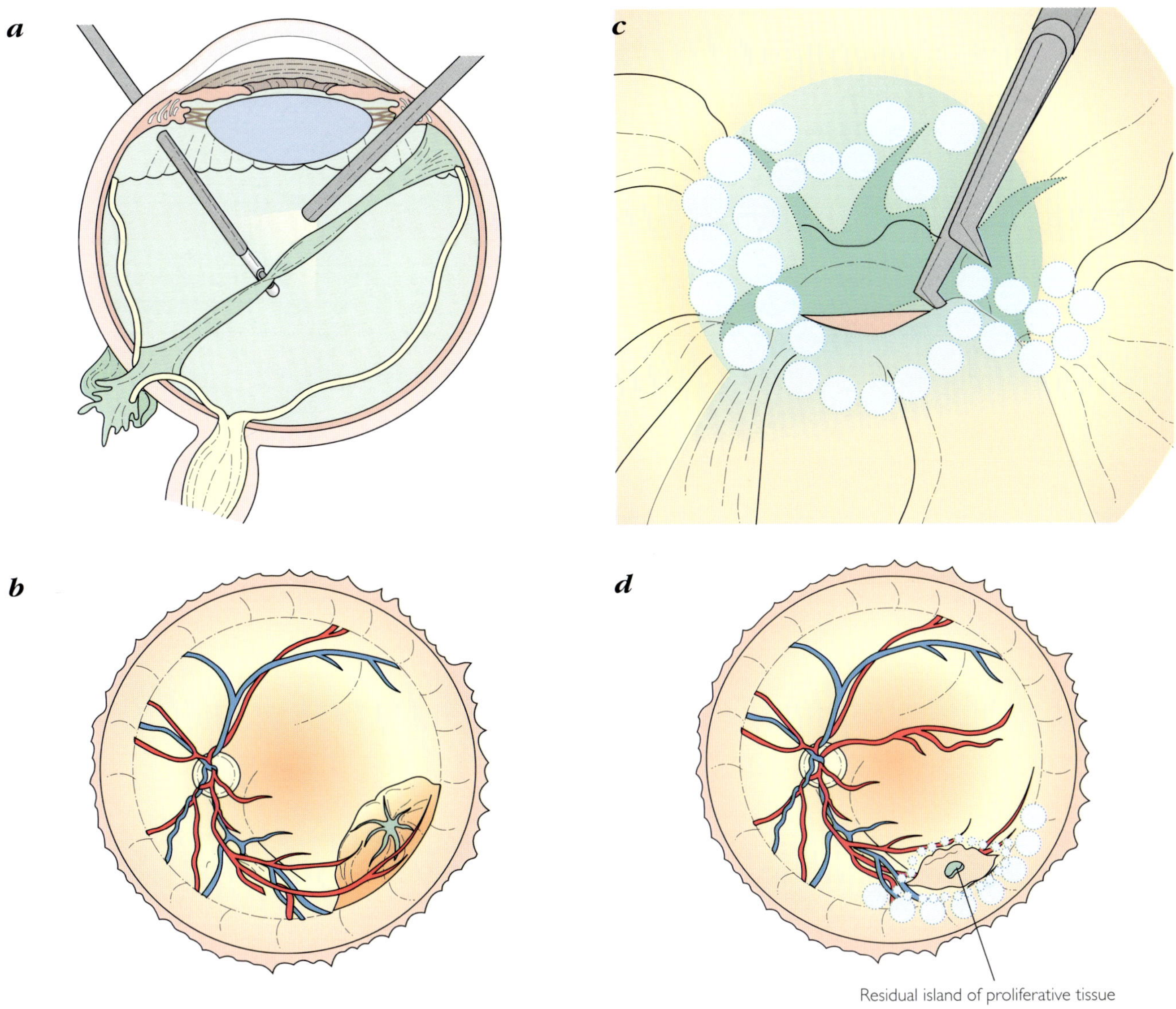

Figure 28.11 *(a) Incarcerated retina should be lysed by patchy retinectomy. (b) Perforating injuries are managed with primary repair of the entry site. Seven to 10 days later, pars plana vitrectomy is performed with removal of the posterior hyaloid. The proliferation growing through the exit site should be reduced to a stump but not eliminated. (c) After diathermy, the retina is cut. (d) The resulting retinal hole is usually large.*

dictated by the size, location and chronicity of the wound. A retinectomy is indicated if the retinal incarceration or contraction prevents reattachment of the retina.

PENETRATING TRAUMA (Fig. 28.11)

A pars plana vitrectomy and exploration of the wound are carried out. Visualization may be reduced in the presence of significant trauma, therefore care must be taken not to enter the subretinal space with the vitrectomy instruments. If the wound is recent and only a focal area of incarceration is involved, the retina may be teased out of the wound. This may be facilitated by the use of a PFCL and direct manipulation of the incarcerated tissue with forceps.

In most cases, if the retinal tissue cannot be dislodged from the wound or if the incarceration is older and the folds are fixed, the incarcerated retina

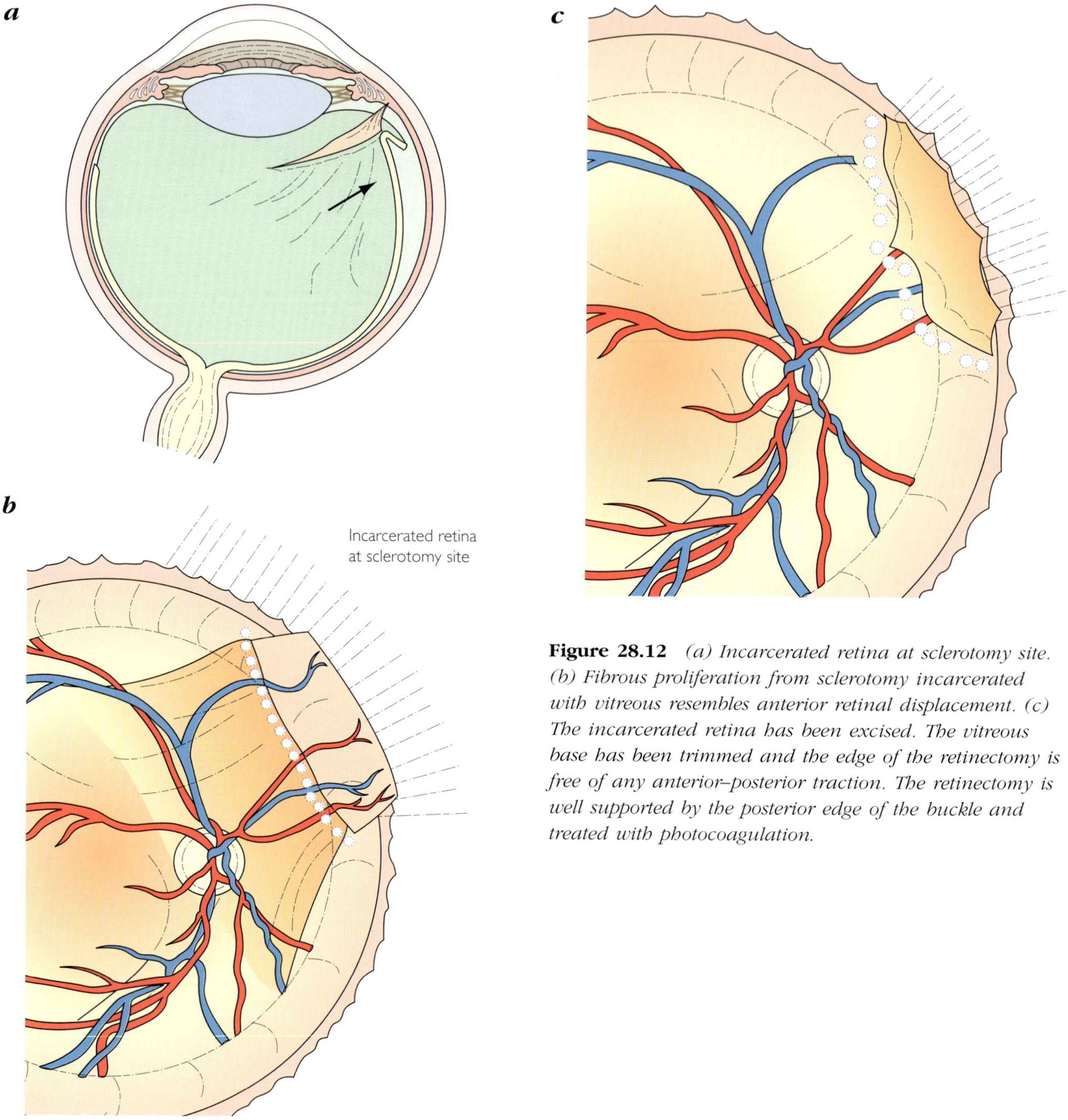

Figure 28.12 *(a) Incarcerated retina at sclerotomy site. (b) Fibrous proliferation from sclerotomy incarcerated with vitreous resembles anterior retinal displacement. (c) The incarcerated retina has been excised. The vitreous base has been trimmed and the edge of the retinectomy is free of any anterior–posterior traction. The retinectomy is well supported by the posterior edge of the buckle and treated with photocoagulation.*

must be excised. Diathermy is applied to the immediate area around the incarceration site, taking care to cauterize the larger vessels thoroughly. After diathermy, the scissors blade or a membrane pick usually can be placed tangentially through the necrotic retina into the subretinal space. The retina should be lifted away from the RPE before cutting. The retina may be cut in a lamellar fashion with reapplication of diathermy as needed until the retina has been incised for 360° around the wound site.

PFCL may be injected over the posterior pole to stabilize any bullous retina that may be detached around the incarceration site. The retinal defect created by the retinectomy should be treated with laser endophotocoagulation and the eye filled with a long-acting tamponading agent.

a

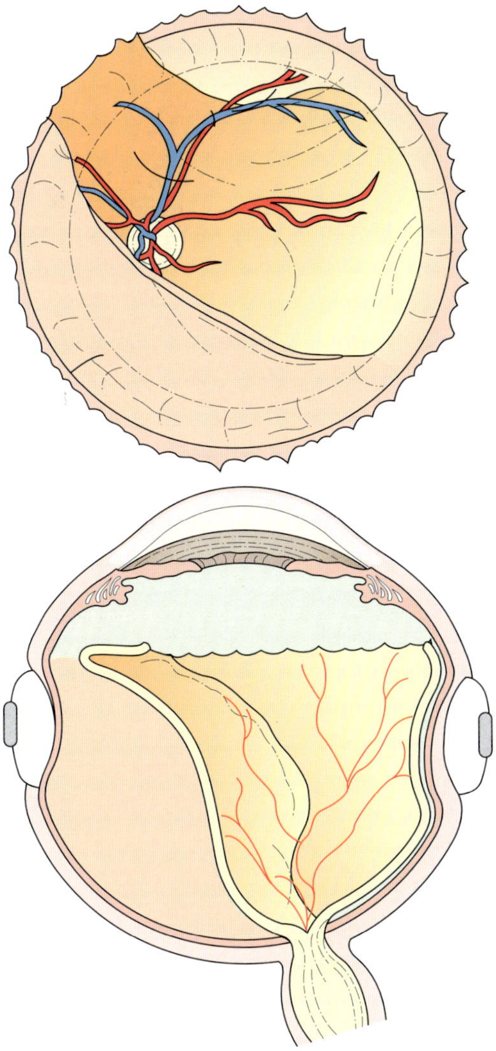

b

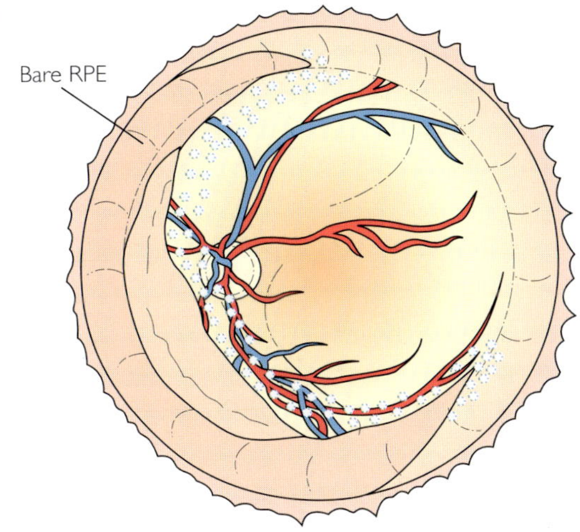

Figure 28.13 *Distal retinal incarceration. (a) The retina is torn and incarcerated in the wound on the opposite side of globe. (b) The retina has been excised from the incarceration site. The retinectomy has been carried out into the adjacent healthy retina and well treated with photocoagulation. Nasally, the bare retinal pigment epithelium can be seen anterior to the edge of the retinectomy.*

SURGICAL SCLEROTOMY SITE (Fig. 28.12)

In a mechanism very similar to traumatic incarceration, surgical intervention creates a potential incarceration site. This may occur intraoperatively with inadvertent perforation while draining subretinal fluid during a scleral buckle procedure. It may occur at the conclusion of a routine pars plana vitrectomy if vitreous is incarcerated in the sclerotomy site. Incarceration may occur postoperatively if a traumatic injury is severe enough to rupture the wound.

DISTAL RETINAL INCARCERATION (Fig. 28.13)

Distal retinal incarceration may occur occasionally and will result in a very large defect when the retina is excised from the wound. These eyes may require up to a 360° retinectomy to separate the retina from the wound. These instances may be managed much like a GRT. PFCL is usually required to stabilize the posterior retina before manipulation.

POTENTIAL PITFALLS WITH ANTERIOR RETINECTOMIES

The major complications of retinotomy are hemorrhage, inability to unfold and reattach the retina, hypotony, visual field loss, recurrent fibrous proliferation from the retinotomy site and persistent traction leading to retinal detachment when the retinotomy is too small.

Hemorrhage may result from inadequate diathermy of the vessels. Application of excessive diathermy can result in tissue necrosis. In some cases, there may be oozing from smaller vessels and capillaries. Because of the potential for oozing and later hemorrhage, we prefer to treat the retina with a continuous row of diathermy before cutting.

Intraoperative hemorrhage usually can be controlled by raising the infusion bottle temporarily, causing an increase of intraocular pressure. Use of a combination diathermy and a fiberoptic light source or a three-function tissue manipulator will provide readily available diathermy in the event of hemorrhage during a retinectomy. If significant persistent hemorrhage occurs, thrombin can be infused into the eye to control bleeding.[16]

Complete hemostasis is essential because inadequately diathermized vessels may lead to significant postoperative hemorrhage, resulting in severe fibrin formation and fibrous proliferation. This type of fibrous reproliferation may bridge the edge of the cut retina and the more anterior structures and lead to retinal redetachment.

Hypotony is seen in some eyes after large retinotomies. In the report by Morse et al,[17] hypotony (intraocular pressure less than 5 mmHg) developed in 43% of reattached eyes. This complication is probably most often related to fibrosis and detachment of the ciliary body associated with anterior proliferation. Another possible etiology of hypotony is increased absorption of intraocular fluid from the large area of exposed RPE. Whether the latter is a significant factor in the production of hypotony is unknown.

Persistent traction leading to retinal detachment occurs when the retinectomy is too small and residual proliferative tissue is left behind. It is imperative to extend the retinectomy well into normal retina in all directions in order to release all potential traction.

SURGICAL RESULTS

The selective use of relaxing retinectomies has permitted successful retinal attachment in eyes that have proven refractive to less aggressive conventional modalities. In 1986, Machemer et al[2] reported the results of relaxing retinotomies in 56 eyes that were considered to be inoperable by the standards of that time. At the end of a 6-month follow-up period, the retina was attached in 18 of 45 eyes (40%). Visual acuity was 5/200 or better in 3 of 18 eyes (6.7%).

Since its inception, the indications for relaxing retinotomy have expanded and the postoperative anatomical and functional results have improved. In a series by Han et al,[18] 54 consecutive eyes underwent relaxing retinotomy (42 for PVR (78%) and 12 for trauma (22%)). After a 6-month minimum follow-up, anatomic success (retina attached posterior to the scleral buckle and an intraocular pressure of 3 mmHg or more) was achieved in 35 eyes (64%). Visual outcome of 5/200 or better was achieved in 14 eyes (26%). Factors that favorably influenced visual outcome were a superior location of the relaxing retinotomy and preoperative visual acuity of hand motions or better.

Morse et al[17] reported a retrospective study of 100 eyes followed for a minimum of 6 months. At the end of 6 months, 58% were completely attached and 8% were partially attached (macula attached). At the final follow-up, visual acuity was 5/200 in 29% of eyes, 20/200 or better in 17% and 20/100 or better in 5%. In this study the length of the retinotomy did not appear to influence the success rate. However, they did note that the poorest visual results were associated with a relaxing retinotomy involving the entire temporal quadrant or a radial relaxing retinotomy.

The Silicone Study[19] was a multicentered, randomized clinical trial that evaluated the efficacy of silicone oil and long-acting gas in eyes with severe vitreoretinopathy. The study was divided into two groups: Group 1 (no previous vitrectomy) and Group 2 (previous vitrectomy). There were 100 eyes in Group 1 and 2 combined that underwent retinotomy with either perfluoropropane gas (C_3F_8) or silicone oil. At the end of 6 months, 58 eyes (58%) had complete retinal reattachment, 38 eyes (38%) achieved visual acuity of 5/200 or better, 31% were hypotonus and 35% were noted to have corneal opacities. Reoperation rates appeared similar between those eyes undergoing retinectomy (30 of 102 eyes, 29%) and those not requiring retinotomy (77 of 238, 32%).

CONCLUSION

Retinectomies are performed when all other, less-aggressive surgical maneuvers fail to reattach the retina. The original surgical reports demonstrated some visual potential for eyes that would have otherwise been lost. Over the last decade, with improved surgical techniques, instruments and adjuvants, success rates have improved accordingly.

In most instances, tractional forces can be relieved by placing an encircling scleral buckle and by performing aggressive membrane dissection. In eyes with persistent retinal foreshortening, these areas can be removed. Retinectomies are most often performed in the presence of PVR or proliferative vascular retinopathy or because of retinal incarceration in a traumatic or surgical wound.

Circumferential retinotomies are preferred over radial retinotomies. Giant tears and resultant large retinectomies are best managed with intraoperative PFCL, followed by endophotocoagulation and prolonged tamponade with either long-acting gas or silicone oil.

Complications of retinectomies can be serious and eyes requiring such aggressive surgical intervention will have some resultant decline in visual function. However, with appropriate management, cases that would have been previously lost can now obtain some useful visual function. The enhanced rates of anatomic and functional success are multifactorial, reflecting both greater experience with the procedures as well as wider indications.

ACKNOWLEDGMENTS

Supported in part by the National Institutes of Health P30 EY06360 Departmental Core Grant, Research to Prevent Blindness, Inc. and Heed Ophthalmic Fellowship Foundation (M.D.B.).

REFERENCES

1. Machemer R. Retinotomy, *Am J Ophthalmol* (1981) **92:**768–74.
2. Machemer R, McCuen BW II, de Juan E Jr. Relaxing retinotomies and retinectomies, *Am J Ophthalmol* (1986) **102:**7–12.
3. Zivojnovic R, Mertens DAE, Peperkamp E. Das flüssige Silikon in der Amotio Chirurgie (II). Bericht über 280 Falle-weitere Entwicklung der Technik, *Klin Monatsbl Augenheilkd* (1982) **181:**444–52.
4. Zivojnovic R. *Silicone Oil in Vitreoretinal Surgery* (Martinus Nijhoff/Dr W Junk: Dordrecht, The Netherlands, 1987): 19–22, 52–60.
5. Parke DW II, Aaberg TM. Intraocular argon laser photocoagulation in the management of severe proliferative vitreoretinopathy, *Am J Ophthalmol* (1984) **97:**434–43.
6. Aaberg TM. Management of anterior and posterior proliferative vitreoretinopathy: XLV Edward Jackson Memorial Lecture, *Am J Ophthalmol* (1988) **106:**519–32.
7. Machemer R, Aaberg TM, Freeman HM, et al. An updated classification of retinal detachment with proliferative vitreoretinopathy, *Am J Ophthalmol* (1991) **112:**159–65.
8. The Retina Society Terminology Committee. The classification of retinal detachment with proliferative vitreoretinopathy, *Ophthalmology* (1983) **90:**121–5.
9. Michels RG, Thompson JT, Rice TA, Freund D. Effect of scleral buckling on vector forces caused by epiretinal membranes, *Am J Ophthalmol* (1986) **102:**449–51.
10. Lewis H, Aaberg TM. Causes of failure after repeat vitreoretinal surgery for recurrent proliferative vitreoretinopathy, *Am J Ophthalmol* (1991) **111:**15–19.
11. Lewis H, Aaberg TM, Abrams GW. Causes of failure after initial vitreoretinal surgery for severe proliferative vitreoretinopathy, *Am J Ophthalmol* (1991) **111:**8–14.
12. Lewis H, Aaberg TM, Abrams GW, et al. Management of the lens capsule during pars plana lensectomy, *Am J Ophthalmol* (1987) **103:**109–10.
13. Zivojnovic R. *Silicone Oil in Vitreoretinal Surgery* (Martinus Nijhoff/Dr W Junk: Dordrecht, The Netherlands, 1987): 19–22, 90.
14. Lewis H, Abrams GW, Foos RY. Clinicopathologic findings in anterior hyaloidal fibrovascular proliferation after diabetic vitrectomy, *Am J Ophthalmol* (1987) **104:**614–18.
15. Lewis H, Abrams GW, Williams GA. Anterior hyaloidal fibrovascular proliferation after diabetic vitrectomy, *Am J Ophthalmol* (1987) **104:**607–13.
16. Thompson JT, Glaser BM, Michels RG, de Bustros S. The use of intravitreal thrombin to control hemorrhage during vitrectomy, *Ophthalmology* (1986) **93:**279–82.
17. Morse LS, McCuen BW II, Machemer R. Relaxing retinotomies: analysis of anatomic and visual results, *Ophthalmology* (1990) **97:**642–8.
18. Han DP, Lewis MT, Kuhn EM, et al. Relaxing retinotomies and retinectomies: surgical results and predictors of visual outcome, *Arch Ophthalmol* (1990) **108:**694–7.
19. Blumenkranz MS, Azen SP, Aaberg TM, et al. Relaxing retinectomy with silicone oil or long-acting gas in eyes with severe proliferative vitreoretinopathy: Silicone Study Report 5, *Am J Ophthalmol* (1993) **116:**557–64.

Chapter 29 Posterior relaxing retinotomy

Stephen A Meffert and Gholam A Peyman

INTRODUCTION

In certain complex retinal detachments, even after apparently complete removal of epi- and/or subretinal membranes, the retina fails to relax sufficiently to permit reattachment. In such cases, a relaxing retinotomy may be necessary for release of traction and successful retinal attachment. Relaxing retinotomies involve transection of the neurosensory retina and the associated vascular supply. This procedure is only undertaken when the inherent loss of retinal function caused by the retinotomy is outweighed by an increased probability of the posterior retina remaining attached, leading to stabilization of ocular status. Retinotomy is only performed late in the procedure after other techniques to release retinal traction, such as scleral buckling and peeling or transecting epi- and subretinal membranes, have been unsuccessful or insufficient.

The concept of relaxing retinotomy was initially described by Machemer.[1–3] Zivojnovic emphasized the use of retinotomy for release of retinal traction and in conjunction with silicone oil tamponade.[4] Subsequent authors have defined its role in proliferative vitreoretinopathy (PVR),[5–9] proliferative vasculopathies[6–10] and traumatic or surgical retinal incarceration.[1,2,6,11] Anatomic and visual results have been evaluated in case series of patients requiring relaxing retinotomy for various indications.[7,12–15]

Relaxing retinotomy may be indicated in patients with PVR, proliferative vascular retinopathy and traumatic retinal incarceration. In a series advocating aggressive removal of anterior traction in PVR, a higher relaxing retinotomy rate was still associated with a higher single-operation success rate.[17] Although primarily a procedure of last resort, our impression is that relaxing retinotomy may offer an improvement in the single-operation success rate that may offset the inherent drawbacks of retinal transection.

Relaxing retinotomies are performed in a variety of orientations, extents and locations. They may be radial, oblique or circumferential and encompass various degrees from small sectors to 360°. The selection of the proper orientation and extent of a retinotomy is determined on a case-by-case basis. Simple circumscribing retinotomies may be useful in retinal incarceration or to isolate a focal area of traction. Radial retinotomies are effective in releasing some localized traction, but are seldom sufficient and may extend posteriorly during air–fluid exchange. Circumferential retinotomies are most commonly employed because they release the anterior–posterior vector force of retinal traction. Combinations of circumferential and radial or oblique orientations may be indicated in certain cases.

The location of a circumferential retinotomy may be anterior or posterior. In general, retinotomies should be posterior to unrelieved retinal traction. However, some surgeons prefer to place the retinotomy as anteriorly as possible, while others prefer to use a posterior location consistently. The advantage of using an anterior site is the possible preservation of greater peripheral retinal function and decreased risk of significant hemorrhage. An anterior retinotomy is, however, slightly more difficult technically, difficult to tamponade inferiorly with currently available long-term vitreous substitutes and usually requires lens removal and anterior retinectomy.

A posterior relaxing retinotomy has the advantages of being technically simpler, easily tamponaded by silicone oil or gas (Fig. 29.1) and usually does not require lensectomy or retinectomy.[16] A posterior retinotomy also commonly allows reattachment of peripheral retina anterior to the retinotomy site. Anterior reattachment is more likely because there is a greater length of relaxed anterior retina available to appose the retinal pigment epithelium (RPE). This chapter will describe the surgical technique for posterior relaxing retinotomy.

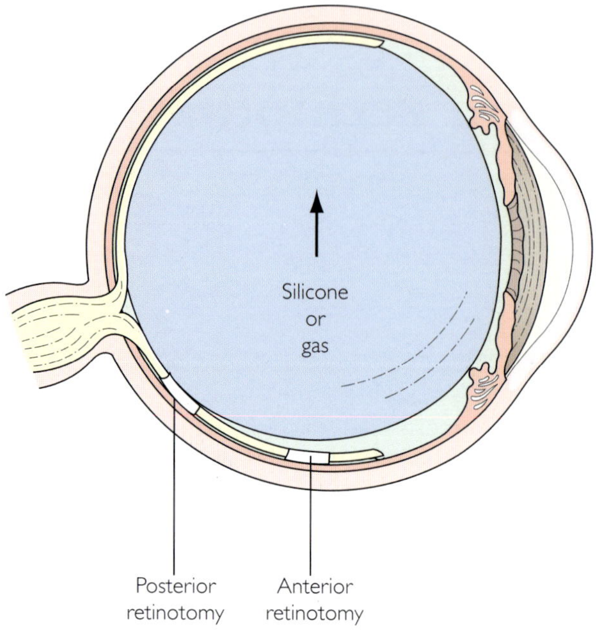

Figure 29.1 *Relative locations of anterior (peripheral) and posterior relaxing retinotomies. Note that the posterior retinotomy is more readily tamponaded by the silicone oil or gas bubble.*

INDICATIONS

The indications for posterior relaxing retinotomy are similar to the anterior relaxing retinotomy. It is primarily a last option for a retina that cannot be flattened by other means. An inability to flatten the retina during air–fluid exchange after complete membrane removal indicates the need for a relaxing retinotomy; the surgeon can judge this by assessing the compliance of the retina and its ability to appose the concave surface of the eye wall.

PREOPERATIVE EVALUATION

Preoperative evaluation should include a complete eye examination. If the use of silicone oil is considered, the iris and lens should be inspected to determine if an adequate barrier to anterior migration of the silicone oil exists and to assess any potential difficulties in placing an inferior peripheral iridotomy (e.g. iatrogenic or traumatic iris damage, interference of intraocular lens haptic). If the need for a relaxing retinotomy is anticipated, particular emphasis should be placed on a careful analysis of the location, direction and extent of retinal traction.

A comprehensive evaluation of the components of retinal traction is often possible in the preoperative examination. Meticulous indirect ophthalmoscopy with scleral depression is essential. B-scan ultrasonography is useful in patients with media opacity. Computerized tomography is occasionally indicated in patients presenting after trauma to evaluate an intraocular foreign body and may be helpful in assessing liquefaction of subretinal or suprachoroidal hemorrhage.[17] Time spent in careful preoperative planning will be rewarded by efficiency in the operating room.

If the patient is referred from another institution, the complete medical record, including operative reports, should be obtained. Knowledge of prior procedures, particularly scleral buckling and type of tamponading agents used, will affect the surgical plan.

INSTRUMENTATION

- Standard three-port vitrectomy equipment and instrumentation.
- Intraocular monopolar diathermy.
- Vertical scissors.
- Angled horizontal scissors.
- Extrusion or flute needle with soft or hard tip.
- Laser (endolaser and/or indirect laser).

Optional or for specific indications:

- Perfluorocarbon liquids.
- Perfluorocarbon gas.
- Silicone oil.
- Wide-angle viewing system.

SURGICAL TECHNIQUE

After a conjunctival peritomy is made, an infusion cannula is placed through a sclerotomy carefully located to avoid bullously detached retina or areas of anterior retinal displacement. A 4-mm infusion cannula is used in phakic eyes and a 6-mm cannula is used in aphakic or pseudophakic patients. A standard three-port pars plana vitrectomy is performed. The posterior hyaloid and all significant epiretinal membranes are removed. Subretinal membranes that prevent the retina from attaching must also be transected or removed. At this point, a relaxing retinotomy may be considered if the retina fails to develop sufficient laxity to allow reattachment.

In selected cases, an early relaxing retinotomy may be the best option in patients with anterior PVR requiring extensive dissection of the vitreous base. Although it is necessary to release all major areas of traction, particularly traction bands to the ciliary body or posterior iris surface, an extremely meticulous anterior dissection extends operating time significantly. It may also increase retinal trauma, and a relaxing retinotomy is often necessary despite complete dissection. We feel that a shortened operating time is undervalued in the literature, but is of significant benefit to the patient provided that surgical goals are met. Certainly, complete relief of anterior traction is a desirable goal and the majority of traction must be released. It should be cautioned that the decision to perform retinotomy is not a casual one, and extensive surgical experience is helpful in deciding appropriate intraoperative timing.

The location and extent of retinotomy are determined by examining the traction forces preventing retinal reattachment. Regardless of location, it is of fundamental importance to extend the retinotomy past all areas of remaining traction. Some authors feel that perfluorocarbon liquid (PFCL) may help to identify areas of remaining traction and determine the extent of retinotomy necessary.[18] We have found that, in general, the surgeon can accurately judge the extent of retinotomy needed. PFCLs are helpful in keeping the posterior retina attached.

The most common error of surgeons learning the technique is insufficient retinotomy, and the most common location of recurrent or persistent retinal detachment after retinotomy is at the ends of the previously performed retinotomy, where retinal traction remains. Wide-angle viewing systems are extremely useful in gaining a global impression of retinal traction and ensuring adequate relief of anterior proliferation.[19] The most common type of retinotomy that we perform is a posterior inferior circumferential retinotomy of 180–270°. The posterior location of the retinotomy should not be closer than two disc diameters from the nasal aspect of the optic disc and arcade vessels and should not be closer than five disc diameters from the temporal aspect of the optic disc. The technique of performing this type of retinotomy will be discussed and variations will be described.

The first step in performing a posterior relaxing retinotomy is to ensure hemostasis along the intended extent of the retinotomy. This may be accomplished by avoiding major vessels and using unipolar diathermy to cauterize the retina along the intended path of the retinotomy. Diathermy also provides a chorioretinal adhesion at the retinotomy edge. Diathermy is usually effective in closing even large vessels, such as second-order vascular branches. If bleeding occurs, infusion pressure should be increased and aspiration of blood and additional diathermy should be performed as indicated. Diathermy is traditionally done in a double row (Fig. 29.2a). A single row of larger burns also may be used and is preferred by the authors (Fig. 29.2b). It is important to place two or three extra burns along the course of larger vessels crossing the retinotomy to ensure closure.

Frequently, diathermy will become ineffective after a coagulum of tissue accumulates on the tip of the probe. This accumulation may be removed, without removing the probe from the eye, by using the light pipe or a lighted pick to scrape the tip. It is important to ensure that diathermy is complete and that no untreated areas remain that may bleed during transection of the retina.

The diathermy probe also may be used to cut the retina, thus performing retinotomy in one step (Fig. 29.2c). The ease with which the retina is transected is related to its structural integrity. Thinned, atrophic retina in diabetics or chronic retinal detachment can be cut easily with diathermy. Although faster, this technique often requires higher diathermy power or longer application and may result in greater retinal trauma. When using diathermy to create the retinotomy, thin bridges of retina may be left across the retinotomy, which must be transected with scissors to ensure complete relief of traction.

Vertical or horizontal intraocular scissors are commonly used to transect the retina either between or peripheral to the diathermy marks, depending on the technique used (Fig. 29.3). Care must be taken to avoid trauma to the underlying RPE and choroid. Damage to the choroid can result in massive hemorrhage. Usually, the retinotomy is located in detached retina and a plane beneath the retina is easily established. Techniques for retinotomy in attached retina

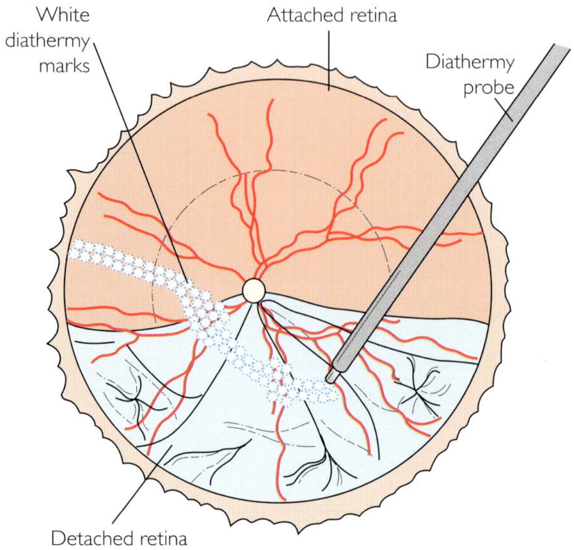

a

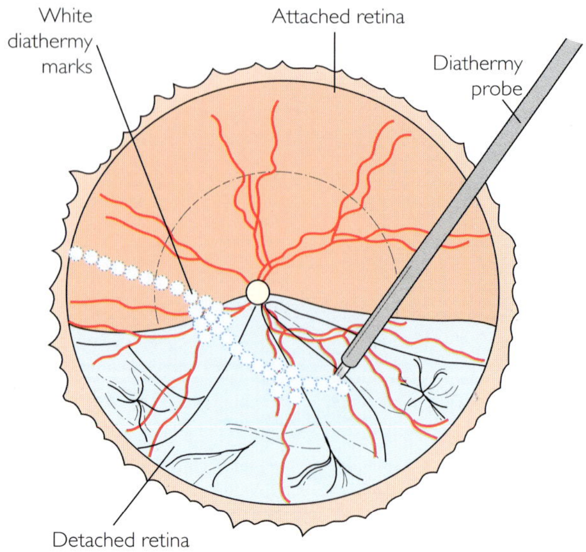

b

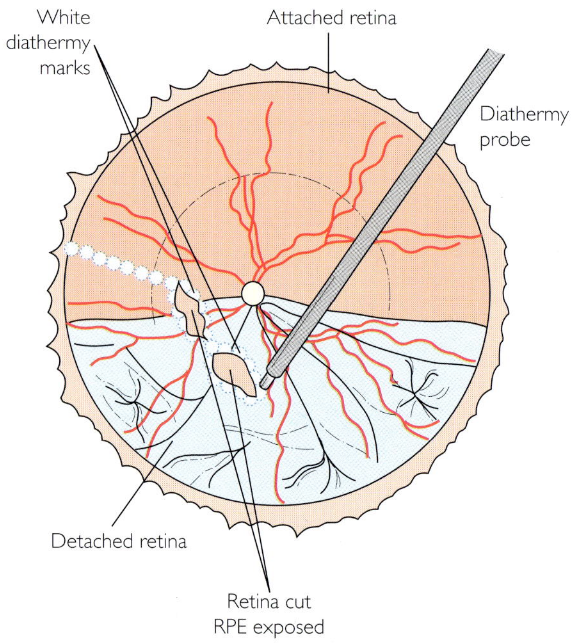

c

Figure 29.2 *(a) Intraocular unipolar diathermy is used along the intended path of the retinotomy in a double row or (b) in a single row. Extra diathermy is placed on major retinal vessels to ensure closure. (c) Diathermy may be used to create the retinotomy. This is most effective in thinned, atrophic retina.*

will be discussed later. The retina should not be lifted excessively, because an inadvertent extension of the retinotomy or retinal tear may result. Upon completion of the planned extent of the retinotomy, the retina should be inspected for any remaining areas of traction, with particular attention to the ends of the retinotomy. It is critical that no retinal traction remains at the lateral extents of the retinotomy. If residual traction is noted, additional diathermy should be applied and the retinotomy extended.

Once the relaxing retinotomy is deemed adequate, air–fluid exchange may be performed. We prefer to use a hard-tipped flute needle, but soft-tipped flute needles or extrusion needles also may be used. It is

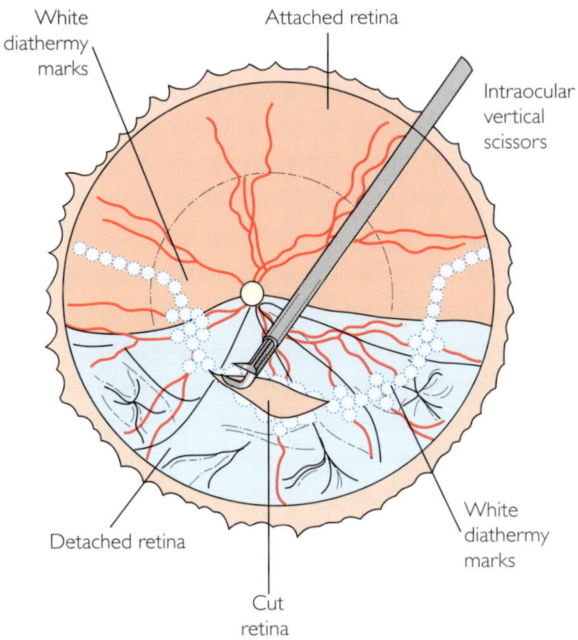

Figure 29.3 *Intraocular scissors are used to create the retinotomy within the margins of the previously applied diathermy. The retinotomy is begun in more highly detached retina and extended toward areas of shallowly detached or attached retina.*

important to place the tip of the aspiration device in close proximity to the RPE exposed by the retinotomy. This placement will ensure complete evacuation of the subretinal fluid and avoid inadvertent aspiration of the mobile edges of the retinotomy. Retinal slippage or inversion of the retinotomy edge almost never occurs with a posterior retinotomy, but may be problematic with a more anterior retinotomy. A PFCL may be used to stabilize the posterior edge of the retinotomy if rolling or slippage occurs.[20]

After complete air–fluid exchange, the retina is inspected. If the retina posterior to the retinotomy fails to flatten completely at this point, it usually means that the extent of the retinotomy is insufficient and must be extended. When the retina is completely flat, two or three rows of endolaser or indirect laser are applied to all edges of the retinotomy, and scatter treatment is performed to all attached retina anterior to the retinotomy. One of the advantages of a posterior retinotomy is a greater probability of reattachment of the retina anterior to the retinotomy. This anterior flap is usually apposed to the RPE, and photocoagulation can be applied. If there is severe contraction of the anterior retina, preventing apposition, it may be resected with the vitreous cutter, but this maneuver is usually not necessary.

When the retina is reattached and laser retinopexy has been applied, perfluorocarbon gas or silicone oil is selected as a tamponading agent. If oil is selected, a large inferior peripheral iridectomy is performed with the vitreous cutter in aphakic and pseudophakic eyes. Silicone oil can provide a stable long-term retinal tamponade, but it must be removed in 3–6 months for maximal visual recovery. Although some surgeons favor perfluorocarbon gas, we prefer to use silicone oil after relaxing retinotomy. Details of silicone oil injection technique are covered in Chapter 19. The advantages of oil are:

- Faster visual recovery, particularly in monocular and low vision patients.
- Better fundus visualization and ability to add laser retinopexy as indicated.
- No possibility of perfluorocarbon gas dilutional error resulting in over- or underfill.
- No need for additional postoperative air–fluid exchanges.
- Prolonged complete tamponade (even when upright) of the posterior retinotomy site.

We feel that for cases requiring posterior retinotomy, silicone oil tamponade may offer a higher single-operation success rate and improved visual outcome than gas tamponade, although this has not been demonstrated in a prospective, randomized study.

ADDITIONAL TECHNIQUES

POSTERIOR RETINOTOMY UNDER SILICONE OIL

For recurrent, usually inferior, retinal detachment after silicone oil tamponade, a retinotomy may be performed without the need for silicone oil removal.[21] We favor air infusion during removal of subretinal fluid; however, a technique has been described that uses a silicone oil pump to inject oil through the infusion cannula during aspiration of subretinal fluid.[22] The high pressure needed for silicone oil injection and a rapid rise in intraocular pressure may complicate this maneuver. When evacuation of subretinal fluid is complete, an intraocular pressure spike can occur because of the relative incompressibility of oil. This pressure spike can drive silicone oil through retinal breaks into the subretinal space.[23]

We currently utilize a standard three-port vitrectomy set-up, with the infusion initially turned to either air or fluid. Using fluid maintains excellent visibility, but may result in the loss of some silicone oil through the sclerotomies. The retinotomy location and extent are determined and diathermy is applied as described above.

After completion of the retinotomy, a hard-tipped flute needle or extrusion cannula is inserted while carefully avoiding aspiration of silicone oil, which will obstruct the needle. The tip is placed adjacent to exposed RPE between the edges of the retinotomy in the fluid layer beneath the silicone oil. Once in position, the infusion is turned to air, and both subretinal fluid and the meniscus of fluid beneath the silicone oil are evacuated (Fig. 29.4). Aspiration is complete when the silicone oil is apposed to the retina and the retinotomy site. This results in complete posterior tamponade of the retina by the silicone oil and an anterior layer of air. One superior sclerotomy is then closed and the other is prepared for silicone oil injection. The air is then replaced by silicone oil by injecting the oil through a sclerotomy site while allowing the air pump to maintain normal intraocular pressure. Laser retinopexy then is applied to the edges of the retinotomy.

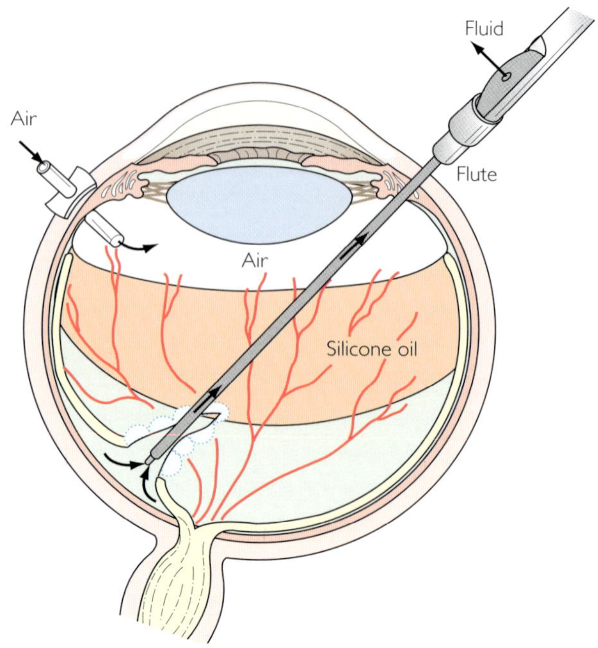

Figure 29.4 *Air is infused as fluid is aspirated beneath the silicone oil bubble with the tip of the flute needle in close proximity to the retinal pigment epithelium exposed by the retinotomy. Aspiration concludes as all subretinal fluid and fluid beneath the silicone oil is evacuated. The retina is then flat and silicone oil tamponades the retinal surface. Additional silicone oil is injected to replace the overlying air bubble.*

POSTERIOR RETINOTOMY AIDED BY PFCL

In patients with extensive tractional retinal detachment resulting from PVR, PFCL is often used to stabilize and reattach the posterior retina after dissection of posterior membranes. The PFCL acts as a 'third hand', providing countertraction and aiding anterior dissection and appreciation of remaining areas of traction. Despite a complete anterior dissection, a relaxing retinotomy is necessary to reattach the retina because of residual traction, stiffness or shortening of the retina in approximately one-third of cases.[7,16]

When a retinotomy is performed before removal of PFCL, operative maneuvers and time are reduced while attachment of the posterior retina is maintained under the PFCL, thus preventing folding or slippage of the posterior retinotomy edge. By maintaining posterior retinal attachment in all areas not under traction, the PFCL helps the surgeon to determine the extent of retinotomy that is necessary to relax the retina adequately before air–fluid exchange. This maneuver may save additional cycles of air–fluid exchange for adjustment of retinotomy size or location. However, it should be cautioned that, because of its higher specific gravity, the PFCL may flatten areas of clinically significant retinal traction, resulting in insufficient retinotomy. The retina immediately anterior to the PFCL is usually flat or very shallowly detached. Intraocular scissors that are commonly used to perform retinotomy in attached retina can cause massive hemorrhage if the choroid is penetrated inadvertently. We have reported a technique using diathermy combined with a silicone-tipped cannula that allows a safe retinotomy in attached retina before removal of PFCL.[24]

Our technique involves the following steps. After injection of the desired volume of PFCL and completion of anterior dissection, the appropriate location of the relaxing retinotomy is determined. The retinotomy site is usually located in attached retina just

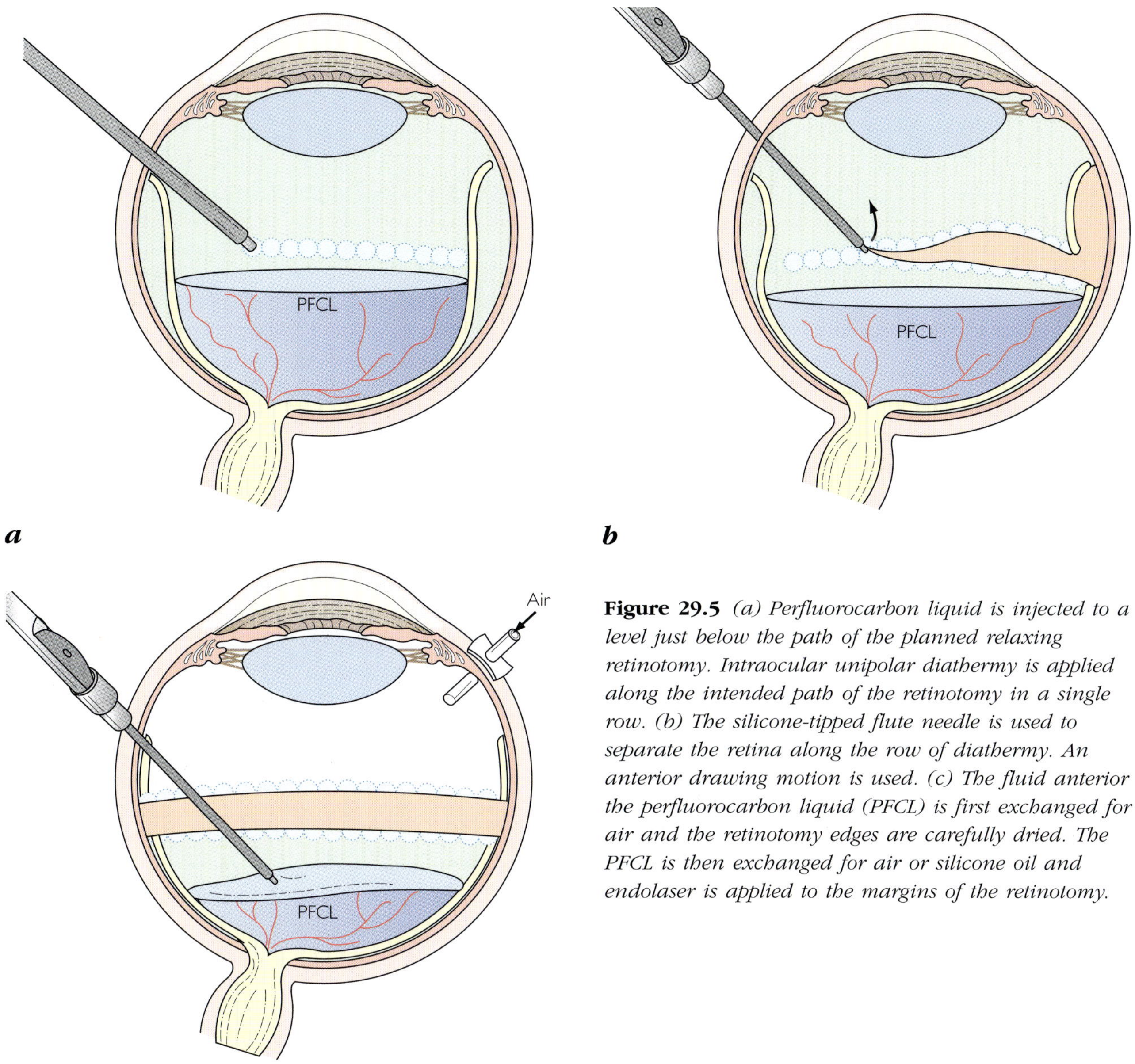

a *b* *c*

Figure 29.5 *(a) Perfluorocarbon liquid is injected to a level just below the path of the planned relaxing retinotomy. Intraocular unipolar diathermy is applied along the intended path of the retinotomy in a single row. (b) The silicone-tipped flute needle is used to separate the retina along the row of diathermy. An anterior drawing motion is used. (c) The fluid anterior to the perfluorocarbon liquid (PFCL) is first exchanged for air and the retinotomy edges are carefully dried. The PFCL is then exchanged for air or silicone oil and endolaser is applied to the margins of the retinotomy.*

anterior to the level of the PFCL. Intraocular diathermy is applied to the retina in a line of adjacent spots at the desired location of the retinotomy (Fig. 29.5a). A silicone-tipped flute needle is used to create the retinotomy instead of intraocular scissors or the vitreous cutter. While the PFCL provides stabilization of the posterior retinotomy edge, the flute needle is used in an anterior drawing motion to apply tangential traction to the retina immediately anterior to the diathermy (Fig. 29.5b). As gentle anterior traction is applied, the retina separates along the row of diathermy. This technique works in much the same way as separating the serrated edges of postage stamps.

Following the retinotomy, two or three rows of endolaser retinopexy are applied to all edges of the retinotomy. Laser is applied through the PFCL to the posterior edge of the retinotomy. A PFCL–air exchange is then performed, with careful attention paid to removing all fluid above the PFCL before removing the PFCL itself (Fig. 29.5c). Much as in giant retinal tears, this sequence of removal prevents slippage or inversion of the retinotomy edge. Silicone oil or perfluorocarbon gas is then selected as a tamponading agent.

COMPLICATIONS

The complications of performing a relaxing retinotomy include those of any pars plana vitrectomy. A loss of peripheral retinal function and consequent loss of visual field are the expected results of retinotomy. Complications secondary to retinotomy include hemorrhage, hypotony, reproliferation, perisilicone proliferation and recurrent retinal detachment. Minor hemorrhage along the retinotomy site is the most common intraoperative complication.[8] Bleeding usually occurs when large retinal vessels are severed after inadequate diathermy. Rarely, trauma to the choroid with scissors during the retinotomy may induce a large hemorrhage. Bleeding can be controlled almost always by raising the infusion pressure and performing additional diathermy. Postoperative hemorrhage, likely caused by continued oozing from the edge of the retinotomy, also may occur rarely. A less common complication of retinotomy is a choroidal neovascular membrane, presumably as a result of disturbance of the RPE–choroid complex.[25]

Hypotony has been reported as a complication of relaxing retinotomy, and may occur in as many as 43% of patients.[12,13] In the Silicone Study, a higher incidence of hypotony was found in those patients who required a relaxing retinotomy than in controls without retinotomy.[7] Perfluorocarbon gas tamponade also was associated with increased risk of hypotony in these eyes. It remains unclear whether the hypotony is caused by the greater preoperative pathology, particularly anterior traction with involvement of the ciliary body, or if it is secondary to the retinotomy itself. It is possible that additional trans-RPE outflow of aqueous fluid occurs at the retinotomy site.

Angiographic study supports the clinical impression that retinotomies cause no significant damage in the attached retina.[25] Retinal perfusion is unaffected, and there is no breakdown of the blood–retinal barrier. Notably, angiography did not show evidence of significant fibrovascular reproliferation.

SURGICAL RESULTS

Alturki et al described the results of posterior retinotomy in 15 consecutive patients with complicated retinal detachment.[15] Eleven patients had PVR, two had trauma and two had an inflammatory retinopathy. The retina was tamponaded with silicone oil in 14 patients. Three patients had short-term tamponade with perfluoroperhydrophenanthrene (Vitreon, Vitrophage Inc., Lyons, IL) followed by silicone oil injection. One patient received sulfur hexafluoride gas. With a minimum follow-up of 6 months, 80% of the retinas remained attached, which is similar to results reported for anterior retinotomy (63–82%).[8,12–14] Visual acuity improved in 53%, remained unchanged in 20% and decreased in 27%. Of the 11 eyes that had stable or improved vision, five (45%) achieved 20/400–20/25 vision, five achieved count fingers perception and one patient remained stable at hand motion perception.

Recently, a retrospective chart review was undertaken of 39 consecutive cases of posterior relaxing retinotomy with greater than 6 months follow-up.[26] Each patient underwent relaxing retinotomy using the technique described in this chapter. Twenty-eight patients were male and 11 were female. Mean age was 48 years, with a range of 2–90 years. Five eyes had no prior surgery, 19 eyes had one previous surgery, eight had two prior surgeries and two eyes had three earlier surgeries. The etiology of unrelieved retinal traction necessitating retinotomy was PVR in all cases. The two most common initiating events were rhegmatogenous retinal detachment in 16 eyes and trauma in eight eyes (three with intraocular foreign bodies). The remaining eyes had proliferative diabetic retinopathy, retinal dialysis, giant retinal tear and retinal incarceration; one eye had juvenile retinoschisis.

Relaxing retinotomy was 90–180° in 34 cases, 270–360° in one case and limited to 2–3 clock-hours in the three cases of retinal incarceration. The central location of the retinotomy was inferior in 26 cases, nasal or temporal in 10 cases and superior in two cases (excluding the patient with 360° retinotomy). All eyes received silicone oil tamponade. Intraoperative reattachment was achieved in all cases.

With a single retinotomy and an average of 2.4 years of follow-up, 87% of cases had retinal reattachment posterior to the retinotomy site. Redetachment occurred in 13% (five eyes). Eight percent (three eyes) required reoperation with extension of the retinotomy to achieve retinal attachment.

Evaluation of functional outcome revealed that 71% (28 eyes) achieved hand motion or better vision. Seven eyes had a visual acuity of 20/40–20/400. Visual acuity was counting fingers in eight eyes, hand motion in 13 eyes and light perception in eight eyes. Three eyes had no light perception.

CONCLUSIONS

Relaxing retinotomy is primarily a procedure of last resort when other methods of reducing retinal traction have failed or are insufficient. Relaxing retinotomy commonly allows reattachment of retinas that are otherwise irreparable. When performing a relaxing retinotomy, it is essential to evaluate the vectors of retinal traction carefully in order to design the most limited retinotomy that will allow complete retinal reattachment. Relaxing retinotomies are most commonly performed circumferentially and may be anterior or posterior. A posterior location may sacrifice some visual field if the anterior retina is functional, in comparison to a more anterior location. However, a posterior retinotomy has the advantages of being technically simpler, faster and being more likely to allow retention of the crystalline lens. A posterior retinotomy is more easily tamponaded in the upright position. It is the opinion of the authors that silicone oil tamponade is preferable in operations requiring posterior relaxing retinotomy.

Single-procedure success rates are difficult to compare between series involving relaxing retinotomy because of differing preoperative characteristics and etiologies of retinal detachment. Our recent data suggest a single-operation success rate of 87% for the technique described in this chapter. It is clear that many different techniques of relaxing retinotomy offer reasonably high rates of anatomic and functional success, given the severity of the pre-existing retinal pathology. Posterior retinotomy is a valuable technique when applied judiciously in complex retinal detachments.

REFERENCES

1. Machemer R. Schneiden der Netzhaut: Eine Behandlungsmoglichkeit zur Weideranlegung der Netzhaut, *Klin Monatsbl Augenheilkd* (1979) **175:**597–601.
2. Machemer R. Retinotomy, *Am J Ophthalmol* (1981) **92:**768–74.
3. Machemer R, McCuen BW II, de Juan E Jr. Relaxing retinotomies and retinectomies, *Am J Ophthalmol* (1986) **102:**7–12.
4. Zivojnovic R, Mertens DAE, Peperkamp E. Das flussige Silikon in der Amotiochirurgie (II). Bericht uber 280 Falle-weitere Entwicklung der Technik, *Klin Monatsbl Augenheilkd* (1982) **181:**444–52.
5. Michels RG. Surgery of retinal detachment with proliferative vitreoretinopathy, *Retina* (1984) **4:**63–83.
6. Abrams GW. Retinotomies and retinectomies. In: Ryan SJ, Glaser BM, eds, *Retina*, 2nd edn, Vol. 3 (CV Mosby: St Louis, 1994): 2203–37.
7. Blumenkranz MS, Azen SP, Aaberg T, et al. Relaxing retinotomy with silicone oil or long-acting gas in eyes with severe proliferative vitreoretinopathy: Silicone Study Report 5, *Am J Ophthalmol* (1993) **116:**557–64.
8. Federman JL, Eagle RC Jr. Extensive peripheral retinectomy combined with posterior 360 degree retinotomy for retinal reattachment in advanced proliferative vitreoretinopathy cases, *Ophthalmology* (1990) **97:**1305–20.
9. McDonald HR, Johnson RN, Madeira D, Schatz H. Surgical results for proliferative vitreoretinopathy, *Eur J Ophthalmol* (1994) **4:**211–17.
10. Han DP, Pulido JS, Mieler WF, Johnson MW. Vitrectomy for proliferative diabetic retinopathy with severe equatorial fibrovascular proliferation, *Am J Ophthalmol* (1995) **119:**563–70.
11. Han DP, Mieler WF, Abrams GW, Williams GA. Vitrectomy for traumatic retinal incarceration, *Arch Ophthalmol* (1988) **106:**640–5.
12. Morse LS, McCuen BW II, Machemer R. Relaxing retinotomies: analysis of anatomic and visual results, *Ophthalmology* (1990) **97:**642–8.
13. Han DP, Lewis MT, Kuhn EM, et al. Relaxing retinotomies and retinectomies: surgical results and predictors of visual outcome, *Arch Ophthalmol* (1990) **108**:694–7.
14. Iverson DA, Ward TG, Blumenkranz MS. Indications and results of relaxing retinotomy, *Ophthalmology* (1990) **97**:1298–304.
15. Alturki WA, Peyman GA, Paris CL, et al. Posterior relaxing retinotomies: analysis of anatomic and visual results, *Ophthalmic Surg* (1992) **23**:685–8.
16. Coll GE, Chang S, Sun J, et al. Perfluorocarbon liquid in the management of retinal detachment with proliferative vitreoretinopathy, *Ophthalmology* (1995) **102**:630–9.
17. Gremillion CM, Peyman GA. Posterior relaxing retinotomy, *Ophthalmic Surg* (1989) **20**:655–7.
18. Peyman GA, Schulman JA. *Intravitreal Surgery: Principles and Practice*, 2nd edn (Appleton & Lange: Norwalk, CT, 1994): 489–549.
19. Lesnoni G, Billi B, Rossi T, Stirpe M. The use of panoramic viewing system in relaxing retinotomy and retinectomy, *Retina* (1997) **17**:186–90.
20. Han DP, Rychwalski PJ, Mieler WF, Abrams GW. Management of complex retinal detachment with combined relaxing retinotomy and intravitreal perfluoro-*n*-octane injection, *Am J Ophthalmol* (1994) **118**:24–32.
21. Kertes P, Peyman GA. Drainage of subretinal fluid under silicone oil, *Can J Ophthalmol* (1997) **32**:445–6.
22. Zivojnovic R. *Silicone Oil in Vitreoretinal Surgery* (Martinus/Dr W Junk Publishers: Dordrecht, The Netherlands, 1987): 146–52.

23. Lean JS. Use of silicone oil as an additional technique in vitreoretinal surgery. In: Ryan SJ, Glaser BM, eds, *Retina*, 2nd edn, Vol. 3 (CV Mosby: St Louis, 1994): 2151–64.
24. Greve MDJ, Peyman GA, Millsap CM. Relaxing retinotomy under perfluorocarbon liquid, *Ophthalmic Surg Lasers* (1996) **27**:154–5.
25. Bopp S, Laqua H, Lucke K. Fluoreszenzangiographische Befunde nach Retinotomien und Retinektomien, *Klin Monatsbl Augenheilk* (1991) **199**:170–6.
26. Meffert SA, Fenton J, Chou F, et al. Posterior retinotomy for proliferative vitreoretinopathy, *Invest Ophthalmol Vis Sci* (1998) **39** (Suppl): S1006 (abst).

Chapter 30 Vitreoretinal surgery for idiopathic epiretinal membranes

H Richard McDonald, Robert N Johnson and Everett Ai

INTRODUCTION

Epiretinal membranes (ERMs) have been recognized since the 1930s, and have been referred to by a multitude of synonyms.[1–17] They have been associated with a vast array of ocular conditions and diseases.[8,10,11,17–38] When ERMs form in the absence of these entities, they are termed idiopathic ERMs, although the great majority are caused by posterior vitreous detachment.[10,11,22,32] Most patients with idiopathic ERMs are asymptomatic and have near-normal vision. However, in some eyes ERMs may cause visually disabling metamorphopsia, diplopia and significantly reduced vision. In these eyes, vitreoretinal surgery has been used to remove membranes and restore vision.[17,20,22,38–42]

INDICATIONS

Vision is decreased in eyes with ERMs for a variety of reasons: one or more full-thickness retinal folds; a trampoline-like sensory foveal elevation (table-top-like traction); foveal ectopia created by an eccentric ERM; retinal vascular leakage causing macular edema; the presence of an opaque, dense membrane directly over the fovea; or traction-induced stasis of axoplasmic flow.[10] These findings may be present, individually or in combination, in eyes with visually significant ERMs. The goal of surgery is to relieve the traction caused by the ERM.

The indications for surgery vary by individual, but usually are reserved for those cases in which the vision has been decreased to the 20/60 level. Eyes with 20/50 vision are occasionally considered for surgery if the primary complaint is diplopia or if the patient suffers debilitating metamorphopsia and requires better vision for employment.

PREOPERATIVE EVALUATION

Eyes being considered for vitrectomy and epiretinal membrane stripping need a careful preoperative evaluation to determine whether the visual loss is caused strictly by the membrane, or is secondary to some other retinal pathologic state such as an impending or early full-thickness macular hole, choroidal neovascularization, postcataract extraction macular edema, macular telangiectasis, cataract, macular ischemia associated with retinal vascular occlusion or peripheral retinal vascular abnormalities or vasoproliferative tumors.[10,28,29] Additional information that may be helpful in accurately assessing risks of surgery include the presence of peripheral breaks or lattice degeneration, the presence of partial posterior vitreous detachment as part of the vitreomacular traction syndrome and the degree of nuclear sclerosis.

SURGICAL PROGNOSIS

There are several factors considered to be of prognostic value in predicting visual recovery following vitrectomy and ERM removal. In a study of eyes with ERMs of various etiologies, eyes with poor preoperative vision tended to improve more frequently and to a greater extent than did eyes with better preoperative vision.[40] However, those eyes with lower levels of preoperative vision usually had poorer final vision than those eyes with better preoperative visual levels, despite having picked up more Snellen lines on acuity testing.

Retinal vascular leakage with cystoid macular edema has been found by some authors to be a relatively poor prognostic factor.[40,42,43] Although not all studies evaluating ERM surgery have agreed, most surgeons feel that significant or long-standing leakage carries a poor prognosis.[20,22] Some of these eyes may have retinal pigment epithelium atrophy associated with leakage. Retinal pigment epithelium (RPE) disruption, from any etiology, is a poor prognostic finding. In most cases, removal of traction diminishes the macular edema.[44,45] In some eyes, however, the traction has caused the retinal capillaries to become permanently incompetent; leakage and edema continue to cause visual impairment postoperatively. In this regard, preoperative fluorescein angiography may aid in determining which eyes will benefit most from surgery.

The etiology of the ERM influences the surgical outcome. Eyes with membranes following retinal detachment fare worse than those with idiopathic ERMs.[50] In a study evaluating vision after membrane removal following retinal detachment or retinal breaks, factors associated with better postoperative vision included the presence of a thin ERM and a macula-on status during the previous detachment.[46]

In a similar study of idiopathic ERMs, factors associated with better postoperative visual results included an initial vision of 20/60 or better, a short duration of blurred vision, a thin ERM and no traction retinal detachment.[41]

It has been suggested that eyes with transparent ERMs achieve better vision after surgery than eyes with opaque membranes.[47] However, others have reported that eyes with opaque membranes do equally well as those with translucent, nonopaque membranes.[22,40]

TIMING OF SURGERY

Surgery for macular puckers following retinal detachment is performed when the membrane has matured and stopped actively contracting, ideally within 2 months of the onset of symptoms.[40,42,45,50] For eyes with idiopathic ERM, the membrane growth is usually slowly progressive, and it is often difficult to determine the onset of symptoms. Surgery is performed when the vision has decreased significantly. This delay does not seem to adversely affect the probability of a good visual outcome. Significant visual improvement has been seen after the removal of membranes present for years before surgery.[40,42,45] However, several studies have indicated that the potential for improvement is reduced if the membrane has been present for an especially prolonged time.[42,45]

SURGICAL PROCEDURE

Surgery for idiopathic ERMs is usually performed under local anesthesia with intravenous sedation administered by an anesthesiologist. A peribulbar injection is performed with a short 23-gauge needle, administering a 5-ml bolus of a 50:50 mixture of 2% Xylocaine (with 1 ml of Wydase) and 0.75% Marcaine. This is followed by a 5-ml injection using the same needle to perform the O'Brien facial nerve block. Two winged conjunctival peritomies are created at the 3 o'clock and 9 o'clock positions to allow sclerotomy sites to be placed 4.0 mm posterior to the surgical limbus in phakic eyes and 3–3.5 mm posterior in pseudophakic eyes. With a pars plana vitrectomy, as much vitreous is removed as is easily and safely possible, without endangering the crystalline lens or peripheral retina.

Approximately 90% of eyes with idiopathic ERM have a posterior vitreous detachment. Eyes with the vitreomacular traction syndrome may have an ERM in association with persistent vitreomacular adhesion.[27,48] In eyes without a posterior vitreous detachment, the vitreous is separated from the posterior pole and the posterior hyaloid face is stripped anteriorly. However, no aggressive attempts are made to strip the vitreous cortex anteriorly to the posterior vitreous base insertion if tenacious adhesions are present.

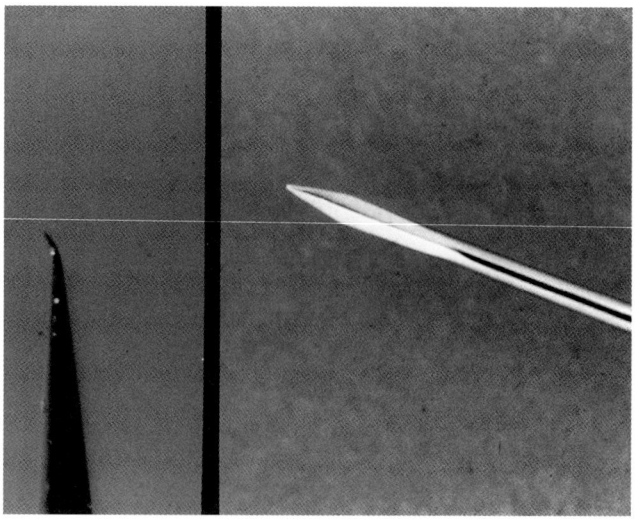

Figure 30.1 *The microvitreoretinal blade has been bent to an approximately 45° angle.*

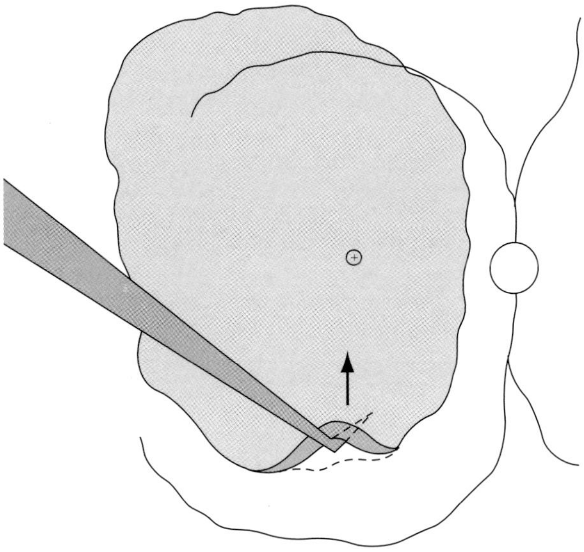

Figure 30.2 *The microvitreoretinal (MVR) blade is used to engage the edge of the epiretinal membrane or to create an edge by dragging the downwardly curved edge of the barbed MVR blade along the surface of the membrane.*

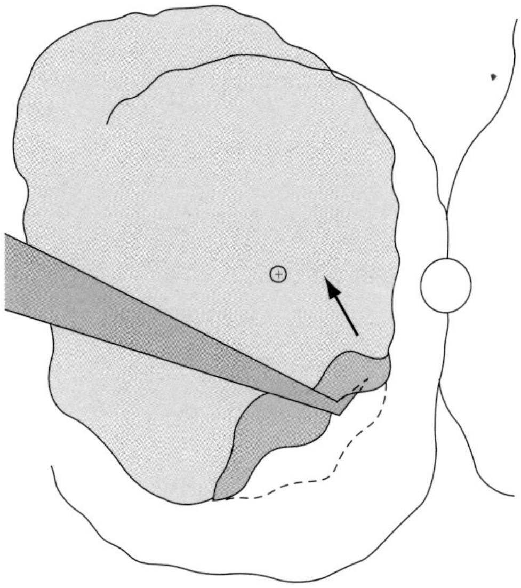

Figure 30.3 *The microvitreoretinal blade is used to elevate the membrane at different areas near the initial dissection point. At each location the membrane is pulled for only a short distance in an effort to avoid shredding the membrane.*

Attention is then directed toward the membrane. If the membrane is thick and fibrotic, it may be possible to grasp the membrane directly with an intraocular foreign-body forceps and lift it from the macular surface. A variety of instruments have been developed to aid in the initiation and completion of epiretinal membrane removal.[52–54] In most cases, however, a barbed microvitreoretinal (MVR) blade (Fig. 30.1) is employed to engage the membrane at its edge and elevate it from the retinal surface (Fig. 30.2). The blade then is used to remove connections to the retina on the edge of the membrane where the dissection was initiated (Fig. 30.3). A 'front' of elevated membrane is created, avoiding fragmenting the membrane by pulling too hard or too long in any one direction (Fig. 30.4). Some surgeons employ a blunt-tipped pick once a broad edge of membrane has been raised, because this may decrease the chance of tearing the membrane and having to find a new edge.

A variety of instruments can be used to begin the dissection, to elevate a broad area of membrane, to remove distal connections and to preserve a 'one-piece' removal of the membrane. Once an entire side of the membrane has been elevated, fine-tipped vitreous

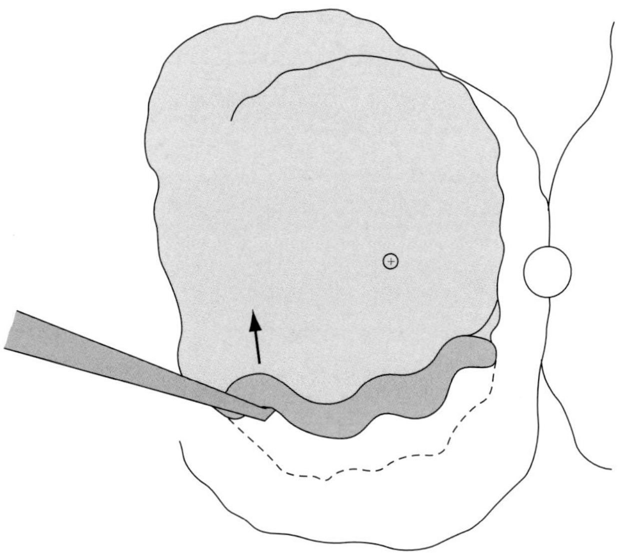

Figure 30.4 *A 'front' of membrane is elevated. Attention is directed to the advancing line of membrane–retinal adhesion. The surgeon memorizes the area over which the membrane has been removed.*

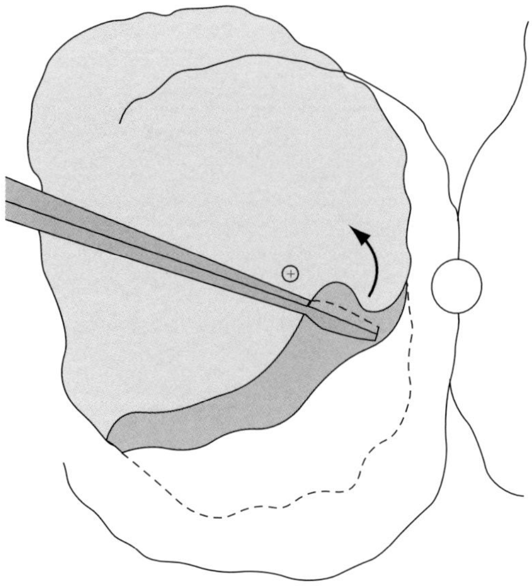

Figure 30.5 *Once a side of epiretinal membrane has been elevated, a fine-tipped, end-gripping foreign-body forceps is used to engage the membrane at multiple sites along the edge of residual adhesion, pulling the membrane toward the fovea.*

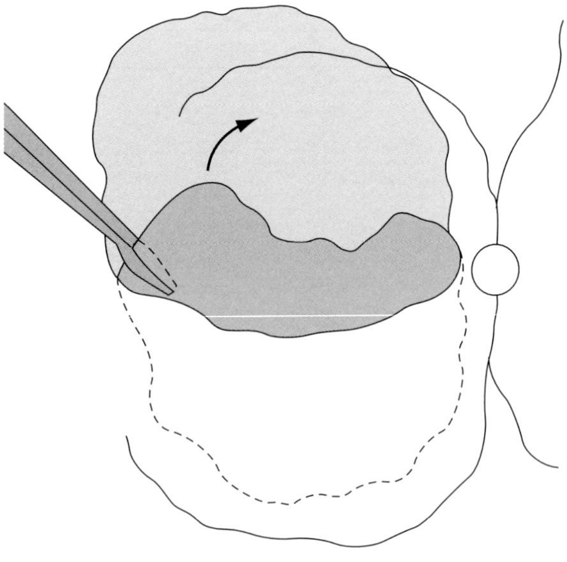

Figure 30.6 *Multiple 'regraspings' of the membrane should take place as close to the membrane–retina interface as possible, to decrease shredding and allow better control of the dissection.*

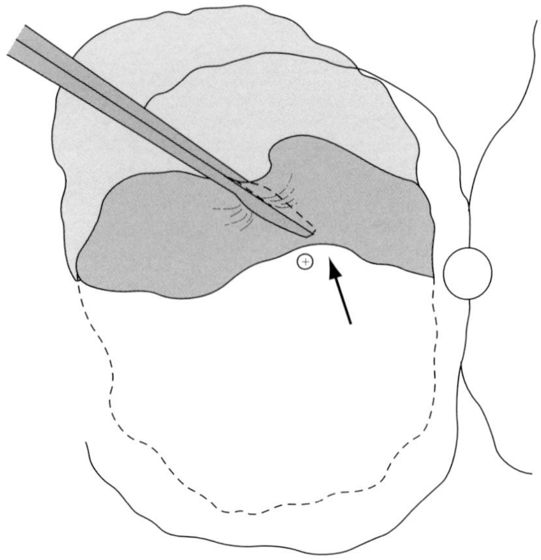

Figure 30.7 *Once the advancing edge comes close to the fovea, the membrane is grasped near the fovea so that it can be observed clearly peeling over and free of all macular connections.*

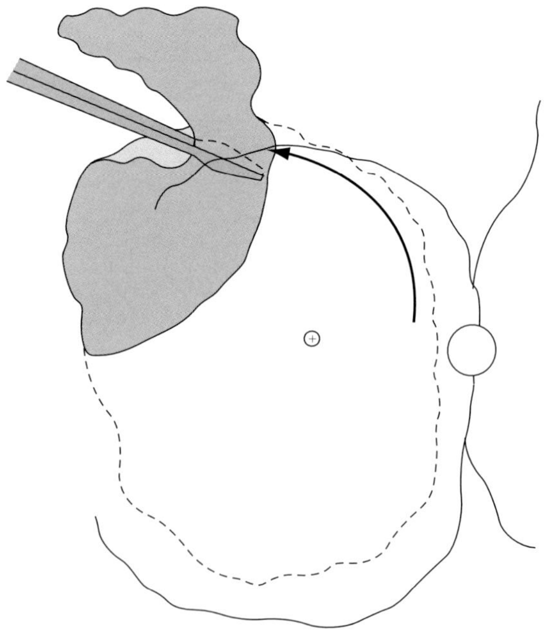

Figure 30.8 *The distal portions of the membrane are wheeled centrally after the membrane has been stripped away from the macula.*

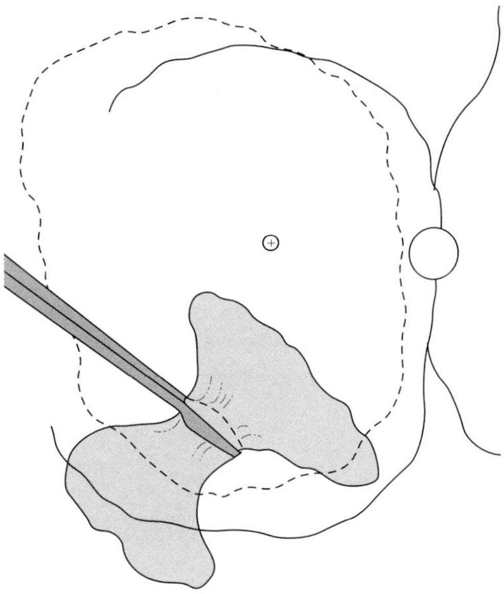

Figure 30.9 *The membrane then can be stripped entirely away from the retina and removed 'en bloc' from the eye.*

forceps are used to elevate the membrane at multiple sites along the advancing edge of residual adhesion (Fig. 30.5). These multiple 'regraspings' should take place as close to the membrane–retina interface as possible (Fig. 30.6). Once this advancing edge approaches the fovea, the membrane is grasped near the fovea so that the fovea can be observed clearly as the membrane is peeled free of all macular connections (Fig. 30.7). The distal portions of the membrane are wheeled centrally after the membrane has been stripped from the central macula (Fig. 30.8). The membrane can then be stripped entirely away from the retina and removed from the eye (Fig. 30.9).

Occasionally, an unusual area of membrane adherence is encountered and the retina may separate from the RPE as traction on the membrane is increased. The membrane should be regrasped and stripped toward this area of adhesion from another direction.

With idiopathic ERMs, there is often no clearly identifiable edge. The barbed MVR blade can be used to develop an edge by dragging its downwardly curved edge along the membrane surface. This dissection should be started over the thickest part of the membrane (or at least the most highly refractile portion of the membrane), but not over a major blood vessel. The membrane is engaged and gently elevated. Often during this 'drag-and-snag' technique it is difficult to know what tissues have been engaged, and the surgeon must examine the tissue that has been elevated. ERMs come up away from the retina as smooth, uniform sheets; internal limiting membrane has a sticky, more adherent quality. It appears glossy and fragments easily. The nerve-fiber layer, when elevated, appears fluffy and is often associated with small hemorrhages.

Some have advocated using a soft-tipped extrusion needle to aspirate the membrane and start the dissection.[49] Others feel that the membrane can be grasped on its surface by a pair of fine-tipped forceps, bypassing the need for finding or developing an edge.[50] In those eyes in which a membrane cannot be elevated otherwise, this 'pinch' technique can be used to remove a membrane. With the tips of the intraocular forceps opened slightly, the membrane–retina complex is pressed down. The fine-tipped forceps are closed and gentle tangential traction is applied. The elevated tissue is analyzed and, in our experience, usually consists of ERM and internal limiting membrane. This tissue then is stripped away from the retina using the forceps. Obviously, there are potential problems with this technique, including RPE trauma and retinal break formation.

ERMs may be associated with cotton-wool spots, usually broad areas of axoplasmic stasis on an edge of the membrane. The membrane is always tenaciously adherent to the retina at these areas of retinal whitening and membrane dissection should not be started in this region. The fluffy nature of the retina, combined with the tight attachment to the membrane, make it difficult to 'snag' an edge while dragging the barbed MVR blade. If an attempt is made to start the dissection at an area of axoplasmic stasis, the result often will be multiple elevations of fluffy clumps of nerve-fiber layer, coupled with numerous hemorrhages at the point of initial engagement. This axoplasmic stasis resolves within 1 week of membrane removal.

Once a membrane is stripped from the surface of the retina, the underlying retina may exhibit a whitish sheen. This occurs in tightly adherent membranes, and frequently in longstanding membranes. Some feel that intense whitening of the retina is a sign that the 'membrane' elevated is actually a sheet of internal limiting membrane.[51] It is essential to memorize the area over which the ERM has been removed, or the surgeon may mistake the whitened retina for residual membrane and attempt to remove it.

Invariably, some thin or idiopathic membranes will shred and the surgeon will have to restart the dissection. This is not a problem if the initial tearing of the membrane has left a slight residual sheet of elevated membrane near the retina. Otherwise, a sharp instrument once again must be employed to raise an edge. If this maneuver must be performed over the fovea, the chances for a posterior break increase. Before scraping for edges, however, an attempt can be made to engage the shredded edge of the membrane with a fine-toothed forceps. The membrane usually has a minimally elevated edge somewhere along the length of its front of dissection (although it may be difficult to visualize). A minute jerk-like motion will result in a sudden movement of the intraocular portion of the forceps. This 'flick' movement produces a wafting of the residual elevated edge of membrane that appears as a subtle shadow 'bobbing' at the fragmented edge of membrane. The surgeon then may grasp this region with forceps and avoid the potential damage of engaging the fovea with the MVR blade.

ERMs puckering the macula following retinal detachment surgery are usually thick, well localized and tightly adherent. They often fill a crevasse-like depression between ridges of tractionally elevated retina. Any of several blunt picks or sharp instruments can be passed through the crevasse to engage the membrane. Once the edge is elevated, the dissection may be almost finished. If the pucker has been longstanding, the elevated retina may be somewhat atrophic and the adhesion firm. The membrane may have to be regrasped and pulled from several directions to ensure a safe removal.

However, idiopathic ERMs cover a far larger area than would have been guessed at preoperative evaluation. The full extent of the membrane may not be appreciated fully until the time of surgery. There are no proven guidelines on how much of the membrane should be removed, but most surgeons feel that the area within the vascular arcades should be free of traction. It is reasonable to strip the membrane as far as necessary in any direction without endangering the retina. If peripheral membrane dissection is undertaken, it should be done under direct visualization. Membranes elevated from the posterior pole should not be grasped and pulled if persistent peripheral adhesions remain.

With tenacious membranes, it is not uncommon for a thin, curvilinear region of retina to be elevated as the membrane is being peeled away. This is often seen after forceps have been used to 'pinch' the membrane directly. Some surgeons feel that this is indicative of stripped internal limiting membrane, but it may be seen also with ERMs. With this degree of traction, there is potential for a posterior retinal break. This risk must be accepted if the membrane being stripped is within the arcades, and there is danger of persistent macular traction if dissection is aborted. However, these risks are usually not acceptable if the area of extreme traction is present outside the arcades.

Rarely, while peeling a membrane from the macula, a surgeon notes that the retina is becoming elevated away from the RPE, indicating that additional force is necessary to remove the membrane. However, additional force may tear the macula. This situation is usually seen in longstanding membrane puckering and atrophic retina. At this point, the membrane should be re-engaged at another site, and a different directional vector force used to strip the membrane. If this technique is not successful, it may be possible to use illuminated forceps in one hand, to stabilize the membrane–retina complex, and another pair of forceps in the other hand to shred and fragment the membrane in order to reduce its tractional effect on the macula. Occasionally, this technique allows complete removal of a membrane that could not be removed otherwise using the traditional 'one-handed' approach.

Along this line, there are a variety of illuminated forceps and illuminated picks that can help to stabilize and 'bimanually' dissect ERMs. None the less, there are rare cases where the membranes cannot be removed, and horizontal scissors are used to truncate the membrane close to the retina. The residual traction usually precludes significant visual improvement.

These techniques enable the surgeon to remove the ERM in virtually all cases. During these dissections, it is inevitable that fragments of internal limiting membrane will be removed along with the ERM.[55] It has been suggested that removal of internal limiting membrane may be associated with a decreased chance of visual improvement.[44] Others have argued that the removal of portions of internal limiting membrane has little adverse effect on vision.[47,50] Most surgeons make no special effort to avoid stripping membrane that may be inner limiting membrane. Despite the near certainty that ERM stripping will occasionally result in large areas of inner limiting membrane being removed, visual results of membrane removal are good.[55]

After the ERM is removed from the eye, indirect ophthalmoscopy is used to examine the peripheral retina for breaks; if encountered, cryotherapy or endolaser photocoagulation is placed and air–fluid exchange is performed. It is always important to examine the peripheral retina prior to air–fluid exchange, because small retinal breaks may be

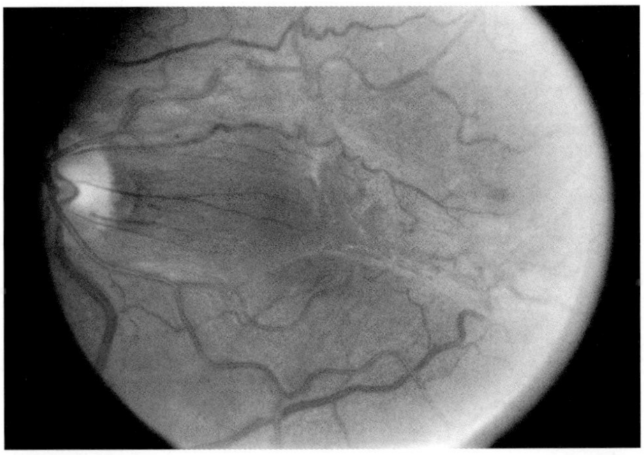

a

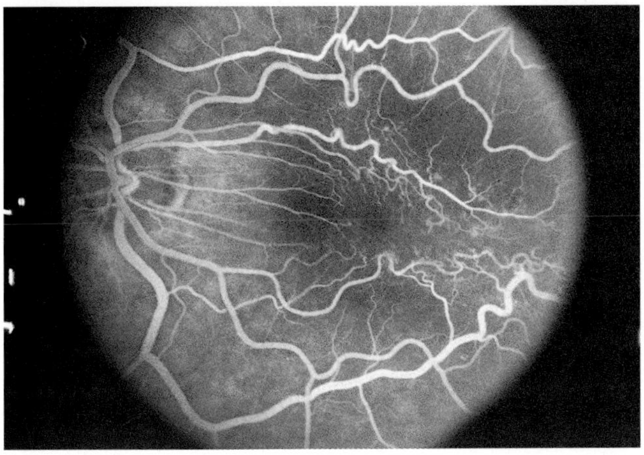

b

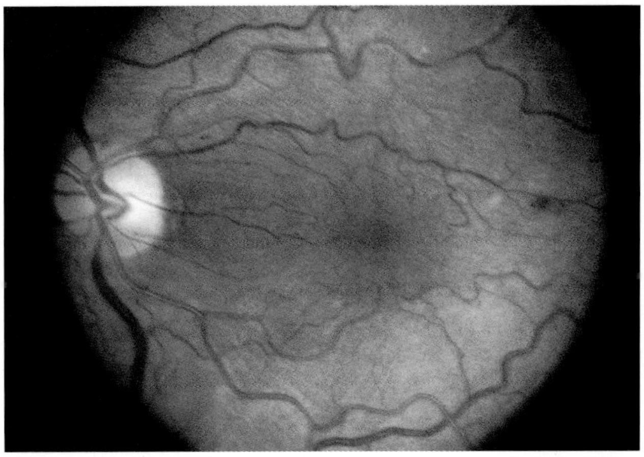

c

Figure 30.10 *(a) Preoperative photograph with epiretinal membrane causing decreased vision to 20/128. Note the sharply defined edge inferior to the fovea, which is an excellent area to begin dissection. (b) Preoperative fluorescein angiogram. Note the retinal vascular tortuosity but there is no retinal vascular leakage. (c) Postoperative photograph, vision 20/40.*

closed under air and overlooked. Sclerotomy sites and conjunctival incisions are closed with 7-0 polyglactin sutures. Patients receive prophylactic subconjunctival cephalosporin antibiotic injections (100 mg) as well as subconjunctival Decadron (24 mg). The eye is patched until the morning after surgery.

RESULTS

Immediately after the removal of an ERM, traction on the underlying retina may be visually decreased. This is more common for macular pucker developing after retinal detachment. The flattening of the macula following removal of an idiopathic membrane is not as dramatic. During the early postoperative period, areas of white retina will disappear and the retina will smooth out considerably. However, in many cases, minimal residual striae will remain indefinitely, despite complete membrane removal.

Vision remains poor for several weeks following surgery; it usually takes several weeks for a patient's vision to improve to the preoperative level. Despite this, patients will note improvement in metamorphopsia during the first month after vitrectomy.

ERM stripping results in significant visual improvement in a great majority of eyes (Figs 30.10–30.13). In eyes undergoing vitrectomy for idiopathic ERMs, vision improves by two or more Snellen lines in roughly 80–90% of cases.[20,22,41,42,46]

Those eyes undergoing surgery for macular pucker after retinal tears or retinal detachment improve by at least two Snellen lines in 65–90% of cases.[42,46]

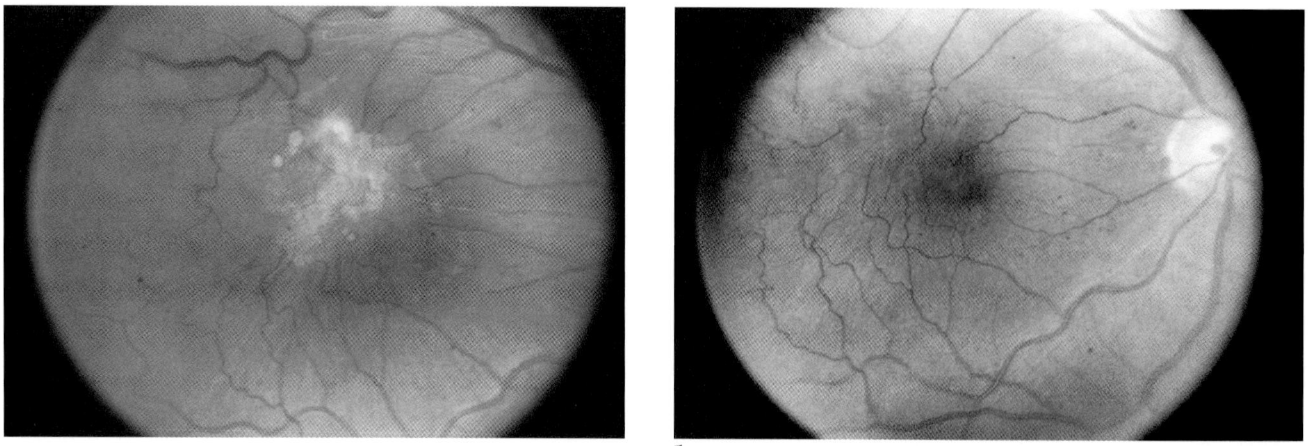

a *b*

Figure 30.11 *(a) Preoperative photograph showing epiretinal membrane, vision 20/160. Clear edge is seen superotemporal to fovea. (b) Postoperative photograph shows smoother macula, vision 20/50.*

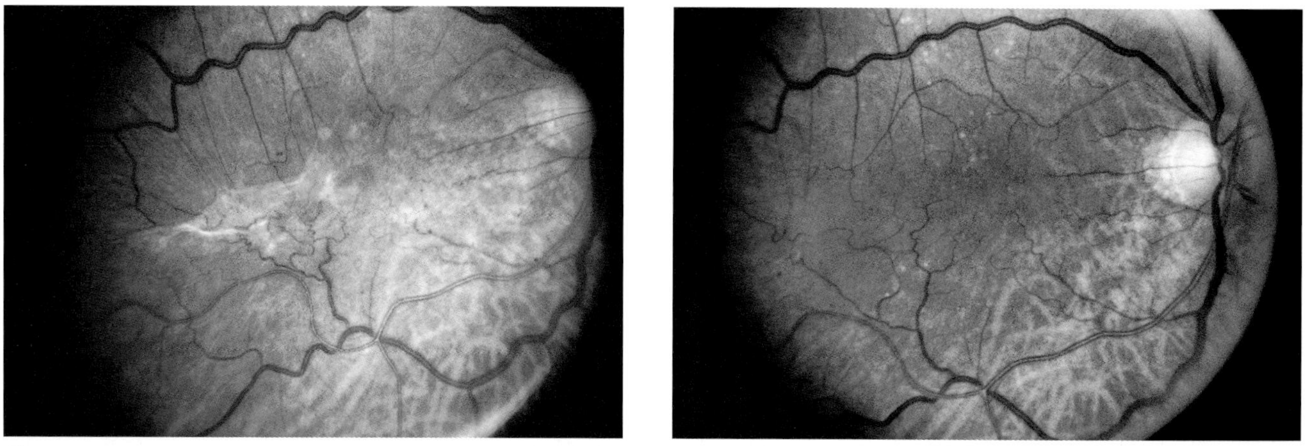

a *c*

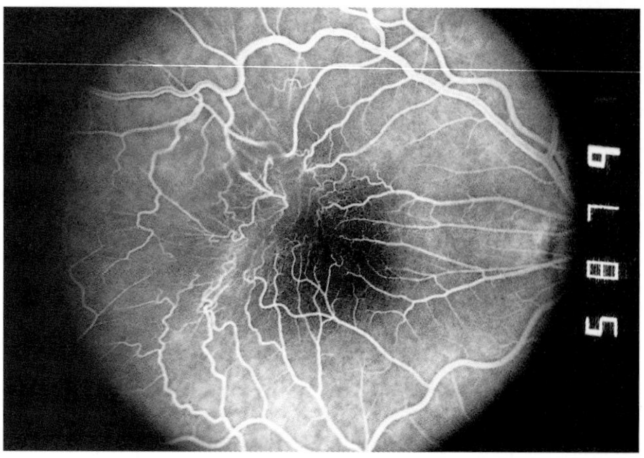

b

Figure 30.12 *(a) Preoperative photograph with epiretinal membrane dragging macula inferotemporally, causing diplopia and decreased vision to 20/100. (b) Preoperative fluorescein angiogram showing retinal vascular tortuosity and minimal leakage. (c) Postoperative photograph. Vision has improved to 20/30.*

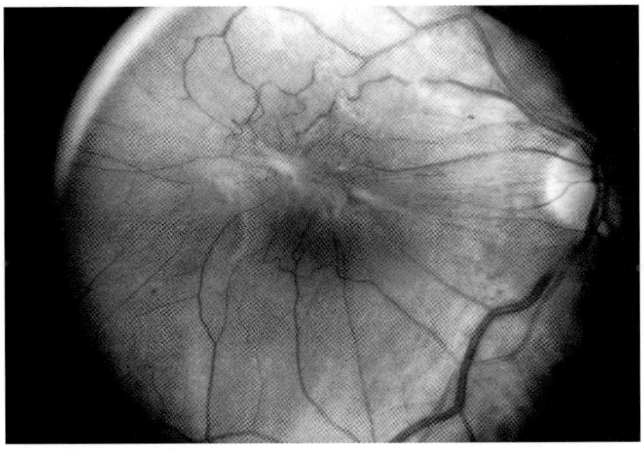

a

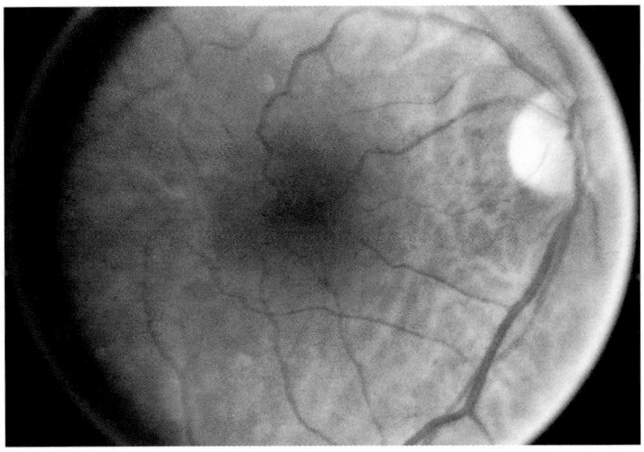

b

Figure 30.13 *(a) Preoperative photograph with epiretinal membrane decreasing vision to 20/100. (b) Postoperative photograph. Retinal tortuosity is greatly diminished, the macula is smooth and vision is 20/30.*

Obviously, better vision in these eyes is closely associated with whether there was a previous macular detachment.[23,56] In the largest series examining this type of macular pucker, 88% of eyes improved; 75% of eyes in which the macula had not been detached achieved postoperative vision of 20/60 or better, whereas only 24% achieved this level of vision if prior detachment involved the macula.[50,57]

Although ERM stripping usually results in significant visual improvement, and in a great majority of eyes metamorphopsia is diminished or eliminated, few eyes regain 20/20 vision. Patients with idiopathic membranes may expect to regain approximately half of the vision lost because of development of the membrane, resulting in final vision of 20/40 or better in 25–50% of operated eyes.[20,22,41,42,46] Therefore, the preoperative vision is a good indicator of eventual visual recovery. Most of this visual recovery occurs 2–3 months following surgery. Vision may continue to improve for 6–12 months postoperatively.

COMPLICATIONS

The most common complication of vitrectomy and ERM stripping surgery is cataract formation. Indeed, increasing nuclear sclerosis is considered a guaranteed side-effect of surgery in older individuals. It has been described in 12–68% of postoperative phakic eyes;[20,22,41,42,58,59] the longer the follow-up period, the greater the incidence of progressive lens opacity. In many eyes, vision improves for 6–9 months and then slowly begins to decline as progressive lens opacity begins. Usually, patients will not experience their best postoperative vision until cataract surgery is performed.

Initially, postvitrectomy cataracts do not have the classic yellowish-brown appearance of significant nuclear sclerosis. Rather, there is subtle pale greenish-gray opalescence. Patients usually begin to require increasingly myopic refractive correction 6–12 months before the cataract becomes obvious. Posterior subcapsular cataracts are not seen following surgery in the absence of iatrogenic lens damage or gas–fluid exchange. The cause of postoperative nuclear sclerosis remains unclear.

Retinal breaks occur in 1–6% of cases, almost exclusively in the periphery.[22,41,42,46,59] Posterior breaks are infrequently seen; when encountered, they are treated with air–fluid exchange and postoperative prone positioning without the need for endolaser photocoagulation. These breaks usually are the result of poor visualization and aggressive initial attempts at membrane engagement. Peripheral breaks are treated with cryotherapy or endolaser photocoagulation followed by air or gas exchange. These breaks may be created by instruments inserted through the vitreous base, or stripping of posterior hyaloid out toward the vitreous base insertion in cases with incomplete vitreous detachment. In eyes with an idiopathic ERM and a complete posterior vitreous detachment, the incidence of peripheral retinal breaks is reduced.

Retinal detachment (seen in 1–7% of eyes) is usually the result of overlooked breaks present at the end of surgery.[20,22,23,41,42,46,59] Late detachment, occurring several weeks after surgery, probably occurs in conjunction with contraction of vitreous incarcerated in sclerotomy sites. These detachments can be treated with scleral buckling or pneumatic retinopexy.

Visually significant, recurrent ERMs occur in up to 5% of eyes.[20,22,41,46,59] Many eyes may develop subtle ERMs following surgery, but rarely do they make a significant impact on visual improvement or require reoperation. Retinal phototoxicity has been reported as a complication of coaxial illumination from the operating microscope and/or the fiberoptic endoilluminator.[22,60,61] Endophthalmitis has been reported as a rare complication of ERM stripping surgery.[23]

Although the chances for visual improvement following vitrectomy and ERM stripping are excellent, patients and their families must understand that complications may occur and result in poor vision, the need for reoperation and even the loss of the eye. Each individual must weigh the risks against the benefits and decide if surgery is the best course for them.

ACKNOWLEDGMENTS

Supported by the Retina Research Fund of St Mary's Medical Center, San Francisco, California, and by a grant from the Wayne and Gladys Valley Foundation, Oakland, California, USA.

REFERENCES

1. Anderson JR. *Detachment of the Retina* (Cambridge University Press: Cambridge, 1931): 94.
2. Lyle DJ. Detachment of the internal limiting membrane of the retina (hyaloid membrane), *Trans Am Acad Ophthalmol Otolaryngol* (1934) **39:**201–17.
3. Gass JDM. Lamellar macular hole: a complication of cystoid macular edema after cataract extraction, *Arch Ophthalmol* (1976) **94:**793–800.
4. Gass JDM. *Stereoscopic Atlas of Macular Diseases: Diagnosis and Treatment* (CV Mosby: St Louis, 1987): 694–712.
5. Hamilton AM. Pre-retinal traction membranes, *Trans Ophthalmol Soc UK* (1972) **92:**387–93.
6. Hansen RI, Friedman AH, Gartner S, Henkind P. The association of retinitis pigmentosa with preretinal macular gliosis, *Br J Ophthalmol* (1977) **61:**597–600.
7. Kleinert H. Primare Netzhautfaltelung im Macula Bereich, *Graefes Arch Clin Exp Ophthalmol* (1954) **155:**350–8.
8. Maumenee AE. Further advances in the study of the macula, *Arch Ophthalmol* (1967) **78:**151–65.
9. Maumenee AE. Doyne Memorial Lecture. Fluorescein angiography in the diagnosis and treatment of lesions of the ocular fundus, *Trans Ophthalmol Soc UK* (1969) **88:**529–56.
10. McDonald HR, Aaberg TM. Idiopathic epiretinal membranes. *Semin Ophthalmol* (1986) **1:**189–95.
11. Noble KG, Carr RE. Idiopathic preretinal gliosis, *Ophthalmology* (1982) **89:**521–3.
12. Reeser FH, Aaberg TM. Vitreous humor. In: Records RE, ed, *Physiology of the Human Eye and Visual System* (Harper & Row: Hagerstown, MD, 1979): 284–327.
13. Roth AM, Foos RY. Surface wrinkling retinopathy in eyes enucleated at autopsy, *Trans Am Acad Ophthalmol Otolaryngol* (1971) **75:**1047–58.
14. Schatz H. *Essential Fluorescein Angiography: a Compendium of 100 Classic Cases* (Pacific Medical Press: San Francisco, 1982).
15. Scudder MJ, Eifrig DE. Spontaneous surface wrinkling retinopathy, *Ann Ophthalmol* (1975) **7:**333–41.
16. Wise GN. Macular changes after venous obstruction, *Arch Ophthalmol* (1957) **58:**544–57.
17. Wise GN. Congenital preretinal macular fibrosis, *Am J Ophthalmol* (1975) **79:**363–5.
18. Carney MD, Jampol LM. Epiretinal membranes in sickle cell retinopathy, *Arch Ophthalmol* (1987) **105:**214–17.
19. Lobes LA Jr, Burton TC. The incidence of macular pucker after retinal detachment surgery, *Am J Ophthalmol* (1978) **85:**72–7.
20. Margherio RR, Cox MS Jr, Trese MT, et al. Removal of epimacular membranes, *Ophthalmology* (1985) **92:**1075–83.
21. McDonald HR, Abrams GW, Burke JM, Neuwirth J. Clinicopathologic results of vitreous surgery for epiretinal membranes in patients with combined retinal and retinal pigment epithelial hamartomas, *Am J Ophthalmol* (1985) **100:**806–13.
22. McDonald HR, Verre WP, Aaberg TM. Surgical management of idiopathic epiretinal membranes, *Ophthalmology* (1986) **93:**978–83.
23. Michels RG. Vitrectomy for macular pucker, *Ophthalmology* (1984) **91:**1384–8.
24. Mills PV. Preretinal macular fibrosis, *Trans Ophthalmol Soc UK* (1979) **99:**50–3.
25. Schachat AP, Shields JA, Fine SL, et al. Combined hamartomas of the retina and retinal pigment epithelium, *Ophthalmology* (1984) **91:**1609–15.
26. Tanenbaum HL, Schepens CL, Elzeneiny I, Freeman HM. Macular pucker following retinal detachment surgery, *Arch Ophthalmol* (1970) **83:**286–93.
27. McDonald HR, Johnson RN, Schatz H. Surgical results in the vitreomacular traction syndrome, *Ophthalmology* (1994) **101:**1397–403.
28. McDonald HR, Schatz H, Johnson RN, et al. Vitrectomy in eyes with peripheral retinal angioma associated with traction macular detachment. *Ophthalmology* (1996) **103:**329–35.
29. Laatikainen L, Immonen I, Summanen P. Peripheral retinal angiomalike lesion and macular pucker, *Am J Ophthalmol* (1989) **108:**563–6.

30. Appiah AP, Hirose T. Secondary causes of premacular fibrosis, *Ophthalmology* (1989) **96:**389–92.
31. Saran BR, Brucker AJ. Macular epiretinal membrane formation and treated retinal breaks, *Am J Ophthalmol* (1995) **120:**480–5 [published erratum appeared in *Am J Ophthalmol* (1996) **121:**334].
32. Wise GN. Preretinal macular fibrosis (an analysis of 90 cases), *Trans Ophthalmol Soc UK* (1972) **92:**131–40.
33. Barr CC, Michels RG. Idiopathic nonvascularized epiretinal membranes in young patients: report of six cases, *Ann Ophthalmol* (1982) **14:**335–41.
34. Han DP, Wilkinson WS. Late ophthalmic manifestations of the shaken baby syndrome, *Ophthalmology* (1988) **95:**(Suppl):180(abst).
35. Kimmel AS, Weingeist TA, Blodi CF, Wells KK. Idiopathic premacular gliosis in children and adolescents, *Am J Ophthalmol* (1989) **108:**578–81.
36. Laatikainen L, Punnonen E. 'Idiopathic' preretinal macular fibrosis in young individuals, *Int Ophthalmol* (1987) **10:**11–14.
37. Polk TD, Gass JD, Green WR, et al. Familial internal limiting membrane dystrophy, *Arch Ophthalmol* (1997) **115:**878–85.
38. Smiddy WE, Michels RG, Gilbert HD, Green WR. Clinicopathologic study of idiopathic macular pucker in children and young adults, *Retina* (1992) **12:**232–6.
39. Machemer R. A new concept for vitreous surgery: two instrument techniques in pars plana vitrectomy, *Arch Ophthalmol* (1974) **92:**407–12.
40. Rice TA, de Bustros S, Michels RG, et al. Prognostic factors in vitrectomy for epiretinal membranes of the macula, *Ophthalmology* (1986) **93:**602–10.
41. De Bustros S, Thompson JT, Michels RG, et al. Vitrectomy for idiopathic epiretinal membranes causing macular pucker, *Br J Ophthalmol* (1988) **72:**692–5.
42. Poliner LS, Olk RJ, Grand MG, et al. Surgical management of premacular fibroplasia, *Arch Ophthalmol* (1988) **106:**761–4.
43. Trese MT, Chandler DB, Machemer R. Macular pucker: 1. Prognostic criteria, *Graefes Arch Clin Exp Ophthalmol* (1983) **221:**12–15.
44. Michels RG. Vitreous surgery for macular pucker, *Am J Ophthalmol* (1981) **92:**628–39.
45. Michels RG. A clinical and histopathologic study of epiretinal membranes affecting the macula and removed by vitreous surgery, *Trans Am Ophthalmol Soc* (1982) **80:**580–656.
46. De Bustros S, Rice TA, Michels RG, et al. Vitrectomy for macular pucker: use after treatment of retinal tears or retinal detachment, *Arch Ophthalmol* (1988) **106:** 758–60.
47. Trese M, Chandler DB, Machemer R. Macular pucker. II. Ultrastructure, *Graefes Arch Clin Exp Ophthalmol* (1983) **221:**16–26.
48. Melberg NS, Williams DF, Balles MW, et al. Vitrectomy for vitreomacular traction syndrome with macular detachment, *Retina* (1995) **15:**192–7.
49. Garretson BR, de Bustros S, Packo KH. Suction elevation of epiretinal membranes (letter), *Arch Ophthalmol* (1992) **110:**449.
50. Sjaarda RN, Michels RG. Macular pucker, In: Ryan SJ, ed, *Retina* (CV Mosby: St Louis, 1994): 2301–11.
51. Morris R, Witherspoon CD, Kuhn F, Preister B. Internal limiting membrane (ILM) maculorhexis for traction maculopathy, *Vitreoret Surg Technol* (1997) **8:**1–4.
52. Peyman GA. A combination pick and flute needle, *Arch Ophthalmol* (1989) **107:**1687.
53. Meredith TA. Epiretinal membrane delamination with a diamond knife, *Arch Ophthalmol* (1997) **115:**1598–9.
54. Tano diamond dusted membrane scraper (product announcement), *Retina* (1997) **17:**365.
55. Sivalingam A, Eagle RC Jr, Duker JS, et al. Visual prognosis correlated with the presence of internal-limiting membrane in histopathologic specimens obtained from epiretinal membrane surgery, *Ophthalmology* (1990) **97:**1549–52.
56. Michels RG, Gilbert HD. Surgical management of macular pucker after retinal reattachment surgery, *Am J Ophthalmol* (1979) **88:**925–9.
57. Clarkson JG, Green WR, Massof D. A histopathologic review of 168 cases of preretinal membrane, *Am J Ophthalmol* (1977) **84:**1–17.
58. De Bustros S, Thompson JT, Michels RG, et al. Nuclear sclerosis after vitrectomy for idiopathic epiretinal membranes, *Am J Ophthalmol* (1988) **105:**160–4.
59. Ciulla TA, Pesavento RD. Epiretinal fibrosis, *Ophthalmic Surg Lasers* (1997) **28:**670–9.
60. McDonald HR, Irvine AR. Light-induced maculopathy from the operating microscope in extracapsular cataract extraction and intraocular lens implantation, *Ophthalmology* (1983) **90:**945–51.
61. McDonald HR, Harris MJ. Operating microscope-induced retinal phototoxicity during pars plana vitrectomy, *Arch Ophthalmol* (1988) **106:**521–3.

Chapter 31 Surgical treatment of macular holes

Kamal Kishore and Robert T Wendel

INTRODUCTION

Full-thickness macular holes are defects involving all layers of the retina, from the internal limiting membrane through the outer segment of the retinal photoreceptors. Lamellar holes involve only a portion of retinal layers. Idiopathic macular holes predominantly affect emmetropic patients in the sixth or seventh decade of life, more often women at a ratio of 2:1–3:1.[1,2] The prevalence has been estimated to be 3.3 per 1000.[3] Other causes of macular holes include trauma, high myopia, cystoid macular edema, inflammation, solar retinopathy, vitreomacular traction syndrome, traction from epiretinal membranes and degenerative conditions of the retina. Idiopathic macular holes are bilateral in about 16% of patients. Our understanding of etiopathogenesis, natural history and surgical management of idiopathic macular holes has improved significantly over the past decade and will be reviewed in this chapter.

PATHOGENESIS

Traumatic macular holes may result from immediate contusive injury to the retina, avulsion of retinal tissue from trauma-induced posterior vitreous detachment (PVD) or breakdown of cystoid change.[1,4,5] Tangential traction caused by shrinkage of premacular vitreous cortex is currently believed to be responsible for idiopathic macular hole formation.[6–8] The process typically begins in eyes with liquefied pockets of premacular vitreous and no PVD.

Gass described four stages of macular holes (Fig. 31.1).[8] Stage 1 or impending macular hole is characterized by foveolar detachment resulting in a yellow spot (stage 1-A) or a yellow ring (stage 1-B). Vision

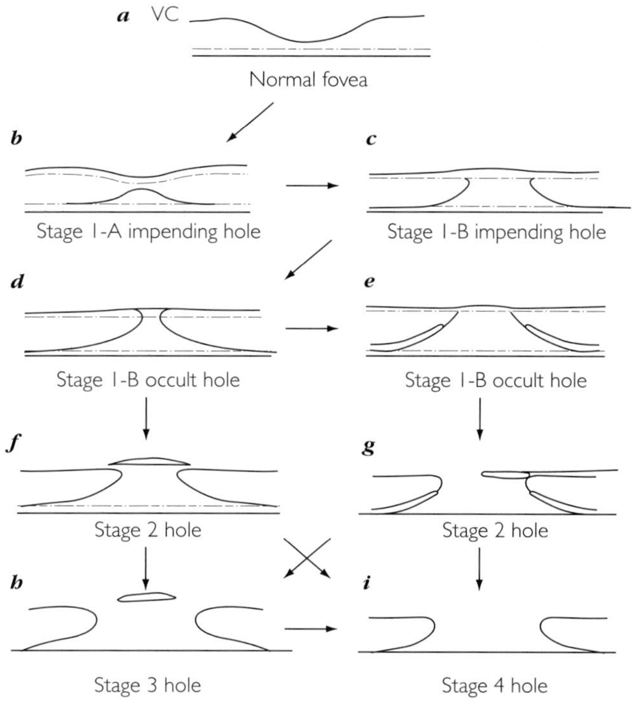

Figure 31.1 *Stages of development of a senile macular hole. (a) Normal fovea, with layer of vitreous cortex lying on internal limiting membrane of retina. (b) Stage 1-A impending hole: early contraction of outer part of vitreous cortex with foveolar detachment. (c) Stage 1-B impending hole: further vitreous contraction and condensation of the prefoveolar vitreous cortex with foveal detachment. (d, e) Stage 1-B occult hole: dehiscence of the retinal receptor layer at the umbo with centrifugal retraction of the retinal receptors. (f) Stage 2 hole with early separation of condensed prefoveolar vitreous cortex, with formation of pseudo-operculum that is larger than the hole. (g) Stage 2 hole with tear in vitreous cortex at junction of the prefoveolar vitreous cortex and edge of macular hole. (h) Stage 3 hole with pseudo-operculum. (i) Stage 4 hole after posterior vitreous separation. (Adapted with permission from Gass JD. Reappraisal of biomicroscopic classification of stages development of a macular hole,* Am J Ophthalmol *(1995)* ***119****:752–9.*[8]*)*

is in the 20/25 to 20/70 range. Stage 1 lesions may be asymptomatic or the patient may notice the sudden onset of metamorphopsia, especially if the other eye has impaired vision. The yellow spot measures about 100–200 μm in diameter and has been attributed to increased visibility of xanthophyll resulting from a shallow foveolar detachment. The yellow spot, however, is not pathognomonic for macular holes because it may be seen also in cystoid macular edema, central serous retinopathy, vitreomacular traction syndrome, solar retinopathy, macular drusen, adult vitelliform dystrophy, pigment epithelial detachment and any other condition causing foveolar detachment.[8,9] Other lesions mistaken for stage 1 holes include lamellar holes, aborted stage 1 holes with pseudo-operculum, stage 2 holes, epiretinal membranes and juxtafoveal telangiectasia.[9] Biomicroscopy reveals a loss of foveal reflex, but no PVD. Fluorescein angiography may be normal or show slight hyperfluorescence centrally.[10]

Stage 1-B lesions result from further elevation of foveolar retina to the level of the surrounding thick perifoveal retina, leading to stretching of retinal tissue in the center. The yellow ring is the result of foveal thinning in the center, which causes the xanthophyll to assume a ring configuration (Fig. 31.2). Progression from a yellow spot to a yellow ring is pathognomonic for macular holes. Many stage 1-B lesions may be caused by tiny breaks in the photoreceptors in the center of the foveola, but with intact internal limiting membrane (occult macular hole).[8] The change from 'impending' stage 1-B lesions to 'occult' stage 1-B lesions cannot be detected biomicroscopically. Fluorescein angiography may show hyperfluorescence of variable intensity in the center of the fovea.[10]

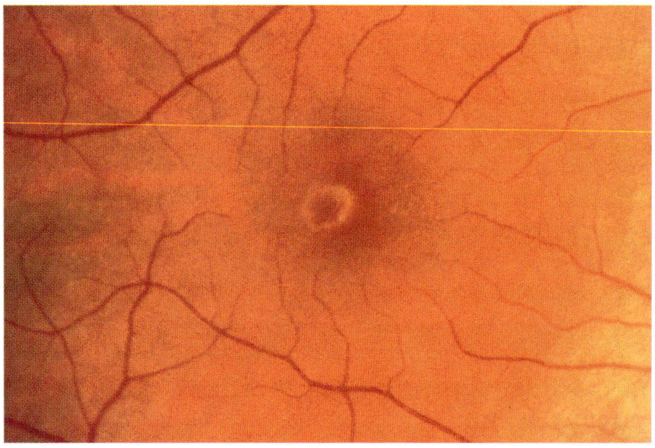

Figure 31.2 *Stage 1-B macular hole, right eye. Vision 20/40.*

Stage 1 lesions are transient. They may resolve within a few weeks owing to spontaneous vitreofoveal separation. Resolution may be accompanied by improvement of vision and metamorphopsia. A semitranslucent premacular opacity may be visible biomicroscopically, representing contracted vitreous cortex. A lamellar macular hole may also result if vitreofoveal separation causes avulsion of the inner retinal layers.

Approximately 40% of impending macular holes progress to full-thickness macular holes.[9,11–13] The yellow ring enlarges progressively because of continued traction. Contracted prefoveal vitreous usually remains tightly adherent to the retinal surface as a semitransparent opacity, or may remain transparent and invisible. Gass believes that most cases of enlargement of the yellow ring result from the formation of an occult tear in the foveolar umbo,[8] structurally the weakest part of the fovea, and progressive centrifugal displacement of retinal receptors. Loss of retinal receptors does not occur in the majority of the eyes. Such a hole remains occult (stage 1-B) because of opacification of the prefoveal vitreous cortex. Vitreofoveal separation at this stage results in formation of a pseudo-operculum in front of the retina, which is much larger than the hole itself. Very rarely, a true operculum may form from avulsion of retinal tissue. Most commonly, no retinal tissue is present in the prefoveal opacity on histopathological examination.[14] The inner edge of the yellow ring may be serrated, presumably corresponding to the edge of the occult retinal hole.

Stage 2 begins with a visible full-thickness break that is first seen usually at the inner edge of the yellow ring, most commonly in the temporal or superior macula. Yellow pigmentation fades in this area because of possible diffusion of xanthophyll out of the retina, and serration of the inner edge disappears presumably as a result of relief of traction. This break is in the contracted prefoveal vitreous bridging around the retinal hole, and not in the retinal tissue, as previously believed.[8] Infrequently, a small round hole in the center of the yellow ring may be the first indicator of full-thickness hole formation (Fig. 31.3). Intravenous fluorescein angiography may show intense hyperfluorescence in the area of the full-thickness defect and may help to differentiate these lesions from stage 1 holes.[9]

The macular hole enlarges over a period of days to weeks. Johnson and Gass followed 10 eyes with stage 2 macular holes and showed that progression to stage 3 or 4 holes occurred within 6 months.[7]

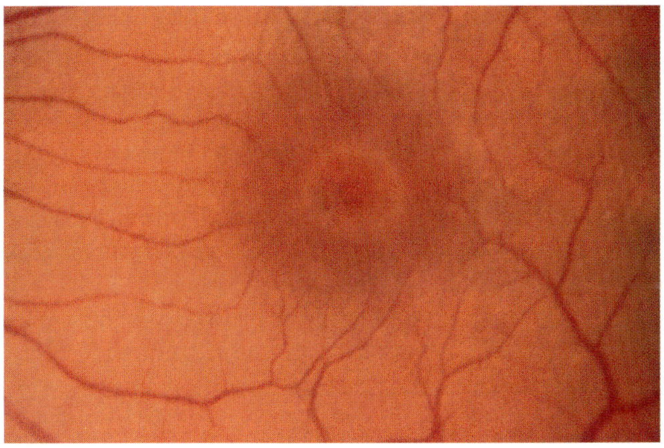

Figure 31.3 *Stage 2 macular hole, left eye. Note round 125-μm defect in the center of the yellow ring. Vision 20/80.*

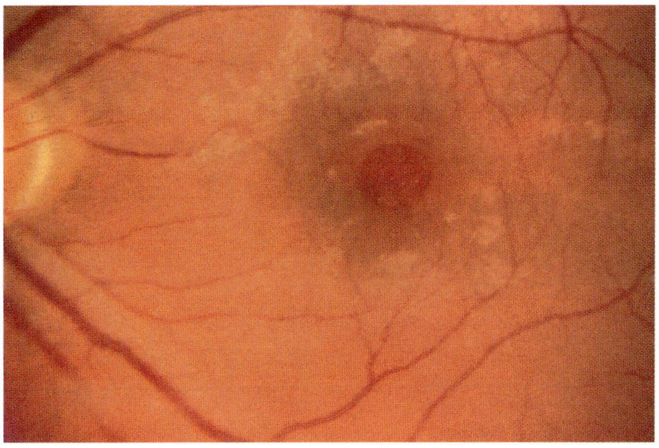

Figure 31.4 *Stage 4 macular hole. Note translucent epiretinal membrane surrounding the hole.*

Fourteen of 19 (75%) eyes with stage 2 holes followed by the Vitrectomy for Macular Hole Study Group progressed to stage 3 or 4 holes within 1 year.[15]

Eyes with eccentric holes and those with pericentral hyperfluorescence were more likely to progress than those with centric holes. Progression is believed to involve additional contraction of prefoveal vitreous, which causes a 360° tear in the condensed vitreous cortex at the edge of the retinal hole.[8] The underlying retinal hole also continues to enlarge, presumably because of centrifugal retraction of retinal tissue. All stages of enlargement are considered to be stage 2. Because fully developed holes usually measure between 400 and 600 μm, Gass has suggested that all holes less than 400 μm in diameter without PVD should be considered stage 2 lesions.[8] An 'operculum' is demonstrable in 25–75% of fully developed holes.

Stage 3 is characterized by a fully developed macular hole, but without PVD. Mean visual acuity is 20/200, with a range of 20/40 to 5/200. The hole is a round, sharply defined defect measuring 400–600 μm with a surrounding 1000–1500 μm rim of retinal detachment. The patient describes metamorphopsia on an Amsler grid. A gap in the narrow slit beam (positive Watzke–Allen test) is seen in 95% of patients. A scotoma is demonstrated within the hole in virtually 100% of patients using a 50-μm aiming beam of an argon or krypton laser. Thinning and depigmentation of retinal pigment epithelium (RPE) occurs within the area of the macular hole, contributing to hyperfluorescence on fluorescein angiography. Multiple yellow opacities are seen at the level of the RPE within most holes. These opacities change in number and distribution over time. The retina near the margin of the hole may show microcystic changes. Wrinkling of the inner retinal surface caused by an epiretinal membrane may be seen in 10–20% of cases. Vitreofoveal separation exists in the foveal area, resulting in an operculum-like structure in 75–85% of patients, but there is no evidence of PVD in the retina.[10]

After separation of the vitreous from the entire macular surface and the disc, the hole is classified as stage 4, regardless of size (Fig. 31.4). Operculum-like opacity may be seen on the posterior hyaloid surface temporal to the Weiss ring. Visual acuity stabilizes at about 20/200 in stage 4 holes. Spontaneous closure is rare, but may be caused by growth of an epiretinal membrane.[12,16]

ADDITIONAL THEORIES OF MACULAR HOLE FORMATION

Morgan and Schatz implicated involutional macular thinning (IMT) in the pathogenesis of idiopathic macular holes,[17] characterized by a thin, atrophic fovea that had lost its normal architecture. Lesions characterized as IMT had an abnormal depression of the fovea, appeared red, had a yellow ring around them and/or showed hyperfluorescence on intravenous fluorescein angiography. Twenty-six of 93 eyes (27%) with IMT developed a macular hole on follow-up. Morgan and Schatz believed that compromised choroidal circulation was the initiating event,

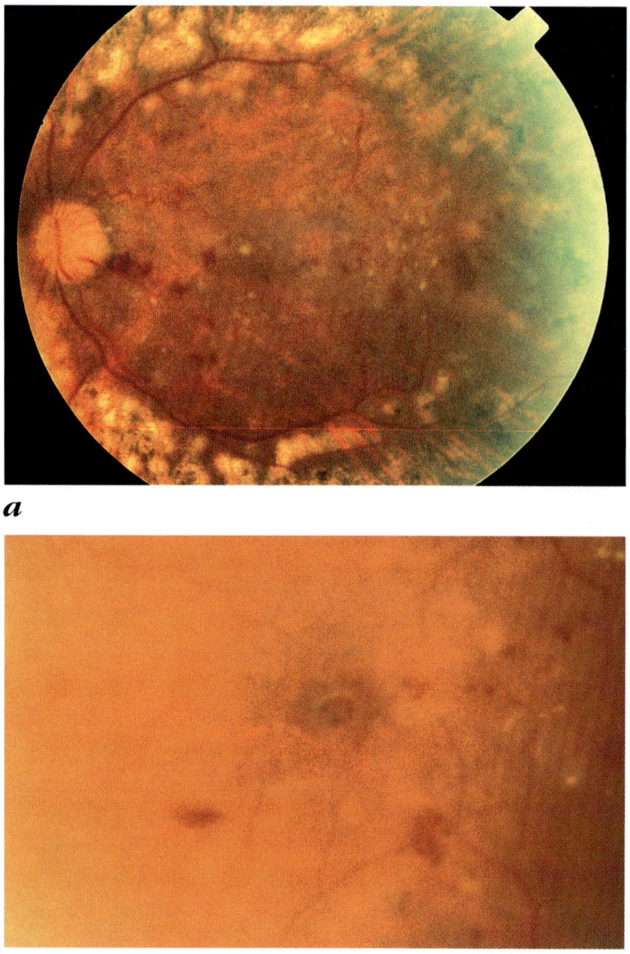

a

b

Figure 31.5 *(a) Left eye. Six weeks after a pars plana vitrectomy for proliferative diabetic retinopathy with traction retinal detachment. Note yellow spot (stage 1-A macular hole) in the center of the fovea. (b) The same eye 6 months later. A full-thickness macular hole measuring 400 μm in diameter has formed.*

whereas traction on a thinned fovea during spontaneous PVD served as the final step.

Macular holes have been described in atypical situations, such as eyes with well-documented PVD,[18] after repair of rhegmatogenous retinal detachment by pneumatic retinopexy,[19] or scleral buckling[18,20–22] and after pars plana vitrectomy (Fig. 31.5).[23] To explain the formation of macular holes in these atypical cases and also possibly in typical cases, Lipham and Smiddy have offered an alternative hypothesis that formation of an atrophic hole in the foveal center as a result of degenerative change may serve as the initiating event.[23] Glial proliferation on the posterior surface of the overlying cortical vitreous may cause closure of foveolar dehiscence, giving the appearance of a stage 1-B hole in the classification of Gass. However, if glial proliferation spreads along the inner retinal surface, its subsequent contraction will cause edges of umbo dehiscence to be pulled centrifugally and the typical configuration of macular hole will result. This degenerative theory also explains why pars plana vitrectomy for impending macular holes does not eliminate the risk of formation of full-thickness holes.[24]

RISK TO FELLOW EYE

Approximately 25% of patients with macular holes will have posterior vitreous separation from the optic nerve and the macula in the fellow eye and are therefore at very low risk for developing a macular hole in the fellow eye. Reported risk of macular hole formation in the fellow eye ranges from 3% to 29%.[2,12,25–30] According to Gass,[10] it is probably 10–15% if the fellow eye does not have a PVD, but reduces to less than 1% in the presence of PVD. In most patients, the second eye is involved within 2 years.[2] A prospective study involving 114 normal fellow eyes without PVD found a 15.6% cumulative incidence of developing a full-thickness macular hole over a 5-year period. None of the eyes developed a full-thickness macular hole after occurrence of PVD. The authors emphasized the need for careful evaluation of the status of the vitreous in the fellow eye in order to provide an accurate risk assessment to the patient.[30]

DIFFERENTIAL DIAGNOSIS

Differential diagnosis of macular holes includes epiretinal membranes with pseudoholes, impending macular holes, lamellar macular holes and macular degeneration.[31] Important features differentiating true macular holes from 'pseudoholes' are a surrounding cuff of subretinal fluid, drusen-like yellowish deposits in the base of the hole, a distinct and circular margin around the hole and an 'operculum.' A positive Watzke–Allen test and absolute scotoma on the aiming beam of the argon or krypton laser are also considered fairly specific for full-thickness macular holes.[32] Intravenous fluorescein angiography alone is not reliable in differentiating full-thickness macular holes from lamellar holes. The majority of patients with true macular holes will have a visual acuity of less than 20/80, or will drop to this level within a few weeks. Limiting surgery to patients with vision less than this level in doubtful cases may prevent unnecessary surgery.[31] Microperimetry using a scanning laser ophthalmoscope may show an absolute scotoma corresponding to the macular hole and may allow differentiation from pseudoholes.[33]

HISTOPATHOLOGY

The edges of holes are typically rounded with some cystic changes in the outer plexiform and inner nuclear layers. Cellular proliferation commonly extends from the edges of the hole to the inner retinal surface. Nodular proliferations of RPE probably account for yellowish deposits in the base of the macular holes seen biomicroscopically.[14,34]

Tissue removed during surgery for idiopathic macular holes has demonstrated internal limiting membrane in 11 of 12 eyes.[35] Cellular proliferation on the internal limiting membrane and cells with myofibroblastic differentiation were also noted in many stage 3 and 4 eyes.[35] Histopathology of eyes after successful macular hole surgery showed closure of the macular hole, reattachment of the macula and return of xanthophyll to the center of the macula. Proliferation of glial or Mueller cells was noted in two of the three eyes; one eye showed hole closure and near-normal return of retinal anatomy without any evidence of glial proliferation.[36,37] Contractile cells have been identified in the vitreous of patients undergoing surgery for impending macular holes.[38]

Fibroglial tissue has been identified in the operculum removed during macular hole surgery.[39] Ezra et al studied ultrastructural characteristics of opercula removed from 18 eyes undergoing surgery for idiopathic stage 3 macular holes.[40] All opercula had glial cells. Fragments of internal limiting membrane were noted in 61% of specimens. Neurites and synaptic complexes resembling those of photoreceptors were observed in 39%. The anatomic success rate was much lower in eyes containing neurites in the opercula than those that demonstrated only glial cells (14% vs 82%), but the final visual outcome in eyes with a successful anatomic result was similar in both groups. The authors concluded that opercula containing neurites were true opercula resulting from a full-thickness foveal tear and were correlated with poor prognosis for initial surgery.[40]

SURGICAL TREATMENT OF MACULAR HOLES

Laser treatment to the edge of the macular hole to flatten surrounding localized retinal detachment has been suggested,[41] but has found little acceptance because of retinal damage from laser application. Pars plana vitrectomy with gas tamponade has been used with success in the treatment of retinal detachment caused by macular holes.[42–44] A multicenter clinical trial evaluated the benefits of vitrectomy in patients with stage 1 holes. A full-thickness macular hole developed in 37% of eyes in the vitrectomy group compared to 40% of those randomized to the observation group, suggesting that any benefit from vitrectomy in eyes with stage 1 macular hole was probably minimal. A conservative approach was therefore recommended for such lesions.[24]

Apart from reports of treatment of macular holes associated with retinal detachment, idiopathic macular holes were generally considered inoperable. Kelly and Wendel[45] in 1991 published the first report of successful closure of idiopathic macular holes in 30 of 52 eyes (58%) with pars plana vitrectomy, removal of adherent cortical vitreous, stripping of epiretinal membranes, total air–fluid exchange, and tamponade with a nonexpansile concentration of sulfur hexafluoride (SF_6) gas. Vision improved by two or more lines in 22 of 30 (73.3%) eyes in which the macular hole was successfully closed.[45] Several authors have since reported surgical results with closure of macular holes ranging from 58% to 94% (Table 31.1).[45–59] Surgical treatment is currently indicated for stage 2, 3 and 4 macular holes. Visual improvement depends on successful closure of the hole and duration of symptoms. Eyes with symptoms of less than 6 months' duration have a better visual prognosis. Improved anatomic and functional success was associated with smaller hole size, shorter duration of symptoms and better initial acuity.[46,60–62] Visual improvement for up to three years has been noted after successful macular hole surgery.[63] Patients with proliferative diabetic retinopathy may have a worse prognosis.[64]

Table 31.1 Gas tamponade and adjuvants in surgery for macular holes

Study	*Year*	*Hole closure rate*	*Visual acuity improved by more than 2 lines among those with hole closed*	*Gas tamponade*	*Adjuvant*
Kelly and Wendel[45]	1991	30/52 (58%)	75%	20% SF_6	None
Wendel et al[46]	1993	125/170 (73%)	76%	20% SF_6	None
Orellana and Lieberman[47]	1993	7/12 (58%)	100%	20% SF_6	None
Lansing et al[48]	1993	22/23 (96%)	86.36%	16% C_3F_8	TGF-β
Smiddy et al[49]	1993	53/58 (91.3%)	NA	16% C_3F_8	TGF-β
Gaudric et al[50]	1995	19/20 (95%)	89.5%	17% C_2F_6	Autologous platelet concentration
Liggett et al[51]	1995	11/11 (100%)	11/11 (100%)	16% C_3F_8	Autologous serum
Vine and Johnson[52]	1996	20/25 (80%)	NA		Thrombin
Thompson et al[53]	1996	85/90 (94.4%)	NA	16% C_3F_8	None
		19/30 (63.3%)	NA	10% C_3F_8	None
		19/29 (65.5%)	NA	5% C_3F_8	None
Wells and Gregor[54]	1996	29/44 (67%)	NA		Autologous serum
Polk et al[55]	1996	60/71 (85%)	58/60 (96%)	16% C_3F_8	TGF-β
Korobelnik et al[56]	1996	7/8 (85.5%)	4/7 (57.1%)	15% C_3F_8	Autologous platelet concentrate
Freeman et al[58]	1997	36/53 (69%)	11/32 (30.5%)	16% C_3F_8	None
Smiddy et al[59]	1997	39/43 (91%)	28/39 (71%); improved >3 lines	16% C_3F_8	None

SURGICAL TECHNIQUE

Surgery is performed under local or general anesthesia. A standard three-port pars plana vitrectomy is performed. A PVD is created and adherent vitreous cortex is removed in cases with stage 2 and 3 holes. This may be accomplished by using a silicone-tipped extrusion needle attached to active suction. The needle is swept gently over the retinal surface near the temporal arcades or just temporal to the fovea. Engagement of vitreous cortex in the tip causes it to flex ('fish strike' sign, Fig. 31.6). Continued aspiration and traction will cause PVD. Alternatively, the vitrectomy instrument may be used at high suction to engage the cortical vitreous nasal to the nerve (Fig. 31.7). Suction of 150–400 mmHg may be applied as needed. Once engaged, PVD is created by lifting the vitrectomy instrument straight upward into the midvitreous cavity. The cutter is activated to

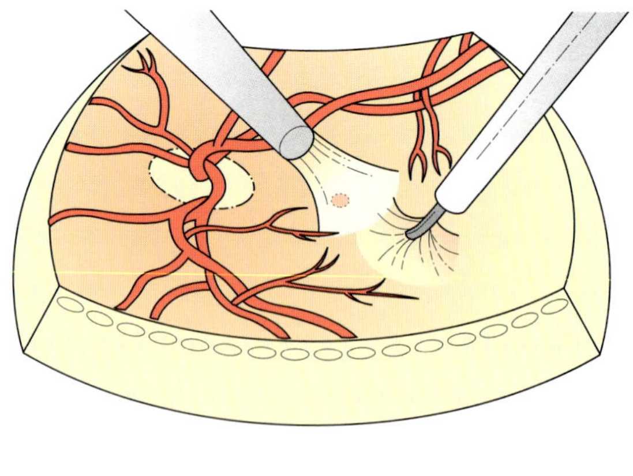

Figure 31.6 *Surgical technique sweeping silicone-tipped extrusion needle over the retinal surface to identify adherent cortical vitreous ('fish strike') sign. (Adapted with permission from Kelly NE, Wendel RT. Vitreous surgery for idiopathic macular holes: results of a pilot study,* Arch Ophthalmol *(1991)* ***109****:654–9.*[45] *Copyright © 1991, American Medical Association.)*

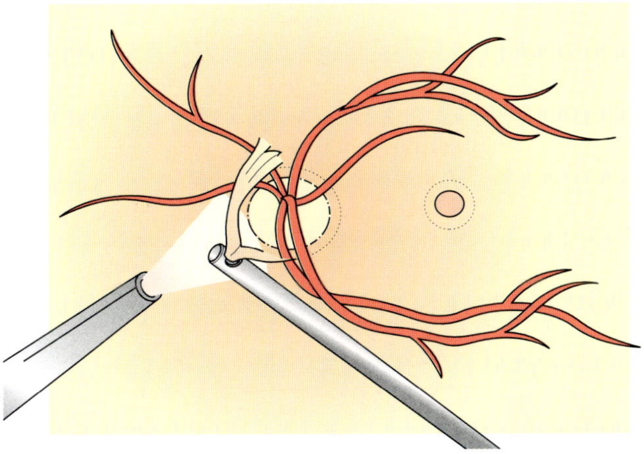

Figure 31.7 *Vitreous cortex is engaged with the vitrector nasal to the optic nerve. Posterior vitreous detachment is created by lifting the vitrector straight up into the midvitreous cavity.*

remove peeled vitreous cortex and to avoid unnecessary traction on the peripheral retina. The vitrector may minimize traction while removing vitreous cortex, allows immediate reflux if needed and reduces the necessity for exchange of instruments. It is currently our favored technique for creating a PVD. The edges of the macular hole should be observed carefully to prevent enlargement of the hole during this step.

Sharp dissection with a membrane pick or barbed microvitreoretinal (MVR) blade may be performed to create an opening in the posterior hyaloid near the disc margin either nasally or just inside the temporal arcades. A blunt 90° pick may be inserted through this opening and the posterior hyaloid peeled by a combination of anterior, centrifugal and circumpapillary movements.[65] Bimanual techniques using an extrusion needle in one hand and an illuminated spatula in the other hand may also be used.[66] Once the posterior hyaloid is engaged near the optic nerve with a silicone-tipped cannula, continuous suction is applied while an illuminated spatula is introduced beneath the posterior hyaloid to facilitate its separation.[67] Alternatively, an illuminated spatula may be passed through the engaged posterior hyaloid, thus allowing fluid to go through these holes to facilitate detachment of posterior hyaloid (Fig. 31.8).

Autologous plasmin has been used with success in inducing a PVD in pediatric traumatic macular holes.[68] A total dose of 0.4 IU of autologous plasmin

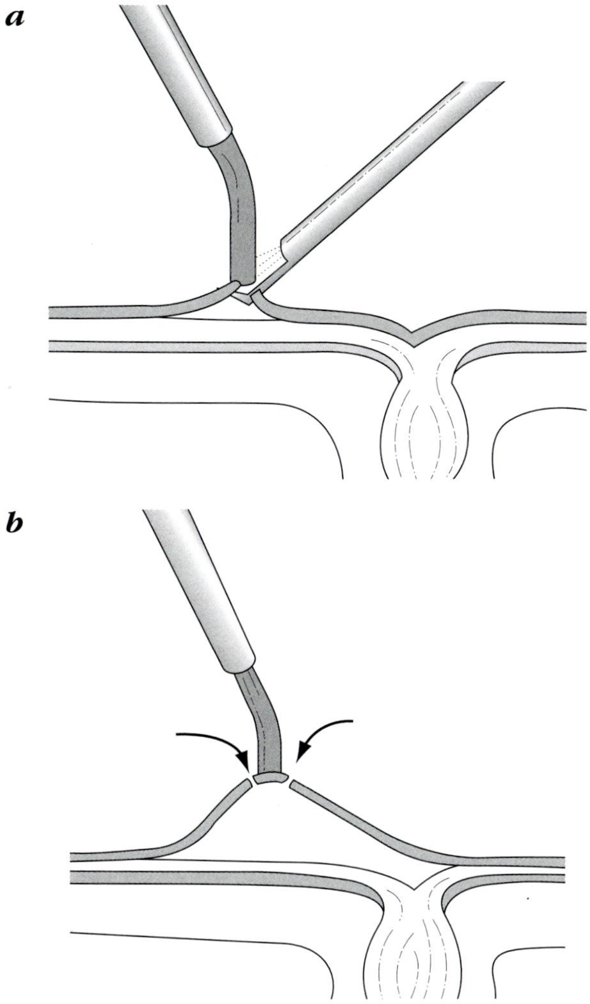

Figure 31.8 *(a) Posterior segment illustration showing the flexible cannula with posterior hyaloid impaled in the tip. The illuminated spatula goes through just beneath the tip of the silicone cannula. (b) Posterior segment illustration showing elevation of the posterior hyaloid with the cannula letting the irrigation fluid go through the two orifices made in the posterior hyaloid, facilitating the complete separation. (Adapted with permission from Ruiz-Moreno JM, Pérez-Santonja JJ. Dissection of the posterior hyaloid,* Arch Ophthalmol *(1998)* ***116****:1392–3.[67])*

was injected into the vitreous cavity 15 minutes prior to vitrectomy. According to the investigators, this allowed rapid and atraumatic separation of posterior hyaloid from the retina. All four eyes where plasmin was used had a successful closure of the hole. Instillation of a few drops of autologous blood has been reported to facilitate visualization of posterior cortical vitreous.[69]

PEELING OF EPIRETINAL MEMBRANES

Significant epiretinal membranes are seen clinically in only 10–20% of eyes; however, they are found histologically in 75% of eyes with full-thickness macular holes. These membranes tend to be friable and difficult to remove. Meticulous dissection of all visible epiretinal membranes is currently recommended.[23,46,49] These membranes may be removed with standard techniques using a barbed MVR blade, pick or vitreous forceps (Figs 31.9–31.11). Prolonged dissection of epiretinal membranes should be avoided because it may cause damage to the internal limiting membranes or retina and may cause phototoxicity. A diamond-dusted silicone cannula may facilitate removal of epiretinal membranes.[70]

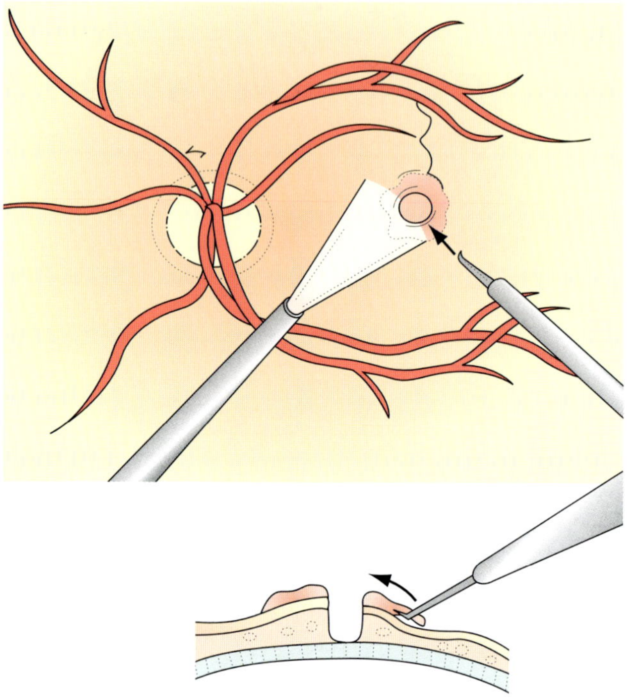

Figure 31.9 *A slit is made in the most prominent part of the epiretinal membrane with a barbed microvitreoretinal blade.*

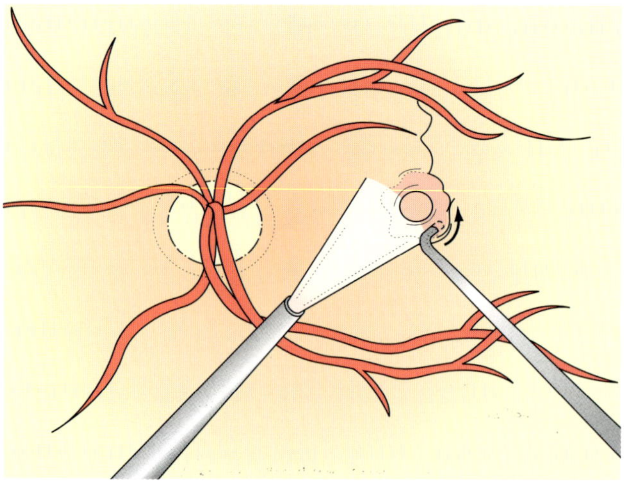

Figure 31.10 *A blunt vitreoretinal pick is introduced beneath the epiretinal membrane and peeling is begun in a circumferential fashion.*

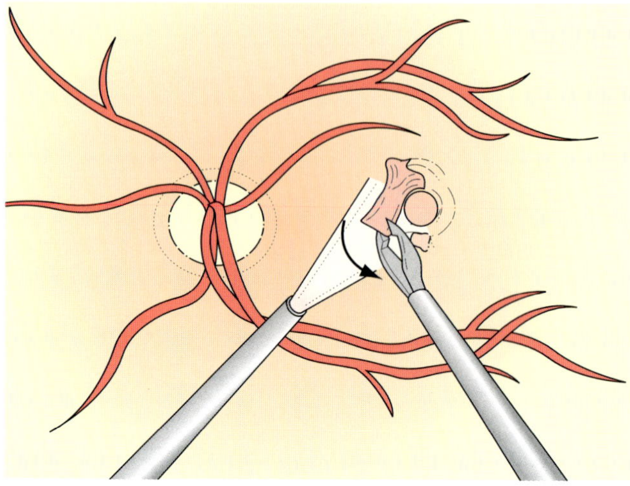

Figure 31.11 *The flap of the epiretinal membrane is grasped with a microforceps to complete peeling for 360°.*

AIR–FLUID EXCHANGE

The peripheral retina should be examined carefully for any tears before air–fluid exchange. Fluid is removed just anterior to the optic nerve or over the nasal peripapillary retina with a flute needle or extrusion cannula during air–fluid exchange. Subretinal fluid surrounding the macular hole may be removed; however, its removal may be complicated by enlargement of the hole and usually is not necessary. After waiting for 10–15 minutes, residual fluid may be removed from the posterior pole to ensure maximal dehydration,[71] but this step usually is not necessary. Gas is flushed to replace air with gas. Face-down positioning for 1–2 weeks is required postoperatively and should be discussed with the patient and family before surgery to ensure compliance.

A study by Thompson et al showed a higher hole closure rate with a prolonged tamponade using 16% perfluoropropane (C_3F_8) as compared to 10% and 5% C_3F_8.[53] The authors did not remove epiretinal membranes in their study. However, an excellent success rate has been observed with 20% SF_6 gas. Silicone oil has been used with success in patients unable to maintain a prone position postoperatively.[72] Most surgeons do not use silicone oil for tamponade because it mandates a second operation for the removal of oil. Rarely, droplets of silicone oil may be trapped inside the hole and prevent its closure (Fig. 31.12).

Simultaneous cataract surgery in phakic eyes undergoing repair of a macular hole has been suggested.[73,74] Tornambe et al[74] achieved hole closure in 26 of 33 eyes (79%) with such an approach. Most patients in their study did not have a visually significant cataract. Complications included intraocular lens capture in two eyes, posterior synechiae in four, iris incarceration in the cataract wound in one eye and retinal detachment in three eyes. The authors performed meticulous dissection to remove all visible epiretinal membranes. The patients were not required to maintain 'face-down' positioning postoperatively. Because the gas bubble does not exert any force toward the macula when the head is upright, the surgical success may depend more on direct relief of tangential traction by removal of epiretinal membranes.[75] The primary purpose of the gas bubble in this situation may be to isolate the vitreous fluid and allow a glial membrane to form across the hole.[76]

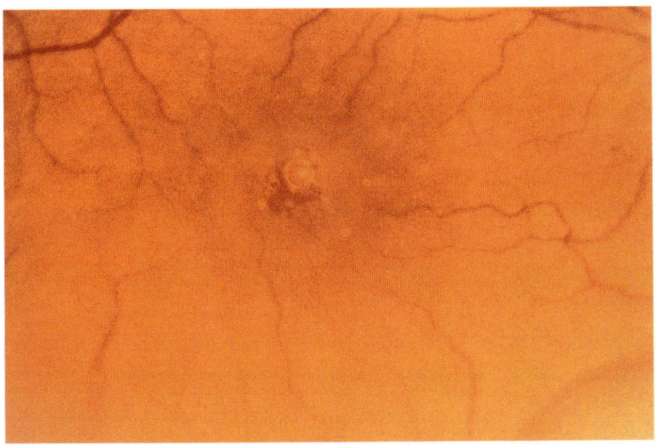

Figure 31.12 *Droplets of silicone oil trapped within the macular hole prevent its closure. Repeat surgery consisting of silicone oil removal, stripping of epiretinal membrane and tamponade with 16% perfluoropropane gas results in successful closure of the hole.*

Subsequent contraction of the membrane leads to closure of the hole. However, if tangential traction from epiretinal membranes is not relieved completely, 'face-down' positioning may permit buoyant pressure from the gas bubble to be exerted against the macular hole. This pressure may keep the edges of the macular hole firmly in contact with the pigment epithelium and promote its closure.[75]

Removal of the internal limiting membrane may relieve the tractional component on the retinal surface and improve anatomic success.[77,78] Eckardt and associates achieved a 92% hole closure rate following removal of 'membrane limitans interna' and found myofibroblasts on electron microscopy.[77] The authors recommended routine removal of the internal limiting membrane in all cases.

Removal of RPE cells from the base of the macular hole by aspiration with either a silicone-tipped cannula or a blunt-tipped 27-gauge needle has been suggested to improve the anatomic and functional success rate.[79] Hypertrophy of the RPE was noted in 14% of eyes, but was not associated with adverse visual effects.[79] Min and associates performed endolaser treatment to the base of the macular hole after pars plana vitrectomy and peeling of membranes.[80] A curved probe was used to avoid the edges of the macular hole, using a power setting of 50–200 mW and 0.05–0.2 seconds' duration to give a single, mild, gray burn. All eight eyes achieved successful closure of the macular hole. Mild pigmentary disturbance corresponding to the laser burn was noted but was not associated with adverse visual outcome.[80]

Peyman and associates inserted an absorbable plug made from partially cross-linked gelatin into the macular hole after pars plana vitrectomy and peeling of membranes.[81] The patients were required to maintain a face-down position for only 2–3 days. The hole was closed in all 19 eyes. The authors, however, recommend its use only in recurrent macular holes and those in highly myopic eyes.

ADJUVANTS

Several adjuvants such as bovine or recombinant transforming growth factor beta-2 (TGF-β_2), bovine thrombin and autologous fibrinogen, autologous platelet concentrate, autologous serum, tissue glue, cyanoacrylate, mussel adhesive protein and plasma–thrombin mixture have been used during macular hole surgery (Table 31.1). The adjuvant TGF-β_2 has been studied most extensively with excellent results, but a randomized study by Thompson et al failed to demonstrate any significant benefit.[82] Bovine thrombin was associated with increased intraocular inflammation and hypopyon formation in 28% of eyes.[52] Hole closure was achieved in 80% of eyes in that study, which is similar to the rate achieved without adjuvants. Use of autologous blood products may be associated with higher risk of endophthalmitis. Most retina surgeons do not use adjuvants for macular hole surgery at this time. Excellent surgical results have been obtained without the use of adjuvants; however, they may have a role in the management of chronic macular holes and in patients with a prior failed surgery.[62,83,84]

COMPLICATIONS OF MACULAR HOLE SURGERY

In addition to general complications associated with vitreous surgery, such as the progression of cataract,[85] retinal detachment, suprachoroidal hemorrhage, high intraocular pressure, vascular occlusion, epiretinal membrane formation, cystoid macular edema and endophthalmitis, surgery for macular holes has some unique complications, including pigment epithelial changes, retinal tear and detachment, visual field defects and late reopening of the hole. Some of these unique complications may be related to surgical manipulations required for creating a PVD and removal of membranes around the macular hole. In addition, prolonged face-down positioning may cause exacerbation of cervical disc and ulnar nerve palsy, and bed rest may be complicated by deep vein thrombosis and pulmonary embolism. High intraocular pressure may be seen in the first or second postoperative weeks in eyes with long-acting gas tamponade. Elevation of intraocular pressure was most marked in patients receiving recombinant TGF-β.[86]

CHANGES IN RPE

Poliner and Tornambe described alterations in RPE in 75% of 16 eyes following macular hole surgery.[87] Other authors have also described similar changes with incidences ranging from 5.3%[46] to 75%.[87–91] In nine eyes described by Wendell et al,[46] visual acuity improved from the preoperative level by two lines or more in three eyes (33%), remained unchanged in four (44%) and was worse in the remaining two eyes.

Alterations in RPE were seen in 31 of 95 eyes (33%) in the Vitrectomy for Macular Hole Study.[91] Eighty-four percent of these eyes had successful closure of the macular hole. Three types of RPE alterations were described: 'facet' lesions in 65%, 'phototoxicity lesions' in 23% and 'scattered hyperfluorescence' in 7%. Facets were well-defined localized areas of RPE hyper- or hypopigmentation measuring 501.7±55 μm. They were associated with hyper- or hypofluorescence or late staining on fluorescein angiogram. Phototoxicity lesions were larger, had a round or oval shape and were characterized by diffuse stippling throughout the macula, with angiography showing widespread hyperfluorescence and late staining.

Visual acuity as measured by potential acuity meter (PAM) was significantly worse in eyes with RPE alteration than in those without (20/80 vs 20/50). Eyes with phototoxicity lesions had significantly worse visual acuity than those with facet lesions (20/160 vs 20/80). Facets may have been caused by mechanical trauma during removal of the hyaloid or subretinal fluid or by compromised choriocapillaris perfusion from prolonged postoperative gas tamponade.

RETINAL TEARS AND DETACHMENT

Retinal breaks and detachment are well-known complications of pars plana vitrectomy. The incidence of retinal detachment after surgery for epiretinal membranes ranges from 1% to 7%.[92,93] Only one of 27 eyes undergoing surgery for impending (stage 1) holes developed postoperative retinal detachment.[24] The incidence of retinal detachment following surgery for full-thickness macular holes ranges from 1.1%[46] to 14%,[90] and was 11% in 95 eyes in the Vitrectomy for Macular Hole Study.[91] Retinal detachments were seen 2–15 weeks (mean 6.7) after surgery in the Vitrectomy for Macular Hole Study and involved the macula in 60%. All eyes with 'macula-on' detachment had a closed macular hole. Six eyes (60%) had inferior retinal detachments, one (10%) had a superior retinal detachment, one (10%) had a localized retinal detachment within the posterior pole and two eyes (20%) had total detachment. Eyes with retinal detachment had worse visual acuity at 12

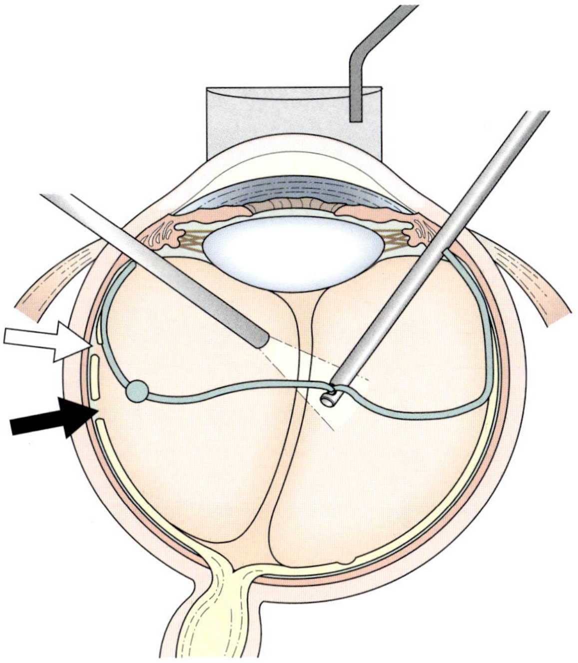

Figure 31.13 *Surgically induced posterior vitreous detachment may create intraoperative iatrogenic retinal breaks; the break may be an operculated hole (dark arrow) or a horseshoe tear (white arrow). (Adapted with permission from Sjaarda RN, Glaser BM, Thompson JT, et al. Distribution of iatrogenic retinal breaks in macular hole surgery,* Ophthalmology *(1995)* ***102****:1387–92.*[95]*)*

months as compared to preoperative visual acuity. Inferior detachments in the study were seen in eyes without PVD, possibly suggesting the role of iatrogenic trauma during creation of the PVD (Fig. 31.13). Traction on the inferior retina could also result from a gas bubble in an incompletely vitrectomized eye as seen after pneumatic retinopexy.[94]

In another study, 73% of all iatrogenic breaks were located in the two temporal quadrants and 60% were in the two inferior quadrants after macular hole surgery (Fig. 31.14).[95] It is important to examine the vitreous base carefully with the indirect ophthalmoscope or a microscope-based wide-angle viewing system with scleral depression before air–fluid exchange, because air may impair the view of the peripheral vitreous and cause flattening of retinal breaks, making their detection difficult (Fig. 31.15).

Prophylactic treatment of lattice degeneration also has been recommended.[96] Late-onset retinal detachments also may occur from progressive contracture of vitreous incarcerated in sclerotomy sites.[90] Akduman and associates observed postoperative inferior retinal detachment in 6/73 (8.2%) eyes undergoing macular hole surgery.[97] Two eyes had inferior retinal breaks and underwent further surgery to repair the retinal detachment. No retinal breaks could be identified in the remaining four eyes, and retinal detachment resolved spontaneously in each of those four eyes.

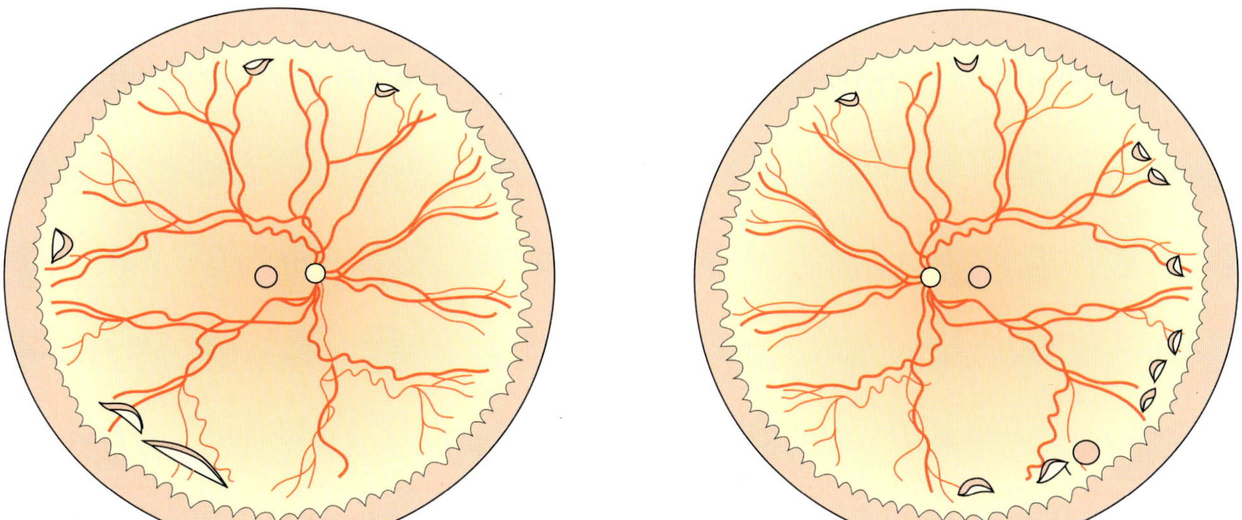

a ***b***

Figure 31.14 *Distribution of retinal breaks in right and left eyes following macular hole surgery: (a) five breaks occurred in 4/75 right eyes; (b) 10 breaks occurred in 6/106 left eyes. Breaks occurred less often near the surgeon's right-hand sclerotomy and more often in the two temporal quadrants. (Adapted with permission from Sjaarda RN, Glaser BM, Thompson JT, et al. Distribution of iatrogenic retinal breaks in macular hole surgery,* Ophthalmology *(1995)* ***102****:1387–92.*[95]*)*

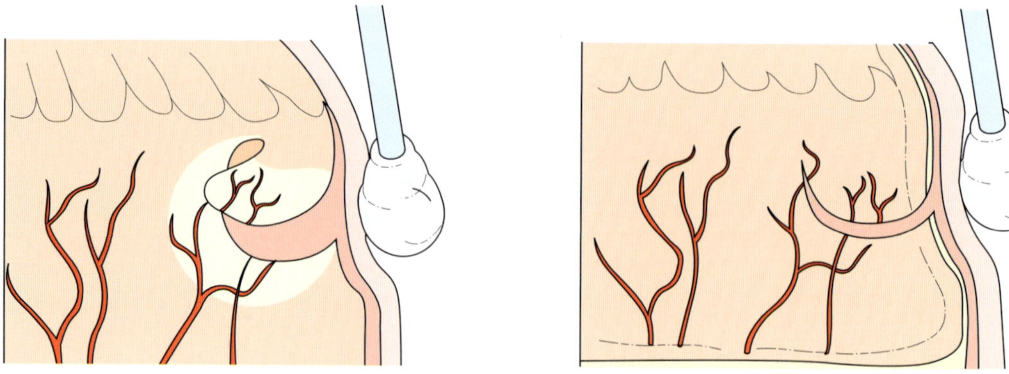

a *b*

Figure 31.15 *Examination of peripheral retina. (a) examination before fluid–gas exchange allows detection of peripheral retinal tear; (b) examination after fluid–gas exchange may allow the tear to go undetected. (Adapted with permission from Sjaarda RN, Glaser BM, Thompson JT, et al. Distribution of iatrogenic retinal breaks in macular hole surgery,* Ophthalmology *(1995)* ***102***:*1387–92.*[95]*)*

The authors recommended a period of observation for postoperative retinal detachments following macular hole surgery where no break could be identified.

VISUAL FIELD DEFECTS

Melberg and Thomas described the occurrence of visual field defects after pars plana vitrectomy for macular hole.[98] Other authors subsequently reported similar cases.[99–105] Field defects are seen mostly as absolute scotomas in the inferior or temporal field (Fig. 31.16) and may be accompanied by segmental optic nerve pallor, relative afferent pupillary defect[101] and decreased nerve-fiber layer thickness in the affected segment.[102] The incidence of peripheral visual field loss was 16% in a retrospective study.[100]

Anterior ischemic optic neuropathy and branch retinal arteriolar occlusion have accounted for visual field loss in some eyes.[100] In others, proposed mechanisms are elevated intraocular pressure, fluctuation of intraocular pressure, optic nerve damage from retrobulbar injection, direct mechanical trauma to the nerve or indirect damage to the nerve-fiber layer during suction in the creation of a PVD. Welch suggested that dehydration of the nerve-fiber layer opposite the site of air infusion may be responsible for visual defects.[103] Air from an infusion cannula secured in the inferotemporal quadrant flows directly to the superonasal retina and may cause dehydration damage in that location. Welch secured the infusion cannula at the 12 o'clock position in eight eyes and found a visual field defect in the superior quadrant in four.[103]

Ohji and associates passed air through water before instilling it into the eye for a fluid–air exchange in 33 eyes undergoing macular hole surgery; they found a visual field defect in none of the eyes compared with 9/39 (23%) control eyes. The authors concluded that humidified air for fluid–air exchange may prevent postoperative visual field loss.[104]

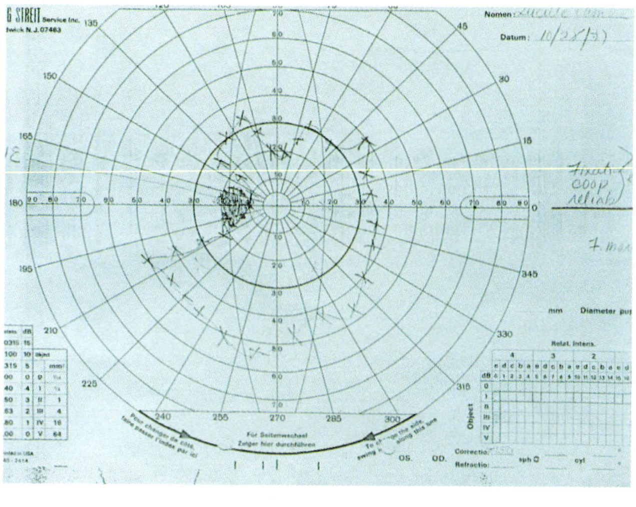

Figure 31.16 *Temporal field defect after macular hole surgery.*

In a prospective study involving 30 eyes, postoperative visual field loss was noted in seven eyes (23%).[105] Four eyes (13%) developed peripheral scotoma, and arcuate field loss was noted in three (10%). Elevated intraocular pressure was found in three eyes that developed an arcuate field loss. The authors suggested that increased intraocular pressure might have caused arcuate field defects.[105]

LATE REOPENING OF MACULAR HOLES

Late reopening of macular holes as a result of the formation of epiretinal membranes has been reported.[106–108] A retrospective review of 167 eyes with initially successful macular hole surgery showed reopening of the macular hole with acute diminution of vision in eight eyes (4.8%) after a period of two to 22 months (mean 12.5) after initial surgery.[107] A repeat operation was successful in two of three eyes in achieving hole closure with improvement of vision. A case of the opening of a macular hole after cataract surgery complicated by a dropped nucleus has been described. This patient had successful hole closure and excellent visual acuity after reoperation.[63]

Paques et al prospectively followed 72 eyes with successful macular hole surgery.[108] Late reopening was observed in five eyes (7%) during a mean follow-up of 12.3 months. In four eyes, it occurred soon after otherwise uncomplicated cataract surgery. Visible epiretinal membranes were observed in four eyes (80%). Successful hole closure was achieved in all three eyes that underwent a repeat procedure.

FAILED MACULAR HOLE SURGERIES

Failed macular hole surgery was associated with an enlargement of the hole diameter by a mean of 22%, an increase in size of the cuff of subretinal fluid by a mean of 36% and a decrease in visual acuity by a mean of 0.71 Early Treatment of Diabetic Retinopathy Study (ETDRS) line. Successful hole closure by repeat surgery was obtained in 17 of 23 eyes (65%) and was associated with an improvement in visual acuity by a mean of 3.7 ETDRS lines.[109]

Macular hole persisting after initial vitrectomy may be treated by an outpatient fluid–gas exchange. Johnson and associates performed outpatient fluid–gas exchange on 23 eyes with failed macular hole surgery one to eight weeks after vitrectomy and obtained successful closure of the hole in 17 (74%) eyes.[110] Laser photocoagulation to the macular hole bed followed by fluid–gas exchange for a recurrent macular hole was first reported by Del Priore and associates.[111] Seven spots of krypton laser at the setting of 50 μm size, 0.1 second duration and 80 mW power were given to bare RPE at the base of the hole in a C-pattern, avoiding the foveal center and edges of neural retina. The patient underwent fluid–gas exchange 2 hours later. The hole closed and the patient regained 20/40 vision postoperatively. Mild RPE disturbance at the site of application of the laser burn was observed.

Ikuno and associates applied a single spot of argon green/blue-green laser to the bed of a macular hole followed by fluid–gas exchange in 13 eyes with macular holes persisting after initial vitrectomy.[112] They achieved anatomic closure in 12/13 eyes (92%) and visual acuity improved by two or more lines in 6/13 eyes (46%). Stimulation of the RPE in the bed of the macular hole is believed to release cytokines, such as platelet-derived growth factor and TGF-β, which may promote gliosis and lead to closure of the hole.

Other reported complications of macular hole surgery have included choroidal neovascular membrane formation,[49,60,91] epiretinal membrane formation,[106] vascular occlusion,[45] cystoid macular edema,[91] endophthalmitis[90] and flat anterior chamber.[55]

SUMMARY

This chapter describes the etiopathogenesis, clinical features and surgical treatment of macular holes, including complications. Macular holes are an important cause of visual loss in the elderly. Approximately 75–85% of macular holes can be closed with vitreous surgery and 55–65% of patients may be expected to show improvement in visual acuity by two or more lines. Long-term improvement in vision for up to 3 years may occur. Smaller holes and those with a duration of less than 6 months have a better prognosis.

Silicone oil tamponade may be useful in patients unable to maintain a postoperative face-down position. Complications of surgery are associated with adverse visual prognosis and are more likely to occur in patients with larger holes.[91] It is expected that with further understanding of the mechanisms of these complications and refinement of surgical technique, the complication rate will be reduced.

REFERENCES

1. Aaberg TM. Macular holes: a review, *Surv Ophthalmol* (1970) **15**:139–62.
2. Aaberg TM, Blair CJ, Gass JD. Macular holes, *Am J Ophthalmol* (1970) **69**:555–62.
3. Fine S. Macular holes (discussion), *Ophthalmology* (1993) **100**:871.
4. Garcia-Arumi J, Corcostegui B, Cavero L, Sararols L. The role of vitreoretinal surgery in the treatment of posttraumatic macular hole, *Retina* (1997) **17**:372–7.
5. Madreperla SA, Benetz BA. Formation and treatment of a traumatic macular hole, *Arch Ophthalmol* (1997) **115**:1210–11.
6. Gass JDM. Idiopathic senile macular hole: its early stages and pathogenesis, *Arch Ophthalmol* (1988) **106**:629–39.
7. Johnson RN, Gass JD. Idiopathic macular holes: observations, stages of formation, and implications for surgical intervention, *Ophthalmology* (1988) **95**:917–24.
8. Gass JD. Reappraisal of biomicroscopic classification of stages of development of a macular hole, *Am J Ophthalmol* (1995) **119**:752–9.
9. Gass JD, Joondeph BC. Observations concerning patients with suspected impending macular holes, *Am J Ophthalmol* (1990) **109**:638–46.
10. Gass JDM. *Stereoscopic Atlas of Macular Diseases; Diagnosis and Treatment*, 4th edn (CV Mosby: St Louis, 1997): 916–36.
11. De Bustros S, Wendel RT. Vitrectomy for impending and full-thickness macular holes, *Int Ophthalmol Clin* (1992) **32**:139–52.
12. Guyer DR, de Bustros S, Diener-West M, Fine SL. Observations on patients with idiopathic macular holes and cysts, *Arch Ophthalmol* (1992) **110**:1264–8.
13. Akiba J, Yoshida A, Trempe CL. Risk of developing a macular hole, *Arch Ophthalmol* (1990) **108**:1088–90.
14. Frangieh GT, Green WR, Engel HM. A histopathologic study of macular cysts and holes, *Retina* (1981) **1**:311–36.
15. Kim JW, Freeman WR, El-Haig W, et al. Baseline characteristics, natural history, and risk factors to progression in eyes with stage 2 macular holes: results from a prospective randomized clinical trial, *Ophthalmology* (1995) **102**:1818–29.
16. Lewis H, Cowan GM, Straatsma BR. Apparent disappearance of a macular hole associated with development of an epiretinal membrane, *Am J Ophthalmol* (1986) **102**:172–5.
17. Morgan CM, Schatz H. Involutional macular thinning: a pre-macular hole condition, *Ophthalmology* (1986) **93**:153–61.
18. Gordon LW, Glaser BM, Ie D, et al. Full-thickness macular hole formation in eyes with a pre-existing complete posterior vitreous detachment, *Ophthalmology* (1995) **102**:1702–5.
19. Hejny C, Han DP. Vitrectomy for macular hole after pneumatic retinopexy, *Retina* (1997) **17**:356–7.
20. Smiddy WE. Atypical presentation of macular holes, *Arch Ophthalmol* (1993) **111**:626–31.
21. Brown GC. Macular hole formation following rhegmatogenous retinal detachment repair, *Arch Ophthalmol* (1988) **106**:765–6.
22. Green WR, Kengon KR, Michels RG, et al. Ultrastructure of epiretinal membranes causing macular pucker after retinal re-attachment surgery, *Trans Ophthalmol Soc UK* (1979) **99**:65–77.
23. Lipham WJ, Smiddy WE. Idiopathic macular hole following vitrectomy: Implications for pathogenesis, *Ophthalmic Surg Lasers* (1997) **28**:633–9.
24. De Bustros S, Vitrectomy for Prevention of Macular Hole Study Group. Vitrectomy for prevention of macular holes: Results of a randomized multicenter clinical trial, *Ophthalmology* (1994) **101**:1055–60.
25. McDonnell PJ, Fine SL, Hillis AI. Clinical features of idiopathic macular cysts and holes, *Am J Ophthalmol* (1982) **93**:777–86.
26. Bronstein MA, Trempe CL, Freeman HM. Fellow eyes of eyes with macular holes, *Am J Ophthalmol* (1981) **92**:757–61.
27. Morgan CM, Schatz H. Idiopathic macular holes, *Am J Ophthalmol* (1985) **99**:437–44.
28. Fisher YL, Slakter JS, Yannuzzi LA, Guyer DA. A prospective natural history study and kinetic ultrasound evaluation of idiopathic macular holes, *Ophthalmology* (1994) **101**:5–11.
29. Lewis ML, Cohen SM, Smiddy WE, Gass JD. Bilaterality of idiopathic macular holes, *Graefes Arch Clin Exp Ophthalmol* (1996) **234**:241–5.
30. Ezra E, Wells JA, Gray RH, et al. Incidence of idiopathic full-thickness macular holes in fellow eyes: a 5-year prospective natural history study, *Ophthalmology* (1998) **105**:353–9.
31. Smiddy WE, Gass JD. Masquerades of macular holes, *Ophthalmic Surg* (1995) **26**:16–24.
32. Martinez J, Smiddy WE, Kim J, Gass JD. Differentiating macular holes from macular pseudoholes, *Am J Ophthalmol* (1994) **117**:762–7.
33. Tsujikawa M, Ohji M, Fujikado T, et al. Differentiating full thickness macular holes from impending macular holes and macular pseudoholes, *Br J Ophthalmol* (1997) **81**:117–22.
34. Guyer DR, Green WR, de Bustros S, Fine SL. Histopathologic features of idiopathic macular holes and cysts, *Ophthalmology* (1990) **97**:1045–51.
35. Yooh HS, Brooks HL Jr, Capone A Jr, et al. Ultrastructural features of tissue removed during idiopathic macular hole surgery, *Am J Ophthalmol* (1996) **122**:67–75.
36. Funata M, Wendel RT, de la Cruz Z, Green WR. Clinicopathologic study of bilateral macular holes treated with pars plana vitrectomy and gas tamponade, *Retina* (1992) **12**:289–98.
37. Madreperla SA, Geiger GL, Funata M, et al. Clinicopathologic correlation of a macular hole treated by cortical vitreous peeling and gas tamponade, *Ophthalmology* (1994) **101**:682–6.
38. Campochiaro PA, van Niel E, Vinores SA. Immunocytochemical labeling of cells in cortical vitreous from patients with premacular hole lesions, *Arch Ophthalmol* (1992) **110**:371–7.
39. Madreperla SA, McCuen BW II, Hickingbotham D, Green WR. Clinicopathologic correlation of surgically removed

macular hole opercula, *Am J Ophthalmol* (1995) **120**:197–207.
40. Ezra E, Munro PM, Charteris DG, et al. Macular hole opercula: ultrastructural features and clinicopathological correlation, *Arch Ophthalmol* (1997) **115**:1381–7.
41. Schocket SS, Lakhanpal V, Miao XP, et al. Laser treatment of macular holes, *Ophthalmology* (1988) **95**:574–82.
42. Gonvers M, Machemer R. A new approach to treating retinal detachment with macular hole, *Am J Ophthalmol* (1982) **94**:468–72.
43. Blankenship GW, Ibanez-Langlois S. Treatment of myopic macular hole and detachment: intravitreal gas exchange, *Ophthalmology* (1987) **94**:333–6.
44. Bidwell AE, Jampol LM, Goldberg MF. Macular holes and excellent visual acuity: case report, *Arch Ophthalmol* (1988) **106**:1350–1.
45. Kelly NE, Wendel RT. Vitreous surgery for idiopathic macular holes: results of a pilot study, *Arch Ophthalmol* (1991) **109**:654–9.
46. Wendell RT, Patel AC, Kelly NE, et al. Vitreous surgery for macular holes, *Ophthalmology* (1993) **100**:1671–6.
47. Orellana J, Lieberman RM. Stage III macular hole surgery, *Br J Ophthalmol* (1993) **77**:555–8.
48. Lansing MB, Glaser BM, Liss H, et al. The effect of pars plana vitrectomy and transforming growth factor-beta 2 without epiretinal membrane peeling on full-thickness macular holes, *Ophthalmology* (1993) **100**:868–72.
49. Smiddy WE, Glaser MB, Thompson JT, et al. Transforming growth factor beta-2 significantly enhances the ability to flatten the rim of subretinal fluid surrounding macular holes: preliminary anatomic results of a multicenter prospective randomized study, *Retina* (1993) **13**:296–301.
50. Gaudric A, Massin P, Paques M, et al. Autologous platelet concentrate for the treatment of full-thickness macular holes, *Graefes Arch Clin Exp Ophthalmol* (1995) **233**:549–54.
51. Liggett PE, Skolik S, Horio B, et al. Human autologous serum for the treatment of full-thickness macular holes: a preliminary study, *Ophthalmology* (1995) **102**:1071–6.
52. Vine AK, Johnson MW. Thrombin in the management of full thickness macular holes, *Retina* (1996) **16**:474–8.
53. Thompson JT, Smiddy WE, Glaser BM, et al. Intraocular tamponade duration and success of macular hole surgery, *Retina* (1996) **16**:373–82.
54. Wells JA, Gregor ZJ. Surgical treatment of full-thickness macular holes using autologous serum, *Eye* (1996) **10**:593–9.
55. Polk TD, Smiddy WE, Flynn HW Jr. Bilateral visual function after macular hole surgery, *Ophthalmology* (1996) **103**:422–6.
56. Korobelnik JF, Hannouche D, Belayachi N, et al. Autologous platelet concentrate as an adjunct in macular hole healing: a pilot study, *Ophthalmology* (1996) **103**:590–4.
57. Kim JW, Freeman WR, Azen SP, et al. Prospective randomized trial of vitrectomy or observation for stage 2 macular holes, *Am J Ophthalmol* (1996) **121**:605–14.
58. Freeman WR, Azen SP, Kim JW, et al. Vitrectomy for the treatment of full-thickness stage 3 or 4 macular holes: results of a multicentered randomized clinical trial, *Arch Ophthalmol* (1997) **115**:11–21.
59. Smiddy WE, Pimental S, Williams GA. Macular hole surgery without using adjunctive additives, *Ophthalmic Surg Lasers* (1997) **28**:713–17.
60. Ryan E Jr, Gilbert HD. Results of surgical treatment of recent-onset full-thickness idiopathic macular holes, *Arch Ophthalmol* (1994) **112**:1545–53.
61. Willis AW, Garcia-Cosio JF. Macular hole surgery: comparison of longstanding versus recent macular holes, *Ophthalmology* (1996) **103**:1811–14.
62. Thompson JT, Sjaarda RN, Lansing MB. The results of vitreous surgery for chronic macular holes, *Retina* (1997) **17**:493–501.
63. Leonard RE II, Smiddy WE, Flynn HW Jr, Feuer W. Long-term visual outcome in patients with successful macular hole surgery, *Ophthalmology* (1997) **104**:1648–52.
64. Flynn HW Jr. Macular hole surgery in patients with proliferative diabetic retinopathy (letter), *Arch Ophthalmol* (1994) **112**:877–8.
65. Han DP, Abrams GW, Aaberg TM. Surgical excision of the attached posterior hyaloid, *Arch Ophthalmol* (1988) **106**:998–1000.
66. Mein CE, Flynn HW Jr. Recognition and removal of the posterior cortical vitreous during vitreoretinal surgery for impending macular hole, *Am J Ophthalmol* (1991) **111**:611–13.
67. Ruiz-Moreno JM, Pérez-Santonja JJ. Dissection of the posterior hyaloid, *Arch Ophthalmol* (1998) **116**:1392–3.
68. Margherio AR, Margherio RR, Hartzer M, et al. Plasmin enzyme-assisted vitrectomy in traumatic pediatric macular holes, *Ophthalmology* (1998) **105**:1617–20.
69. Ryan EA, Lee S, Chern S. Use of intravitreal autologous blood to identify posterior cortical vitreous in macular hole surgery, *Arch Ophthalmol* (1995) **113**:822–3.
70. Lewis JM, Park I, Ohji M, et al. Diamond-dusted silicone cannula for epiretinal membrane separation during vitreous surgery, *Am J Ophthalmol* (1997) **124**:552–4.
71. Rubin JS, Thompson JT, Sjaarda RN, et al. Efficacy of fluid–air exchange during pars plana vitrectomy, *Retina* (1995) **15**:291–4.
72. Goldbaum MH, McCuen BW, Hanneken AM, et al. Silicone oil tamponade to seal macular holes without position restrictions, *Ophthalmology* (1998) **105**:2140–8.
73. Miller JH Jr, Googe JM Jr, Hoskins JC. Combined macular hole and cataract surgery, *Am J Ophthalmol* (1997) **123**:705–7.
74. Tornambe PE, Poliner LS, Grote K. Macular hole surgery without face-down positioning: a pilot study, *Retina* (1997) **17**:179–85.
75. Berger JW, Brucker AJ. The magnitude of the bubble buoyant pressure: implications for macular hole surgery (letter), *Retina* (1998) **18**:84–6.
76. Tornambe PE. Response (letter), *Retina* (1998) **18**:86.
77. Eckardt C, Eckardt U, Groos S, et al. Entferung der Membrana limitans interna bei Makulalochern: Klinische und morphologische Befunde, *Ophthalmologe* (1997) **94**:545–51.
78. Olsen TW, Sternberg P Jr, Capone A Jr, et al. Macular hole surgery using thrombin-acivated fibrinogen and selective removal of the internal limiting membrane, *Retina* (1998) **18**:322–9.
79. Nao-i N, Sawada A. Effect of debridement of the retinal pigment epithelium in full-thickness macular hole surgery, *Acta Ophthalmol Scand* (1998) **76**:234–7.
80. Min WK, Lee JH, Ham DI. Macular hole surgery in conjunction with endolaser photocoagulation, *Am J Ophthalmol* (1999) **127**:306–11.

81. Peyman GA, Daun M, Greve MDJ, et al. Surgical closure of macular hole using an absorbable macular plug, *Int Ophthalmol* (1997) **21**:87–91.
82. Thompson JT, Smiddy WE, Williams GA, et al. Comparison of recombinant transforming growth factor-beta-2 and placebo as an adjunctive agent for macular hole surgery, *Ophthalmology* (1998) **105**:700–6.
83. Smiddy WE, Sjaarda RN, Glaser BM, et al. Reoperation after failed macular hole surgery, *Retina* (1996) **16**:13–18.
84. Ezra E, Aylward WG, Gregor ZJ. Membranectomy and autologous serum for the retreatment of full-thickness macular holes, *Arch Ophthalmol* (1997) **115**:1276–80.
85. Thompson JT, Glaser BM, Sjaarda RN, Murphy RP. Progression of nuclear sclerosis and long-term visual results of vitrectomy with transforming growth factor beta-2 for macular holes, *Am J Ophthalmol* (1995) **119**:48–54.
86. Thompson JT, Sjaarda RN, Glaser BM, Murphy RP. Increased intraocular pressure after macular hole surgery, *Am J Ophthalmol* (1996) **121**:615–22.
87. Poliner LS, Tornambe PE. Retinal pigment epitheliopathy after macular hole surgery, *Ophthalmology* (1992) **99**:1671–7.
88. Duker JS. Retinal pigment epitheliopathy after macular hole surgery (letter), *Ophthalmology* (1993) **100**:1604–5.
89. Charles S. Retinal pigment epithelial abnormalities after macular hole surgery (letter), *Retina* (1993) **13**:176.
90. Park SS, Marcus DM, Duker JS, et al. Posterior segment complications after vitrectomy for macular hole, *Ophthalmology* (1995) **102**:775–81.
91. Banker AS, Freeman WR, Kim JW, et al. Vision-threatening complications of surgery for full-thickness macular holes, *Ophthalmology* (1997) **104**:1442–53.
92. Novak MA. Vitrectomy for epiretinal membranes, *Semin Ophthalmology* (1994) **9**:29–46.
93. Margherio RR, Cox MS Jr, Trese MT, et al. Removal of epimacular membranes, *Ophthalmology* (1985) **92**:1075–83.
94. Hilton GF, Tornambe PE, The Retinal Detachment Study Group. Pneumatic retinopexy: an analysis of intraoperative and postoperative complications, *Retina* (1991) **11**:285–94.
95. Sjaarda RN, Glaser BM, Thompson JT, et al. Distribution of iatrogenic retinal breaks in macular hole surgery, *Ophthalmology* (1995) **102**:1387–92.
96. Blumenkranz MS. Discussion: vision threatening complications of surgery for full thickness macular holes, *Ophthalmology* (1997) **104**:1452–3.
97. Akduman L, Del Priore LV, Kaplan HJ. Spontaneous resolution of retinal detachment occurring after macular hole surgery, *Arch Ophthalmol* (1998) **116**:465–7.
98. Melberg NS, Thomas MA. Visual field loss after pars plana vitrectomy with air/fluid exchange, *Am J Ophthalmol* (1995) **120**:386–8.
99. Boldt HC, Munden PM, Folk JC, Mehaffrey MG. Visual field defects after macular hole surgery, *Am J Ophthalmol* (1996) **122**:371–81.
100. Pendergast SD, McCuen BW II. Visual field loss after macular hole surgery, *Ophthalmology* (1996) **103**:1069–77.
101. Kerrison JB, Haller JA, Elman M, Miller NR. Visual field loss following vitreous surgery, *Arch Ophthalmol* (1996) **114**:564–9.
102. Hutton WL, Fuller DG, Snyder WB, et al. Visual field defects after macular hole surgery: a new finding, *Ophthalmology* (1996) **103**:2152–9.
103. Welch JC. Dehydration injury as a possible cause of visual field defect after pars plana vitrectomy for macular hole, *Am J Ophthalmol* (1997) **124**:698–9.
104. Ohji M, Nao-i N, Saito Y, et al. Prevention of visual field defect after macular hole surgery by passing air used for fluid–air exchange through water, *Am J Ophthalmol* (1999) **127**:62–6.
105. Paques M, Massin P, Santiago PY, et al. Visual field loss after vitrectomy for full-thickness macular holes, *Am J Ophthalmol* (1997) **124**:88–94.
106. Fekrat S, Wendel RT, de la Cruz Z, Green WR. Clinicopathologic correlation of an epiretinal membrane associated with a recurrent macular hole, *Retina* (1995) **15**:53–7.
107. Duker JS, Wendel RT, Patel AC, Puliafito CA. Late re-opening of macular holes after initially successful treatment with vitreous surgery, *Ophthalmology* (1994) **101**:1373–8.
108. Paques M, Massin P, Santiago PY, et al. Late reopening of successfully treated macular holes, *Br J Ophthalmol* (1997) **81**:658–62.
109. Leonard RE II, Smiddy WE, Flynn HW Jr. Visual acuity and macular hole size after unsuccessful macular hole closure, *Am J Ophthalmol* (1997) **123**:84–9.
110. Johnson RN, McDonald HR, Schatz H, Ai E. Outpatient postoperative fluid–gas exchange after early failed vitrectomy surgery for macular hole, *Ophthalmology* (1997) **104**:2009–13.
111. Del Priore LV, Kaplan HJ, Bonham RD. Laser photocoagulation and fluid-gas exchange for recurrent macular hole, *Retina* (1994) **14**:381–2.
112. Ikuno Y, Kamei M, Saito Y, et al. Photocoagulation and fluid–gas exchange to treat persistent macular holes after prior vitrectomy: a pilot study, *Ophthalmology* (1998) **105**:1411–18.

Part VII Subretinal Surgery Techniques

Chapter 32 Surgical removal of subretinal hemorrhage

Alan E Kimura

INTRODUCTION

Recombinant tissue plasminogen activator (tPA) has been used systemically in the management of acute myocardial infarction since 1984.[1] Ophthalmic usage in postvitrectomy anterior chamber fibrin formation began in 1988.[2] Its usage has evolved into management of submacular hemorrhage, with a variety of options currently being debated and refined. Current controversy centers around a safe dosage of intravitreal tPA which avoids toxicity of the vehicle, and whether or not the retina imposes a barrier on the movement of intravitreal tPA into the subretinal space. Still to be answered is whether or not the subretinal blood is liquefied or solid preoperatively. The answer to this question would clarify the need for, the timing of, and the dosage of tPA.

Our understanding of the intricate physiologic relationships of tissue-type plasminogen activator in the eye is limited. A balance between tissue-type plasminogen activator and tissue plasminogen inhibitor has been studied in cultured human trabecular meshwork cells[3] and in human aqueous humor following extracapsular cataract extraction and polymethymethacrylate lens implantation,[4] as well as bovine aqueous and vitreous humor.[5] Further studies in human ocular fluids and tissues may lead to a refinement in the therapeutic use of recombinant tPA in various pathologies. Dosage, timing of injection and route of administration are undergoing refinement.

Human recombinant tPA has been used to lyse fibrin clots in the anterior chamber following cataract extraction and lens implantation, with one study relating a larger incision and longer operating time with a higher incidence of postoperative fibrin formation.[6] Other reported uses include the treatment of fibrin formation following penetrating keratoplasty,[7] glaucoma filtering surgery or post-traumatic total hyphema.[8] Postvitrectomy fibrin clot lysis with recombinant tPA also has been described.[9] Pupillary block[10] and maintenance of an inferior peripheral iridectomy in conjunction with intravitreal silicone oil tamponade are other applications of recombinant tPA.[11]

Side-effects and complications of intracameral tPA include hyphema, corneal stromal thickening, elevated intraocular pressure, breakthrough vitreous hemorrhage, endophthalmitis, retinal break with detachment, subretinal rebleed, and exudative retinal detachment with pigmentary retinopathy following spontaneous resolution. To minimize the rate of rebleed, lower doses of recombinant tPA have been advocated with a suggestion of comparable success rates, although repeat injections may be necessary. The creation of fibrin-degradation products as a result of the plasminogen cascade is theoretically toxic and some argue for their removal by washout following the use of tPA,[12] but this practice is uncommon.

New indications for removal of submacular hemorrhage that employ intravitreal or subretinal instillation of recombinant tPA will be discussed in this chapter.

RATIONALE FOR SUBMACULAR SURGERY TO REMOVE SUBMACULAR HEMORRHAGE

Submacular surgery is performed to remove submacular hemorrhage because the natural untreated history of a thick submacular hemorrhage leads to poor vision.[13,14] The presence of submacular hemorrhage causes a rapid deterioration of the retina, when fibrin contraction from the clot may cause shearing of the photoreceptors.

RATIONALE FOR USE OF tPA

Tissue plasminogen activator is a serine protease that converts plasminogen to plasmin. Plasmin in turn lyses fibrin into soluble degradation products. When bound to fibrin, tPA has a markedly increased affinity for plasminogen, thus effectively confining the activity to the surface of the fibrin clot. Subretinal irrigation with tPA induces subretinal clot lysis and facilitates clot removal.

PREPARATION OF tPA FOR INTRAOCULAR INJECTION

Details regarding preparation of recombinant tPA for intraocular administration and storage are provided by Jaffe et al.[15] Recommendations for preparation and storage were updated and reviewed by Johnson in the Annual AAO Vitreoretinal Update 1999.[16]

SURGICAL TECHNIQUES

As in any rapidly evolving field, there are many approaches to achieve the same goal,[17] yet the various techniques share a common 'critical path' illustrated below. The following brief sections show the progression of the surgical management of submacular hemorrhage, beginning with the least invasive procedure and ending with the most invasive.

OBSERVATION

The natural history of hemorrhage is poor for subretinal heme secondary to hemorrhagic age-related macular degeneration (ARMD). Some believe that submacular hemorrhage from retinal arteriolar macroaneurysm may be observed for spontaneous resolution.

PNEUMATIC DISPLACEMENT WITH PRONE POSITIONING

Ohji et al.[18] recommend the intravitreal injection of 0.4–0.5 ml pure perfluoropropane gas initially with prone positioning to displace subretinal hemorrhage.

PNEUMATIC DISPLACEMENT WITH INTRAVITREAL tPA, FOLLOWED BY PRONE POSITIONING

Heriot first proposed the concept of pneumatic displacement of subretinal hemorrhage and incorporated intravitreal tPA as part of the procedure.[19]

INTRAVITREAL tPA, VITRECTOMY WITH PERFLUOROCARBON LIQUID (PFCL) ROLLING TAMPONADE, FOLLOWED BY SUBRETINAL IRRIGATION/ASPIRATION OF tPA

Kimura et al.[20] described preoperative intravitreal tPA, followed by vitrectomy and rolling perfluorooctane (PFO) tamponade to displace liquefied subretinal blood through a retinotomy. Subretinal instillation of tPA followed for non-mobilized, submacular solid clots of blood. Kamei et al. reported larger numbers of patients.[21]

VITRECTOMY, SUBRETINAL IRRIGATION/ASPIRATION OF tPA

Peyman et al.[17,22] and Lewis et al.[23] favor subretinal irrigation of tPA, followed by 20–45 minutes to allow for enzymatic action, followed by subretinal aspiration. Millsap et al. use separate retinotomy sites for subretinal irrigation and aspiration.[22]

LARGE RETINAL INCISION FOLLOWED BY SUBRETINAL DISSECTION

This technique was originally proposed to gain access to the subretinal space and remove large submacular clots. The unacceptably high incidence of postoperative failure from detachment and proliferative vitreoretinopathy from retinal incision led to a search for less invasive approaches.

CASE SELECTION

The most important step in management is proper case selection. Consideration of the patient's underlying pathology is of paramount importance. The untreated natural history of a thick submacular hemorrhage from age-related macular degeneration carries a worse prognosis than a similar hemorrhage from a retinal arterial macroaneurysm or trauma. The anatomic location of the blood also portends the likelihood of performing a relatively atraumatic surgery or one that denudes a large patch of retinal pigment epithelium (RPE). A subretinal hemorrhage is easier to remove than a subretinal pigment epithelial hemorrhage, which may be accompanied by removal of a geographic patch of the RPE.

REMOVAL OF VITREOUS

The second critical step is the removal of vitreous to create working space and to allow stripping of the posterior hyaloid (to reduce the chances of preretinal membrane formation and subsequent macular puckering). This is usually accomplished by a three-port pars plana vitrectomy (Fig. 32.1) followed by stripping of the posterior hyaloid (Fig. 32.2). A soft-tipped, flexible silicone needle is useful in stripping the posterior hyaloid by looking for the 'fish-strike sign'; the vitrectomy handpiece or sharp dissection with a bent needle or the subretinal pick provide alternative instrumentation for this task.

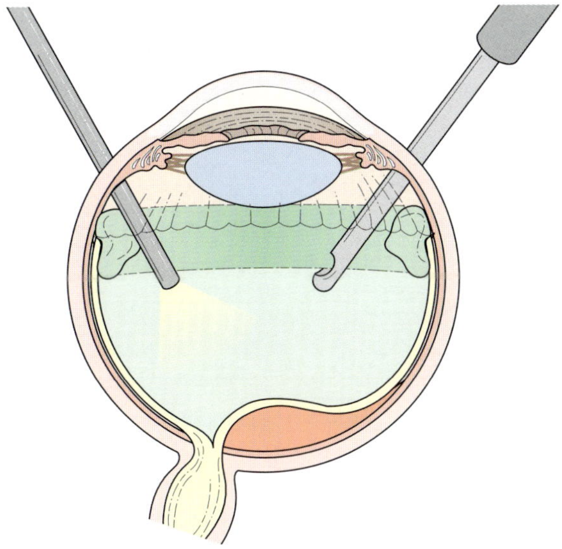

Figure 32.1 *A three-port pars plana core vitrectomy is performed.*

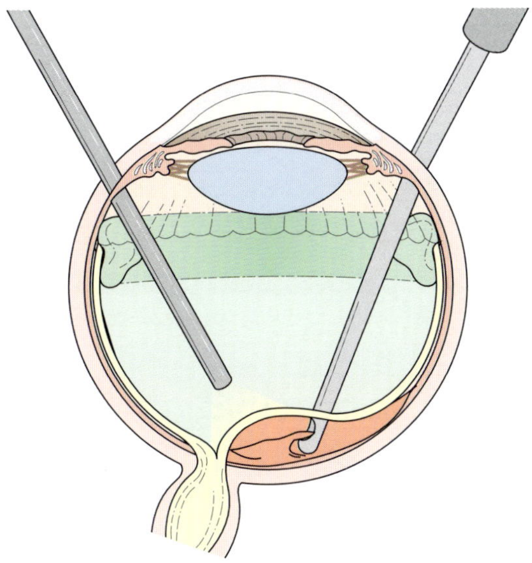

Figure 32.2 *A soft-tipped, flexible silicone needle is useful in stripping the posterior hyaloid by looking for the 'fish-strike sign'. An illuminated light pick in the other hand can impale the elevated hyaloid face. Alternative instrumentation includes a vitrectomy handpiece (shown), sharp dissection with a bent needle or the subretinal pick.*

RETINOTOMY

Most surgeons now favor a small retinotomy. The early surgical technique included diathermy to the retinotomy site prior to opening the retina. However, this is generally not required. Additionally, endolaser of the retinotomy site is no longer necessary at the conclusion of surgery, unless a large retinotomy was created during subretinal manipulations.

A retinotomy is created at the edge of the hemorrhage away from the foveola to allow manipulation of instrumentation in the subretinal space without creating undue traction on the retinotomy site. Some surgeons advocate the use of multiple retinotomy sites to allow greater flow and drainage from the subretinal space.[22] Many surgeons will inject fluid through the retinotomy into the subretinal space and thus balloon up the retina overlying the clot. Occasionally this extends beyond the clot into unaffected retina. Precise microliter infusion control during this technique theoretically could produce less trauma to the photoreceptors.

INJECTION OF tPA

In a pilot study, 6 µg/0.1 ml of intravitreally administered tPA appeared to be effective in producing clot lysis for moderate to small hemorrhages.[18] Further experience suggests that higher doses are required for larger clot lysis. An exact dosage that is proven to be safe and effective has not been established in

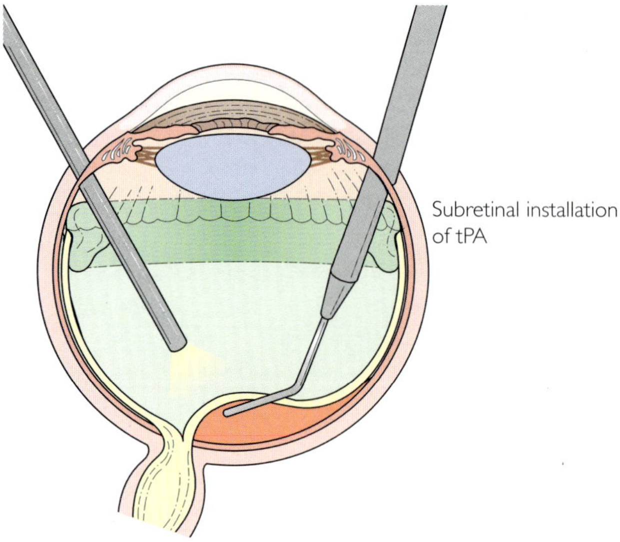

Figure 32.3 *Using an angled subretinal cannula, tissue plasminogen activator is slowly injected into the subretinal space. Sequential injections may be required for total lysis and removal of the clot. A mandatory intraoperative waiting time of 20–45 minutes is required while the drug liquefies the clot.*

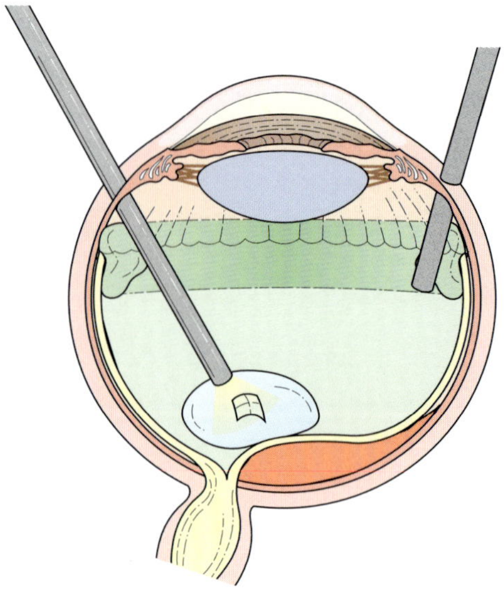

Figure 32.4 *Rolling premacular PFCL bubble. Perfluorocarbon liquids may be instilled intravitreally overlying the liquefied subretinal clot in sufficient amount to flow over the clot and express it toward the retinotomy site.*

humans. We now use 25 μg/0.1 cc of tPA intravitreally, followed by a concentration of 10 μg/0.1 ml subretinally as needed. A fluorescein strip may be dipped into the solution prior to instillation to detect reflux back into the vitreous cavity.

Experimental work has produced inconclusive results regarding the efficacy of subretinal clot lysis. In pigs, intravitreal tPA did not appear to produce clot lysis.[24] In cats, intravitreal instillation appeared to produce reliable clot lysis in the artificially created subretinal space.[25]

We favor subretinal instillation of tPA through the retinotomy site directly into the subretinal space (Fig. 32.3). This technique delivers the drug directly into the area of the clot, but requires a mandatory intraoperative waiting time of 20–45 minutes while the drug liquefies the clot. Using an angled subretinal cannula, tPA is slowly injected into the subretinal space. Sequential injections may be required for total lysis and removal of the clot.

CLOT REMOVAL

Aspiration can be achieved with a passive, soft-tipped, flexible cannulated flute needle or an extrusion needle connected to active aspiration (Grizzard cannula, Visitec). The fluted needle with a backflush reservoir allows expression of inadvertently aspirated retinal tissue and solid clots that block the aspiration port. Perfluorocarbon liquids may be instilled intravitreally overlying the liquefied subretinal clot in sufficient amount to flow over the clot and express it toward the retinotomy site (Fig. 32.4). Too small a bubble will prevent flow with the surgeon's hand rotation, and too large a bubble will tamponade the retinotomy site and prevent steamrolling of the clot.

Multiple retinotomy sites may facilitate the expression of the subretinal hemorrhage (Fig. 32.5).[21] A double-barreled needle may be inserted through the retinotomy site into the subretinal space to encourage break-up of the clot and aspiration from within the subretinal space. A compromise between a more vigorous and effective double-barrel needle technique and its attendant trauma is another consideration.

If a subretinal neovascular membrane has been identified preoperatively or intraoperatively, extraction may be considered. I have seen some neovascular membranes apparently involute postoperatively following submacular drainage of hemorrhage with tPA without extraction or thermal ablation.

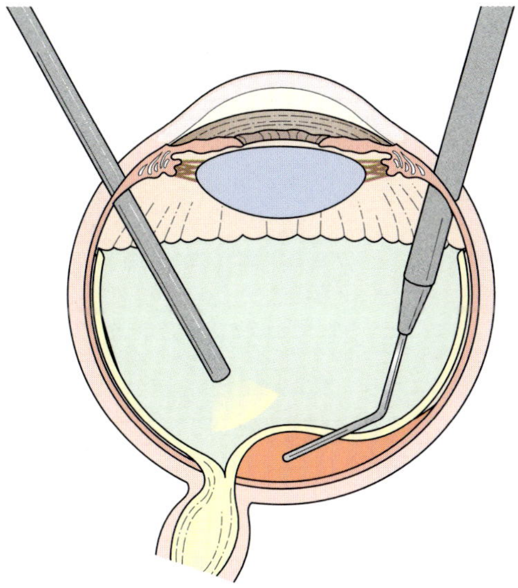

Figure 32.5 *Active aspiration of subretinal hemorrhage.*

LASER PHOTOCOAGULATION

If the retinotomy site remains small with sealed edges, without traction or intervening hemorrhage between the retina and RPE, then I choose not to endolaser the site and risk a small pucker. The posterior pole has a good capacity to dehydrate the subretinal space, even in the face of a retinotomy.

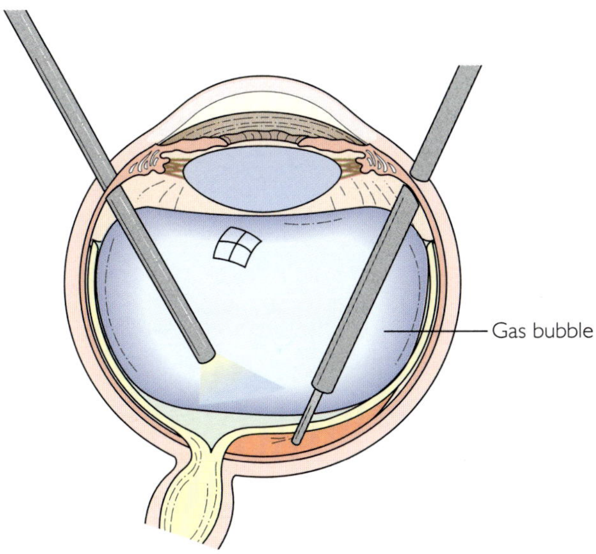

Figure 32.6 *An air–fluid exchange is performed to tamponade the retina.*

If, on the other hand, there is a fairly large extension of the retinotomy, the moderate application of laser is warranted. Care should be taken to avoid creation of inadvertent retinal breaks by overly intense laser, particularly in areas of blood. A gas–fluid exchange with room air is usually sufficient to tamponade the retinotomy and 'iron out' the retina.

Before the air–fluid exchange (Fig. 32.6), it is prudent to examine the sclerotomy sites with indirect ophthalmoscopy for retinal complications arising from sharp, angular instrument insertion. Face-down positioning in the recovery room places the air against the macula and its retinotomy site. Finally, the usual precautions against Valsalva maneuvers (both during extubation and in recovery if general endotracheal tube anesthesia is employed) and restrictions on vigorous activity common to other delicate vitrectomy surgery are in order.

POSTOPERATIVE COMPLICATIONS

Postoperatively, vitreous hemorrhage and even hyphema may occur from continued drainage of the submacular space, or conceivably from an effect of the residual recombinant tPA within the eye, although this is conjecture. Depending upon the severity of the rebleed, observation, outpatient gas–fluid exchange or repeat vitrectomy are options. Secondary glaucoma may accompany the postoperative rebleed and should be treated appropriately. Secondary retinal breaks and retinal detachment should be diagnosed and treated immediately, as should proliferative changes inducing traction upon the retinotomy site.

INTRAVITREAL INJECTION OF tPA

Continual evolution of technique seeks to minimize tissue trauma to the retina and RPE. Work under investigation seeks to eliminate the manipulations in the subretinal space by injecting intravitreally (25 μg/0.1 ml), followed by intravitreal gas injection (0.3 ml of 100% perfluoropropane) and prone-positioning 6 hours after injection for the next 24 hours.[26] This technique is followed by inferior displacement of the hemorrhage out of the center of the macula.

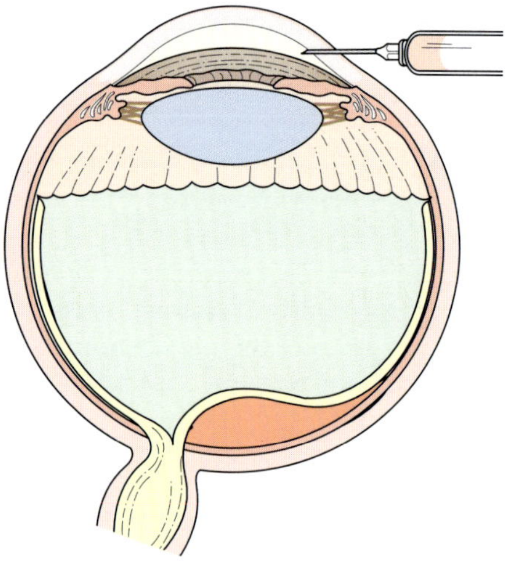

Figure 32.7 *Anterior chamber paracentesis is performed before intravitreal injection of tissue plasminogen activator.*

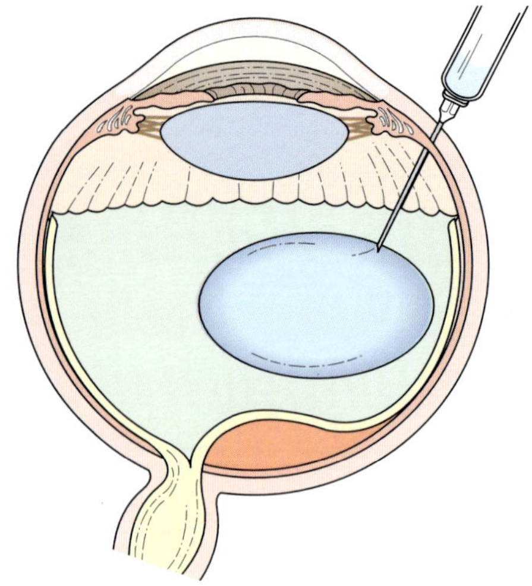

Figure 32.9 *Perfluorocarbon gas (C_3F_8, 0.4 ml) is injected into the vitreous cavity.*

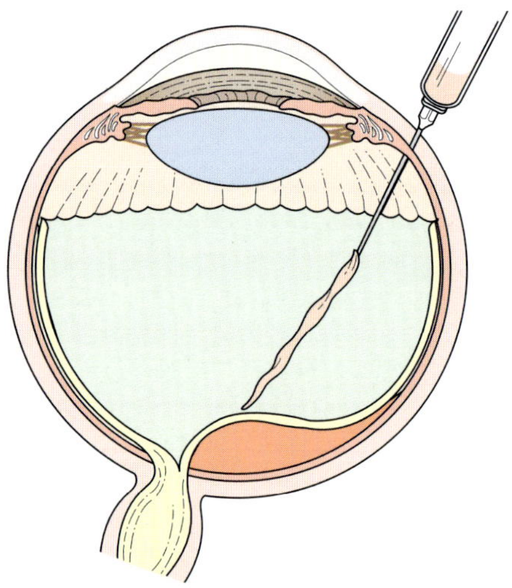

Figure 32.8 *Tissue plasminogen activator is injected intravitreally with the bevel of the needle facing up.*

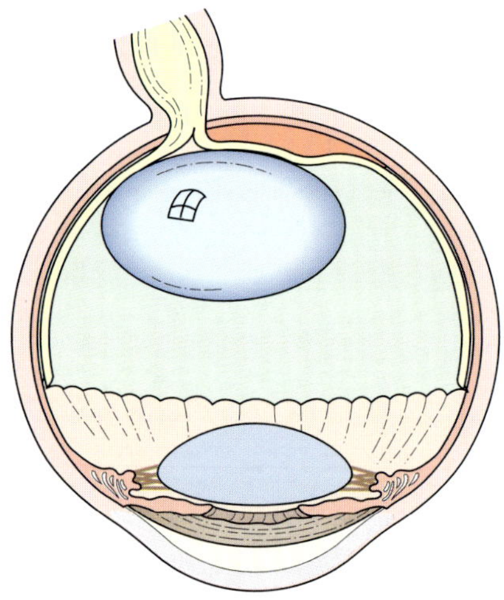

Figure 32.10 *The subretinal hemorrhage is displaced by the gas bubble after face-down positioning.*

Refinement in technique suggests the need for anterior chamber paracentesis (Fig. 32.7) before the intravitreal injections of gas and recombinant tPA (Figs 32.8–32.10). The choice of gas involves a compromise between the more effective but longer-lasting perfluoropropane gas versus a possibly less effective but shorter acting sulfur hexafluoride gas bubble.

Although effective in displacing subretinal hemorrhage inferiorly below the macula, visual acuity remains at a level of legal blindness because of the pre-existing macular pathology of age-related macular degeneration. Better ambulatory vision is reported by many patients.

SUMMARY

Currently, the optimal management of submacular hemorrhage from age-related macular degeneration would appear to be the injection of a gas bubble intravitreally in an attempt to displace the hemorrhage pneumatically. This is likely to be effective in some cases, and if this maneuver fails, it would be reasonable to inject tPA intravitreally and re-attempt pneumatic displacement. Should this prove ineffectual, pars plana vitrectomy would be the next step, in order to access the subretinal space via retinotomy. A rolling PFCL displacement may displace liquefied blood through a retinotomy. If this is still ineffectual in clearing the submacular space, subretinal irrigation of tPA should be performed with single or multiple retinotomies to clear the subretinal space. Large incision retinotomies are no longer in favor.

It must be remembered that a dramatic recovery of central visual acuity is still elusive, whatever the current approach.

REFERENCES

1. Collen D, Topol EJ, Tiefenbrunn AJ, et al. Coronary thrombolysis with recombinant human tissue-type plasminogen activator: a prospective, randomized, placebo-controlled trial, *Circulation* (1984) **70:**1012–17.
2. Williams GA, Lambrou FH, Jaffe GA, et al. Treatment of postvitrectomy fibrin formation with intraocular tissue plasminogen activator, *Arch Ophthalmol* (1988) **106:**1055–8.
3. Shuman MA, Polansky JR, Merkel C, Alvarado JA. Tissue plasminogen activator in cultured human trabecular meshwork cells: predominance of enzyme over plasminogen activator inhibitor, *Invest Ophthalmol Vis Sci* (1988) **29:**401–5.
4. Yoshitomi F, Utsumi E, Hayashi M, et al. Postoperative fluctuations of tissue plasminogen activator (t-PA) in aqueous humor of pseudophakes, *J Cataract Refract Surg* (1991) **17:**543–6.
5. Hayashi K, Nakashima Y, Sueishi K, Tanaka K. Fibrinolytic activity and localization of plasminogen activator in bovine vitreous body and aqueous humor, *Jpn J Ophthalmol* (1989) **33:**66–75.
6. Muller-Jensen K, Zimmermann H. Zu Risikofaktoren, Prophylaxe und Therapie von Fibrinreaktionen nach IOL-Implantation, *Klin Monatsbl Augenheilkd* (1995) **207:**287–91.
7. Heidemann DG, Williams GA, Blumenkranz MS. Tissue plasminogen activator and penetrating keratoplasty, *Ophthalmic Surg* (1990) **21:**364–5.
8. Laatikainen L, Mattila J. The use of tissue plasminogen activator in post-traumatic total hyphaema, *Graefes Arch Clin Exp Ophthalmol* (1996) **234:**67–8.
9. Jaffe GJ, Abrams GW, Williams GA, Han DP. Tissue plasminogen activator for postvitrectomy fibrin formation, *Ophthalmology* (1990) **97:**184–9.
10. Jaffe GJ, Lewis H, Han DP, et al. Treatment of postvitrectomy fibrin pupillary block with tissue plasminogen activator, *Am J Ophthalmol* (1989) **108:**170–5.
11. MacCumber MW, McCuen BW II, Toth CA, et al. Tissue plasminogen activator for preserving inferior peripheral iridectomy patency in eyes with silicone oil, *Ophthalmology* (1996) **103:**269–73.
12. Maeno T, Maeda N, Ikeda T, Tano Y. Tissue plasminogen activator treatment of postvitrectomy pupillary fibrin membrane, *Nippon Ganka Gakkai Zasshi* (1991) **95:**1124–8.
13. Lim JI, Subretinal hemorrhage, *Int Ophthalmol Clin* (1995) **35:**95–104.
14. Bennett SR, Folk JC, Blodi CF, Klugman M. Factors prognostic of visual outcome in patients with subretinal hemorrhage, *Am J Ophthalmol* (1990) **109:**33–7.
15. Jaffe GJ, Green GD, Abrams GW. Stability of recombinant tissue plasminogen activator, *Am J Ophthalmol* (1989) **108:**90–1.
16. Johnson MW. Pneumatic displacement of submacular hemorrhage. Presented at the Annual AAO Vitreoretinopathy Update: Orlando, FL, 1999.
17. Peyman GA, Nelson NC Jr, Alturki W, et al. Tissue plasminogen activating factor assisted removal of subretinal hemorrhage, *Ophthalmic Surg* (1991) **22:**575–82.
18. Ohji M, Saito Y, Hayashi A, et al. Pneumatic displacement of subretinal hemorrhage without tissue plasminogen activation, *Arch Ophthalmol* (1998) **116:**1326–32.
19. Heriot WJ. Further experience in management of submacular hemorrhage with intravitreal tPA. In: *Proceedings of the 1997 Update on Macular Surgery.* San Francisco: American Academy of Ophthalmology (1997), 82–4.
20. Kimura AE, Reddy CV, Folk JC, Farmer SG, Removal of subretinal hemorrhage facilitated by preoperative intravitreal tissue plasminogen activator, *Retina* (1994) **14:**83–4.
21. Kamei M, Tano Y, Maeno T, et al. Surgical removal of submacular hemorrhage using tissue plasminogen activator and perfluorocarbon liquid, *Am J Ophthalmol* (1996) **121:**267–75.
22. Millsap MC, Peyman GA, Greve MDJ. Subretinal hemorrhage removal with multiple retinotomy sites in age-related macular degeneration, *Ophthalmic Surg* (1994) **25:**723–5.
23. Lewis H. Intraoperative fibrinolysis of submacular hemorrhage with tissue plasminogen activator and surgical drainage, *Am J Ophthalmol* (1994) **118:**559–68.
24. Boone DE, Boldt HC, Ross RD, et al. The use of intravitreal tissue plasminogen activator in the treatment of experimental subretinal hemorrhage in the pig model, *Retina* (1996) **16:**518–24.
25. Coll GE, Sparrow JR, Marinovic A, Chang S. Effect of intravitreal tissue plasminogen activator on experimental subretinal hemorrhage, *Retina* (1995) **15:**319–26.
26. Hrach CJ, Johnson MW, Hassan AS, et al. Retinal toxicity of commercial intravitreal tissue plasminogen activator solution in cat eyes, *Arch Ophthalmol* (2000) **118:**659–63.

Chapter 33 Surgical removal of choroidal neovascular membranes

Nancy M Holekamp and Matthew A Thomas

INTRODUCTION

In 1991 the first report of the successful removal of subfoveal choroidal neovascularization (CNV) in two patients with ocular histoplasmosis ushered in the modern era of submacular surgery.[1] The surgical technique was revolutionary, introducing small retinotomies and small-gauge subretinal instruments. Since 1991, the surgical technique for removing subfoveal CNV has become well established. In contrast, clear indications for the procedure have yet to be defined. Both aspects of submacular surgery will be discussed.

INDICATIONS

SUBFOVEAL CHOROIDAL NEOVASCULARIZATION

The surgical removal of subfoveal CNV has not been proven beneficial for any disease entity. However, this surgical technique has been applied to many types of subfoveal CNV with varying results, some favorable and others not. To date, the most experience with this type of surgery has been in eyes with subfoveal CNV caused by:

- Ocular histoplasmosis
- Idiopathic causes
- Multifocal choroiditis
- Trauma
- High myopia
- Angioid streaks
- Macular dystrophies
- Age-related macular degeneration (ARMD).

Case selection is the single most important determinant of potential surgical success.[2] A subfoveal choroidal neovascular membrane (CNVM) that lies beneath the neurosensory retina but anterior to a healthy retinal pigment epithelium (RPE) has the best visual prognosis, because preservation of RPE is crucial in reestablishing photoreceptor function. The following factors describe a subfoveal CNV with a favorable surgical prognosis:[3]

- Patient age less than 50 years.
- Subretinal pigmented halo around the CNV.
- Sharply defined borders and plaque-like elevation to the CNV.
- No biomicroscopic or stereoscopic angiographic evidence of RPE elevation.
- The fellow eye is normal.

Other favorable prognostic factors in selecting subfoveal CNV for surgery include:

- Good visual potential (i.e. no prior subfoveal laser).
- Short duration of foveal involvement.
- Origin of CNV away from the foveal center.
- Few adhesions of CNV to the retina or adjacent scars.

NONSUBFOVEAL CNV

Clearly, the same surgical techniques for removing subfoveal CNV can be used for removing nonsubfoveal CNV. In fact, the first successful case of using these surgical techniques for the removal of an extrafoveal CNVM caused by ARMD was described in 1994.[4] More recently, successful experience has been reported in the removal of large peripapillary CNV[5] and juxtafoveal CNV.[6] Surgery occasionally may be considered in the following selected cases of nonsubfoveal CNV:

- Large, exudative extrafoveal CNV.
- Large peripapillary CNV.
- Juxtafoveal CNV.

Table 33.1 Surgical results: a single surgeon's experience in 247 cases

Disease	*Postop visual acuity*			*Postop change in visual acuity*			*Recurrence rate*	*Mean follow-up* (months)
	≥20/40	20/50–20/100	≤20/200	Better ≥ 3 lines	Same ± 2 lines	Worse ≤ 3 lines		
Ocular histoplasmosis (n = 120)	35%	30%	35%	40%	44%	16%	42%	13
Multifocal choroiditis (n = 17)	59%	29%	12%	65%	29%	6%	18%	8
Idiopathic (n = 19)	21%	26%	53%	42%	53%	5%	37%	10
ARMD (n = 60)	3%	13%	84%	15%	65%	20%	32%	13
High myopia (n = 17)	12%	41%	47%	12%	65%	23%	53%	10
Angioid streaks (n = 5)	0	20%	80%	0	100%	0	100%	6

ARMD, age-related macular degeneration

Again, subretinal surgery is not proven to be beneficial for the removal of any type of CNV. Surgery should only be considered in the above cases if laser photocoagulation is not indicated according to current guidelines or if laser is thought to be potentially damaging to visual acuity or visual field.

SURGICAL RESULTS

SUBFOVEAL CNV

The Submacular Surgery Trials are currently evaluating the benefit of submacular surgery for eyes with subfoveal CNV caused by histoplasmosis, idiopathic causes and ARMD. Until the surgical results of that prospective, randomized study are known, the largest experience with subfoveal surgery reported to date was presented by Matthew A Thomas in the 1995 Macula Society Rosenthal Lecture.[7]

Thomas reviewed the surgical results of 247 cases of subfoveal surgery for the following disease entities: ocular histoplasmosis (120 eyes), ARMD (60 eyes), idiopathic causes (19 eyes), multifocal choroiditis (17 eyes), high myopia (17 eyes), angioid streaks (5 eyes) and miscellaneous causes (9 eyes). The results are shown in Table 33.1.

Table 33.2 summarizes the results in Table 33.1. It is evident that eyes with subfoveal CNV resulting from a focal disease of the RPE, such as ocular histoplasmosis, multifocal choroiditis and idiopathic causes, have a more favorable surgical outcome. In these eyes, subfoveal RPE is usually preserved during surgery. In contrast, eyes with subfoveal CNV caused by diffuse and/or degenerative disease of the RPE, such as ARMD, high myopia or angioid streaks, have a less favorable surgical outcome. In these eyes, subfoveal RPE is usually lost during surgery.

Table 33.2 Summary of surgical results

Better surgical results in focal disease	*Poor surgical results in diffuse disease*
Ocular histoplasmosis	Age-related macular degeneration
Idiopathic	High myopia
Multifocal choroiditis	Angioid streaks
Often subfoveal RPE is preserved	*Usually subfoveal RPE is lost*

Table 33.3 Surgical results for juxtafoveal CNV in 35 cases

Postop visual acuity			*Postop change in visual acuity*			*Recurrence rate*	*Mean follow-up (months)*
≥ 20/40	*20/50–20/100*	*≤20/200*	*Better ≥ 3 lines*	*Same ± 2 lines*	*Worse ≤ 3 lines*		
51%	26%	23%	57%	26%	17%	49%	14

NONSUBFOVEAL CNV

Nonsubfoveal CNV is usually treated successfully with laser photocoagulation. Occasionally, extrafoveal CNV does not fit within current treatment guidelines. In one such example, a large exudative macular detachment resolved after surgical removal of a poorly defined extrafoveal CNVM. Visual acuity improved from 20/200 to 20/25 with 18 months of follow-up.[4]

Peripapillary CNV also is usually treated successfully with laser photocoagulation. However, in a review by Atebara and colleagues[5] of 19 cases of submacular surgery for large non-ARMD peripapillary CNV, four eyes were found to have nonsubfoveal CNV that did not meet Macular Photocoagulation Study (MPS) criteria for laser photocoagulation. After submacular surgery, postoperative visual acuity was 20/25 or better in all four cases. These types of cases are rare, but may be best managed by submacular surgery.

Juxtafoveal CNV also is usually treated with laser photocoagulation. As an alternative to laser surgery, Joseph and Thomas[6] reviewed 35 cases of submacular surgery for juxtafoveal CNV resulting from a variety of causes: ocular histoplasmosis (18 eyes), idiopathic (13 eyes), ARMD (6 eyes), myopia (4 eyes) and miscellaneous causes (3 eyes).[6] Although the results from this small study (Table 33.3) are encouraging, laser photocoagulation is still the only treatment shown to be beneficial for juxtafoveal CNV.

COMPLICATIONS

Eyes undergoing submacular surgery are at risk for the same types of complications seen with other macular surgery. These include endophthalmitis, retinal tear, retinal detachment and progression of cataract. Potential complications unique to submacular surgery include foveal dehiscence during subretinal balanced salt solution (BSS) infusion, subretinal hemorrhage, persistently open retinotomy postoperatively and CNV at the retinotomy site. The most prevalent postoperative problem is recurrent CNV, which can be expected to occur in 40–50% of cases.[8]

PREOPERATIVE EVALUATION

Three important questions must be answered preoperatively:

- The etiology of the CNV.
- The location of the CNV as subfoveal or nonsubfoveal.
- The health of the RPE surrounding the CNV.

Therefore, in addition to the standard preoperative evaluation of any surgical candidate, eyes to be considered for submacular surgery should undergo the following:

- Refracted visual acuity.
- Slit-lamp biomicroscopy.
- Fluorescein angiography.

Slit-lamp biomicroscopy can be used to check the patient's central fixation as well as to assess whether the CNV lies anterior to the RPE. A high-quality fluorescein angiogram may identify a subfoveal versus nonsubfoveal CNVM and detect any abnormality of the surrounding RPE.

SURGICAL TECHNIQUE

INSTRUMENTATION

Submacular surgery requires the same vitrectomy set-up and instrumentation used for other types of macular surgery in addition to the following:[9]

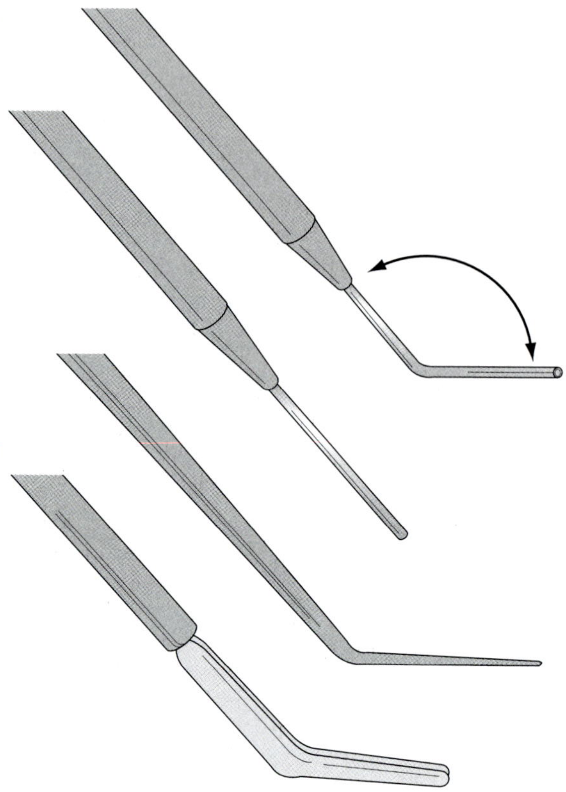

Figure 33.1 *Additional instruments used for submacular surgery: (a) 130° angled 33-gauge infusion cannula (the tip of the instrument is beveled up at 45°); (b) straight 33-gauge cannula; (c) 130° angled 36-gauge subretinal pick; (d) 130° angled horizontal subretinal forceps.*

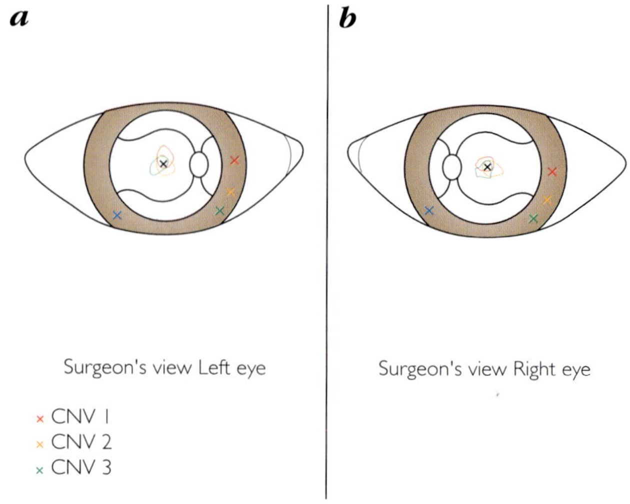

Figure 33.2 *Sclerotomy location for a right-handed surgeon. (a) Surgeon's view, left eye: red, CNV 1; yellow, CNV 2; green, CNV 3, (b) surgeon's view, right eye: red, CNV 1; yellow, CNV 2; green, CNV 3.*

- 130° Angled 36-gauge subretinal pick.
- 130° Angled 33-gauge subretinal infusion cannula.
- 130° Angled horizontal subretinal forceps.
- Straight 33-gauge cannula. (Fig. 33.1).

Small-gauge instruments on 20-gauge shafts allow subretinal manipulation through small, self-sealing retinotomies. A long tapering tip on each instrument permits the retinotomy to be made as far from the fovea as possible. A 130° bend from the shaft allows manipulation at the tip of the instrument without striking the heel against the RPE or choroid.

PROCEDURE

SCLEROTOMY LOCATION

Most surgeons prefer to perform subretinal membrane dissection and removal with their dominant hand. When setting up a standard three-port pars plana vitrectomy, site selection for the dominant hand sclerotomy is important (Fig. 33.2). A sclerotomy should be placed so that the CNV can be reached directly without going over a previous laser scar or risking extensive manipulation under the fovea. It is helpful to bring a copy of the preoperative angiogram to the operating room so that the precise location of the CNV is known.

- Location of CNV 1 inferior to the fovea (Fig. 33.2) requires placement of a sclerotomy in position 1 along the horizontal meridian.
- Location of CNV 2 centered on the fovea allows sclerotomy placement in standard position 2. If a pre-existing laser scar were to make a temporal approach difficult, then the sclerotomy may have to be shifted.
- Location of CNV 3 on the far side of the fovea from the dominant hand may require placement of a sclerotomy in position 3 along the vertical meridian.

As a general rule, a straight line should exist between the sclerotomy, retinotomy and point of desired contact with the CNV while avoiding the fovea or pre-existing laser scars.

Nonlasered, small retinotomies placed in the papillomacular bundle do not create postoperative visual

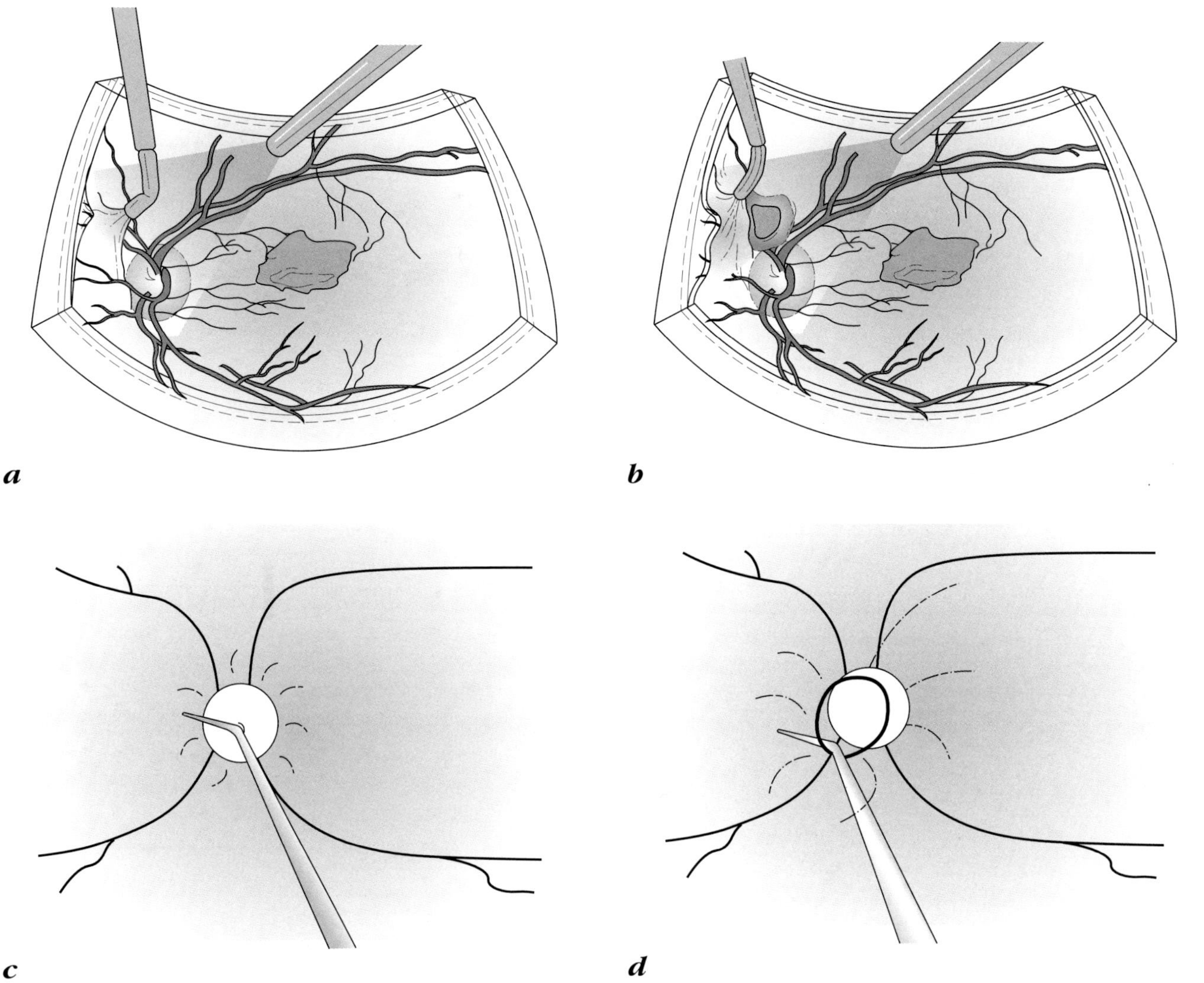

Figure 33.3 *(a,b) Soft-tipped extrusion needle is used to engage posterior hyaloid near disc. (c,d) A 130° angled short, flat pick called the 'hyaloid lifter' is used to lift the Weiss ring in a controlled manner.*

field defects. Therefore, a right-handed surgeon may use the dominant hand when operating on a left eye, and a left-handed surgeon may use the dominant hand when operating on a right eye.

Occasionally it is helpful to turn the microscope and operate from the temporal side if adequate access to the CNV is blocked by laser scars, etc.

CORE VITRECTOMY

A core vitrectomy is carried out in the standard fashion.

POSTERIOR HYALOID STRIPPING

A soft-tipped cannula with active extrusion is used to assess the location of the posterior hyaloid (Fig. 33.3a,b). A 'fish strike' sign indicates that the hyaloid membrane is attached to the retinal surface. One may also check for the absence of fluid dripping into the vitrectomy cassette when the hyaloid membrane is engaged with active aspiration.

If the posterior hyaloid is attached, tangential and anterior traction using continuous suction with the soft-tipped cannula is applied to create separation. In young individuals the attachment may be so strong that suction pressures of 200–300 mmHg may be required.

We now prefer using a 130° angled short, flat pick called the 'hyaloid lifter' to lift the Weiss ring in a more controlled manner (Fig. 33.3c,d). Beginning at the outer margin of the optic nerve head and moving the pick just over the retinal surface outward in a radial direction, the Weiss ring can be engaged and lifted. A 'wave' of posterior hyaloidal separation can be seen to spread over the retinal surface centrifugally as the Weiss ring is elevated to the midvitreous cavity. This technique is particularly useful in patients under the age 50 years in whom aspiration may not easily achieve hyaloidal separation.

Posterior hyaloid separation is not confirmed until a Weiss ring is seen. One may also use a soft-tipped cannula to verify separation. It is important that no hyaloidal attachment remain in the area of the planned retinotomy.

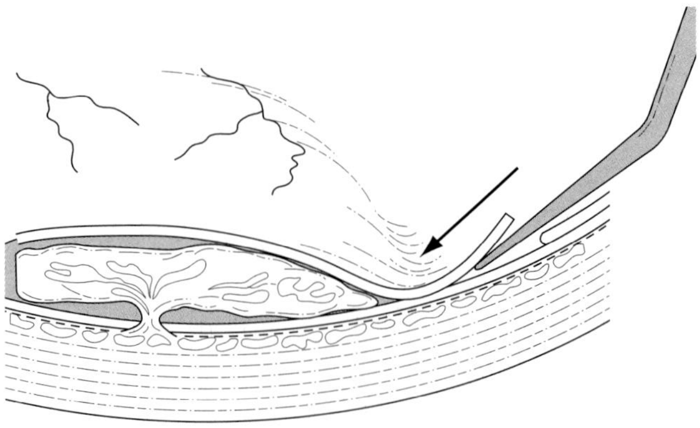

Figure 33.4 *The ideal retinotomy location is on the line between the point of contact with the choroidal neovascularization and the sclerotomy, as far from the foveal center as possible while allowing adequate access. It is away from visible macular vessels. The arrow indicates the vector force when making the retinotomy.*

PERIPHERAL VITRECTOMY

A complete peripheral vitrectomy is carried out. It is important to remove vitreous posterior to the dominant hand sclerotomy to minimize complications associated with bringing the angled pick, infusion cannula, forceps and scissors in and out of the eye.

RETINOTOMY: SELECTION, TECHNIQUE, COMPLICATIONS

A retinotomy that allows instrument access to the subfoveal space must, of necessity, be quite near the fovea. Minimizing the size of this hole, placing it as far from the fovea as possible and avoiding complications are important considerations in preserving paracentral visual function.

An ideal retinotomy is located on the line between the point of contact with the CNV and the sclerotomy (Fig. 33.4) and is as far from the foveal center as possible while allowing adequate access. Visible macular vessels are avoided.

The tip of the 36-gauge pick can be pushed through neurosensory retina to achieve a tiny retinotomy. As the pick is advanced obliquely through the retina, a small hemorrhage may occur as retinal capillaries are cut, but this bleeding always responds to increased intraocular pressure. The precise location of the retinotomy should be noted as the pick is withdrawn, so that the 33-gauge infusion needle subsequently can be introduced through the same hole.

Small choroidal hemorrhages can form if the pick pierces Bruch's membrane. Postoperatively, CNV has occurred at retinotomy sites where the RPE and Bruch's membrane have been scraped. Therefore, a slight lifting motion as the pick perforates the neurosensory retina avoids scraping underlying RPE and Bruch's membrane.

CREATION OF A NEUROSENSORY DETACHMENT

A 5-ml syringe filled with BSS is connected via silicone tubing to a 33-gauge angled infusion cannula. It is important to verify that no air bubbles are present in the tip or the line by ejecting fluid while lightly tapping the cannula held in an upright position before placing it in the eye.

As the surgeon holds the tip of the 33-gauge cannula in the mouth of the retinotomy, the surgical assistant applies minimal pressure on the syringe, slowly injecting fluid into the subretinal space. The surgeon carefully advances the cannula through the retinotomy. The angled tip allows the surgeon to direct the stream of fluid over the CNV (Fig. 33.5). Often hydrodissection can produce complete separation of the CNV from the overlying retina. This limited neurosensory detachment gives the surgeon working space between the CNV and the retina.

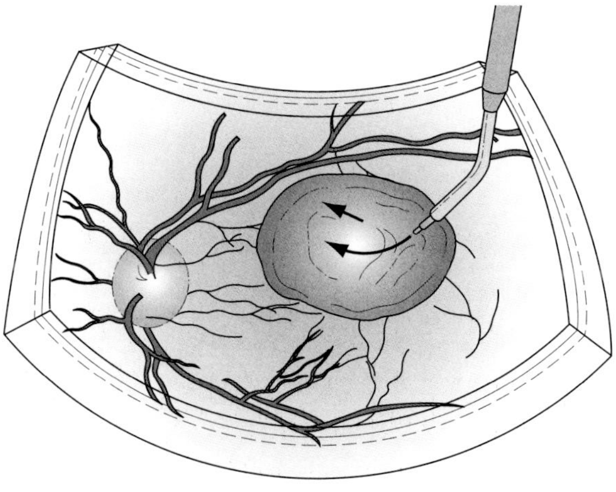

Figure 33.5 *Balanced salt solution is injected beneath the neurosensory retina with an angled blunt infusion cannula.*

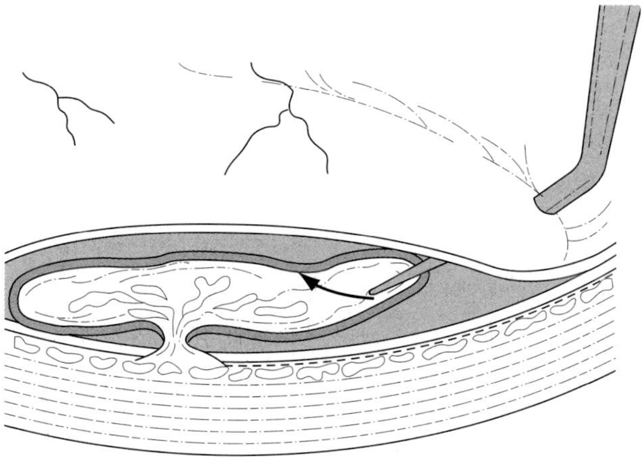

Figure 33.6 *After the pick has been passed over the retina to determine that no adhesions remain, the pick is used to elevate the edge of the membrane from the underlying retinal pigment epithelium.*

Care must be taken to avoid tearing the neurosensory retina with the infusion of fluid. A bolus infusion can blow a hole through the foveal center or tear the retina at points of adhesion (e.g. laser scars, fibrotic CNV). A large volume of fluid can create a retinal detachment.

MEMBRANE DISSECTION WITH PICK: SELECTION, TECHNIQUE, COMPLICATIONS

Membrane dissection begins with passing the pick over the entire surface of the CNV to verify that no anterior connections to the retina exist (Fig. 33.6). If pressure from the pick fails to break remaining adhesions, then the horizontal subretinal scissors are introduced through the retinotomy and tissue is cut close to the membrane's surface.

Once the CNV is free from overlying retina, an edge of the membrane must be separated from the underlying RPE. The tip of the pick is nudged along the leading edge of the CNV until a plane of cleavage is identified. A larger, thin white fibrin rim often will separate along with the smaller, thicker, pigmented CNV. Once the cleavage plane is found, gentle upward pressure is exerted as the pick is rotated beneath the surface of the membrane.

Parallax induced by the neurosensory fluid as well as turbidity of fluid will make depth perception difficult. Care is required to avoid pushing posteriorly into the RPE or choroid with the sharp tip of the pick. The intraocular pressure should be raised immediately at any evidence of hemorrhaging during these manipulations.

REMOVAL WITH FORCEPS: SELECTION, TECHNIQUE, COMPLICATIONS

Once an edge of the CNV has been elevated sufficiently to grasp with forceps and a good portion of the CNV has been mobilized, the horizontal subretinal forceps are introduced through the retinotomy in a closed position. The intraocular pressure is maximally elevated. The forceps are slowly opened to grasp the full-thickness membrane at its elevated edge or to grasp the ingrowth stalk beneath the CNV (Fig. 33.7a). Gentle, continuous traction toward the retinotomy is maintained as the surgeon watches for evidence of retinal tearing or RPE loss. If either occurs, traction should be stopped and additional pick manipulation carried out.

No bleeding should occur with the intraocular pressure elevated. As the CNV is disconnected, only a trace amount of hemorrhage collects in the subretinal space at the site of the severed stalk.

The disconnected membrane is pulled through the retinotomy, which stretches to accommodate (Fig. 33.7b). Similarly, the CNV will mold to fit through the retinotomy. Thus, very large membranes can fit through very small retinotomies.

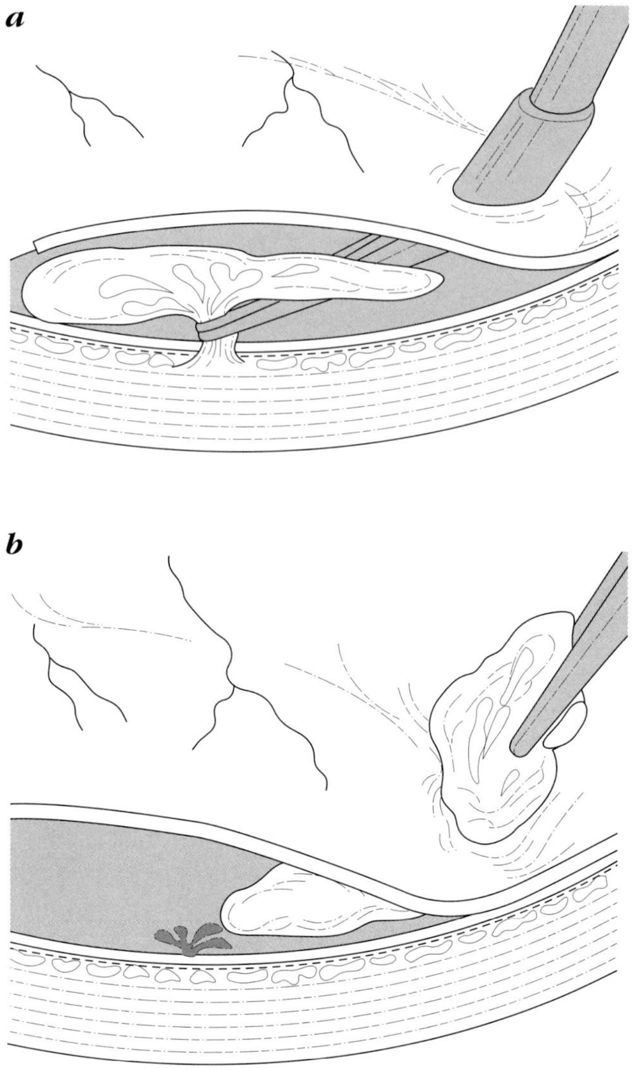

Figure 33.7 *(a) Subretinal forceps are used to grasp the ingrowth stalk from the choroid. (b) After the membrane has broken free, it can be extracted from the subretinal space through the small retinotomy.*

HEMOSTASIS

The membrane is simply held in the midvitreous cavity as the surgeon focuses attention on the macula for signs of bleeding. The intraocular pressure remains elevated for at least 1 minute, but is slowly lowered at intervals as the surgeon continues to look for bleeding. Should bleeding occur, the infusion pressure is maximally elevated and the process starts over. Several attempts may be required to lower the intraocular pressure before adequate hemostasis is achieved.

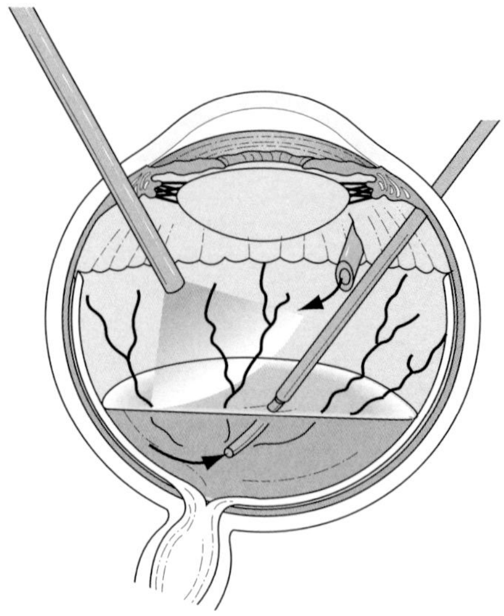

Figure 33.8 *A fluid–air exchange is performed by aspirating over the disc. No aspiration is performed in the retinotomy.*

The CNV is either removed from the eye through the pars plana or cut and aspirated with the vitrectomy instrument.

PERIPHERAL RETINAL EXAMINATION

Indirect ophthalmoscopy with scleral depression for 360° is performed to rule out peripheral retinal tears.

AIR–FLUID EXCHANGE

A complete air–fluid exchange is carried out using a silicone-tipped extrusion needle to aspirate over the optic nerve (Fig. 33.8). To avoid enlarging the retinotomy, aspiration is usually not done in or through the retinotomy itself. A 33-gauge cannula may be used to aspirate the fluid directly overlying the retinotomy, resulting in complete retinal reattachment.

PARTIAL AIR–FLUID EXCHANGE

In eyes with a small retinotomy, the vitreous cavity is refilled with fluid (Fig. 33.9) using a soft-tipped cannula connected with silicone tubing to a 5-ml syringe containing BSS, leaving only a 10–25% air-fill.

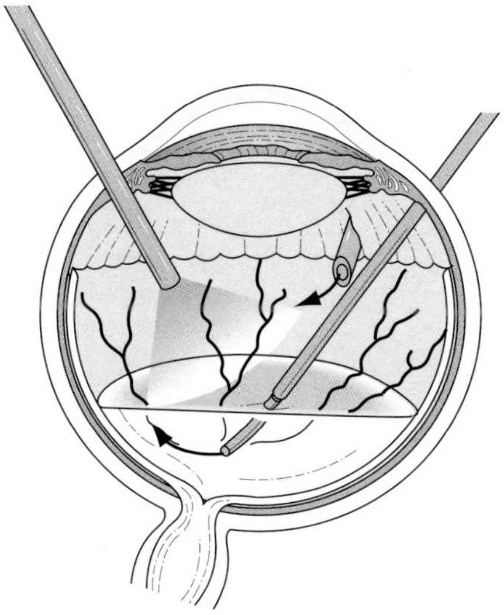

Figure 33.9 *The vitreous cavity is partially refilled with fluid leaving only a 10–25% air-fill.*

In eyes with a large, irregular retinotomy or in patients who will not be able to maintain prone positioning, a 100% air-fill is permissible. Nonexpansile, long-acting intraocular gas is rarely used.

POSTOPERATIVE CARE

FACEDOWN POSITIONING

Patients are asked to maintain a strict facedown position until they are examined 1 day postoperatively, allowing the small intraocular air bubble to close the macular retinotomy. The retinotomy generally seals overnight (it becomes invisible within 1 month). On the first postoperative day, if the retinotomy is closed (it still may be visible) and the air bubble is small (25% or less), then facedown positioning is discontinued. Postoperative medications and instructions are the same as for other macular surgery.

FOLLOW-UP

The recurrence rate approaches 50% for some types of subfoveal CNV. In one study of 117 eyes with ocular histoplasmosis, 57% of all recurrences occurred within 3 months after surgery and 86% within 6 months after surgery.[8] Therefore, the single most important aspect of postoperative care is vigilant surveillance for recurrent neovascularization.

We recommend that a baseline fluorescein angiogram be obtained at the 1-week postoperative visit. It is unlikely that it will show recurrence (the earliest time to recurrence is about 2 weeks). However, postsurgical angiograms are often difficult to interpret, and this one can be used for future comparison. Angiograms should be obtained every 2 weeks for the next 6 weeks, and then every month for the next 3 months. Recurrences are common, and prompt recognition allows laser treatment outside the fovea and a good visual outcome.[9]

INDICATIONS FOR REOPERATION

CNV can recur in the subfoveal location in up to 66% of eyes, as shown in one study.[8] There are no clear indications for reoperation. In that same study, of 51 eyes with recurrences, 17 eyes underwent repeat submacular surgery. Although several eyes did well, with better than 20/40 postoperative visual acuity, mean and median visual acuities were not as good as those in eyes that were observed or treated with laser in this nonrandomized, retrospective study. In general, only eyes that initially recovered good postoperative visual acuity before developing recurrence and eyes that have recurrent CNV with favorable prognostic features should be considered for repeat submacular surgery.

REFERENCES

1. Thomas MA, Kaplan HJ. Surgical removal of subfoveal neovascularization in the presumed ocular histoplasmosis syndrome, *Am J Ophthalmol* (1991) **111:**1–7.
2. Thomas MA, Dickinson JD, Melberg NS, et al. Visual results after surgical removal of subfoveal choroidal neovascular membranes, *Ophthalmology* (1994) **101:**1384–96.
3. Gass JD. Biomicroscopic and histopathologic considerations regarding the feasibility of surgical excision of subfoveal neovascular membranes, *Am J Ophthalmol* (1994) **118:**285–98.
4. Connor TB Jr, Wolf MD, Arrindell EL, Mieler WF. Surgical removal of an extrafoveal fibrotic choroidal neovascular membrane with foveal serous detachment in age-related macular degeneration, *Retina* (1994) **14:**125–9.

5. Atebara NH, Thomas MA, Holekamp NM, et al. Surgical removal of large non-AMD peripapillary choroidal neovascular membranes, *Ophthalmology* (1998) **105:**1598–605.
6. Joseph DJ, Thomas MA. Surgical treatment of juxtafoveal choroidal neovascularization, *Invest Ophthalmol Vis Sci* (1997) **38** (Suppl): S457 (abst).
7. Thomas MA. Vitrectomy surgery for choroidal neovascularization, Macula Society Rosenthal Lecture, Boca Raton, FL, 1995.
8. Melberg NS, Thomas MA, Dickinson JD, Valluri S. Managing recurrent neovascularization after subfoveal surgery in presumed ocular histoplasmosis syndrome, *Ophthalmology* (1996) **103:**1064–8.
9. Thomas MA, Ibanez HE. Instruments for submacular surgery, *Retina* (1994) **14:**84–7 [published erratum appears in *Retina* (1994) **14:**190].

Part VIII Surgical Techniques of Posterior Segment Tumors

Chapter 34 Fine-needle biopsy of intraocular tumors

Patrick E Ma and Mandi D Conway

INTRODUCTION

The techniques of intraocular biopsy have developed since the early 1970s.[1–4] Eye-wall resection,[5–8] chorioretinal biopsy[9–11] and fine-needle aspiration[12] have progressed, with the introduction of smaller instruments and the accumulation of surgical experience, to become safer and more widely used. Ophthalmic surgeons have the ability to examine intraocular pathology directly by clinical examination, unlike other disciplines of medicine. However, in patients with diagnostic dilemmas, biopsy techniques are important, especially when decisions on patient care and alternative therapy are needed.

Biopsy techniques must be minimally invasive to the delicate structures of the eye and have low complication rates to preserve vision. Modified eye-wall resections, particularly the techniques of lamellar sclerectomy described by Peyman[7] and Shields,[13] have been useful and curative in many ciliary body and choroidal melanoma cases. Fine-needle biopsy techniques allow diagnostic samples for pathologic assessment[14,15] but the techniques require skill and co-ordination between the surgeon and a trained cytopathologist in the preparation, handling and interpretation of the small specimens. Histopathologic tissue diagnosis may assist in clinical treatment decisions as adjuncts to external plaque radiotherapy, proton beam therapy and thermotherapy.[12]

Preoperative preparation and planning are important in patients requiring intraocular biopsy. Informed consent should state the goals of therapy, complications and risks, and should be discussed with the patient and the family. Discussions regarding anticipated pathologic results and how they affect treatment options can often be addressed with patients to avoid delays in intraoperative treatment decisions.

Prior to radiotherapy or resection, noninvasive techniques are used to image the lesion; such techniques include fluorescein and indocyanine green angiography, ultrasound, computed tomography or magnetic resonance imaging. Fine-needle aspiration may add to this diagnostic armamentarium and assist in therapeutic decision-making in some cases.

The most common biopsy is the vitreous tap employed in acute endophthalmitis (see Chapter 43). Solid tumor biopsies are more difficult to perform and require proper needle tip placement visualization and control to obtain the sample and prevent complications. Hemorrhages in the tumor and vitreous are the most common complications and usually do not require surgical intervention unless excessive. Fine-needle biopsy is especially useful in eyes with suspected metastatic carcinoma when there is no clear evidence of other metastatic disease or a primary source.

Good visualization of the tumor is important to the success of fine-needle aspiration. It is critical to avoid areas of retinal detachment into which hemorrhage may track, which inhibits visualization of the lesion and encourages proliferative vitreoretinopathy or iatrogenic rhegmatogenous retinal detachment. Tumors may be approached through the sclera directly overlying the tumor or transvitreally (Figs 34.1 and 34.2).[15]

Solid tumor fine-needle aspiration requires high suction and care must be taken to adjust the needle size, tubing and syringe size to optimize the desired suction and enhance suction control. Vitreous traction, which can produce a retinal detachment, must be avoided.

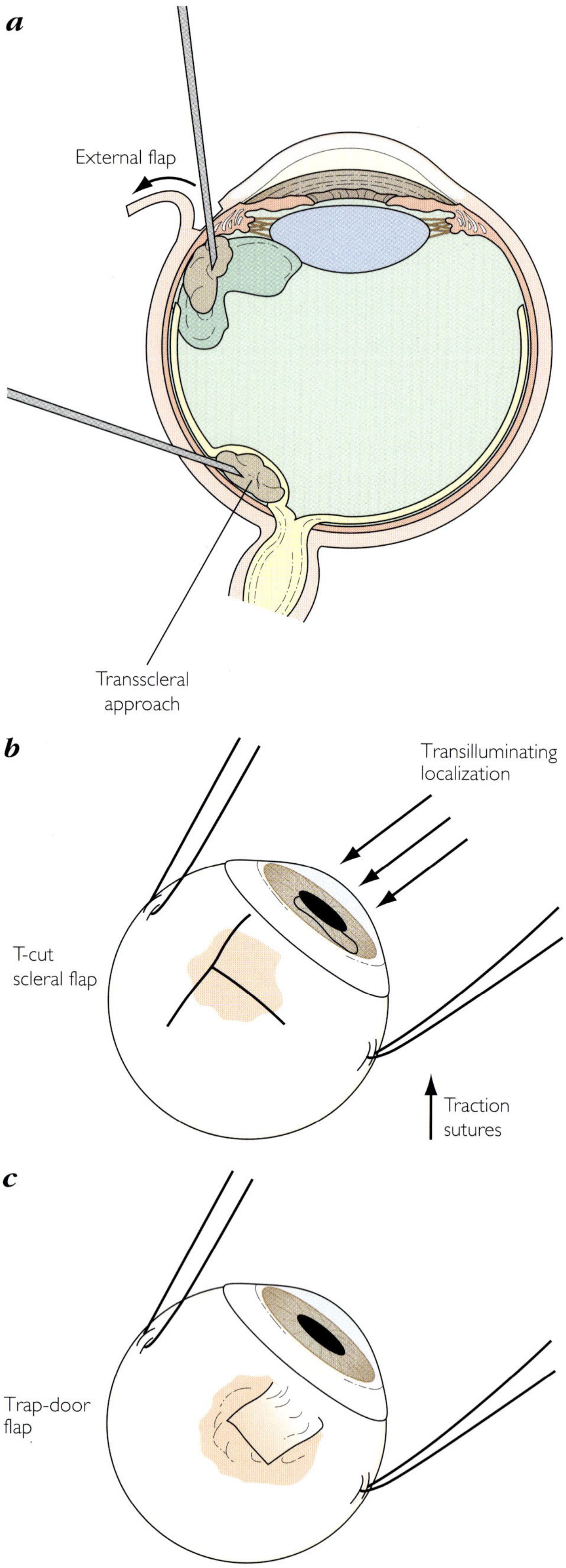

Figure 34.1 *Direct approach of fine-needle aspiration biopsy in the phakic eye. (a) An external scleral flap is made. The tumor is approached transsclerally. An operating microscope is used to localize the tumor. A partial-thickness flap in a (b) T-shaped fashion or (c) a trap-door fashion is created prior to the needle biopsy.*

EQUIPMENT

A 20- to 25-gauge one-inch to 1.5-inch needle is connected by extension tubing (with a luer-lock) to a 10-ml syringe. Suction is activated by the assistant or a mechanical device (Fig. 34.3).

TECHNIQUE

The placement of the biopsy needle and the approach to the tumor depend on the ease of visualization and the lens status of the eye. Limbal approaches for anterior lesions are done with viscoelastic maintenance of the anterior chamber and visualization through an operating microscope.

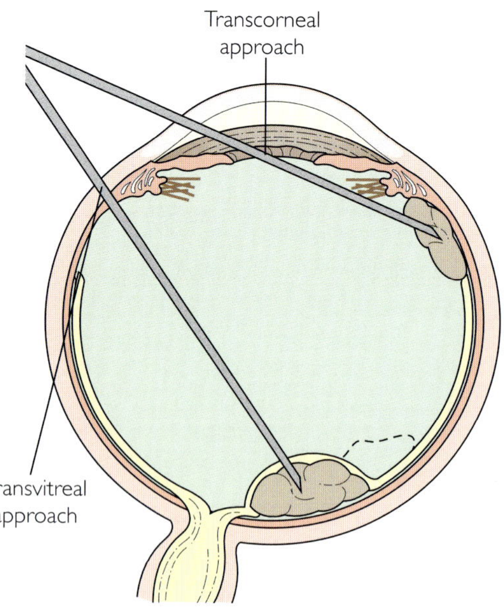

Figure 34.2 *The aphakic eye is entered either through the cornea or through the pars plana. Areas of retinal detachment must be avoided. The tumor is approached transvitreally.*

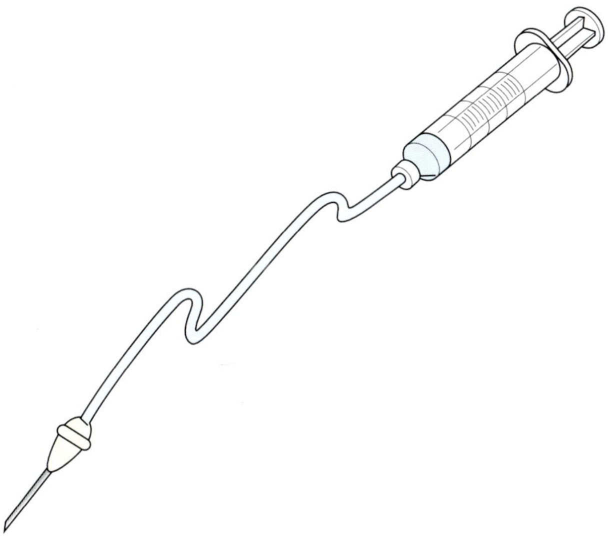

Figure 34.3 *A 20- to 25-gauge 1-inch to 1.5-inch needle is connected by extension tubing (with a luer-lock) to a 10-ml control syringe. Suction is activated by the assistant or a mechanical device.*

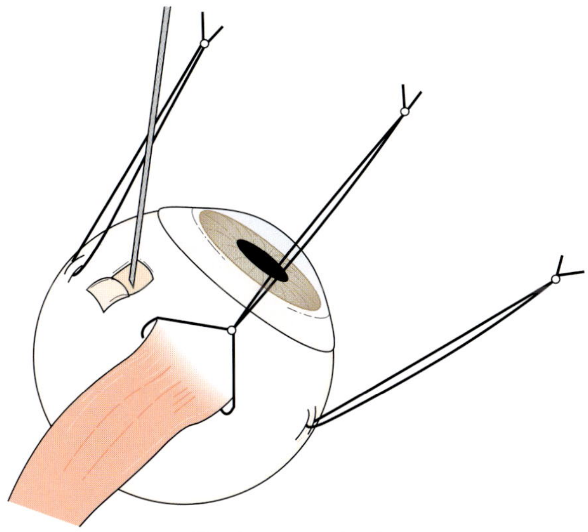

Figure 34.4 *Stabilization of the eye during fine-needle aspiration biopsy is achieved using traction sutures placed behind the recti muscles or sutured to the sclera.*

Stabilization of the globe during fine-needle aspiration (Fig. 34.4) can be achieved by a limited conjunctival opening at the desired quadrant, the use of traction sutures behind the recti muscles and the use of scleral sutures for traction.

A pars plana approach with a wide-angle viewing system attached to the microscope allows the surgeon to use bimanual instrumentation. Indirect ophthalmoscopy requires one hand to hold the condensing lens. Extension tubing permits safe aspiration of the tumor without needle movements. Stabilization of the eye by the surgeon, retraction sutures or an assistant are equally important.

When choroidal tumors are biopsied transvitreally, the retina must be penetrated. Retinal holes are often self-sealing when created in attached retina where there is no vitreous traction. If an overlying retinal detachment exists, these areas should be avoided for single fine-needle aspiration but may be accessible using vitrectomy techniques.

The needle is placed into the tumor, followed by an abrupt aspiration of tumor. The needle is then advanced further. The needle tip can be bent to avoid posterior scleral perforations but it needs a large sclerostomy entrance wound. The advancement–aspiration cycle is repeated two to three additional times before the needle is removed from the tumor. Suction is allowed to equilibrate before the needle is withdrawn, to prevent vitreous incarceration, tumor seeding and expulsion of the needle's contents before its removal from the eye. Tumor samples should be confined to the needle lumen only. The sample must be flushed from the needle with 1–2 ml of normal saline for prompt delivery to the pathologist. Alcohol- or air-dried fixation should not be attempted in the operating room. Cryopexy or laser photocoagulation can be placed around retinotomy sites to prevent retinal detachment. Complications such as retinal detachments can be treated with scleral buckling, vitrectomy or, less frequently, with pneumatic techniques.

MECHANICAL ASPIRATION

Mechanical aspiration can be performed using a 5–10-ml syringe with extension tubing. There is no need to see the fluid.

AUTOMATED ASPIRATION DEVICES (VITRECTOMY MACHINE)

Vitrectomy machines can generate 300–400 mmHg of vacuum. The surgeon must be watchful of continued aspiration to avoid unexpected retinal or vitreous incarceration.

COMPLICATIONS OF FINE-NEEDLE BIOPSY

Fine-needle biopsy can be complicated by retinal perforation, tear, retinal hemorrhage, rhegmatogenous retinal detachment, proliferative vitreoretinopathy, vitreous hemorrhage, tumor hemorrhage, subretinal hemorrhage tracking into macular area, tumor seeding into vitreous or scleral tunnel, choroidal hemorrhage and endophthalmitis.

REFERENCES

1. Peyman GA, Diamond JG, Axelrod AJ. Sclero-chorio-retinal (SCR) resection in humans, *Ann Ophthalmol* (1974) **6:**1347–52.
2. Peyman GA, Meisels HI, Batko KA, Vlchek JK. Full thickness eye wall biopsy: I. An experimental approach to the tissue diagnosis and study of choroidal and retinal lesions, *Invest Ophthalmol* (1975) **14:**484–7.
3. Peyman GA, Fishman GA, Sanders DR, Vlchek JK. Histopathology of Goldmann–Favre syndrome obtained by full-thickness eye-wall biopsy, *Ann Ophthalmol* (1977) **9:**479–84.
4. Peyman GA, Juarez CP, Raichand M. Full-thickness eye-wall biopsy: long-term results in 9 patients, *Br J Ophthalmol* (1981) **65:**723–6.
5. Peyman GA, Dodich NA. Full thickness eye wall resection: an experimental approach for treatment of choroidal melanoma. I. Dacron-graft, *Invest Ophthalmol* (1972) **11:**115–21.
6. Peyman GA, Apple DJ. Local excision of choroidal malignant melanoma: full thickness eye wall resection, *Arch Ophthalmol* (1974) **92:**216–18.
7. Peyman GA, Rednam KVR. Juarez CP. Improvement of eye wall resection technique, *Ophthalmic Surg* (1983) **14:**588–90.
8. Peyman GA, Juarez CP, Diamond JG, Raichand M. Ten years experience with eye wall resection for uveal malignant melanomas, *Ophthalmology* (1984) **91:**1720–5.
9. Peyman GA, Cohen SB. Ab interno resection of uveal melanoma, *Int Ophthalmol* (1986) **9:**29–36.
10. Peyman GA, Charles H. Internal eye wall resection in the management of uveal melanoma, *Can J Ophthalmol* (1988) **23:**219–23.
11. Lee KJ, Peyman GA, Raichand S. Internal eye wall resection for posterior uveal melanoma, *Jpn J Ophthalmol* (1993) **37:**287–92.
12. Shields JA, Shields CL, Ehya H, et al. Fine-needle aspiration biopsy of suspected intraocular tumors: the 1992 Urwick Lecture, *Ophthalmology* (1993) **100:**1677–84.
13. Shields JA, Shields CL, Shah P, Sivalingam V. Partial lamellar sclerouvectomy for ciliary body and choroidal tumors, *Ophthalmology* (1991) **98:**971–83.
14. Augsburger JJ, Shields JA. Fine needle aspiration biopsy of solid intraocular tumors: indications, instrumentation and techniques, *Ophthalmic Surg* (1984) **15:**34–40.
15. Char DH, Miller TR, Ljung BM, et al. Fine needle aspiration biopsy in uveal melanoma, *Acta Cytol* (1989) **33:**599–605.
16. Ma PE, Peyman GA. Uveal biopsy. In: Tasman W, Jaeger EA, eds, *Duane's Clinical Ophthalmology* (JB Lippincott: Philadelphia, 1993): 1–13.

Chapter 35 Chorioretinal biopsy

Kamal Kishore and Gholam A Peyman

INTRODUCTION

Ophthalmologists traditionally have relied on the ophthalmoscopic appearance of retinal lesions, combined with results of systemic evaluation and laboratory tests, to reach a diagnosis in patients with intraocular inflammatory disorders. In as many as 33% of patients with intraocular inflammation, a specific etiologic diagnosis cannot be established,[1] and many posterior uveitides may present without pathognomonic features.[2] Further confusion occurs because malignant processes confined to the eye may present with inflammation, and pathologic evaluation of the tissue may be necessary to attain the correct diagnosis. Inflammation caused by infectious agents may be clinically indistinguishable from that caused by noninfectious agents. In such cases, tissue diagnosis may be required to institute specific antimicrobial therapy and to limit the patient's exposure to potentially harmful therapy.

THE WORK-UP

A thorough systemic evaluation, including examination of spinal fluid, if indicated, may provide a diagnosis in many cases of ocular inflammation and should be considered before proceeding with more invasive procedures, such as chorioretinal biopsy.

Indications for chorioretinal biopsy are: the worsening of intraocular inflammation despite empiric therapy; and to exclude a diagnosis of malignancy or specific microbiologic etiology. Biopsy for inflammatory conditions should be performed only if it is believed that the findings will significantly alter the patient's therapy and should, in general, be considered only for macula-threatening lesions unresponsive to therapy.[3] Patients with bilateral inflammation of unknown etiology may be considered for biopsy in the eye with worse vision.

Diagnostic chorioretinal biopsy is justified only if the support of an experienced immunopathologist and the necessary laboratory capabilities, including immunohistochemistry, electron microscopy and tissue- and viral-culture techniques are available.[3] Preoperative consultation with an ocular pathologist (including previous therapy, medical history and suspected diagnoses) is valuable in planning appropriate processing of delicate specimens.

Proper handling of specimens is critical to obtain a diagnosis. The biopsy sample will be small and must be divided into several pieces for histopathologic, immunohistochemical, molecular biological studies and culture.

VITREOUS BIOPSY

Diagnostic vitrectomy can provide a sample for microbiologic and cytopathologic analysis without significant damage to the eye.[4] A vitreous tap may be performed by inserting a 23- or 25-gauge needle into the midvitreous cavity through the pars plana and removing 0.1–0.2 ml of vitreous fluid. This technique is primarily used for endophthalmitis (see Chapter 43). A battery-powered portable vitrector may be used to collect a vitreous sample in an outpatient setting.[5]

In vitreous biopsy cases, a larger vitreous sample may be required for culture, cytology, immunohistochemical staining and other investigations to evaluate the inflammatory condition. Therefore, the use of a vitrectomy instrument is usually preferred in these cases. A diagnostic vitrectomy may be performed through a self-sealing pars plana incision using a 23-gauge vitrector developed by Peyman[6] or a similar 25-gauge instrument developed by de Juan.[7]

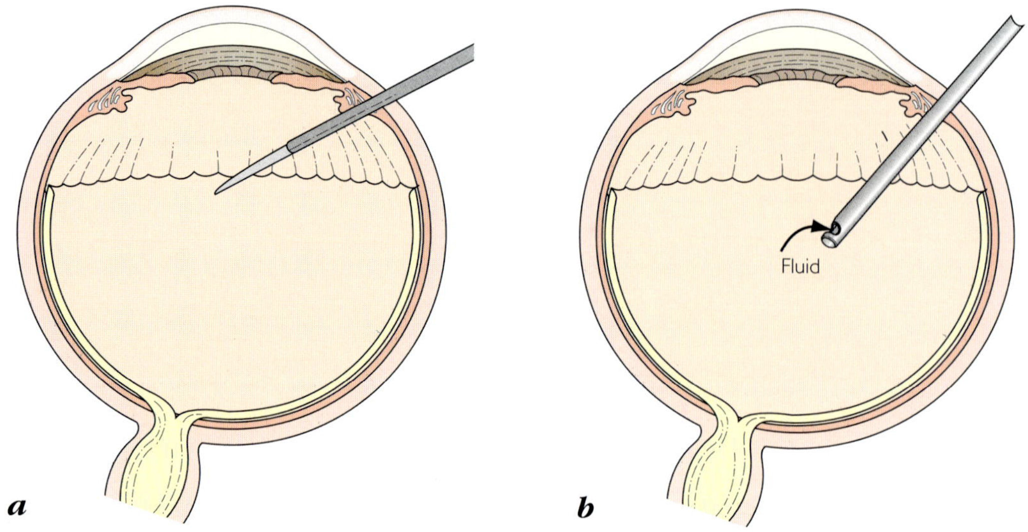

Figure 35.1 *(a) Penetration of sclera with Ziegler blade before vitreous tap. (b) Vitreous biopsy performed with microinstrumentation.*

To perform this technique, a small conjunctival incision is made over the pars plana. A Ziegler knife is used to create a sclerotomy for insertion of the miniaturized vitrector (Figs 35.1–35.3). Manual aspiration is performed into a syringe attached to the aspiration tube. Indirect ophthalmoscopy allows safe introduction of the needle and safe injection of air to maintain the intraocular pressure through a separate pars plana site with a 30-gauge needle, which avoids dilution of the vitreous sample. A 1–2-ml aliquot of vitreous may be removed safely and rapidly by this technique with minimal ocular trauma. Only one self-sealing incision

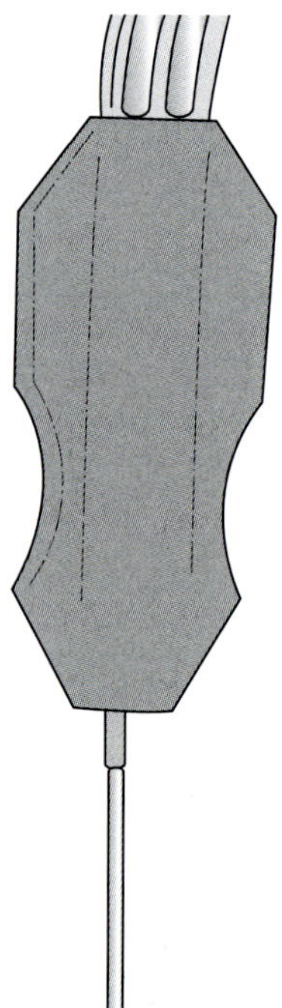

Figure 35.2 *The 23-gauge vitrectomy instrument.*

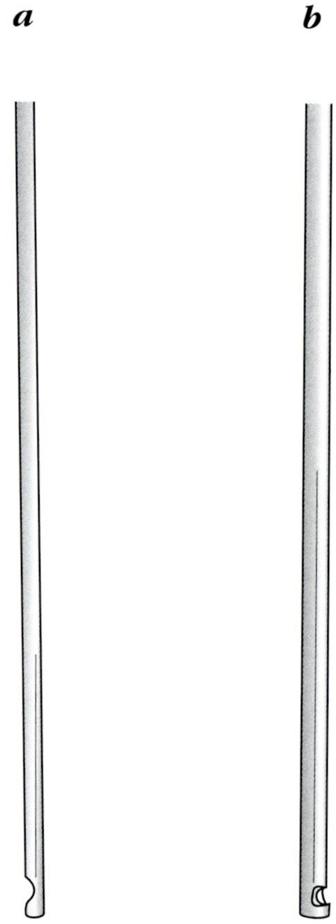

Figure 35.3 *The tip of the miniaturized instrument (a) and the tip of a standard 20-gauge instrument (b).*

is required and the procedure may be performed in an outpatient setting. Intraocular antibiotics and steroids may be injected as indicated.

Alternatively, a conventional three-port vitrectomy may be performed to obtain a vitreous biopsy. A three-way stopcock should be attached to the aspiration line between the handpiece and collection cassette. A syringe connected to the stopcock allows collection of undiluted vitreous fluid at the beginning of the vitrectomy. An air pump attached to the infusion line injects air, maintains the intraocular pressure and prevents dilution of the vitreous sample.[8] Some surgeons use a millipore filter to collect vitreous cells and bacteria. Material retained on the millipore filter may be cultured or stained for cytology.

Davis et al[9] performed immunocytochemical analysis of vitreous cells in 14 eyes with ocular inflammation. Immunocytochemical staining was used as an adjunct to routine cytology for more precise identification of inflammatory cells. An initial 10-ml specimen of diluted core vitreous was collected in a separate syringe while fluid was infused through an infusion cannula. Fluid accumulated in the vitrectomy cassette was also handled as a separate specimen. Both specimens were centrifuged at 1000 rpm for 8 minutes at 4°C. Cells were resuspended in tissue culture medium to an appropriate volume. Slides were made by one of two methods. Slides were prepared using the cytocentrifuge after resuspending cells in 4 ml of medium. The apparatus was primed with bovine serum albumin to reduce cell loss. Five to ten slides were made after cytocentrifugation. Alternatively, cells were resuspended in 1 ml of tissue culture medium and 50 µl drops were placed directly on gelatinized slides and allowed to air dry. No significant difference was noted with either method, although cytocentrifugation tended to give a more dispersed specimen.

Two slides from each method were stained by Gram, Giemsa or Diff Quick® stains for cytology. The remaining slides were fixed by submersing in acetone for 7 minutes; immunohistochemical staining was performed using the avidin–biotin immunoperoxidase technique. Monoclonal antibodies were used as indicated in Table 35.1.

Davis et al[9] found that intraocular infections demonstrated more numerous macrophages and neutrophils. Primary lymphomas showed restriction of staining for either kappa or lambda light chains, indicating monoclonal origin of malignant B lymphocytes, and inflammatory uveitis was characterized by the predominance of T lymphocytes. Thus, different patterns of immmunocytochemical staining were useful in differentiating these three broad categories of intraocular inflammation.

Table 35.1 Monoclonal antibodies for immunocytochemical staining of vitreous cellular infiltrates[9]

Lymphocyte markers	
CD3	Pan T cell
CD4	T-Helper/inducer subset
CD8	T-Suppressor/cytotoxic subset
CD19, 20, 22	B Cell
Macrophage markers	
CD11b, c: 64, 68	Macrophage/monocyte
Activation markers	
HLA-Dr	
CD25	IL-2 receptor
Lymphoma panel	
Giemsa and Diff Quick	Hematologic stain
CD3	Pan T cell
L26	B Cell
Kappa	Monoclonal and polyclonal light-chain constant region
Lambda	Monoclonal and polyclonal light-chain constant region

Primary intraocular lymphoma, previously known as reticulum cell sarcoma, is a subtype of non-Hodgkin's lymphoma predominantly affecting the eye and central nervous system. Approximately 85% of cases arise from B cells.[10] Patients are usually in the sixth to seventh decade of life at the time of presentation. The most common initial manifestation is a chronic posterior uveitis caused by vitreous infiltration by lymphoma and inflammatory cells. The majority of patients develop multiple subretinal pigment epithelium infiltrates, which typically enlarge to form sharply defined, large, yellowish-white subretinal pigment epithelial masses. The surface of these tumors shows a characteristic speckling of pigment, producing a leopard-skin pattern. One or both eyes may be affected at presentation, but involvement becomes bilateral in more than 80% of patients, often after a delay of months to years.[10–13]

Friedman found that approximately 20% of patients had central nervous system involvement at the time of presentation,[14] which eventually occurs in 80%.[14,15]

Central nervous system involvement is usually multicentric and is the most common cause of death in these patients. Lymphoma cells are present in the vitreous and subretinal pigment epithelial space and only secondarily involve the choroid. Other retinal manifestations include retinal vasculitis,[12] an acute retinal necrosis-like picture,[12,16] retinal vascular occlusion,[12,17] optic nerve infiltration,[17,18] anterior uveitis and neovascular glaucoma.[15,19] Vitreous biopsy may be necessary to establish the diagnosis and some patients may require more than one biopsy.[20–25]

Char et al[23] retrospectively reviewed immunologic and cytologic analysis on pars plana vitreous aspirates obtained with 20-gauge needles in nine patients with intraocular lymphoma. In three patients, cytologic details from a second sample obtained during vitrectomy from the aspiration reservoir were compared with the material obtained from needle aspiration. They found that cytologic evaluation was more accurate than immunologic marker studies and that morphologic details were better defined when cells were obtained from a needle aspirate rather than from the aspiration reservoir.

Intraocular non-Hodgkin's lymphoma may occur in patients with acquired immunodeficiency syndrome. Diagnosis may be complicated by the simultaneous presence of ocular infection and lymphoma. Sometimes biopsy of associated intracranial lesions or a spinal tap may provide a presumptive diagnosis of intraocular lymphoma in these patients. Vitreous biopsy or chorioretinal biopsy may be needed in other cases.[26,27]

Other applications of diagnostic vitreous biopsy include intraocular metastasis,[28–30] intraocular nematodes,[31,32] amyloidosis[33] and myiasis.[34]

CHORIORETINAL BIOPSY

In many cases of intraocular lymphoma, cells recovered from vitrectomy may be inflammatory in nature and may not accurately reflect the disease process.[35,36] Therefore, recovery of inflammatory cells alone from a vitreous biopsy specimen should not rule out lymphoma in suspected cases.[12,14,15,35,36] Of five patients with intraocular lymphoma reported by Ridley and associates,[12] only two had positive vitreous biopsy results. Two patients required a retinal biopsy for correct diagnosis. In some patients, the disease process may be confined to the outer retina and choroid.

Manifestations of various disease processes may be atypical in immunocompromised individuals. The correct diagnosis is required to institute appropriate therapy, to protect or treat the fellow eye and, in some cases, to treat a life-threatening systemic condition.[37,38] The following techniques may be used, as dictated by the location of the disease process.

EXTERNAL CHORIORETINAL BIOPSY

Peyman et al first described an experimental technique for chorioretinal biopsy in 1975[39,40] and subsequently reported their clinical experience in patients.[41,42] Six eyes had chorioretinal degenerations of unknown etiology, whereas the remaining three had ocular inflammation of unknown etiology. Other investigators subsequently reported their experience with chorioretinal biopsy.[3,37,43–49]

Surgical technique

Surgery can be performed under local or general anesthesia. A 360° limbal peritomy is performed and the four rectus muscles are isolated with 4-0 silk sutures. The Peyman eye basket is sutured to the sclera around the proposed site of biopsy (Fig. 35.4a, b). An 8-mm corneal trephine is used to incise approximately a half-thickness of the sclera (Fig. 35.4c). An infusion cannula is inserted but infusion is not commenced until the biopsy is completed. Two superior pars plana sclerotomies are created for the subsequent pars plana vitrectomy (Fig. 35.4d).

The partial-thickness scleral flap is dissected with a no. 64 beaver blade and left hinged so that it can be retracted from the surgical field (Fig. 35.4e). A 4-mm skin trephine is then used to mark the site of biopsy within the bed of the remaining half-thickness sclera (Fig. 35.4f). The biopsy site margins are treated with surface diathermy followed by penetrating diathermy. The 4-mm specimen is then excised with sharp scissors (Fig. 35.4g). A partial vitrectomy is performed through the biopsy site where the scleral button was removed (Fig. 35.4h). The hinged partial-thickness scleral flap is laid back in place and sutured with 9-0 nylon sutures (Fig. 35.4i). The ocular volume is reconstituted by commencing infusion through the preplaced infusion cannula (Fig. 35.4j). The pars plana vitrectomy is then performed through the preplaced sclerotomy sites (Fig. 35.4k) and endolaser is applied around the biopsy site.

Martin et al[3] used a modified approach for chorioretinal biopsy. After peritomy and isolation of

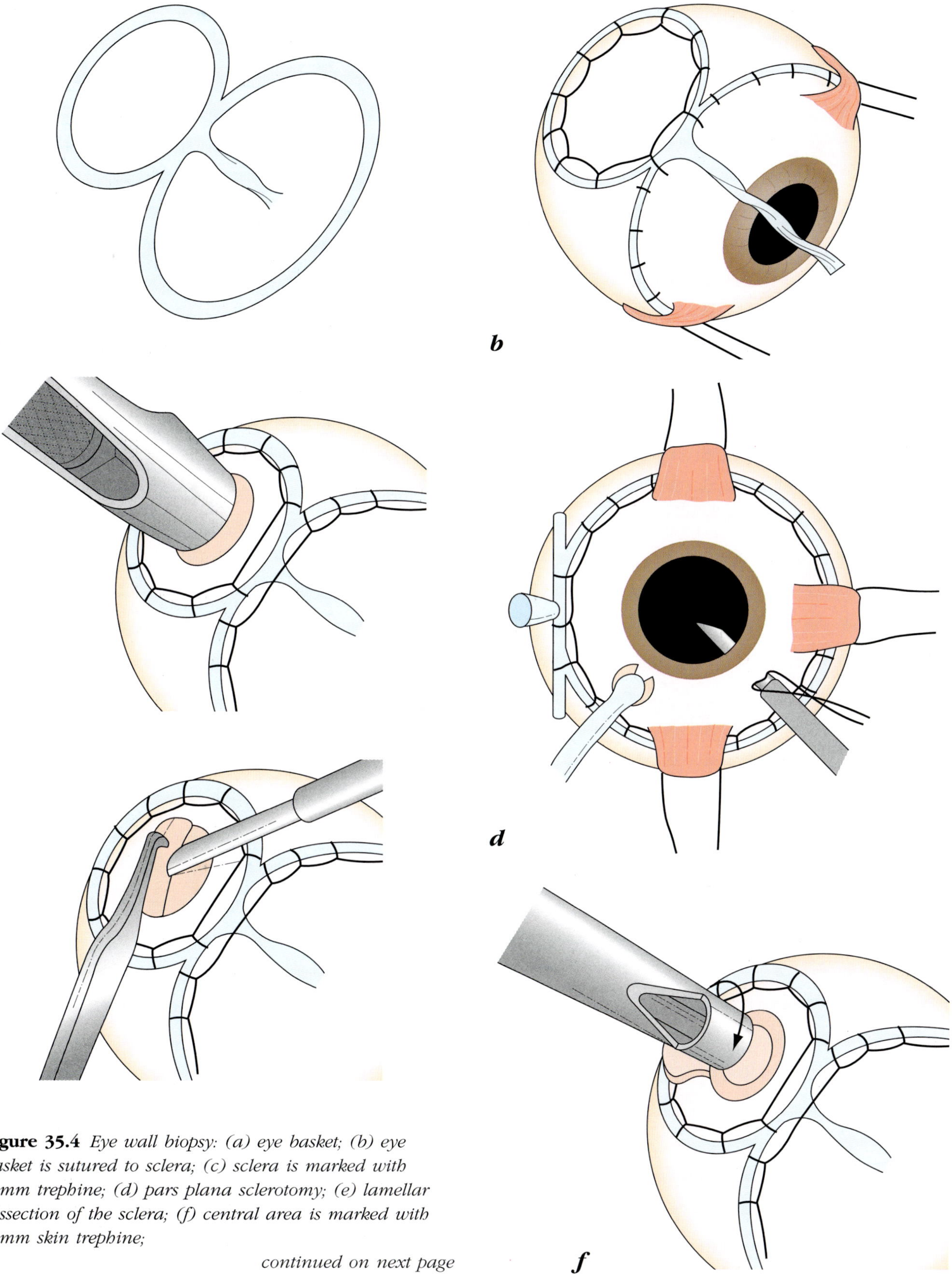

a

b

c

d

e

f

Figure 35.4 *Eye wall biopsy: (a) eye basket; (b) eye basket is sutured to sclera; (c) sclera is marked with 8-mm trephine; (d) pars plana sclerotomy; (e) lamellar dissection of the sclera; (f) central area is marked with 4-mm skin trephine;*

continued on next page

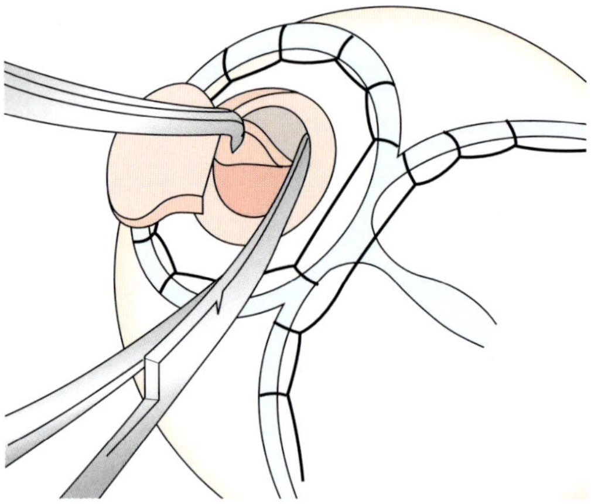

g

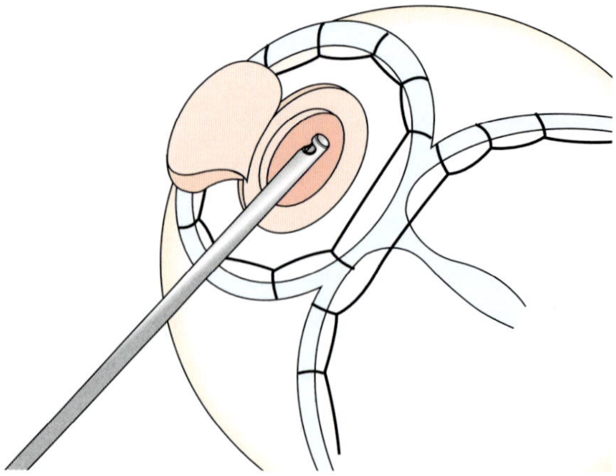

h

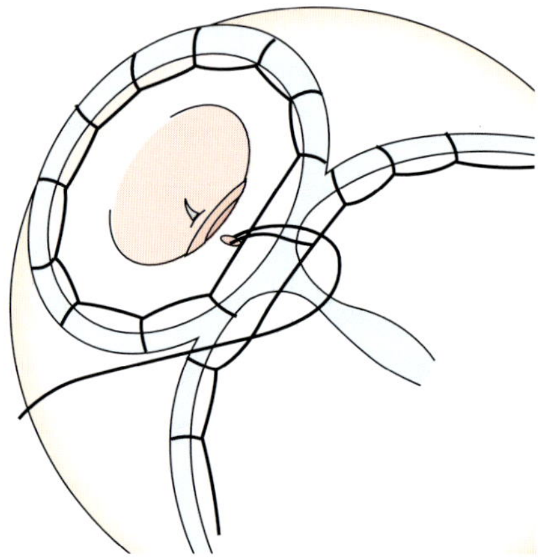

i

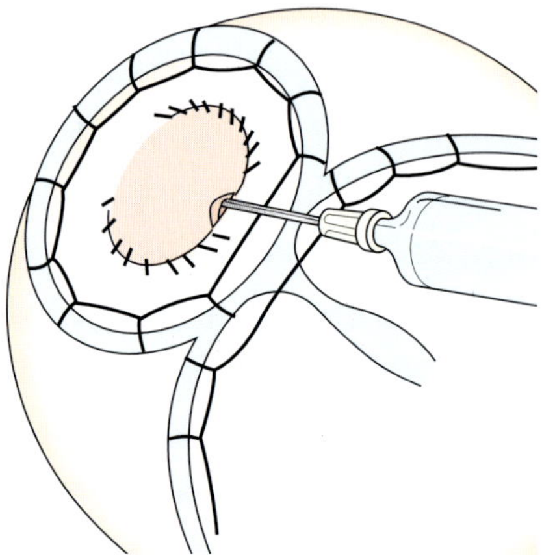

j

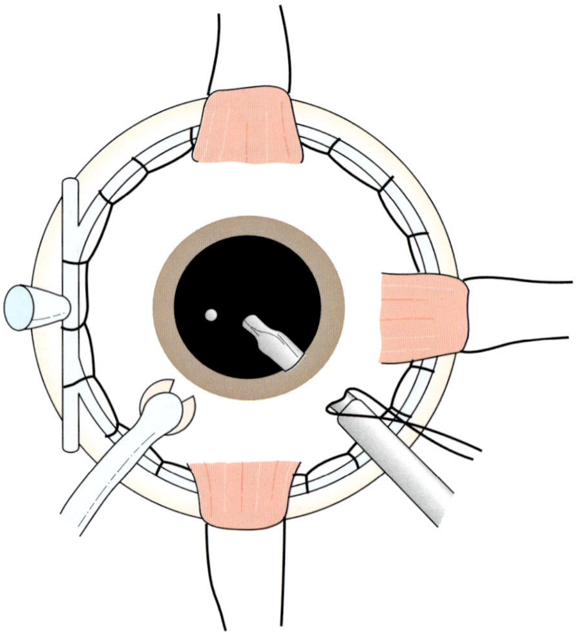

k

Figure 35.4 *Eye wall biopsy continued. (g) Surface and penetrating diathermy applied and sclera, choroid and retina excised; (h) limited vitrectomy performed; (i) sclera is closed; (j) air injected through scleral incision; (k) repeat pars plana vitrectomy and air–fluid exchange performed.*

muscles, a standard three-port pars plana vitrectomy was performed and the vitreous sample was submitted for culture and cytologic analysis. If the clarity of media allowed, preoperative laser photocoagulation was applied 1–3 days before surgery in a wide zone surrounding the biopsy site. Otherwise, endolaser treatment was applied during surgery. The biopsy site was marked on the sclera and markings for a 6-mm × 6-mm scleral flap were outlined, beginning 5–6 mm posterior to the limbus. The infusion line was left running as a nearly full-thickness scleral flap, hinged posteriorly, was dissected. The flap was retracted, exposing nearly bare choroid. Two rows of penetrating diathermy were placed through the choroid and retina along the margins of the wound. After the infusion line was turned off, a no. 75 blade was used to make two incisions parallel to the limbus (approximately 4 mm apart) through the choroid and retina. Vannas scissors were used for complete removal of the block by grasping one edge with 0.12-mm forceps to ensure that both choroid and retina were contained within the forceps. The biopsy specimen was given to the pathologist. Any presenting vitreous was removed from the wound with a vitreous cutter. The scleral flap was closed with interrupted 9-0 nylon sutures. A fluid–gas exchange was performed with either 20% sulfur hexafluoride or 15% perfluoropropane.

COMPLICATIONS AND RESULTS

Peyman et al[50] reported 12 years of experience with chorioretinal biopsy in 11 eyes. Minor intraoperative choroidal bleeding was controlled easily with diathermy. One patient developed early postoperative vitreous hemorrhage that cleared within 3 weeks. One patient developed a cataract and another developed a localized traction retinal detachment postoperatively.

In contrast, all seven patients described by Martin et al[3] developed a visually significant cataract in the postoperative period after an average time interval of 9 months. One patient developed peripheral retinal neovascularization that regressed following cryotherapy. One patient developed a retinal detachment from multiple breaks in the zone of previous retinitis; the biopsy site remained attached. One eye became phthisical. No vitreous hemorrhage or expulsive hemorrhage occurred and no exacerbation of ocular inflammation was observed. As a result of information gleaned from the biopsy, therapy was altered in five of seven patients.

Rutzen et al[37] reported on nine patients who underwent external chorioretinal biopsy using a technique similar to that of Martin.[3] Complications included one persistent retinal detachment, a recurrent retinal detachment and mild postoperative vitreous hemorrhage in two patients. Biopsy results led to a change of therapy in three of nine patients in their series.

ENDORETINAL BIOPSY AND CHORIORETINAL BIOPSY *AB INTERNO*

Endoretinal biopsy is performed when the primary disease process is located within the retina. It is performed in conjunction with a pars plana vitrectomy, and posterior segment scissors are used to obtain a retinal specimen.

Freeman et al[51] performed endoretinal biopsies on 13 eyes with infectious or inflammatory retinitis associated with retinal detachment. After pars plana vitrectomy, diathermy was applied contiguously along the posterior border of the intended biopsy site. A retinotomy site was created with the blade of the vertical scissors. If necessary, gentle irrigation of fluid through the retinotomy site was performed to ensure adequate separation between the retina and choroid to prevent inadvertent damage to the choroid. The specimen then was excised with vertical scissors by initially making a 3–6-mm long cut along the posterior border. The incision was extended anteriorly for 2–4 mm. A rectangular piece was excised, leaving a small area attached to the remainder of the retina to prevent it from slipping into the subretinal space. The specimen then was grasped with intraocular forceps and pulled toward the sclerotomy site to break its attachment to the retina. After the forceps were withdrawn, the intraocular pressure was elevated to float the tissue specimen into the sclerotomy, where it was gently grasped with fine-tissue forceps and withdrawn. An air–fluid exchange was performed using the biopsy site for internal drainage. Silicone oil was injected in nine eyes, sulfur hexafluoride in two eyes and perfluoropropane in two eyes. Macular reattachment was obtained in all eyes. Three eyes demonstrated acute retinal necrosis, nine had cytomegalovirus retinitis and one had immune complex retinal vasculitis. Two eyes developed retinal detachment resulting from proliferative vitreoretinopathy; one retina was successfully reattached using silicone oil.

Peyman performed internal retinal biopsy in 14 eyes.[52] A three-port pars plana vitrectomy was performed. Repair of any retinal detachment preceded retinal biopsy. Encircling endodiathermy was applied around the area to be biopsied (Fig. 35.5a). A square piece of retina was incised with vitreous scissors and removed with intraocular forceps. Endolaser treatment was applied around and inside the biopsied area (Fig. 35.5b,c). No significant complications were noted. A similar technique may be used to perform retinochoroidal biopsy.[53] Hypotensive anesthesia to maintain the systolic pressure around 100 mmHg may be employed to reduce bleeding, but care should be taken to avoid prolonged hypotension in elderly patients and those with cardiovascular diseases.

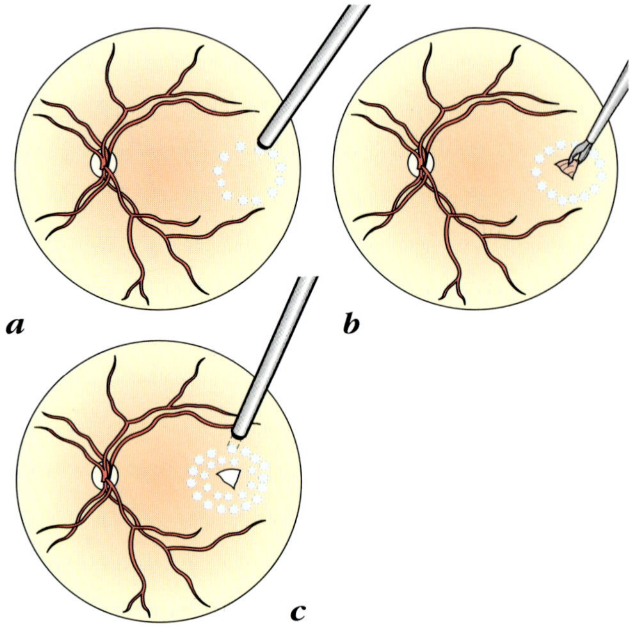

Figure 35.5 *Retinal biopsy. The retina is attached or surgically reattached before biopsy. (a) After complete vitrectomy, two rows of diathermy or laser coagulation are applied around a 1.5-disc diameter area of retina. (b) Specimen is cut, separated completely from its attachment and removed with forceps. (c) Endolaser coagulation applied to bed and border of biopsy site.*

Rutzen et al[37] reported their experience with 24 endoretinal biopsies using a technique described by Freeman et al.[51] Retinal biopsy specimens were 1–4 mm^2 in area and an attempt was made to perform biopsy in the area of transition between normal and affected retina. The biopsy was obtained successfully in all eyes. However, it led to a change in therapy in only one patient. Complications included persistent retinal detachment in two eyes, recurrent retinal detachment in three eyes, postoperative glaucoma in one eye and development of cataract in two eyes.

This chapter provides indications, techniques and complications of the various modalities that may be employed to obtain a biopsy specimen from the eye. Vitreous biopsy is the least invasive of these techniques and may be sufficient to provide a diagnosis in many cases. Multiple vitreous biopsies may be needed in some cases and special staining techniques in consultation with a pathologist may improve diagnostic yield. External chorioretinal biopsy is useful for lesions anterior to the equator, whereas posterior lesions are better approached by internal techniques. An attempt should be made to obtain the biopsy at the junction of involved healthy tissue. An exhaustive systemic evaluation should precede chorioretinal biopsy and a prior consultation with a pathologist is needed for appropriate processing of the delicate specimen.

REFERENCES

1. Henderly DE, Genstler AJ, Smith RE, Rao NA. Changing patterns of uveitis, *Am J Ophthalmol* (1987) **103**:131–6.
2. Freeman WR, Stern WH, Gross JG, et al. Pathologic observation made by retinal biopsy, *Retina* (1990) **10**:195–204.
3. Martin DF, Chan CC, de Smet M, et al. The role of chorioretinal biopsy in the management of posterior uveitis, *Ophthalmology* (1993) **100**:705–14.
4. Carroll DM, Franklin RM. Vitreous biopsy in uveitis of unknown cause, *Retina* (1981) **1**:245–51.
5. Josephberg RG. *Vitreous Society Meeting*, New Orleans, LA, 1997.
6. Peyman GA. A miniaturized vitrectomy system for vitreous and retinal biopsy, *Can J Ophthalmol* (1990) **25**:285–6.
7. De Juan E Jr, Hickingbotham D. Refinements in microinstrumentation for vitreous surgery, *Am J Ophthalmol* (1990) **109**:218–20.
8. Tamai M, Nakazawa M. A collection system to obtain vitreous humor in clinical cases (letter), *Arch Ophthalmol* (1991) **109**:465–66.
9. Davis JL, Solomon D, Nussenblatt RB, et al. Immunocytochemical staining of vitreous cells: indications, techniques, and results, *Ophthalmology* (1992) **99**:250–6.
10. Freeman LN, Schachat AP, Knox DL, et al. Clinical features, laboratory investigations, and survival in ocular reticulum cell sarcoma, *Ophthalmology* (1987) **94**:1631–9.
11. Char DH, Ljung BM, Miller T, Phillips T. Primary intraocular lymphoma (ocular reticulum cell sarcoma): diagnosis and management, *Ophthalmology* (1988) **95**:625–30.
12. Ridley ME, McDonald HR, Sternberg P Jr, et al Retinal manifestations of ocular lymphoma (reticulum cell sarcoma), *Ophthalmology* (1992) **99**:1153–61.
13. Gass JDM, Sever RJ, Grizzard WS, et al. Multifocal pigment epithelial detachments by reticulum cell sarcoma: a characteristic funduscopic picture, *Retina* (1984) **4**:135–43.
14. Friedman AH. Uveitis affecting the retina and posterior segment. In: Freeman WR, ed, *Practical Atlas of Retinal Diseases and Theory* (Raven Press: New York, 1993): 37–70.
15. Siegel MJ, Dalton J, Friedman AH, et al. Ten-year experience with primary ocular 'reticulum cell sarcoma' (large cell non-Hodgkin's lymphoma), *Br J Ophthalmol* (1989) **73**:342–6.
16. Gass JDM, Trattler HL. Retinal artery obstruction and atheromas associated with non-Hodgkin's large cell lymphoma (reticulum cell sarcoma), *Arch Ophthalmol* (1991) **109**:1134–9.
17. Guyer DR, Green WR, Schachat AP, et al. Bilateral ischemic optic neuropathy and retinal vascular occlusions associated with lymphoma and sepsis: clinicopathologic correlation, *Ophthalmology* (1990) **97**:882–8.

18. Kattah JC, Suski ET, Killen JY, et al. Optic neuritis and systemic lymphoma, *Am J Ophthalmol* (1980) **89**:431–6.
19. Goldey SH, Stern GA, Oblon DJ, et al. Immunophenotypic characterization of an unusual T-cell lymphoma presenting as anterior uveitis: a clinicopathologic case report, *Arch Ophthalmol* (1989) **107**:1349–53.
20. Michels RG, Knox DL, Erozan YS, Green WR. Intraocular reticulum cell sarcoma: diagnosis by pars plana vitrectomy, *Arch Ophthalmol* (1975) **93**:1331–5.
21. Minckler DS, Font RL, Zimmerman LE. Uveitis and reticulum cell sarcoma of brain with bilateral neoplastic seeding of vitreous without retinal or uveal involvement, *Am J Ophthalmol* (1975) **80**:433–9.
22. Parver LM, Font RL. Malignant lymphoma of the retina and brain: initial diagnosis by cytologic examination of vitreous aspirate, *Arch Ophthalmol* (1979) **97**:1505–7.
23. Char DH, Ljung BM, Deschenes J, Miller TR. Intraocular lymphoma: immunological and cytological analysis, *Br J Ophthalmol* (1988) **72**:905–11.
24. Wilson DJ, Braziel R, Rosenbaum JT. Intraocular lymphoma: immunopathologic analysis of vitreous biopsy specimens, *Arch Ophthalmol* (1992) **110**:1455–8.
25. Whitcup SM, de Smet MD, Rubin BI, et al. Intraocular lymphoma: clinical and histopathologic diagnosis, *Ophthalmology* (1993) **100**:1399–406.
26. Stanton CA, Sloan DB III, Slusher MM, Greven CM. Acquired immunodeficiency syndrome-related primary intraocular lymphoma, *Arch Ophthalmol* (1992) **110**:1614–17.
27. Kumar SR, Gill PS, Wagner DG, et al. Human T-lymphotropic virus type I-associated retinal lymphoma: a clinicopathologic report, *Arch Ophthalmol* (1994) **112**:954–9.
28. Piro P, Pappas HR, Erozan YS, et al. Diagnostic vitrectomy in metastatic breast carcinoma in the vitreous, *Retina* (1982) **2**:182–8.
29. Young SE, Cruciger M, Lukeman J. Metastatic carcinoma to the retina: case report, *Ophthalmology* (1979) **86**:1350–4.
30. Swartz M, Schumann GB. Acute leukemic infiltration of the vitreous diagnosed by pars plana aspiration, *Am J Ophthalmol* (1980) **90**:326–30.
31. Messner KH, Kammerer WS. Intraocular cysticercosis, *Arch Ophthalmol* (1979) **97**:1103–5.
32. Bathrick ME, Mango CA, Mueller JF. Intraocular gnathostomiasis, *Ophthalmology* (1981) **88**:1293–5.
33. Doft BH, Machemer R, Skinner M, et al. Pars plana vitrectomy for vitreous amyloidosis, *Ophthalmology* (1987) **94**:607–11.
34. Custis PH, Pakalnis VA, Klintworth GK, et al. Posterior internal ophthalmomyiasis: identification of a surgically removed Cuterebra larva by scanning electron microscopy, *Ophthalmology* (1983) **90**:1583–90.
35. Lopez JS, Chan CC, Burnier M, et al. Immunohistochemistry findings in primary intraocular lymphoma (letter), *Am J Ophthalmol* (1991) **112**:472–4.
36. Kennerdell JS, Johnson BL, Wisotzkey HM. Vitreous cellular reaction: association with reticulum cell sarcoma of brain, *Arch Ophthalmol* (1975) **93**:1341–5.
37. Rutzen AR, Ortega-Larrocea G, Dugel PU, et al. Clinicopathologic study of retinal and choroidal biopsies in intraocular inflammation, *Am J Ophthalmol* (1995) **119**:597–611.
38. Morinelli EN, Dugel PU, Riffenburgh R, Rao NA. Infectious multifocal choroiditis in patients with acquired immune deficiency syndrome, *Ophthalmology* (1993) **100**:1014–21.
39. Peyman GA, Meisels HI, Batko KA, Vlchek JK. Full thickness eye wall biopsy. I. An experimental approach to the tissue diagnosis and study of choroidal and retinal lesions, *Invest Ophthalmol* (1975) **14**:484–7.
40. Peyman GA, Homer P, Kasbeer R, Vlchek J. Full thickness eye wall biopsy: II. In primates, *Invest Ophthalmol* (1975) **14**:565–7.
41. Peyman GA, Fishman GA, Sanders DR, et al. Biopsy of human scleral–chorioretinal tissue, *Invest Ophthalmol* (1975) **14**:707–10.
42. Peyman GA, Juarez CP, Raichand M. Full-thickness eye-wall biopsy: long-term results in 9 patients, *Br J Ophthalmol* (1981) **65**:723–6.
43. Constable IJ, Slatter DH, Horne R. Chorioretinal biopsy in dogs, *Invest Ophthalmol Vis Sci* (1980) **19**:603–9.
44. Constable IJ, Chester GH, Horne R, Harriott JF. Human chorioretinal biopsy under controlled systemic hypotensive anesthesia, *Br J Ophthalmol* (1980) **64**:559–64.
45. Taylor D, Day S, Tiedemann K, et al. Chorioretinal biopsy in a patient with leukemia, *Br J Ophthalmol* (1981) **65**:489–93.
46. Grutzmacher RD, Henderson D, McDonald PJ, Coster DJ. Herpes simplex chorioretinitis in a healthy adult, *Am J Ophthalmol* (1983) **96**:788–96.
47. Constable IJ, Thompson D, van Bockxmeer F. The value of rational biopsy: tissue culture of chorioretinal biopsies, *Trans Ophthalmol Soc UK* (1983) **103**:475–9.
48. Palestine AG, Nussenblatt RB, Chan CC, et al. Histopathology of the subretinal fibrosis and uveitis syndrome, *Ophthalmology* (1985) **92**:838–44.
49. Chan CC, Palestine AG, Davis JL, et al. Role of chorioretinal biopsy in inflammatory eye disease, *Ophthalmology* (1991) **98**:1281–6.
50. Peyman GA, Schulman J, Raichand M. Diagnosis and therapeutic surgery of the uvea: Part II. Results, *Ophthalmic Surg* (1987) **18**:310–16.
51. Freeman WR, Wiley CA, Gross JG, et al. Endoretinal biopsy in immunosuppressed and healthy patients with retinitis: indications, utility, and techniques, *Ophthalmology* (1989) **96**:1559–65.
52. Peyman GA. Internal retinal biopsy: surgical technique and results, *Int Ophthalmol* (1990) **14**:101–4.
53. Peyman GA, Barrada A. Retinochoroidectomy ab interno, *Ophthalmic Surg* (1984) **15**:749–51.

Chapter 36 Tumor resection

Gholam A Peyman, Abdulrahman A Alghadyan and John Fenton

INTRODUCTION

Intraocular tumors can be either primary or metastatic. The primary tumors may originate from cells normally present in the eye, such as mesodermal and neuroectodermal cells. The most common metastatic tumor to the eye is breast cancer in females and lung cancer in males.[1] Malignant melanoma is the most common primary tumor in adults whereas retinoblastoma is the most common primary tumor in children.[2] Numerous therapeutic modalities used to treat intraocular tumors aim to save the patient's life (enucleation and exenteration) and vision (cryotherapy, laser, thermotherapy, radiation and local resection). In this chapter, we review the general concept of diagnosis and management of intraocular tumors, with special emphasis on surgical options and techniques used to treat these lesions.

DIAGNOSIS

The work-up of patients with intraocular tumors includes:

- A complete history of ocular and systemic diseases, family predisposition to certain disease processes, pain, flashes of light, floaters and changes in vision.
- A complete physical examination.
- An ocular examination, including visual acuity, visual field, intraocular pressure and pupillary reactions; other findings include the presence of strabismus, ocular inflammation, scleritis, pseudorheumatoid nodules, hyphema, vitreous hemorrhage and proptosis.[3–8]
- A computed tomography (CT) scan and magnetic resonance imaging (MRI) to determine the size, shape and possible extrascleral and optic nerve extension of the lesion.
- A- and B-Scan ultrasounds, to determine the shape, size and thickness of the tumor; the A-scan in malignant melanoma shows high initial spike and low-to-medium internal reflectivity; hemangioma shows high internal reflectivity and possible pulsation of the lesion; cysts demonstrate empty space inside the lesion.
- HLA typing, because there is an association between HLA-B40 and death as a result of metastasis from uveal melanoma.[9]
- Fundus photographs for documentation and follow-up.
- A fluorescein angiogram in malignant melanoma shows multiple pinpoint hyperfluorescences in the early venous phase, enlarging as the study progresses; a double circulation may be seen if Bruch's membrane is penetrated by the tumor; hemangiomas show initial hyperfluorescence whereas metastatic lesions show late hyperfluorescence.
- Retinal and/or choroidal biopsy[10–13] may be done using transvitreal needle aspiration of the intraocular tumors; incisional biopsy also may be performed.

To rule out metastatic disease, the following tests are performed: complete blood count, liver function tests, urinalysis and stool analysis for occult blood, chest X-ray and bone scan.

MANAGEMENT

The management of intraocular tumors depends on size and extent of the tumor, the patient's general condition, the presence or absence of metastases and the status of the other eye.[14,15] Enucleation is still performed for eyes with large intraocular tumors that cannot be treated by other means.[16] Enucleation was thought by some investigators to increase the chance of metastasis[17–21] but this theory was challenged by others.[22] For large intraocular tumors with extensive orbital extension, exenteration and/or radiation may be the therapy of choice. Radiotherapy is discussed in Chapter 37.

Radiation is not without complications,[23–33] therefore the search for a safer modality of therapy continues. Photocoagulation[34–39] was found to be effective in the management of small intraocular tumors of 3 mm or less in thickness[40,41] or as an adjunct to a surgical procedure.[40,42,43] Both irradiation[44,45] and photosensitizers[46] enhance the action of laser photocoagulation. Recurrence after photocoagulation has been reported.[47] Hyperthermia,[43,48,49] which can be induced either by microwave, transpupillary thermotherapy or ultrasound, may destroy the tumor and act synergistically with radiation.

Chemotherapy[15,50–53] is used in the treatment of advanced cases of intraocular tumors with metastasis. Immunotherapy plays a role in cancer therapy.[44,45,54] Retinal ganglion neurotrophic factor–monoclonal antibody (RGNTF–McAb)[44,54] and lymphokine-activated killing (LAK) cells[45] have been shown to be effective in the treatment of retinoblastoma whereas interleukin-2 might be effective in the treatment of malignant melanoma.[55]

RESECTION

Resection of iris and ciliary body tumors was performed with encouraging results.[56,57] The techniques have been refined with time.[58–64] The experimental and clinical work of Peyman and associates made local resection of posterior tumor an acceptable technique.[65–83] Resection of intraocular tumor was performed in humans at a limited number of centers in the world with encouraging results for both anterior and posterior segment tumors.[73,80–86]

Several factors, including the size of the tumor, play an important role in the outcome of surgery. The smaller the tumor, the better is the result of surgery. The eye can tolerate resection of tumors with a diameter of less than 15 mm. Peyman and coworkers studied full-thickness eye-wall resection extensively in animals (rabbits and primates) and found that the animal eyes could tolerate resection of less than 15 × 7 mm.[69–72] The clinical data from Peyman and associates,[65,74] Foulds and Damato, and Shields et al[84,86,92,93] and others support these findings. These techniques may provide an alternative to enucleation of eyes harboring tumors.

The following factors may influence the outcome of surgery:

- The absence of retinal detachment is predictive of a better prognosis; if a detachment is present, the lesser the extent of the detachment, the better the prognosis.[87]
- Tumors involving the optic disc and extending to the sclera carry poor prognoses.[88]
- Tumors located close to the fovea have a poor visual prognosis.[87]
- The clarity of the media.
- The absence of metastatic disease.
- The ability of the patient to tolerate moderate hypotensive (systolic blood pressure 90–110 mmHg) general anesthesia.

TECHNIQUES: ANTERIOR SEGMENT TUMORS

EXTERNAL APPROACH

Iridectomy involves removing the tumor with adequate surrounding normal iris tissue by way of a limbal incision and resuturing the iris, if possible, to create a round pupil.[59,60,89] Iridocyclectomy[58,60,62,85] involves removing the tumor with adequate normal surrounding iris and ciliary body, described first by Zirm in 1911.[58] He used a T-shaped scleral and limbal incision. Friede[61] removed the ciliary body tumor using a limbal incision with parallel radial scleral cuts. Flieringa[62] used a partial-thickness scleral incision around the tumor and a scleral flap hinged to the limbus. The anterior chamber was entered. The limbal incision was extended to both sides of the flap. The scleral flap and the cornea were reflected to expose the tumor. Incision was made at the pupil in both sides of the tumor and carried out through the ciliary body and anterior choroid. Müller[63] removed the tumor using a limbal incision and double scleral cuts, forming a double door in the sclera and the limbus. He suggested that

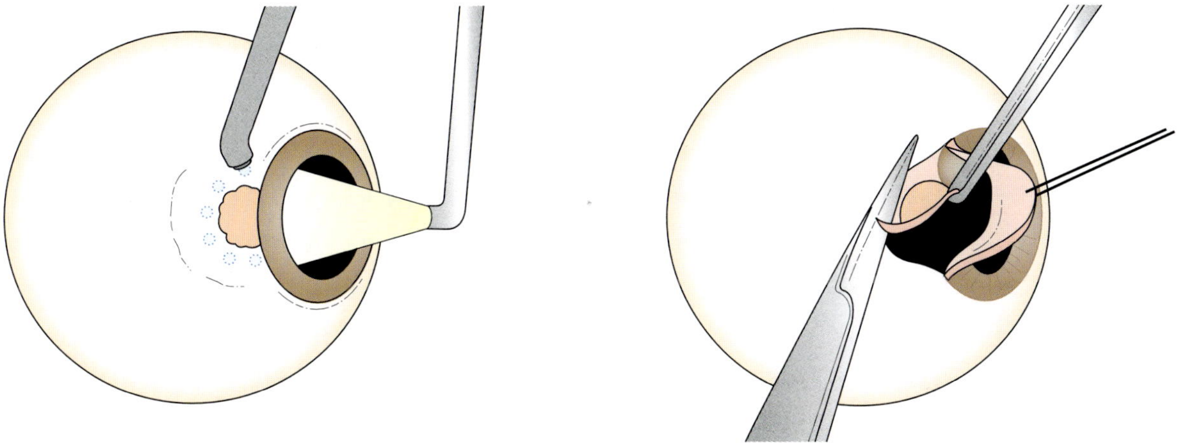

Figure 36.1 *Surgical technique of resection of iris and ciliary body tumor.*

2.5 clock-hours can be removed from the ciliary body safely. Barrada and associates[67] reported that primate eyes could tolerate removal of 6 clock-hours from the ciliary body.

Peyman and associates[90,91] modified the technique (Fig. 36.1). The patient is anesthetized using hypotensive anesthesia, in which systolic pressure is kept to approximately 90 mmHg to minimize bleeding. However, hypotensive anesthesia should be avoided in patients with asthma, a history of carotid occlusive disease, cerebral thrombosis, myocardial ischemia and, to a lesser degree, hypertension, diabetes and pulmonary disease. A 360° limbal peritomy is made and 4-0 black silk sutures are passed under the bellies of the recti muscles. Using transillumination, the tumor is localized and the borders are marked using a marker or a light diathermy effect. This localization should be confirmed with indirect ophthalmoscopy. The globe is supported by suturing a Peyman cyclectomy C-shaped wire on the sclera.[91]

Three sclerotomies are made away from the tumor site; the infusion cannula is introduced through one sclerotomy and the other two are closed temporarily. If the tumor does not involve the sclera, a partial-thickness scleral flap hinged to the limbus is made. If the ciliary body tumor extends to involve the anterior choroid, the removal of the involved part of the choroid and preoperative laser photocoagulation around the tumor are necessary. The scleral flap is elevated and penetrating diathermy is applied around the tumor in the tumor-free area. The anterior chamber is entered at the base of the flap. At the pupillary margin, two radial incisions are made on both sides of the tumor and extended posteriorly to remove the lesion involving the ciliary body and the choroid. The scleral flap is closed using 7-0 Dacron sutures. A vitrectomy, followed by fluid–gas exchange, is performed. The sclerotomies for the light pipe and vitrectomy handpiece are closed. A no. 20 silicone strip is sutured around the globe with 4-0 mattress sutures to create a buckle. The cannula is removed and the sclerotomy is closed. The eye is filled either with a 20% dilution of long-acting gas, such as sulfur hexafluoride (SF_6) or perfluoropropane (C_3F_8) in air, or with silicone oil. The conjunctiva is closed using 8-0 Vicryl sutures. Subconjunctival injections of antibiotic and steroid are given.

Penetrating sclerouveoretinovitrectomy (full-thickness eye-wall resection)

If the sclera and retina are involved by the tumor, then a full-thickness eye-wall resection is probably indicated (Fig. 36.2), provided that the tumor size does not preclude resection. This procedure was used by Meyer-Schwickerath[64] and was studied extensively by Peyman and coworkers.[65–72] In this technique, patients should receive preoperative panretinal photocoagulation with two overlapping rows around the tumor. The surgery is performed 4 to 5 weeks later.

Hypotensive general anesthesia is used to minimize bleeding. A 360° limbal peritomy is performed. The edges of the tumor are marked using light diathermy, with the aid of the transilluminator, and are confirmed using indirect ophthalmoscopy.

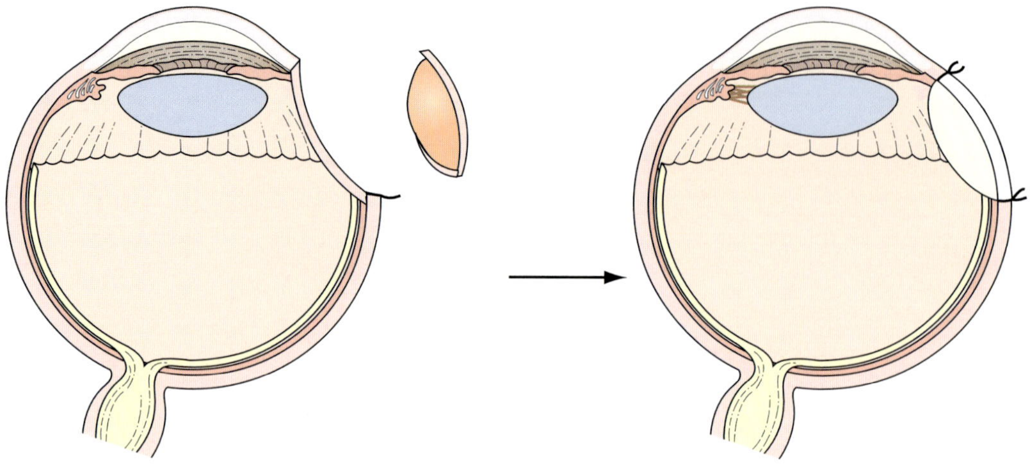

Figure 36.2
External full-thickness resection with donor sclera.

Three sclerotomies are made away from the tumor site: for the infusion cannula, light pipe and vitrectomy handpiece; the latter two are closed with scleral plugs or temporary sutures. A full-thickness scleral incision is made around the tumor about 2 mm from the edge of the tumor; a scleral graft of the same size should be ready before making this scleral incision. The uveal tissue around the tumor is coagulated first with a blunt-tipped diathermy probe and then with a penetrating-tip diathermy. The tumor is excised with the overlying sclera and underlying retina and choroid. The scleral graft is sutured airtight using 7-0 Dacron sutures. A complete vitrectomy is performed followed by fluid–gas exchange and endolaser to the adjacent incision site, and a limited scattered panretinal photocoagulation is performed. The globe is filled with SF_6, C_3F_8 or silicone oil.

Peyman and associates[66] reported a 10-year follow-up of their patients who had undergone full-thickness eye-wall resection; they found that eleven eyes had to be enucleated and two had metastasis; the rest (21 of 34, 62%) had vision ranging between 20/30 and hand motion. A postmortem study of one eye that underwent this procedure for mid-sized malignant melanoma showed excellent preservation of intraocular structures.[92]

Partial sclerouveoretinovitrectomy involves removing the overlying retina with the tumor but preserving the partial thickness of the sclera. The procedure is otherwise the same as that of full-thickness eye wall resection (Fig. 36.2).

The *partial lamellar sclerouvectomy* was used by Flieringa,[62] Stallard,[60] Foulds and Damato[41] and Shields and associates,[93] with some modifications. In this technique, the retina is not excised with the tumor and no penetrating diathermy is used. This will differentiate it from iridocyclectomy described above. The tumor is excised with the choroid and the inner part of the sclera (Fig. 36.3). The outer portion of the sclera is used to close the defect.

INTERNAL APPROACH FOR REMOVAL OF ANTERIOR SEGMENT LESIONS

Peyman recently described this technique for the management of epithelial downgrowth[94] (Fig. 36.4) and a benign leiomyoma.[95] The technique involves transscleral diathermy of the adjacent ciliary body. Three pars plana sclerotomies are performed away from the lesion. One of the sclerotomies is used for the infusion cannula. Using intraocular diathermy, the uninvolved border of the pars plana ciliary body is coagulated. Vitreous scissors are used to cut the tissue. The excised tissue is either removed by forceps or cut and aspirated using a vitrectomy instrument. A complete vitrectomy is done with laser application to the adjacent tissue. The procedure is completed by an air–fluid exchange.

TECHNIQUES: POSTERIOR SEGMENT TUMORS

EXTERNAL APPROACH

Tumors can be removed with adjacent tissue as in full-thickness eye–wall resection (Fig. 36.5a), or with partial thickness of the sclera left to close the defect

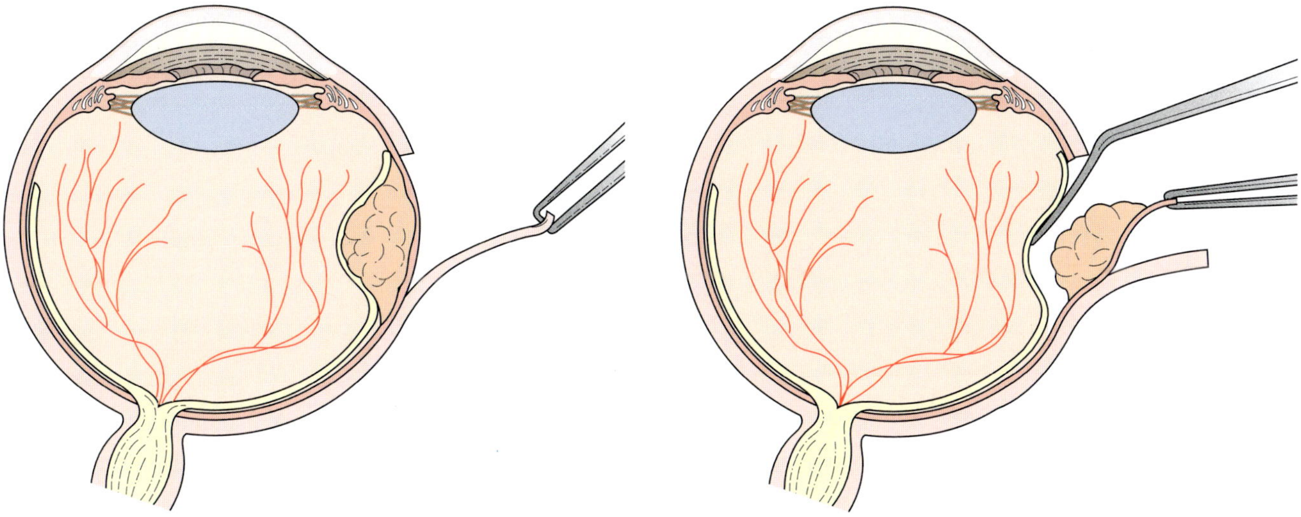

Figure 36.3 *Lamellar scleral flap plus uvectomy.*

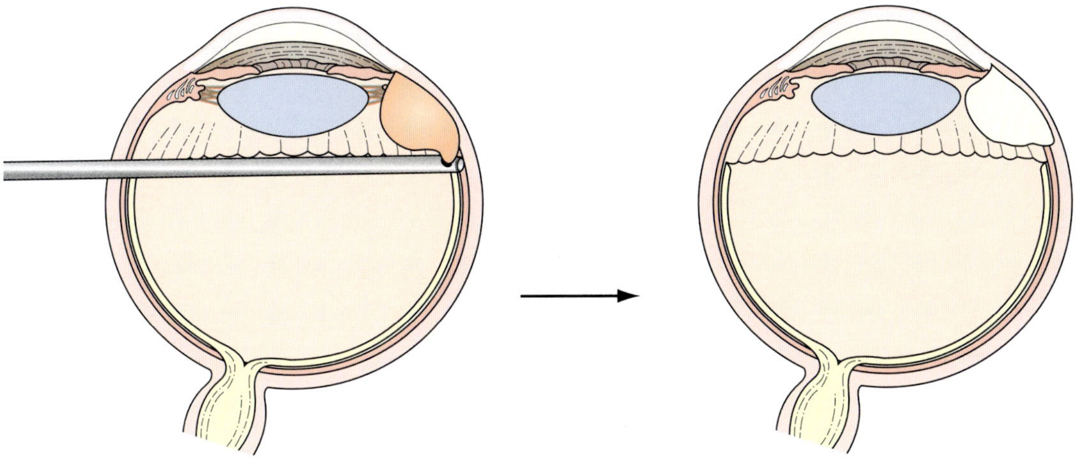

Figure 36.4 *Internal resection of the ciliary body.*

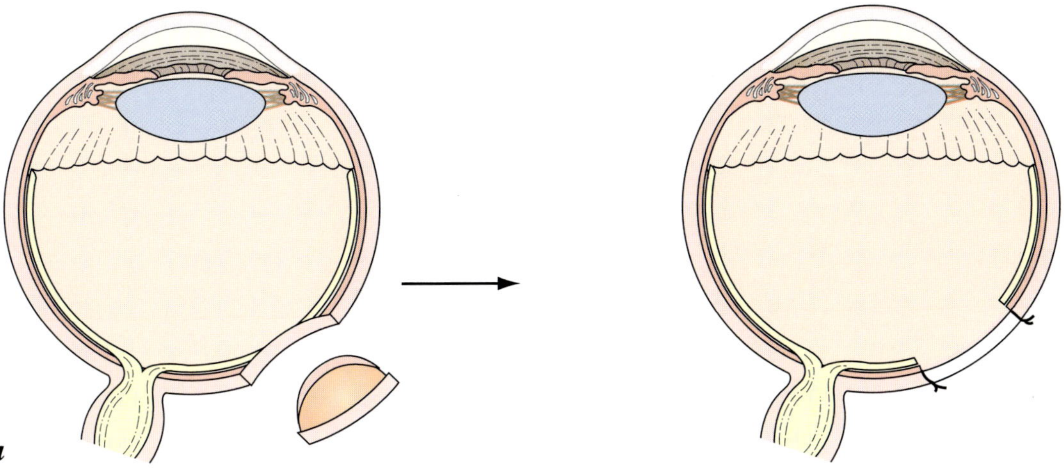

a

Figure 36.5 *(a) Full-thickness eye-wall resection with donor sclera.*

continued overleaf

Figure 36.5 *continued. (b) Full-thickness eye-wall resection. (c) Uvectomy with scleral flap. (d) External sclerochoroidectomy with partial-thickness scleral flap.*

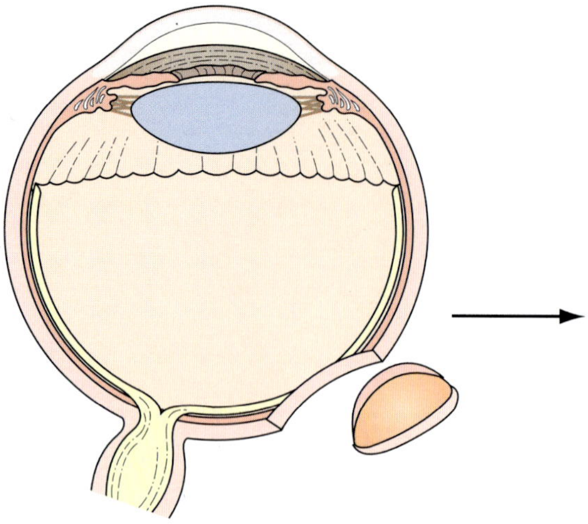

b

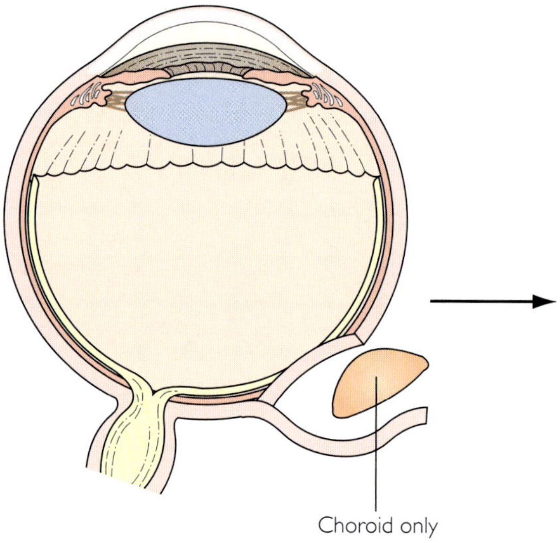

c

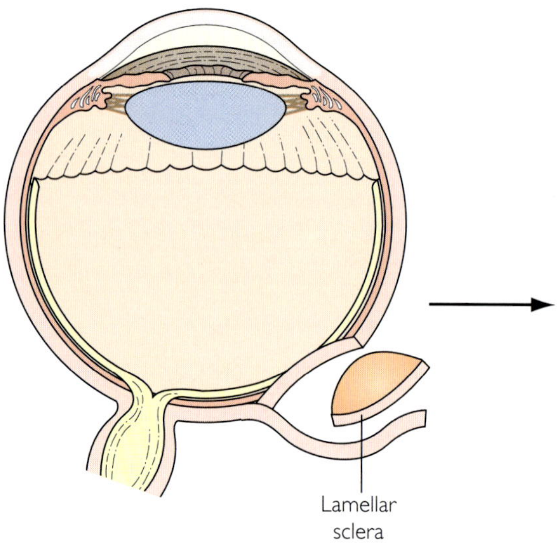

d

(Fig. 36.5b). These procedures require initial transillumination, partial dissection of the sclera and excision of the tumor followed by three-port vitrectomy to remove the vitreous and replace it with silicone oil. However, the uveal tumor can be removed with the choroid only (Fig. 36.5c) or by sparing the retina and the outer part of the sclera (Fig. 36.5d).

INTERNAL RESECTION

SURGICAL CRITERIA

Patient selection for internal resection should be based on the following criteria:

- Malignant melanomas of the choroid with no evidence of optic nerve or extrascleral extension by ophthalmoscopy, CT or MRI, or of metastatic disease after systemic evaluation by an oncologist.
- Posterior margin of melanoma extended no closer than one disk diameter to the optic nerve.
- The patient's general health will allow 3 hours of general anesthesia with possible hypotensive periods.

CASE SELECTION

Critical to the selection of the therapeutic alternatives (observation, radiation, enucleation or limited resection) is the patient's individual informed consent. The age of the patient, the visual potential of the other eye and the occupation and emotional demands of the patient are crucial in agreeing to a treatment strategy. The possible complications and requirement for additional surgery must be explained to the patient. It may be necessary to combine the resection with full-thickness eye-wall resection necessitating scleral grafts.[96]

SURGICAL TECHNIQUE

The technique of internal resection has evolved gradually with changes in instrumentation and indications.[96–98]

INTERNAL RETINOCHOROIDECTOMY

A preoperative photocoagulation is performed around the tumor 3 weeks before surgery. A 360° peritomy is performed and the sclera and vortex veins are examined carefully for extraocular extension of melanoma. If none is found, we proceed with a limited standard posterior three-port pars plana vitrectomy and, if necessary, pars plana lensectomy. Whenever possible, the vitrector and light pipe are positioned opposite the tumor for easy manipulation. The anterior vitreous is retained during the tumor resection to trap tumor cells that might be liberated during the melanoma excision and removal (Fig. 36.6).

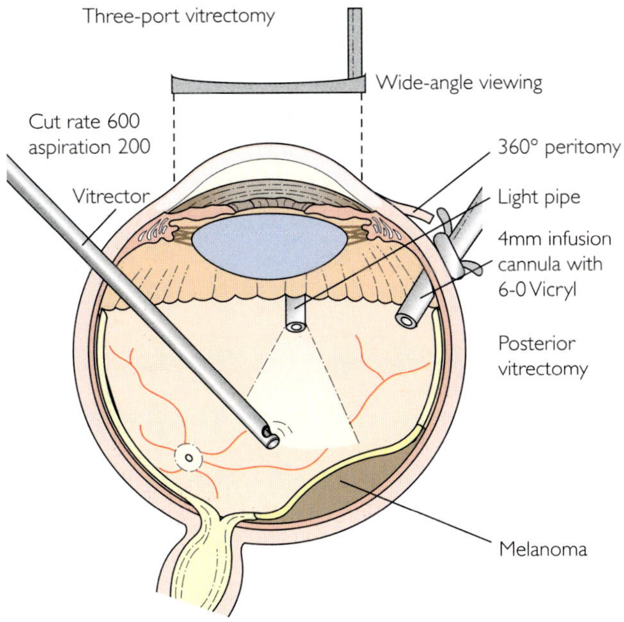

Figure 36.6 *A limited standard posterior three-port pars plana vitrectomy and, if necessary, pars plana lensectomy are performed. The vitrector and light pipe are positioned opposite the tumor, if possible, for easy manipulation. The anterior vitreous is retained during the tumor resection to trap tumor cells that are liberated during the melanoma excision and removal.*

Wide-angle viewing systems may be used, such as a binocular indirect ophthalmoscope (BIOM) for easy visualization of the periphery. Transillumination of the tumor from the side opposite the tumor allows accurate measurement of the margins without errors of parallax.

Extensive laser endophotocoagulation is applied to the tumor (Fig. 36.7). Endodiathermy is applied to the blood vessels around the tumors. The healthy margins of the tumor are heavily treated with diathermy. The tumor is dissected using the vitrector

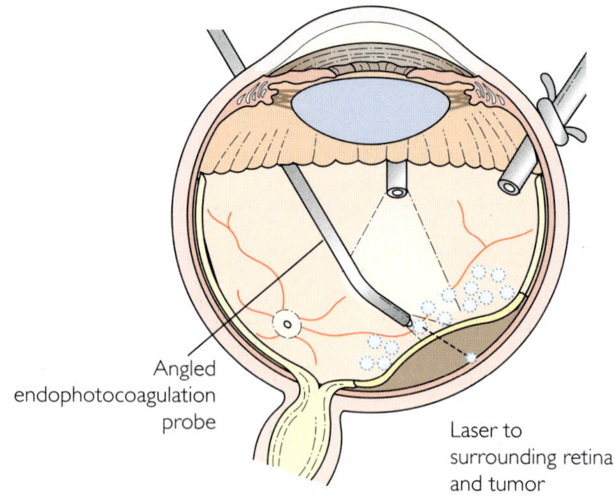

Figure 36.7 *An extensive laser endophotocoagulation is applied to the tumor and surrounding area.*

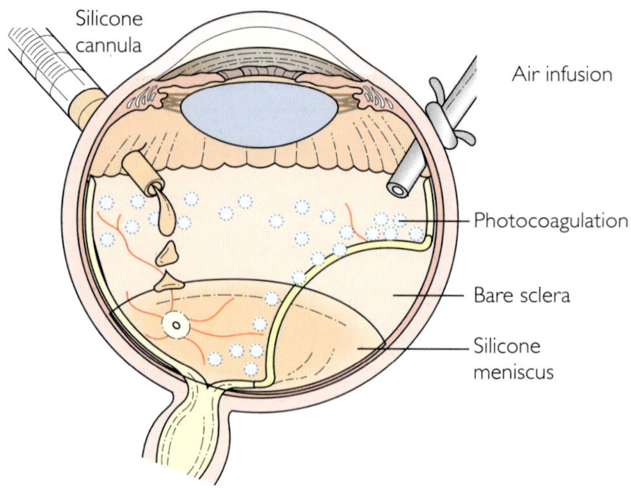

Figure 36.9 *One sclerotomy is enlarged to accept a 16-gauge silicone cannula and the eye is filled with silicone oil, which is usually removed 6–12 months later.*

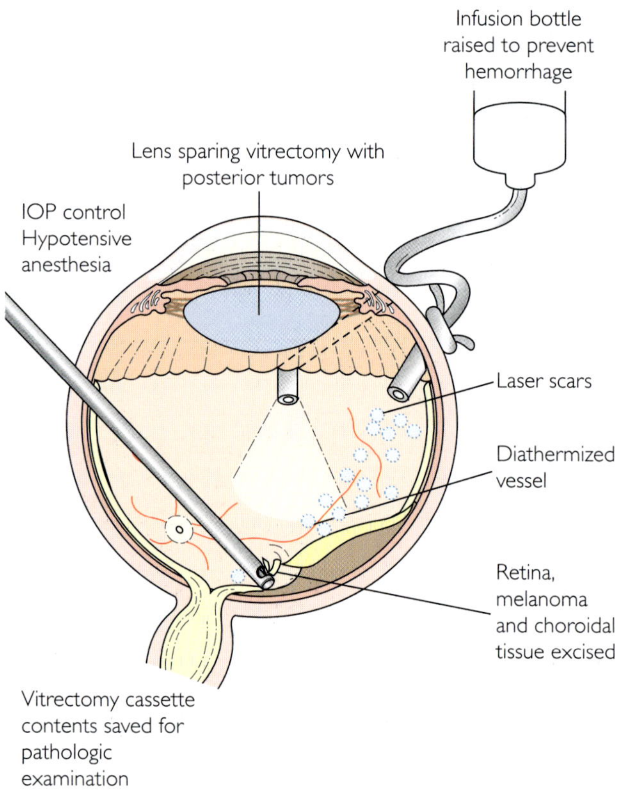

Figure 36.8 *The tumor is dissected using the vitrector or scissors, or a diathermy probe may be used to cut and coagulate the tissue.*

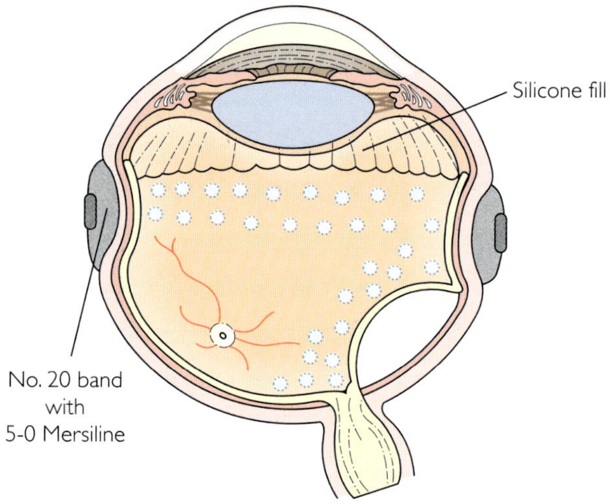

Figure 36.10 *An encircling no. 20 band is placed and secured with previously placed 5-0 Dacron mattress sutures.*

or scissors to cut and diathermy is used to coagulate the tissue (Fig. 36.8). Hemorrhage may be controlled by raising the intraocular pressure (by elevating the infusion bottle) or by hypotensive control of blood pressure to 100 mmHg. After the resection, a complete vitrectomy and a fluid–air exchange are performed, and an additional prophylactic endolaser is applied in the fundus periphery and the scleral bed.

One sclerotomy is enlarged to accept a 16-gauge silicone cannula and the eye is filled with silicone oil, (Fig. 36.9), which is usually removed 6–12 months later. An encircling no. 20 band is placed and secured with previously placed 5-0 Dacron mattress sutures (Fig. 36.10).

RETINA-SPARING INTERNAL RESECTION

Peyman and associates introduced a technique of internal resection under a retinal flap for removal of tumors located close to the optic nerve and fovea (Fig. 36.11).[83] Preoperative laser coagulation is not performed around the tumor. A partial vitrectomy is performed first and arcuate contiguous diathermy lesions are applied 130–180° away from the fovea or the optic nerve (Fig. 36.12).

A 160° retinotomy is made (Fig. 36.12). The retinal flap is dissected and reflected to expose the tumor. The tumor is cut from the surrounding choroid using diathermy and scissors, and removed using the vitrectomy instrument (Fig. 36.13). Laser is applied on the scleral bed and at the tumor margin. The vitrectomy is completed. The retina is reflected back in place and a fluid–air exchange is performed (Fig. 36.14). Laser is applied around the retinotomy. A long-acting gas (20% dilution) or silicone oil is used to fill the eye. The sclerotomies are closed, except those connected to the cannula. A circumferential scleral buckle is applied. The cannula is removed and the sclerotomy is closed. The patient may be advised to continue follow-up examinations along with medical work-ups.

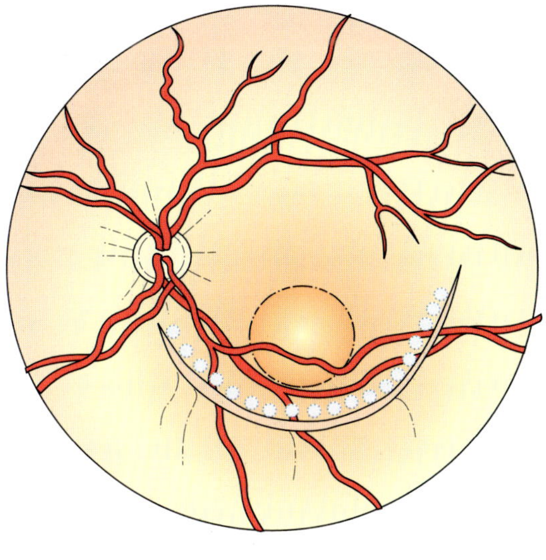

Figure 36.12 *Following endodiathermy, a 160° arcuate retinotomy is performed ensuring a 1 disc diameter tumor-free margin.*

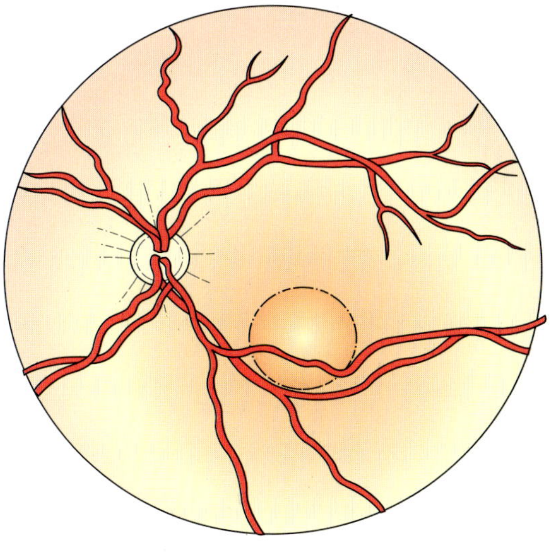

Figure 36.11 *Internal resection under a retinal flap. Uveal melanoma located in the posterior pole within 2 disc diameters of the optic nerve and within 0.5 disc diameters of the fovea.*

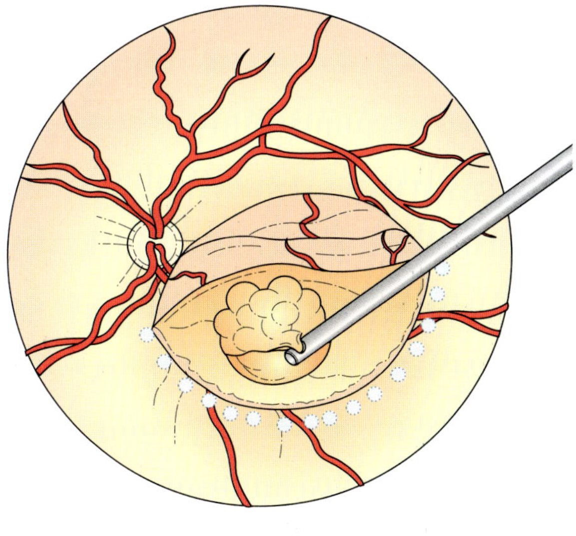

Figure 36.13 *The retinal flap is dissected and the entire tumor exposed. Argon endolaser is applied to both the tumor surface and free margins. Tumor and free margins are then dissected from the surrounding tissue bed and removed.*

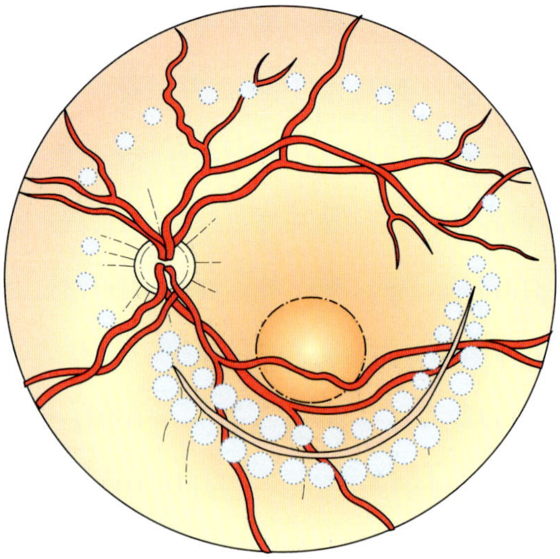

Figure 36.14 *Following tumor removal and complete vitrectomy, the retinal flap is repositioned and an air–fluid exchange performed. Endolaser is applied to the retinotomy edges and the posterior pole.*

The most common postoperative complications in the Kertes series of 32 cases were vitreous hemorrhage (37.5%), cataract (25%), retinal detachment (9%), elevated intraocular pressure (9%), band keratopathy (3%) and hypotony (3%).[97] Retinal detachment occurred in two patients requiring further surgery. Ancillary procedures were necessary with most patients.

Air–fluid exchange may be necessary to improve visualization if a nonclearing vitreous hemorrhage occurs postoperatively. Phakic eyes may require subsequent cataract extraction if lensectomy is not performed initially. Additional laser photocoagulation may be given in the postoperative period. Three (9.4%) of the eyes were enucleated; four (12.5%) have lost light perception.[97]

Ten patients (31.2%) had visual acuities of better than 20/200 and 18 of 32 (56.3%) were between 20/400 and light perception. There was one local recurrence. Three patients developed distant metastasis and died of malignant melanoma. Another developed biopsy-proven adenocarcinoma liver metastasis (mortality and metastatic rate, 12%).

These results must be interpreted in the context that there was a combination of small (4), medium (26) and large (2) tumors by the Collaborative Ocular Melanoma Study protocol and that 90% were within two disc diameters of the fovea or disc. Ninety percent of patients retained their globe, avoiding the emotional, psychological and cosmetic complications attendant with enucleation. With an average of 3.5 years of follow-up, our results are as good as other treatment modalities. Ten years of experience with this technique has proved that internal resection of choroidal tumors can be performed safely and may be particularly suited to treatment of tumors in close proximity to the fovea and disc.

REFERENCES

1. Volpe NJ, Albert DM. Metastases to the uvea. In: Albert DM, Jakobiec FA, eds, *Principles and Practice of Ophthalmology: Clinical Practice*, Vol. 5 (Saunders: Philadelphia, 1994): 3260–70.
2. Cutler SJ, Young JL. Third national cancer survey incidence data, *Nat Cancer Inst Monogr* (1975) **41:**1–454.
3. Petersen RA. Retinoblastoma: diagnosis and nonradiation therapies. In: Albert DM, Jakobiec FA, eds, *Principles and Practice of Ophthalmology: Clinical Practice*, Vol. 5 (Saunders: Philadelphia, 1994): 3279–85.
4. Lakhanpal V, Dogra MR, Aquilla JB. Episcleral pseudorheumatoid nodule with a choroidal mass simulating malignant melanoma, *Ann Ophthalmol* (1992) **24:**152–5.
5. Cunliffe IA, Rennie IG. Choroidal melanoma presenting as vitreous hemorrhage, *Eye* (1993) **7:**711–3.
6. Rőse GE, Hoh HB, Harrad RA, Hungerford JL. Intraocular malignant melanomas, *Eye* (1993) **7:**539–41.
7. Yap EY, Robertson DM, Buettner H. Scleritis as an initial manifestation of choroidal malignant melanoma, *Ophthalmology* (1992) **99:**1693–7.
8. Servodidio CA, Abramson DH. Presenting signs and symptoms of choroidal melanoma: What do they mean? *Ann Ophthalmol* (1992) **24:**190–4.
9. Jager MJ, Volker-Dieben HJ, de Wolff-Rouendaal D, et al. Possible relation between HLA and ABO type and prognosis of uveal melanoma, *Doc Ophthalmol* (1992) **82:**43–7.
10. Peyman GA, Meisels HI, Batko KA, Vlchek JK. Full thickness eye wall biopsy. I. An experimental approach to the tissue diagnosis and study of choroidal and retinal lesions, *Invest Ophthalmol* (1975) **14:**484–7.
11. Peyman GA, Homer P, Kasbeer R, Vlchek J. Full thickness eye wall biopsy. II. In primates, *Invest Ophthalmol* (1975) **14:**565–7.
12. Peyman GA, Fishman GA, Sanders DR, et al. Biopsy of human scleral–chorioretinal tissue, *Invest Ophthalmol* (1975) **14:**707–10.
13. Shields JA, Shields CL, Ehya H, et al. Fine-needle aspiration biopsy of suspected intraocular tumors. The 1992 Urwick lecture, *Ophthalmology* (1993) **100:**1677–84.
14. Shields JA, Shields CL, Donoso LA. Management of posterior uveal melanoma, *Surv Ophthalmol* (1991) **36:**161–95.
15. Albert DM, Niffenegger AS, Willson JK. Treatment of metastatic uveal melanoma: review and recommendations, *Surv Ophthalmol* (1992) **36:**429–38.

16. Olsen KR, Curtin VT. Enucleation and plaque treatment. In: Albert DM, Jakobiec FA, eds, *Principles and Practice of Ophthalmology: Clinical Practice*, Vol. 5 (Saunders: Philadelphia, 1994): 3217–22.
17. Zimmerman LE, McLean IW. An evaluation of enucleation in the management of uveal melanomas, *Am J Ophthalmol* (1979) **87:**741–60.
18. Zimmerman LE, McLean IW, Foster WD. Does enucleation of the eye containing a malignant melanoma prevent or accelerate the dissemination of tumour cells? *Br J Ophthalmol* (1978) **62:**420–5.
19. Packard RBS. In malignant choroidal melanoma will a delay in radical treatment influence prognosis, *Trans Ophthalmol Soc UK* (1983) **103:**49–53.
20. Niederkorn JY. Enucleation-induced metastasis of intraocular melanomas in mice, *Ophthalmology* (1984) **91:**692–700.
21. Niederkorn JY. Enucleation in consort with immunologic impairment promotes metastasis of intraocular melanomas in mice, *Invest Ophthalmol Vis Sci* (1984) **25:**1080–6.
22. Seigel D, Myers M, Ferris F III, Steinhorn SC. Survival rates after enucleation of eyes with malignant melanoma, *Am J Ophthalmol* (1979) **87:**761–5.
23. Shields JA. Cataract surgery after radiotherapy for uveal melanoma (editorial), *Arch Ophthalmol* (1992) **110:**473–4.
24. Kleineidam M, Augsburger JJ, Hernandez C, et al. Cataractogenesis after Cobalt-60 eye plaque radiotherapy, *Int J Radiat Oncol Biol Phys* (1993) **26:**625–30.
25. Gragoudas ES, Egan KM, Seddon JM, et al. Intraocular recurrence of uveal melanoma after proton beam irradiation, *Ophthalmology* (1992) **99:**760–6.
26. Manschot WA, van Strik R. Uveal melanoma: therapeutic consequences of doubling times and irradiation results; a review, *Int Ophthalmol* (1992) **16:**91–9.
27. Abramson DH, Giovinazzo V, Servodidio CA, Weil AR. Visual fields in a successfully radiated retinoblastoma patient, *J Ophthalmic Nurs Technol* (1992) **11:**17–19.
28. Guyer DR, Mukai S, Egan KM, et al. Radiation maculopathy after proton beam irradiation for choroidal melanoma, *Ophthalmology* (1992) **99:**1278–85.
29. Archer DB, Amoaku WM, Kelly G. Choroidoretinal neovascularization following radon seed treatment of retinoblastoma in two patients, *Br J Ophthalmol* (1993) **77:**95–9.
30. Robinson LL, Mertens A. Second tumors after treatment of childhood malignancies, *Hematol Oncol Clin North Am* (1993) **7:**401–15.
31. Helton KJ, Fletcher BD, Kun LE, et al. Bone tumors other than osteosarcoma after retinoblastoma, *Cancer* (1993) **71:**2847–53.
32. Imhof SM, Hofman P, Tan KE. Quantification of lacrimal function after D-shaped field irradiation for retinoblastoma, *Br J Ophthalmol* (1993) **77:**482–4.
33. Kincaid MC, Folberg R, Torczynski E. Complications after proton beam therapy for uveal malignant melanoma: clinical and histopathological study of five cases, *Ophthalmology* (1988) **95:**982–91.
34. Qiang Z, Cairns JD. Laser photocoagulation treatment of choroidal melanoma, *Aust NZ J Ophthalmol* (1993) **21:**87–92.
35. Zhao Q, Cairns JD. Laser photocoagulation treatment of small malignant choroidal melanomas, *Chung Hua Yen Ko Tsa Chih* (1993) **29:**36–9.
36. Foulds WS, Damato BE. Low-energy long-exposure laser therapy in the management of choroidal melanomas, *Graefes Arch Clin Exp Ophthalmol* (1986) **224:**26–31.
37. Shukla M, Gerke E, Bornfeld N, Meyer-Schwickerath G. Tumor regression after photocoagulation of malignant melanomas of the choroid: an ultrasonographic study, *Ophthalmologica* (1987) **194:**119–25.
38. Brancato R, Pratesi R, Leoni G, et al. Semiconductor diode laser photocoagulation of human malignant melanoma, *Am J Ophthalmol* (1989) **107:**295–6.
39. Shields JA, Shields CL, De Potter P. Photocoagulation of retinoblastoma, *Int Ophthalmol Clin* (1993) **33**(3):95–9.
40. Peyman GA, Alghadyan A, Peace JH. A contact Nd:YAG laser to resect large ciliary body and choroidal tumors, *Int Ophthalmol* (1987) **11:**55–61.
41. Foulds WS, Damato BE. Alternatives to enucleation in the management of choroidal melanoma, *Aust NZ J Ophthalmol* (1986) **14:**19–27.
42. Peyman GA, Nelsen PT, Axelrod AJ, et al. Full thickness eye wall resection: evaluation of preoperative photocoagulation, *Invest Ophthalmol* (1973) **12:**262–6.
43. Peyman GA, Axelrod AJ, Graham RO. Full-thickness eye wall resection: an experimental approach for treatment of choroidal melanoma: evaluation of cryotherapy, diathermy and photocoagulation, *Arch Ophthalmol* (1974) **91:**219–22.
44. Zhou MH, Ren F. Growth inhibitory action of RGNTF–McAb on human retinoblastoma cell line Y-79, *Chung Hua Yen Ko Tsa Chih* (1993) **29:**349–52.
45. Yang L, Wang H, Zhang X, et al. Clinical observation of immunotherapy in ocular malignant tumors with lymphokine-activated killing (LAK) cell, *Yen Ko Hsueh Pao* (1993) **9:**51–4.
46. Fisher AM, Murphree AL, Gomer CJ. Clinical and preclinical photodynamic therapy, *Lasers Surg Med* (1995) **17:**2–31.
47. Barr CC, Norton EWD. Recurrence of choroidal melanoma after photocoagulation therapy, *Arch Ophthalmol* (1983) **101:**1737–40.
48. Steeves RA, Murray TG, Moros EG, et al. Concurrent ferromagnetic hyperthermia and 125I brachytherapy in a rabbit choroidal melanoma model, *Int J Hyperthermia* (1992) **8:**443–9.
49. Finger PT. Microwave plaque thermoradiotherapy for choroidal melanoma, *Br J Ophthalmol* (1992) **76:**358–64.
50. Hathirat P, Kunavisarut S, Chuansumrit A, et al. Chemotherapy in patients with retinoblastoma, *J Med Assoc Thai* (1993) **76** (Suppl 2): 85–91.
51. Lee TW, Yang SW, Kim CM, et al. Chemosensitization to adriamycin by cyclosporin A and verapamil in human retinoblastoma cell lines, *J Korean Med Sci* (1993) **8:**104–9.
52. Sanborn G, Niederkorn J, Kan-Mitchell J, Albert D. Prevention of metastasis of intraocular melanoma in mice treated with difluoromethylornithine, *Graefes Arch Clin Exp Ophthalmol* (1992) **230:**72–7.
53. Sanborn GE, Niederkorn JY, Gamel JW. Efficacy of dacarbazine (DTIC) in preventing metastases arising from intraocular melanomas in mice, *Graefes Arch Clin Exp Ophthalmol* (1992) **230:**192–6.
54. Ren F, Zhou MH. Immunotherapy of human retinoblastoma with RGNTF–monoclonal antibody using nude mice as model, *Chung Hua Chung Liu Tsa Chih* (1992) **14:**323–6.
55. Dorval T, Fridman WH, Mathiot C, Pouillart P. Interleukin-2 therapy for metastatic uveal melanoma (letter), *Eur J Cancer* (1992) **28A:**2087.
56. Reese AB, Jones IS, Cooper WC. Surgery for tumors of the iris and ciliary body, *Am J Ophthalmol* (1968) **66:**173–84.
57. Forrest AW, Keyser RB, Spencer WH. Iridocyclectomy for melanomas of the ciliary body: a follow-up study of

pathology and surgical morbidity, *Ophthalmology* (1978) **85:**1237–49.
58. Zirm EK. Über endobulbae Operationen, *Arch F Augenheilk* (1911) **69:**233–6.
59. Stallard HB. Surgery of malignant melanoma of the iris, *Br J Ophthalmol* (1951) **35:**774–83.
60. Stallard HB. Partial choroidectomy, *Br J Ophthalmol* (1966) **50:**660–2.
61. Friede R. Zur operation maligner Geschwülste des Ciliarkörpers, *Ophthalmologica* (1956) **131:**168–78.
62. Flieringa HJ. A method of surgery in the angle of the anterior chamber of the eye, *Trans Ophthalmol Soc UK* (1961) **81:**421–5.
63. Müller HK. Die Partielle Ausschneidung von Iris und Ciliarkörper, *Doc Ophthalmol* (1969) **26:**679–97.
64. Meyer-Schwickerath G. Excision of malignant melanoma of the choroid, *Mod Probl Ophthalmol* (1974) **12:**562–6.
65. Peyman GA, Raichand M. Full thickness eye wall resection of choroidal neoplasm, *Ophthalmology* (1979) **86:**1024–36.
66. Peyman GA, Juarez CP, Diamond JG, Raichand M. Ten years experience with eye wall resection for uveal malignant melanomas, *Ophthalmology* (1984) **91:**1720–5.
67. Barrada A, Peyman GA, Palacio MN. Limitation of iris and ciliary body resection in primates, *Retina* (1984) **4:**119–22.
68. Peyman GA, Rednam KVR, Juarez CP. Improvement in eye wall resection technique, *Ophthalmic Surg* (1983) **14:**588–90.
69. Peyman GA, Dodich NA. Full thickness eye wall resection: an experimental approach for the treatment of choroidal melanoma. I. Dacron-graft, *Invest Ophthalmol* (1972) **11:**115–21.
70. Peyman GA, May DR, Ericson ES, Goldberg MF. Full thickness eye wall resection: an experimental approach for the treatment of choroidal melanoma. II. Homo- and hetero-graft, *Invest Ophthalmol* (1972) **11:**668–74.
71. Peyman GA, Ericson ES, Axelrod AJ, May DR. Full-thickness eye wall resection in primates. An experimental approach to treatment of choroidal melanoma, *Arch Ophthalmol* (1973) **89** (5):410–12.
72. Peyman GA, Koziol J. Limitation of eye wall resection, *Can J Ophthalmol* (1974) **9:**328–37.
73. Peyman GA, Rednam KR, Mottow-Lippa L, Flood T. Treatment of large von Hippel tumors by eye wall resection, *Ophthalmology* (1983) **90:**840–7.
74. Peyman GA, Charles H. Internal eye wall resection in the management of uveal melanoma, *Can J Ophthalmol* (1988) **23:**219–23.
75. Peyman GA, Katoh N, Tawakol M, et al. Contact application of Nd:YAG laser through a fiberoptic and a sapphire tip, *Int Ophthalmol* (1987) **11:**3–12.
76. Yu DY, Cohen SB, Peyman G, Tso MOM. Mesectodermal leiomyoma of the ciliary body: new evidence of neural crest origin, *J Pediatr Ophthalmol Strabismus* (1990) **27:**317–21.
77. Mani H, Peyman GA, Leff SI. Intraocular meningothelial meningiomas, *Int Ophthalmol* (1988) **12:**207–11.
78. Peyman GA, Barrada A. Retinochoroidectomy ab interno, *Ophthalmic Surg* (1984) **15:**749–51.
79. Peyman GA, Hindi M. Ab interno retinochoroidectomy in primates, *Arch Ophthalmol* (1985) **103:**572–5.
80. Lee KJ, Peyman GA, Raichand S. Internal eye wall resection for posterior uveal melanoma, *Jpn J Ophthalmol* (1993) **37:**287–92.
81. Peyman GA, Schulman J, Raichand M. Diagnosis and therapeutic surgery of the uvea, II. Results, *Ophthalmic Surg* (1987) **18:**310–16.
82. Peyman GA, Raichand M, Schulman J. Diagnosis and therapeutic surgery of the uvea, part I. Surgical technique, *Ophthalmic Surg* (1986) **17:**822–9.
83. Peyman GA, Nelson NC Jr, Paris CL, et al. Internal choroidectomy of posterior uveal melanomas under a retinal flap, *Int Ophthalmol* (1992) **16:**439–44.
84. Shields JA, Shields CL, De Potter P. Local resection of posterior uveal tumors, *Int Ophthalmol Clin* (1993) **33:**137–42.
85. Vail DT. Iridocyclectomy: a review, *Am J Ophthalmol* (1971) **71:**161–8.
86. Foulds WS, Damato BE. Surgical resection of choroidal melanomas. In: Ryan S, ed, *Retina*, Vol 1 (CV Mosby, St Louis, 1989): 713–20.
87. Damato BE, Paul J, Foulds WS. Predictive factors of visual outcome after local resection of choroidal melanoma, *Br J Ophthalmol* (1993) **77:**616–23.
88. Yanoff M, Fine SB. *Ocular Pathology: A Text and Atlas.* 2nd edn (Harper & Row: Philadelphia, 1982).
89. Kara GB. Excision of uveal melanomas: a 15–year experience, *Ophthalmology* (1979) **86:**997–1023.
90. Peyman GA, Salzano TC, Green JL, Andrews AH. Role of the CO_2 laser in chorioretino-iridocyclectomy, *Ophthalmic Surg* (1981) **12:**426–31.
91. Peyman GA, Schulman JA. *Intravitreal Surgery: Principles and Practice.* 2nd edn (Appleton & Lange: Norwalk, CT, 1994).
92. Shields JA, Augsburger JJ, Stefanyszyn MA, Connor RW. Sclerochorioretinal resection for choroidal melanoma: a clinicopathologic correlation of a postmortem eye, *Ophthalmology* (1984) **91:**1726–30.
93. Shields JA, Shields CL, Shah P, Sivalingam V. Partial lamellar sclerouvectomy for ciliary body and choroidal tumors, *Ophthalmology* (1991) **98:**971–83.
94. Peyman GA, Peralta E, Ganiban GJ, Kraut R. Endoresection of iris and ciliary body in epithelial downgrowth: a case report, *J Cataract Refract Surg* (1998) **24:**130–3.
95. Peyman GA, Martinez CE, Hew A, et al. Resection of ciliary body leiomyoma, *Can J Ophthalmol* (1998) **33:**32–4.
96. Peyman GA, Gremillion CM, Fang T, Baziuk N, Internal resection of chorioretinal lesions. In: Youn DH, Rhee SW, Lee J, eds, *XII Transactions of the Asia-Pacific Academy of Ophthalmology* (Asia-Pacific Academy of Ophthalmology: Seoul, Korea, 1989): 59–66.
97. Kertes PJ, Johnson JC, Peyman GA. Internal resection of posterior uveal melanoma, *Br J Ophthalmol* (1998) **82:**1147–53.
98. Foulds WS, Damato BE, Burton RL. Local resection versus enucleation in the management of choroidal melanoma, *Eye* (1987) **1:**676–9.

Chapter 37 Ophthalmic brachytherapy: treatment of choroidal melanoma and retinoblastoma

Paul T Finger and A Linn Murphree

INTRODUCTION

BRACHYTHERAPY VERSUS TELETHERAPY

'Brachytherapy' is derived from the Greek term *brachy* meaning 'short' or 'close'. Today the term brachytherapy refers to any interstitial, intracavitary or other implantation of a radiation source into the body, usually planned for a short length of time. In ophthalmic oncology there are rare instances of permanent radioactive source implantation.[1–3] These techniques are not to be confused with 'teletherapy', derived from the Greek term *tele* meaning 'at a distance'. Today the term teletherapy means treatment at a distance or the use of external beam radiation therapy (EBRT). Other well-known forms of EBRT include charged-particle therapy (helium ion and proton beam) and the gamma knife.[1]

RADIATION BIOLOGY

Radiation can work by directly damaging cellular DNA and by producing free radicals (primarily hydroxyl radicals) that secondarily affect tumor DNA and other important cellular structures. Radiation injury can immediately destroy DNA or create mutations that take years to cause the death of tumor cells.[1]

The tumor's vascular system is another target of radiation. While acute radiation-induced vasculitis is common, vascular occlusion is dependent on total dose, dose rate and time. Clinical studies have indicated that radiation has both short- and long-term effects on both tumor and normal tissues.[1]

Local control of intraocular tumors has been defined by radiation oncologists as the cessation of growth or tumor shrinkage. In ophthalmology, this assessment is made by such non-physiologic parameters as ophthalmoscopy and ultrasonography. No one has determined the metastatic potential (if any) of radiotherapy-treated intraocular tumors; in fact, posttreatment histopathologic evaluations of choroidal melanomas have noted both the presence of mitotic figures and some cell cycling.[4,5]

BRACHYTHERAPY IN THE TREATMENT OF CHOROIDAL MELANOMA

HISTORY OF RADIOTHERAPY FOR CHOROIDAL MELANOMA

In 1930, Moore was the first to use brachytherapy to preserve vision for a monocular patient with uveal melanoma.[3] He implanted radon seeds directly into a choroidal melanoma. Stallard tried this technique, but also went on to develop cobalt-60 (^{60}Co) plaque radiotherapy.[6,7] Since then, multiple-case series have been published describing the use of various radiation techniques, including ruthenium-106 (^{106}Ru), iodine-125 (^{125}I), radon seeds in eye plaques, iridium-192 (^{192}Ir), palladium-103 (^{103}Pd) and charged particles (protons and helium ions).[8–13]

The most commonly used form of radiotherapy for treatment of choroidal melanomas is ophthalmic plaque brachytherapy. This technique involves affixing a dish-shaped source, most commonly ^{125}I or

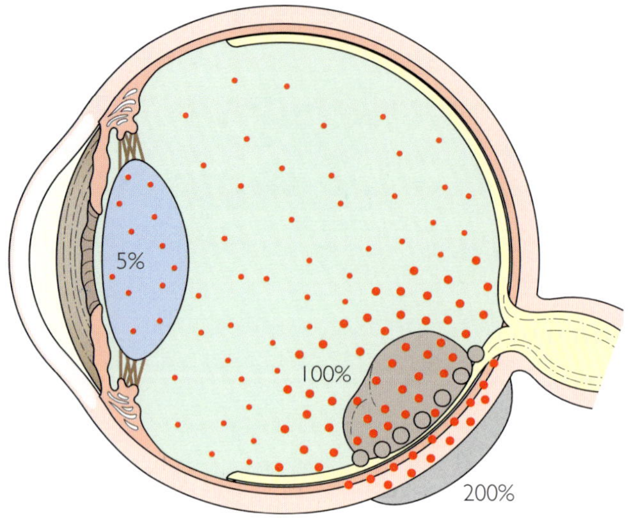

Figure 37.1 *An illustration of a low-energy (^{125}I or ^{103}Pd) episcleral ophthalmic plaque beneath an intraocular tumor. (Adapted with permission from Finger PT. Radiation therapy for choroidal melanoma,* Surv Ophthalmol *(1997)* ***42****:215–32.*[1] *Copyright © 1997, Elsevier Science.)*

^{106}Ru onto the sclera over the base of the intraocular tumor. During eye-plaque therapy, radiation travels through and is sequentially absorbed by the sclera, the tumor, the retina, the vitreous and normal ocular structures as it exits the eye (Fig. 37.1).

SURGICAL CRITERIA AND CASE SELECTION

UVEAL MELANOMA

Before surgery, all patients should be examined for evidence of metastatic disease and for their ability to tolerate the procedures. All patients should be informed that current studies suggest that (on average) 5 years after radiotherapy there is a small (8%) chance that their irradiated tumor may regrow, that irradiated eyes may require secondary enucleation (for tumor regrowth or glaucoma) and that with current techniques only 44% are expected to have vision equal to or better than 20/200 in the treated eye.

The anatomy of most uveal melanomas is ideal for plaque radiotherapy. They are solitary tumors that arise within the uveal tract (choroid, ciliary body and iris) of one eye. They extend from the vascular eye wall and push the retina into the avascular vitreous humor. Because ophthalmic plaques deposit most of their radiation in and around the base of the tumor, they preferentially target its vascular supply (Fig. 37.1).

Although most uveal melanomas are found to form a dome shape, at least 25% demonstrate a collar-button configuration. When Bruch's membrane is intact, it functions as a barrier to leaking of tumor blood vessel components before and after radiation. A large percentage of choroidal melanomas erode through Bruch's membrane and extend into the vitreous or beneath the retina. These tumors are more likely to cause vitreous and subretinal seeding, hemorrhage, retinal invasion and intraretinal exudation. These tumors are also poorer candidates for plaque radiotherapy. Any treatment should consider all sites of melanoma infiltration.

It is generally accepted that in comparison to treatment of small- or medium-sized choroidal melanomas, radiotherapy of large neoplasms (greater than 10 mm in apical height or 16 mm in basal dimension) is associated with worse outcomes for vision and eye retention. Irradiated eyes with large tumors are more likely to develop scleral thinning, neovascular glaucoma, cataract, vitreous hemorrhage, retinal detachment, radiation retinopathy, and radiation optic neuropathy. Also, plaque radiotherapy of anterior uveal melanomas is more likely to induce cataract, while irradiation of posterior tumors is more likely to cause radiation retinopathy.

PLAQUE INSERTION: OVERVIEW

Plaque radiotherapy requires precise tumor localization. In order to include microscopic extension beyond the visible tumor's edge, the bowl-shaped plaque diameters are usually chosen to include a 2-mm 'tumor-free' margin as determined by ophthalmoscopy, ultrasonography and, lastly, by the tumor's transillumination shadow that is measured at surgery. Therefore the targeted '100%' basal zone is typically a minimum of 14 mm for a tumor with a 10-mm base. There will be a variable amount of lateral spread beyond the targeted zone, depending upon which radionuclide (isotope) is used, whether the metallic plaque has sidewalls and how the radioactive seeds are distributed within the plaque.

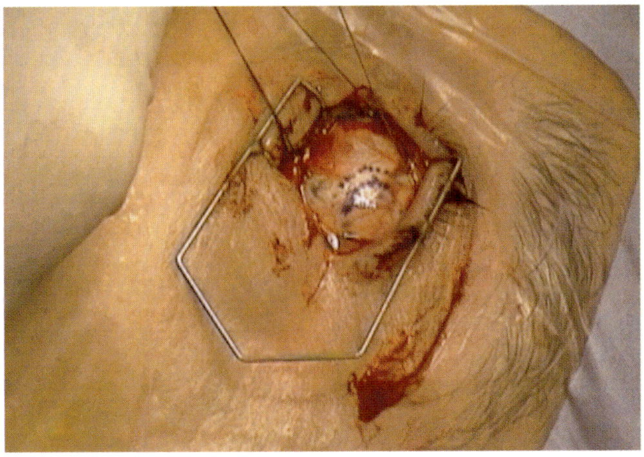

Figure 37.2 *An intraoperative clinical photograph showing episcleral markings after transillumination. Note that the inner markings are at the edges of the tumor shadow; the outer markings represent the 2–3-mm margin.*

The surgical technique requires a conjunctival peritomy. Tenon's fascia is opened in at least two adjacent quadrants. Transillumination is performed to define the tumor's edges. Typically, direct and indirect techniques are used. If the tumor's shadow extends beneath a rectus muscle, the muscle is isolated, sutured, transected from its insertion and allowed to retract, so direct and indirect transillumination is accurate. Pigmented intraocular tumors create a transillumination shadow on the episclera, which is marked with a surgical pen. Then a caliper is used to confirm the size of the tumor's base and act as a guide to mark the 2–3-mm margin around the tumor (Fig. 37.2). Episcleral sutures are used to anchor the radioactive plaque onto the sclera. If rectus muscle disinsertion is required to allow room for the plaque, a temporary reinsertion can be made. This is repaired permanently when the plaque is removed.

In the treatment of small posterior or amelanotic tumors, the transillumination shadow may not be visible. In these cases, scleral indentation along the edge of the plaque during ophthalmoscopy is commonly used for localization. Two-dimensional and three-dimensional intraoperative ultrasonography also can be used to check for proper plaque positioning (Fig. 37.3).[14]

Finger and colleagues have developed a new technique called diode-light transillumination for localization of plaques to cover intraocular tumors. After the plaque is sewn into position, plaque-mounted diode lights can be viewed as a circle around the intraocular tumor. In the treatment of choroidal melanoma, radiation is usually delivered as

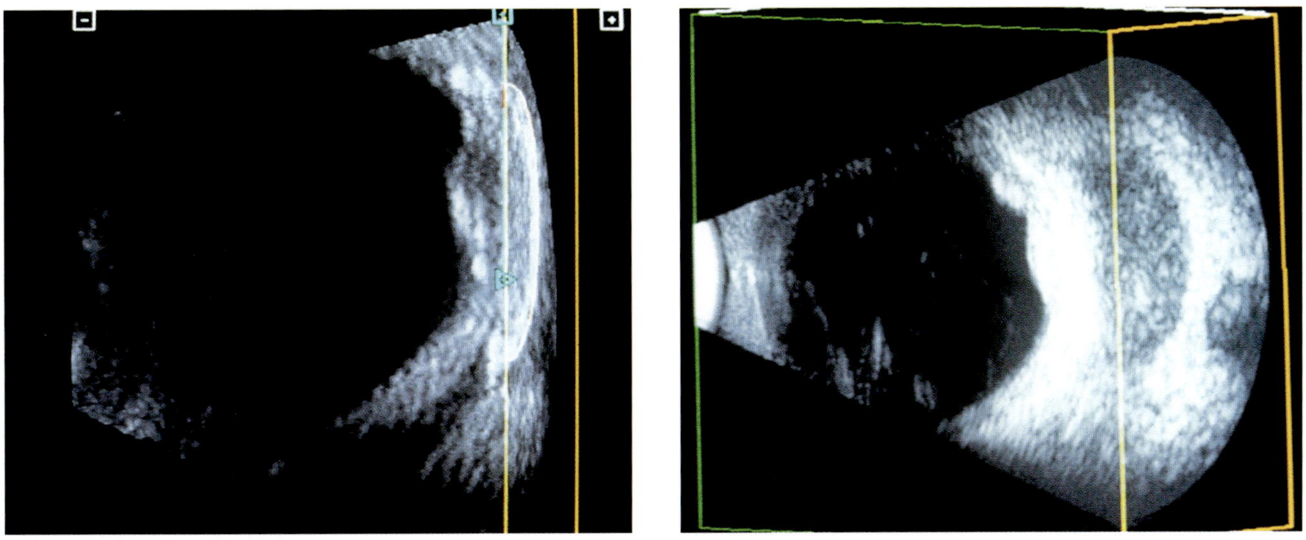

a *b*

Figure 37.3 *(a) A two-dimensional ultrasound scan of an episcleral plaque beneath a choroidal melanoma. (b) A three-dimensional ultrasound scan showing the tumor, the plaque and its orbital shadow, as well as the optic nerve shadow in the posterior orbit.*

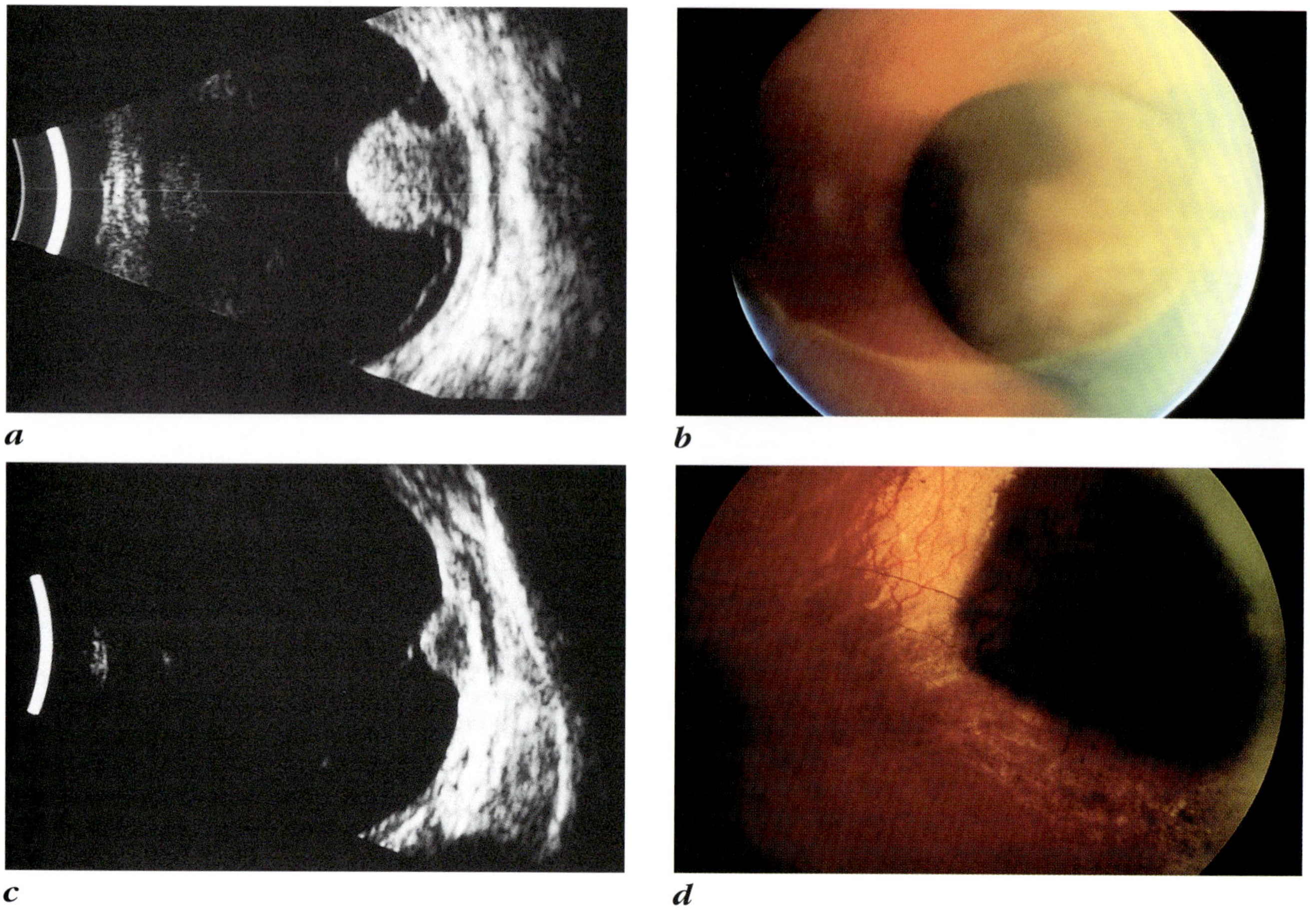

Figure 37.4 *(a, b) Note the collar-button shaped choroidal melanoma prior to ^{103}Pd ophthalmic plaque radiotherapy. (c, d) Note the regression pattern seen several years after treatment.*

an outpatient over 5–7 days, after which the plaque is removed (Fig. 37.4).

PLAQUE INSERTION OVER ANTERIOR UVEAL MELANOMAS

Anterior uveal melanomas can be treated with standard eye plaques (Fig. 37.5). We have found that the cornea is relatively radiation resistant and therefore tolerant of irradiation. Ultrasound biomicroscopy can be used to determine the tumor's apical height or prescription point.

Surgical placement of eye plaques over the limbus presents a unique challenge. The eye wall does not assume a smooth curvature at the limbus, the suture eyelets can be very irritating to the cornea and the plaque is exposed to movements of the eyelids, which can cause displacement. Therefore, the plaque

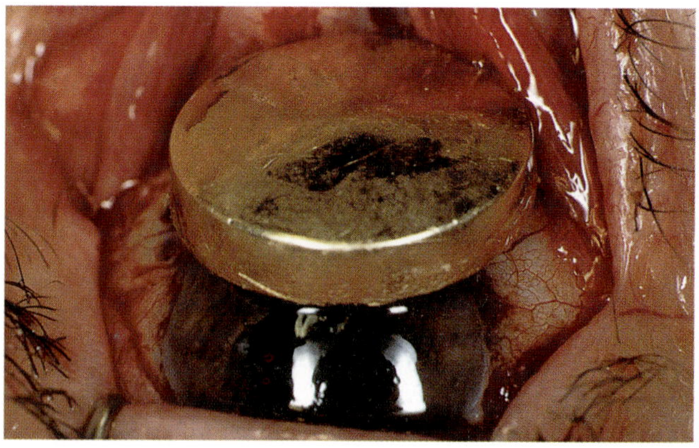

Figure 37.5 *A standard gold eye plaque containing ^{103}Pd seeds sewn to cover a ciliary body melanoma with iris extension. The surface eyelets are sewn to the episclera at the posterior margin of the plaque to avoid corneal irritation. The conjunctiva is brought over to cover the plaque.*

should be attached so that the eyelets do not come in contact with the cornea, and then the conjunctiva should be draped to cover the back of the plaque (as possible). The conjunctival covering will allow the lids to slide over the back of the plaque, decreasing the chance of displacement (Fig. 37.5).

PLAQUE INSERTION FOR JUXTAPAPILLARY CHOROIDAL MELANOMAS

When an intraocular tumor touches the optic nerve, it is physically impossible for an eye plaque to be placed over the tumor's posterior margin (Fig. 37.6).[1] There have been two approaches to this problem. First, modified 'notched' plaques, which have the posterior aspect of the sidewall removed, can be used. This allows radiation to escape the plaque in the direction of the optic nerve. This may or may not be necessary because juxtapapillary plaques have been shown to 'tilt' back as they are pushed against the optic nerve.[14] However, this tilting will decrease the apical tumor dose and must be compensated for in dose calculations. Three-dimensional ultrasonic measurements of the tilted plaque's position (relative to the tumor) will increase the reliability of ophthalmic dosimetry in these challenging cases.[14]

We currently recommend enucleation as treatment of juxtapapillary melanomas in contact with greater than 90° of the optic nerve margin, because juxtapapillary tumors, especially small tumors adjacent to the optic nerve, carry the greatest risk for eye-plaque decentration (geographic miss). Clearly, these cases should be reserved for surgeons with extensive experience of posterior plaque placement. The risks and potential benefits associated with the use of notched plaques or teletherapy are also reviewed with each patient.

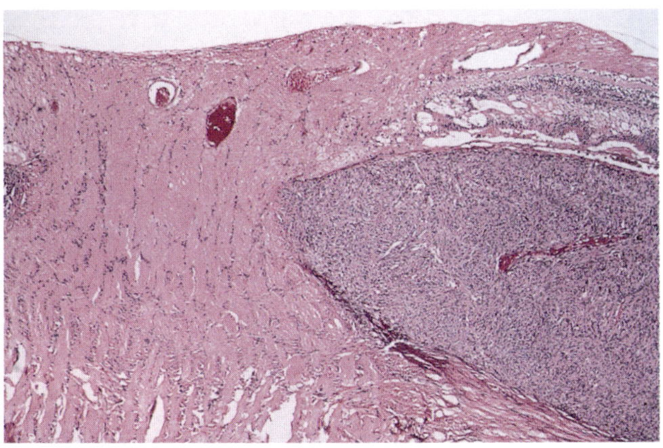

Figure 37.6 *Histopathology of an enucleated melanoma reveals that there is no method of placing an ophthalmic plaque to cover the posterior margin of a juxtapapillary tumor, much less a 2-mm margin.*

Clearly, nonplaque therapies should be considered for treatment of juxtapapillary melanomas and metastatic carcinomas. In general, most metastatic carcinomas to the uvea can be treated with EBRT, which offers excellent local control.

RADIATION COMPLICATIONS

Complications are affected by both radiotherapy-specific factors, (e.g. total dose, dose rate and dose volume) as well as tumor-related factors (e.g. tumor size, location and its biologically variable response to irradiation).[1] Because larger doses are commonly used in the treatment of melanoma versus retinoblastoma, radiation complications are more common in the treatment of choroidal melanomas. Radiation effects are often delayed and therefore the incidence of complications increases over time (follow-up).

Adnexal radiation complications are rarely associated with plaque radiotherapy. Transient eyelid edema and iridocyclitis have been noted. Late anterior segment complications have included dry eye, iris neovascularization, secondary glaucoma and cataract. Acute posterior segment or intraocular radiation complications have included secondary retinal detachment and hemorrhage (vitreous, retinal and/or choroidal). Common late posterior segment complications include both radiation retinopathy and optic neuropathy. Less common complications include strabismus, scleral atrophy and cystoid macular edema. Radiation therapy of choroidal melanomas can also induce (albeit rarely) exudative or hemorrhagic retinochoroidopathy.[1]

PROGNOSIS FOR VISION

Neovascular glaucoma, cataract, vitreous hemorrhage, tumor under the fovea, retinal detachment (primary and secondary), radiation retinopathy, optic neuropathy and secondary enucleation can all affect a patient's vision. Some of these conditions are found before treatment and can affect a patient's outcome after treatment. For example, any patient's vision can be improved when a pre-existing retinal detachment or vitreous hemorrhage resolves, or can be corrected (e.g. removal of cataract) after a tumor has been successfully irradiated. Unfortunately, radiation damage tends to occur after years of functional vision. It is a challenge to predict visual outcomes after ophthalmic radiation therapy.

It is reasonable to assume that treatment of larger tumors increases the size of the targeted zone and the amount of radiation delivered to all surrounding normal ocular structures. Therefore, larger tumors carry a poorer visual prognosis. Nasal tumors shift the targeted zone away from the macula, which decreases the incidence of radiation maculopathy and optic neuropathy. Shifting the targeted zone into the anterior segment (treatment of ciliary body tumors) decreases posterior segment complications.[1]

In general, plaque brachytherapy offers a good visual prognosis in the treatment of anterior tumors, particularly those located in the nasal quadrants. However, many uveal melanomas are located in the posterior pole and most retinoblastomas are either large or multifocal. This underscores the need for further research to decrease the amount of radiation required to treat intraocular tumors.[15–18]

NEW APPLICATIONS

HYPERTHERMIA

Enhancement of radiotherapy with hyperthermia may lead to a reduction in the amount of ionizing radiation needed to treat intraocular tumors.[15,19] This is because heat (hyperthermia) is a known radiation sensitizer.[15,20,21] It is reasonable to assume that dose reductions of adjuvant hyperthermia would decrease the incidence of ionizing radiation-associated complications noted after plaque radiotherapy (e.g. ^{60}Co, ^{106}Ru, ^{125}I, ^{103}Pd).[19]

Plaque-like antennas have been fashioned for placement on the sclera overlying intraocular tumors.[19,21] Two clinical case series reported that hyperthermia with plaque radiotherapy resulted in similar local control and rates of metastasis.[19,21] Complications included chorioretinal infarctions anterior to the tumor's base and lower intraocular pressure after treatment of anterior tumors.[19] Sixty-nine percent of our microwave thermoradiotherapy patients retained vision better than or equal to 20/200 (mean of 5 years' follow-up).[19] This retention of vision may have been related to the lower plaque-radiotherapy dose (average of 56 gray [Gy] to the apex of the tumor) given to those patients who received adjuvant microwave hyperthermia.

BRACHYTHERAPY IN THE TREATMENT OF RETINOBLASTOMA

Brachytherapy plays only a modest part in the treatment of retinoblastoma, in contrast to its major role in the management of medium-sized choroidal melanomas. Radiation physicists load radioactive seeds on the undersurface of a round or curved carrier applicator or plaque using tissue glue or another adhesive substance. The surgeon centers the plaque directly over the tumor and secures it with superficial scleral sutures. The exposure time (number of hours the plaque is in place over the tumor) is the variable in the formula to calculate the total dose delivered. If the particular seeds used have a high dose/rate ratio, then the hours of exposure are short. If the dose/rate ratio is low, then the plaque can be left in place longer to deliver the desired total dose.

The features of the tumor (in the eye to be radiated) are the determining factors in the decision between teletherapy and brachytherapy. In general, brachytherapy is most effectively used in anterior or equatorial focal disease with a relatively smaller tumor volume. In contrast, teletherapy (EBRT) is the treatment of choice when the retinoblastoma is posterior, diffuse, multifocal or large.

HISTORY OF BRACHYTHERAPY IN THE MANAGEMENT OF RETINOBLASTOMA

In 1930, Moore, Stallard and Milner treated an eye with retinoblastoma by inserting a radon seed into the eye through a puncture in the sclera. It is not surprising that this first trial of brachytherapy did not establish a pattern of treatment that was widely accepted for the management of retinoblastoma.[2,3] This group refined the surgical technique and in 1958 Stallard described embedding cobalt seeds in applicators designed to be sewn onto the sclera directly over the tumor.[22] Stallard published two reviews of brachytherapy in the treatment of retinoblastoma (in Britain) in the decade following introduction of what his colleagues called 'Stallard discs'.[23,24] Abramson and colleagues described the American (New York) experience with ^{60}Co plaques for a similar period (1951–1965) in their 1994 publication.[25]

BRACHYTHERAPY VS TELETHERAPY

Recently published data have raised significant questions refuting one argument for the exclusive use of EBRT when radiation of the eye is indicated. Previously, it had been assumed that radiating the whole retina somehow 'sterilized' that organ and prevented the development of new retinoblastoma tumors. However, in a recent series, newly arising tumors were observed 11 times in 34 eyes previously treated with EBRT. These authors comment that the traditional belief that EBRT can prophylactically treat the retina should be questioned seriously.[26]

HISTORY OF TELETHERAPY IN THE MANAGEMENT OF RETINOBLASTOMA

In 1903, Hilgartner made the first documented attempt to treat retinoblastoma with X-rays.[27] Eighty-four treatments of an unknown dose were given. According to Hilgartner, the tumor-filled right eye became phthisical and the small tumor in the left eye 'resorbed'. Good vision was retained for a time but the child was subsequently lost to follow-up.

Schoenberg described the second patient treated with teletherapy in 1919. He used a lateral port (entry site of the radiation is from the side through the lateral wall of the orbit).[28] The radioactive source was radium. Three years after treatment, the tumor had regressed and the vision was good. At 10 years, a cataract had been removed but useful vision was still present.[29] In 1944, however, 25 years after the treatment, Reese reported in his book that a 'scar tissue glioma' developed over the temporal radiation port and the patient died of metastatic disease from a second malignant neoplasm.[30]

Verhoeff described the third patient documented to have been treated with external radiation.[31] The child with bilateral tumors was diagnosed and treated at age 17 months. The right eye was enucleated and the tumor in the left eye was treated with a lateral port. Based on the results in this patient, Verhoeff made the point that it was probably hopeless to destroy a large retinoblastoma with radiation and that enucleation was the better choice of treatment. He suggested, however, that if the tumor in the other eye was smaller, radiation should be tried. Probably because of Verhoeff's pre-eminent position in ophthalmology, his treatment plan in this one patient was followed as a treatment dictum until the last 10 years.

OVERVIEW OF THE CURRENT ROLE OF BRACHYTHERAPY IN PEDIATRIC SOLID TUMORS

Brachytherapy may be underutilized in the management of pediatric solid tumors. In 1994, Fontanesi and colleagues observed that radiotherapy delivered through the use of interstitial, intracavitary or permanent placement of radioactive isotopes in adult oncology had become a common treatment modality based on improved local control and patient survival.[32] In contrast, pediatric oncologists used these same irradiation techniques infrequently in children with cancer, despite properties that allow highly focal irradiation delivery and significant reduction of dose to surrounding tissues.

These authors described their use of brachytherapy in pediatric oncology between the years 1981 and 1992 at St. Jude's Children's Research Hospital in Memphis.[32] They gave 50 brachytherapy sessions to 46 children. The most commonly treated tumor was rhabdomyosarcoma (14 cases), followed closely by soft-tissue sarcoma (10 cases) and retinoblastoma (10 cases). Brachytherapy was used as primary treatment in 11 cases, to boost previously given EBRT in 16 sites and to treat locally recurrent disease, metastatic sites or second malignant neoplasms in 23 sites.

The result of treatment in these 46 children was good. Disease-free intervals of 2–115 months' postimplantation (median of 41 months) were maintained in 43/50 sites. The seven local failures occurred 2–20 months' postimplantation, with a median of 6 months. Severe complications were observed in almost one-quarter of patients (12/43).[32]

RADIOACTIVE SOURCES OF ISOTOPES USED IN RETINOBLASTOMA

BRACHYTHERAPY

In 1930, a radon seed implanted into the vitreous by Moore and colleagues became the first radioactive source used for ophthalmic brachytherapy in the management of retinoblastoma.[2] However, this technique did not achieve wide acceptance. Individual seeds were difficult to handle and to implant. A complicating feature (radiation retinopathy), initially appearing years after radon seed implantation, has been described.[33]

The radioactive isotope ^{60}Co (first introduced in 1963) gradually replaced radon as the source and was to become the dominant isotope in radioactive plaques used to treat retinoblastoma until the early 1980s. The advantage of ^{60}Co was its ease of use and good therapeutic outcome. Its disadvantages included the fact that radiation was delivered to the surgeon's hands as well as to surrounding normal tissue, including orbital bone for 360°, because its radiation could not be shielded easily.

The low-energy radioisotope ^{125}I was first used for retinoblastoma in 1974. By the mid-1980s, Memorial Sloan-Kettering and most other major centers in North America had switched to ^{125}I in an effort to spare normal tissue and lower the rate of complications.[34] The low-energy photons emitted by ^{125}I seeds can be blocked completely by gold. The ^{125}I seeds are loaded on the underside of a gold plaque applicator, which serves as a shield for surrounding normal tissue (including orbital bone). This technique offers great potential benefit for those children with bilateral retinoblastoma who are particularly susceptible to radiation-induced second malignant neoplasms.

Another advantage of the low-energy ^{125}I is the short penetration depth of the radiation. Because most of the radiation has been attenuated before it reaches the opposite eye wall, ^{125}I is safer for surgeons, operating room personnel and the families of radiated children. A malleable oval lead eye-patch approximately 1/8-inch in thickness could be worn over the eye, thus shielding nursing mothers and other caregivers. The states of California and New York, unlike many other states, consider ^{125}I plaque brachytherapy to pose such little risk to the public that plaqued patients are allowed to travel the state highways and be treated as an outpatient for insertion and removal.

Palladium-103 is a low-energy radioisotope with characteristics similar to ^{125}I. Finger and colleagues reported a dosimetry study comparing the radioactive seeds of ^{103}Pd and ^{125}I in ophthalmic plaque therapy.[17] These authors concluded that the slightly lower energy photons (21 keV ^{103}Pd vs 28 keV ^{125}I) were absorbed more completely by the tumor and therefore fewer photons were available to damage normal tissue. Although ^{103}Pd photons have not been used to treat retinoblastoma, based on this information ^{103}Pd photons might have some advantages in this childhood intraocular tumor.

In Europe, two other isotopes, ^{106}Ru and ^{192}Ir have been more widely used than ^{125}I. Ruthenium-106 emits beta particles, which tend to travel a shorter distance (e.g. 5 mm) than ^{125}I or ^{103}Pd photons.[1] Although less radiation should reach the orbital bones in children, the ^{106}Ru source is not encased in or blocked by a gold seed-carrier, and the dose to the base of the tumor can be two to three times higher than with low-energy photons. Iridium-192 is a high-energy gamma emitter, which is available as a radioactive wire. Iridium-192 wire was employed by Madreperla et al to treat recurrent vitreous seeds at the vitreous base.[35]

DELIVERED RADIATION DOSE

TERMINOLOGY AND ABBREVIATIONS

'Rad' is an old term for absorbed radiation dose; 1 rad is equivalent to 0.01 J/kg or 0.01 Gy (gray) or 1 cGy (centigray). The gray (Gy), the current unit for absorbed radiation dose, is defined as the energy deposited in an object by radiation, divided by the mass of the object. The usual radiation dose for retinoblastoma in the old literature, approximately 4000 rads, would be equivalent to 4000 cGy or 40 Gy.

DOSE

Historically, the calculated dose delivered to the apex of a retinoblastoma (being treated primarily with brachytherapy) has been similar to the total dose given for primary EBRT, generally about 4000 cGy with a range of 3500–4500 cGy. A brachytherapy dose of 4000 cGy to the apex of a retinoblastoma means that the base of a 6- or 7-mm high tumor as well as the tumor vessels and retinal vessels in the radiation field receive a dose of nearly 8000 cGy. Although radiation retinopathy can be seen following the primary treatment of retinoblastoma, it is unusual. This is not the case if brachytherapy is used to consolidate a tumor following primary neoadjuvant chemotherapy (chemoreduction). The following section describes the dose adjustment required if brachytherapy follows platinum-based chemotherapy.

BRACHYTHERAPY FOLLOWING CARBOPLATIN-BASED SYSTEMIC CHEMOTHERAPY HAS AN INCREASED COMPLICATION RATE

Brachytherapy is one of the components of sequential additional local therapy (SALT), along with

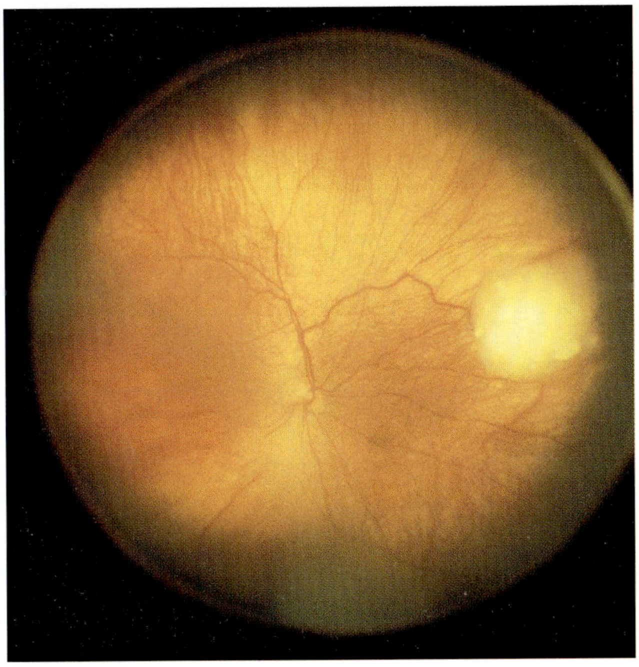

a

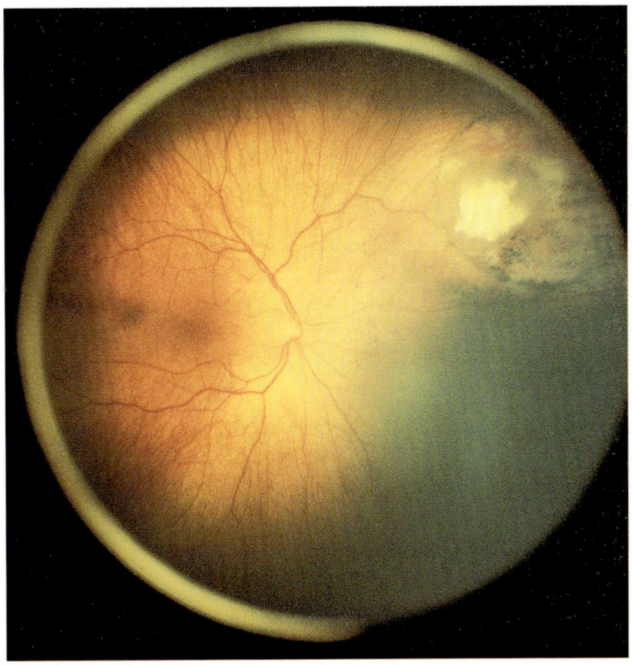

b

Figure 37.7 *(a) A peripheral unifocal retinoblastoma, which is an ideal candidate for brachytherapy. (b) Postplaque regression of the retinoblastoma (photographs taken with the RetCam, Massey Research Laboratories).*

cryotherapy and photocoagulation, currently used following chemoreduction (primary neoadjuvant chemotherapy) to consolidate the tumor kill.[40] Carboplatin is known to potentiate the effects of radiation.[36–40] In the first six eyes in which we used ^{125}I brachytherapy to deliver 4000 cGy to the apex after systemic carboplatin therapy, all six eventually developed significant vision loss from radiation retinopathy.[40] We plan to reduce the dose of delivered radiation to the range of 2500 cGy from 4000 cGy. Other groups treating patients in the same way (including Philadelphia [personal communication]) experienced the same complications. If brachytherapy is used within 1 year after carboplatin therapy, the dose of the radiation should be adjusted downward.

INDICATIONS FOR BRACHYTHERAPY IN INTRAOCULAR RETINOBLASTOMA PRIMARY TREATMENT

Brachytherapy is indicated as primary treatment *only* when there is a solitary retinoblastoma measuring less than 10–15 mm at the base and extending into the vitreous no more than 8–10 mm *and* located outside the posterior pole of the eye *and* vitreous seeding is absent or detectable only within 2 mm of the tumor surface *and* the other eye is not being treated primarily by chemotherapy (Fig. 37.7). In view of these indications, it is not surprising that Balmer and associates treated only six of 153 retinoblastoma eyes primarily with brachytherapy.[41] In Los Angeles, we used brachytherapy as primary treatment in only eight of more than 200 consecutively treated eyes (unpublished data).

RECURRENT DISEASE FOLLOWING EBRT

Brachytherapy has been tried, usually without great success, to salvage eyes with recurrent retinoblastoma following teletherapy (Fig. 37.8). If the EBRT dose is more than 40 Gy, the addition of another 20 or 30 Gy via brachytherapy will lead to radiation retinopathy in the large majority of eyes so treated. In addition, if this generally radiosensitive tumor survives the first radiation treatment, radioresistant tumor clones are likely to be present in the recurrent disease.

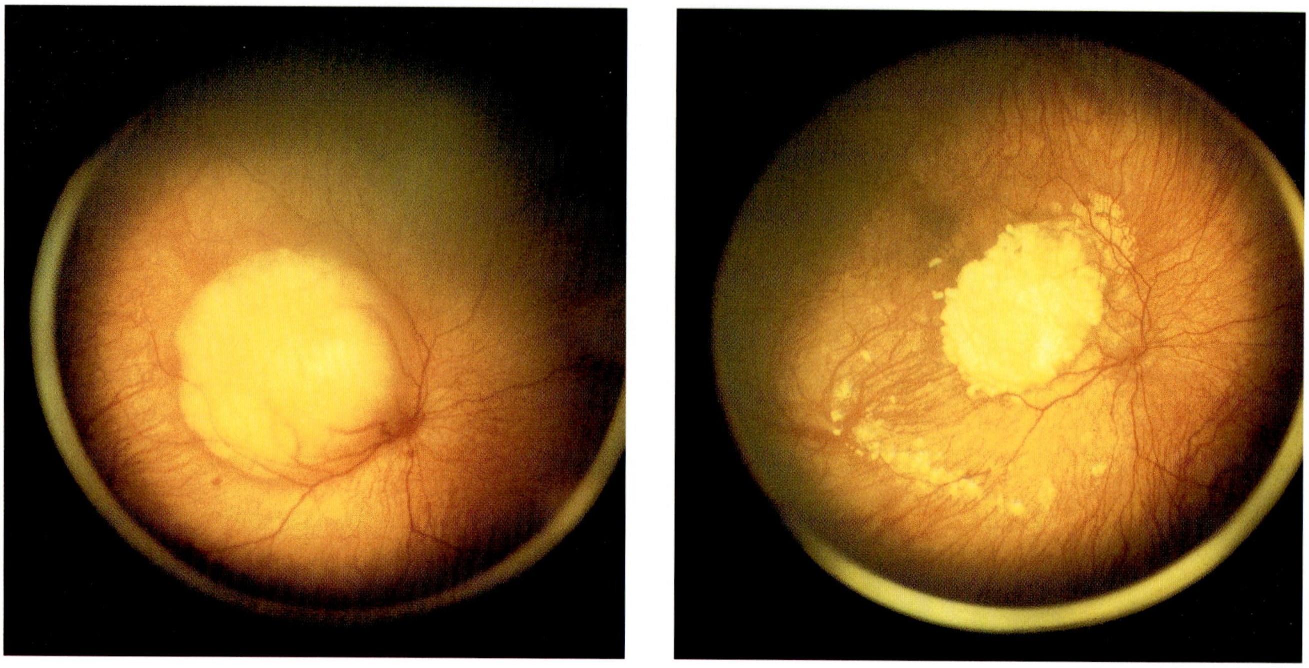

a b

Figure 37.8 *(a) A posterior unilateral recurrent retinoblastoma. (b) Treatment with brachytherapy is an option in this poorly sighted eye. In this case, the parents did not want either external beam radiotherapy or enucleation.*

CONSOLIDATION OR RECURRENT DISEASE FOLLOWING CHEMOREDUCTION

When systemic chemotherapy was first used as primary neoadjuvant therapy to reduce the volume of intraocular tumor, brachytherapy was considered a major modality for successful consolidation with SALT, along with cryotherapy and laser photocoagulation. We were initially surprised to see radiation retinopathy in the first six eyes in which we used ^{125}I radioactive plaques to deliver 40 Gy to the apex of the residual tumor mass as part of SALT, and discontinued the use of standard dose brachytherapy following chemotherapy. Similar experiences were seen in Philadelphia and London.

It is clear that chemotherapy, especially carboplatin, potentiates the effect of radiotherapy: brachytherapy more than teletherapy. To avoid these complications, we have decreased the dose delivered to the apex of the tumor following chemoreduction by almost half, to 25 Gy. Care should be exercised before full doses of brachytherapy are delivered within 1 year of the child having received systemic chemotherapy.

RECURRENT DISEASE FOLLOWING CRYOTHERAPY OR PHOTOCOAGULATION

Perhaps the single most common and safest use of brachytherapy is for recurrent intraocular disease outside the posterior pole. Typically, the recurrence follows the treatment of a small anterior lesion with one to three sessions of cryotherapy. If recurrent disease is associated with localized vitreous seeding, radioactive plaque therapy is the only effective local treatment modality remaining.

INDICATIONS FOR BRACHYTHERAPY IN RECURRENT ORBITAL RETINOBLASTOMA

Brachytherapy has been used to treat orbital retinoblastoma in three innovative ways. In 1993, Bentel and colleagues at Duke implanted a single ^{125}I seed in a methylmethacrylate sphere that was implanted surgically in the orbit to treat locally recurrent orbital disease in the presence of a fellow eye with good vision.[42] Sealy and colleagues in Capetown treated patients with histologic evidence of high risk of recurrent orbital disease with a different orbital implant.[43] The South African implant consisted of six partially shielded tubes around the periphery of the orbit and one unshielded tube in the center. The shields of the peripheral tubes protected the orbital bones from radiation. In Los Angeles, we have positioned individual tubes containing partially shielded ^{125}I seeds under computed tomography control to surround recurrent orbital disease (unpublished data).

INDIVIDUAL CASE PLANNING

DATA GATHERING FOR PREPARATION OF THE TREATMENT PLAN

Once the decision has been made to treat an eye with a radioactive plaque, a specific treatment plan must be prepared. This is done by the radiation physicist, with critical input from the plaquing surgeon. The physicist must have precise information about the size of the eye, the location, shape and size of the tumor and its distance from vital intraocular structures. This information comes from a variety of sources. An accurate retinal drawing is prepared, noting precisely the distance in disc diameters and millimeters of each tumor edge from the optic nerve, the fovea and the lens, as well as the circumferential and radial diameters of the tumor in millimeters.

From the orbital computed tomography scan taken as part of the diagnostic work-up, the exact size of the child's eye can be determined. Ultrasonography provides the height or apex of the tumor and retinal examination and photographs provide the diameter of the base. Before the availability of the wide-angle RetCam© (Massie Research Laboratories, Pleasanton, CA), the 30° Zeiss or Topcon fundus cameras provided little help in documenting retinoblastoma photographically. With the RetCam©, a single 8 × 10 print of a 90–110° view can be used for treatment planning.

BEBIG PLAQUE PLANNING SOFTWARE

The most widely used commercially available software for plaque planning was written by Astrahan and is marketed by the German company BEBIG, GmbH, Berlin.[44,45] The software, written for and running on the Mac OS, allows three-dimensional reconstruction of the patient's eye by the computer. The computed tomography image of the globe is scanned into the software. The digital retinal image from the RetCam© then is applied to the inner surface of the patient's virtual eye. Ultrasonographic measurements allow precise assignment of the tumor apex.

From the three-dimensional model of the patient's eye and tumor, the distances from the tumor to the nerve, fovea, lens and limbus can be calculated precisely. A model of the prepared plaque then can be positioned over the tumor with virtual ^{125}I seeds with activity matching those to be used in the surgery. Isodose curves are calculated and recalculated instantaneously as the seeds are repositioned. The best fit can be determined easily to give the planned radiation dose to the tumor with the smallest dose to the vital structures within the eye.

PLAQUE CONFIGURATION AND PREPARATION

Scleral applicators or 'plaques' are constructed in a great many sizes and shapes. Some centers custom-make plaques for each tumor. Others use different-sized round plaques with or without the plastic spacers commonly used in the Collaborative Ocular Melanoma Study.[46] A posterior notch can be manufactured for treatment of juxtapapillary tumors.

At the University of Southern California we have used a slightly rounded and curved rectangle for ^{125}I ophthalmic brachytherapy for more than 15 years (Fig. 37.9). This plaque has a posterior notch for the

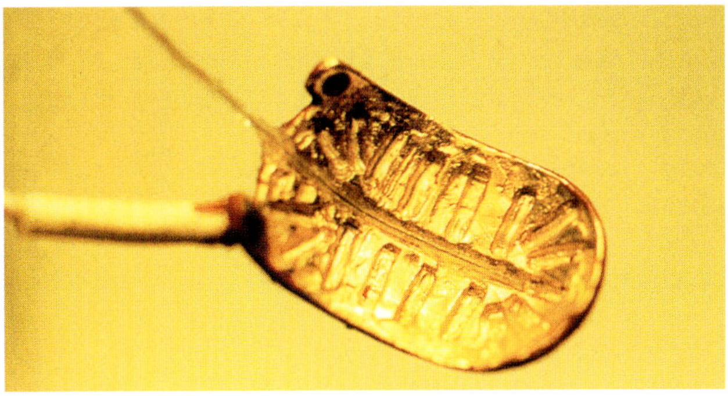

Figure 37.9 *The usual type of eye plaque used at the University of Southern California, with an electrical connector near one suture eyelet and a temperature probe in the center groove. This plaque can deliver ^{125}I with localized current field hyperthermia.[19] The seeds can be loaded in the anterior, middle or posterior slots, depending on the location of the tumor.*

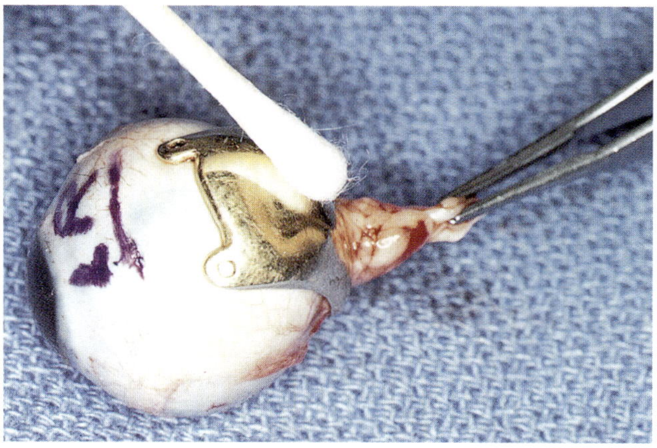

Figure 37.10 *A view of the other side of the type of plaque used at the University of Southern California showing how it would fit on the sclera. In this photograph, there is a notch that fits snugly around the optic nerve (not seen). The anterior eyelets are approximately 6–7 mm posterior to the lateral rectus (LR) insertion in this eye that has just been enucleated for retinoblastoma.*

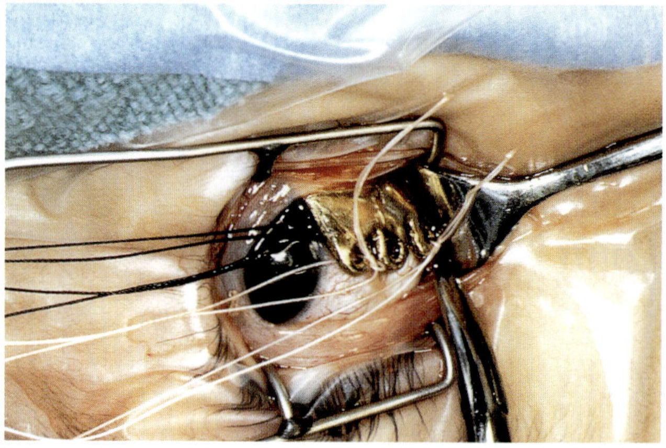

Figure 37.11 *Insertion of the gold plaque loaded with ^{125}I seeds. The plaque is slipped between the elevated conjunctiva and the sclera. It will be tied temporarily until the exact position is achieved.*

optic nerve. In enucleated globes, when the posterior notch is snugly around the optic nerve, the anterior edge of the 10-mm wide plaque lies at the insertion of the medial rectus muscle on the nasal aspect of the globe and at a point 7 mm posterior to the lateral rectus insertion on the temporal side (Fig. 37.10).

Differential loading of the seeds allows the convenience of one plaque to be a useful applicator for many different tumor sizes and locations. With the plaque used at the University of Southern California, an anterior tumor would be approached by loading radioactive seeds only in the anterior slots (Fig. 37.11). Determination of how many seeds and exactly where they should be loaded is part of the plaque planning software described below.

One of the least welcome features of plaque brachytherapy is the extremely high dose of radiation required at the sclera to deliver tumoricidal doses to the apex of the larger tumors. This feature is a result of the additive effect of the ^{125}I photons, which radiate from each seed at an angle greater than 30–45° away from the photons entering the eye perpendicular to the sclera. As the lateral spread of radiation from each seed adds to that from every other seed, the total dose to the base is high and radiation complications increase. A new plaque at the University of Southern California partially solves the problem of overlapping radiation near the plaque surface by sinking the seeds into a deeper slot in the gold plaque.[47] The walls of the deeper slots then serve as a shield to the unwanted lateral spread of photons from each seed, resulting in much better columniation of the radiation from the plaque. Although not perfect, these new slotted plaques go a long way toward delivering no more radiation at the base of a tumor than the apex receives. They should also contribute to significantly less radiation retinopathy associated with ocular brachytherapy.

SURGICAL IMPLANTATION

CONCEPT

The purpose of the surgery is to sew the applicator or plaque loaded with radioactive sources (usually called seeds) temporarily to the episcleral surface centered over the tumor to be radiated. The radioactive seeds are closest to the sclera and in the case of ^{125}I the gold plaque blocks radiation to normal orbital tissue. The length of time the plaque is left in place is calculated by the physicist planning the treatment and will vary depending on the activity of the radioactive seeds.

APPROACH

The surgical approach to implantation of a radioactive plaque in a child with retinoblastoma is little different from the approach used to center the plaque on the sclera directly over choroidal melanomas in adults. There are small differences, however. For obvious reasons, both implantation and removal of the plaque must be done with the infant or small child under general anesthesia. The thick round plaques with the plastic spacers used commonly in adults treated in the Collaborative Ocular Melanoma Study often cannot be used easily because of the small orbit and limited space in children.

A 360° peritomy is recommended for best exposure. Traction sutures are placed beneath the appropriate adjacent rectus muscles if the base of the tumor to be plaqued is localized exactly between them. Most commonly, at least one rectus muscle will need to be removed at its insertion for adequate exposure of the base of the tumor. The same technique and sutures (double arm 6-0 Vicryl) that a strabismus surgeon uses for rectus muscle recessions are appropriate.

DETERMINING THE CORRECT POSITION OF THE PLAQUE

The entire procedure described below to determine the correct position of the plaque on the sclera is done with an unloaded or 'cold' plaque that is identical in size and shape to the 'hot' plaque. The use of a cold (sometimes referred to as a 'dummy') plaque minimizes unnecessary radiation exposure to the patient and to the surgeon. Only after the cold plaque has been sutured temporarily into position and the appropriateness of that position has been checked by scleral depression along each edge of the plaque does the loaded 'hot' plaque replace it.

Once exposure of the sclera overlying the base of the tumor has been accomplished, the technique of transpupillary transillumination is not useful for localizing retinoblastoma. Unlike pigmented choroidal melanoma, retinoblastoma is nonpigmented and does not create a transillumination defect. The surgeon determines the general location of the tumor and, with the use of scleral depression and indirect ophthalmoscopy, outlines the edge of the tumor on the scleral surface with a surgical marking pen. The distance from the limbus to the anterior edge of the tumor as marked on the sclera is checked against the prediction of the pre-prepared software prediction. The surgeon then marks the position of the edge of the plaque and the location of the suture eyelets before passing the preplaced 4-0 or 5-0 nonabsorbable sutures. A spatula needle is used and the sutures are passed in such a way that the needle exits the sclera in the center of the plaque eyelet mark. The surgeon secures the cold plaque with temporary ties of the sutures and then again uses ophthalmoscopy and scleral depression along the edges to confirm correct centering of the plaque over the tumor.

INSERTING THE 'HOT' PLAQUE

Once the correct location has been confirmed, the surgeon removes the dummy plaque and secures the 'hot' plaque with the preplaced sutures. If a rectus muscle has been removed and its insertion is exposed, it can be reattached and allowed to hang back over the plaque during the few days when the plaque is in place. The muscle then is tied temporarily and a considerable length of Vicryl suture is left. Then, upon removal of the plaque, the muscle can be pulled up and tied to its original insertion.

CLOSURE AND POSTOPERATIVE OCULAR CARE

The conjunctiva is pulled forward and secured to the superficial sclera near the limbus. Because the bulk of the plaque may cause tension on the conjunctiva, simply closing the conjunctiva similarly to closure at the end of strabismus surgery may not be adequate to prevent dehiscence and exposure of the plaque.

Subconjunctival antibiotics and steroids are injected/irrigated beneath the conjunctiva at the end of the case. Antibiotic ointment is applied to the corneal surface and the eye patch is closed with at least two eye pads. A malleable 1/8-inch thick oval lead shield is shaped to cover the eye pads and taped into place. The eye patch should be changed and antibiotic/steroid drops instilled into the eye three to four times per day.

PLAQUE REMOVAL

Plaque removal is scheduled as close as possible to the hour when the required dose has been delivered. Because a typical dose/rate ratio for ^{125}I is 50 cGy/hour, removing the plaque 1 or 2 hours on either side of the scheduled time creates no problem. Generally, quick removal of the plaque can be done under topical/local anesthesia with intravenous sedation in an adult. A retrobulbar injection may be difficult or impossible because of the presence of the plaque in the orbit. Good intravenous sedation combined with topical and subconjunctival local anesthesia is usually adequate to open the conjunctiva painlessly for 140–180° and to cut the nonabsorbable sutures. Of course, a child requires general anesthesia. The surgeon grasps the edge of the plaque with heavy forceps and gently slides it from beneath the conjunctiva. If a rectus muscle has been tied temporarily to its insertion and allowed to hang back, it can be untied, advanced to its original position and retied. The conjunctiva is then closed in the usual way. Antibiotics are applied and the eye is covered with a simple patch.

ENSURING THAT ALL RADIOACTIVE SEEDS ARE SUCCESSFULLY REMOVED

The surgeon and radiation physicist must ascertain that all radioactive sources are removed successfully from the patient. Upon removal of the plaque, the surgeon counts the number of implanted seeds before depositing the plaque into its lead carrier or 'pig'. Once the 'pig' is covered and removed from the vicinity of the operating table, the radiation physicist checks the patient with a Geiger counter for evidence of retained radiation sources. Only if this check of the patient and the room is clear can the radiation exposure be certified as completed.

EXTERNAL BEAM RADIATION TREATMENT OUTCOMES FOR COMPARISON WITH BRACHYTHERAPY

Direct comparisons are not possible between EBRT and brachytherapy outcomes because EBRT is generally used to treat more advanced disease (Fig. 37.10). In 1996, Hernandez and colleagues described the outcomes from the Philadelphia series using EBRT.[26] The dose was 45 Gy. Overall, only 44% of 34 eyes were controlled locally with EBRT alone. Minimal disease fared well (local control was obtained in 78% of Reese/Ellsworth Group 1 and Group 2 eyes) whereas more advanced disease outcomes with EBRT alone were dismal (20% of eyes in Reese-Ellsworth Groups 3–5). When EBRT was combined with salvage therapy, including plaque, cryotherapy and photocoagulation, the overall ocular survival rate improved from 44% to 73%.

BRACHYTHERAPY TREATMENT OUTCOMES

Because different isotopes have been used, depending upon timing and location of the patient series, outcomes will be presented separately.

COBALT-60 BRACHYTHERAPY OUTCOMES

In 1983 Buys and colleagues presented the New York experience with ^{60}Co. They treated 31 eyes of 30 patients with plaques. Salvage of the eye was possible in 29 of the 30 patients.[48]

Fass and colleagues described the outcome of treating *only recurrent* retinoblastoma with cobalt plaque.[34] Eighty-five patients were plaqued in their series between 1968 and 1987. Seventy-two of the 85 patients had failed EBRT. Time from initial treatment to failure ranged from 13 to 60 months. The median dose was 40 Gy, with a range of 30–50 Gy. Eyes were salvaged in 55 of the 85 patients. Twenty-two of the 30 enucleated eyes had progression of disease. The other eight eyes had radiation retinopathy with or without progression of the retinoblastoma.

Abramson used a cobalt plaque as primary brachytherapy treatment in only one of 48 patients with conservative management of unilateral retinoblastoma.[49]

IODINE-125 BRACHYTHERAPY OUTCOMES

The same series of 103 eyes treated with ^{125}I plaques from Philadelphia has been described in multiple publications. Hernandez was the senior author of the paper that best described outcomes.[50] Thirty-one of the 103 eyes were treated with primary brachytherapy and five of the 31 (16%) experienced recurrence. In 72 eyes plaqued because of recurrent disease, eight of 72 (11%) had recurrence.

TUMOR REGRESSION PATTERNS FOLLOWING BRACHYTHERAPY

Regression patterns following treatment with ^{60}Co were described in 1983.[48] In 31 treated eyes, 15 (50%) showed Type I regression (calcium only). Only one of the 31 (3%) eyes developed Type II regression (fish-flesh). Five patients (16%) had a combination of calcium and fish-flesh (Type III). Nine patients (29%) had only a flat chorioretinal scar, which the authors labeled type IV.

RADIATION RETINOPATHY FOLLOWING BRACHYTHERAPY

Archer and colleagues reported localized radiation retinopathy many years after radon seed implantation in two patients.[33] In a report of the complications seen following cobalt plaques, Fass and colleagues from New York reported radiation retinopathy in about 10% of 85 plaqued eyes.[34] Seventy-two of those eyes had received previous EBRT. In the series of 103 plaques from Philadelphia, the incidence of radiation retinopathy is not described. In our series of six ^{125}I plaques used as consolidation following chemoreduction, all six eyes developed radiation retinopathy when a dose of 40 Gy was delivered to the apex of the tumor.[40]

POTENTIATION OF THE EFFECT OF BRACHYTHERAPY

Numerous radiosensitizers are known. Low-dose carboplatin is known to increase the effect of radiation. Heat is another well-known radiosensitizer. Liggett and colleagues have combined localized current field hyperthermia and brachytherapy in the treatment of melanoma.[21] We have used their technique in two eyes with retinoblastoma. Laser-generated hyperthermia has been combined with brachytherapy and holds some potential for decreasing the total dose of radiation needed.

DISCUSSION

Plaque radiation therapy can spare vision, both monocular and binocular (central and/or peripheral), and offers the cosmetic benefit of globe retention. No prospective randomized clinical studies have determined the impact of radiotherapy versus enucleation on quality of life, the incidence of metastases or which form of plaque radiotherapy offers the most acceptable complication rate. Ophthalmic plaque radiotherapy offers a method to deliver localized radiation of small- and medium-sized intraocular tumors. Brachytherapy can be useful in controlling the growth of intraocular tumors, retaining useful vision and allowing cosmetic retention of the globe in selected cases.

REFERENCES

1. Finger PT. Radiation therapy for choroidal melanoma, *Surv Ophthalmol* (1997) **42:**215–32.
2. Moore RF. Choroidal sarcoma treated by the intraocular insertion of radon seeds, *Br J Ophthalmol* (1930) **14:**145–52.
3. Moore RF, Stallard HB. Milner JG. Retinal gliomata treated by radon seeds, *Br J Ophthalmol* (1931) **15:**673–96.
4. Kindy-Degnan N, Char DH, Swift P, et al. Bromodeoxyuridine uptake in the assessment of hyperthermic therapy for intraocular tumor, *Arch Ophthalmol* (1989) **107:**746–50.
5. Char DH, Crawford JB, Kaleta-Michaels S, et al. Analysis of radiation failure after uveal melanoma brachytherapy, *Am J Ophthalmol* (1989) **108:**712–16.
6. Stallard HB. Radiotherapy for malignant melanoma of the choroid, *Br J Ophthalmol* (1966) **50:**147–55.
7. Stallard HB. Malignant melanoblastoma of the choroid, *Bibl Ophthalmol* (1968) **7:**16–38.
8. Lommatzsch PK. Results after beta-irradiation (^{106}RU/^{106}RL) of choroidal melanomas: 20 years' experience, *Br J Ophthalmol* (1986) **70:**844–51.
9. Lommatzsch P. ^{106}Ru/^{106}Rh plaque radiotherapy for malignant melanomas of the choroid: with follow-up results more than 5 years, *Doc Ophthalmol* (1988) **68:**225–38.
10. Packer S, Stoller S, Lesser ML, et al. Long-term results of iodine 125 irradiation of uveal melanoma, *Ophthalmology* (1992) **99:**767–74.
11. Gragoudas ES, Seddon JM, Egan K, et al. Long-term results of proton beam irradiated uveal melanomas, *Ophthalmology* (1987) **94:** 349–53.
12. Char DH, Castro JR, Kroll SM, et al. Five-year follow-up of helium ion therapy for uveal melanoma, *Arch Ophthalmol* (1990) **108:**209–14.
13. Finger PT, Moshfeghi DM, Ho TK. Palladium 103 ophthalmic plaque radiotherapy, *Arch Ophthalmol* (1991) **109:**1610–13.
14. Finger PT, Romero JM, Rosen RB, et al. Three-dimensional ultrasonography of choroidal melanomas: localization of radioactive eye plaques, *Arch Ophthalmol* (1998) **116:**305–12.
15. Finger PT. Thermoradiotherapy for eye tumors. In: Seegenschmidt MH, Fessenden P, Vernon CC, eds, *Medical Radiology, Thermoradiotherapy and Thermochemotherapy*, Vol.2 (Springer-Verlag: Berlin, 1996): 175–85.
16. Finger PT, Ho TK, Fastenberg DM, et al. Intraocular radiation blocking, *Invest Ophthalmol Vis Sci* (1990) **31:**1724–30.
17. Finger PT, Lu DF, Buffa A, et al. Palladium 103 versus iodine 125 for ophthalmic plaque radiotherapy, *Int J Rad Oncol Biol Phys* (1993) **27:**849–54.
18. Finger PT, Buffa A, Mishra S, et al. Palladium 103 plaque radiation therapy for uveal melanoma: clinical experience, *Ophthalmology* (1994) **101:**256–63.

19. Finger PT. Microwave thermoradiotherapy for uveal melanoma: results of a 10–year study, *Ophthalmology* (1997) **104:**1794–1803.
20. Coleman DJ, Lizzi FL, Burgess SE, et al. Ultrasonic hyperthermia and radiation in the management of intraocular malignant melanoma, *Am J Ophthalmol* (1986) **101:**635–42.
21. Liggett PE, Ma C, Astrahan M, et al. Combined localized current field hyperthermia and irradiation for intraocular tumors, *Ophthalmology* (1991) **98:**1830–6.
22. Stallard HB. Retinoblastoma treated by radio-active applicators, *Acta XVIII Conc Ophthalmol Belg* (1958) **2:**1360–9.
23. Stallard HB. The treatment of retinoblastoma, *Ophthalmologica* (1966) **151:**214–30.
24. Stallard HB. The treatment of retinoblastoma, *Bibl Ophthalmol* (1968) **75:**149–73.
25. Abramson DH, Niksarli K, Ellsworth RM, Servodidio CA. Changing trends in the management of retinoblastoma: 1951–1965 vs 1966–1980, *J Pediatr Ophthalmol Strabismus* (1994) **31:**32–7.
26. Hernandez JC, Brady LW, Shields JA, et al. External beam radiation for retinoblastoma: results, patterns of failure, and a proposal for treatment guidelines, *Int J Radiat Oncol Biol Phys* (1996) **35:**125–32.
27. Hilgartner HL. Report of a case of double glioma treated with x-ray, *Texas State J Med* (1902–1903) **18:**322.
28. Schoenberg MJ. A case of bilateral glioma of the retina apparently arrested in the non-enucleated eye by radium treatment, *Arch Ophthalmol* (1919) **48:**485–8.
29. Schoenberg MJ. Report on a case of bilateral glioma of the retina cured in the non-enucleated eye by radium treatment, *Arch Ophthalmol* (1927) **56:**221–8.
30. Reese AB. *Tumors of the Eye* (Paul R. Hoeber, Inc: New York, 1951): 67–143.
31. Verhoeff FH. Glioma retinae treated by X-rays with apparent destruction of the tumor and preservation of vision, *Arch Ophthalmol* (1921) **50:**450–6.
32. Fontanesi J, Rao BN, Fleming ID, et al. Pediatric brachytherapy: the St. Jude's Children's Research Hospital experience, *Cancer* (1994) **74:**733–9.
33. Archer DB, Amoaku WM, Kelly G. Choroidoretinal neovascularisation following radon seed treatment of retinoblastoma in two patients, *Br J Ophthalmol* (1993) **77:**95–9.
34. Fass D, McCormick B, Abramson D, Ellsworth R. Cobalt 60 plaques in recurrent retinoblastoma, *Int J Radiat Oncol Biol Phys* (1991) **21:**625–7.
35. Madreperla SA, Hungerford JL, Doughty D, et al. Treatment of retinoblastoma vitreous base seeding, *Ophthalmology* (1998) **105:**120–4.
36. Muderspach LI, Curtin JP, Roman LD. Carboplatin as a radiation sensitizer in locally advanced cervical cancer: a pilot study, *Gynecol Oncol* (1997) **65:**336–42.
37. Ewend MG, Williams JA, Tabassi K. Local delivery of chemotherapy and concurrent external beam radiotherapy prolongs survival in metastatic brain tumor models, *Cancer Res* (1996) **56:**5217–23.
38. Murray TG, Roth DB, O'Brien JM. Local carboplatin and radiation therapy in the treatment of murine transgenic retinoblastoma, *Arch Ophthalmol* (1996) **114:**1385–9.
39. Sciuto R, Maini CL, Tofani A, et al. Radiosensitization with low-dose carboplatin enhances pain palliation in radioisotope therapy with strontium-89, *Nucl Med Commun* (1996) **17:**799–804.
40. Murphree AL, Villablanca JG, Deegan WF 3rd. Chemotherapy plus local treatment in the management of intraocular retinoblastoma, *Arch Ophthalmol* (1996) **114:**1348–56.
41. Balmer A, Gailloud C, Potter P, et al. Treatment of retinoblastoma and results: Lausanne 1963–1989, *Klin Monatsbl Augenheilkd* (1990) **196:**374–6.
42. Bentel GC, Halperin EC, Buckley EG. ^{125}I embedded in an orbital prosthesis for retreatment of recurrent retinoblastoma, *Med Dosim* (1993) **18:**1–5.
43. Sealy R, Stannard C, Shackleton D. Improved cosmesis in retinoblastoma patients treated with iodine-125 orbital irradiation, *Ophthalmic Paediatr Genet* (1987) **8:**95–9.
44. Astrahan MA, Luxton G, Jozsef G, et al. An interactive treatment planning system for ophthalmic plaque radiotherapy, *Int J Radiat Oncol Biol Phys* (1990) **18:**679–87.
45. Astrahan MA, Luxton G, Jozsef G, et al. Optimization of ^{125}I ophthalmic plaque brachytherapy, *Med Phys* (1990) **17:**1053–7.
46. Earle J, Kline RW, Robertson DM. Selection of iodine 125 for the Collaborative Ocular Melanoma Study, *Arch Ophthalmol* (1987) **105:**763–4.
47. Astrahan MA, Luxton G, Pu Q, Petrovich Z. Conformal episcleral plaque therapy, *Int J Rad Oncol Biol Phys* (1997) **39:**505–19.
48. Buys RJ, Abramson DH, Ellsworth RM, Haik B. Radiation regression patterns after cobalt plaque insertion for retinoblastoma, *Arch Ophthalmol* (1983) **101:**1206–8.
49. Abramson DH, Marks RF, Ellsworth RM, et al. The management of unilateral retinoblastoma without primary enucleation, *Arch Ophthalmol* (1982) **100:**1249–52.
50. Hernandez JC, Brady LW, Shields CL, et al. Conservative treatment of retinoblastoma: the use of plaque brachytherapy, *Am J Clin Oncol* (1993) **16:**397–401.

Part IX Surgical Techniques in Trauma

Chapter 38 Management of hyphema, repair of iridodialysis, and repair of corneoscleral lacerations

Thomas M Aaberg Jr and Patrick E Rubsamen

INTRODUCTION

Many factors determine the eventual anatomic and visual outcome of an eye after incurring trauma. A number of these factors are defined by the extent and nature of the injury. However, the outcome may be modified by the surgical approach. This chapter addresses the assessment and surgical management of traumatic hyphema, iridodialysis and corneoscleral lacerations.

TRAUMATIC HYPHEMA

PREOPERATIVE EVALUATION

As with all ocular trauma, a good history of the inciting injury is important in determining the mechanism and extent of the injury. In the setting of traumatic hyphema, critical issues to address in the history are the mechanism of injury (blunt vs sharp or penetrating), the severity (poke vs severe blow to the head) and any medical history of bleeding diatheses (Coumadin use) or hemoglobinopathies (sickle-cell disease).

A complete examination of both eyes and a general examination of the patient's overall health and stability are critical in any trauma patient. Patients with traumatic hyphema may have sustained blunt trauma to the head, potentially resulting in a closed head injury. Particularly in the elderly population, who are prone to falling and predisposed to subdural hematoma, the mental status and a neurologic screening examination are necessary. Once the patient's stability has been established, the ophthalmic examination can be performed. Visual acuity and particularly a pupillary examination may alert the examining physician to more extensive pathology, such as suprachoroidal hemorrhage, occult scleral rupture or traumatic optic neuropathy. Slit-lamp biomicroscopy is essential to characterize better the size and appearance of the hyphema and any concurrent ocular pathology. Because traumatic hyphema results from tearing of iris or ciliary body structures as the eye is compressed and the lens–iris diaphragm is displaced posteriorly, the physician should look specifically for concurrent sphincter ruptures, iridodialysis, cyclodialysis, angle recession and zonular dialysis.

The size of a hyphema can range from a microhyphema (free-floating red blood cells without any significant layering) to a total hyphema (completely filling the anterior chamber). The hyphema color and liquefaction provide information on aqueous circulation and the age of the clot (Fig. 38.1). A black clot ('eight-ball hyphema') suggests deoxygenated

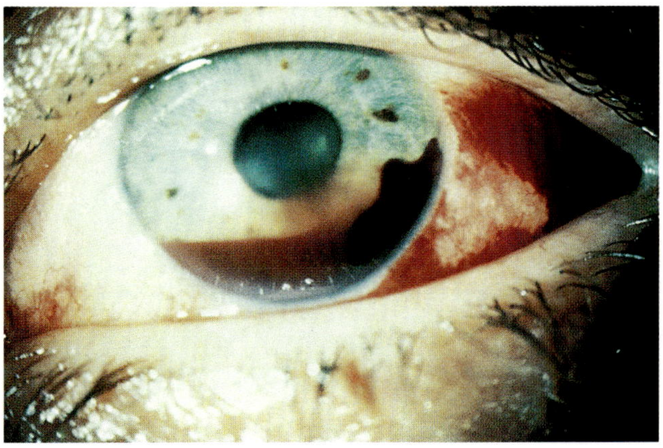

Figure 38.1 *Layered hyphema.*

hemoglobin and poor aqueous circulation; oxygenated blood will be red and implies some degree of aqueous turnover. This information is important in the timing of surgical intervention because 'eight-ball' hyphemas may lead to pressure spikes and corneal bloodstaining sooner. As opposed to a fixed-formed clot, a liquefied clot, which has layers in the most dependent part of the eye and moves freely, has already undergone lysis and probably presents less risk of rebleeding.

If there is a question of more extensive ocular pathology that cannot be assessed because of media opacities, imaging studies may be useful. In many centers, computed tomography (CT) is considered the single most useful imaging study. CT scanning can image scleral abnormalities, intraocular blood, intraocular or orbital foreign bodies and fractures of the bony orbit. The most comprehensive CT scan orbital study includes 1–1.5-mm axial and coronal cuts through the orbits and chiasm. CT is limited, however, by beam hardening artifacts from metal (e.g. foreign body or dental fillings) and poor resolution of plastic and wooden foreign bodies.

Echography is a user-dependent imaging modality that is less expensive, dynamic and readily available. It is particularly useful in assessing the posterior segment of traumatized eyes with media opacities (Fig. 38.2). Echography has resolution up to 1 mm and can detect intraocular foreign bodies, lens rupture, retinal detachment and choroidal hemorrhage. Posterior ruptures can be detected in many cases; however, up to 25% of cases may be missed.[10] Echographic clues that increase the likelihood of a posterior rupture include incarcerated vitreous, retinal thickening, irregular scleral contours, decreased scleral reflectivity and episcleral hemorrhage in the adjacent space.

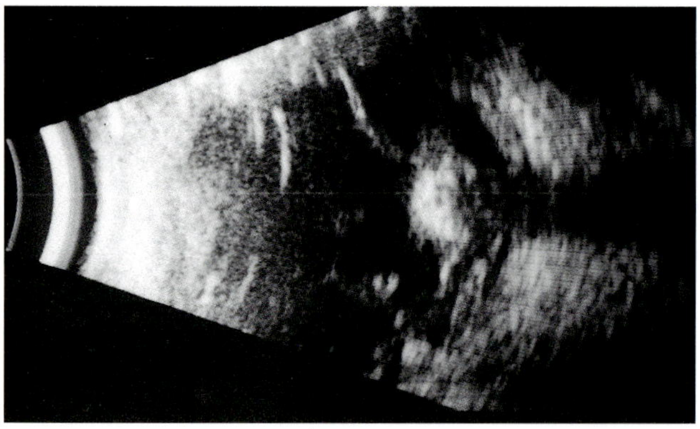

Figure 38.2 *Echo of traumatized eye with vitreous tracking to posterior rupture site, and vitreous hemorrhage.*

Table 38.1 Laboratory tests for selected patients with hyphema

Sickle preparation
Hemoglobin electrophoresis
Prothrombin time
Partial thromboplastin time
Bleeding time

Selected patients with traumatic hyphema should have a directed laboratory work-up (Table 38.1). Black patients who have not been tested for sickle-cell disease should have a sickle preparation or hemoglobin electrophoresis. In patients with a known bleeding diathesis, blood coagulation tests (partial thromboplastin time, prothrombin time, bleeding time, platelet counts and liver function tests) should be considered.

MEDICAL MANAGEMENT

In most cases, medical management is instituted initially and typically includes head-elevated positioning (greater than 30°), bed rest, cycloplegics and topical or systemic steroids, or more recently antifibrinolytic agents (aminocaproic acid and tranexamic acid). Cycloplegics (atropine 1% daily or scopolamine 1/4% four times a day) may add to patient comfort, prevent malignant glaucoma or pupillary block and facilitate posterior segment examination. Steroids (topical prednisolone acetate 1% four times a day or systemic prednisone 0.5–1.0 mg/kg/day) increase patient comfort and theoretically stabilize clot formation, thereby decreasing the rate of rebleeding. Aminocaproic acid (50 mg/kg given orally every 4 hours, not to exceed 30 g/day, for 5 days, or topical aminocaproic acid) is an antifibrinolytic agent that competitively inhibits plasmin from binding to fibrin and prevents clot lysis and consequent rebleeding.

SURGICAL MANAGEMENT

INDICATIONS

When medical management fails, prompt surgical intervention is warranted. Indications for surgery

Table 38.2 Indications for surgical intervention in hyphema

Elevated intraocular pressure
Corneal bloodstaining
Nonclearing, visually significant blood clot

include uncontrolled elevated intraocular pressure (IOP), corneal bloodstaining and persistent nonresorbing blood clot (Table 38.2). For non-sickling patients, IOP limits for surgical intervention are greater than 50 mmHg for 5 days or greater than 35 mmHg for 7 days. These IOP limits may be too high, however, for patients with sickle-cell trait or disease, and patients with pre-existing glaucomatous optic nerve damage or corneal endothelial dysfunction.

Corneal bloodstaining and elevated IOP occur more frequently in traumatic hyphemas that rebleed as compared to those that do not (58% vs 22%, respectively).[4] Rebleeding most commonly occurs 2–5 days after the initial injury. During this time, these patients should be observed daily. If no other serious pathology exists and if the patient can be entrusted to comply with the medical regimen and follow-up, he or she may be seen as an outpatient. However, if psychosocial issues prevent compliance, then hospital admission is recommended. Setting a particular IOP as an intervention point should be based on the clinical situation (e.g. sickle-cell trait or disease and patients with pre-existing glaucomatous optic nerve damage or corneal endothelial dysfunction).

Anterior chamber washout with or without adjuvant thrombolytics is the simplest and safest procedure. If the clot has autolysed, the majority of the blood can be evacuated without the use of thrombolytics. If, however, the clot is organized, thrombolysis with tissue plasminogen activator (tPA, 10–20 μg) may be necessary for adequate clearing of the anterior chamber. For best results, at least 20 minutes are required for enzymatic clot- or fibrinolysis. Therefore, it may be helpful to inject the thrombolytic into the anterior chamber while the patient is in the holding room or in the clinic.

Two limbal paracenteses are created with a no. 75 blade (Fig. 38.3a), typically at the 10 o'clock and 2 o'clock positions. Balanced saline solution is infused into the anterior chamber via a 23- or 25-gauge butterfly cannula or an anterior chamber maintainer. The surgeon can either blot the posterior lip of the opposing paracentesis, allowing aqueous, blood and fibrin to exit passively, or one can actively aspirate with a manual or automated aspiration instrument (Fig. 38.3b). If a significant clot still remains, the vitrectomy cutter can be employed (Fig. 38.3c). However, while operating with the vitrectomy cutter

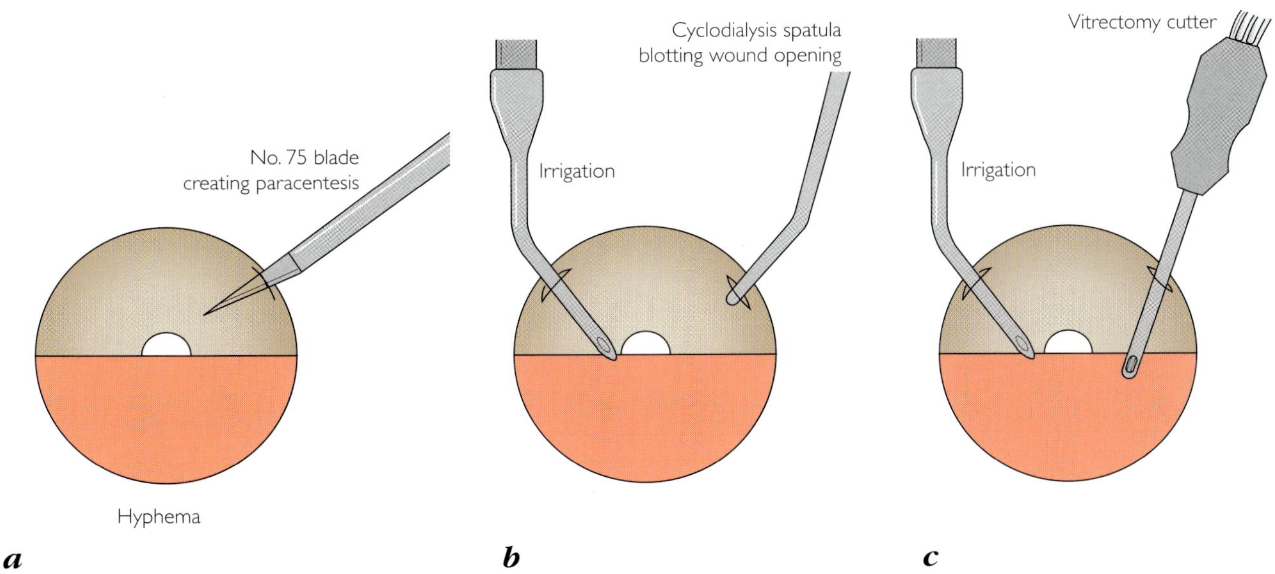

Figure 38.3 *(a) Creating a paracentesis with a no. 75 blade. (b) Irrigating anterior chamber via one paracentesis and blotting the other paracentesis. (c) Irrigating anterior chamber and using vitrectomy cutter.*

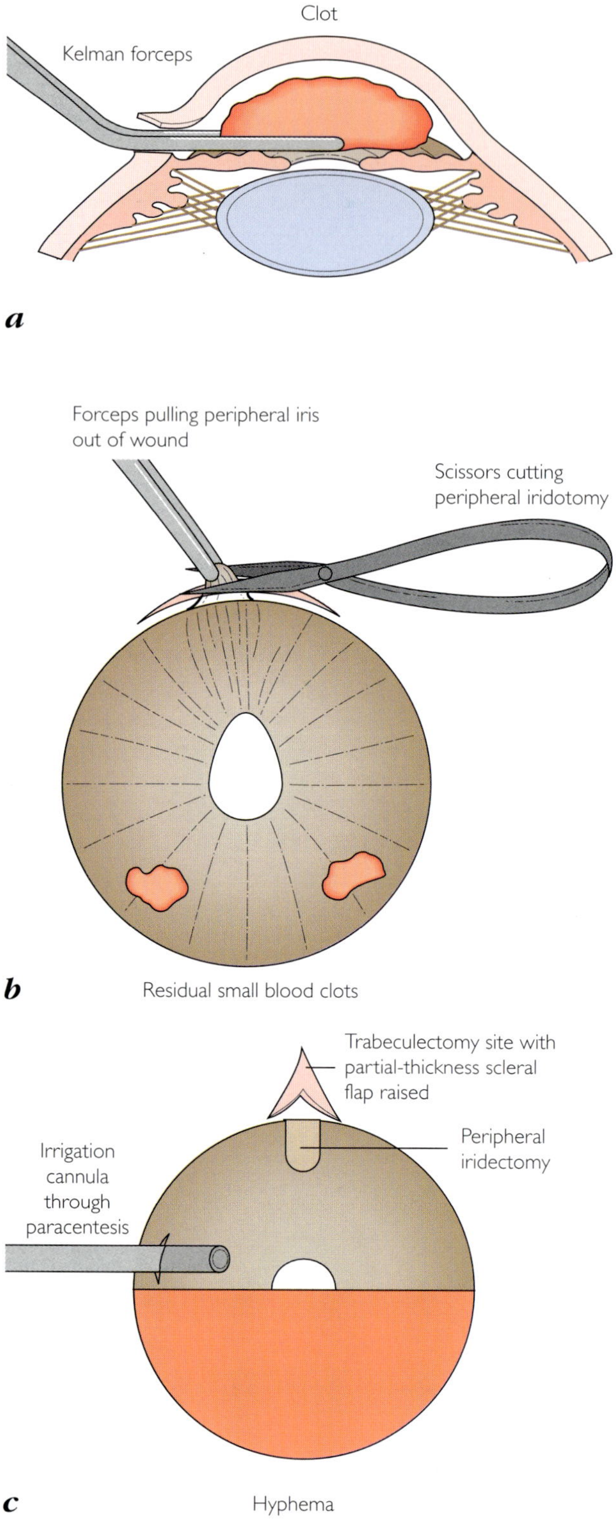

Figure 38.4 *Large clots or significant angle damage. (a) Delivering clot through limbal wound with Kelman forceps. (b) Making peripheral iridotomy. (c) Trabeculectomy may be combined with clot removal.*

in the anterior chamber, the surgeon must be vigilant about the corneal endothelium, iris and lens. The goal should be to remove all free-floating debris and clear the visual axis (thereby improving visual acuity and preventing pupillary block). It is not necessary and in fact may be counterproductive to remove the entire clot. Excessive attempts at removal of all blood may result in recurrent anterior chamber hemorrhage.

Large clots also can be extracted via larger limbal wounds (Fig. 38.4). This technique is best performed when the clot has retracted maximally (4–7 days). A limbal wound is fashioned at the superior margin, approximately 4–5 mm in length. The clot is grasped with intraocular forceps (diamond-dusted microforceps, Kelman–McPherson or Utrata) and removed. A surgical peripheral iridectomy and anterior chamber washout are performed and the wound is closed. This technique has some limitations and potential complications. Without the closed system and bimanual method described above, it is more difficult to control intraocular bleeding. The superior conjunctiva is involved in the surgical wound and scarring may prevent successful filtering surgery in the future. Finally, iris and vitreous may be adherent to the clot as it is expressed, potentially creating greater pathology.

In cases of significant angle damage or total hyphema with elevated IOP, trabeculectomy and peripheral iridectomy in conjunction with anterior chamber washout have been advocated.[12] This procedure provides a convenient entry site to break up any loose clot and remove it with irrigation while alleviating pupillary block and creating a temporary filtration site (which eventually scars). A standard trabeculectomy and peripheral iridectomy are fashioned at the superior limbus. A limbal paracentesis is made in a surgically convenient location and the anterior chamber is gently irrigated with balanced saline solution. The irrigating cannula may be used carefully to dislodge or break up the blood clot; however, aggressive or blind maneuvers should be avoided. By using this surgical technique, none of the patients in the series reported by Weiss and associates experienced surgical complications.[12] The disadvantage of this procedure is that the scarred trabeculectomy site may prevent future filtration surgery in this area.

If recurrent hemorrhage occurs, the surgeon has several options available. When using a closed system, such as bimanual anterior chamber hyphema washout, increased infusion pressure (maintained for several minutes) alone may adequately tamponade the site of hemorrhage. If bleeding persists and visualization allows, intraocular diathermy can be applied directly to the bleeding iris vessel. If the bleeding site cannot be identified, thrombin (100 U/ml) can be injected over the area. The ensuing clot should not be disturbed because recurrent hemorrhage will occur.

IRIDODIALYSIS

PREOPERATIVE EVALUATION

The patient's history is important in the evaluation and management of iridodialysis. Patients with a small dialysis, particularly if it is superior and covered by the upper lid, are often asymptomatic and can be followed without intervention. Symptomatic patients will complain of photophobia, glare and/or monocular diplopia. Patients (particularly those with fair irides) also may be bothered by cosmetically obvious anisocoria. When counseling the patient, the severity of these symptoms must be put in context of the risks and potential complications of each management option.

Because iridodialysis results after trauma or intraocular surgery, concurrent intraocular pathology may exist. Consequently, the clinician must thoroughly examine the eye, looking for other manifestations of blunt or surgical trauma (e.g. angle recession, cyclodialysis, lens damage, zonular rupture, vitreous prolapse and retinal tear or dialysis).

Nonsurgical management of symptomatic iridodialysis is limited and often unrewarding. Cosmetic contact lenses with painted irides are available and can successively decrease symptoms and improve cosmesis in some cases.

SURGICAL MANAGEMENT

Several surgical techniques for the repair of iridodialysis have been described.[3,7,11,13] The choice of surgical technique depends on multiple factors, including the phakic status of the patient, other procedures to be performed and the extent of the dialysis.

When iridodialysis is the only significant anterior segment pathology, repair can be performed with a double-armed McCannell needle, a straight 27-gauge needle with a hole drilled in the bevel (TREK needle, Escalon Medical TR9921, Escalon Medical Corp., Skillman, NJ) or a 30-gauge needle (Fig. 38.5).

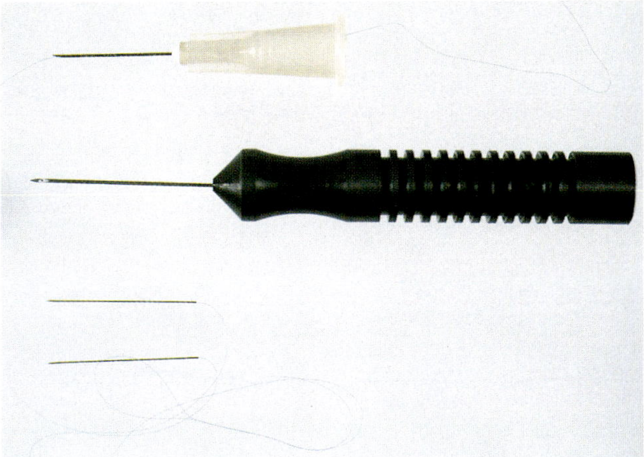

Figure 38.5 *McCannell double-armed suture, TREK needle threaded with 10-0 prolene and 30-gauge needle threaded with 10-0 prolene.*

Because these needles must be passed across the anterior chamber over the lens and iris, there is a risk of damaging the iris and lens, resulting in intraocular hemorrhage or cataract formation. Such complications can be avoided with the use of due caution and viscoelastics (injected into the anterior chamber and a small amount between the iris and lens capsule).

When using a double-armed McCannell needle, a conjunctival limbal peritomy is created over the area of the dialysis and a limbal paracentesis is fashioned 180° away from the middle of the iridodialysis. The first needle is passed through the paracentesis, into and across the anterior chamber and through the base of the iridodialysis (Fig. 38.6a). The needle should exit through the sclera at the level of the iris root, 1–1.5 mm posterior to the limbus. The second needle is passed in a similar fashion (Fig. 38.6b). The use of a 25-gauge needle (Fig. 38.6c) passed through the limbal area closest to the dialysis and placed end-to-end with the McCannell needle can serve as a guide for needle passage. The free ends of the suture are tied over the sclera and the knot is buried. The conjunctiva is closed in a routine fashion. Some clinicians believe that the suture should be placed under a scleral flap, thereby eliminating a potential wick for bacteria and subsequent endophthalmitis.[5,7] However, if the conjunctiva adequately covers the entire suture, and because the knot is buried, there is little risk of overlying conjunctival erosion.

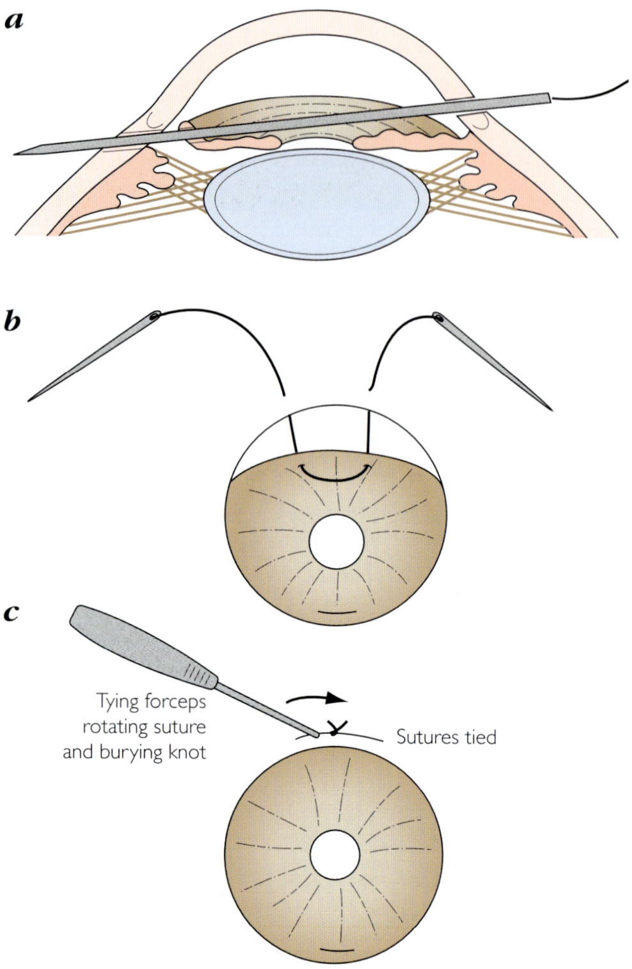

Figure 38.6 *McCannell suture technique. (a) Needle passing through paracentesis, anterior chamber, iris base, iris root and sclera (side view). (b) Second needle passed and externalized (top view). (c) Suture tied over sclera and buried.*

When using a TREK or 30-gauge needle, a 10-0 prolene suture must be placed through the eyelet of the needle tip or through the barrel of the 30-gauge needle initially (Fig. 38.7). A conjunctival limbal peritomy is created over the area of the dialysis. These needles, however, do not require a paracentesis because only one pass through the limbus is necessary. The needle is passed through peripheral cornea 180° away from the middle of the iridodialysis, across the anterior chamber, through the base of the iridodialysis and through the iris root and sclera (Fig. 38.7a). Several centimeters of suture are pulled through the wound (maintaining a threaded needle) and held securely with a locking needle-holder or by the surgical assistant. The needle is retracted back into the anterior chamber (Fig. 38.7b) and back out of the iris base. A second pass through the iris base is made (Fig. 38.7c) and the needle is again brought through the sclera at the level of the iris root. The free ends of the suture are tied over the sclera and the knot is buried. The conjunctiva is closed in a routine fashion.

When the dialysis is large, more than two fixation points may be necessary. This can be accomplished by repeating a similar procedure with a new double-armed McCannell suture or by making extra passes with the TREK or 30-gauge needle (Fig. 38.8). When the latter two needles are used, suture loops are created on each successive pass. The loops are made long enough to cut and tie and the knots are buried. The base of the iridodialysis should be divided equally with the number of fixation points planned: if two fixation points are planned, the iris should be divided into thirds; if four are planned, the iris should be divided into fifths; and so on.

Particularly in large iridodialyses, the edge of the iris base may roll or may be difficult to engage with the needle. Entry into the iris can be facilitated and controlled better with intraocular forceps, such as a microforceps by Grieshaber (supplied in the USA by Alcon Laboratories, Inc., Fort Worth, TX) or the 25-gauge forceps designed by Chang and Coll.[3] When using an intraocular forceps, an additional limbal paracentesis is created in a surgically convenient location; this will enable the surgeon to find and grasp the iris base more easily.

An alternative technique to the closed system offered by the special needle already discussed is to reapproximate the dialysis via a larger limbal wound. This technique is particularly useful if there is a coexistent cataract. The surgeon should fashion a limbal wound through which both iridodialysis repair and cataract extraction can be performed (Fig. 38.9a). In these cases, the iris base can be externalized and fixated sclerally via the iris root under direct visualization. A temporal limbal scleral phacoemulsification incision is fashioned 1.5–2.0 mm posterior to the limbus. The edge of the iridodialysis is grasped and externalized with an intraocular forceps. Each needle of a double-armed 10-0 prolene suture is passed through the iris (anterior to posterior) and then through the iris root 1–1.5 mm posterior to the limbus (Fig. 38.9b). If the surgical wound allows, the spacing between suture bits should be symmetric. Therefore, a 180° iridodialysis with two fixation sutures should have sutures placed 2 clock-hours apart. The free ends are tied over sclera and the knot is buried.

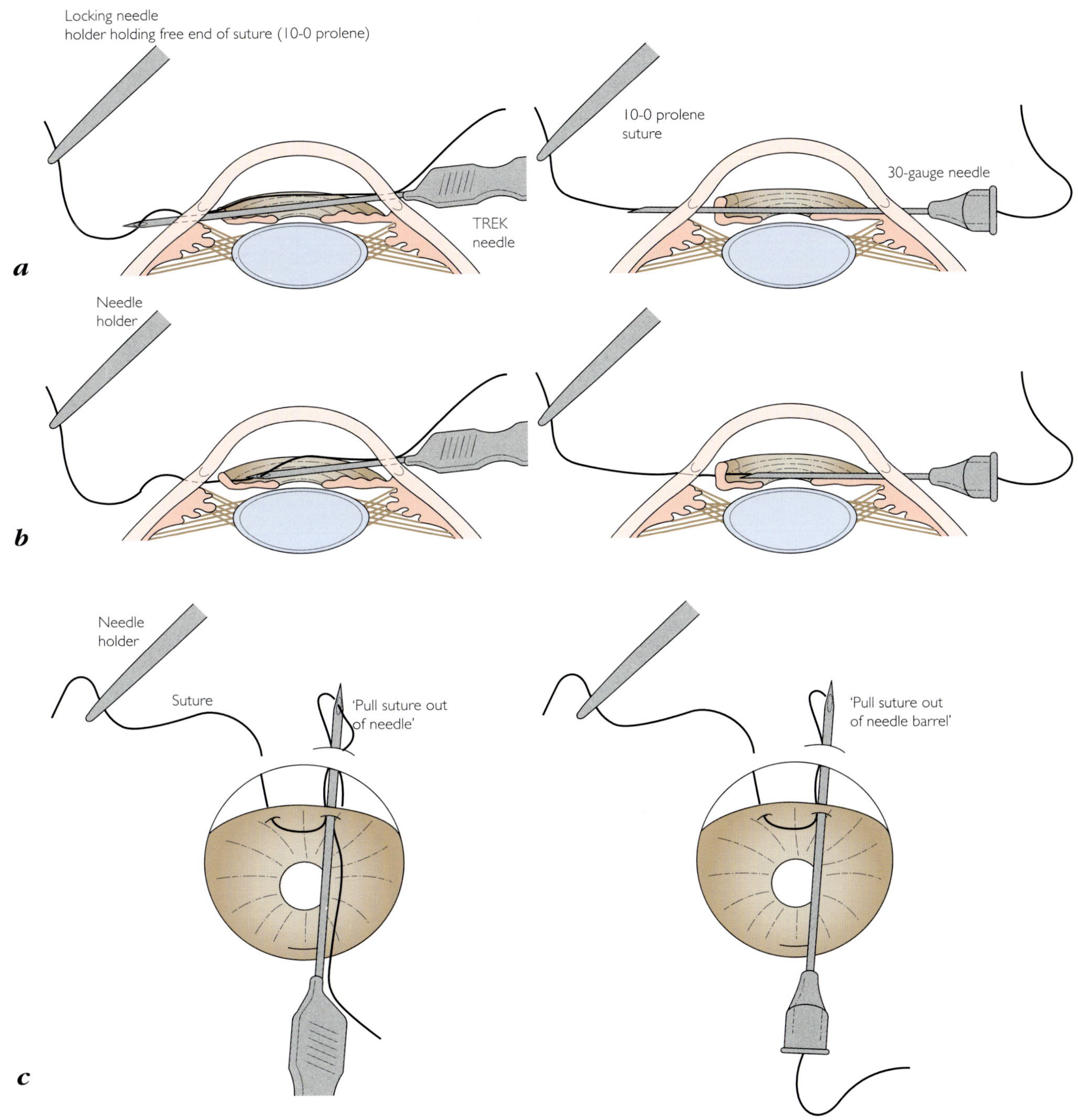

Figure 38.7 *The TREK (left) and 30-gauge (right) techniques. (a) Needle passing through peripheral cornea, anterior chamber, iris base, iris root and sclera with a needle-holder grasping the free end of the suture (side view). (b) Needle retracted back into anterior chamber (side view). (c) Second pass (top view).*

In the setting of coexistent cataract, the surgeon proceeds with cataract extraction in a routine fashion. After the cataract surgery is completed, the scleral flap is sutured back into position, covering the iridodialysis suture. With this technique, direct visualization and manipulation of the iris base and greater visualization of needle placement minimize unintentional trauma to other intraocular structures (lens capsule, trabecular

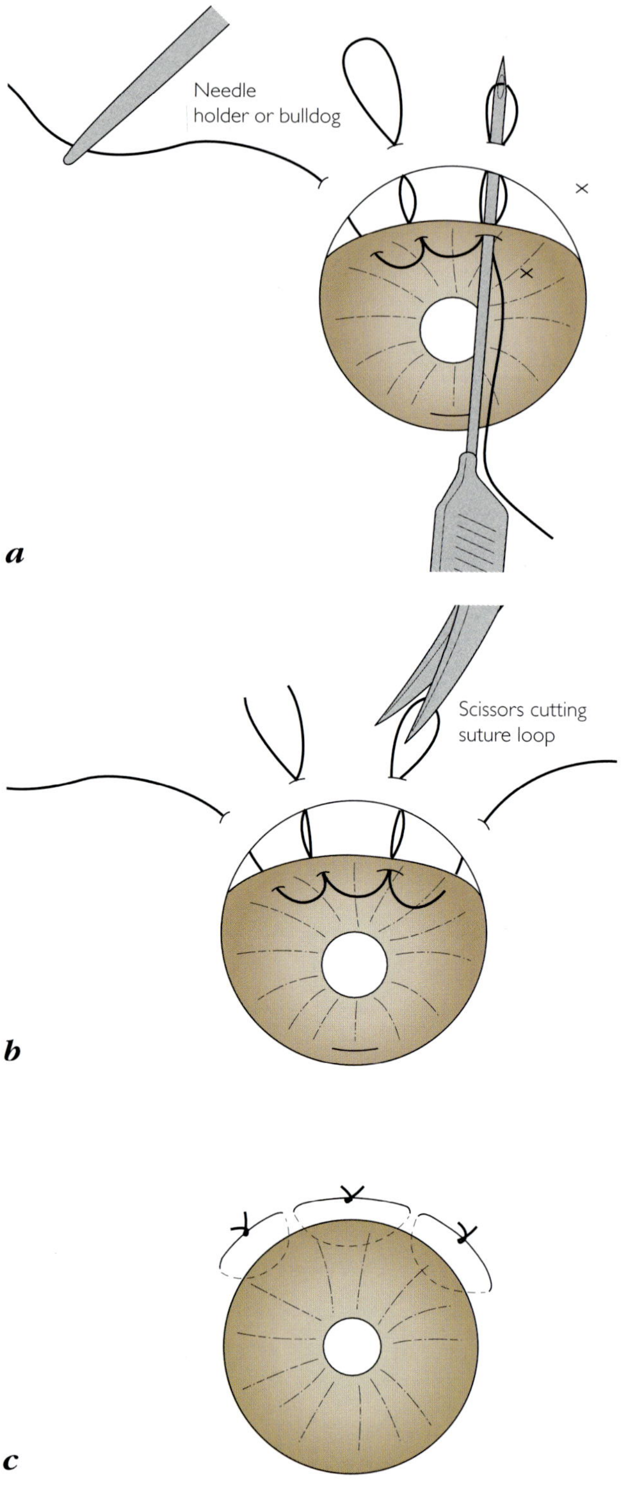

Figure 38.8 *The TREK technique for large dialysis. (a) Two fixation points already done with a loop fashion, third pass being done and grasping suture to make second loop (top view). (b) Cutting suture loop. (c) Tying correct sutures to each other over sclera.*

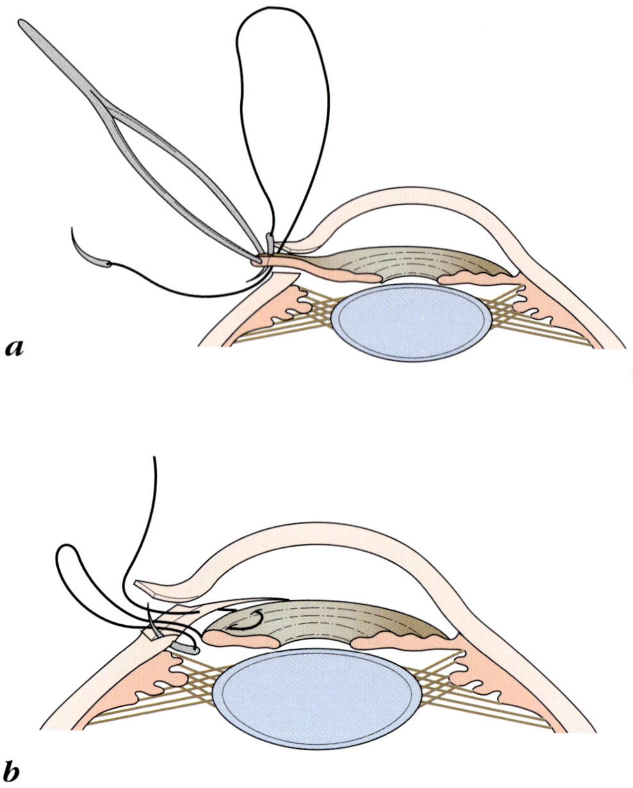

Figure 38.9 *Direct technique. (a) Cataract wound fashioned, iris base held external to the wound and second needle being passed through iris base edge (side view). (b) Passing second needle through iris base and scleral bed (side view).*

meshwork and ciliary body). Consequently, for phakic eyes, where iridodialysis alone is to be repaired, this may still be the preferred surgical technique.

CORNEOSCLERAL LACERATIONS

PREOPERATIVE EVALUATION

The initial evaluation of a patient with a corneoscleral laceration should proceed similarly to that described in the previous sections. In these eyes, however, the extent of the injury, the age of the patient (children) or the presence of alcohol or other psychogenic drugs may prevent a thorough preoperative examination. Attempting to perform a complete examination in an uncooperative patient may result in excessive pressure on the globe and extrusion of intraocular contents. In these instances, a better examination may be deferred until the patient is under general anesthesia.

SURGICAL MANAGEMENT

Suture needles are designed to facilitate proper suture placement with little or no tissue manipulation necessary. Avoiding manipulation of wound edges will minimize tissue maceration and subsequent wound leaks, and inadvertent contact of deeper vascular structures and subsequent intraocular hemorrhage (Table 38.3). Utilizing the arc of a needle, the needle can be passed through the cornea or sclera with a twisting motion alone (Fig. 38.10). If counterpressure is necessary, the limbus or an extraocular muscle can be held with a 0.12 or 0.3 mm forceps. If the wound is gaping such that a single needle pass is difficult, the needle should be passed completely through each wound edge. Sutures should be passed perpendicular to the wound, avoiding the visual axis when possible,

Table 38.3 Principles of suturing corneoscleral lacerations

Minimize manipulation of laceration edges
Utilize the needle arc
Place sutures perpendicular to the laceration
Avoid the visual axis when possible
Longer suture passes are easier to rotate (1 mm to either side of the laceration)
Sutures should pass through 80–90% stromal depth
Suture tension should optimize wound integrity and minimize irregular astigmatic changes

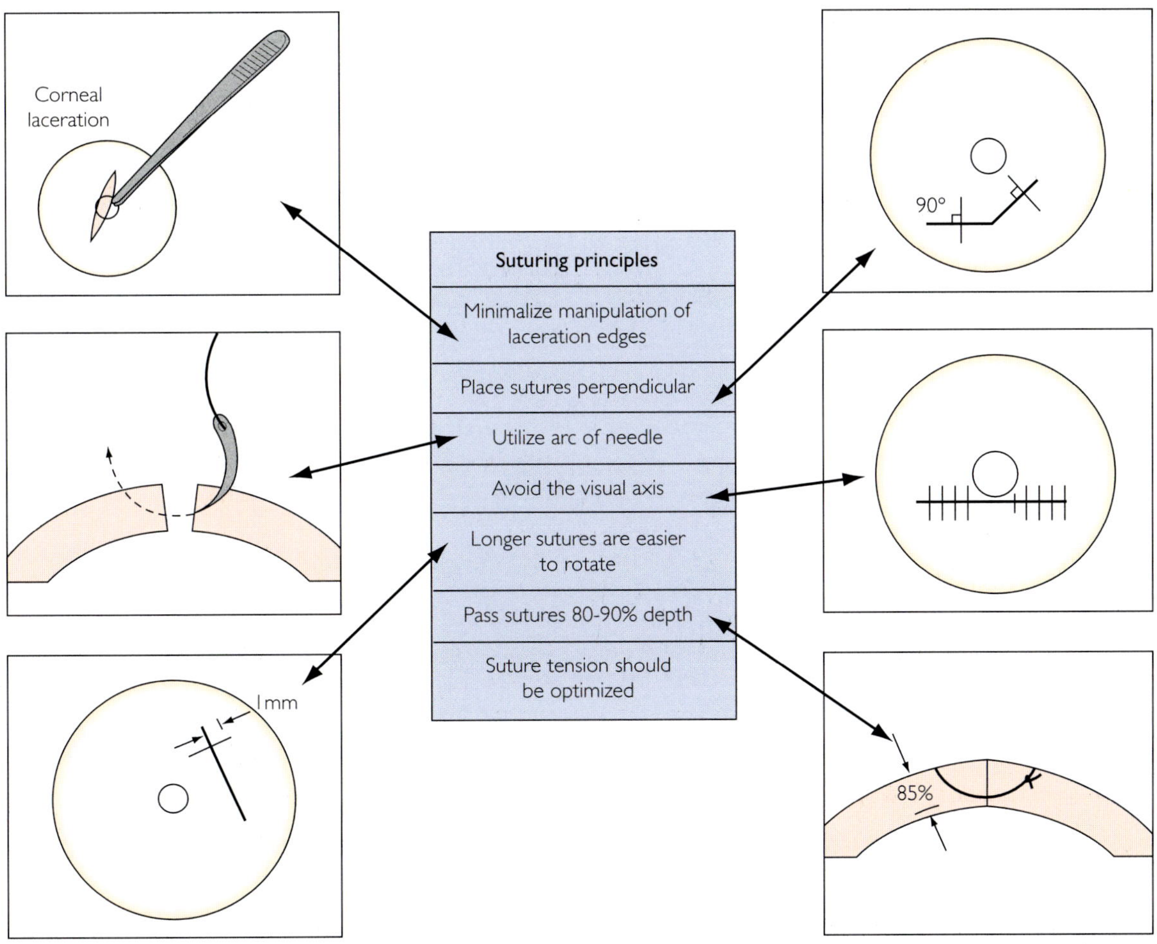

Figure 38.10 *Suturing techniques.*

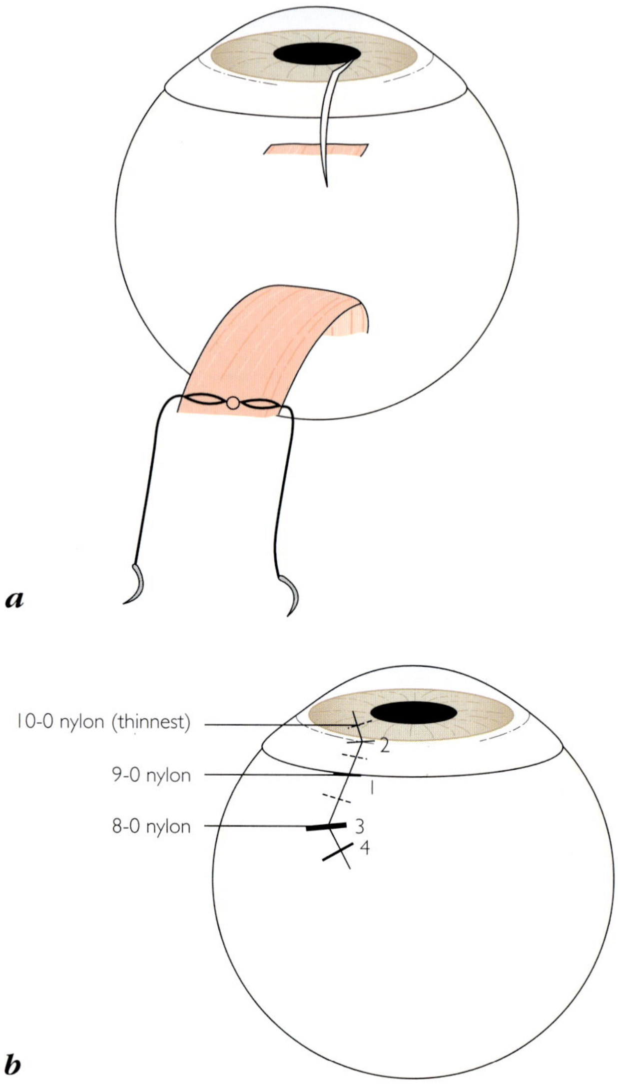

Figure 38.11 *(a) Technique for temporarily removing rectus muscle, conjunctival peritomy, double-armed suture passed and tied to rectus muscle. (b) Corneoscleral wound closed with 10-0, 9-0 and 8-0 nylon with cardinal sutures in place and bisecting one section of laceration.*

entering and exiting 1 mm to either side of the laceration and at 80–90% corneal stroma depth. The orientation, length and depth of the suture pass minimize wound distortion, tissue maceration and endothelial gaping while facilitating suture rotation. Suture tension is also critical. The surgeon seeks a balance between wound integrity and irregular astigmatism. This balance is particularly challenging in soft eyes. In such cases, loose or tight sutures can be replaced once the wound is closed and the eye is reformed, or slip knots can be used and suture tension can be adjusted. Slip knots often are more difficult technically but have the advantage of circumventing multiple needle passes.

When a laceration extends to the limbus or subconjunctival hemorrhage prevents a complete examination, a limbal peritomy and careful inspection of that area are recommended (Fig. 38.11a). If a laceration extends under a rectus muscle that cannot be retracted safely, disinsert the muscle and isolate it on a double-armed 5-0 or 6-0 Vicryl suture (in order to reapproximate it after the laceration is closed). Gently irrigate all wound surfaces with balanced saline solution to debride the wound of possible foreign debris.

Corneal lacerations should be closed with multiple interrupted 10-0 nylon sutures, the limbus should be closed with 9-0 nylon suture and sclera should be closed with 8-0 nylon (Fig. 38.11b). The order in which sutures are placed depends on the configuration and length of the laceration. Linear lacerations are mostly closed physiologically by progressively bisecting the wound until it is closed (i.e. starting in the middle of the wound and then placing a suture halfway to either side and the end of the wound, etc.). Jagged lacerations are common and are best closed by placing cardinal sutures at each corner or bend of the wound, before placing the remaining reinforcing sutures. In some cases, the sclera can be closed nicely with a running shoestring technique, such as is used to close the incision made for a ganciclovir implant.

Stellate corneal and scleral lacerations may be challenging to close (Fig. 38.12). A watertight closure can be difficult to achieve; consequently, a variety of methods have been described to seal such lacerations. Multiple criss-crossing sutures are technically less difficult, but tend to be bulky and ineffective (Fig. 38.12a). Modified horizontal mattress sutures and purse-string sutures with the knot buried in the wound tend to give a better result in some cases (Fig. 38.12b, c).

In other cases a water-tight closure at the intersection point simply cannot be obtained with suturing techniques because of edema, maceration or missing tissue. In these situations, cyanoacrylate tissue adhesive can seal small defects and a corneal or scleral patch graft can be used to seal large defects (Fig. 38.12d). At the conclusion of the case, it is important to bury corneal suture knots to maximize wound healing and patient comfort. If cyanoacrylate glue is used, a soft contact lens should be placed

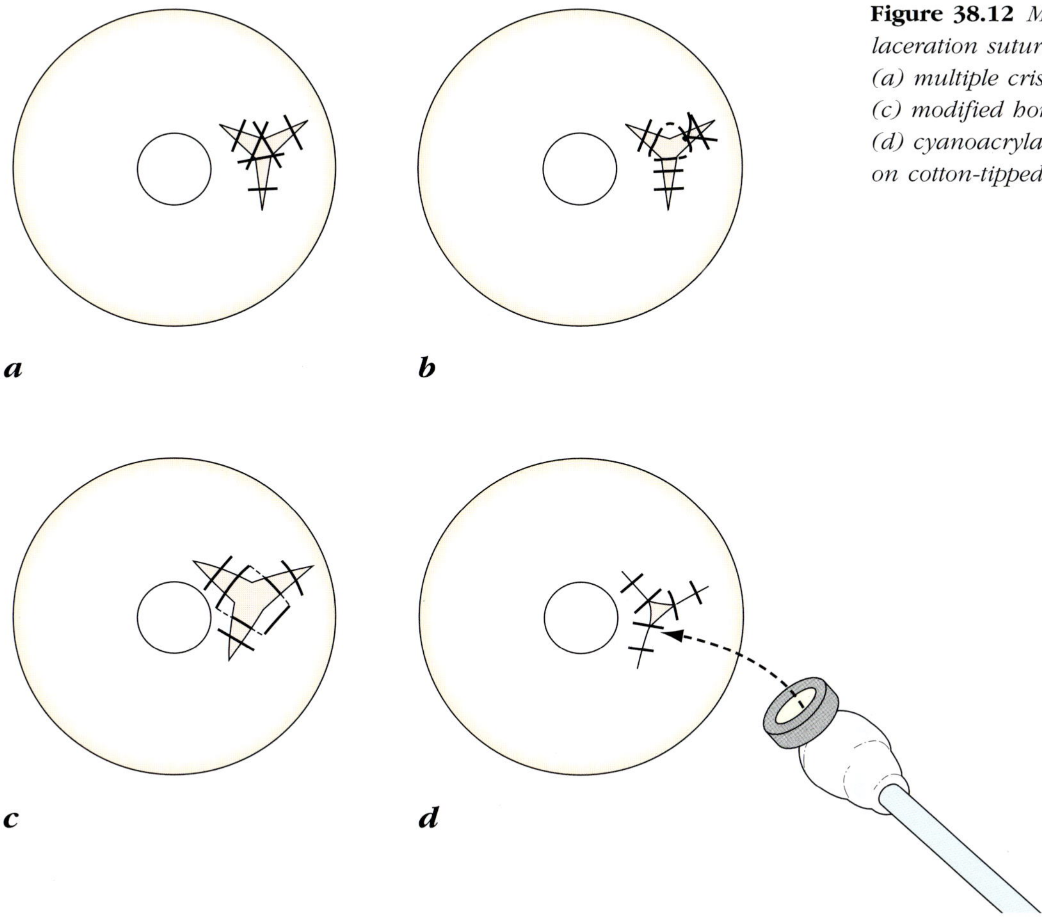

Figure 38.12 *Montage of stellate laceration suturing techniques: (a) multiple criss-cross; (b) purse-string; (c) modified horizontal mattress; (d) cyanoacrylate glue and plastic disc on cotton-tipped applicator.*

over the cornea to minimize patient discomfort from the rough glue edges.

If the uvea has prolapsed, its viability and the presence of an overlying epithelial membrane should be assessed. If the uveal tissue appears necrotic, it should be excised and examined by a pathologist; a sample may be sent to the microbiology department for culture. If the uveal tissue appears viable, any epithelial membrane that has grown over the tissue should be removed and repositioned (Fig. 38.13). Epithelial membranes can be removed with a fine-tipped forceps, a cotton-tipped applicator or a cellulose sponge.

Iris repositioning can be performed pharmacologically, mechanically or both. In selected cases, sterile (previously unopened) miotics or mydriatics may be useful to assist in mechanical repositioning. Surgically, a limbal paracentesis is fashioned at a location that will provide the best lever arm for sweeping iris from the wound (usually perpendicular to the orientation of the wound). The cannula is passed through the paracentesis and positioned between the iris and wound. The iris is either dissected out of the wound by injecting viscoelastic between the wound and iris or is swept from the wound with the cannula while injecting enough

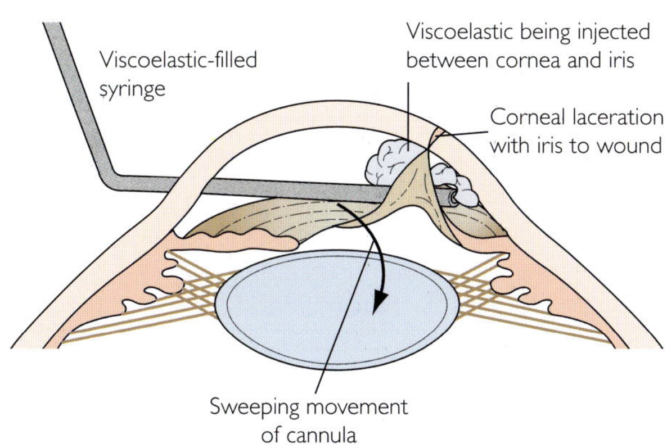

Figure 38.13 *Technique of repositing iris with viscoelastic and 27-gauge cannula.*

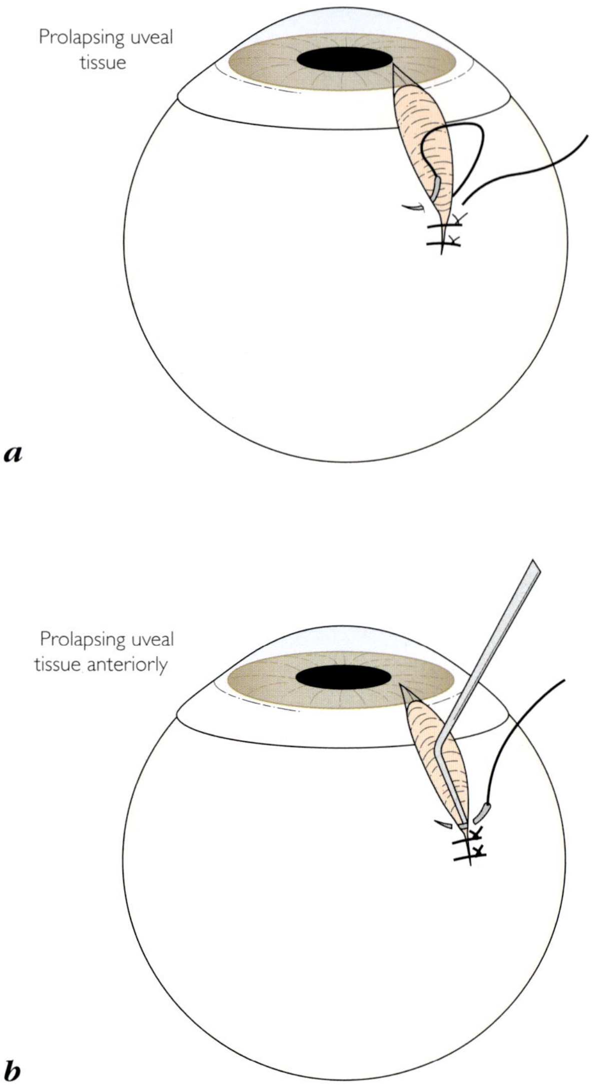

Figure 38.14 *Technique of repositing posterior uveal tissue: (a) oversewing; (b) repositing tissue with cyclodialysis spatula while suturing.*

viscoelastic between the wound and iris to maintain a barrier to future iris prolapse (Fig. 38.13). Too much viscoelastic will cause the wound to gape, making closure difficult.

When the uvea is prolapsing through a posterior wound, the tissue may fall back if it is oversewn and the wound is 'zippered' closed (Fig. 38.14a). Alternatively, an assistant can reposit the tissue with a cyclodialysis spatula while the surgeon places and ties the suture (Fig. 38.14b). If vitreous is incarcerated in the wound, a manual cellulose-sponge vitrectomy or automated vitrectomy around the wound is performed.

Once the integrity of the eye has been restored, it should be reformed by injecting balanced saline solution into the anterior or posterior chambers. The cannula or needle should be visualized always. If the visualization is prevented by media opacities, defer reforming the eye because the cannula or needle may enter the lens or the suprachoroidal or subretinal space. When reforming the eye, all wounds should be monitored carefully for leaks and reinforcing sutures should be placed appropriately. If the sutured wounds are watertight but the eye does not maintain pressure, most likely there is another laceration or rupture site necessitating further exploration.

Patients with traumatic cataract or lens rupture may require lens extraction (Fig. 38.15). If the decision is made to remove the lens at the initial laceration closure, several methods are available. The technique used to remove the lens depends on the preference

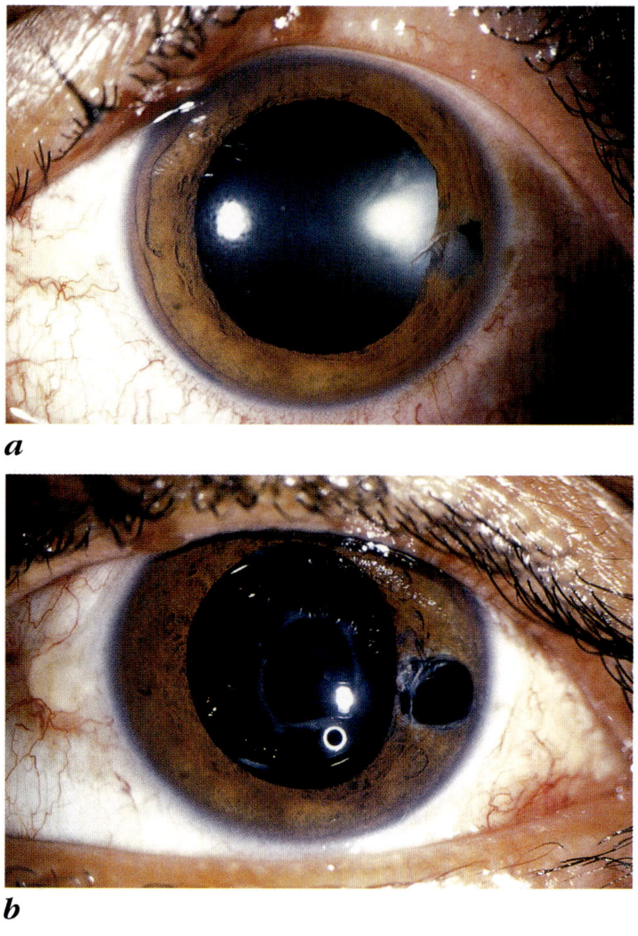

Figure 38.15 *Preoperative (a) and postoperative (b) photos of lens rupture and intraocular lens implantation.*

of the surgeon, the stability of the lens and the age of the patient. In young patients, the lens usually can be aspirated with the automated or manual irrigation/aspiration instrument or a vitrectomy handpiece. In older patients, phacoemulsification of the harder nuclei usually is necessary. Large extracapsular wounds should be avoided in acutely traumatized eyes because there may be increased risk of expulsive choroidal hemorrhage.

Prompt visual rehabilitation with the primary placement of an intraocular lens in selected traumatized eyes is becoming less controversial. In patients who underwent lensectomy and intraocular lens implantation at the time of primary repair of a penetrating ocular injury, 64–87% of patients obtained 20/40 or better visual acuity.[8,9] The potential difficulties in primary intraocular lens placement are proper intraocular lens power selection and poor capsular support.

In eyes with a corneoscleral or scleral laceration and an attached retina, complicated retinal detachment and proliferative vitreoretinopathy occur in 23–27% of cases.[2,6] Subsequent surgical repair of such detachments is challenging and at times ultimately unsuccessful. For this reason, prophylactic scleral buckling of eyes with scleral lacerations, particularly with prolapsed or incarcerated vitreous or uveal tissue, should be considered. Uncontrolled clinical studies have demonstrated that the rate of delayed retinal detachment can be reduced by 43–70% in eyes with prophylactic scleral buckles compared to those that were not buckled.[1,2,6] Theoretically, an encircling scleral buckle reduces the risk of retinal detachment by reducing the circumferential contraction of the vitreous base and anteroposterior traction of the fibroproliferative tissue. If a scleral buckle is placed, an encircling element should be used and should be positioned optimally to support the vitreous base (Fig. 38.16).

It must be kept in mind that the primary goal in ocular trauma is to restore the integrity of the globe. Other considerations such as lens rupture or dislocation, iridodialysis and choroidal hemorrhage are secondary and may be addressed at future surgical procedures when circumstances are more controlled.

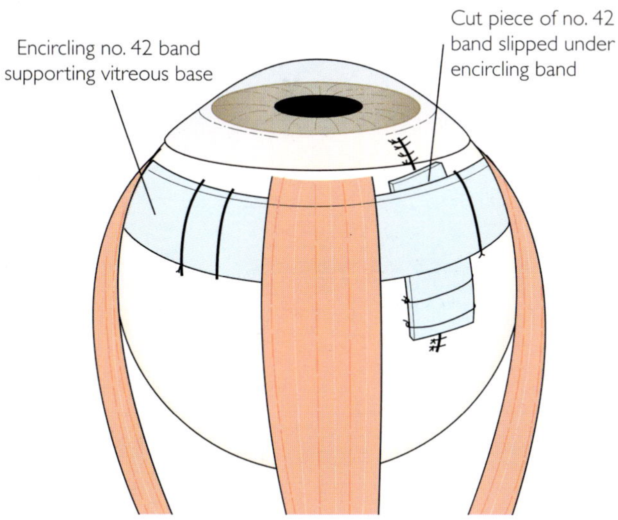

Figure 38.16 *Encircling scleral buckle supporting vitreous base, with radial element over scleral laceration.*

CONCLUSION

Ocular trauma creates significant personal, financial, societal and medical burdens. An ophthalmologist's greatest role in minimizing this burden should be as an educator of preventive medicine and eye protection. However, for those eyes that have sustained significant ocular trauma, the prognosis continues to improve as we advance our understanding of the pathophysiology of ocular trauma, medicines, instrumentation and surgical techniques.

REFERENCES

1. Ahmadieh H, Soheilian M, Sajjadi H, et al. Vitrectomy in ocular trauma: factors influencing final visual outcome, *Retina* (1993) **13:**107–13.
2. Brinton GS, Aaberg TM, Reeser FH, et al. Surgical results in ocular trauma involving the posterior segment, *Am J Ophthalmol* (1982) **93:**271–8.
3. Chang S, Coll GE. Surgical techniques for repositioning a dislocated intraocular lens, repair of iridodialysis, and secondary intraocular lens implantation using innovative 25-gauge forceps, *Am J Ophthalmol* (1995) **119:**165–74.
4. Edwards WC, Layden WF. Traumatic hyphema: a report of 184 consecutive cases, *Am J Ophthalmol* (1973) **75:**110–16.
5. Heilskov T, Joondeph R, Olsen KR, Blankenship GW. Late endophthalmitis after transscleral fixation of a posterior chamber intraocular lens, *Arch Ophthalmol* (1989) **107:**1427.
6. Hutton WL, Fuller DG. Factors influencing final visual results in severely injured eyes, *Am J Ophthalmol* (1984) **97:**715–22.
7. Kervick GN, Johnston SS. Repair of inferior iridodialysis using a partial-thickness scleral flap, *Ophthalmic Surg* (1991) **22:**354–5.

8. Koenig SB, Ruttum MS, Lewandowski MF, Schultz RO. Pseudophakia for traumatic cataracts in children, *Ophthalmology* (1993) **100:**1218–24.
9. Rubsamen PE, Irvin WD, McCuen BW II, et al. Primary intraocular lens implantation in the setting of penetrating ocular trauma, *Ophthalmology* (1995) **102:**101–7.
10. Rubsamen PE, Cousins SW, Winward KE, Byrne SF. Diagnostic ultrasound and pars plana vitrectomy in penetrating ocular trauma, *Ophthalmology* (1994) **101:**809–14.
11. Wachler BB, Krueger RR. Double-armed McCannell suture for repair of traumatic iridodialysis, *Am J Ophthalmol* (1996) **122:**109–10.
12. Weiss JS, Parrish RK, Anderson DR. Surgical therapy of traumatic hyphema, *Ophthalmic Surg* (1983) **14:**343–5.
13. Zeiter JH, Shin DH, Shi DX. A closed chamber technique for repair of iridodialysis, *Ophthalmic Surg* (1993) **24:**476–80.

Chapter 39 Management of traumatic lens subluxation and dislocation

Sundeep Dev and Dennis P Han

INTRODUCTION

Damage to the crystalline lens frequently occurs in association with ocular trauma. Both blunt and penetrating trauma can cause lens injury resulting in opacification, subluxation, dislocation, disruption or total expulsion of the crystalline lens. The greater the extent of lens damage, the poorer the visual prognosis in eyes with penetrating injuries.[1] The prognosis is worsened if the lens is displaced or expelled.[1,2]

The term 'subluxation' refers to a partial dislocation, whereas 'dislocation' refers to a total displacement of the lens. Ocular penetration with direct injury to the lens usually results in rapid opacification and often gross lens disruption into either the vitreous or anterior chamber. Violation of the lens capsule can result in marked intraocular inflammation and phacogenic glaucoma. Zonular compromise in contusion injuries allows vitreous to prolapse around the lens and into the anterior chamber. Such forces can be severe enough to cause concomitant scleral ruptures and posterior segment injuries.

SURGICAL INDICATIONS

In most cases, removal of the lens should be avoided at the time of initial injury. The exception to this is when gross disruption of the lens occurs, resulting in free lens material in the eye. Such disruption results in a severe inflammatory reaction and glaucoma; however, small breaks in the lens capsule may spontaneously seal with subsequent development of only a focal cataract.

In general, traumatic lacerations are closed primarily to allow the eye to reform. Delaying more extensive intraocular surgery often gives concomitant corneal edema, hyphema and inflammation a chance to resolve. It also allows the surgeon to assess better the extent of the injury, the overall visual prognosis and to develop a more detailed surgical plan with the patient's consent. Lens surgery in the setting of posterior segment injury may be delayed for 7–10 days after the initial injury.[3–8]

In some cases, a displaced lens is well tolerated and surgery may be avoided. Glaucoma is one of the most common indications for lens removal after lens trauma. Damage to the lens capsule causes intense intraocular inflammation, resulting in phacogenic glaucoma. A subluxated lens can result in pupillary block glaucoma. In one series of traumatic lens dislocation, 56% had a preoperative elevation of intraocular pressure (IOP).[9] Vitreous prolapse into the anterior chamber may cause corneal decompensation and a secondary form of open-angle glaucoma. Other indications for removal of a subluxated lens include the presence of a cataract, optical disturbance from the lens edge, uncorrectable astigmatism from the abnormal lens position and marked lens instability and phacodonesis.

Indications for removal of dislocated lenses include cystoid macular edema, excessive mobility of the dislocated lens which can result in retinal injury, and obscuration of the optical axis. Associated complications of retinal detachment, proliferative vitreoretinopathy and recurrent vitreous hemorrhage necessitate removal of the lens.

The management of subluxated and dislocated lenses has been improved dramatically with the development of modern vitreoretinal microsurgical techniques. Previous techniques, including cryoextraction, lens extraction with forceps or lens loops and passage of needles through the pars plana, were associated with a high incidence of complications.[10–18] Pars plana vitrectomy and lensectomy techniques eliminate complications arising from excessive vitreous traction during attempted lens removal. The large scleral incision required to remove the lens during cryoextraction or removal with a lens loop is not necessary with vitrectomy and lensectomy. A small entry site may reduce the risk of intraoperative expulsive hemorrhage and postoperative wound astigmatism and instability.

PREOPERATIVE EVALUATION

The symptoms of a patient with a displaced lens depend on the position of the lens. The patient may complain of decreased vision caused either by acquired astigmatism and refractive shift or acquired aphakia in cases of dislocation. Other symptoms are glare and monocular diplopia from the lens edge. A cataract will result in decreased visual acuity and contrast sensitivity (Fig. 39.1). Inflammation, glaucoma and corneal edema can result in pain and photophobia. In cases of blunt injury, one must maintain a high degree of suspicion for an occult rupture. Special attention is given to the visual acuity, the corneal status, the degree of intraocular inflammation and the IOP. Lens subluxation is occasionally subtle. Zonular dehiscence is marked by the presence of iridodonesis and phacodonesis. The anterior chamber should be examined carefully for the presence of vitreous. The lens itself should be examined for breaks in the anterior and posterior capsule, along with the presence of cataract. One should also carefully evaluate the vitreous and retina for vitreous hemorrhage, retinal tears and detachments and the presence of cystoid macular edema. Ultrasonography can be very helpful in evaluating the status of the retina and vitreous in eyes with opaque media, and a dislocated lens is easily diagnosed (Fig. 39.2). Computed tomography also may be helpful in evaluating the possibility of a dislocated lens.[19]

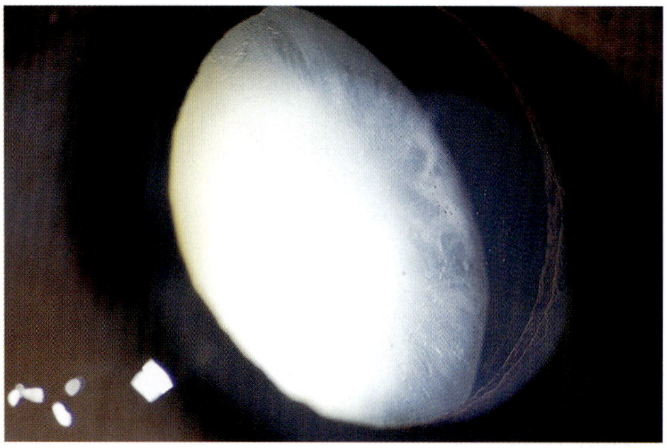

Figure 39.1 *Subluxated cataractous lens in a patient with a remote history of blunt trauma.*

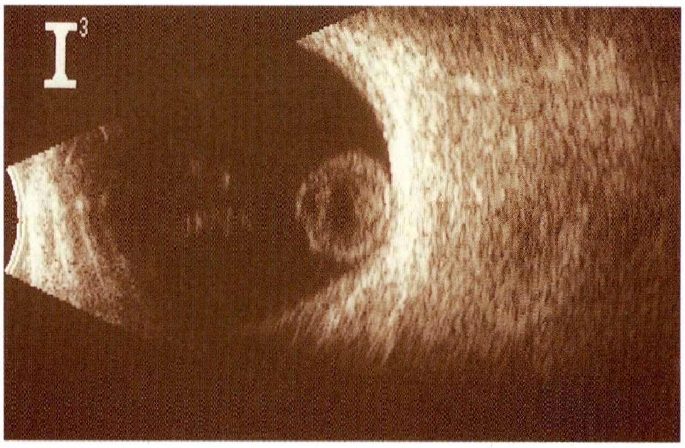

Figure 39.2 *B-Scan echography demonstrating a totally dislocated crystalline lens after trauma.*

SURGICAL TECHNIQUE AND INSTRUMENTATION

SUBLUXATED LENSES

A 360° conjunctival peritomy should be created to rule out an occult scleral rupture. Silk sutures (2-0) can be looped around the recti muscles to increase surgical exposure and provide greater maneuverability. If adequate pupillary dilation is not achieved with preoperative mydriatics, iris retractors through the limbus may be used. An infusion cannula should be placed through a 20-gauge sclerotomy created 3.0 mm posterior to the limbus in the inferotemporal quadrant of the eye. This quadrant is preferred because the ora serrata is located further posterior inferotemporally and the exterior portion of the cannula is less likely to impact the eyelid margins when maneuvering the eye. It is essential to visualize the cannula prior to turning the infusion on, to avoid a suprachoroidal infusion. In cases of densely cataractous lenses, one should not activate the primary infusion until sufficient lens removal is performed so that the cannula can be visualized. Following the placement of the infusion cannula, superior sclerotomies are made 3.0 mm from the limbus.

A 20-gauge bent needle is generally placed as a secondary infusion to provide irrigating solution if the primary infusion cannot be visualized, as commonly occurs in such cases. This needle may be placed through the pars plana with the tip directed into the anterior chamber or through the corneal limbus, providing infusion during the initial removal of prolapsed vitreous.

Zonular loss and vitreous extruding around the subluxated lens often occur. The prolapsed vitreous is cut away by introducing the vitrector in the area of zonular loss and into the anterior chamber (Fig. 39.3). An extensive core vitrectomy is not performed because the visualization is often poor through a cataractous lens and the vitreous can help to support the lens and fragments during the lensectomy. We generally use a cutting rate of 600 cuts per minute (cpm) and a suction setting of 150 mmHg to perform the vitrectomy. Then a 20-gauge microvitreoretinal (MVR) blade is reintroduced through the sclerotomy (on the side where the lens is less subluxated), penetrating directly into the substance of the lens. The blade is rotated 180° to create a passage into the lens. Next, an infusion needle is introduced into this passage into the lens. This infusion needle is used to fixate and soften the lens during phacofragmentation (Fig. 39.3). The needle may be used to bring the posteriorly subluxated lens back into its anatomic position.

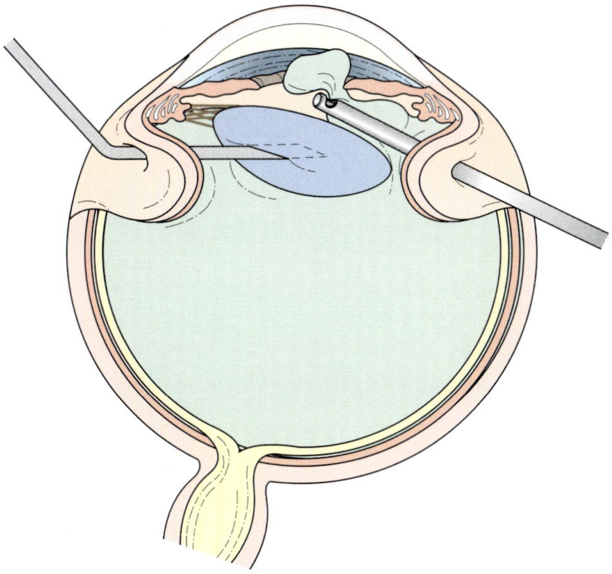

Figure 39.3 *Schematic diagram demonstrating fixation of a subluxated lens with a 20-gauge needle and removal of anteriorly prolapsed vitreous using a pars plana approach.*

In cases in which the lens is tipped quite far back or the lens is easily disrupted, making stabilization with the needle difficult, intraocular pick-forceps can be used to grasp the capsule and stabilize the lens in its usual anatomic position. A phacofragmatome is introduced into the lens. The power setting is dependent on the unit used and the density of the lens. The linear phaco mode is used. The phacofragmatome is activated only as the tip is moved in a forward direction. Division of the lens into several fragments should be avoided in order to reduce the risk of losing the fragments posteriorly. The nucleus should be sculpted until the lensectomy is complete (Fig. 39.4). If some lens fragments fall into the vitreous cavity, these should be addressed after the bulk of the lens has been removed and after a core vitrectomy has been performed.

Zonular support is usually inadequate in cases of subluxated lenses to support placement of an intraocular lens. The residual capsule should be removed to avoid difficulties with late capsular opacification and adhesion to the iris; removal is easily accomplished using the vitrector at a slow cutting rate (200–300 cpm). Diamond-dusted end-grabbing forceps or pick-forceps are useful in grasping the capsule from under the iris (Fig. 39.5). Additionally, gentle scleral depression can be used to help visualize and remove peripheral capsular or lenticular remnants with the vitrectomy unit (Fig. 39.6). After all lens material has been removed, a vitrectomy is performed. Small residual lens particles often may be removed with the vitrectomy unit. The light pipe can be used to help guide the lens pieces into the cutting port. Larger, denser pieces may require the use of a fragmatome.

The posterior hyaloid face should be removed whenever possible. Post-traumatic eyes are usually inflamed; leaving the hyaloid face can result in late retinal traction and can provide a scaffold for proliferative membrane formation and contraction. Often a posterior vitreous detachment can be created by increased suction (250–350 mmHg) with the vitrector or a soft-tipped extrusion cannula over the optic nerve head, with simultaneous brief elevation of the infusion bottle. Alternatively a barbed MVR blade or other fine retinal pick can be used to lift the hyaloid

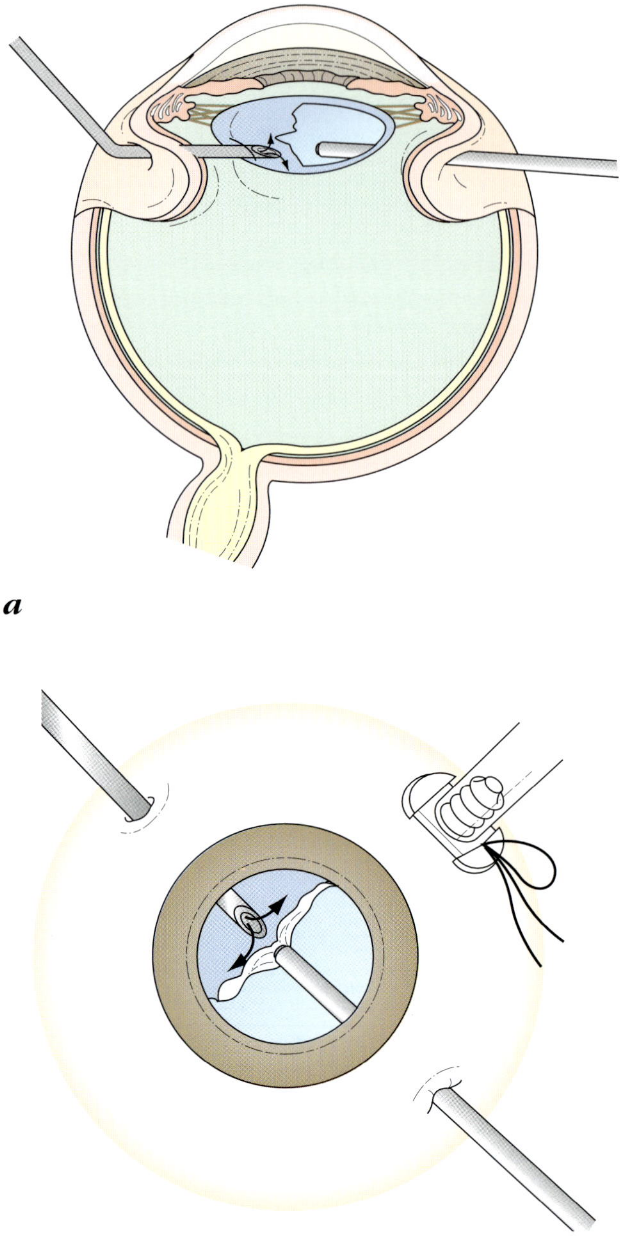

a

b

Figure 39.4 *Schematic diagram demonstrating the technique of pars plana lensectomy using a 20-gauge needle for the stabilization of the subluxated lens. (a) Note that the nucleus is sculpted out using the phacofragmatome to retain the lens in a single large piece until the lensectomy is complete. (b) Surgeon's view of the eye with residual lens (needle in it through the scleral opening) and the phaco coming from the lower right to remove the residual lens. Lens material on the right has previously been removed.*

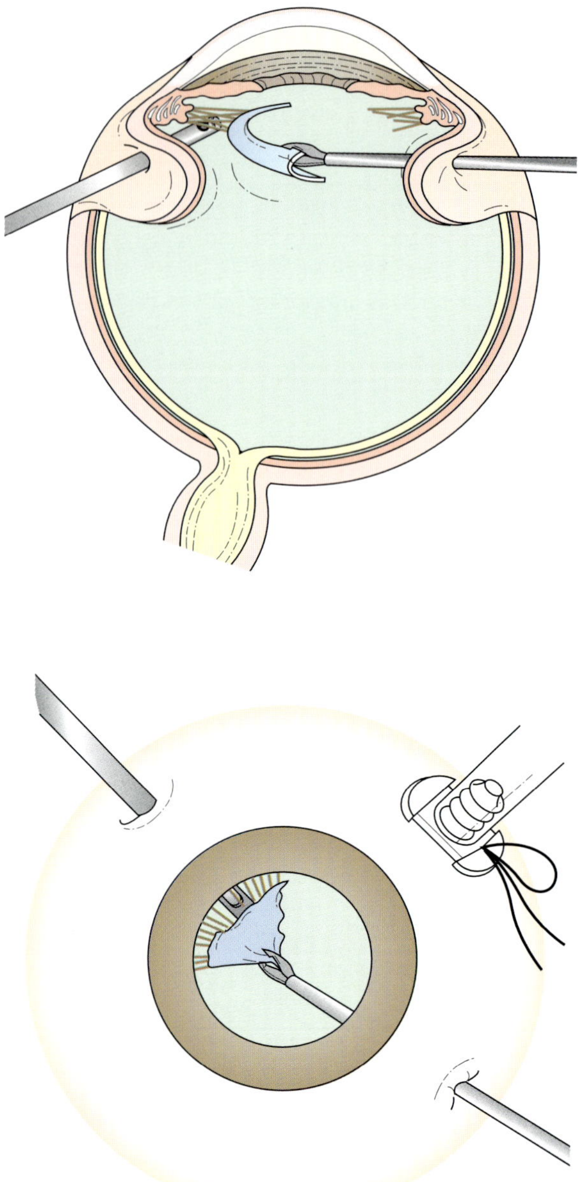

a

b

Figure 39.5 *Schematic diagram demonstrating removal of peripheral capsular remnants after the lensectomy is complete. (a) Note that end-grabbing forceps are used to pull the capsule centrally into the pupillary space and the vitrector is then used to cut it free and remove it. (b) Surgeon's view showing capsule being pulled by forceps while the vitrector 'eats' the zonules and capsular case from the upper left of the diagram.*

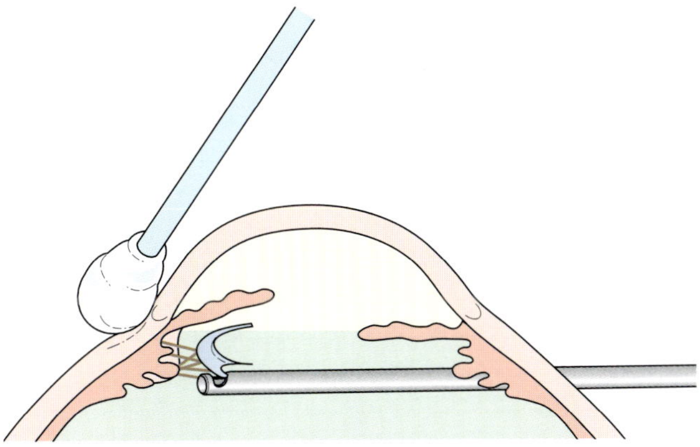

Figure 39.6 *Scleral depression can be used to assist in removal of far peripheral capsular and lenticular remnants.*

face from the retina at the edge of the optic nerve head.

After the vitrectomy is complete, plugs are placed into the sclerotomies. The eye is examined with indirect ophthalmoscopy and scleral depression. Lens particles are often present in the vitreous base. If only an occasional small piece (less than 1 mm in size) is present, retrieval is not necessary because these pieces often clear spontaneously and there is a risk of an inadvertent retinal break when pursuing them. If the vitreous base contains a significant number or size of lens fragments, these should be removed using the vitrector. A wide-field viewing system or gentle peripheral scleral depression from a skilled assistant will greatly facilitate this process.

A Weck-cell vitrectomy should be performed at each of the sclerotomies before closure. The sclerotomies are closed with a figure-of-eight 8-0 Vicryl suture. The conjunctiva is reapposed and sutured together with the 8-0 Vicryl as well. We prefer to leave the eye slightly soft because it may develop some inflammation and subsequent pressure rise. We place a drop of scopolamine and apply some erythromycin ointment to the eye and patch it with a hard shield overlying the patch.

DISLOCATED LENSES

After the sclerotomies are created as above, a core vitrectomy is performed, making sure to free vitreous from around the dislocated lens, where it can be particularly adherent. If possible a vitreous detachment should be created, if not already present (see above). We usually remove any remaining capsule and cortical material that may be present at this point, as described above. Before removing the lens, a small amount of perfluorocarbon liquid may be injected beneath the lens to protect the macula from impact by the lens during the phacofragmentation. This maneuver is particularly useful for dense nuclei. The fragmatome unit is inserted. The infusion bottle is raised moderately to accommodate the higher suction forces from this unit. Attention to the retinal perfusion status is important and, in our experience, the infusion bottle height does not have to be raised above the level where perfusion is compromised. Infusion bottle height should be decreased when fragmentation is not being performed.

The phaco power setting is proportionally increased with increasing lens nucleus density. It is important that the minimum effective power should be used because heat from the fragmentation unit is transmitted all along its shaft and can cause retinal/scleral burns and retinal breaks. To avoid these complications, the fragmatome is placed in aspiration mode only to engage the lens and draw it into the midvitreous cavity. While continuing to aspirate, the phaco is enabled (Fig. 39.7). We usually use pulse mode to decrease fragment dispersion, allowing the

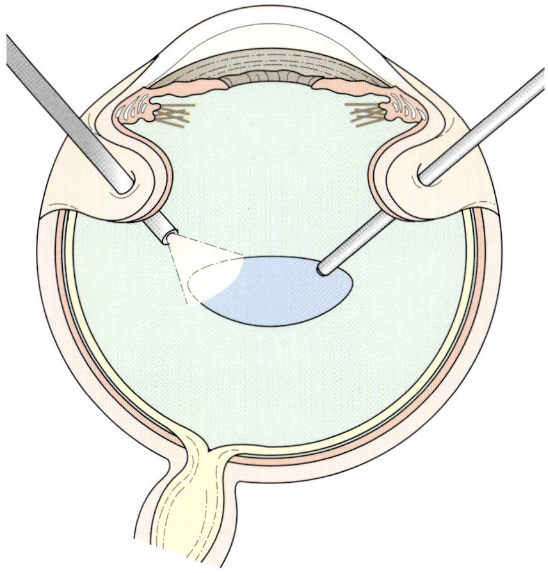

Figure 39.7 *Schematic diagram demonstrating aspiration of the lens into the midvitreous cavity using the phacofragmatome unit. This is done prior to using any phaco power to avoid thermal damage to the retina.*

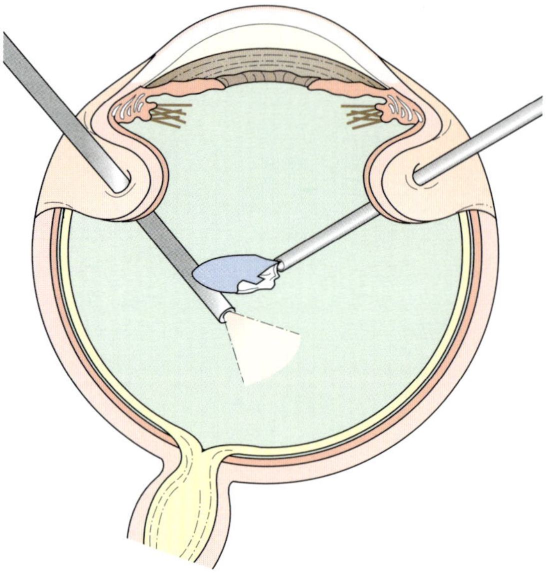

Figure 39.8 *Schematic diagram demonstrating the use of the vitreous light pipe to stabilize lens fragments during phacofragmentation of dislocated lens material.*

nucleus to stay intact while slowly decreasing in size. This maneuver provides the most efficient lens removal with minimum phaco time, and avoids the need to retrieve multiple small lens fragments.

While performing the phaco, it is important that the lens is engaged by the phaco tip at all times. If contact is lost, the aspiration and phaco should be deactivated and the lens re-engaged and brought to the midvitreous cavity. The light pipe may be used under the lens to provide additional support and to help push the lens into the fragmatome (Fig. 39.8). Once the nucleus is removed, any smaller fragments may be retrieved in the same manner. The phaco power should be lowered with smaller pieces because otherwise they will shoot away from the phaco needle, making retrieval more difficult. If a vitreous detachment is not present, posterior hyaloid stripping should be performed before retrieving small pieces from the macula because often subsequently they become mobilized and will be easier to remove. The eye should be examined by indirect ophthalmoscopy with scleral depression before closing.

Several authors advocate the use of perfluorocarbon liquid to 'float' the lens up into the anterior chamber to be removed by a limbal wound.[20–23] This approach may be most useful in cases of very dense, hard nuclei, which may otherwise require long amounts of phaco time at high power.

The most common complication to occur during this surgery is the formation of a retinal break from instrument manipulations or from the heat of the fragmatome unit itself. Small peripheral retinal breaks (often near sclerotomy sites) should be treated with cryopexy or laser. Larger breaks may require the addition of a scleral buckle. If a retinal detachment is present, perfluorocarbon liquid may flatten the retina during lens removal and allow laser retinopexy. We also place a scleral buckle in such cases. An injection of intraocular gas to help further tamponade the detachment or break is sometimes necessary, especially with breaks and detachments in which the break is not adequately flattened at the end of the case.

Another common intraoperative complication is bleeding during the vitrectomy. Post-traumatic eyes are generally inflamed with engorged vessels. Bleeding, which can occur from the sclerotomy sites or from areas of retinal vascular injury, is usually managed by temporarily raising the infusion pressure and removing the blood with an extrusion cannula. In some instances, endodiathermy may be needed. Careful cauterization of scleral blood vessels at the sclerotomy sites is also important.

Corneal edema may occur during the operation, especially when surgery is attempted soon after the initial traumatic episode. Visibility is essential to the successful outcome of surgery and the surgeon should not hesitate to scrape the central corneal epithelium when needed. In mild cases, a wet cotton-tipped applicator may be rolled over the cornea to help reduce edema.

In general, we do not place a primary intraocular lens in the setting of acute trauma. The risks of endophthalmitis, postoperative inflammation and/or glaucoma, synechiae formation, retinal detachment and the possibility of the need for future surgery in these injured eyes are reasons to wait. Younger trauma patients may tolerate contact lens rehabilitation or a short, second operation at a later, safer time point for the insertion of a secondary intraocular lens. However, in certain scenarios, primary intraocular lens placement should be considered. In a quiet stable eye with a more remote history of trauma, we routinely place an anterior chamber lens after vitrectomy. Malinowski et al have shown that open-loop, flexible, anterior chamber lenses are well tolerated in patients undergoing combined lensectomy–vitrectomy and represent a viable alternative to the more difficult and potentially higher risk placement of scleral or iris-fixated posterior chamber lenses.[24] It is important to perform a peripheral iridectomy at the time of surgery to avoid the risk of acute angle-closure glaucoma. Also, in acute cases with undamaged retina, a low risk of subsequent retinal detachment and clearly good visual potential, one should consider primary lens placement as well.

POSTOPERATIVE CARE

Patients are examined on postoperative day 1. Careful attention is paid to ocular inflammation, eye pressure and retinal status. The patient is begun on prednisolone drops six times per day, scopolamine twice per day, a broad-spectrum antibiotic drop or ointment four times per day and topical ketorolac four times a day as a prophylaxis against cystoid macular edema. If the examination is satisfactory, the patient is asked to return in approximately 5 days, at which time we begin tapering the steroids. The ketorolac is usually given for a minimum of 6 weeks and often for a 3-month course. In young children, aggressive visual rehabilitation and patching should be performed in the early postoperative period to help minimize the effects of amblyopia.

POSTOPERATIVE COMPLICATIONS

The postoperative complications from dislocated lens surgery are similar to those of vitrectomy. Persistent lens fragments may result in prolonged inflammation, glaucoma and cystoid macular edema. Endophthalmitis should always be a concern, particularly in cases of penetrating trauma. The development of retinal breaks and detachments should be evaluated carefully and treated with appropriate surgery. Many patients will develop angle-recession glaucoma[19,16,25,26] and will require life-long follow-up.

Surgery in this setting, especially in inflamed eyes, can result in postoperative hyphema and vitreous hemorrhage, most of which are self-limiting.[26] In cases of persistent hyphema, we generally only intervene surgically for persistent, uncontrolled rises in IOP (especially in patients with sickle-cell trait) or corneal blood staining. Vitreous hemorrhages should be followed carefully with serial ultrasounds to rule out retinal detachment. If no coexisting problems develop, we generally manage the hemorrhage conservatively and intervene only after it has had an adequate opportunity to clear (approximately 3 months).

Some patients may develop epiretinal membranes, especially if the posterior hyaloid face was not removed at the time of surgery. These membranes are subsequently removed when they become visually significant.

SURGICAL RESULTS

Although there are several reports of the use of vitrectomy and lensectomy techniques in cases of congenital or hereditary lenticular dislocation and dislocations as a result of complicated cataract surgery, there are only very limited data on surgical results using these techniques in the traumatic setting. Peyman and associates reported results for 13 dislocated lenses secondary to trauma in 1979.[26] Other than minimal bleeding in one case, no intraoperative complications occurred. Postoperative complications included transient corneal edema in one patient and persistently elevated IOP in three patients with diagnosed angle-recession glaucoma. Two of these latter patients lost vision, with one eye becoming phthisical. All eyes with phacolytic glaucoma had normal IOP after surgery. Nine of the other 11 patients had marked improvements in visual acuity, with the other two limited by macular degeneration. Ten eyes in this series had subluxated lenses; eight were from unknown causes and two were associated with Marfan's syndrome. All ten had good results with visual acuity returning to at least 20/200 in all eyes and better than 20/100 in eight eyes. No complications occurred in these patients. These authors also reported results of five eyes with lens dislocation associated with perforating injuries. Although they were able to achieve media clarity and reformation of the globes, four eyes with no light perception vision preoperatively remained at this level. The one other eye improved from light perception to 20/25. Postoperative complications were directly related to the preoperative status, including the presence of a traumatic laceration, retinal detachment or uncontrollable glaucoma.

Other authors also have shown that the presence of a dislocated crystalline lens in the setting of penetrating ocular trauma carries a poorer prognosis.[1,2] Sternberg reported that patients with a normal or cataractous lens without evidence of dislocation had an odds ratio of 5.22 for predicting a visual outcome of 20/800 or better.[2] De Juan et al reported that only 2.2% of patients with a subluxated or expelled lens were able to obtain a final visual acuity of 20/50 or better, whereas 35% of cases with an intact cataractous lens and 45% with a clear lens at presentation obtained this level of final vision.[1] Other series also have shown promising results using similar pars plana techniques for nontraumatic subluxated lenses.[27,28]

A few authors also have reported successful use of high-density vitreous substitutes as an adjunct to pars plana vitrectomy techniques for the management of traumatically induced lens dislocation. We generally reserve this technique of 'floating' the dislocated lens to the anterior chamber to be removed for cases of extremely hard lenses or with coexisting retinal detachment. Liu et al used fluorosilicone oil and perfluorocarbon liquid to manage three cases of traumatically dislocated lenses with hard nuclei.[22] Postoperative complications included a residual oil droplet in the anterior chamber of one eye and persistent cystoid macular edema in the other. Lewis et al used perfluorocarbon liquids in two cases of traumatically dislocated lenses and retinal detachments.[23] In both cases the retinas were successfully attached and visual acuities improved over 6–9 months of follow-up.

REFERENCES

1. De Juan E Jr, Sternberg P Jr, Michels RG. Penetrating ocular injuries: types of injuries and visual results, *Ophthalmology* (1983) **90:**1318–22.
2. Sternberg P Jr, De Juan E Jr, Michels R, Auer C. Multivariate analysis of prognostic factors in penetrating ocular injuries, *Am J Ophthalmol* (1984) **98:**467–72.
3. Mieler WF, Mittra RM. The role and timing of pars plana vitrectomy in penetrating ocular trauma (editorial), *Arch Ophthalmol* (1997) **115:**1191–2.
4. Meredith TA, Gordon PA. Pars plana vitrectomy for severe penetrating injury with posterior segment involvement, *Am J Ophthalmol* (1987) **103:**549–54.
5. Conway BP, Michels RG. Vitrectomy techniques in the management of selected penetrating ocular injuries, *Ophthalmology* (1978) **85:**560–83.
6. Ryan SJ, Allen AW. Pars plana vitrectomy in ocular trauma, *Am J Ophthalmol* (1979) **88** (3 Pt 1): 483–91.
7. Gregor Z, Ryan SJ. Complete and core vitrectomies in the treatment of experimental posterior penetrating eye injury in the rhesus monkey. 1. Clinical features, *Arch Ophthalmol* (1983) **101:**441–5.
8. Brinton GS, Aaberg TM, Reeser FH, et al. Surgical results in ocular trauma involving the posterior segment, *Am J Ophthalmol* (1982) **93:**271–8.
9. Rosenbaum LJ, Podos SM. Traumatic ectopia lentis: some relationships to syphilis and glaucoma, *Am J Ophthalmol* (1967) **64:**1095–8.
10. Calhoun FP Jr, Hagler WS. Experience with the Jose Barraquer method of extracting a dislocated lens, *Am J Ophthalmol* (1960) **50:**701–15.
11. Barraquer J. Surgery of the dislocated lens, *Trans Am Acad Ophthalmol Otolaryngol* (1972) **76:**44–59.
12. Demmler U, Sautter U. Surgery in subluxated lenses in adults, *Dev Ophthalmol* (1985) **11:**162–5.
13. Zaidman GW. The surgical management of dislocated traumatic cataracts, *Am J Ophthalmol* (1985) **99:**583–5.
14. Bode D, Lloyd WC III, Griffith DG. The use of a trochar to fixate a dislocated lens, *Ann Ophthalmol* (1986) **18:**14–15.
15. Chandler PA. Choice of treatment in dislocation of lens, *Arch Ophthalmol* (1964) **7:**765.
16. Jarrett WH III. Dislocation of the lens: a study of 166 hospitalized cases, *Arch Ophthalmol* (1967) **78:**289–96.
17. Jensen AD, Cross HE. Surgical treatment of dislocated lenses in the Marfan syndrome and homocystinuria, *Trans Am Acad Ophthalmol Otolaryngol* (1972) **76:**1491–9.
18. Liesman N. Congenital cataract and ectopia lentis: An analysis of 152 patients treated in 1943–1967, *Acta Ophthalmol* (1972) **112** (Suppl): 13–79.
19. Seigel RS, Sell J, Magnus DE. CT appearance of traumatic dislocated lens, *Am J Neuroradiol* (1988) **9:**390.
20. Greve MDJ, Peyman GA, Mehta NJ, Millsap CM. Use of perfluoroperhydrophenanthrene in the management of posteriorly dislocated crystalline and intraocular lenses, *Ophthalmic Surg* (1993) **24:**593–7.
21. Shapiro MJ, Resnick KI, Kim SH, Weinberg A. Management of the dislocated crystalline lens with a perfluorocarbon liquid, *Am J Ophthalmol* (1991) **112:**401–5.
22. Liu KR, Peyman GA, Chen MS, Chang KB. Use of high-density vitreous substitutes in the removal of posteriorly dislocated lenses or intraocular lenses, *Ophthalmic Surg* (1991) **22:**503–7.
23. Lewis H, Blumenkranz MS, Chang S. Treatment of dislocated crystalline lens and retinal detachment with perfluorocarbon liquids, *Retina* (1992) **12:**299–304.
24. Malinowski SM, Mieler WF, Koenig SB, et al. Combined pars plana vitrectomy–lensectomy and open-loop anterior chamber lens implantation, *Ophthalmology* (1995) **102:**211–16.
25. Rodman HI. Chronic open angle glaucoma associated with traumatic dislocation of the lens: a new pathogenic concept, *Arch Ophthalmol* (1963) **69:**445–54.
26. Peyman GA, Raichand M, Goldberg MF, Ritacca D. Management of subluxated and dislocated lenses with the vitrophage, *Br J Ophthalmol* (1979) **63:**771–8.
27. Girard LJ, Canizales R, Esnaola N, Rand WJ. Subluxated (ectopic) lenses in adults: long-term results of pars plana lensectomy–vitrectomy by ultrasonic fragmentation with and without a phacoprosthesis, *Ophthalmology* (1990) **97:**462–5.
28. Hakin KN, Jacobs M, Rosen P, et al. Management of the subluxed crystalline lens, *Ophthalmology* (1992) **99:**542–5.

Chapter 40 Removal of intraocular foreign bodies

William J Wirostko, William F Mieler and Cathleen M McCabe

INTRODUCTION

Intraocular foreign bodies (IOFB) are both a common and serious problem in traumatic ocular injuries. They occur in up to 40% of open globes and put an eye at risk for infection, retinal detachment and metallosis.[1,2] They represent a true emergency and can produce blindness even with the best of treatment. Most IOFB afflict young productive members of society while hammering, drilling or grinding in the workplace.[3–7] Consequently, IOFB injuries are very costly, both economically and personally.

With appropriate treatment, most eyes maintain or recover good vision. In a recent study, approximately 80% of eyes recovered visual acuity to 5/200 or better and 60% of eyes achieved at least 20/40.[3,5] Removal of the IOFB is integral for good visual rehabilitation. Ideally, this should be done urgently, either at the time of primary wound closure or as soon as possible thereafter. Good anatomic and visual recovery is the product of many factors, including a detailed history and examination, appropriate ancillary testing, a minimally traumatic IOFB removal, repair of associated ocular damage and vigilant follow-up. Occasionally, however, the IOFB leads to damage that cannot be overcome.

INDICATIONS FOR IOFB REMOVAL

The majority of IOFB should be removed on an emergent basis. A delay of greater than 24 hours produces a fourfold greater risk for endophthalmitis and a worsened visual prognosis.[2] Furthermore, the IOFB may be more difficult to extract because of the formation of encapsulating fibrous tissues, fibrovascular membranes, an organized vitreous or a rhegmatogenous retinal detachment.[8] An urgent extraction also limits ocular toxicity from metallic IOFB. The authors recognize that, rarely, a closed globe may present with an incidental IOFB, and that for these eyes IOFB removal may be more disruptive than observation. The decision to extract the IOFB from these eyes must be made on an individual basis, and if the IOFB is left in place one must be certain that it comprises an inert substance.

PREOPERATIVE EVALUATION

While obtaining a history of an injured eye, one must remain suspicious for an IOFB. It is helpful to consider that all traumatized eyes, especially open globes, contain an IOFB until proven otherwise. Suspicion must be greatest whenever a history of hammering, drilling, grinding or an explosion is elicited. These activities produce the majority of IOFB.[3–6] Other mechanisms for IOFB include motor vehicle accidents,[9] assault,[10] lawn mower accidents[11] and bee stings.[12] One should ascertain the circumstances of the injury, the elapsed time since the injury and the composition and magnetic properties of any potential IOFB. The history can be quite helpful for suggesting the presence of an IOFB when media opacity prevents a thorough examination. The use of safety glasses does not preclude the possibility of an IOFB.

All eyes suspected to contain an IOFB need a complete examination. Important baseline information includes visual acuity, pupillary reaction, intraocular pressure, iris color and lens status. The anterior segment should be inspected for evidence of an open globe injury. In most cases, the entrance site involves the cornea (65%), but other sites include the limbus (10%) and sclera (25%).[3–6] One must remember that a wound may be self-sealing and that mild pressure asymmetry may be all that

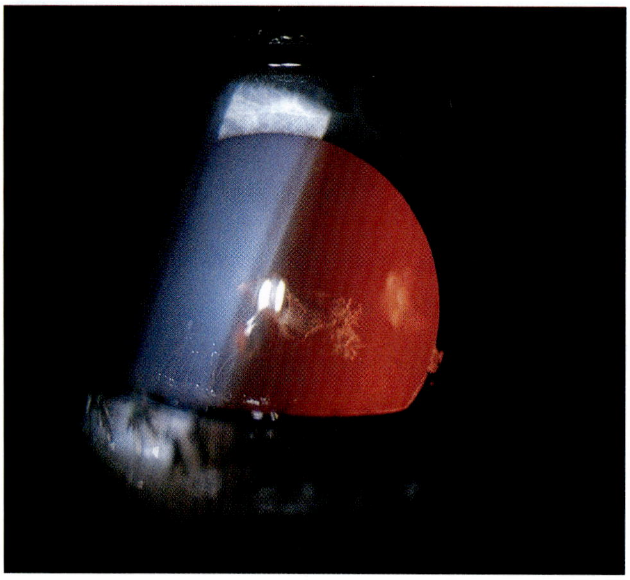

Figure 40.1 *Lenticular laceration caused by intraocular foreign body.*

suggests an open globe injury with an IOFB. All intraocular structures must be searched for incarcerated IOFB. Common resting locations include the vitreous (61%), anterior chamber (15%), retina (14%), lens (8%) and subretinal space (5%).[3] IOFB should have their location, shape, number, size and composition recorded. If the IOFB is difficult to find, the location of an iris or lenticular laceration (Fig. 40.1) may be helpful in suggesting a trajectory. All posterior segment trauma, including media opacities, retinal tears and retinal detachments, should be described in full detail because progressive media opacification may limit future examinations. During the examination, one should be careful not to prolapse any intraocular contents out of the globe because this usually worsens the prognosis.

Ancillary tests may be necessary to document the IOFB or determine the extent of associated ocular trauma. They are most valuable when intraocular hemorrhage, cataracts or other media opacities limit the clinical examination. Common diagnostic tests include computed tomography (CT), echography, magnetic resonance imaging (MRI) and plain film radiology (PFR).

CT is the diagnostic modality of choice. It is highly sensitive and offers the ability to locate any IOFB accurately without extensive patient co-operation or globe manipulation.[13] Also, it can suggest the composition of an IOFB by measuring its radiodensity.[14] CT is most sensitive when thin cuts of less than 1.5 mm are obtained in both an axial and coronal orientation.[15] However, even this technique may miss IOFB smaller than 0.7 mm,[14] IOFB located adjacent to the sclera[10] or IOFB composed of wood.[16,17] Helical scanning demonstrates no significant benefit over conventional axial techniques.[18] CT is the modality of choice for ruling out a metallic IOFB before MRI studies are performed.

Ocular echography is another valuable modality. It demonstrates high diagnostic sensitivity and can detect both radiolucent and radiopaque IOFB through reverberation and acoustic shadowing. In one study of 46 eyes, echography demonstrated 100% sensitivity for detecting all IOFB, including a cilium.[19] Echography can be performed in the office and is helpful for assessing associated ocular damage, including retinal detachment, choroidal hemorrhage and vitreous hemorrhage.[19,20] It may be the only modality capable of demonstrating a subtle posterior exit wound, a violation of the posterior lens capsule or the exact location of an IOFB lying adjacent to sclera. Disadvantages of echography include the requirements of patient co-operation and ocular manipulation. The risk for expelling intraocular contents from an open globe may be minimized by performing the examination through closed lids or by completing the study intraoperatively after the globe has been closed. Echography has poor specificity and should be interpreted always in conjunction with other testing. This will prevent mistaking minute intraocular air bubbles for multiple small metallic IOFB. If greater accuracy regarding an IOFB is sought, as is often the case with anterior chamber IOFB,[21] high-frequency echography can be used.

MRI is helpful for documenting nonmetallic IOFB. It is typically ordered when a wood or plastic IOFB is suspected and other studies are nondiagnostic.[22,23] MRI should not be used as a screening test. It employs high magnetic forces and is capable of inducing ocular damage through movement of occult metallic IOFB.[24] A negative CT scan to exclude the presence of a metallic IOFB is required before any MRI study is obtained.

PFR has limited value in the diagnosis of IOFB. It is grossly insensitive and is by itself a poor test for ruling out the presence of an IOFB. In one study, PFR failed to demonstrate an IOFB in 60% of eyes known to contain foreign material.[25,26] Even if PFR is negative, CT should be obtained if an IOFB is suspected.

The preoperative evaluation for an IOFB concludes with arranging for emergency surgery with removal of the IOFB. A medical history is obtained in preparation for surgery and the patient's tetanus immunity status is updated. The open globe is covered with a protective shield and intravenous antibiotics are given for infection prophylaxis, especially if surgery is to be delayed. Agents with a broad spectrum of activity and good ocular penetration are best, such as vancomycin and ceftazidime. The use of antibiotics is discussed further in the following sections on ancillary surgical treatment and postoperative follow-up.

INSTRUMENTATION

Instrumentation for IOFB removal involves magnets and forceps. Magnets offer many advantages and should be employed whenever possible. They automatically align a magnetic IOFB along its long axis and present its smallest cross-section to the wound for transscleral passage.[27–29] Currently, two types of magnets exist: external magnets and rare-earth magnets (Fig. 40.2). External magnets generate great force but are large, bulky and offer imprecise IOFB control. They are restricted to use outside of the eye. Internal magnets are small, delicate and precise. They generate less force and are best used within the eye, where they can be placed in close approximation to the IOFB. Their use in the posterior segment requires a pars plana vitrectomy (PPV).

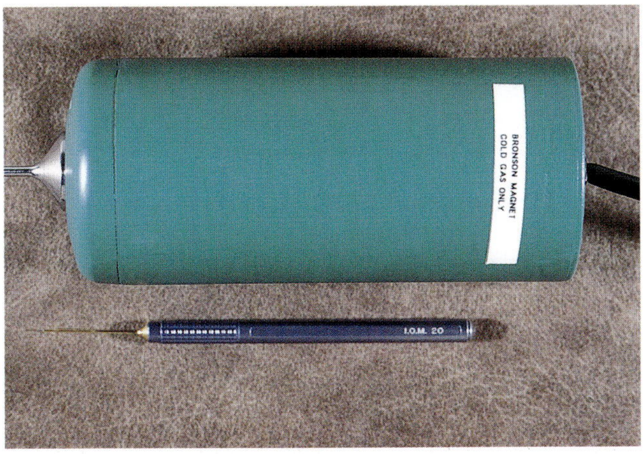

Figure 40.2 *Bronson external magnet (above) and rare-earth intraocular magnet (below).*

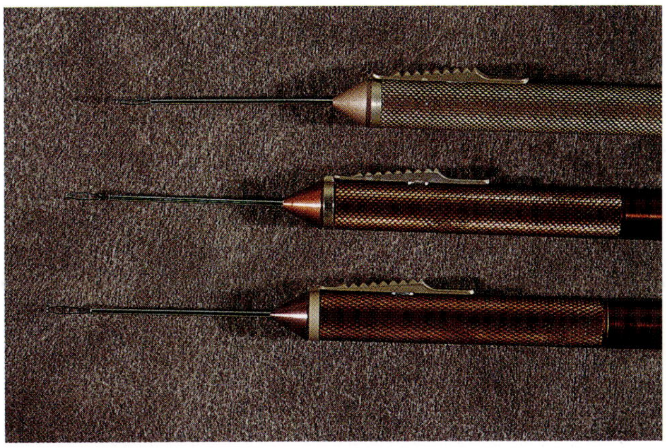

Figure 40.3 *A collection of intraocular foreign body forceps.*

The use of all magnets requires accurate IOFB localization. Failure to do so can produce ocular damage through unwanted impaction of the IOFB into lens or retina or by traction from the IOFB on ocular structures, including the retina and vitreous.[27]

In cases of nonmagnetic IOFB, intraocular forceps should be employed (Fig. 40.3). Forceps also should be used for passing the IOFB across the ocular wall, even if a magnet was used initially. Forceps generate greater holding power than magnets and are less likely to drop the IOFB back into the eye, where it may hit the macula. If concern exists about dropping the IOFB, perfluorocarbon liquid can be injected posteriorly to dampen the impact and to protect the retina.[8] IOFB delivery is easiest when the IOFB is delivered across the ocular wall in the orientation of smallest cross-section. The use of heavy extraocular forceps to grasp the IOFB once it becomes exposed also facilitates delivery.

ROUTE OF IOFB EXTRACTION

The appropriate route for extraction depends on the size, composition and location of the IOFB, as well as the presence of associated ocular damage. In all cases, the route offering greatest IOFB control and producing the least amount of extraction trauma should be chosen. A minimally traumatic extraction is the product of an accurate IOFB assessment, a properly prepared extraction site and proper instrumentation. Most IOFB are best removed at the time

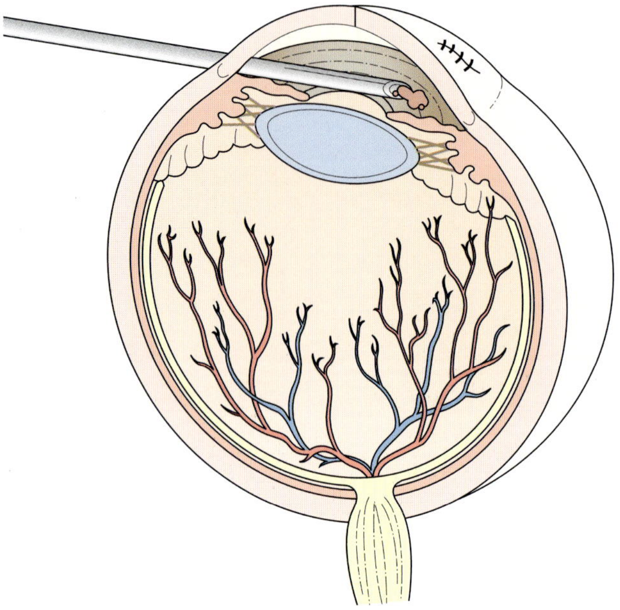

Figure 40.4 *Schematic diagram depicting extraction of an anterior segment intraocular foreign body through a limbal incision after repair of the traumatic laceration.*

of repair of the penetrating ocular wound. This offers repair of the injury, along with restoration of ocular integrity, in a single operation.

IOFB located in the anterior chamber are best removed through a secondary limbal incision after the traumatic laceration has been repaired (Fig. 40.4). This limits the trauma to the original laceration and facilitates instrumentation. The secondary incision should be placed 90° away from the IOFB to avoid traversing instruments over the lens capsule. Additional lenticular protection is possible by pharmacologically inducing miosis. The IOFB can be engaged with either intraocular forceps or a rare-earth magnet, while viscoelastics maintain the anterior chamber. Viscoelastic dissection may be helpful for removing IOFB from the iris. Lens extraction usually is necessary if the IOFB is embedded in the lens.[30] Removing the lens *in toto* helps to prevent

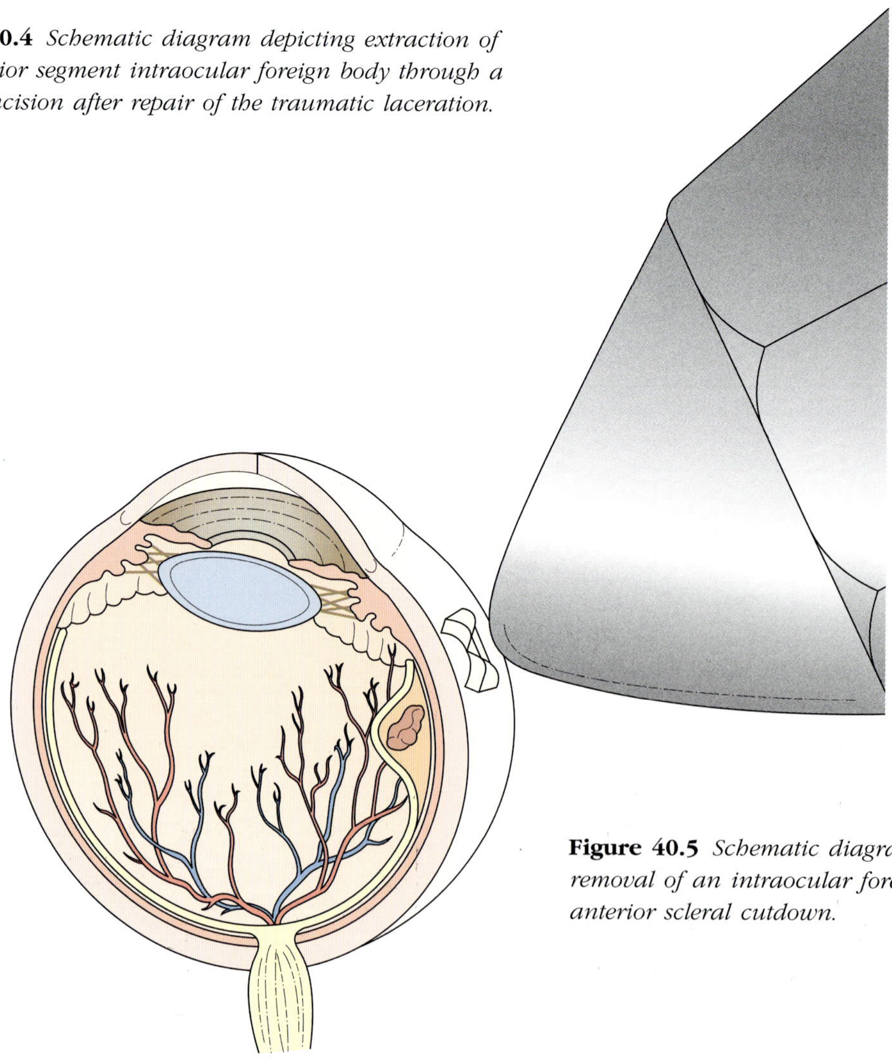

Figure 40.5 *Schematic diagram demonstrating the removal of an intraocular foreign body through an anterior scleral cutdown.*

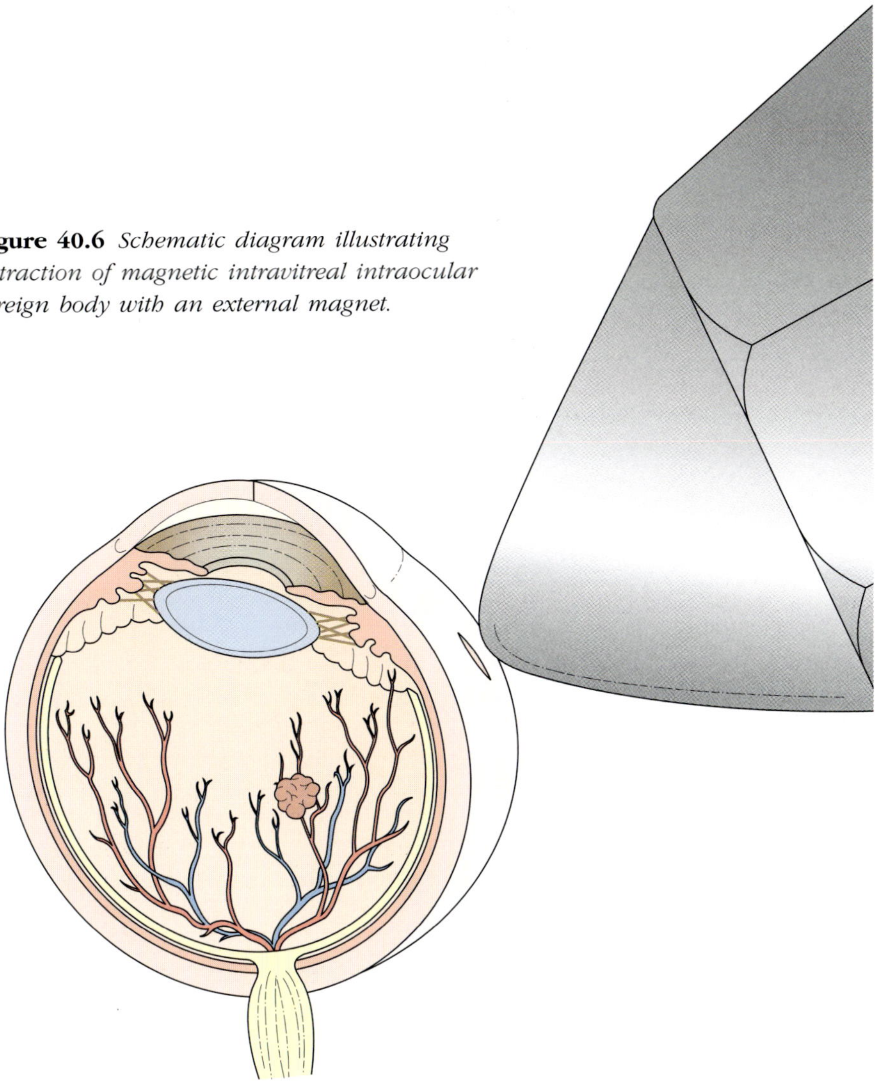

Figure 40.6 *Schematic diagram illustrating extraction of magnetic intravitreal intraocular foreign body with an external magnet.*

dropping the IOFB into the posterior segment. If the intralenticular IOFB can be grasped, IOFB extraction should be performed before cataract extraction. The anterior capsular laceration often can be converted into a capsulorhexis and the cataract removed by aspiration. Intraocular lens implantation can be performed concurrently, depending upon the extent of the trauma and the risk of infection.

Magnetic IOFB located both anterior to the equator and in the subretinal or intraretinal space can be removed through a scleral cutdown (Fig. 40.5). This involves extracting the IOFB through a T-shaped scleral and uveal incision with an external magnet. The flap should be created after indirect ophthalmoscopy has localized the IOFB, and diathermy should be applied to the surrounding uveal bed to limit the risk of hemorrhage. Transpupillary laser photocoagulation retinopexy may be placed around the IOFB site. Both treatments are best placed prior to transuveal passage because hemorrhage may limit further treatment. After extraction is complete, the sclerotomies are sutured closed. A scleral buckle may be placed, especially if the retina is incarcerated in the wound.

Intravitreal magnetic IOFB that are clearly visible and free of incarcerated tissue can be removed through a pars plana sclerostomy with an external magnet (Fig. 40.6). The pars plana incision should be created in a location that offers the shortest and most direct route of extraction while minimizing the chance of IOFB impaction into the lens and retina. Diathermy can be applied to the sclerotomy, as well

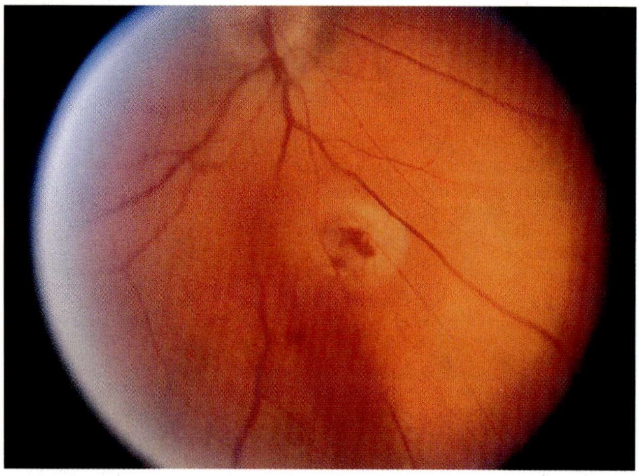

Figure 40.7 *Fundus photograph of intraocular foreign body retinal impaction site. (Courtesy of Thomas B Connor Jr MD, Milwaukee, WI.)*

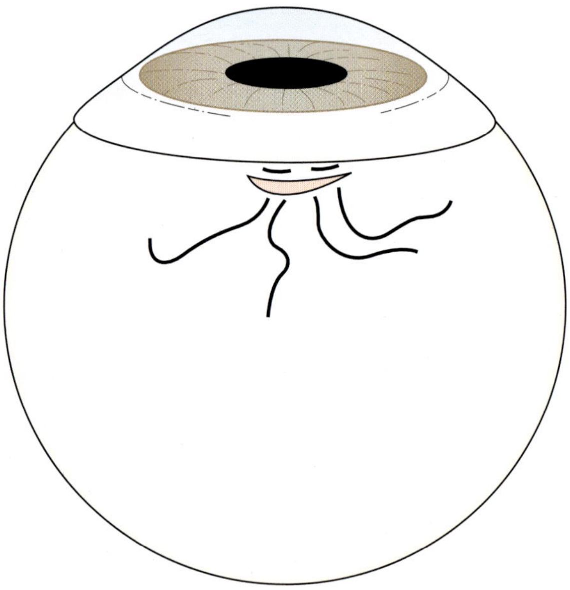

Figure 40.8 *Schematic diagram demonstrating preplaced horizontal mattress sutures across pars plana sclerotomy.*

as laser photocoagulation to any IOFB impaction site (Fig. 40.7). Preplaced horizontal mattress sutures allow rapid closure of large sclerotomies (Fig. 40.8). IOFB extraction is best achieved with the assistant holding the external magnet while the surgeon controls the magnet's foot pedal and visualizes the IOFB with the indirect ophthalmoscope. A simple conical tip on the external magnet works well in most cases. It is not necessary to insert the tip through the sclerotomy. The authors do not perform PPV routinely in these eyes. Studies suggest that PPV adds little benefit other than a slightly decreased risk of endophthalmitis.[1,3,13] However, these studies were nonrandomized and contained selection bias.

Posterior segment IOFB that are nonmagnetic, too large for pars plana delivery, obscured by media opacity or embedded in the posterior segment will require PPV for extraction. The authors recommend an IOFB cross-section size limit of approximately 5 mm for pars plana extraction, although it is not known precisely if even larger IOFB can be removed safely through the pars plana.

PPV allows the use of intraocular forceps and rare-earth magnets (Fig. 40.9). The latter are especially helpful for achieving a delicate dissection of the IOFB from the retina and fibrous tissue.[31,32] Thick fibrous capsules may require incision with a myringotomy blade. PPV enables the creation of retinotomies or retinectomies for access to subretinal IOFB[32] and allows the passage of large IOFB across the pupil into the anterior chamber for a limbal extraction (Fig. 40.10). Ureter stone forceps can be employed for very large IOFB (Fig. 40.11);[33] these can be introduced through a pars plana or limbal incision. Posterior segment damage can be repaired, vitreous hemorrhages can be cleared, disrupted lens may be removed and retinal detachments may be repaired. For potentially infected eyes, PPV provides large vitreous samples, decreases the intraocular bacterial load, irrigates toxins from the eye and possibly decreases the risk of endophthalmitis.[13] Finally, PPV allows the posterior hyaloid to be separated in cases with intraretinal IOFB.[34] This separation is achieved by engaging the hyaloid under suction with either a soft-tipped extrusion cannula or vitrectomy instrument and peeling it anteriorly with a pick. A posterior hyaloidectomy should be performed also if a retinal detachment develops during the extraction of an IOFB. Retinal tears should be free of all adherent vitreous.

All IOFB and any available aqueous or vitreous should be sent for bacterial and fungal cultures because positive cultures could influence treatment if endophthalmitis develops.[35] Cultures are ideally performed on various media to guarantee identification of a possible organism. The absence of clinical endophthalmitis should not prevent microbiologic studies because 40% of infected eyes have a delayed presentation and display no signs of infection at presentation.[3] Culture results must be interpreted in

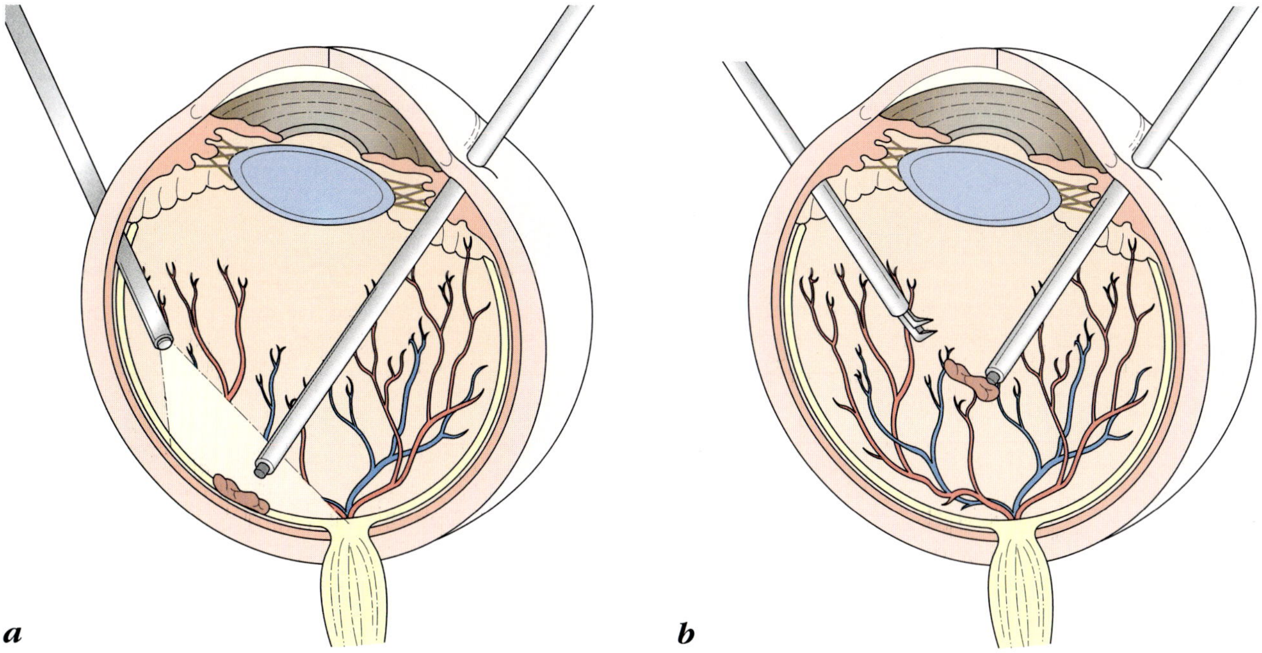

Figure 40.9 *(a) Schematic diagram showing the use of rare-earth magnet to free intraretinal foreign body. (b) Once the foreign body has been freed of adhesions, it is transferred to forceps for transscleral delivery.*

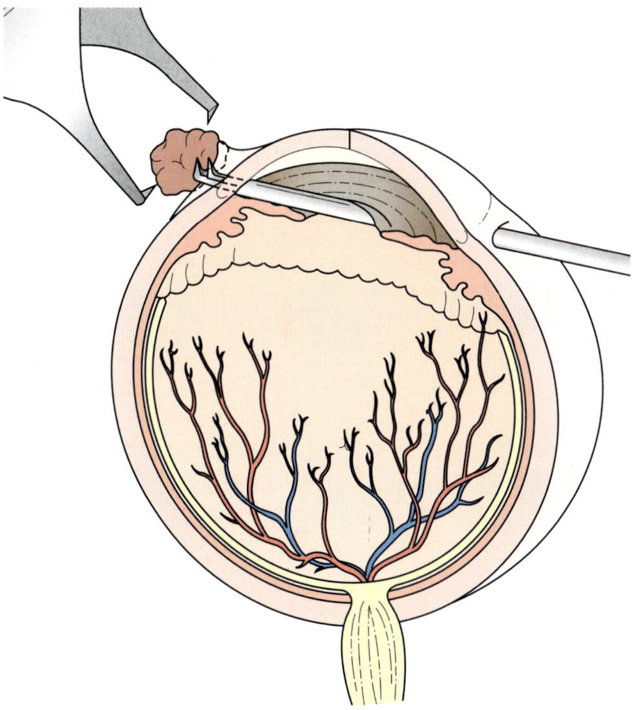

Figure 40.10 *Schematic diagram depicting passage of large intraocular foreign body through limbal incision after transpupillary passage into anterior chamber.*

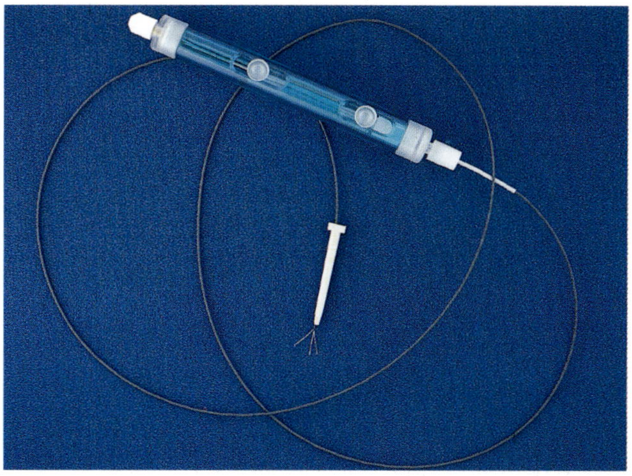

Figure 40.11 *Ureter stone forceps.*

conjunction with clinical examination. Not all infected eyes will have positive cultures and, conversely, the isolation of an organism does not guarantee that clinical signs of infection will develop. Up to 65% of IOFB are associated with positive cultures, whereas only 8–13% of eyes develop endophthalmitis.[2,13]

ANCILLARY SURGICAL TREATMENT

Various anterior and posterior segment procedures may be employed to repair the associated ocular damage caused by an IOFB. Common interventions include retinopexy, retinal reattachment procedures, cataract extractions and intravitreal injections.

Retinopexy involves using either laser photocoagulation or cryotherapy to create a chorioretinal adhesion around a retinal break or the IOFB impaction site. It should be placed around all retinal tears occurring distant to an IOFB impaction site. Its placement at impaction sites, however, remains controversial. Two rows of adjacent laser photocoagulation placed around all IOFB impaction sites before removal have been recommended (Fig. 40.12).[36] This was shown to be 100% effective for preventing retinal detachment in a series of 36 patients. Either indirect argon or diode photocoagulation may be used. Some surgeons allow the retinopexy to mature before IOFB extraction.[34,37–39] However, this delay in IOFB removal invites other complications. Other clinicians claim that no retinopexy is needed at the impaction site.[37,40] They propose that IOFB impaction produces a spontaneous chorioretinal adhesion and that additional adhesive therapy is potentially harmful with no supplemental benefit.

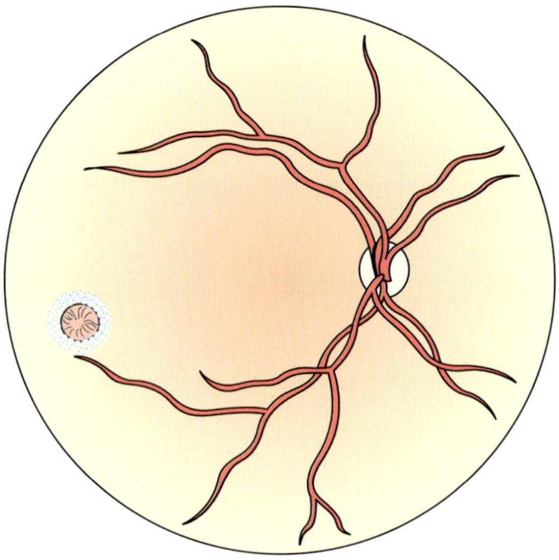

Figure 40.12 *Schematic diagram demonstrating laser retinopexy around intraocular foreign body impaction site.*

All authors agree that retinal breaks need treatment once a retinal detachment occurs. Retinal reattachment procedures include scleral buckling, PPV and/or gas tamponade. Recently, primary silicone oil tamponade was shown to be valuable for treating IOFB-related retinal detachments.[41] Prophylactic scleral buckles may be placed around these eyes with a high risk for detachment. Although this provides no proven benefit, a possible protective effect has been described.[42] Retinal tears with adherent vitreous should be supported with a scleral buckle.

Cataract surgery may be required if the lens is lacerated, dislocated or subluxated. Lens extraction clears a view to the posterior segment and decreases the risk for phacoantigenic endophthalmitis and glaucoma.[30] Furthermore, it removes a potential nidus for infectious endophthalmitis. One could consider a limbal approach if both good zonular support and an intact posterior capsule are present, but otherwise a pars plana approach should be employed. Removing the traumatized lens also simplifies the differential diagnosis of postinjury inflammation in an eye at risk for infection. It must be stated that not all lenticular injuries are progressive and that a good visual outcome may be possible with lens preservation.[43] Aphakia can be managed with either an immediate or delayed intraocular lens placement. The latter is the traditional and probably safer method. However, it leaves the eye aphakic and requires additional surgery. In contrast, immediate intraocular lens placement offers quick visual rehabilitation but risks the placement of foreign material in a potentially infected eye. It also potentiates the chance for using the wrong intraocular lens power. None the less, good results have been reported[39,44,45] and immediate intraocular lens placement may be considered if there is a low risk for endophthalmitis. Appropriate informed consent is essential in both strategies.

The proper use of prophylactic intravitreal antibiotics remains controversial. Some clinicians advocate their use with all IOFB injuries.[39,46] They quote the high rate of infection with IOFB injuries and the guarded prognosis after endophthalmitis as justification. Others, including the authors of this chapter, recognize that intravitreal antibiotics, especially aminoglycosides, are not always benign and can produce untoward side-effects, including retinal toxicity, allergic reactions and the development of resistant bacteria.[47] The authors recommend using intravitreal antibiotics only when the eye demonstrates signs of infection or is at high risk for endophthalmitis, such as in the setting of organic matter contamination.

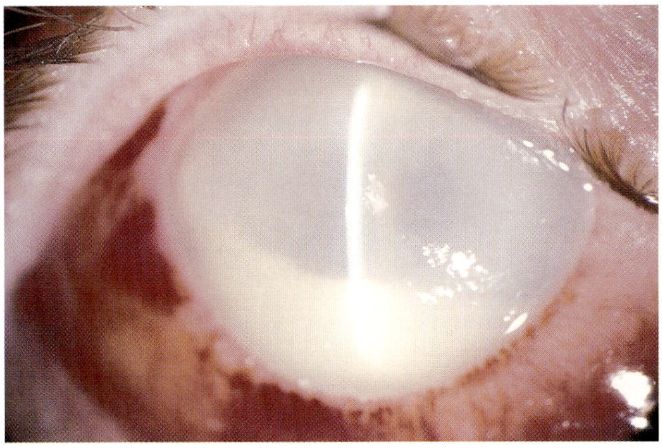

Figure 40.13 *Hypopyon secondary to endophthalmitis in eye with intraocular foreign body.*

Eyes with hypopyon formation (Fig. 40.13), vitritis, retinitis or vasculitis should definitely receive intravitreal antibiotics, because these are signs commonly associated with infection. The most commonly employed intravitreal antibiotics are vancomycin (1 mg) combined with either amikacin (200–400 μg) or ceftazidime (2.25 mg). Subconjunctival and fortified topical antibiotics usually are employed in all cases. Also, a short course of systemic antibiotics is used, although the true benefit of systemic antibiotics in the setting of trauma has never been proven; it is considered the standard of care. Specific recommendations for these antibiotics are outlined in the next section on postoperative follow-up. The use of intraocular corticosteroids is quite controversial and is also discussed in the next section. There is an increasing tendency to treat endophthalmitis in an outpatient setting; thus, rather than utilizing intravenous vancomycin or a cephalosporin for 1–3 days, often a quinolone such as ciprofloxacin is given orally for approximately 7 days.

POSTOPERATIVE FOLLOW-UP

Close follow-up after IOFB removal is necessary for the timely diagnosis and management of any postoperative complication, which may present in an immediate or delayed fashion and be visually devastating. Common complications include endophthalmitis, proliferative vitreoretinopathy (PVR), retinal detachment, metallosis and subretinal neovascularization.

ENDOPHTHALMITIS

Infectious endophthalmitis should be suspected whenever increased intraocular inflammation develops after an IOFB injury. A high index of suspicion is mandatory because infections develop in 8–13% of IOFB injuries[2,3] and can produce blindness in 66% of eyes.[46] One must be extremely suspicious when the IOFB is organic in composition or is soil contaminated. In these eyes, endophthalmitis develops in up to 30% of cases and tends to be very aggressive because infection with Bacillus species ranges up to 50%.[13,46,48] Other risk factors for endophthalmitis include the presence of a retained IOFB for more than 24 hours,[2] a patient older than 50 years[2] and an IOFB comprised of steel.[3,46,48] Bacterial strains most commonly identified include bacillus, staphylococcus and streptococcus.[2,13,49] Bacillus endophthalmitis carries the worst prognosis because it produces phthisis, and leads to enucleation or total vision loss in 75% of cases.[49] It is common with organic or soil-contaminated IOFB.[48]

Treatment for endophthalmitis associated with an IOFB involves emergently removing the foreign body, obtaining complete bacterial cultures and administering intravitreal, subconjunctival, topical and possibly intravenous antibiotics. Administration of intravitreal antibiotics is the most important factor by far in successfully suppressing the infection. This can produce a good result, even in the presence of Bacillus endophthalmitis.[50,51] Delaying the intravitreal antibiotic injection beyond 24 hours leads to a worsened prognosis.[3]

The ideal injectable should be safe and provide broad Gram-negative and Gram-positive coverage. As noted in the ancillary surgical treatment section, the authors recommend vancomycin (1.0 mg) in combination with either ceftazidime (2.25 mg) or amikacin (200–400 μg). An advantage of ceftazidime over amikacin is its lower retinotoxicity.[52,53] However, amikacin does possess a synergistic bactericidal ability with vancomycin and may be preferred when Bacillus species are suspected,[54] although most cases of Bacillus are sensitive to vancomycin alone. One should allow 24–48 hours before assessing any treatment response. This interval will help to differentiate inflammation from infection. Reinjection can be done whenever intravitreal treatment is considered inadequate or incomplete.

Intravitreal antibiotic levels can be prolonged with intravenous agents. Intravenous cefazolin (1 g every 8 hours, adult dose),[55] ceftazidime (1 g every 8 hours, adult dose), [39,56] vancomycin (1 g every 12 hours, adult dose)[57] and ciprofloxacin (400 mg every 12 hours, adult dose)[58] all cross the blood–ocular barrier and provide broad coverage. The authors recommend intravenous vancomycin in combination with a third-generation cephalosporin or ciprofloxacin for 1–3 days. Oral ciprofloxacin (750 mg every 12 hours, adult) achieves therapeutic levels but requires multiple doses over several days.[59] The authors discourage the use of intravenous aminoglycosides such as gentamicin because they do not consistently achieve therapeutic intravitreal levels[55,60] and there is significant morbidity.

Although the current standard of care for retained IOFB includes intravenous antibiotics, a trend is developing toward outpatient management, increased use of oral agents and shorter duration of treatment. Subconjunctival injection and topical application are two additional routes for antibiotic administration. Antibiotics given by these routes, however, including vancomycin, cephalosporins and aminoglycosides, produce bactericidal levels only in the anterior chambers.[61]

Treatment for endophthalmitis often involves a PPV when inflammation is severe. This procedure decreases the infectious load,[13,49] obtains material for cultures and allows better antibiotic distribution within the posterior segment. It may also irrigate bacteria and toxins from the eye.[13] Clinicians must realize that traumatic endophthalmitis is different from postoperative endophthalmitis and that the conclusions of the Endophthalmitis Vitrectomy Study (EVS) regarding vitreous tap versus vitrectomy are not applicable.

The proper use for corticosteroids in endophthalmitis remains unknown and controversial. One postoperative clinical study has suggested a beneficial effect of intravitreal corticosteroids in the setting of *Staphylococcus aureus*,[63] although an experimental model in rabbits using *Staphylococcus aureus* documented a worsened outcome and corticosteroids administered systemically offered no apparent advantage.[64] Although corticosteroids may be beneficial for decreasing inflammation and potentially limiting ocular damage, they can also potentiate an infection. Currently, their use depends on surgeon preference. If employed, the following dosages are commonly used: intravitreal dexamethasone 400 µg/0.1 ml, periocular Decadron 4–12 mg and systemic prednisone 0.7–1.0 mg/kg/day.

RETINAL DETACHMENT

Retinal detachment with PVR is common following an IOFB injury. In up to 8% of IOFB injuries, visual loss to at least 5/200 occurs as a result of retinal detachment, epiretinal membrane formation or development of subretinal fibrosis.[3] Its severity is exacerbated by the presence of an intraretinal IOFB. For these eyes, the rate of PVR-related retinal detachment and visual loss to 5/200 appears to be as high as 50% and 40%, respectively.[34,38] Other risk factors for PVR include the presence of vitreous hemorrhage, a retinal break, persistent intraocular inflammation and multiple surgeries.[34,39,65] The best defense against PVR appears to be PPV, with removal of the posterior hyaloid and meticulous attention to any and all retinal breaks. The introduction of this procedure corresponds with a drop in the rate of retinal detachment from 87% in 1972[66] to 50% in 1982.[34] The authors recommend PPV with removal of the posterior hyaloid in all eyes with an intraretinal IOFB.

SIDEROSIS BULBI

Siderosis bulbi develops when iron is retained within the eye. Its rate of development and its degree of severity depend upon the content and location of the iron. Larger and more posterior ferrous IOFB have the worst prognosis.[67] Histopathologically, siderosis is characterized by the accumulation of iron within metabolically active cells. Cells of the retinal pigment epithelium, pars plana, trabecular meshwork, corneal epithelium, lens epithelium and pupillary constrictor muscle all may be affected.[67,68]

Clinical signs of siderosis include reduced visual acuity, mydriasis, iris heterochromia, brown deposits beneath the anterior lens capsule and cataract formation.[67] Electrophysiological changes include an abnormal electroretinogram (ERG) and dark-adaptation study. These abnormalities usually precede visual loss and may be progressive despite removal of the iron.[67,69] The classic ERG change is a supernormal signal initially, followed by a decrease in the b-wave amplitude with time. The implicit time remains unchanged.[29]

The visual prognosis for siderosis is good and most eyes retain 20/40 vision or better.[69] However, the authors advocate removal of the intraocular iron whenever possible. If extraction is deferred, serial ERGs are helpful for monitoring the retinal degeneration. IOFB extraction should be entertained if ERG deterioration is noted.[69] The cataract can be removed by a standard limbal approach.[67]

CHALCOSIS

Chalcosis develops from retained intraocular copper. Its severity and ability to produce visual loss depend primarily on the copper concentration in the IOFB. IOFB containing over 95% copper can induce a severe, rapidly progressive purulent endophthalmitis that frequently produces phthisis.[70] Copper alloys between 85% and 95% typically produce visual loss through the deposition of copper in Descemet's membrane, the anterior lens capsule, the vitreous cavity and the internal limiting membrane of the retina.[70] This is seen clinically as Kayser–Fleischer rings, anterior subcapsular sunflower cataracts, a greenish discoloration of the vitreous and greenish refractile deposits in the internal limiting membrane, respectively.[29,71] The prognosis with these changes is good and 90% of eyes maintain vision at a level of 20/60 or better.[71] IOFB containing less than 85% copper usually produce no detectable changes.[71]

SUBRETINAL NEOVASCULARIZATION

A subretinal neovascularization may develop after IOFB injuries.[39] It typically arises in locations where Bruch's membrane is disrupted, either from direct trauma or from a focally destructive foreign-body granuloma.[72] Laser photocoagulation may be attempted but the efficacy of this treatment remains unknown.

SURGICAL RESULTS

The visual outcome of surgery for retained IOFB is primarily influenced by the initial injury. Eyes with a poor initial visual acuity (less than 5/200), an afferent pupillary defect, a large laceration (greater than 10 mm), a wound extending posterior to the spiral of Tillaux or a blunt mechanism of injury typically have a poor outcome, as do eyes with an intraretinal IOFB, lenticular disruption or a dense vitreous hemorrhage.[3,34,72,73] In contrast, eyes with an initial visual acuity of 20/200 or better, a sharp mechanism of injury, a laceration of less than 10 mm and an anterior wound location suffer less visual impairment.[74]

Certain IOFB characteristics often present a poor prognosis. Blunt IOFB, such as BB pellets (a type of shot 0.18" in diameter), require great energy for transcorneal or transscleral passage and consequently inflict much damage during penetration. They commonly produce retinal tears, retinal dialysis, choroidal ruptures and choroidal detachments, as well as optic nerve avulsions and ciliary body necrosis.[3,73,75] In one study, no patients who sustained a BB-gun injury achieved a visual acuity greater than 5/200, and 86% of the eyes were enucleated.[75] Retained BB pellets can also produce visual loss through metallosis, because they classically contain a steel core with copper or zinc plating. Air pellets are usually 98% lead. Standard BB caliber is 4.5 mm. Nonmetallic IOFB also convey a poor prognosis through their typical blunt edges and by their association with high-energy activities, such as explosions, gun shots and trauma.[4] Organic IOFB place an eye at risk for endophthalmitis.[48] Magnetic IOFB may convey toxicity through one of their substances, including iron, copper, lead or zinc.[70,71]

In contrast, IOFB that are metallic, nonmagnetic and sharp have a better prognosis. Metallic IOFB are generally sharp and penetrate the globe with little disruption.[76] Also, they are commonly produced by low-energy activities, such as hammering or grinding.[4] Nonmagnetic IOFB are typically inert substances, including aluminum, gold, platinum, silver, glass, stone and plastic. These are generally well tolerated by the eye.

In the majority of IOFB injuries, a good final vision is achieved. Eighty percent of eyes will obtain a visual acuity of at least 5/200, and 60% will recover to 20/40 or better.[3,5] Interestingly, the percentage of eyes recovering vision to 20/40 or better has changed very little over the last 25 years, despite the development of vitreous surgery.[3] Explanations include the possibility that the initial injury is the limiting factor for visual recovery, or that eyes recovering vision to 20/40 usually do not require PPV. The advent of PPV has decreased the enucleation rate, however.[3,77]

PREVENTION

Although our skills for removal of IOFB have leapt forward, our ability to prevent an IOFB injury has lagged behind. In recent studies, only 6% of workers used safety glasses.[78] This is unfortunate, because prevention is the most effective therapy. Possible routes to improving prevention include increasing public awareness, imposing stricter workplace regulations, enforcing seat-belt regulations and curbing illicit drug use.

CONCLUSION

IOFB are common in open-globe injuries, causing an assortment of adverse problems, many of them leading to severe visual loss. Clinicians must remain suspicious of a possible IOFB in any traumatized eye. The greatest chance for visual rehabilitation occurs with a timely diagnosis and extraction. Several routes are available for IOFB removal, but the correct one depends on various factors, including IOFB location, composition, magnetic properties and associated ocular damage. Close follow-up after IOFB injuries is essential to monitor for any complications, including endophthalmitis, PVR, retinal detachment, metallosis and subretinal neovascularization. In most cases, the IOFB can be extracted successfully and a good visual outcome achieved.

REFERENCES

1. Shock JP, Adams D. Long-term visual acuity results after penetrating and perforating ocular injuries, *Am J Ophthalmol* (1985) **100:**714–18.
2. Thompson JT, Parver LM, Enger CL, et al. Infectious endophthalmitis after penetrating injuries with retained intraocular foreign-bodies: National Eye Trauma System, *Ophthalmology* (1993) **100:**1468–74.
3. Williams DF, Mieler WF, Abrams GW, Lewis H. Results and prognostic factors in penetrating ocular injuries with retained intraocular foreign bodies, *Ophthalmology* (1988) **95:**911–16.
4. Khani SC, Mukai S. Posterior segment intraocular foreign bodies, *Int Ophthalmol Clin* (1995) **35**(1):151–61.
5. Behrens-Baumann W, Praetorius G. Intraocular foreign bodies: 297 consecutive cases, *Ophthalmologica* (1989) **198:**84–8.
6. Armstrong MF. A review of intraocular foreign body injuries and complications in N. Ireland from 1978–1986, *Int Ophthalmol* (1988) **12:**113–17.
7. Schwartz JG, Somerset JS, Harrison JM, et al. Eye injuries with metal missiles presenting to an emergency center: a three year study, *Am J Emerg Med* (1991) **9:**313–17.
8. Sternberg P Jr. Trauma: principles and techniques of treatment. In: Ryan SJ, ed, *Retina*, 2nd edn (CV Mosby: St Louis, 1994): 2351–78.
9. Nanda SK, Mieler WF, Murphy ML. Penetrating ocular injuries secondary to motor vehicle accidents, *Ophthalmology* (1993) **100:**201–7.
10. Dannenberg AL, Parver LM, Fowler CJ. Penetrating eye injuries related to assault: The National Eye Trauma System Registry, *Arch Ophthalmol* (1992) **110:**849–52.
11. John G, Witherspoon CD, Feist RM, Morris R. Ocular lawnmower injuries, *Ophthalmology* (1988) **95:**1367–70.
12. Gilboa M, Gdal-On M, Zonis S. Bee and wasp stings of the eye: retained intralenticular wasp sting: a case report, *Br J Ophthalmol* (1977) **61:**662–4.
13. Mieler WF, Ellis MK, William DF, Han DP. Retained intraocular foreign bodies and endophthalmitis, *Ophthalmology* (1990) **97:**1532–8.
14. Zinreich SJ, Miller NR, Aguayo JB, et al. Computed tomographic three-dimensional localization and compositional evaluation of intraocular and orbital foreign bodies, *Arch Ophthalmol* (1986) **104:**1477–82.
15. Spierer A, Tadmor R, Treister G, et al. Diagnosis and localization of intraocular foreign bodies by computed tomography, *Ophthalmic Surg* (1985) **16:**571–5.
16. Topilow HW, Ackerman AL, Zimmerman RD. Limitations of computerized tomography in the localization of intraocular foreign bodies, *Ophthalmology* (1984) **91:**1086–91.
17. Specht CS, Varga JH, Jalali MM, Edelstein JP. Orbitocranial wooden foreign body diagnosed by magnetic resonance imaging: dry wood can be isodense with air and orbital fat by computed tomography, *Surv Ophthalmol* (1992) **36:**341–4.
18. Chacko JG, Figueroa RE, Johnson MH, et al. Detection and localization of steel intraocular foreign bodies using computed tomography: a comparison of helical and conventional axial scanning, *Ophthalmology* (1997) **104:**319–23.
19. Rubsamen PE, Cousins SW, Winward KE, Byrne SF. Diagnostic ultrasound and pars plana vitrectomy in penetrating ocular trauma, *Ophthalmology* (1994) **101:**809–14.
20. Wilhelm JL, Zakov ZN, Weinstein ME, et al. Localization of suspected intraocular foreign bodies with a modified Delta 2020 scanner, *Ophthalmic Surg* (1981) **12:**633–41.
21. Nouby-Mahmoud G, Silverman RH, Coleman DJ. Using high-frequency ultrasound to characterize intraocular foreign bodies, *Ophthalmic Surg* (1993) **24:**94–9.
22. Williamson TH, Smith FW, Forrester JV. Magnetic resonance imaging of intraocular foreign bodies, *Br J Ophthalmol* (1989) **73:**555–8.
23. LoBue TD, Deutsch TA, Lobick J, Turner DA. Detection and localization of nonmetallic intraocular foreign body by magnetic resonance imaging, *Arch Ophthalmol* (1988) **106:**260–1.
24. Kelly WM, Paglen PG, Pearson JA, et al. Ferromagnetism of intraocular foreign body causes unilateral blindness after MR study, *Am J Neuroradiol* (1986) **7:**243–5.
25. Bryden FM, Pyott AA, Bailey M, McGhee CN. Real time ultrasound in the assessment of intraocular foreign bodies, *Eye* (1990) **4**(Pt 5):727–31.
26. Watson A, Hartley DE. Alternative methods of intraocular foreign-body localization, *Am J Roentgenol* (1984) **142:**789–90.
27. Coleman DJ, Lucas BC, Rondeau MJ, Chang S. Management of intraocular foreign bodies, *Ophthalmology* (1987) **94:**1647–53.

28. Hadden OB, Wilson JL. The management of intraocular foreign bodies, *Aust NZ J Ophthalmol* (1990) **18:**343–51.
29. De Bustros S. Posterior segment intraocular foreign bodies. In: Shingleton BJ, Hersh PS, Kenyon KR, eds, *Eye Trauma*, (Mosby Year Book: St Louis, 1991): 226–37.
30. O'Neill E, Eagling EM. Intraocular foreign bodies: indications for lensectomy and vitrectomy, *Trans Ophthalmol Soc UK* (1978) **98:**47–8.
31. Coleman DJ. A suction tip for controlled removal of nonmagnetic intraocular foreign bodies, *Am J Ophthalmol* (1978) **85:**255–6.
32. Joondeph BC, Flynn HW Jr. Management of subretinal foreign bodies with a cannulated extrusion needle, *Am J Ophthalmol* (1990) **110:**250–3.
33. McCarthy MJ, Pulido JS, Soukup B. The use of ureter stone forceps to remove a large intraocular foreign body, *Am J Ophthalmol* (1990) **110:**208–9.
34. Slusher MM, Sarin LK, Federman JL. Management of intraretinal foreign bodies, *Ophthalmology* (1982) **89:**369–73.
35. Rubsamen PE, Cousins SW, Martinez JA. Impact of cultures on management decisions following surgical repair of penetrating ocular trauma, *Ophthalmic Surg Lasers* (1997) **28:**43–9.
36. Smiljanic NS, Vicic DO. Combat eye injuries: laser photocoagulation prophylaxis of retinal deatchment, *J Trauma: Injury, Infection, Critical Care* (1996) **40**(3 Suppl):S157–8.
37. Ambler JS, Meyers SM. Management of intraretinal foreign bodies without retinopexy in the absence of retinal detachment, *Ophthalmology* (1991) **98:**391–4.
38. Slusher MM. Intraretinal foreign bodies: management and observations, *Retina* (1990) **10** (Suppl 1):S50–4.
39. Ahmadieh H, Sajjadi H, Azarmina M, et al. Surgical management of intraretinal foreign bodies, *Retina* (1994) **14:**397–403.
40. Spalding SC, Sternberg P Jr. Controversies in the management of posterior segment ocular trauma, *Retina* (1990) **10** (Suppl 1):S76–82.
41. Spiegel D, Nasemann J, Nawrocki J, Gabel VP. Severe ocular trauma managed with primary pars plana vitrectomy and silicone oil, *Retina* (1997) **17:**275–85.
42. Hutton WL, Fuller DG. Factors influencing final visual results in severely injured eye, *Am J Ophthalmol* (1984) **97:**715–22.
43. Pieramici DJ, Capone A, Rubsamen PE, Roseman RL. Lens preservation after intraocular foreign body injuries, *Ophthalmology* (1996) **103:**1563–7.
44. Koenig SB, Mieler WF, Han DP, Abrams GW. Combined phacoemulsification, pars plana vitrectomy, and posterior chamber intraocular lens insertion, *Arch Ophthalmol* (1992) **110:**1101–4.
45. Rubsamen PE, Irvin WD, McCuen BW II, et al. Primary intraocular lens implantation in the setting of penetrating ocular trauma, *Ophthalmology* (1995) **102:**101–7.
46. Seal DV, Kirkness CM. Criteria for intravitreal antibiotics during surgical removal of intraocular foreign bodies, *Eye* (1992) **6** (Pt 5):465–8.
47. Alfonso EC, Flynn HW Jr. Controversies in endophthalmitis prevention: the risk for emerging resistance to vancomycin (editorial), *Arch Ophthalmol* (1995) **113:**1369–70.
48. Boldt HC, Pulido JS, Blodi CF, et al. Rural endophthalmitis, *Ophthalmology* (1989) **96:**1722–6.
49. Alfaro DV, Roth D, Liggett PE. Posttraumatic endophthalmitis: causative organisms, treatment, and prevention, *Retina* (1994) **14:**206–11.
50. Foster RE, Martinez JA, Murray TG, et al. Useful visual outcomes after treatment of *Bacillus cereus* endophthalmitis, *Ophthalmology* (1996) **103:**390–7.
51. Mieler WF, Glazer LC, Bennett SR, Han DP. Favourable outcome of traumatic endophthalmitis with associated retinal breaks or detachment, *Can J Ophthalmol* (1992) **27:**348–52.
52. Aaberg TM, Flynn HW Jr, Murray TG. Intraocular ceftazidime as an alternative to the aminoglycosides in the treatment of endophthalmitis, *Arch Ophthalmol* (1994) **112:**18–19.
53. Conway BP, Campochiaro PA. Macular infarction after endophthalmitis treated with vitrectomy and intravitreal gentamicin, *Arch Ophthalmol* (1986) **104:**367–71.
54. Kervick GN, Flynn HW Jr, Alfonso E, Miller D. Antibiotic therapy for *Bacillus* species infections, *Am J Ophthalmol* (1990) **110:**683–7.
55. Alfaro DV, Pince K, Park J, et al. Systemic antibiotic prophylaxis in penetrating ocular injuries: an experimental study, *Retina* (1992) **12:**S3–6.
56. Schech JM, Alfaro DV II, Laughlin RM, et al. Intravenous gentamicin and ceftazidime in penetrating ocular trauma: a swine model, *Retina* (1997) **17:**28–32.
57. Meredith TA, Aguilar HE, Shaarawy A, et al. Vancomycin levels in the vitreous cavity after intravenous administration, *Am J Ophthalmol* (1995) **119:**774–8.
58. Alfaro DV, Hudson SJ, Rafanan MM, et al. The effect of trauma on the ocular penetration of intravenous ciprofloxacin, *Am J Ophthalmol* (1996) **122:**678–83.
59. El Baba FZ, Trousdale MD, Gauderman WJ, et al. Intravitreal penetration of oral ciprofloxacin in humans, *Ophthalmology* (1992) **99:**483–6.
60. El-Massry A, Meredith TA, Aguilar HE, et al. Aminoglycoside levels in the rabbit vitreous cavity after intravenous administration, *Am J Ophthalmol* (1996) **122:**684–9.
61. Mauger TF. Antimicrobials. In: Mauger TF, Craig EL, eds, *Havener's Ocular Pharmacology*, 6th edn (CV Mosby: St. Louis, 1994): 234–349.
62. Mao LK, Flynn HW Jr, Miller D, Pflugfelder SC. Endophthalmitis caused by *Staphylococcus aureus*, *Am J Ophthalmol* (1993) **116:**584–9.
63. Meredith TA, Aguilar HE, Drews C, et al. Intraocular dexamethasone produces a harmful effect on treatment of experimental *Staphylococcus aureus* endophthalmitis, *Trans Am Ophthalmol Soc* (1996) **94:**241–52.
64. Aguilar HE, Meredith TA, Drews C, et al. Comparative treatment of experimental *Staphylococcus aureus* endophthalmitis, *Am J Ophthalmol* (1996) **121:**310–17.
65. Cardillo JA, Stout JT, LaBree JL, et al. Post-traumatic proliferative vitreoretinopathy: the epidemiologic profile, onset, risk factors, and visual outcome, *Ophthalmology* (1997) **104:**1166–73.
66. Percival SP. Late complications from posterior segment intraocular foreign bodies, with particular reference to retinal detachment, *Br J Ophthalmol* (1972) **56:**462–8.
67. Hope-Ross M, Mahon GJ, Johnston PB. Ocular siderosis, *Eye* (1993) **7:**419–25.
68. Talamo JH, Topping TM, Maumenee AE, Green WR. Ultrastructural studies of cornea, iris, and lens in a case of siderosis bulbi, *Ophthalmology* (1985) **92:**1675–80.

69. Weiss MJ, Hofeldt AJ, Behrens M, Fisher K. Ocular siderosis: diagnosis and management, *Retina* (1997) **17:**105–8.
70. Rao NA, Tso MO, Rosenthal AR. Chalcosis in the human eye: a clinicopathologic study, *Arch Ophthalmol* (1976) **94:**1379–84.
71. Rosenthal AR, Marmor MF, Leuenberger P, Hopkins JL. Chalcosis: a study of natural history, *Ophthalmology* (1979) **86:**1956–72.
72. Wilson MW, Grossniklaus HE, Heathcote JG. Focal posttraumatic choroidal granulomatous inflammation, *Am J Ophthalmol* (1996) **121:**397–404.
73. De Juan E Jr, Sternberg P Jr, Michels RG. Penetrating ocular injuries: types of injuries and visual results, *Ophthalmology* (1983) **90:**1318–22.
74. Pieramici DJ, MacCumber MW, Humayun MU, et al. Open-globe injury: update on types of injuries and visual results, *Ophthalmology* (1996) **103:**1798–803.
75. Sternberg P Jr, de Juan E Jr, Green WR, et al. Ocular BB injuries, *Ophthalmology* (1984) **91:**1269–77.
76. Potts AM, Distler JA. Shape factor in the penetration of intraocular foreign bodies, *Am J Ophthalmol* (1985) **100:**183–7.
77. De Juan E Jr, Sternberg P Jr, Michels RG, Auer C. Evaluation of vitrectomy in penetrating ocular trauma: a case-control study, *Arch Ophthalmol* (1984) **102:**1160–3.
78. Dannenberg AL, Parver LM, Brechner RJ, Khoo L. Penetrating eye injuries in the workplace: The National Eye Trauma System Registry, *Arch Ophthalmol* (1992) **110:**843–8.

Chapter 41 Penetrating and perforating injuries

Dennis P Han and Sundeep Dev

INTRODUCTION

Management of penetrating and perforating globe injuries represents a challenge to the vitreoretinal surgeon because of the complexity and variation in presentation that may occur. However, basic principles apply to the repair of such injuries. These include: preoperative evaluation to assess the extent and type of damage, including the use of appropriate imaging studies; restoration of the integrity of the globe by identification and closure of corneal and scleral lacerations; establishment of a clear visual axis; removal of intraocular foreign bodies (IOFB); repair and prophylaxis of retinal detachment; and prevention of infection.

Since the introduction of vitrectomy techniques in the 1970s, the role of vitrectomy in penetrating trauma has been defined experimentally[1–5] and clinically.[6–10] These studies have established the essential role of the vitreoretinal surgeon in the management of posterior segment penetrating injury. Three main aspects of trauma management are facilitated by vitrectomy. These include:

- Interruption of intraocular proliferative processes. Fibrovascular ingrowth of tissue from entry and exit wounds may develop along the tract of injury through the vitreous cavity. Vitrectomy eliminates the scaffold for such ingrowth and has been shown experimentally to prevent retinal detachment from this process. Vitrectomy has been associated with a favorable trend toward improved outcome in perforating injuries, providing clinical evidence that such an effect may exist.[6]
- Removal of intraocular debris and clearing of the visual axis. Vitrectomy allows removal of disrupted lens material, traumatic cataract, vitreous–lens admixture and vitreous hemorrhage. Contaminated material within the eye is also removed, reducing the risk of intraocular infection.[11] Vitrectomy allows the removal of IOFB and will be discussed separately.
- Treatment of retinal detachment and retinal tears. Clearing the visual axis and removal of the formed vitreous humor relieves vitreous traction and allows the use of laser photocoagulation and intraocular tamponade. With these techniques, detached retinas may be repaired in a timely fashion.

Vitrectomy is most commonly required in injuries with significant posterior segment involvement, such as posteriorly extending scleral lacerations, deep corneal lacerations with lens and retinal damage, perforating globe injuries and retained IOFB. Specific indications for vitrectomy in penetrating trauma are listed in Table 41.1.

Table 41.1 Indications for vitrectomy in penetrating trauma

- Traumatic cataract with disrupted posterior capsule
- Vitreous–lens admixture in the anterior chamber or vitreous cavity
- Severe vitreous loss
- Severe or nonclearing vitreous hemorrhage
- Retinal detachment (tractional, rhegmatogenous or hemorrhagic), retinal tears, dialyses or incarceration
- Perforating globe injury ('double penetrating' injury)
- Retained intraocular foreign body
- Post-traumatic endophthalmitis

PREOPERATIVE EVALUATION

A careful history should be obtained as to the circumstances of the injury (motor-vehicle accident, assault, occupational, etc.) and the type of object striking the eye (sharp or blunt, organic versus inorganic). The onset of visual loss, the place of injury (home versus workplace) and whether the patient had been using spectacles or protective eye wear at the time of the injury should be recorded. A history of striking metal on metal should alert the examiner to search for an occult penetrating wound and evaluate for a retained IOFB. Previous visual loss, amblyopia or strabismus should also be noted in the medical record.

Visual acuity measurement should be obtained if possible in all cases, because it is strongly predictive of final visual outcome.[12] A pupillary examination to assess for a relative afferent pupillary defect may help to determine whether optic nerve damage is present. Slit-lamp examination is performed to evaluate the extent of the globe laceration, the presence of uveal prolapse or vitreous incarceration and the integrity of the lens. Indirect ophthalmoscopy should be attempted early in the patient's course, before worsening of media opacity, to determine whether a retinal detachment is present or to localize retinal tears or retained IOFB.[13]

In an eye with opaque media, radiographic studies to rule out IOFB should be obtained. Orbital plain-film x-rays are adequate to rule out metallic IOFB in low-risk cases. In patients with a high likelihood of harboring a retained intraocular or intraorbital foreign body, computed tomography (CT) scanning is recommended to provide more accurate localization. Magnetic resonance imaging (MRI) scanning should be avoided because of the risk of ocular damage from migration of retained ferromagnetic IOFB. Ultrasonography may be performed for precise localization of IOFB and is particularly useful for detection of radiolucent IOFB. It is also useful to assess for retinal or choroidal detachment, and for posterior exit wounds in cases of suspected globe perforation manifested by a discontinuity in the scleral wall (see later section on perforating globe injuries). However, ultrasonography should be performed in eyes that have been repaired primarily or that have small, self-sealing wounds in order to avoid prolapsing intraocular tissue by inadvertent pressure on the globe that may occur during the examination.

Electrophysiologic tests have been used to determine visual potential in cases of penetrating injury with posterior segment involvement. The bright-flash visual evoked potential (VEP) has been determined to be predictive of visual outcome. Its usefulness is attributed to its ability to measure both macular and optic nerve integrity, which are both critical for central visual function.[14] The flash electroretinogram (ERG) has also been evaluated, but its disadvantages are that it requires placement of a contact lens and is less predictive of visual outcome than the flash VEP. Unlike the flash VEP, the flash ERG measures a mass response from the photoreceptors that does not necessarily reflect central visual function. The authors currently use electrophysiologic testing to confirm a poor visual prognosis in severely injured eyes with absent light perception in which surgical repair is not planned or in which enucleation is being considered.

TIMING OF INTERVENTION

The optimal timing of vitrectomy in trauma remains controversial. In some retrospective studies, intervention within 72 hours of injury has been associated with a more favorable prognosis.[6,9] However, a delay of several days may reduce the risk of severe intraocular bleeding that has been attributed to uveal congestion developing immediately after the initial injury.[15] After several days, a spontaneous separation of the posterior hyaloid may also occur, making vitrectomy easier to perform.[16]

In eyes with retained IOFB, early vitreoretinal surgery should be considered because of the increased risk of endophthalmitis if the IOFB is retained for more than 24 hours from the time of injury.[17]

In perforated globes with a posterior exit wound that is not accessible for primary repair, deferral for several days allows fibroblastic tissue growth to close the wound spontaneously.[1] Such wound closure may reduce the risk of tissue extrusion through the wound during vitrectomy.

Large hemorrhagic choroidal detachments may interfere with safe introduction of instruments through the pars plana. Drainage of choroidal hemorrhage may be necessary and is more easily accomplished after liquefaction occurs, which may require several days. Similarly, large subretinal hemorrhages are more easily removed after liquefaction.[18]

The presence of hyphema or clotted blood in the anterior chamber may also prevent visualization of the posterior segment and the crystalline lens. If the lens is intact, deferral of vitrectomy for a number of days may allow the anterior chamber blood to clear or become liquefied. Alternatively, anterior chamber washout, hydraulic manipulation of hemorrhage or excision of clotted blood may be attempted (see below). If the lens is damaged, the blood may be removed surgically in conjunction with lensectomy. If the visual potential is limited, the importance of retaining an intact crystalline lens is significantly lessened.

Severe corneal injury may interfere with visualization of the posterior segment during vitrectomy and may require a period of observation for corneal edema to clear. If corneal involvement is limited or does not involve the visual axis, viewing the posterior segment through the uninvolved portion of the cornea by way of a well-dilated pupil may be possible. In cases of severe corneal involvement interfering with posterior visualization, placement of a temporary keratoprosthesis may be required (see below).

The authors' preference is to operate within 10 days of injury if possible, so that if an eye proves irreparable at surgery, preparations for enucleation within 14 days of injury may be made to limit the risk of sympathetic ophthalmia in the uninjured eye.

ADJUNCTIVE TECHNIQUES

Scleral buckling should be considered for eyes with retinal detachment or evidence of peripheral retinal damage. It may be useful as an adjunct to primary repair of the globe alone or in conjunction with pars plana vitrectomy for more complex injuries. The role of prophylactic scleral buckling in penetrating injury is controversial. Several studies have shown a reduced risk of postoperative retinal detachment in association with prophylactic scleral buckling,[8,10,14] whereas others have not.[19] Retinal cryotherapy applied to posterior scleral lacerations during primary repair is of uncertain benefit and may be potentially harmful because of possible release of retinal pigment epithelial cells into the vitreous cavity[20] and breakdown of the blood–ocular barrier[21] that may stimulate intraocular fibroblastic proliferation.

Perfluorocarbon liquids, by virtue of their increased density relative to water or saline, are useful as intraoperative tools for retinal reattachment.[22,23] Their use is generally limited to repair of coexisting rhegmatogenous retinal detachment. However, they may be useful to remove liquefied subretinal blood, by displacing it through a peripheral break or retinotomy into the vitreous cavity where it may be removed. Similarly, removal of liquefied suprachoroidal blood through an external sclerotomy may be facilitated. Following injection of perfluorocarbon liquid and retinal reattachment, laser photocoagulation of retinal breaks, fluid–air exchange and injection of long-acting gas or silicone oil tamponade may be performed.

MANAGEMENT OF ANTERIOR CHAMBER HEMORRHAGE BEFORE PARS PLANA VITRECTOMY

After exploration and repair of corneoscleral lacerations, opacities in the anterior segment often must be removed prior to posterior vitrectomy. In some instances, a thin layer of liquefied blood may coat the anterior surface of an intact crystalline lens, making posterior visualization difficult. In such cases, hydraulic displacement of the blood using viscoelastic material may permit satisfactory visualization of the posterior segment without the need for lensectomy (Fig. 41.1).

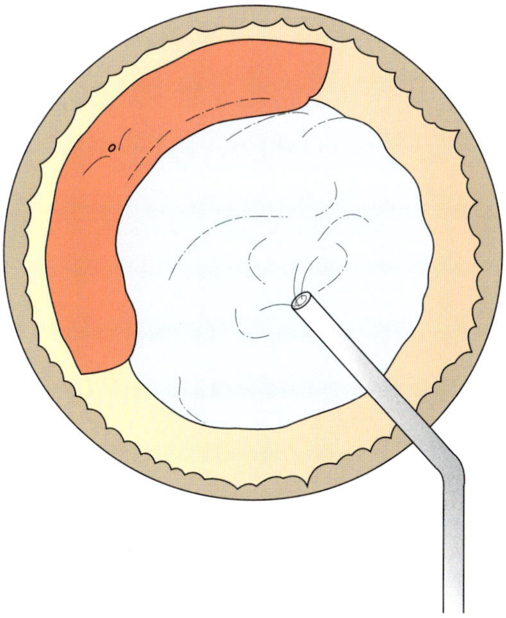

Figure 41.1 *Viscoelastic manipulation of clot. Transparent viscoelastic fluid pushes blood toward periphery of angle to allow clear visual axis.*

INSTRUMENTATION

- Ziegler blade.
- Viscoelastic material.
- 27-Gauge blunt cannula.
- Vitrectomy probe or 20-gauge tapered cannula for aspiration.
- 20-Gauge needle for infusion of balanced salt solution.
- 10-0 Nylon suture.

SURGICAL TECHNIQUE

A thin layer of mobile red blood cells coating the anterior surface of the crystalline lens may obscure fundus viewing and may be displaced hydraulically by injecting viscoelastic material into the anterior chamber. A paracentesis tract is made at the limbus with a Ziegler blade, at a site opposite the most dense accumulation of blood. The viscoelastic material is injected through a 27-gauge blunt cannula at the edge of the pupil and is allowed to spread across the lens, maneuvering the red blood cells to the opposite side of the anterior chamber. If the anterior chamber becomes excessively deep or severe intraocular pressure elevation occurs, a second paracentesis tract is made opposite the first to allow egress of fluid. After completion of posterior segment surgery, the viscoelastic material must be removed to prevent severe postoperative intraocular pressure elevation. The limbal incisions are enlarged and the material is aspirated with a vitrectomy probe or non-tapered 20-gauge cannula. Balanced salt solution is infused simultaneously via a 20-gauge cannula or needle to prevent anterior chamber collapse. Limbal incisions are closed with single 10-0 nylon sutures.

REMOVAL OF DISRUPTED LENS MATERIAL, VITREOUS–LENS ADMIXTURE AND ANTERIOR VITREOUS HEMORRHAGE

Disrupted lens material (Fig 41.2a), vitreous–lens admixture and hemorrhage in the pupillary region may obscure posterior viewing during vitrectomy and must be removed before posterior vitrectomy. During this stage of the procedure, precautions are necessary to avoid inadvertent suprachoroidal infusion. Drainage of pre-existing choroidal hemorrhage and confirmation that cannulae for infusion are positioned within the vitreous cavity may reduce the risk of this complication (Fig. 41.2b). A hand-held infusion should be used until the tip of a presutured pars plana infusion cannula can be visualized within the vitreous cavity.

During clearing of opacities and disrupted lens material, the integrity of the residual peripheral lens capsule may be assessed and retained if sufficient for support of intraocular lens implantation in the ciliary sulcus (Fig. 41.2c). Implantation may be considered as a primary or secondary procedure in eyes with good visual prognoses.

INSTRUMENTATION

- Measuring calipers.
- 20-Gauge needle or blunt cannula for infusion.
- 20-Gauge microvitreoretinal blade.
- Vitrectomy cutter/aspirator.
- Phacofragmentation/aspiration needle.
- 4-mm Infusion cannula (pars plana).
- 5-0 Nylon or similar gauge suture for fixation of pars plana infusion cannula.

SURGICAL TECHNIQUE

If significant disruption of the posterior capsule is suspected, pars plana lensectomy may reduce the risk of further vitreous loss. Posteriorly dislocated lens material during lens extraction also may be removed more easily via a pars plana approach (see Fig. 41.2a).

Traumatic cataract, vitreous–lens admixture, and anterior vitreous hemorrhage may be removed via a pars plana approach, often during the initial phase of posterior vitrectomy (see Fig. 41.2b). Sclerotomy sites initially are made through the pars plana 2.5–3.0 mm posterior to the limbus. Sclerotomy incisions should be placed at least 2 or 3 mm from the penetrating wound in order to avoid extension of the incisions into the wound during subsequent surgical manipulations and loss of globe integrity. For initial infusion, an angled 20-gauge needle or cannula attached to the infusion is positioned in the pupillary space, where its tip can be identified. Removal of disrupted lens material and hemorrhagic retropupillary membranes may be accomplished with a vitrectomy cutter/aspirator during simultaneous infusion through the cannula.

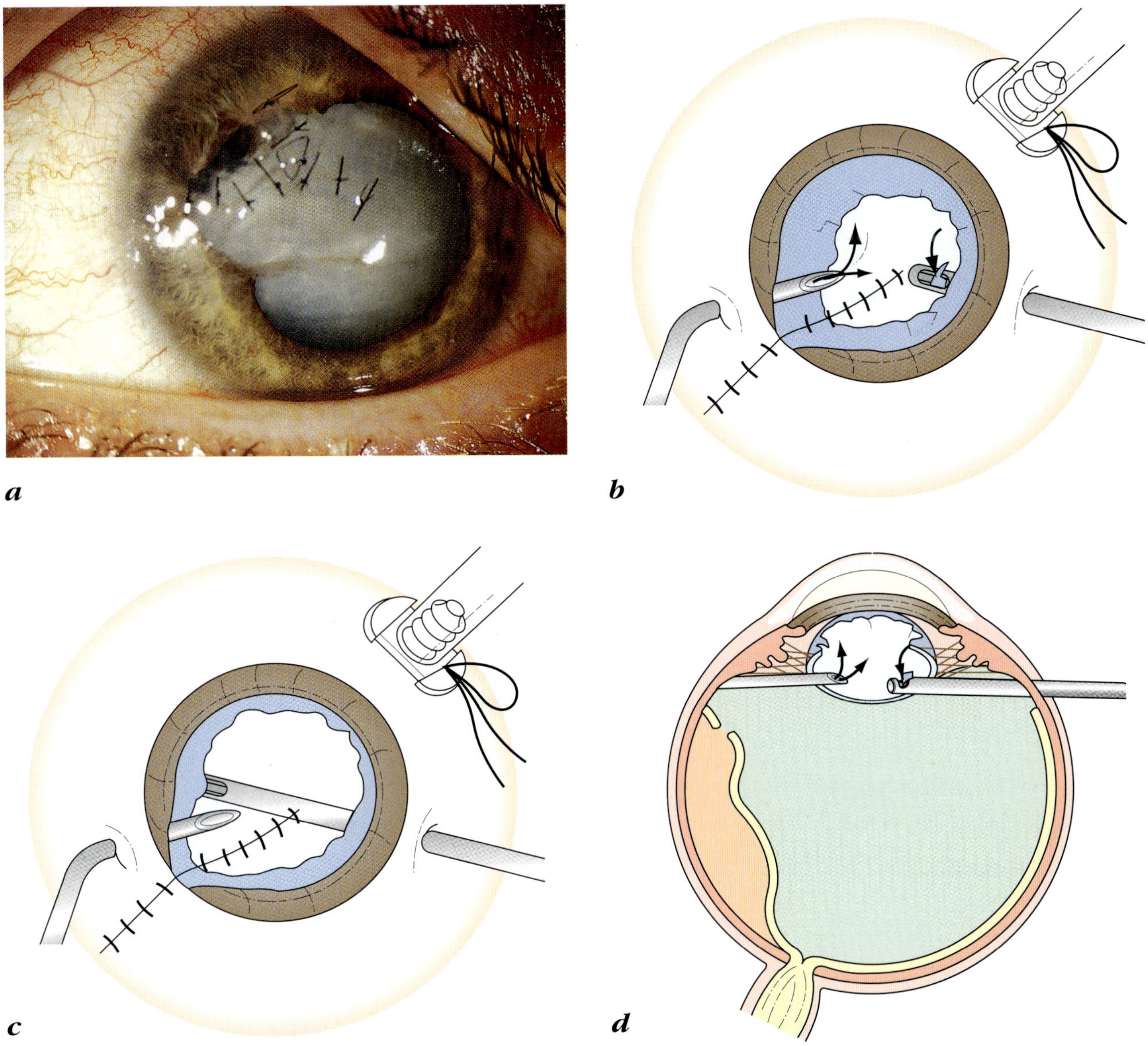

Figure 41.2 *(a) External photograph demonstrating disrupted lens material, vitreous–lens admixture and hemorrhage in the pupillary region obscuring fundus posterior view. (b) An angled 20-gauge needle or cannula is used as initial infusion until presewn pars plana infusion cannula tip is confirmed to be within the vitreous cavity. The angled cannula tip is brought into the anterior chamber for visualization. (c) The vitrectomy cutter is used for removal of anterior capsule. (d) Side view of the procedure.*

In adults, phacofragmentation may be required to remove the lens nucleus. The angled needle or cannula is used until infusion through a preplaced pars plana infusion cannula can be performed safely. A preplaced 4-mm infusion cannula allows full-thickness penetration of both the sclera and edematous or minimally detached uvea at the pars plana, reducing the risk of inadvertent suprachoroidal infusion. In the event that there is a large suprachoroidal hemorrhage or effusion that detaches the pars plana portion of the ciliary body, drainage of suprachoroidal blood or fluid must be performed (see Chapter 42). A limbal approach may permit a limited anterior vitrectomy/lensectomy in such cases.

Following removal of cortex and nucleus, residual capsular material may be excised with the vitrectomy cutter/aspirator (see Fig. 41.2c,d). The capsule may be removed entirely or, in selected cases, a rim of capsule may be retained for subsequent support of a posterior chamber intraocular lens. Once the disrupted lens material and retropupillary membranes are removed, the pars plana infusion cannula may be visualized more easily and a standard three-port vitrectomy may be initiated.

VITRECTOMY FOR REMOVAL OF DENSE VITREOUS HEMORRHAGE

Removal of dense vitreous hemorrhage may be challenging because the retina, particularly if it is detached, may lie in close proximity to the hemorrhage. Inadvertent retinal damage may occur because of poor visualization of the retina during excision of the hemorrhage. After removal of anterior vitreous hemorrhage (Fig. 41.3a) and initiation of a three-port vitrectomy, a staged approach is required to minimize inadvertent excision of retinal tissue during posterior vitrectomy (Fig. 41.3b–e).

INSTRUMENTATION

- 20-Gauge vitrectomy cutter/aspirator.
- 20-Gauge silicone-tipped aspiration cannula, tapered to 23-gauge.
- Endoilluminator pole.
- Vitrectomy contact lens, or alternative viewing system.

VITRECTOMY CONSOLE SETTINGS

- For removal of clotted blood: suction 100–150 mmHg, cutting 400–700 cpm.
- For removal of layered blood (posterior hyphema): suction 50–100 mmHg.

SURGICAL TECHNIQUE

Eyes with dense vitreous hemorrhage may require anterior vitrectomy to allow visualization of the pars plana infusion cannula. The vitrectomy is performed using the angled 20-gauge cannula and vitrectomy cutter/aspirator (see Fig. 41.3a). Alternately, an infusion-endoilluminator may be used in concert with the vitrectomy cutter/aspirator. Once infusion through the pars plana is established, the 20-gauge hand-held infusion cannula is no longer needed and can be exchanged with an endoillumination probe, and posterior vitrectomy can be initiated.

During posterior vitrectomy, dense vitreous hemorrhage must be removed carefully to avoid inadvertent retinal damage by the vitrectomy cutter, particularly if the retina is detached. The axial vitreous is first excised to avoid the peripheral retina. The vitrectomy begins anteriorly and proceeds posteriorly toward the region of the optic nerve head along a path least likely to encounter the detached retina (see Fig. 41.3b, dotted outline of vitrectomy cutter). Constant visual contact with the end of the vitrectomy cutter is critical to avoid damage to the retina and is facilitated in hazy media by holding the endoilluminator close to the cutter tip and by keeping the operating microscope continuously in focus.

Once the retina or optic nerve head is visualized, a plane can be defined that allows separation of the retina from the hemorrhage for safer removal (see Fig. 41.3c). Removal is facilitated by gently elevating and excising the posterior vitreous centrally to peripherally, while simultaneously monitoring the position of the retina relative to the vitrectomy cutter tip.

Layered posterior blood (posterior hyphema) should be removed as soon as possible to avoid dispersion and loss of visualization; the blood is removed using a silicone-tipped aspiration cannula attached to the vitrectomy console at low-to-moderate suction (50–100 mmHg). This procedure also prevents mobile red blood cells from migrating into the anterior chamber and settling on the surface of the crystalline lens (see Fig. 41.3d).

EXCISION OF THE POSTERIOR HYALOID DURING VITRECTOMY

For severe injuries, induction of a posterior vitreous separation is important to allow removal of vitreous hemorrhage that remains 'plastered' against the retina, potentially obscuring retinal breaks near entrance and exit wounds and preventing laser treatment. It also eliminates a scaffold by which subsequent proliferation

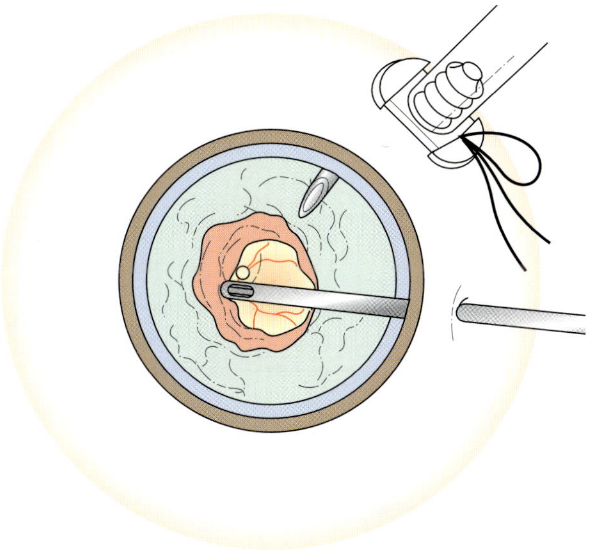

a

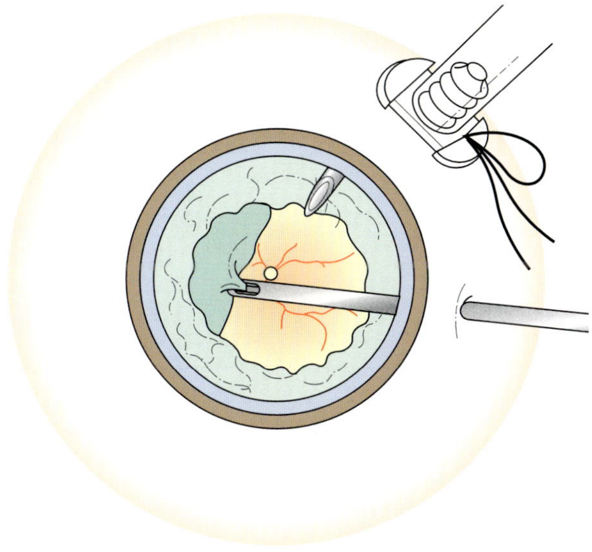

b

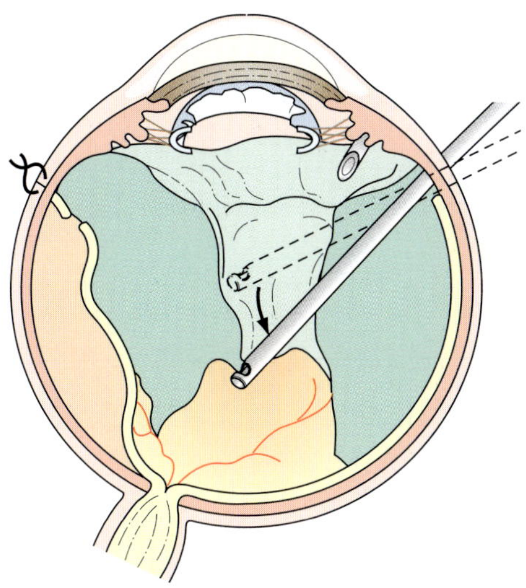

c

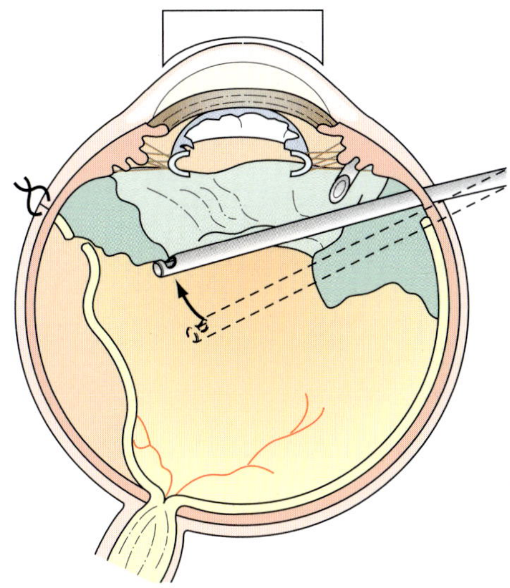

d

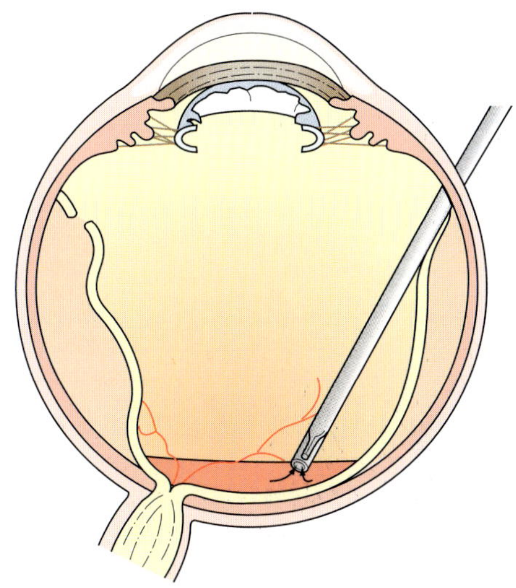

e

Figure 41.3 *(a) In initial phase of vitrectomy, vitrectomy probe tip is kept close to visual axis of globe and (b) moved posteriorly to optic nerve head to allow early identification of retinal location and to avoid damage to detached retina obscured by and adherent to vitreous hemorrhage. (c, d) After retina is identified posteriorly, the posterior vitreous is elevated and excised from posterior to anterior, keeping the retina in view. (e) Aspiration of residual hemorrhage and layered blood.*

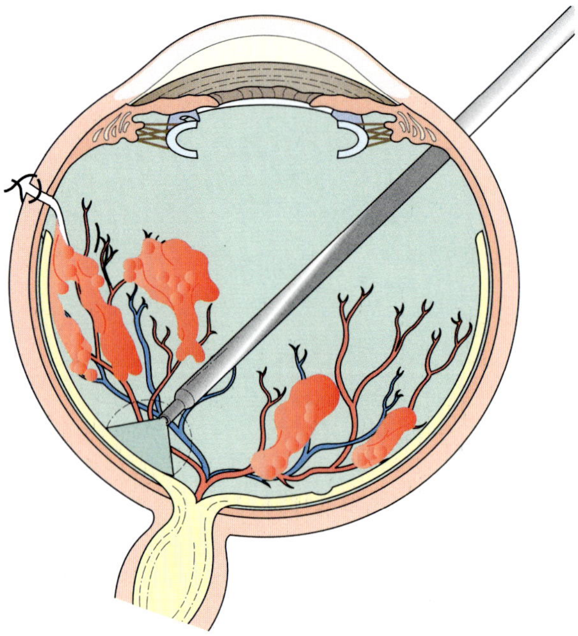

a

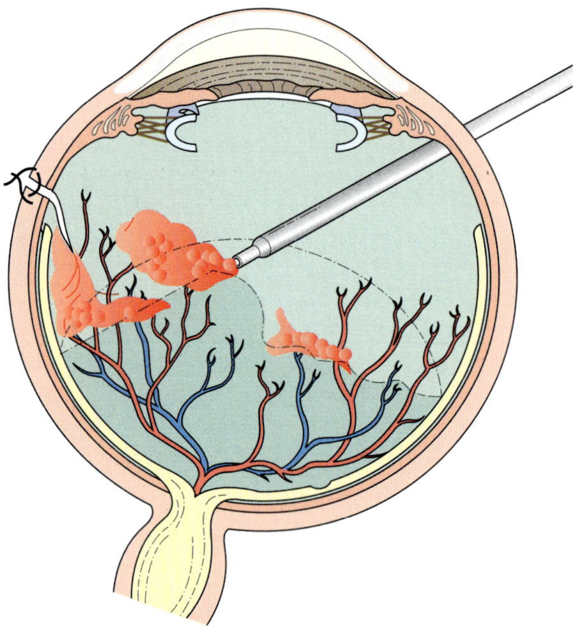

b

Figure 41.4 *(a) Separation of posterior hyaloid and excision of blood clots. Clotted blood emanates from the wound. Scleral laceration extends from area of sutured wound. Blood clots are adherent to the retina. Posterior hyaloid is engaged near the disc with a silicone-tipped cannula. (b) Cross-section of blood as it elevates with posterior hyaloid. 'Ring' of peripheral part of posterior hyaloid is seen where it remains attached. Blood separates from proximity of wound as posterior hyaloid is elevated.*

of membranes and contraction along the retinal surface may occur. Inner retinal striae and multiple small clots that remain adherent to the retina after a nearly complete posterior vitrectomy are signs of an attached posterior vitreous cortex (Figs 41.4a,b).

INSTRUMENTATION

Same as for vitrectomy for dense vitreous hemorrhage:

- 20-Gauge vitrectomy cutter/aspirator.
- 20-Gauge silicone-tipped aspiration cannula, tapered to 23-gauge.

VITRECTOMY CONSOLE SETTINGS

- For engaging posterior vitreous cortex: suction 250–300 mmHg, infusion bottles partially elevated.

SURGICAL TECHNIQUES

The strongest posterior adhesion of the vitreous cortex to the fundus is at the optic nerve head. This adhesion often must be broken with relatively focal traction first, after which the remainder of the vitreous cortex separates more easily. The infusion bottles are elevated briefly, and the suction on the vitrectomy console is set to 250–300 mmHg. The posterior vitreous cortex is engaged near the disc with a silicone-tipped cannula or vitrectomy cutter set on aspiration only. Once engaged, the cortex is pulled slowly anteriorly, breaking its adhesions to the disc (see Fig. 41.4a). Alternatively, sharp dissection of the vitreous cortex from the region of the optic nerve head to initiate separation of the posterior vitreous may be performed using a barbed microvitreoretinal blade or a more specialized pick.

Preretinal hemorrhage separates from the retina along with the vitreous cortex, making its removal easier. Once separated, blood and vitreous surrounding the wound can be excised more easily (Fig. 41.4b). The vitreous cortex usually remains tightly adherent to ocular wounds, and excessive traction on the vitreous attached to these areas may induce or exacerbate retinal breaks or detachment. Instead, the separated vitreous cortex and vitreous hemorrhage are truncated with the vitrector at the site of attachment to the wounds. The infusion bottles and vitrectomy suction and cutting settings then are returned to the standard settings and the separated vitreous cortex is excised with the vitrectomy cutter.

PERFORATING GLOBE INJURIES

The term perforating globe injury, also known as 'double penetrating' injury, refers to the injury that results in both entrance and exit wounds through full-thickness cornea or sclera. Such injuries are usually caused by high-velocity missiles, such as those fired from shotguns or pellet guns (Fig. 41.5) or from spear-like objects striking the eye (Fig. 41.6). They are complicated by retinal damage at the exit wound, transvitreal traction between the two wounds and the sequelae of blunt trauma, such as hyphema, *commotio retinae*, choroidal rupture or subretinal hemorrhage, all of which result from the high-velocity nature of the injury. If the exit wound involves the macula or optic nerve head, visual function may be severely affected (Fig. 41.7).

Orbital imaging may provide definitive evidence of a perforating globe injury. The presence of an anterior penetrating wound of the globe in conjunction with imaging studies showing a retained retrobulbar foreign body without IOFB suggests a perforating globe injury with a posterior exit wound (Fig. 41.8). B-Scan echography or CT scanning may identify a discontinuity of the posterior sclera, defining more exactly the location of the exit wound. Exit wounds located postequatorially may not be visible at the time of primary repair, even with globe exploration. A waiting period of several days between primary globe repair and secondary intervention with vitrectomy is important to allow sealing of the exit wound and reduce the risk of iatrogenic prolapse of tissues.[1]

In perforating globe injuries, vitrectomy should include excision of the vitreous tract that extends from the entrance and exit wounds, as well as vitreous attachments to the wounds (Figs 41.9a,b). These

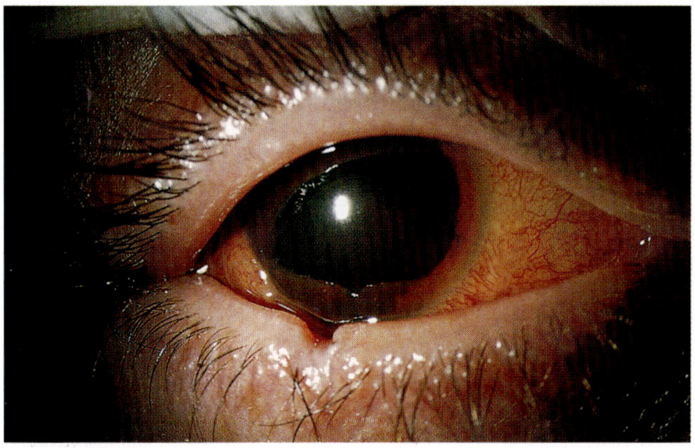

Figure 41.5 *Perforating globe injury from BB gun. External examination shows lid margin defect over the site of the globe's entrance wound.*

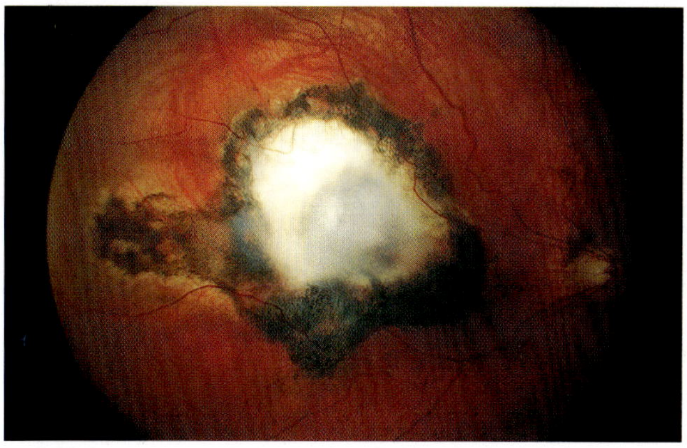

Figure 41.7 *Perforating globe injury from BB gun following pars plana vitrectomy, lensectomy, scleral buckle and fluid–gas exchange. Visual acuity with aphakic correction was 20/400 with eccentric viewing, as a result of a large macular exit wound. The sclera is visible and surrounds a central scleral defect sealed with fibrous tissue.*

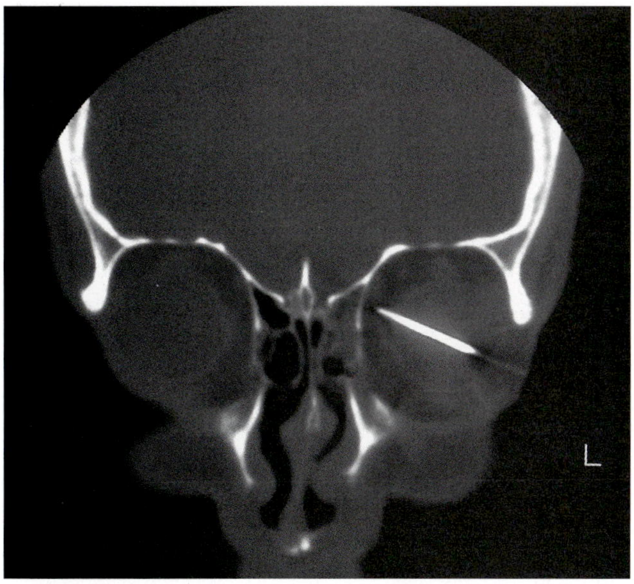

Figure 41.6 *CT scan of a perforating globe injury induced by a wire projectile. A posterior exit wound is present through which the wire foreign body protrudes.*

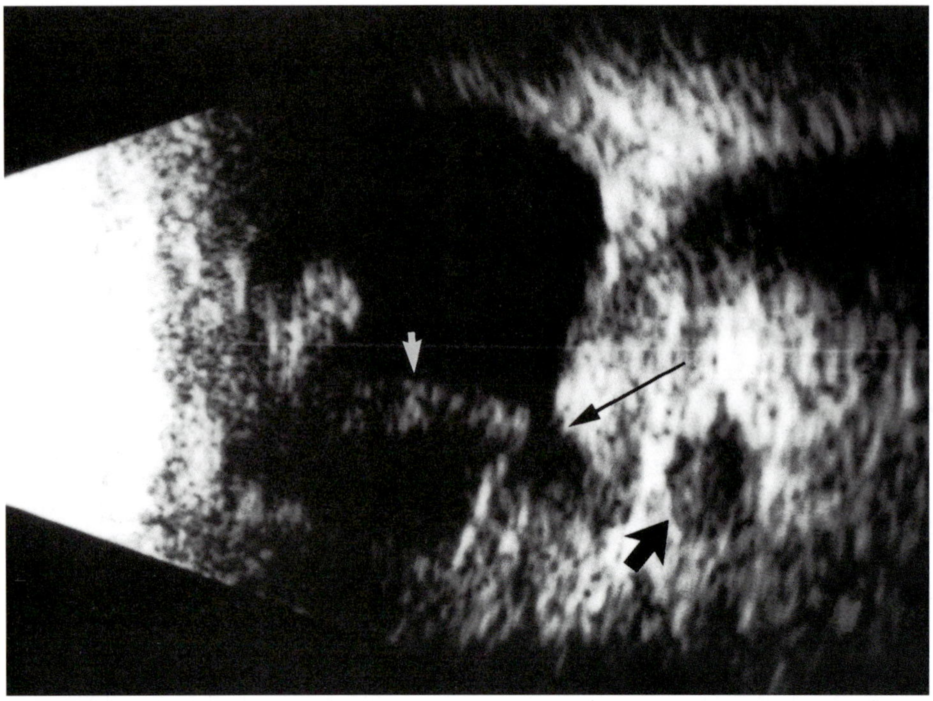

Figure 41.8 *Ultrasonogram of a perforated globe caused by a BB gun demonstrates posterior scleral defect (long arrow) with a hemorrhagic tract extending transvitreally (small arrowhead). Foreign body is visible posterior to the globe (large arrowhead).*

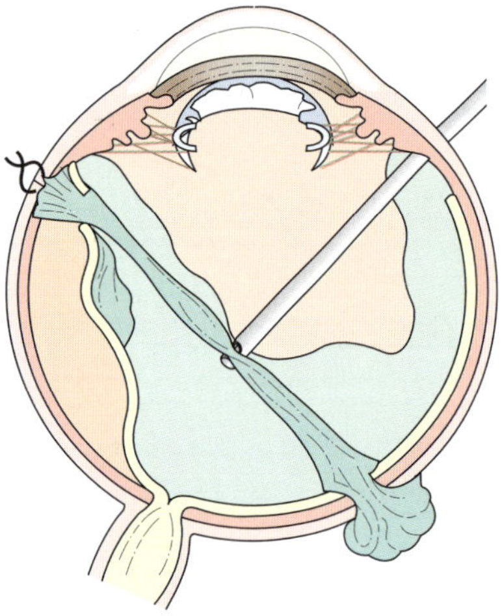

a

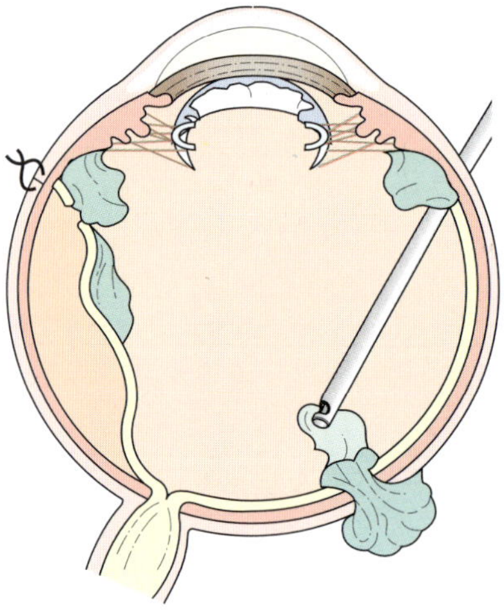

b

Figure 41.9 *(a) Cross-section of a perforating eye injury demonstrating a fibrovascular tract through the vitreous. After an anterior vitrectomy, the tract is transected. (b) Excision of hyaloid from area of wound, total posterior vitrectomy and excision of proliferation at the exit site.*

measures may reduce the risk of transvitreal proliferation and secondary retinal detachment.[1,2]

PENETRATING TRAUMA AND RETINAL DETACHMENT

Retinal detachment from penetrating trauma may assume a variety of configurations. Intraoperative indirect ophthalmoscopy performed after clearing of the visual axis is an essential diagnostic technique for recognizing the cause of retinal detachment in individual cases and instituting appropriate therapy. Rhegmatogenous retinal detachment may result from retinal breaks associated with the ocular wound or from breaks in other locations induced by vitreous traction.

The presence of bullous or mobile retinal detachment usually indicates that an open retinal break is present. Hemorrhagic retinal detachment may result

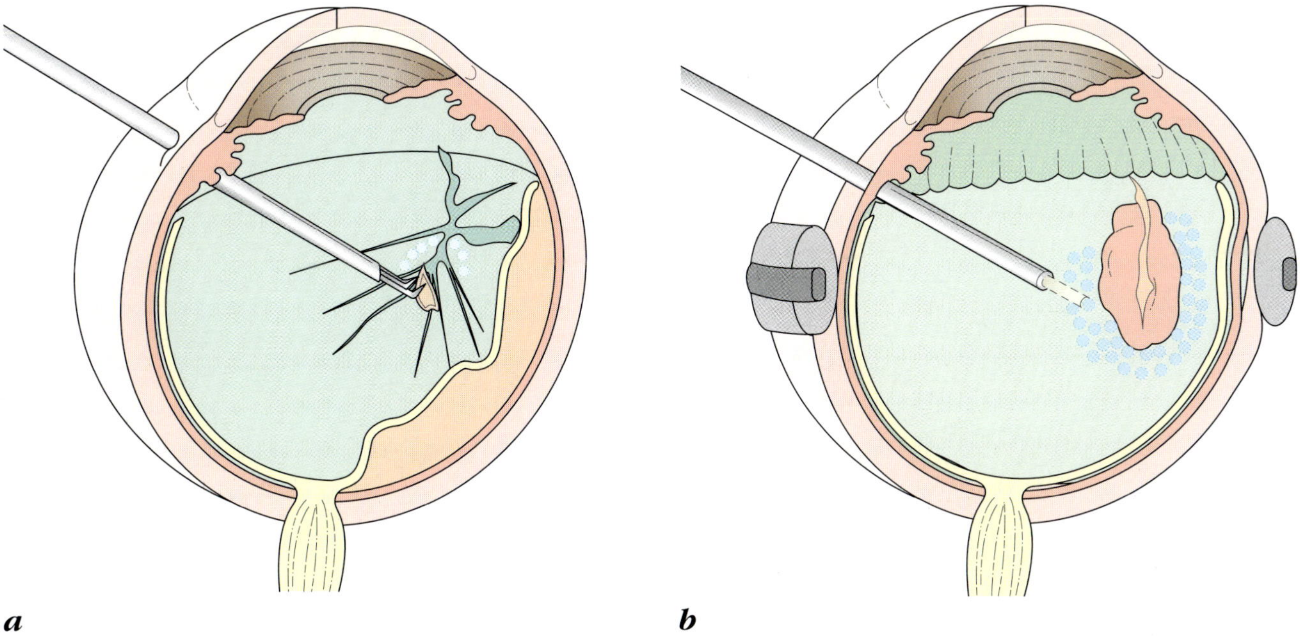

Figure 41.10 *(a) Retina incarcerated into scleral wound demonstrates immobile retinal folds radiating from wound. (b) Relaxing retinotomy usually creates a large retinal defect. Following fluid–gas exchange or perfluorocarbon liquid injection, laser photocoagulation is placed around the defect. If perfluorocarbon liquid is used to flatten the retina, a perfluorocarbon–air or perfluorocarbon–silicone oil exchange may be performed.*

from severe bleeding from rupture of the choroid or the penetrating wound itself. The presence of clotted blood producing a solid elevation of the retina is diagnostic. Removal of subretinal blood may be indicated if it forms a thick layer beneath the macula, if it prevents adequate retinopexy or if it detaches a large area of the fundus.

Traction retinal detachment occurs if there is massive retinal or vitreous incarceration in the wound, or if proliferative vitreoretinopathy (PVR) develops. Wound dehiscence during vitrectomy may also exacerbate retinal incarceration and traction retinal detachment. Subretinal membrane formation with secondary retinal traction is a classic manifestation of PVR following penetrating trauma, possibly caused by choroidal damage or subretinal hemorrhage that often accompanies such injuries.

Rhegmatogenous retinal detachment and PVR are handled with standard vitreoretinal surgical techniques (see Chapters 13, 14 and 27). These include vitrectomy, removal of proliferative epiretinal membranes, fluid–air exchange, scleral buckling of the peripheral retina and long-acting tamponade. However, retinal detachments associated with severe retinal incarceration into the traumatic wound may require special measures to relieve retinal traction, including scleral buckling of retinal incarceration sites and relaxing retinotomy or retinectomy[24] (Figs 41.10a,b). In hemorrhagic retinal detachments, removal of subretinal hemorrhage may be necessary to permit retinopexy around retinal breaks or to preserve macular function from secondary effects of persistent submacular hemorrhage. Large hemorrhagic detachments also may justify surgical removal of subretinal hemorrhage[18] (Figs. 41.11a–c). Closure and treatment of retinal breaks, relief of retinal traction and removal of visually significant subretinal hemorrhage are primary surgical goals during vitrectomy for retinal detachment.

VITRECTOMY FOR RETINAL INCARCERATION

INSTRUMENTATION

- Vitrectomy cutter or vertical cutting scissors (MPC scissors).

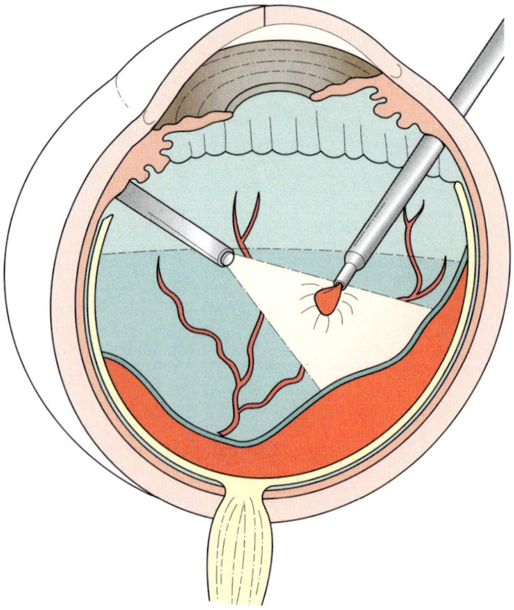

a

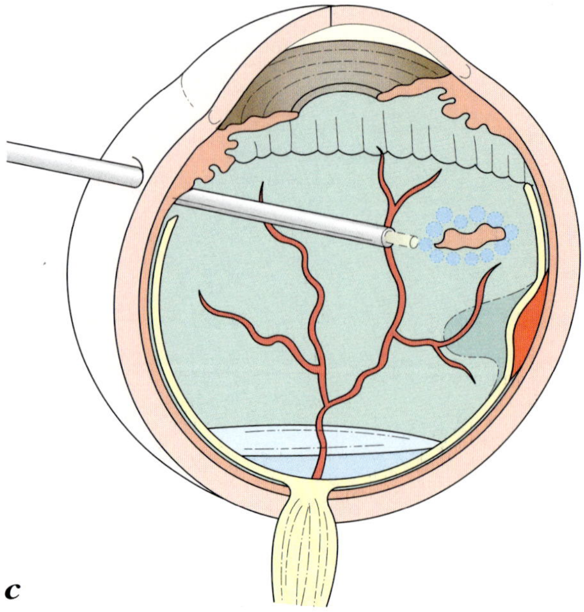

c

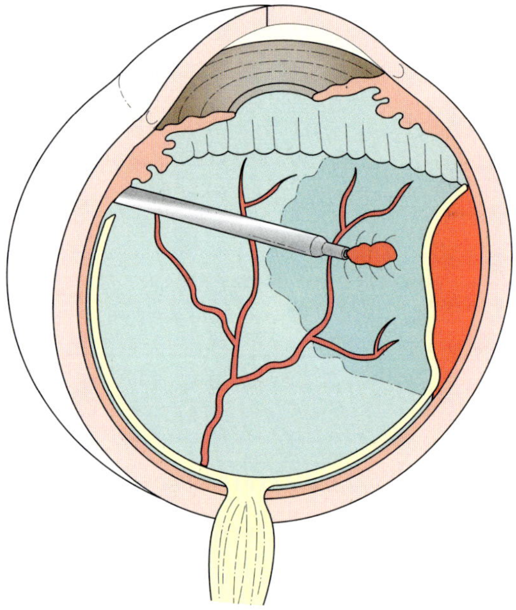

b

Figure 41.11 *(a) A massive subretinal hemorrhage and internal drainage of subretinal blood. A posterior drainage retinotomy is placed outside the macular region, closest to the area of maximal retinal elevation. Suction or forceps may be required to remove liquefied or clotted blood. Once a drainage retinotomy is created, removal of as much blood as possible is required to achieve adequate retinopexy around the drainage site. (b) Hemorrhagically elevated retinal tear and internal drainage of localized subretinal blood. Sufficient blood should be removed to allow adequate retinopexy around the tear. Care must be taken not to extend the detachment by exerting minimal traction and performing fluid–air exchange immediately after drainage. (c) After sufficient subretinal blood is removed, fluid–air exchange and subsequent endophotocoagulation around the tear are performed. A small amount of subretinal blood outside the macula and away from the tear may remain without ill effect. Parts (a)–(c) adapted with permission from Han DP, Mieler WF, Schwartz DM, Abrams GW. Management of traumatic hemorrhagic retinal detachment with pars plana vitrectomy,* Arch Ophthalmol *(1990)* ***108***:*1281–6. Copyright © 1990, American Medical Association.*

- Silicone-tipped aspiration cannula (20-gauge tapered to 23-gauge).
- Endodiathermy.
- Perfluorocarbon liquid.
- Air pump attached to sutured pars plana infusion cannula.
- Laser with endophotocoagulator probe or indirect ophthalmoscope laser.
- Scleral buckling elements.
- 5-0 Nylon or Dacron sutures for scleral buckle fixation.
- Light source: fiberoptic endoilluminator.
- Biconcave contact lenses or alternative vitrectomy viewing system.
- Long-acting gas tamponade or silicone oil.
- Silicone oil injector (viscous fluid injector).

SURGICAL TECHNIQUE

Retina incarcerated into a scleral wound demonstrates immobile retinal folds radiating from the wound (see Fig. 41.10a). Extensive vitreous traction from severe vitreous loss also is usually present. If there is a retinal detachment caused by severe retinal traction to the wound that cannot be relieved by scleral buckling, relaxing retinotomy is indicated. The retina is incised with a vitrectomy cutting instrument or with vertical intraocular scissors, as peripherally and as close to the site of incarceration as possible. Large retinal vessels near the retinotomy edge must be diathermized before cutting in order to avoid severe bleeding.

Relaxing retinotomy usually creates a large retinal defect. Following fluid–gas exchange or perfluorocarbon liquid injection, laser photocoagulation is placed around the defect (see Fig. 41.10b). If perfluorocarbon liquid is used to flatten the retina, a perfluorocarbon–air or perfluorocarbon–silicone oil exchange may be performed.[25] Scleral buckling of the defect, if possible, and of the surrounding vitreous base may prevent subsequent retinal detachment if PVR and vitreous base contraction were to develop. Intravitreal injection of a perfluoropropane gas mixture or silicone oil usually is needed to achieve an adequately long retinal tamponade to obtain permanent closure of the retinal defect.

REMOVAL OF SUBRETINAL HEMORRHAGE

Indications for removal of subretinal blood in penetrating trauma include massive hemorrhagic retinal detachment (see Fig. 41.11a), hemorrhagically elevated retinal tears (see Figs 41.11b,c) and bullous retinal detachment with associated subretinal hemorrhage. Localized, extramacular hemorrhagic retinal detachment not associated with retinal breaks or bullous elevation may be observed and usually resolves spontaneously.[18]

INSTRUMENTATION

As listed above for retinal incarceration.

SURGICAL TECHNIQUE

A massive subretinal hemorrhagic retinal detachment may require internal drainage of subretinal blood. In the presence of an open peripheral break, perfluorocarbon liquid injection may permit liquefied blood to migrate into the vitreous cavity through the break, where it can be removed subsequently. However, if this fails, a posterior drainage retinotomy may be placed peripheral to the macular region, closest to the area of maximal retinal elevation (see Fig. 41.11a). Suction or forceps may be required to remove the blood. Once a drainage retinotomy is created, removal of as much blood as possible is required to achieve adequate retinopexy around the drainage site. Postoperative laser treatment then may be performed around the drainage site.

A hemorrhagically elevated retinal tear requires internal drainage of subretinal blood to achieve adequate retinopexy (see Fig. 41.11b). Sufficient blood should be removed to allow adequate retinopexy. Exerting minimal traction on the retina and performing fluid–air exchange immediately after drainage should reduce the risk of extending the detachment. The use of perfluorocarbon liquid also may assist in hydraulically displacing the hemorrhage from the subretinal space into the vitreous cavity.

After removal of a sufficient amount of subretinal blood, fluid–air exchange and laser photocoagulation around the tear are performed (see Fig. 41.11c). A small amount of subretinal blood outside the macula and away from the tear may remain, without ill effect.

VITRECTOMY WITH PLACEMENT OF A TEMPORARY KERATOPROSTHESIS FOR EYES WITH SEVERE CORNEAL DAMAGE

The use of temporary keratoprostheses is an important management technique for severely injured eyes with extensive corneal injury.[26,27] If a large area of the central cornea is damaged or distorted, or there is corneal tissue loss, temporary placement of a keratoprosthesis may be needed to allow posterior visualization (Figs 41.12–41.14). In most such instances, the lens has been damaged and the eye must be rendered aphakic during vitrectomy to allow posterior repair. Penetrating keratoplasty is performed following completion of the vitrectomy.

Placement of a temporary keratoprosthesis usually is performed as a secondary procedure in conjunction with posterior vitrectomy. Although obtaining a watertight seal around the prosthesis is ideal, a very small amount

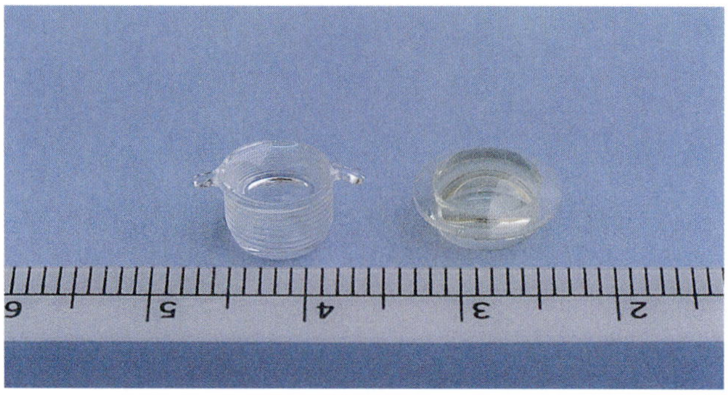

Figure 41.12 *Temporary keratoprostheses for use during vitrectomy.* (Left) *Landers–Foulks keratoprosthesis, constructed of polymethylmethacrylate.* (Right) *Eckardt keratoprosthesis, constructed of silicone rubber.*

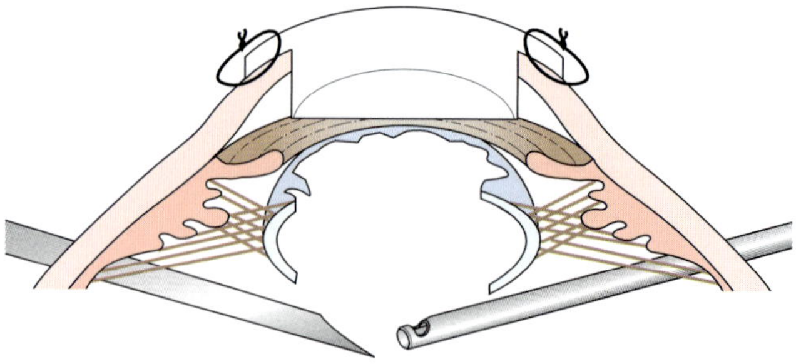

Figure 41.14 *Side view of Eckardt temporary keratoprosthesis for posterior segment viewing through severely injured cornea.*

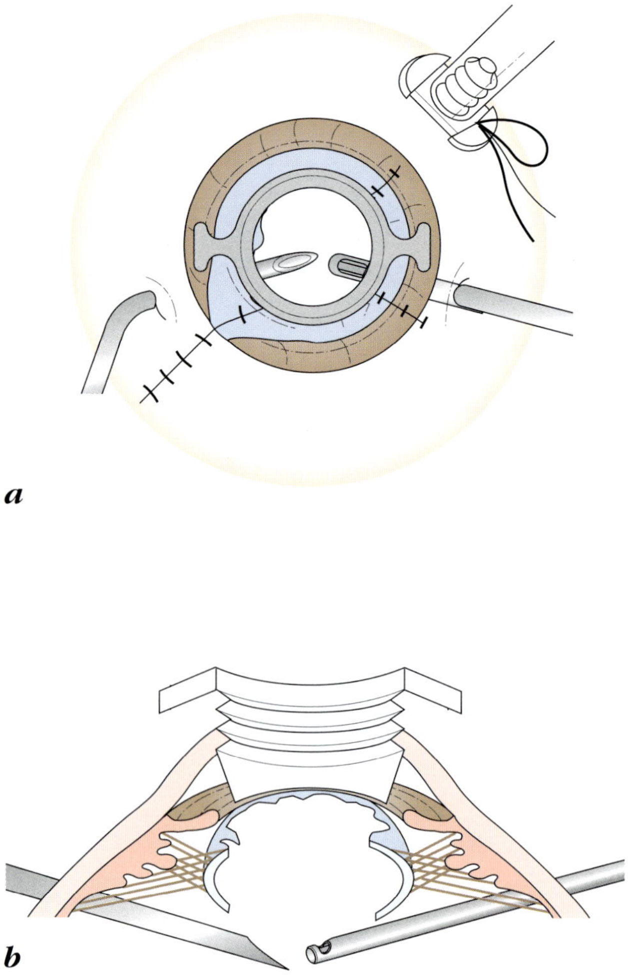

Figure 41.13 *Positioning of the Landers–Foulks temporary keratoprostheses during vitrectomy. (a) Top view. (b) Side view.*

of seepage around the device can be tolerated as long as it is securely positioned and leakage does not increase significantly during transient intraocular pressure elevations. After placement of the keratoprosthesis, extensive manipulation of the globe should be performed with extreme caution. Scleral buckling, if anticipated, should be performed prior to trephination of the cornea.

SURGICAL TECHNIQUE

Following previous closure of the corneal wound, a corneal bed is trephined and the prosthesis is inserted into the corneal opening. The Landers–Foulks prosthesis is secured easily by rotating it into the wound so that the threads at its outer aspect firmly engage the corneal tissue (see Fig. 41.13). Suture fixation is required at only two sites. No additional contact lens is required for posterior segment viewing. Viewing of the fundus periphery through the microscope is difficult, and indirect ophthalmoscopy is not possible. Several diameter sizes are available. The corneal bed diameter should be slightly smaller than the prosthesis diameter, and the graft diameter should be slightly larger than the prosthesis diameter. (Example: if the prosthesis used has a diameter of 6.2 mm, the trephined corneal bed diameter is 6.0 mm and the donor graft is 6.5 mm.)

Positioning of the Eckardt prosthesis (see Fig. 41.14) requires fixation at least at four sites, using 10-0 nylon sutures placed through the silicone rubber substance of the prosthesis and the abutting host corneal tissue. A vitrectomy contact lens is required for microscopic viewing of the fundus. Good visualization of the fundus periphery may be obtained with the operating microscope or indirect ophthalmoscope. Its flatter configuration allows retention of intraocular lenses, if present. Its diameter at the junction of the cornea and prosthesis is 7.0 mm. The host cornea opening is made with a trephine of diameter 6.5 mm. Because insertion of the keratoprosthesis dilates the corneal opening, a slightly oversized graft (7.2 mm diameter) is recommended for permanent keratoplasty.

PROPHYLAXIS OF ENDOPHTHALMITIS AFTER PENETRATING TRAUMA

Post-traumatic endophthalmitis occurs in 2–7% of penetrating posterior segment injuries[28] and in 7–13% of cases with retained IOFB.[28–30] An increased risk of endophthalmitis also has been observed in eyes with disruption of the crystalline lens.[13] Bacillus species are a common cause of endophthalmitis after penetrating trauma, and may be associated with a fulminant endophthalmitis and poor visual prognosis.[31] Unfortunately, a delay in diagnosis is common because the presence of media opacity and coexisting poor visual acuity make diagnosis difficult. Pars plana vitrectomy itself may have a protective effect against the development of endophthalmitis by removing infectious material from the eye before clinical infection occurs.[11]

The role of prophylactic intravitreal injection of antibiotics after penetrating trauma to prevent endophthalmitis is controversial. However, it may be considered in high-risk patients, such as those with retained IOFB or those involving contamination with organic material. The currently advocated antimicrobial agents for prophylactic intravitreal injection include vancomycin 1.0 mg and ceftazidime 2.2 mg. An aminoglycoside, such as amikacin 400 μg, may also be considered but its use is less suited to prophylaxis because of a possible increased risk of macular toxicity. Inclusion of Gram-negative coverage with ceftazidime or amikacin may be of greater potential benefit in eyes contaminated with organic material, such as those injured in a rural setting.[32] Postoperative prophylaxis is discussed below.

POSTOPERATIVE MANAGEMENT

Postoperative management consists of topical cycloplegics, antibiotics and corticosteroids beginning immediately postoperatively. A course of prophylactic systemic antibiotic therapy should be continued for 5–7 days after initial injury. The authors usually initiate a broad-spectrum cephalosporin (e.g. intravenous cefazolin 1 g every 6 hours) during the initial hospitalization for primary repair and then switch immediately to an oral quinolone agent (e.g. ciprofloxacin 750 mg orally, twice daily) at discharge. Intraocular pressure elevation is managed with nonmiotic topical antiglaucoma agents as necessary. In patients in whom significant inflammation is likely, a brief (5–7 day) course of systemic corticosteroid therapy also may be considered.

Follow-up examination is performed within 24–48 hours of surgery, 5–7 days later and every 1–4 weeks until stable, after which visits can occur at longer intervals of 2–6 months. Closer follow-up is indicated for cases at high risk for retinal detachment, endophthalmitis or sustained intraocular pressure elevation.

Patients with retained silicone oil tamponade require monitoring for possible side-effects from the silicone oil. Patients are advised to return to the clinic if they notice reduced vision, pain, photopsia, floaters or a new visual field defect.

In spite of advances in surgical technique, late complications of penetrating trauma represent a significant threat to visual outcome. These include the development of delayed retinal detachment, fibrous ingrowth, cataract, glaucoma, severe hypotony and sympathetic ophthalmia. For these reasons, long-term follow-up examinations on a yearly basis are generally recommended for any patient having sustained a penetrating globe injury.

SURGICAL RESULTS

Using pars plana vitrectomy and the adjunctive techniques described above, the reported rates of obtaining functional visual acuity of 5/200 or better range from approximately 50% to 75% in large series of eyes with penetrating trauma.[8,9,14,19,33–35] However, the visual prognosis in individual cases varies considerably according to the type of injury and associated complications. Blunt penetrating injuries[35] were associated with a 38% rate of functional success, compared to 67% for sharp penetrating injuries.[35] An extremely poor visual prognosis has been reported in association with perforating and air rifle injuries,[12,14] large lacerations,[14] massive subretinal hemorrhage,[14,18] retinal detachment[35] or retinal incarceration.[24]

SUMMARY

Management of penetrating and perforating ocular trauma requires a complete armamentarium of vitreoretinal surgical techniques. Nevertheless, even the most complex ocular injuries may be handled appropriately by adhering to the basic principles of ocular trauma management. Pars plana vitrectomy may advance these principles by interrupting intraocular proliferation, removing vitreous opacities and treating complications such as retinal detachment or endophthalmitis. By using these techniques, success rates of up to 75% may be obtained in penetrating posterior segment injury, and excellent outcomes are possible.

REFERENCES

1. Topping TM, Abrams GW, Machemer R. Experimental double-perforating injury of the posterior segment in rabbit eyes: the natural history of intraocular proliferation, *Arch Ophthalmol* (1979) **97:**735–42.
2. Abrams GW, Topping TM, Machemer R. Vitrectomy for injury: the effect on intraocular proliferation following perforation of the posterior segment of the rabbit eye, *Arch Ophthalmol* (1979) **97:**743–8.
3. Cleary PE, Ryan SJ. Vitrectomy in penetrating eye injury: results of a controlled trial of vitrectomy in an experimental posterior penetrating eye injury in the rhesus monkey, *Arch Ophthalmol* (1981) **99:**287–92.
4. Gregor Z, Ryan SJ. Complete and core vitrectomies in the treatment of experimental posterior penetrating eye injury in the rhesus monkey. I. Clinical features, *Arch Ophthalmol* (1983) **101:**441–5.
5. Gregor Z, Ryan SJ. Complete and core vitrectomies in the treatment of experimental posterior penetrating eye injury in the rhesus monkey. II. Histologic features, *Arch Ophthalmol* (1983) **101:**446–50.
6. De Juan E Jr, Sternberg P Jr, Michels RG, Auer C. Evaluation of vitrectomy in penetrating ocular trauma: a case control study, *Arch Ophthalmol* (1984) **102:**1160–3.
7. Coleman DJ. Pars plana vitrectomy: the role of vitrectomy in traumatic vitreopathy, *Trans Am Acad Ophthalmol Otolaryngol* (1976) **81** (3 Pt 1):406–13.
8. Brinton GS, Aaberg TM, Reeser FH, et al. Surgical results in ocular trauma involving the posterior segment, *Am J Ophthalmol* (1982) **93:**271–8.
9. Coleman DJ. Early vitrectomy in the management of the severely traumatized eye, *Am J Ophthalmol* (1982) **93:**543–51.
10. Miyake Y, Ando F. Surgical results of vitrectomy in ocular trauma, *Retina* (1983) **3:**265–8.
11. Mieler WF, Ellis MK, Williams DF, Han DP. Retained intraocular foreign bodies and endophthalmitis, *Ophthalmology* (1990) **97:**1532–8.
12. Sternberg P, de Juan E, Michels RG. Multivariate analysis of prognostic factors in penetrating ocular injuries, *Am J Ophthalmol* (1984) **98:**467–72.
13. Thompson WS, Rubsamen PE, Flynn HW Jr, et al. Endophthalmitis after penetrating trauma: risk factors and visual acuity outcomes, *Ophthalmology* (1995) **102:**1696–1701.
14. Hutton WL, Fuller DG. Factors influencing final visual results in severely injured eyes, *Am J Ophthalmol* (1984) **97:**715–22.
15. Conway BP, Michels RG. Vitrectomy techniques in the management of selected penetrating ocular injuries, *Ophthalmology* (1978) **85:**560–83.
16. Ryan SJ, Allen AW. Pars plana vitrectomy in ocular trauma, *Am J Ophthalmol* (1979) **88:**483–91.
17. Thompson JT, Parver LM, Enger CL, et al. Infectious endophthalmitis after penetrating injuries with retained intraocular foreign bodies, *Ophthalmology* (1993) **100:**1468–74.
18. Han DP, Mieler WF, Schwartz DM, Abrams GW. Management of traumatic hemorrhagic retinal detachment with pars plana vitrectomy, *Arch Ophthalmol* (1990) **108:**1281–6.
19. Hermsen V. Vitrectomy in severe ocular trauma, *Ophthalmologica* (1984) **189:**86–92.
20. Campochiaro PA, Kaden IH, Vidaurri-Leal J, Glaser BM. Cryotherapy enhances intravitreal dispersion of viable retinal pigment epithelial cells, *Arch Ophthalmol* (1985) **103:**434–6.
21. Jaccoma EH, Conway BP, Campochiaro PA. Cryotherapy causes extensive breakdown of the blood–retinal barrier: a comparison with argon laser photocoagulation, *Arch Ophthalmol* (1985) **103:**1728–30.
22. Thompson JT. Use of perfluorocarbon liquids in vitreoretinal surgery. In: Ryan SJ, ed, *Retina* 2nd edn Vol. 3. (Mosby-Yearbook: St Louis, 1994): 2191–201.
23. Peyman GA, Schulman JA, Sullivan B. Perfluorocarbon liquids in ophthalmology, *Surv Ophthalmol* (1995) **39:**375–95.
24. Han DP, Mieler WF, Abrams GW, Williams GW. Vitrectomy for traumatic retinal incarceration, *Arch Ophthalmol* (1988) **106:**640–5.
25. Han DP, Rychwalski PJ, Mieler WF, Abrams GW. Management of complex retinal detachment with combined relaxing retinotomy and intravitreal perfluoro-*n*-octane injection, *Am J Ophthalmol* (1994) **118:**24–32.
26. Landers MB III, Foulks GN, Landers DM, et al. Temporary keratoprosthesis for use during pars plana vitrectomy, *Am J Ophthalmol* (1981) **91:**615–19.
27. Eckardt C. A new temporary keratoprosthesis for pars plana vitrectomy, *Retina* (1987) **7:**34–7.
28. Brinton GS, Topping TM, Hyndiuk RA, et al. Posttraumatic endophthalmitis, *Arch Ophthalmol* (1984) **102:**547–50.
29. Williams DF, Mieler WF, Abrams GW, Lewis H. Results and prognostic factors in penetrating ocular injuries with retained intraocular foreign bodies, *Ophthalmology* (1988) **95:**911–16.
30. Punnonen E, Laatikainen L. Prognosis of perforating eye injuries with intraocular foreign bodies, *Acta Ophthalmol* (1989) **67:**483–91.
31. Parrish CM, O'Day DM. Traumatic endophthalmitis, *Int Ophthalmol Clin* (1987) **27:**112–19.
32. Boldt HC, Pulido JS, Blodi CF, Folk JC, et al. Rural endophthalmitis, *Ophthalmology* (1989) **96:**1722–6.

33. Faulborn J, Atkinson A, Olivier D. Primary vitrectomy as a preventive surgical procedure in the treatment of severely injured eyes, *Br J Ophthalmol* (1977) **61:**202–8.
34. Cupples HP, Whitmore PV, Wertz FD III, Mazur DO. Ocular trauma treated by vitreous surgery, *Retina* (1983) **3:**103–7.
35. Meredith TA, Gordon PA. Pars plana vitrectomy for severe penetrating injury with posterior segment involvement, *Am J Ophthalmol* (1987) **103:**549–54.

Chapter 42 Suprachoroidal hemorrhage

Uday R Desai

LIMITED SUPRACHOROIDAL HEMORRHAGE

The diagnosis of limited suprachoroidal hemorrhage is subjective; there is no consensus on its definition. Patients who have choroidal elevation that is less than that required to have retinal apposition could be considered to have limited hemorrhage. Patients with limited suprachoroidal hemorrhage may have only one quadrant involved or multiple quadrants with low-lying choroidal elevation. These patients characteristically do not have vitreous in the anterior segment. It is important to identify a limited hemorrhage because these patients require no intervention. The choroidal hemorrhages resolve spontaneously over a period of weeks to months.[1–3] While these patients are being observed, it should be noted that although gradual resolution is the rule, it is possible for limited hemorrhage to progress into massive suprachoroidal hemorrhage, necessitating surgical intervention.[4]

MASSIVE SUPRACHOROIDAL HEMORRHAGE

The term massive suprachoroidal hemorrhage is also subjective and is not constrained by any rigid definition; typically, retinal apposition (kissing choroidals) is present. The term may be applied also in cases without retinal apposition but with other conditions that mandate surgical intervention, such as ocular pain or secondary glaucoma. Although massive suprachoroidal hemorrhage may resolve spontaneously in some patients,[5] surgical intervention is generally required.

MASSIVE SUPRACHOROIDAL HEMORRHAGE WITHOUT VITREOUS IN THE ANTERIOR SEGMENT

Careful preoperative evaluation should determine if there is vitreous in the anterior segment. Gonioscopy also may be necessary to confirm the absence of vitreous in the angle or in the surgical wound in patients who have undergone keratoplasty, cataract extraction or glaucoma filtering surgery. The vitreous may be seen easily in aphakic patients. Care must be taken to identify any vitreous that enters the anterior chamber through dehisced zonules in patients who are either phakic or pseudophakic with a posterior chamber intraocular lens (PC-IOL). The vitreous also should be visualized in patients with an anterior chamber intraocular lens (AC-IOL) if the vitreous penetrates the pupil and extends anterior to the AC-IOL. If vitreous is not visible in the anterior segment of aphakic patients, the following management techniques may be applied. Management of cases in phakic or pseudophakic eyes will be discussed later.

Preoperative medical management of intraocular pressure (IOP) may decrease the risk of rebleeding during surgery. Systemic steroids given preoperatively may stabilize the choroidal vasculature; we place patients on 1 mg/kg/day of oral prednisone in the preoperative period. A 2-week interval before surgical intervention will allow the greatest egress of suprachoroidal blood because clot lysis will have occurred.[5,6]

Surgery may be performed under general or local anesthesia. General anesthesia has been implicated in postoperative suprachoroidal hemorrhage as a result of postoperative vomiting; however, with modern general anesthesia techniques we feel relatively secure in proceeding with general anesthesia. The conjunctiva is opened 360° and the muscles are

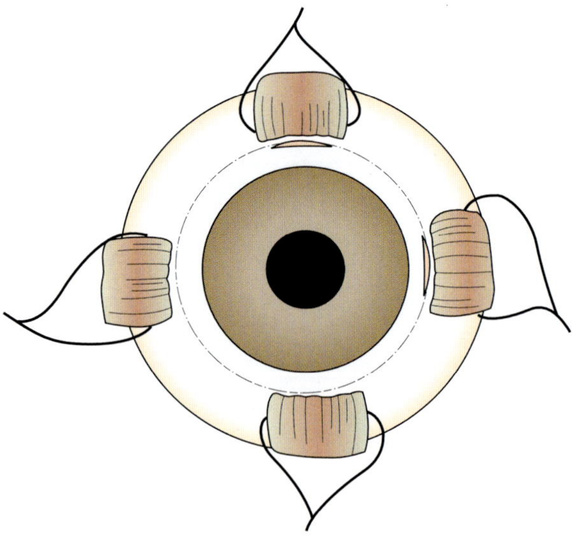

Figure 42.1 *A 360° peritomy is made with radial relaxing incisions at 3 o'clock and 9 o'clock, with 4-0 silk sutures around rectus muscles.*

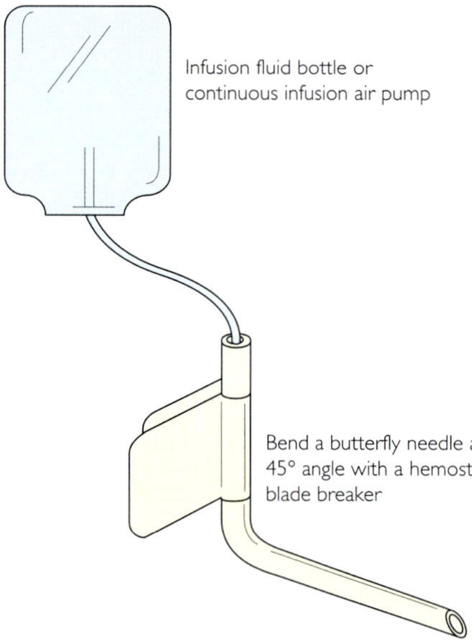

Figure 42.2 *Infusion fluid bottle or continuous infusion air pump. Bend butterfly needle at 45° angle with a hemostat or blade breaker.*

tagged using 4-0 silk suture (Fig. 42.1). A 23-gauge butterfly needle is prepared by bending it to a 45° angle; the needle is connected to the infusion solution and the bottle is raised to a level that allows a steady stream of infusion fluid (Fig. 42.2). The tubing is then clamped. Alternatively, the infusion fluid can be

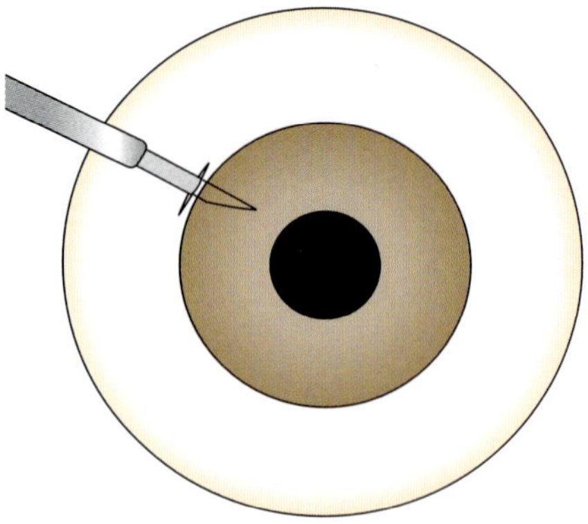

Figure 42.3 *A 15° blade is used to make a self-sealing incision at the limbus in a location that is convenient for the assistant.*

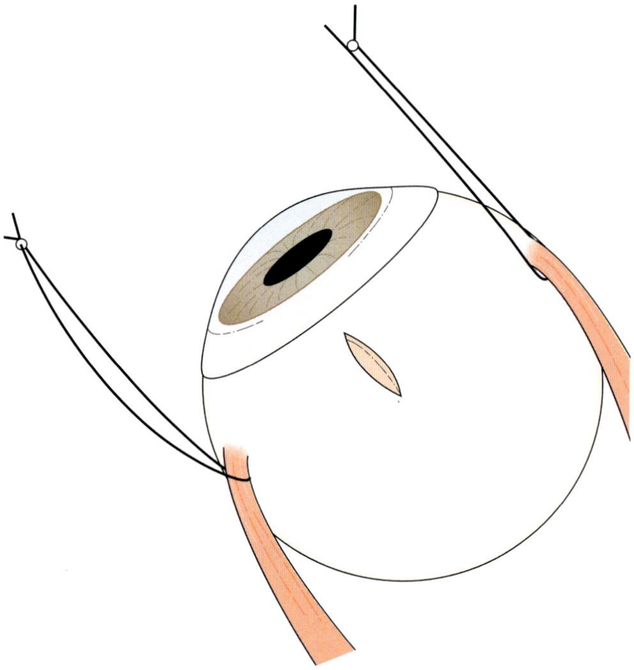

Figure 42.4 *A quadrant is exposed and cautery is applied for hemostasis. A blade is used to make a scleral cut down in a radial fashion. Stop before going through the sclera to full thickness. Apply cautery or diathermy to the edges to keep the scleral edges apart.*

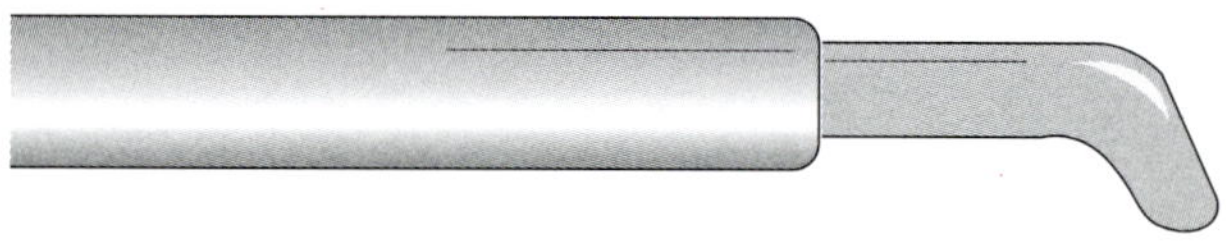

Figure 42.5 *Grieshaber 'hockey stick' blade.*

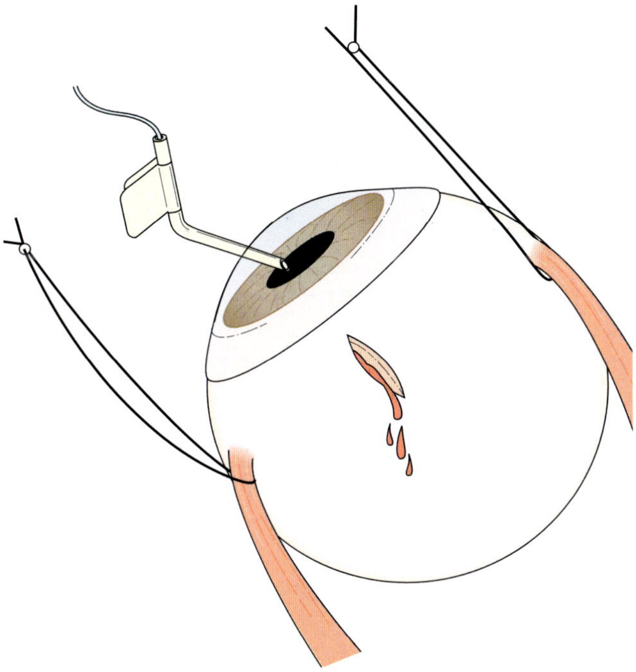

Figure 42.6 *The butterfly needle is placed in the anterior chamber with infusion off. Final layers of sclera are penetrated. As blood drains and the eye begins to soften, the infusion is opened to keep a steady intraocular pressure.*

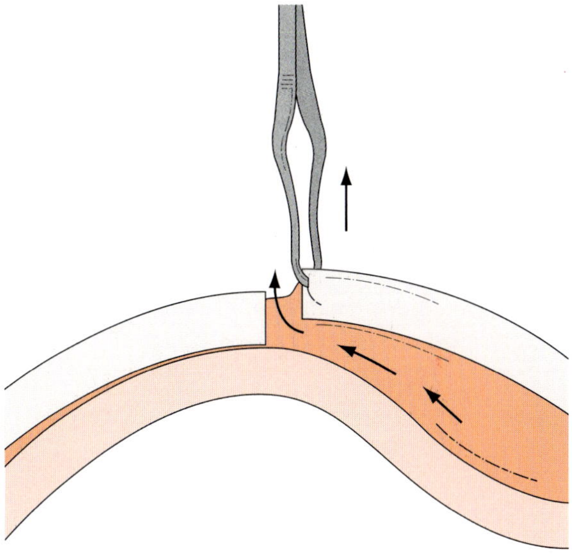

Figure 42.7 *If blood stops flowing, lifting the scleral lip with 0.3-mm forceps may allow trapped blood to egress.*

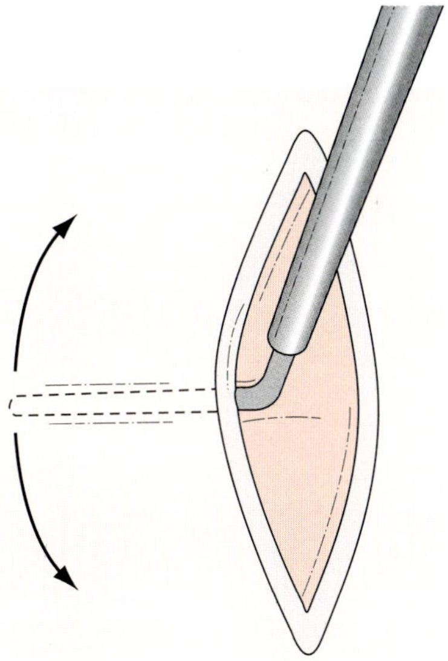

Figure 42.8 *Placing a cyclodialysis spatula in the plane of the suprachoroidal space and sweeping back and forth in an arc-like motion will help to release loculated areas of suprachoroidal blood.*

connected to a continuous pressure air pump so that the pressure remains between 20 and 25 mmHg.[6]

A 15° blade is used to make a paracentesis at the limbus closest to the assistant (Fig. 42.3). The sclerotomy will be placed in the quadrant with the greatest suprachoroidal hemorrhage. Using a Grieshaber blade, a radial sclerotomy is made in the middle of the quadrant. The sclerotomy should be 3–4 mm in length and extend posteriorly starting 4 mm behind the limbus (Figs 42.4 and 42.5). Before the sclerotomy is made, cautery should be applied to the sclera and episclera. When the sclerotomy is almost full thickness, the assistant places the 23-gauge needle with the infusion turned off in the paracentesis. The infusion is initially left off to avoid elevating the IOP excessively before entering the suprachoroidal space.

The surgeon cuts through the remaining sclera and suprachoroidal blood is allowed to egress (Fig. 42.6). As soon as the blood begins to drain from the sclerotomy, the infusion fluid is turned on. If the blood stops flowing, the edges of the sclerotomy can be grasped with 0.3-mm forceps and elevated away from the choroid (Fig. 42.7). If this maneuver does not permit resumed flow of the suprachoroidal blood, a cyclodialysis spatula is placed in the suprachoroidal space through the sclerotomy and swept back and forth on both sides of the sclerotomy for approximately 5 mm (Fig. 42.8). If the blood has stopped flowing, the indirect ophthalmoscope is used to evaluate the status of the choroidals while

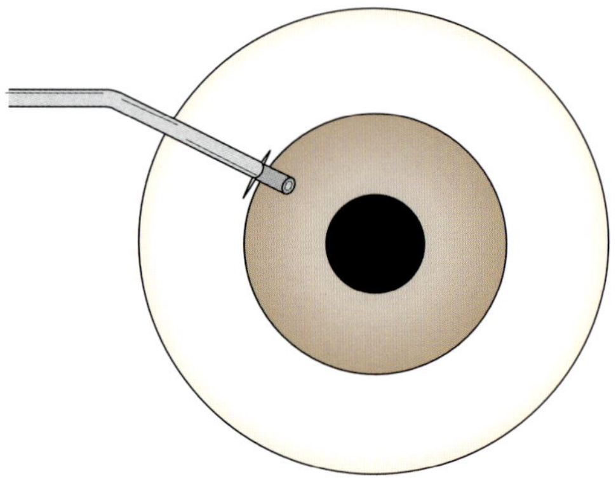

Figure 42.9 *A self-retaining anterior chamber maintainer will allow the assistant's hands to be free.*

the assistant maintains the butterfly needle in the anterior segment. If the choroidals are significantly reduced, the surgery can be terminated. If choroidals are still present, the following technique can be attempted:

- Cotton-tipped applicators are rolled over the sclera in an attempt to bring residual suprachoroidal blood to the existing sclerotomy.
- If this maneuver does not work, additional sclerotomies are made in other quadrants.

Once the choroidals are adequately drained, the butterfly needle is removed from the anterior chamber. The sclerotomy may be left open or closed with 6-0 or 7-0 Vicryl interrupted sutures. Muscle sutures are removed and the conjunctiva is closed using interrupted 6-0 plain catgut.

An alternative that can be used for infusing fluid into the anterior chamber is the self-retaining anterior chamber maintainer (Fig. 42.9). This device can be secured at the limbus and it may free the assistant to help with other parts of the surgery.[7]

SIGNIFICANT CHOROIDAL HEMORRHAGE WITH VITREOUS IN ANTERIOR SEGMENT

When vitreous protrudes into the anterior segment, there is a risk that it is adherent to anterior segment structures, such as the iris or cornea. Very high suspicion of adherence should be given to cases that have vitreous going to the surgical wound. Adherent vitreous may cause tearing of the retina where it is attached at the vitreous base if the adherent vitreous is not relieved before the choroidal blood is drained.

The vitreous must be removed from its anterior connections before significant drainage of the choroidal hemorrhage to prevent tearing of the retina. The fullness of the anterior chamber determines whether to first drain suprachoroidal blood or remove anterior segment vitreous. If the anterior chamber is moderately deep and retina is not present in the anterior chamber, vitrectomy in the anterior chamber before drainage of the suprachoroidal blood is best.[8] Two paracentesis sites are made at the limbus with a 15° blade. The incisions are made slightly closer to the horizontal meridians at the 9:30 and 2:30 clock positions. This lateral displacement will allow access to any vitreous located at the 12 o'clock position. The 23-gauge bent butterfly needle is placed in one of the paracentesis sites and the vitrectomy instrument is placed in the other (Fig. 42.10). The butterfly needle is initially used to sweep vitreous from the surgical wound (Fig. 42.11); excessive force that could be transmitted to the vitreous base must be avoided. In cases of tightly adherent vitreous, the vitrector (600 cuts per minute, 100 mmHg aspiration) is used to sever the connections to the anterior segment. Once the vitreous is separated from the cornea and the corneoscleral angle, attention is addressed to the pupillary margin. Vitreous that is attached to the pupil may be swept gently by the 23-gauge needle in an attempt to free any connections. The vitrector, set on aspiration

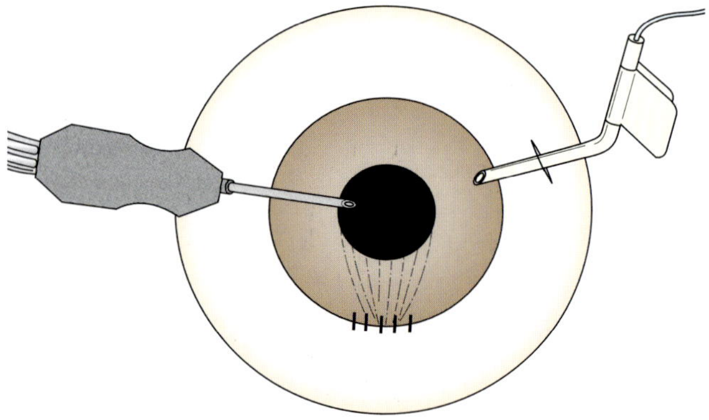

Figure 42.10 *Vitreous in the surgical wound. An infusion needle may be used to sweep the vitreous gently out of the wound.*

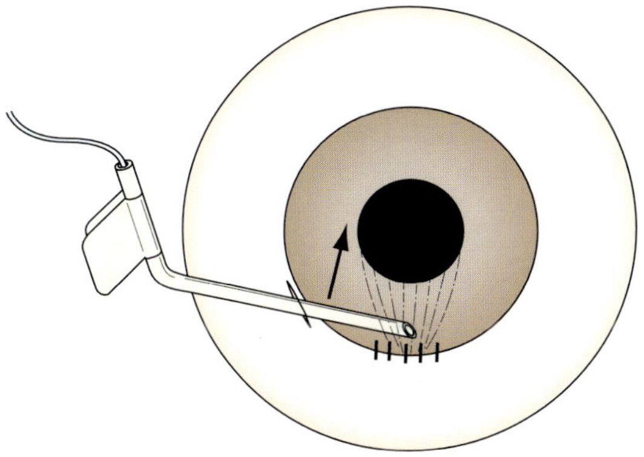

Figure 42.11 *If the infusion needle cannot sweep the vitreous from the wound, the vitrector is used to cut the vitreous as close to the wound as possible.*

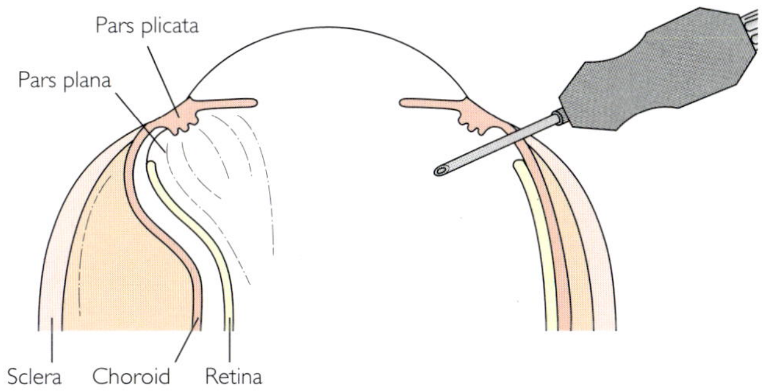

Figure 42.12 *Vitrector placed through the sclerotomy 2.5 mm from limbus. Attachment of vitreous to back side of iris may cause retinal tears as suprachoroidal blood is cleared. Infusion continues through the limbus with the 23-gauge cannula.*

mode, may also be used to aspirate the vitreous gently and free it from connection to the pupil. The released vitreous then is removed using the cutting and aspiration mode on the vitrector. The process of sweeping the vitreous free of any iris connection and removing the vitreous with the vitrector may be carried out under the iris but excessive excursions should be avoided because the retina may be in close proximity to the posterior iris.

Once the anterior segment–vitreous connections are severed, drainage of suprachoroidal blood is carried out as described in the previous section. During drainage, the posterior segment should be examined frequently with the indirect ophthalmoscope to ensure that vitreous traction does not appear between the vitreous base and the posterior iris. If traction is not present and the retina is attached, choroidal blood drainage can continue until adequate amounts of blood are removed.

If traction is present, retinal tearing may result as the choroidal drainage continues. Vitreous connections must be severed between the vitreous base and the posterior iris to prevent tearing. The vitrector must be introduced into the posterior chamber. A microvitreoretinal (MVR) blade is used to enter through the pars plana 2.5 mm posterior to limbus. The opening is made in the superior quadrant on the side of the dominant hand and located to allow access to the site of vitreous traction (Fig. 42.12).

Vitrectomy is used to remove vitreous behind the iris; the more peripheral vitreous may be removed by having the assistant depress the sclera with a cotton-tipped applicator. Once all apparent vitreous traction has been relieved, additional suprachoroidal hemorrhage is removed. As more blood is removed, the indirect ophthalmoscope is used to detect any additional areas of traction. These steps are repeated if traction remains and are continued until all residual traction is relieved and adequate amounts of choroidal hemorrhage are removed. The sclerotomy site for the vitrector is closed with 8-0 nylon suture and the drainage sclerotomy is either left open or closed with 6-0 or 7-0 Vicryl suture. Conjunctiva is reapposed with interrupted 6-0 plain catgut. The paracentesis sites should be self-sealing; if not, they are closed with 9-0 or 10-0 nylon.

ROLE OF PHAKIC STATUS IN ALTERING MANAGEMENT

When suprachoroidal blood is drained, simultaneous replacement of the vitreous is ideal. This prevents the occurrence of hypotony and subsequent risk of rebleeding. In aphakic eyes, the anterior and posterior segments are decompartmentalized and vitreous replacement can proceed through the anterior segment as described above.

In patients who are pseudophakic with an AC-IOL, the eye is still decompartmentalized and there should not be any alteration in management. In patients who are phakic or pseudophakic with a PC-IOL, the intact lens zonules should allow perfusion of infusion fluid into the posterior segment. Infusion into the anterior segment can be achieved with a 23-gauge butterfly needle or a self-retaining anterior chamber

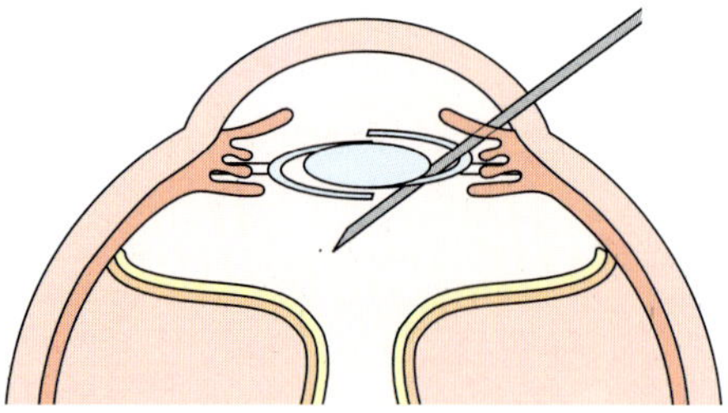

Figure 42.13 *A 23- or 25-gauge butterfly needle may be passed through the limbus, anterior capsule and posterior capsule, allowing the needle to go around the optic for infusion.*

maintainer. Special care should be taken in the phakic patient not to touch the anterior capsule.

During the drainage of suprachoroidal blood, the infusion bottle and the anterior chamber depth should be monitored. As long as the suprachoroidal blood continues to drain, the infusion bottle continues to drip and the anterior chamber does not become excessively deep, the zonules are allowing the infusion fluid to enter the vitreous cavity. Because the zonules will afford some resistance, the infusion pressure or bottle height should not be too high because there is a risk of displacing the lens posteriorly.

In patients with a PC-IOL in which the anterior segment-to-posterior segment flow is limited, it may be necessary to enter the posterior segment through the limbus by passing a 23- to 25-gauge butterfly needle through the anterior capsule, around the optic and through the posterior capsule (Fig. 42.13).[9]

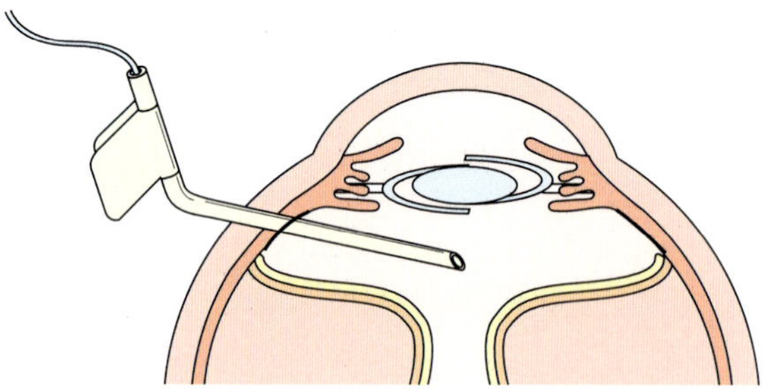

Figure 42.14 *The infusion needle is placed behind the crystalline lens or the posterior chamber intraocular lens. The sclerotomy should be 2.5–3.0 mm behind the limbus. The angle of the needle should be relatively flat in order to avoid the structures in the posterior segment. Care must be taken to avoid hitting the crystalline lens.*

Alternatively, an MVR blade can be passed superonasally or superotemporally 3 mm behind the limbus and directed either parallel or slightly anteriorly, to end up behind the posterior capsule. A 23-gauge butterfly needle connected to the infusion is subsequently passed along the same tract and infusate is allowed to enter the vitreous cavity.

This maneuver also may be necessary in phakic patients. The angle of the MVR blade and the infusing butterfly needle should be chosen to avoid the posterior lens capsule as well as the retina (Fig. 42.14). Once drainage of the choroidal is completed in these patients with pars plana infusion, the periphery should be examined adequately to ensure that no retinal tears have been induced.

If lens touch and cataract formation have occurred in phakic patients, the status of the retina will determine the management. If the retina is detached or the view is indeterminate, the lens is removed via the pars plana by phacofragmentation using a closed system. If the cataract allows the physician to determine that the retina is attached, the surgery is terminated and the cataract is managed on a subsequent occasion.

MANAGEMENT IN EYES UNDERGOING PARS PLANA VITRECTOMY

The incidence of choroidal hemorrhaging associated with pars plana vitrectomy is approximately 2%.[10] Factors that place the eye at risk during vitrectomy surgery include advanced age, elevated preoperative IOP, preoperative diagnosis of rhegmatogenous retinal detachment, aphakic or pseudophakic status and scleral buckle procedure during the vitrectomy.

Placement of broad posterior scleral buckles, intraoperative hypotony and excessive cryopexy also have been suggested as precipitating factors for suprachoroidal hemorrhage during vitrectomy.[11]

Because there is a great potential for poor visual outcome in patients who develop suprachoroidal hemorrhage during vitrectomy, avoidance is the best management technique; knowing the risk factors is important in avoiding this complication. The poorest outcomes appear to occur in patients who have drainage sclerotomies made acutely at the time of the initial surgery. Continued bleeding seems to be a predominant feature of patients undergoing sclerotomies acutely; we recommend terminating the procedure once a massive suprachoroidal hemorrhage occurs. Attempts at lowering the IOP should include aggressive medical management, including hyperosmotics and acetazolamide. A period of 2–3 weeks should elapse before repeated surgical intervention with drainage of suprachoroidal hemorrhage is attempted.

MANAGEMENT OF THE FILTERING BLEB IN GLAUCOMA PATIENTS WHO DEVELOP SUPRACHOROIDAL HEMORRHAGE

Glaucoma-filtering surgery has a high incidence of developing delayed postoperative suprachoroidal hemorrhage when compared to other ocular surgeries; prolonged hypotony is the cause. In patients who develop suprachoroidal hemorrhage, management primarily involves drainage of the hemorrhage in addition to simultaneous vitreous volume replacement. If the volume replacement does not occur, then hypotony associated with hemorrhage drainage may result in recurrent hemorrhage.

Hemorrhage is a potential problem in patients who have a functioning filter because volume replacement with balanced salt solution may be difficult in these patients. If the intraocular space is divided by the crystalline lens or a PC-IOL, a paracentesis is done at the limbus. A 25-gauge cannula is used to inject a viscoelastic substance into the anterior chamber (Fig. 42.15). This will generally displace through the filter to some degree. The anterior chamber, however, should remain formed. Drainage of suprachoroidal hemorrhage is accompanied by infusion through the pars plana, as has been described before.

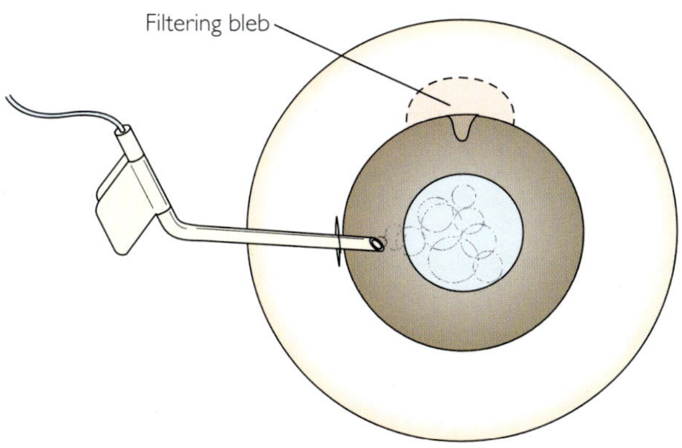

Figure 42.15 *Viscoelastic substance is injected into the anterior chamber. Some may displace into the filtering bleb. This should prevent rapid efflux of infusion fluid and keep the intraocular pressure stable during suprachoroidal blood drainage.*

In eyes that are aphakic or have an AC-IOL, infusion (whether through the limbus or pars plana) will still drain out the filter; maintaining IOP may be impossible. In these cases, sacrificing the filter may be the only alternative. The conjunctiva over the filter is removed and the flap is secured with interrupted 10-0 nylon sutures. The drainage and reformation proceed, as has been described. The potentially high postoperative IOP is managed medically and additional glaucoma surgery is performed as warranted, as the eye stabilizes.

ROLE OF PERFLUOROCARBON LIQUIDS

The removal of suprachoroidal hemorrhage is ideally accompanied by simultaneous vitreous replacement with infusion fluid. Infusion fluid is well tolerated by the eye and allows good visualization. Other modes of vitreous replacement include air,[12] viscoelastic substances,[9] silicone oil[13] and perfluorocarbon liquid.[14] Among these other modalities, air and viscoelastic have the disadvantage of poorer visualization than infusion fluid, and silicone has the disadvantage of more difficult injection.

Perfluorocarbon liquid can be injected easily and allows excellent visualization. In general, it is advisable not to use perfluorocarbon liquid as a first-line vitreous replacement in the management of massive suprachoroidal hemorrhage. There is the risk of leaving perfluorocarbon liquid in the eye, which could have serious consequences over extended periods. Perfluorocarbon liquids may be useful in those rare cases in which suprachoroidal blood is not extruded easily and especially if the suprachoroidal blood remains in the posterior aspect of the globe.

Once it is determined that vitreous and/or retina are not incarcerated in the anterior segment, perfluorocarbon liquid is injected at the limbus or in the pars plana with a 25-gauge needle. The drainage sclerotomies should have been made already, as described above. The perfluorocarbon liquid is injected until the eye is

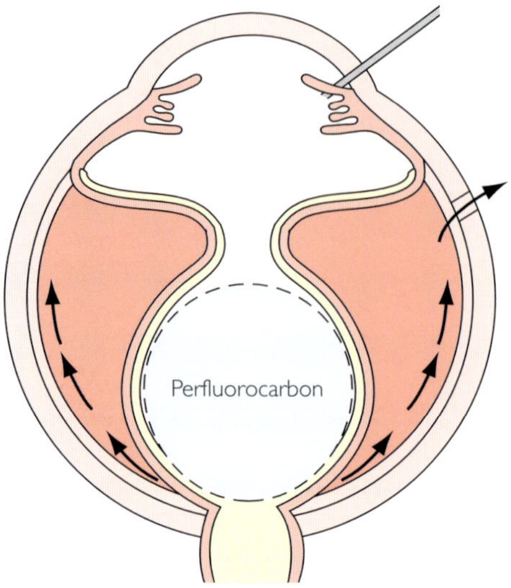

Figure 42.16 *The high specific gravity of the perfluorocarbon liquid allows it to sink to the back of the eye. The lysed suprachoroidal blood travels more anteriorly toward the sclerotomies. Cotton-tipped applicators may be used to massage the blood toward the sclerotomies.*

firm but not hard (Fig. 42.16). Cotton-tipped applicators are used to massage the suprachoroidal fluid toward the existing sclerotomies. Additional sclerotomies are made if the blood does not egress. As blood is removed, additional perfluorocarbon liquid is injected to replace the vitreous volume. This procedure is repeated until all removable blood has been removed. The infusion cannula is placed in the inferotemporal quadrant and superonasal and superotemporal sclerotomies are made to perform anterior, core and peripheral vitrectomy. The perfluorocarbon liquid is removed using passive or active aspiration. The instruments and infusion cannula are removed and the sclerotomies are closed with interrupted sutures.

MANAGEMENT OF SUPRACHOROIDAL HEMORRHAGE ASSOCIATED WITH RETINAL DETACHMENT

Patients who develop a retinal detachment in association with a massive suprachoroidal hemorrhage have been shown to be at risk for a poor visual outcome from the formation of proliferative vitreoretinopathy as well as the formation of large or irregular retinal breaks.[15,16]

Pars plana vitrectomy is generally indicated in eyes with associated retinal detachment. Drainage of suprachoroidal blood is begun with concomitant vitreous replacement with infusion fluid. Initial drainage will allow some space to develop in the anterior portion of the eye. Vitreous attachments in the anterior segment can be relieved with the vitrector in the limbus or in the pars plana. After relief of anterior traction, additional suprachoroidal hemorrhage is drained. A 6-mm infusion cannula is placed after adequate hemorrhage has been cleared. During the process of draining all mobile suprachoroidal hemorrhage, the retina should be evaluated repeatedly to ensure that no additional vitreous traction remains. If traction is seen, additional vitrectomy is completed. Any preretinal and subretinal membranes are removed after vitreous traction is relieved. A mobile retina should remain; in most cases the retina is completely detached. Retinal breaks are marked with diathermy. A posterior drainage retinotomy is made and a fluid–air exchange allows flattening of the retina. Laser photocoagulation is applied surrounding all retinal breaks as well as to treat the pre-equatorial retina 360°. An encircling buckle is placed, which can vary from 4 to 7 mm in diameter, depending on the extent of the retinal breaks. Perfluoropropane gas (12–18%) is flushed through the eye by injecting it through a 30-gauge needle attached to a 60-ml syringe. For eyes with extensive breaks, silicone oil may be injected.

MANAGEMENT OF CHOROIDAL EFFUSION

Choroidal effusion occurs when there is extravasation of serous fluid from the choroidal circulation. This fluid fills the extravascular spaces in the choroid and the suprachoroidal space. This process has been shown to occur in patients undergoing scleral buckling procedures as well as those undergoing anterior segment surgery. Patients who experience this complication after scleral buckling do so because of rapid drainage of subretinal fluid or as a result of outflow obstruction of the vortex veins by the scleral buckle. Patients who undergo anterior segment surgery may develop choroidal effusion as a result of hypotony from wound leaks, overfiltration or ciliary body clefts.

Choroidal effusion may develop acutely or subacutely. The decision to treat choroidal effusions is made when either the macula is detached or there is central retinal apposition and there is no response

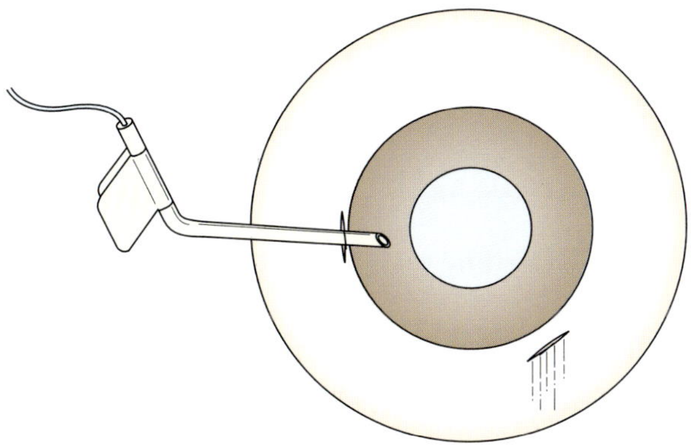

Figure 42.17 *A circumferential sclerotomy is made 3.5–4.0 mm behind the limbus. Straw-colored fluid indicates choroidal effusion. Fluid is replaced with infusion fluid through a 30-gauge needle.*

to high-dose steroids (prednisone 1 mg/kg orally daily for 1–2 weeks).

A limited conjunctival peritomy is made with relaxing incisions. The extent of the peritomy should include the quadrants with the most extensive choroidal detachment. Cautery is used to achieve hemostasis. A 30-gauge needle is fitted to a 3-ml syringe filled with balanced salt solution and is set aside to be used for volume replacement. A circumferential scleral incision is made 3.5–4.0 mm behind the limbus (Fig. 42.17). The length of the incision should be 2–3 mm. Straw-colored suprachoroidal fluid will begin to drain after the suprachoroidal space is entered. As the eye becomes soft, the syringe with the 30-gauge needle is used to replace the volume either through the limbus or the pars plana. Indirect ophthalmoscopy is used to identify any remaining fluid after drainage ceases; if excess fluid remains, additional sclerotomies may be made. After adequate drainage has occurred, the sclerotomies are closed with 6-0 or 7-0 Vicryl sutures.

SUPRACHOROIDAL HEMORRHAGE WITH EXPULSION OF INTRAOCULAR CONTENTS (EXPULSIVE HEMORRHAGE)

ACUTE MANAGEMENT

Expulsive hemorrhage is defined as suprachoroidal hemorrhage with associated expulsion of intraocular contents. Although this complication may occur in cases of traumatic globe rupture, we will limit our discussion to cases occurring during intraocular surgery. Because the incidence of expulsive hemorrhage is so low, the surgeon may not be prepared for its occurrence; this is one reason why these cases may have such a bad prognosis.

Eyes with wounds left open for extended periods with associated hypotony are at risk for developing expulsive hemorrhage. If risk factors for expulsive hemorrhage are present, attempts should be made to keep the wound as small as possible and limit the time of hypotony. Newer techniques of cataract extraction with smaller incisions, tunnel incisions and volume replacement during phacoemulsification probably decrease the incidence of expulsive hemorrhage. Preplacement of a 7-0 or 8-0 silk suture may help to close the wound quickly in cases at risk for expulsive hemorrhage (Fig. 42.18).

In cases in which expulsive hemorrhage occurs, the primary goal is to close the eye as quickly as possible in order to allow as little as possible of the intraocular contents to extrude from the eye. Once suprachoroidal hemorrhage with extrusion is recognized, the wound should be tamponaded with the surgeon's or assistant's finger or a Byrne lens if available. Pressure should be maintained for 1–10 minutes to allow closure of the bleeding vessel and prevent further loss of intraocular contents. The wound is then closed with interrupted 7-0 or 8-0 silk sutures.

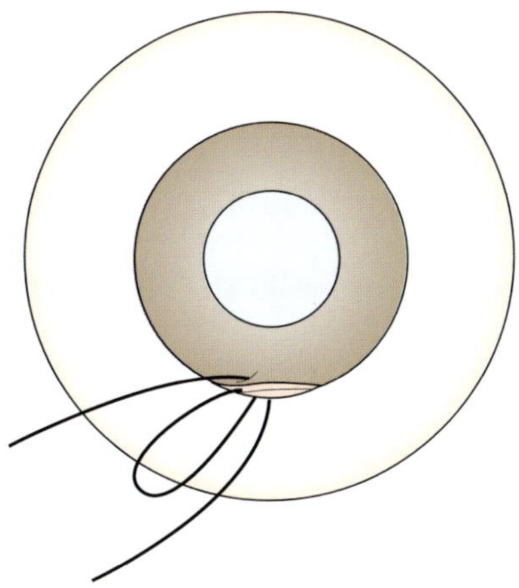

Figure 42.18 *In cases at high risk for expulsive hemorrhage, preplacement of a 7-0 or 8-0 silk suture through the limbal wound may allow rapid closure in case of hemorrhaging. Use of a tunnel incision also may be protective.*

If bleeding continues but the assistant is able to maintain pressure on part of the wound, the surgeon may close the unobstructed wound with interrupted sutures, gradually closing the whole wound. If bleeding is excessive and closure at the wound is not possible, posterior sclerotomies are made with any available blade in the quadrants that appear to harbor the most suprachoroidal blood. Additional sclerotomies are made, as necessary, to ensure extraction of suprachoroidal blood. Sclerotomies are made radially extending from the level of the muscle insertion to 3–4 mm posteriorly. As blood extrudes from the sclerotomies, pressure is relieved from the wound, allowing closure with interrupted sutures. Once the wound is closed the sclerotomies are closed with 6-0 Vicryl suture, if bleeding has not stopped, to tamponade the bleeding vessels.

REFERENCES

1. Hoffman P, Pollack A, Oliver M. Limited choroidal hemorrhage associated with intracapsular cataract extraction, *Arch Ophthalmol* (1984) **102:**1761–5.
2. Frenkel RE, Shin DH. Prevention and management of delayed suprachoroidal hemorrhage after filtration surgery, *Arch Ophthalmol* (1986) **104:**1459–63.
3. Ruderman JM, Harbin TS Jr, Campbell DG. Postoperative suprachoroidal hemorrhage following filtration procedures, *Arch Ophthalmol* (1986) **104:**201–5.
4. Gressel MG, Parrish RK II, Heuer DK. Delayed nonexpulsive suprachoroidal hemorrhage, *Arch Ophthalmol* (1984) **102:**1757–60.
5. Chu TG, Cano MR, Green RL, et al. Massive suprachoroidal hemorrhage with central retinal apposition: a clinical and echographic study, *Arch Ophthalmol* (1991) **109:**1575–81.
6. Lakhanpal V, Schocket SS, Elman MJ, Nirankari VS. A new modified vitreoretinal surgical approach in the management of massive suprachoroidal hemorrhage, *Ophthalmology* (1989) **96:**793–800.
7. Eller AW, Adams EA, Fanous MM. Anterior chamber maintainer for drainage of suprachoroidal hemorrhage (letter), *Am J Ophthalmol* (1994) **118:**258–9.
8. Davison JA. Vitrectomy and fluid infusion in the treatment of delayed suprachoroidal hemorrhage after combined cataract and glaucoma filtration surgery, *Ophthalmic Surg* (1987) **18:**334–6.
9. Baldwin LB, Smith TJ, Hollins JL, Pearson PA. The use of viscoelastic substances in the drainage of postoperative suprachoroidal hemorrhage, *Ophthalmic Surg* (1989) **20:**504–7.
10. Piper JG, Han DP, Abrams GW, Mieler WF. Perioperative choroidal hemorrhage at pars plana vitrectomy: a case-control study, *Ophthalmology* (1993) **100:**699–704.
11. Lakhanpal V, Schocket SS, Elman MJ, Dogra MR. Intraoperative massive suprachoroidal hemorrhage during pars plana vitrectomy, *Ophthalmology* (1990) **97:**1114–19.
12. Abrams GW, Thomas MA, Williams GA, Burton TC. Management of postoperative suprachoroidal hemorrhage with continuous-infusion air pump, *Arch Ophthalmol* (1986) **104:**1455–8.
13. Alexandridis E. Silicone oil tamponade in the management of severe hemorrhagic detachment of the choroid and ciliary body after surgical trauma, *Ophthalmologica* (1990) **200:**189–93.
14. Desai UR, Peyman GA, Chen CJ, et al. Use of perfluoroperhydrophenanthrene in the management of suprachoroidal hemorrhages, *Ophthalmology* (1992) **99:**1542–7.
15. Welch JC, Spaeth GL, Benson WE. Massive suprachoroidal hemorrhage: follow-up and outcome of 30 cases, *Ophthalmology* (1988) **95:**1202–6.
16. Reynolds MG, Haimovici R, Flynn HW Jr, et al. Suprachoroidal hemorrhage: clinical features and results of secondary surgical management, *Ophthalmology* (1993) **100:**460–5.

Part X Management of Endophthalmitis

Chapter 43 Management of endophthalmitis

Mandi D Conway and Gholam A Peyman

INTRODUCTION

Endophthalmitis, one of the most challenging ocular diseases, is also among the most variable in terms of visual outcome; some eyes retain useful reading vision and some are lost. The origin and causative organisms account for this variability in visual and anatomic outcome. Herein, we discuss the pathogenesis and causative organisms of postoperative, traumatic, and endogenous endophthalmitis and describe current diagnostic and management techniques.

DISEASE DESCRIPTION AND ORGANISMS

Endophthalmitis is an inflammatory response to bacterial, fungal, parasitic or viral invasion of the eye. The microbiology varies depending on the etiology. Four major categories are:

- Postoperative.
- Bleb-associated.
- Trauma-associated.
- Endogenous (metastatic).

These major categories are summarized in Table 43.1.[1]

Table 43.1 Major categories of endophthalmitis

Category of endophthalmitis	*Incidence of endophthalmitis*
Postoperative	62%
Bleb-associated	25%
Trauma-associated	10%
Endogenous (metastatic)	<5%

ACUTE ENDOPHTHALMITIS

Bacterial endophthalmitis is a disastrous complication of any intraocular surgery or antecedent trauma. The majority of infectious cases occur during the acute postoperative period. The normal flora colonizing the lids and lashes are the primary source of bacteria in postoperative endophthalmitis. As many as 76–97% of cataract patients may have positive preoperative conjunctival cultures;[2] *Staphylococcus aureus* and streptococci have been cultured from lids of normal patients and are responsible for most cases of postoperative endophthalmitis.[3] Other sources of postoperative endophthalmitis include contaminated irrigation solutions,[4] donor corneas,[5,6] contaminated intraocular lenses (IOLs), hyaluronic acid and aerosols in the operating suite.[7]

Complicating surgical occurrences, such as vitreous loss and wound abnormalities, also carry increased risk of postoperative endophthalmitis. Prolene IOL haptics also have been reported as independent risk factors.[8,9] Intraoperatively, the introduction of bacteria occurs through the surgical wound; postoperatively, however, the opportunity may present as a suture abscess, vitreous wick,[10] corneal ulcer,[11] corneoscleral wound, radial keratotomy incision[12,13] or the incision in sutureless cataract surgery.[14,15]

Bacterial endophthalmitis also occurs (rarely) after secondary IOL implantation. It is associated with: diabetes; transscleral suture fixation of posterior chamber IOLs; polypropylene haptics; preoperative eyelid abnormalities; re-entry into the eye through a

Table 43.2 Microbiology of endophthalmitis

Organism	*Postoperative*[a] (n = 63) (%)	*Bleb-associated*[b] (n = 30) (%)	*Traumatic*[c] (n = 30) (%)
Staphylococcus epidermidis	38	0	20
Staphylococcus aureus	21	7	0
Streptococcus species	11	57	13
Bacillus species	0	0	27
Haemophilus influenzae	3	23	0
Other Gram-negative species	13	7	20
Fungi	8	3	17
Other	6	3	3
Mixed flora	2	0	11

[a] Data from Driebe WT Jr, Mandelbaum S, Forster RK, Schwartz LK, Culbertson WW. Pseudophakic endophthalmitis: diagnosis and management, *Ophthalmology* (1986) **93:** 442–8.
[b] Data from Mandelbaum S, Forster RK, Gelender H, Culbertson W. Late onset endophthalmitis associated with filtering blebs, *Ophthalmology* (1985) **92:** 964–72.[24]
[c] Data from Affeldt JC, Flynn HW Jr, Forster RK, et al. Microbial endophthalmitis resulting from ocular trauma, *Ophthalmology* (1987) **94:** 407–13.

Table 43.3 Causative organism in 102 cases of metastatic bacterial endophthalmitis

Organism	*No. of cases*
Meningococcus	56
Pneumococcus	14
Staphylococcus	11
Streptococcus	9
Escherichia	4
Pseudomonas	2
Proteus	2
Paracolon	1
Klebsiella	1
Bacillus	1
Clostridium	1

Adapted with permission from Shammas HF, Endogenous *E. coli* endophthalmitis, *Surv Ophthalmol* (1977) **21:** 429–35.

previous wound; and postoperative wound defects. When cultured, many of the eyes grow *Staphylococcus epidermidis*. This is easily treated, and subsequent visual outcomes are generally good.[16] Although endophthalmitis is rare after closed vitrectomy (0.14%), it has a very poor prognosis in diabetic patients.[17,18] The major bacterial organisms are summarized in Tables 43.2 and 43.3.[19]

PATIENT SYMPTOMS

Patient symptoms indicative of endophthalmitis include ocular pain, diminished vision and headache with associated drowsiness. Although pain is an important symptom, it is not universal;[20] nearly 25% of patients in the Endophthalmitis Vitrectomy Study (EVS) reported no pain (and slightly more than 30% also had negative cultures).[21]

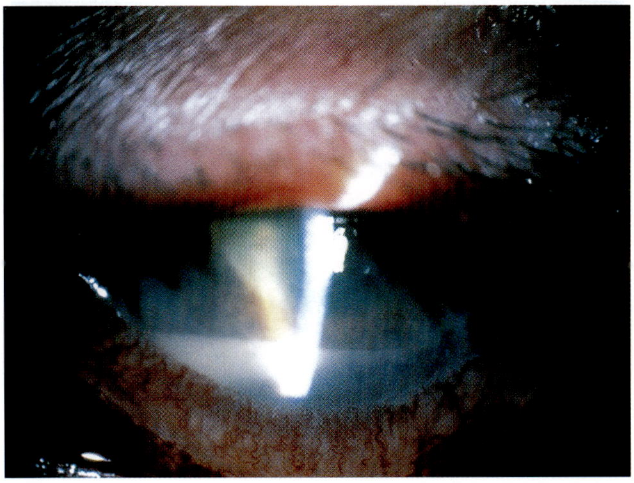

Figure 43.1 *Photograph of a patient with postoperative endophthalmitis. Note the clinical signs of lid edema, conjunctival injection, corneal haziness and a layered hypopyon.*

Frequently the clinician must decide early in the postoperative period whether the eye is infected or has 'sterile' postoperative inflammation. The vitreoretinal surgeon may need to review the recent intraoperative procedure with the operating surgeon to determine if the inflammatory reaction in the eye is unusually severe. Contributing factors such as prolonged operating time, retained lenticular material, pre-existing anterior chamber inflammation, excessive iris manipulation or underlying disease such as diabetes must be integrated with the presenting clinical picture. Occasionally, several cases can be traced to a common source. The epidemiology of this occurrence is important for medicolegal purposes.

Clinical signs may include upper eyelid edema, marked conjunctival hyperemia and intense chemosis, purulent discharge, corneal edema, endothelial precipitates, hypopyon with anterior chamber inflammation (Fig. 43.1) and vitreous haze. The red reflex may be yellowish or absent. In severe cases, proptosis, periorbital swelling, low-grade fever and leukocytosis may be present.

Quick diagnosis and prompt action are essential for successful treatment. Diagnostic sampling techniques, intravitreal pharmaceutical choices and management of unusual scenarios such as melting scleral flaps and endophthalmitis in eyes with silicone oil are discussed in detail in the following text.

BLEB-ASSOCIATED ENDOPHTHALMITIS

Bleb-associated endophthalmitis is a special case of acute postoperative endophthalmitis that occurs any time following filtration surgery; its presentation is similar to that of acute postoperative infection.[22,23] The predisposing factor for this type of endophthalmitis is a longstanding filtering bleb through which organisms gain access to the eye.[24] In early bleb-associated endophthalmitis *S. epidermidis* is isolated in 67% of cases, whereas in later onset bleb-associated endophthalmitis the most commonly isolated species are *Streptococcus* species and *Hemophilus* (although Gram-positive organisms are also seen).[23] The incidence of endophthalmitis immediately after glaucoma procedures is low (0.06–0.2%). However, late bleb leaks occur more frequently following trabeculectomy combined with adjunctive antimetabolites; in these cases, the incidence of endophthalmitis increases to 9% and higher.[25–27] Inferiorly located trabeculectomies carry a higher risk of endophthalmitis, particularly if they are performed with adjunctive mitomycin C.[28]

Because blebitis may progress to endophthalmitis, aggressive antimicrobial therapy is warranted and may include oral quinolones. Moreover, diligent follow-up to detect extension into the vitreous cavity for prompt intravitreal treatment is important. The clinician should not extrapolate the results of the EVS to postfiltration surgery endophthalmitis cases, given the differing pathogenesis and unique spectrum of organisms.[23]

CHRONIC ENDOPHTHALMITIS

Eyes with chronic endophthalmitis do not present with a fulminant clinical picture. Many exhibit waxing and waning of symptoms with a gradual decrease in visual acuity. The inflammation is often totally or partially responsive to topical corticosteroids but recurs following steroid withdrawal or taper. Chronic or low-grade endophthalmitis is most commonly associated with *Propionibacterium acnes* and *S. epidermidis*,[29,30] *Corynebacterium* species and fungi.[31] The inflammation may appear several weeks to many months after cataract surgery.[32]

Propionibacterium acnes, an anaerobic organism introduced from the periocular flora, creates a granulomatous reaction with: keratic precipitates; IOL precipitates; white plaques on both the implant and the capsular bag, typically at the junction of the optic and haptic; and low-grade anterior chamber reaction. Occasionally, beaded white strands of fibrin are seen. The anaerobic metabolism is thought to allow the organisms to survive within the capsular bag, where they are protected from topical and intraocular antimicrobial therapy.[33]

Winward et al[30] reported 22 patients with pseudophakic *P. acnes* endophthalmitis: two eyes presenting acutely were treated with intraocular antibiotic injection alone and experienced no recurrent inflammation. Of the remaining 20 eyes with delayed-onset pseudophakic *P. acnes* endophthalmitis, eight were managed initially with injection alone and seven of these eight developed recurrent endophthalmitis. The other 12 had surgery initially (either pars plana vitrectomy or IOL exchange). Although 4/12 eyes experienced recurrent endophthalmitis, the eyes undergoing capsulectomy as part of the initial management experienced the lowest rate of recurrent endophthalmitis. Of eight eyes eventually undergoing total capsulectomy and IOL explantation, none experienced recurrent endophthalmitis; seven eyes had persistent bacterial colonization of the lens capsular remnants on pathologic examination.[30]

IOL exchange with complete capsular removal during active endophthalmitis was not associated with recurrent or persistent endophthalmitis. The recurrent *P. acnes* endophthalmitis is likely to be due to persistence of viable organisms sequestered within capsular remnants; initial therapy should be directed toward surgical removal of these sequestered organisms.[30]

Further evidence that negative cultures do not preclude bacterial infection was reported by Busin et al[34] regarding IOLs removed from eyes with chronic low-grade endophthalmitis and the capsular remnants that were concomitantly removed; all showed bacteria by scanning electron microscopy, despite negative aqueous humor cultures. This suggests that primary IOL removal with partial or total capsulectomy is indicated in eyes with chronic low-grade endophthalmitis not responsive to medical therapy.

Thach et al[35] have advocated an *en bloc* capsulectomy to obtain culture material for diagnosis of an infectious etiology of refractory chronic recurrent pseudophakic endophthalmitis. They found that surgical removal of the entire lens capsule and its internal contents facilitated isolation and eradication of the causative pathogen in a patient with endophthalmitis refractory to previous vitrectomy, posterior capsulectomy and intravitreal antibiotic injection.

MEDICAL AND SURGICAL THERAPY OF CHRONIC ENDOPHTHALMITIS

The chronicity of the inflammation along with a characteristic appearance of a white plaque on the posterior capsule and white or brown multiple precipitates on the IOL helps to determine the diagnosis and how aggressively to treat chronic endophthalmitis.

INITIAL RESPONSE TO TREATMENT

Initially, one may treat with topical antibiotics and steroids, and although most eyes with chronic endophthalmitis respond with a decrease in inflammation, it recurs once these medications are stopped.

The next approach is an intravitreal tap and injection of vancomycin or clindamycin and aminoglycoside plus dexamethasone. It has been advocated that direct injection of antibiotics into the capsule may enhance clearing of the infection and allow the IOL and capsule to be retained.[36] Whether an intracapsular injection or standard intravitreal approach is preferred, intraocular antibiotics are injected, the eye is followed closely for 4–6 weeks and its condition is precisely documented.

The decision to perform more therapeutic surgery is serious because the treatment must include total removal of the capsule and the IOL. If the initial vitreous culture is positive, the decision is easier. However, often the culture is not positive due to the fastidious nature of the organism in culture media (the culture must be kept for 6 weeks), requiring a good clinical assessment of the eye and of the consequences of removing the IOL and capsule.

SURGICAL REMOVAL OF IOL AND ENTIRE CAPSULE IN *P. ACNES* ENDOPHTHALMITIS

- Open conjunctiva nasally from horizontal meridian to 12:00 and extend temporally to below level where the infusion cannula sclerotomy will be created (Fig. 43.2).

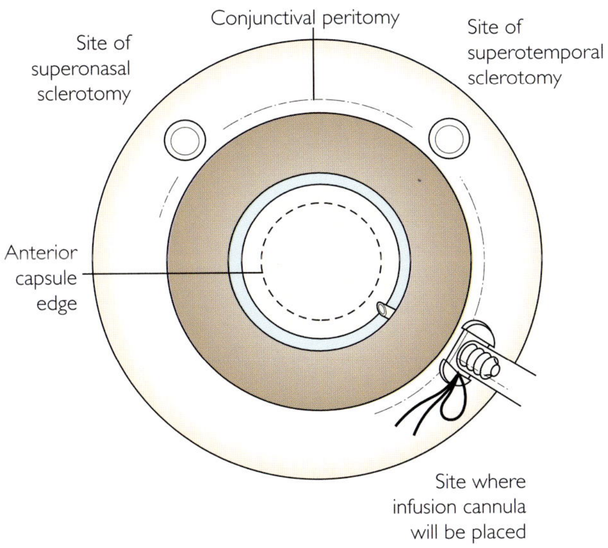

Figure 43.2 *Diagram depicting removal of a posterior chamber intraocular lens (PC-IOL) in an eye with* Propionibacterium acnes *endophthalmitis. This figure depicts creation of a conjunctival peritomy in order to explant a PC-IOL in an eye with* P. acnes *endophthalmitis. The conjunctival peritomy is created from the horizontal meridian nasally to below the level where the infusion cannula will be placed. This is to accommodate a large cataract-type incision to remove the IOL and allow a subsequent vitrectomy.*

- The plan is to make a large cataract incision superiorly to remove the IOL.
- Place the posterior infusion inferotemporally as usual; visualize the tip of the cannula but do not commence infusion at this time to avoid posterior pressure during IOL removal.
- Create both superior sclerotomies and plug them.
- Make a groove for a cataract-type incision with the crescent blade superiorly, creating a wound of sufficient length to remove the IOL (Fig. 43.3).
- Create a paracentesis into the anterior chamber with a sharp blade (via the cataract groove) and fill the anterior chamber with viscoelastic.
- Use a Sinsky hook inserted through the paracentesis to snag the IOL haptics and dial them into the anterior chamber. In fact, snagging only one is probably sufficient to allow it to be grasped with a long McPherson forceps and the IOL can be dialed into the anterior chamber. The eye remains a closed chamber at this point and intraocular pressure is controlled to avoid bleeding and choroidals (Fig. 43.4).

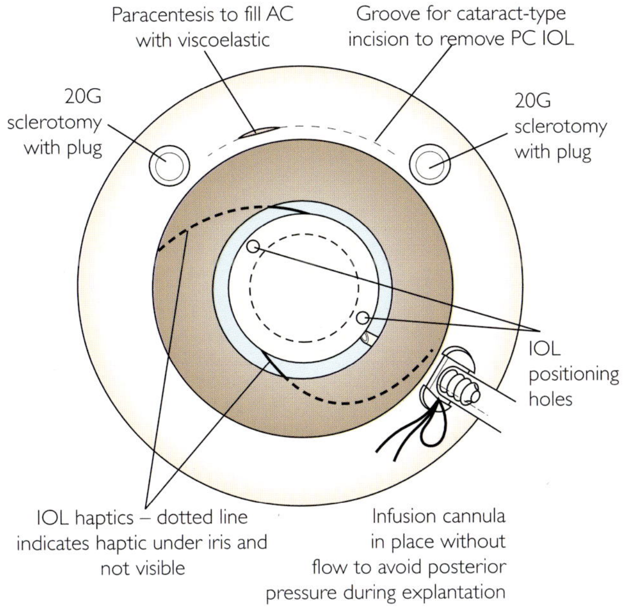

Figure 43.3 *Diagram depicting removal of a posterior chamber intraocular lens (PC-IOL) in an eye with* Propionibacterium acnes *endophthalmitis. This diagram depicts the sequence of events in removing the PC-IOL. The infusion cannula is placed but the infusion is not commenced. If the superior sclerotomies are created at this time, they should be plugged. A groove for a cataract-type incision is created, a paracentesis is created and the anterior chamber (AC) is filled with viscoelastic. A Sinsky hook is used to dial the IOL in the bag to allow one haptic to be prolapsed into the anterior chamber.*

- The full length of the cataract wound is opened.
- Using a rocking motion, the IOL is teased out of the capsule with long McPherson forceps and dialed into the anterior chamber and extracted from the eye (Fig. 43.5).
- Close the cataract wound with 9-0 nylon to provide tensile strength for the subsequent vitrectomy. Replacement of the IOL with an anterior chamber lens or sewn-in posterior chamber lens is not recommended at this stage.
- Some surgeons recommend injection of alpha-chymotrypsin behind the iris to chemodissect the zonules. Unfortunately, this agent is no longer readily available.
- Turn on the posterior infusion under direct visualization.
- Perform an anterior and posterior vitrectomy to remove adherent vitreous (Fig. 43.6).

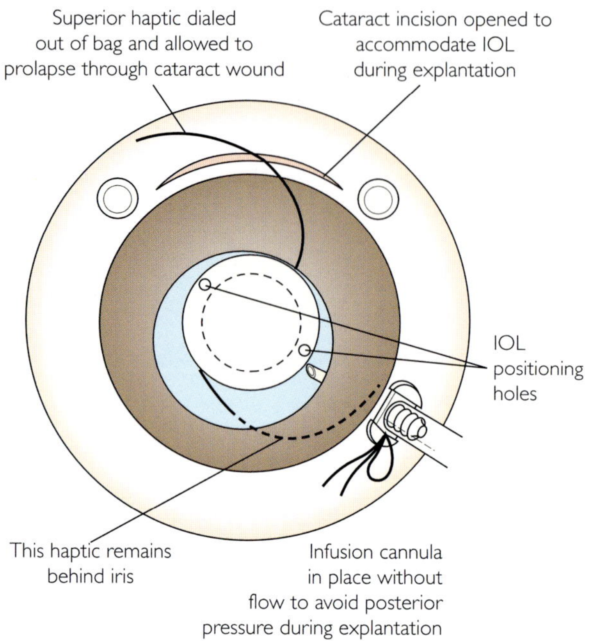

Figure 43.4 *Diagram depicting removal of a posterior chamber intraocular lens (PC-IOL) in an eye with* Propionibacterium acnes *endophthalmitis. The next step is to open the cataract wound and infuse enough viscoelastic to maintain a formed anterior chamber. The IOL haptic in the anterior chamber is allowed to prolapse out of the eye through the wound.*

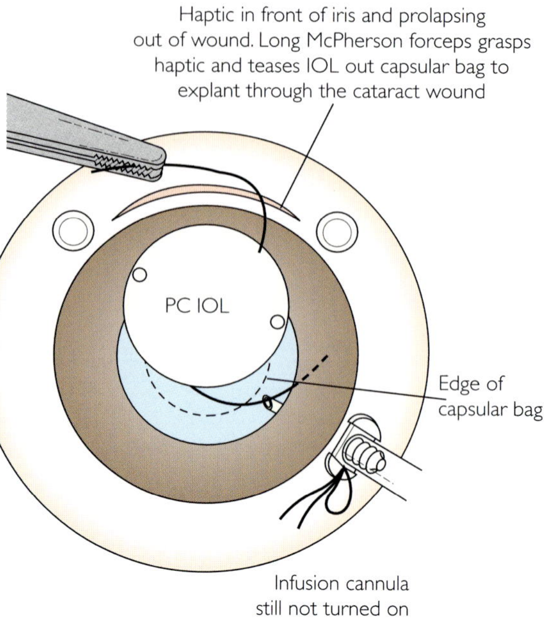

Figure 43.5 *Diagram depicting removal of a posterior chamber intraocular lens (PC-IOL) in an eye with* Propionibacterium acnes *endophthalmitis. Then, using a long McPherson forceps, the haptic is grasped and the IOL is dialed out of the capsular bag and gently extracted from the eye. Note that the posterior infusion is still not turned on.*

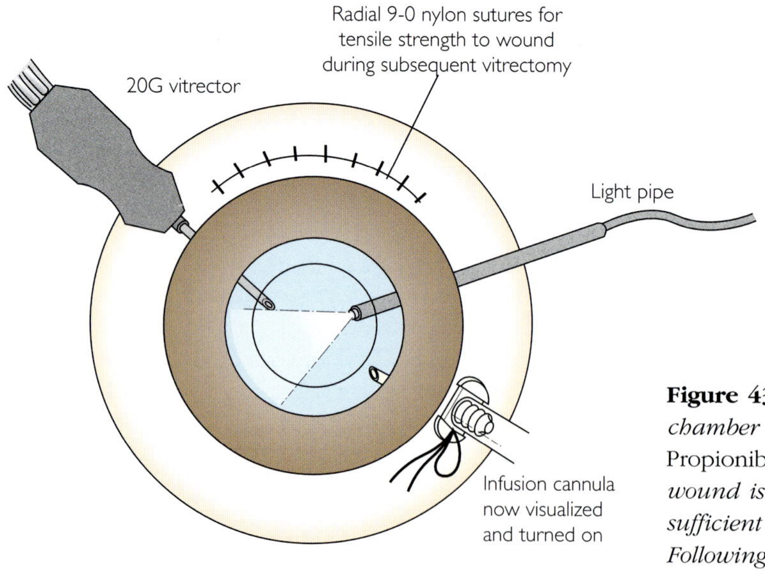

Figure 43.6 *Diagram depicting removal of a posterior chamber intraocular lens (PC-IOL) in an eye with* Propionibacterium acnes *endophthalmitis. The cataract wound is closed with radial 9-0 nylon sutures to provide sufficient tensile strength during the subsequent vitrectomy. Following closure of this wound, the posterior infusion is turned on and a complete vitrectomy is performed. We prefer to use low-dose antibiotics and steroids in the infusion fluid during the vitrectomy (see text).*

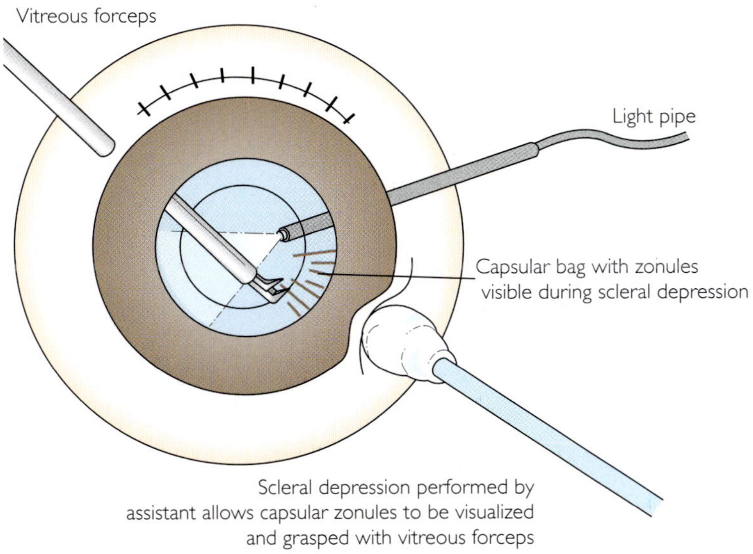

Figure 43.7 *Diagram depicting removal of posterior capsule in an eye with* P. acnes *endophthalmitis. After a complete vitrectomy is performed, the assistant uses scleral depression to allow the surgeon to visualize the capsular zonules. The zonules are grasped with a vitreous forceps and the attachments are gently teased from the ciliary body. If they cannot be separated easily, vitreous scissors may be needed to cut them. The capsule is then separated from the ciliary body and removed from the eye with a vitrector or through the sclerotomy in small pieces.*

- Try to employ a vitreous forceps to grasp the lens capsule while the assistant performs scleral depression. If the capsule easily detaches, extract it through the sclerotomy site with a vitreous forceps. If the capsule is adherent, consider using the vitrector and scleral depression and remove the capsule and zonules from the ciliary body 1 clock-hour at a time under direct visualization (Fig. 43.7).
- If the vitrectomy has not been completed, it can be finished at this time with scleral depression.
- The peripheral retina must be examined carefully and peripheral tears treated with laser or cryopexy. Scleral buckling is optional, depending on the location and extent of any tears.
- Intravitreal antibiotics can be injected prior to closing the infusion site. Use one-tenth of the dose of intravitreal antibiotics recommended for a nonvitrectomized eye (see rationale in the later section on antibiotic selection) and dexamethasone (1 mg).

TRAUMATIC ENDOPHTHALMITIS

Although post-traumatic endophthalmitis is a rare complication of penetrating eye injuries, it can blind potentially salvageable eyes.[37]

Eyes with traumatic endophthalmitis present with similar symptoms to eyes with acute postoperative infections: often intensely red and painful. Here, it is important to suspect an infection because the trauma and immediate surgical repair may induce erythema and pain. In an analysis of endophthalmitis after penetrating trauma, risk factors and visual outcomes were identified. Eyes with a lacerating injury had an increased relative risk of infection when the crystalline lens was disrupted. The prognosis for useful vision (20/400 or better) in eyes with traumatic endophthalmitis is better when less-virulent organisms, such as coagulase-negative staphylococci, are encountered.[38] Of 36 eyes with post-traumatic endophthalmitis in one report, the most common isolates were *Staphylococcus* species (26.5%), *Streptococcus* species (20.6%) and *Bacillus* species (14.7%).[39] *Bacillus* and mixed flora infections (27.8%) are especially common after trauma, and certain toxins elaborated by the organisms may contribute to their particular virulence.[40] The combination of intravitreal clindamycin (or vancomycin) and gentamicin can be effective therapy in *Bacillus* species infections if used early in the course of the disease and combined with vitrectomy and systemic and periocular antibiotics.[41,42]

The microbiology of pediatric post-traumatic endophthalmitis differs from the adult disease with streptococcal species as the most common infecting organisms.[43]

Although Gram-positive isolates are most commonly found singly or as mixed infections in traumatic endophthalmitis, the incidence of Gram-negative infections is higher following trauma than in postoperative endophthalmitis settings. Exogenous endophthalmitis caused by rare organisms is usually a result of penetrating injuries, such as metallic intraocular foreign bodies or animal bites.[44]

Table 43.4 Intravitreal drug preparation

Gentamicin (100 µg) in 0.1 ml of NaCl for injection USP
- One vial is filled with gentamicin 80 mg/2 ml
- Withdraw 0.25 ml in syringe 1 (10 mg)
- Empty contents of syringe 1 into a second 10-ml syringe and add 9.75 ml of 0.9% NaCl for injection USP (preservative free) to make 10 ml of solution (1 mg/ml)
- Withdraw 0.1 ml from syringe 2 into tuberculin (TB) syringe. This will contain 100 µg/0.1 ml of gentamicin

Amikacin (200 µg) in 0.1 ml of NaCl for injection USP
- One vial is filled with amikacin 100 mg/2 ml
- Withdraw 0.4 ml into TB syringe 1, which will contain 20 mg of amikacin
- Empty contents of syringe 1 into a second 10-ml syringe and add 9.6 ml of 0.9% NaCl for injection USP (preservative free) to make 10 ml of solution (2 mg/ml)
- Withdraw 0.1 ml from syringe 2 into TB syringe. This will contain 200 µg/0.1 ml of amikacin

Vancomycin (1 mg) in 0.1 ml of NaCl for injection USP
- One vial of vancomycin powder (500 mg) is diluted with 10 ml of 0.9% NaCl for injection USP (preservative free) (50 mg/ml)
- Withdraw 1 ml into syringe 1 (50 mg/ml)
- Empty contents of syringe 1 into a second syringe and add 4 ml of 0.9% NaCl for injection USP (preservative free) to make 5 ml of solution (10 mg/ml)
- Withdraw 0.1 ml from syringe 2 into TB syringe. This will contain 1 mg/0.1 ml of vancomycin

Clindamycin (450 µg) in 0.1 ml of NaCl for injection USP
- Clindamycin is available in vials containing 150 mg/ml
- Withdraw 0.3 ml into syringe 1, which will contain 45 mg clindamycin
- Empty contents of syringe 1 into a second 10-ml syringe and add 9.7 ml of 0.9% NaCl for injection USP (preservative free) to make 10 ml of solution (4.5 mg/ml)
- Withdraw 0.1 ml from syringe 2 into TB syringe, which will contain 450 µg/0.1 ml of clindamycin

Ceftazidime (1 mg) in 0.1 ml of NaCl for injection USP
- One vial of ceftazidime powder (500 mg) is diluted with 10 ml of 0.9% NaCl for injection USP (preservative free) (50 mg/ml)
- Withdraw 1 ml into syringe 1 (50 mg/ml)
- Empty contents of syringe 1 into a second syringe and add 4 ml of 0.9% NaCl for injection USP (preservative free) to make 5 ml of solution (10 mg/ml)
- Withdraw 0.1 ml from syringe 2 into TB syringe, which will contain 1 mg/0.1 ml of ceftazidime

Dexamethasone (400 µg) (may inject up to 1 mg)
- Withdraw 0.1 ml in a TB syringe from a vial of dexamethasone containing 4 mg/1 ml and inject intravitreally

Amphotericin B (5 µg) in 0.1 ml of sterile water
- One vial of amphotericin B containing 50 mg is diluted with 10 ml of sterile water for injection USP (preservative free) (5 mg/ml)
- Withdraw 0.1 ml (500 µg) in a TB syringe
- Add contents of TB syringe to a syringe containing 9.9 ml of sterile water for injection USP (50 µg/ml)
- Withdraw 0.1 ml in a TB syringe, which will contain 5 µg/0.1 ml of amphotericin B, and inject intravitreally

Adapted with permission from Peyman GA, Schulman JA, *Intravitreal Surgery: Principles and Practice*, 2nd edn (Appleton & Lange:, Norwalk, CT, 1994).[1]

Table 43.5 Maximum nontoxic doses of antibiotics in infusion fluid

Agent	*Nontoxic dose (μg/ml)*
Single	
Chloramphenicol	10
Clindamycin	9
Amikacin	10
Tobramycin	10
Gentamicin	8
Dexamethasone	64
Methicillin	20
Imipenem	16
Lincomycin	10
Teicoplanin	8
Oxacillin	10
Penicillin	80
Amphotericin B methyl ester	75[a]
Netilmicin	4
Ceftazidime	40
Vancomycin	30
Combination	
Gentamicin+oxacillin	8 + 10
Clindamycin+gentamicin	9 + 8
Methicillin+gentamicin	20 + 8
Penicillin+gentamicin	80 + 8

[a] Recommended dose is 10 μg/ml

Note: Following pars plana vitrectomy, the doses should be decreased to one-tenth of the nonvitrectomized eye doses because the vitreous is not present to protect the retina from the medication. *In a nonvitrectomized eye, when antibiotics are combined, we recommend only one-half of the nontoxic dose*

Adapted with permission from Peyman GA. Intraocular drug delivery and treatment of endophthalmitis (interview), *EyeWorld* (1998) **3:** 35–7.

Prompt diagnosis and early treatment with intraocular and systemic antibiotics are important in the successful management of post-traumatic endophthalmitis. The importance of intravitreal antibiotics and corticosteroids with or without vitrectomy has been recognized as a sight-saving maneuver.[45] Table 43.4 describes the preparation of intravitreal drugs.

The use of pars plana vitrectomy has been associated with good visual outcomes in selected cases with limited retinal injury.[39] Adding appropriate antibiotics and steroids to the vitrectomy infusion fluid provides safe, low-dose irrigation of the vitreous cavity intraoperatively, which can be prophylactic against infection (Table 43.5).

Primary posterior chamber IOL implantation following removal of a traumatic cataract with an intact or incomplete posterior capsule has been advocated but remains controversial if endophthalmitis is suspected.[46]

ENDOGENOUS ENDOPHTHALMITIS

Endogenous endophthalmitis presents with underlying systemic infections and immunosuppression in high-risk patients. Those at risk include AIDS patients, organ transplant patients, cancer patients and others on immunosuppressive therapy. Also at risk are patients undergoing recent surgery, patients who sustained recent massive trauma and patients with cardiac anomalies.[47] Additional predisposing factors include: intravenous drug abuse; the presence of a catheter for chronic intravenous access;[48] and patients with poor natural defenses, such as diabetics, chronic alcoholics and asplenic individuals.[49]

Unusual bacteria and fungi, isolated from the vitreous in endogenous endophthalmitis, usually stem from septicemia caused by intrathoracic or intra-abdominal procedures. Other sources are meningitis, osteomyelitis, otitis, phlebitis, endocarditis, ruptured diverticuli, infected transplanted organs, renal lithotripsy, burns, prostatitis and other infections leading to blood-borne pathogens.[50–61]

Although the presenting symptoms may be sudden and frequently fulminant, onset is more insidious with a mildly red eye and diminished vision. Initially the infectious organisms may invade the iris or the choroid, induce breaks in Bruch's membrane and invade the retina and cause vitreous seeding. Endogenous endophthalmitis is usually treated in conjunction with an infectious disease specialist and requires cultures of blood, urine, wounds and, at times, cerebrospinal fluid to detect the source. The disease process can produce highly destructive intraocular infectious foci and requires aqueous and vitreous cultures and occasionally a chorioretinal biopsy. The differential diagnosis of endogenous endophthalmitis includes:

- Cytomegalovirus retinitis.
- Acute retinal necrosis (herpes simplex or herpes zoster).
- Toxoplasmosis.

- Miliary tuberculosis (in underdeveloped countries).
- Toxocara.
- Neoplastic disorders (reticulum cell sarcoma).

The principles of treating endogenous endophthalmitis are:

- Find and eradicate the source.
- Treat systemically.
- If chorioretinitis only, systemic treatment may suffice.
- If vitreous infiltrates are present, a pars plana vitrectomy with antibiotics or antifungals and low-dose dexamethasone in the vitrectomy infusion fluid may be necessary (Tables 43.4 and 43.5).

FUNGAL ENDOPHTHALMITIS

Fungal endophthalmitis is seen in both endogenous and exogenous categories. The disease process can produce highly suggestive but not pathognomonic ocular signs that help the clinician to reach the correct diagnosis. Intraocular inflammation, especially if it is granulomatous, should suggest a possible fungal infection. Usually endogenous cases are associated with illicit drug use, a local foci of fungal infection[61] or systemic immunosuppressive therapy.[62] Exogenous cases have been reported after trauma and in post-operative cases involving contamination of IOLs, intraocular infusion fluids[63] or donor corneas.[64,65]

Endogenous fungal endophthalmitis has increased in the last 20 years due to the widespread use of antibiotics and indwelling catheters.[66] *Candida* species are the most common endogenous pathogens[55] but other fungal pathogens are *Aspergillus* species, *Coccidioides, Blastomyces, Cryptococcus, Sporothrix, Fusarium*, and *Histoplasma capsulatum*. Granulomatous intraocular inflammation and the risk factors outlined previously should raise the index of suspicion of a fungal etiology for endophthalmitis. The retina and vitreous may be involved primarily because the fungal elements gain access through the retinal vasculature. If the diagnosis remains unknown, a vitreous biopsy may be necessary.

Prompt therapy following early diagnosis will improve the visual outcome in most cases of fungal endophthalmitis. Although no particular therapeutic regimen has been established prospectively, strong arguments can be made to treat nearly all *endogenous* fungal endophthalmitis with a systemic antifungal such as amphotericin B or fluconazole.[66–68] Vitrectomy and intravitreal amphotericin (with or without intravitreal corticosteroid) should be considered in cases of endogenous fungal endophthalmitis with significant vitreous involvement or clear progression of disease, despite initial systemic antifungal therapy.[66]

Exogenous fungal endophthalmitis is treated with intravitreal amphotericin B. Severe vitreous involvement requires vitrectomy in addition to intravitreal antifungals. Intravitreal corticosteroids are useful in salvaging vision as adjunctive treatment of exogenous bacterial and fungal endophthalmitis.[69,70]

Factors associated with a poor visual outcome in all types of endophthalmitis include decreased vision on presentation, a positive bacterial culture, a virulent organism and trauma. Another critical factor is the amount of time between the onset of symptoms and the initiation of treatment.[71]

LABORATORY PROCEDURES

Laboratory procedures to confirm the diagnosis include:

- Lid and conjunctival cultures on blood agar, enriched chocolate agar, thioglycolate broth and Sabouraud's media.
- Cultures of the infected bleb, conjunctival flap or corneal wound on the same media.
- Smear of exudate from infected areas on glass slides for Gram, Giemsa and KOH or other fungal stains (Gomori methenamine silver).
- Anterior chamber tap for cultures and stains.
- Vitreous tap for cultures and stains.

The vitreous is the best source of organisms, presumably because it allows better bacterial nutritional support and a greater volume of culture inoculum.[72,73]

HOW TO PERFORM THE ANTERIOR CHAMBER TAP

The anterior chamber tap is similar to a paracentesis and is done *after* the eye surface has been cultured.

- Topical anesthetic should be placed onto the cornea and into the conjunctival cul-de-sac.
- The eye surface can be sterilized with dilute 5–10% povodine–iodine after surface cultures have been taken.

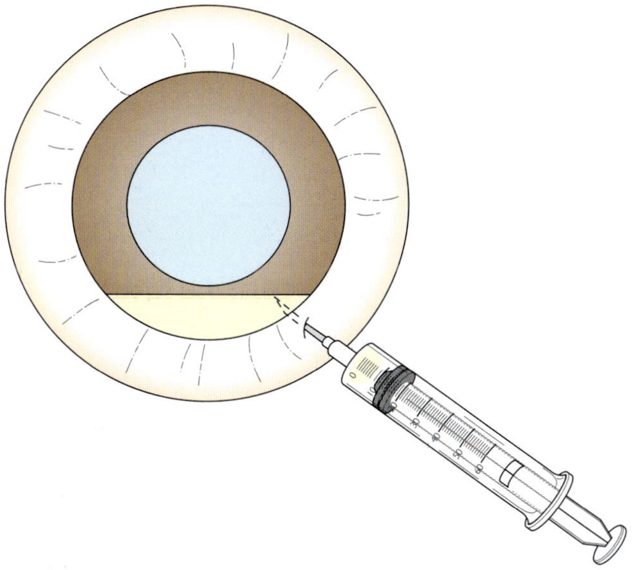

Figure 43.8 *Performance of an anterior chamber tap for diagnostic purposes. This diagram depicts an eye with acute postoperative endophthalmitis. There is a layered hypopyon inferiorly. Prior to performing a diagnostic tap, the eye is cleansed with a dilute solution of Betadine (5%). A paracentesis is performed with a 27- or 30-gauge needle on a tuberculin syringe. Care must be taken to avoid disturbing the hypopyon and the needle should be kept over the iris at all times to avoid touching the lens. A small amount of the aqueous (0.1–0.2 cc) should be aspirated into the sterile syringe. This can be used for Gram stain, culture or other studies.*

- The eye is stabilized with a cotton-tipped applicator or forceps.
- The sample is taken with a 27- or 30-gauge needle attached to a tuberculin syringe.
- The needle should be placed into the anterior chamber from the limbus and kept over the iris in order to avoid lens trauma (Fig. 43.8).
- A sample of approximately 0.2 ml should be taken (if possible).
- Avoid disturbing any hypopyon to retain a view of the posterior pole (if possible) for visualization of the needle tip when injecting antibiotics or performing a vitrectomy.
- A vitreous tap is obtained and then the appropriate antibiotics are injected (Fig. 43.9).

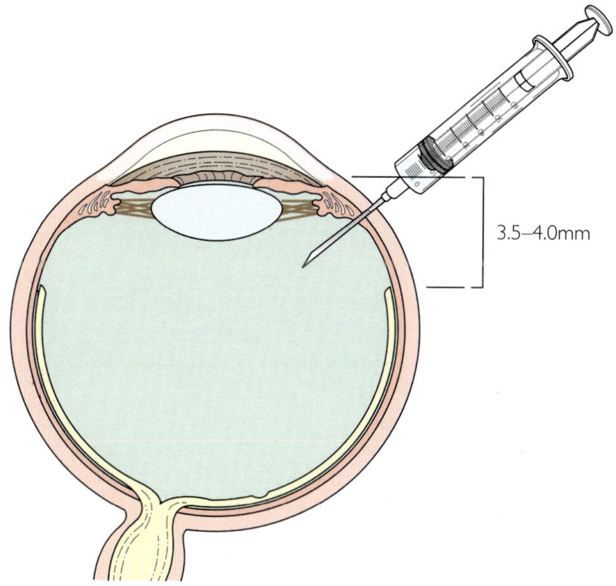

Figure 43.9 *Performance of a vitreous tap for diagnostic purposes with a needle and syringe. This diagram depicts an eye with endophthalmitis from which the vitreous sample is needed. The samples are obtained with a 25- or 23-gauge needle attached to a tuberculin (TB) syringe. The eye is entered 3.5–4.0 mm from the limbus. This distance can be measured with the barrel of a TB syringe: The inner diameter of the barrel measures approximately 4.0 mm. This can be laid on the sclera and a mark made with pressure to give the distance from the limbus. The needle should be placed perpendicular to the sclera and the tip of the needle should be visualized in the pupil if possible, prior to obtaining any sample. The sample is aspirated slowly and in a controlled manner. It is important to obtain a sufficient volume for investigational studies (at least 0.1-0.2 cc). If a sufficient sample cannot be obtained with this instrument, it may be necessary to use a Ziegler knife (to make a larger sclerotomy) and a vitrectomy instrument (to get a sufficient amount of vitreous). We prefer to use a separate syringe for injection of antibiotics, so the original needle used to obtain the sample should be withdrawn and a new needle with a TB syringe and antimicrobials attached should be inserted at the appropriate distance from the limbus. Remember to visualize the needle in the pupil, if possible, and have the bevel of the needle pointed toward the cornea. It is important to inject slowly to avoid a jet stream of drug shooting toward the retina.*

HOW TO PERFORM THE VITREOUS TAP

- The eye should remain anesthetized following the anterior chamber tap, when the eye will be slightly soft.
- The sample should be obtained with a 25-gauge needle attached to a tuberculin syringe.
- The eye is stabilized with a cotton-tipped applicator or forceps.
- The needle should be positioned perpendicular to the eye wall (Fig. 43.9).
- The distance from the limbus at which to enter the eye is 3.5–4.0 mm, depending on lens status. This distance can be approximated using the width of the hub of a sterile tuberculin syringe, which can be placed on the sclera to make a mark.
- The needle should be visualized in the pupil prior to aspirating the sample.
- The largest amount of vitreous that easily enters the syringe (0.2 ml) without undue aspiration pressure should be aspirated. The needle is then withdrawn.
- It is not always possible to obtain vitreous through a 25-gauge needle, and a small sclerotomy with a Ziegler knife may be required to allow a 23-gauge needle access. If it is not possible to obtain a sample, a vitrector may be needed. The vitrector is placed into a sclerotomy site and the sample is aspirated into a 3–6-ml syringe attached to the aspiration port of the vitrector (Fig. 43.10). An assistant provides gentle aspiration while the surgeon visualizes the cutter in the pupil (see later section on vitrectomy for endophthalmitis).
- Do not attempt to reattach a syringe with antibiotics to the original vitreous biopsy needle because it is too difficult to stabilize an unsecured needle in the eye and too easy to traumatize the retina. A safer method is simply to withdraw the biopsy needle and re-enter the eye with the new needle attached to the antibiotic syringe to deliver intravitreal therapy.
- Injection of intravitreal antimicrobial treatment immediately follows the vitreous tap with the bevel of the needle toward the anterior segment. The medication is injected slowly to prevent a jet stream of drug squirting toward the retina (Fig. 43.9).

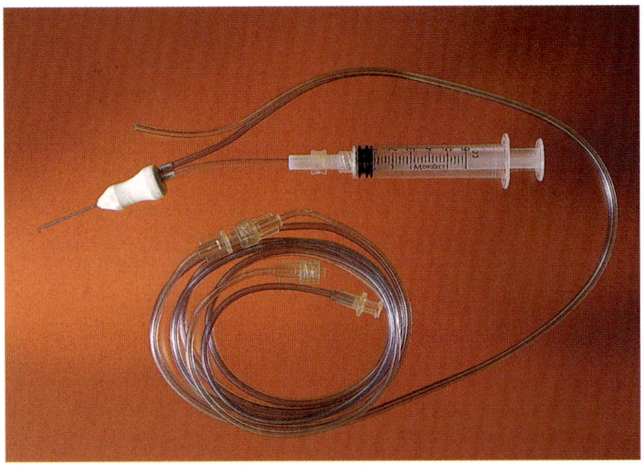

Figure 43.10 *Performance of a vitreous tap for diagnostic purposes with a vitrector. This photograph is of a vitrectomy instrument from which the aspiration tubing has been removed. It has been replaced with a short piece of sterile tubing attached to a 6-cc syringe. As the vitrectomy instrument cuts the vitreous, the sample is aspirated gently into the syringe. If a large sample is desired, the volume in the vitreous cavity can be replaced with sterile air. It is important not to dilute the sample with sterile saline. After the sample is obtained, the original aspiration tubing is replaced on the hub of the vitrector, which can be used to complete the vitrectomy if needed. We prefer to use a separate syringe for injection of antibiotics.*

THERAPY

Endophthalmitis is a potentially devastating disease that requires aggressive management. Although a great deal has been written about its management, current knowledge is based on experience with the most common forms of endophthalmitis:

- Postoperative cases caused by coagulase-negative staphylococci, *S. aureus* and *Streptococcus pneumoniae*.
- Endogenous cases caused by nongroup B streptococci, *Staphylococcus* species, *Candida* species and other fungi.

Previously, antibiotics administered topically, by intravenous infusion and by intramuscular injection were the mainstays of therapy for endophthalmitis. To provide better penetration, frequent subconjunctival antibiotic injections were recommended but ocular penetration issues remained. This has changed, however, and the current mainstay of endophthalmitis treatment is *intravitreal injection of appropriate antimicrobials.*[74–98] This procedure should be initiated as quickly as possible following the diagnosis of endophthalmitis because bacterial colony reproduction occurs every 15–20 minutes. Of course, cultures always should be obtained prior to any antimicrobial treatment. Regardless of the comprehensive ophthalmologist's intention to refer the patient to a vitreoretinal specialist for management, the sight-saving measure of obtaining cultures and instilling antimicrobials immediately following diagnosis of endophthalmitis allows antibiotic activity while the patient is traveling to the vitreoretinal specialist. This strategy should be encouraged.

GUIDELINES FOR INTRAVITREAL INJECTION OF ANTIMICROBIAL THERAPY (Table 43.4)

- Injection of drugs should be contained in the smallest volume possible.
- If intravitreal dexamethasone is planned, note that dexamethasone and vancomycin cannot be placed in the same syringe because they will precipitate.
- Aminoglycosides and dexamethasone can be used in the same syringe.
- The eye should remain anesthetized following the anterior chamber and vitreous tap(s) (Figs 43.3 and 43.9). Remember that the eye will be slightly soft following the anterior chamber and vitreous taps. If the patient is anxious or uncooperative, retrobulbar anesthesia with 2% lidocaine without epinephrine should be considered prior to tapping. It is not advisable to attempt a retrobulbar injection once the eye is softened by the withdrawal of aqueous and vitreous. General anesthesia is preferred for children and patients with open ocular wounds.

ADJUNCTIVE TOPICAL THERAPY

Topical antimicrobial treatment should begin immediately following the injection of the intravitreal drugs and should be continued at least hourly for several days. Although commonly used, subconjunctival therapy is probably not mandatory unless there is a wound infection or an infected filtering bleb.

ANTIBIOTIC SELECTION

Early diagnosis and appropriate treatment with intraocular antibiotics are important factors in the successful management of endophthalmitis. Emerging resistance of organisms to standard antibiotic therapy has forced clinicians to evaluate continually the best intraocular antibiotics for the treatment of endophthalmitis. Although drug combinations are necessary to cover the full range of bacteria causing endophthalmitis, antimicrobial synergy is probably less important in endophthalmitis treatment because of the high intravitreal concentrations of individual antibiotics achieved by intravitreal injection. Acute postoperative endophthalmitis is treated by a combination of broad-spectrum antibiotics (either vancomycin or clindamycin with either amikacin or ceftazidime), which are administered intravitreally, subconjunctivally and topically. *In vitrectomized eyes, the dose of antibiotic must be reduced to one-tenth of the nonvitrectomized dose* (Table 43.5). This is recommended because antibiotic toxicity has been evaluated most often in the nonvitrectomized eye, where the vitreous prevents rapid diffusion of antibiotics toward the retina. The vitreous reduces the concentration of antibiotic that reaches the retina, while allowing the antibiotic to be cleared through the anterior chamber. The recommended doses of common antibiotics are shown in Table 43.5.

ADJUNCTIVE SYSTEMIC THERAPY

Because of the first report of the EVS,[21] some surgeons may defer administration of systemic antibiotics in postoperative endophthalmitis. However, we recommend it for 3–5 days until the vitreous abscess is controlled in postoperative cases and particularly in traumatic and endogenous endophthalmitis. This is especially true if systemic steroids are to be used as advocated by the EVS.[21] It is important to stress that the EVS recommendations do not apply to endogenous, traumatic and bleb-associated cases of endophthalmitis, and that systemic antibiotics are useful adjuncts in these cases.

VITRECTOMY FOR ENDOPHTHALMITIS

When vision in endophthalmitis diminishes to light perception (as recommended by the EVS[21]) or the vitreous haze precludes a view of the disc or a large vessel,[99] pars plana vitrectomy is indicated.[99] If cultures have not been taken, they may be obtained in the operating room before vitrectomy.

It is important to culture the external eye and proceed with wound closure prior to anterior chamber and vitreous taps and/or vitrectomy. The eye can be inflated with sterile air prior to tapping. Alternatively, sterile saline may be used, although this may minimally dilute the sample. Either way, returning the intraocular pressure (IOP) to near normal greatly decreases the chances for producing choroidal detachments. We prefer infusion of air through the infusion line to maintain the IOP if the tip of the infusion cannula can be seen. Following the anterior chamber tap, the eye pressure should be normalized before making sclerotomies for vitrectomy.

- The safest way to perform a vitrectomy in the absence of a posterior view is to insert an anterior chamber maintainer or a bent 23-gauge needle to infuse sterile balanced saline solution or air.
- To obtain diagnostic vitreous samples, use the 23-gauge pneumovitrector[100] (Fig. 43.11) or the 25-gauge vitreous microinstrumentation.[101] Both instruments allow vitreous biopsy without significant traction on the peripheral retina. A complete vitrectomy can be performed immediately after the sample is obtained, or it can be delayed.
- The anterior infusion (using either air or saline) can be turned on promptly after the vitreous sample is obtained. In this way, the IOP may be maintained without sample dilution.
- The vitrector aspiration port is attached to a sterile syringe and manual aspiration is applied as the surgeon performs the vitreous biopsy (Fig. 43.10).
- In a pseudophakic eye with a posterior chamber IOL, the vitrector can be placed just behind the IOL, allowing safe vitreous cutting.
- In a traumatized eye with a cataract, care must be taken to avoid the retina if the view is impaired.
- One useful instrument is a lighted infusion cannula (Fig. 43.12), which can be inserted through a superior sclerotomy and seen through the pupil. This provides adequate illumination for visualization of the vitrector during the vitreous biopsy.
- Following vitreous biopsy, the vitrectomy can be continued using the same lighted infusion cannula to provide both light and infusion during the early vitrectomy.
- A separate infusion cannula should be placed early in the procedure, but the surgeon should wait to commence infusion until the tip of the cannula can be seen in the vitreous cavity. The core vitrectomy then can be completed with the separate infusion on.
- In summary, obtaining a vitreous sample, removing anterior vitreous debris and instilling antibiotics may be accomplished with the two-port vitrectomy, employing the lighted infusion cannula and the vitrector (Fig. 43.12). A conventional three-port vitrectomy may be required to remove inflammatory debris in the posterior vitreous cavity. Manipulations very close to the retina should be avoided. The safest course may be to refrain from performing a complete vitrectomy at

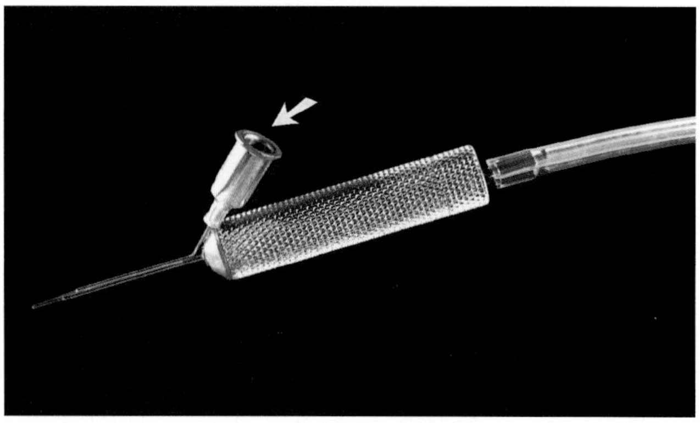

Figure 43.11 *Performance of a vitreous tap for diagnostic purposes with a Microvit vitrector. Shown here is a photograph of a 25-gauge vitrector that was developed for vitreous sampling. Note that there is a convenient air infusion port to which a syringe may be attached (arrow). This vitrector allows safe cutting and aspiration of vitreous through a small-gauge incision. Microvit vitrectors can be used either in the operating room or an outpatient setting. Again, it is important to replace the aspirated volume in the vitreous cavity with sterile air through the same sclerotomy (using a 25-gauge butterfly needle attached to a syringe with a filter). This prevents dilution of the sample and maintains the globe.*

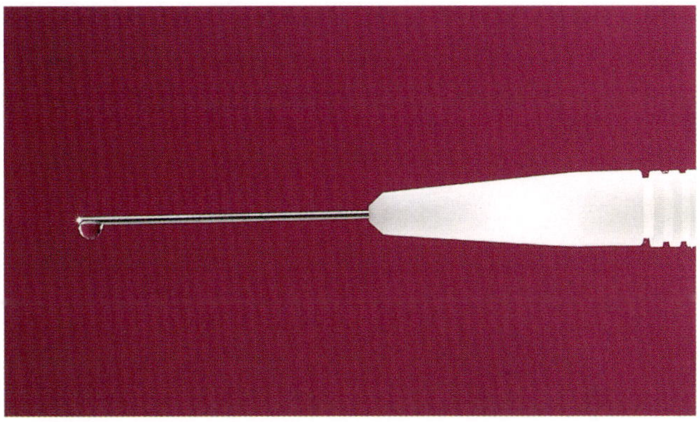

Figure 43.12 *Use of lighted infusion cannula in initial vitrectomy for endophthalmitis. This photograph shows the infusion light pipe, which is a very useful instrument for obtaining a vitreous sample or doing a limited vitrectomy in an eye with endophthalmitis that has a compromised view into the vitreous cavity due to vitreous opacities. Often it is impossible to visualize the posterior infusion cannula. It is, however, possible to place the posterior infusion cannula but refrain from turning it on. The two superior sclerotomies are created as usual. The vitrector is placed in one sclerotomy and the infusion light pipe into the second one. This provides both infusion and light, allowing the anterior vitreous cavity to be debrided. Frequently, the tip of the infusion cannula then can be visualized and posterior infusion can be commenced safely to allow completion of the vitrectomy.*

the first operation, unless this can be accomplished quickly without compromising the retina.

- A poststerilization vitrectomy can be timed to remove vitreous debris and to prevent further enzymatic degradation of the retina. Epiretinal membranes commonly develop after endophthalmitis because of incomplete posterior hyaloid removal, and they require judicious surgical removal. In the EVS, the need for additional procedures was correlated with more severe infections.[102]
- In chronic bacterial postoperative endophthalmitis, if antibiotic treatment is unsuccessful, a pars plana vitrectomy including removal of the IOL and the posterior capsule should be performed.[103]
- In postoperative mycotic endophthalmitis, antimycotics (amphotericin B or fluconazole) are administered intravitreally. If the inflammation is severe, a pars plana vitrectomy should be performed with possible removal of the posterior capsule and the IOL.
- In endogenous mycotic endophthalmitis, antimycotics (amphotericin B or fluconazole) are administered systemically and intravitreally. If the inflammation is severe in these eyes, a pars plana vitrectomy should be performed and antimycotics given intravitreally. These patients are often gravely ill, and the surgical goal may be debridement and intravitreal drug therapy.
- Endogenous bacterial endophthalmitis also is seen frequently in critically ill patients. The clinical course often is rapidly progressive and, despite local and systemic treatment, the eyes may be lost. This is particularly difficult if the patient is too ill to tolerate surgery. In these cases, a pneumovitrectomy at the bedside may allow some vitreous debridement and obtain a satisfactory sample for culture and histopathologic examination.[100] Immediate systemic and intravitreal broad-spectrum antibiotic therapy should be given as necessary.
- In traumatic injuries with intraocular foreign bodies, endophthalmitis prevention is the surgical goal. Acute post-traumatic endophthalmitis is treated by intravitreal antibiotic administration (vancomycin and amikacin, or ceftazidime) in combination with pars plana vitrectomy and removal of the foreign body. Treatment is supplemented by systemic, subconjunctival and topical antibiotic administration. Intravitreal steroids decrease tissue damage and inflammation, although their use is not universal.[69]

PREOPERATIVE HYPOTONY

Surgery in eyes with either wound dehiscence or bleb infections can be complicated by preoperative hypotony. Wound and suture dehiscences must be addressed initially. In bleb infections, surgical excision of the infected leaking bleb and a full-thickness scleral graft may be considered to repair the scleral defect and close the eye.[104]

RETREATMENT

The need for reinjection of antibiotics or a poststerilization vitrectomy for debris is decided on a case-by-case basis. If the eye does not recover after initial treatment, if vision decreases or if the cultures show unusual organisms not covered by the initial broad-spectrum antibiotics, a case can be made for reinjection of another appropriate antibiotic, or for immediate vitrectomy and antibiotic instillation either in the infusion fluid or at the end of the case (one-tenth of the dose recommended for the nonvitrectomized eye).[74–98]

INFUSION FLUID ADDITIVES

Whenever a vitrectomy is performed for endophthalmitis, we recommend adding antibiotics and steroids to the infusion fluid. The doses are provided in Table 43.5.

ENDOPHTHALMITIS IN SILICONE-FILLED EYES

In silicone oil-filled eyes with suspected endophthalmitis, anterior chamber and vitreous taps for culture should be performed initially and then an intravitreal injection of antibiotic dose (one-tenth of the dose recommended for the nonvitrectomized eye) and dexamethasone (1 mg) should be given. If there is purulent exudate in the vitreous cavity, consider removing the silicone using infusion fluid with antibiotics and steroids (8 µg/ml of gentamicin, 9 µg/ml of clindamycin, 20 µg/ml of vancomycin and 64 µg/ml of dexamethasone). Silicone can be reinjected immediately or following resolution of the inflammation. Aggressive management of endophthalmitis in an eye requiring silicone oil tamponade may salvage useful vision.[105] Systemic antibiotics may be used as adjunctive therapy.

COMPLICATIONS OF ENDOPHTHALMITIS

The most dreaded complication of endophthalmitis is loss of the central vision or loss of the eye from the inflammatory process. This is more likely when the treatment has been delayed and when more virulent organisms cause the endophthalmitis.

Extraocular extension of the infectious process is related to those same variables, and to the patient's immune status. The use of systemic antibiotics is helpful in preventing this complication.

Excessive intraocular inflammation (despite control of the infection) can lead to phthisis bulbi and the loss of the eye.

Surgical complications include:

- Iatrogenic retinal holes.
- Postoperative epiretinal membrane formation.
- Postoperative retinal detachment.
- Postoperative proliferative vitreoretinopathy if there is a retinal detachment.
- Postoperative cataract formation.
- Postoperative hypotony and phthisis bulbi.

SUMMARY

Infectious endophthalmitis is a dreaded complication of ocular surgery and trauma. It often induces a substantial reduction in visual acuity and occasionally the loss of the eye, despite modern surgical and pharmaceutical therapy. Acute postoperative endophthalmitis is treated by a combination of broad-spectrum antibiotics (vancomycin, clindamycin and amikacin) administered intravitreally, subconjunctivally and topically, combined with systemic antibiotics (vancomycin and either an aminoglycoside or ceftazidime) for 3–5 days. If vision is diminished to light perception or the vitreoretinal surgeon cannot see the retinal vessels or disc, a pars plana vitrectomy is indicated.[21,99]

Treatment of postoperative endophthalmitis with delayed onset (secondary to a complication such as wound dehiscence) is treated according to the same guidelines outlined for acute postoperative endophthalmitis.

In chronic postoperative endophthalmitis caused by *P. acnes*, antibiotics (vancomycin and either an aminoglycoside or clindamycin) are administered intravitreally. If antibiotic treatment is unsuccessful, a pars plana vitrectomy must be performed including removal of the IOL and the posterior capsule. To reduce ocular destruction caused by inflammation, systemic and intravitreal administration of steroids is recommended in all postoperative and post-traumatic endophthalmitis conditions.

Treatment of endogenous endophthalmitis requires collaboration with an internist. Systemic therapy with antibiotics or antimycotics is obligatory. In addition, broad-spectrum antibiotics (vancomycin and either an aminoglycoside or ceftazidime) or an antimycotic (amphotericin B) are administered topically and intravitreally in some cases. In severe infections, a pars plana vitrectomy is indicated.

To reduce the risk of infection, patients with infectious eye disease should be excluded from elective surgery. Eyes with penetrating or perforating injuries are treated prophylactically with systemic and intravitreal antibiotics during the surgical repair.

The key to controlling endophthalmitis is a high level of suspicion in at-risk eyes, early intervention with cultures and appropriate antimicrobials and steroids, if indicated, and vigilant follow-up.

REFERENCES

1. Peyman GA, Schulman JA. *Intravitreal Surgery: Principles and Practice,* 2nd edn (Appleton & Lange: Norwalk, CT, 1994): 922.
2. Apt L, Isenberg SJ, Yoshimori R, Spierer A. Outpatient topical use of povidone–iodine in preparing the eye for surgery, *Ophthalmology* (1989) **96:**289–92.
3. Speaker MG, Milch FA, Shah MK, et al. Role of external bacterial flora in the pathogenesis of acute operative endophthalmitis, *Ophthalmology* (1991) **98:**639–49.
4. Sherwood DR, Rich WJ, Jacobs JS, et al. Bacterial contamination of intraocular and extraocular fluids during extracapsular cataract extraction, *Eye* (1989) **3** (3):308–12.
5. Leveille AS, McMullan FD, Cavanagh HD. Endophthalmitis following penetrating keratoplasty, *Ophthalmology* (1983) **90**:38–9.
6. Guss RB, Koenig S, De La Pena W, et al. Endophthalmitis after penetrating keratoplasty, *Am J Ophthalmol* (1983) **95:**651–8.
7. Morbidity and Mortality Weekly Report. Outbreaks of postoperative bacterial endophthalmitis caused by intrinsically contaminated ophthalmic solutions–Thailand, 1992, and Canada, 1993, *Morb Mortal Wkly Rep* (1996) **45**(23):491–4.
8. Raskin EM, Speaker MG, McCormick SA, et al. Influence of haptic materials on the adherence of staphylococci to intraocular lenses, *Arch Ophthalmol* (1993) **111:**250–3.
9. Javitt JC, Vitale S, Canner JK, et al. National outcomes of cataract extraction: endophthalmitis following inpatient surgery, *Arch Ophthalmol* (1991) **109:**1085–9.
10. Lindstrom RL, Doughman DJ. Bacterial endophthalmitis associated with vitreous wick, *Ann Ophthalmol* (1979) **11:** 1775–8.
11. Brenner M. Bacterial corneal ulcer, endophthalmitis, and embolic phenomena, *Ann Ophthalmol* (1984) **16:**334–40.
12. Gelender H, Flynn HW Jr, Mandelbaum SH. Bacterial endophthalmitis resulting from radial keratotomy, *Am J Ophthalmol* (1982) **93:**323–6.
13. McLeod SD, Flowers CW, Lopez PF, et al. Endophthalmitis and orbital cellulitis after radial keratotomy, *Ophthalmology* (1995) **102:**1902–7.
14. Maxwell DP, Diamond JP. Infectious endophthalmitis following sutureless cataract surgery (letter), *Arch Ophthalmol* (1992) **110:**915.
15. Oxford KW, Abbott RL, Fung WE, Ellis DS. *Aspergillus* endophthalmitis after sutureless cataract surgery, *Am J Ophthalmol* (1995) **120:**534–5.
16. Scott IU, Flynn HW Jr, Feuer W. Endophthalmitis after secondary intraocular lens implantation: a case-report study, *Ophthalmology* (1995) **102:**1925–31.
17. Ho PC, Tolentino FI. Bacterial endophthalmitis after closed vitrectomy, *Arch Ophthalmol* (1984) **102:**207–10.
18. Cohen SM, Flynn HW Jr, Murray TG, Smiddy WE. Endophthalmitis after pars plana vitrectomy: the Postvitrectomy Endophthalmitis Study Group, *Ophthalmology* (1995) **102:**705–12.
19. Peyman GA, Schulman JA. *Intravitreal Surgery: Principles and Practice,* 2nd edn (Appleton & Lange: Norwalk, CT, 1994): 853–5.
20. Deutsch TA, Goldberg MF. Painless endophthalmitis after cataract surgery, *Ophthalmic Surg* (1984) **15:**837–40.
21. Endophthalmitis Vitrectomy Study Group. Results of the Endophthalmitis Vitrectomy Study: a randomized trial of immediate vitrectomy and of intravenous antibiotics for the treatment of postoperative bacterial endophthalmitis, *Arch Ophthalmol* (1995) **113:**1479–96.
22. Katz LJ, Cantor LB, Spaeth GL. Complications of surgery in glaucoma: early and late bacterial endophthalmitis following glaucoma filtering surgery, *Ophthalmology* (1985) **92:**959–63.
23. Ciulla TA, Beck AD, Topping TM, Baker AS. Blebitis, early endophthalmitis, and late endophthalmitis after glaucoma-filtering surgery, *Ophthalmology* (1997) **104:**986–95.
24. Mandelbaum S, Forster RK, Gelender H, Culbertson W. Late onset endophthalmitis associated with filtering blebs, *Ophthalmology* (1985) **92:**964–72.
25. Parrish RK II, Schiffman JC, Feuer WJ. The Fluorouracil Filtering Surgery Study. In: Kertes PJ, Conway MD, eds, *Clinical Trials in Ophthalmology: a Summary and Practice Guide* (Williams & Wilkins: Baltimore, MD, 1998): 321–34.
26. Collignon-Brach J. Surgery for glaucoma and endophthalmitis, *Bull Soc Belge Ophtalmol* (1996) **260:**73–7.
27. Lipman RM, Deutsch TA. Late-onset *Moraxella catarrhalis* endophthalmitis after filtering surgery, *Can J Ophthalmol* (1992) **27:**249–50.
28. Higginbotham EJ, Stevens RK, Musch DC, et al. Bleb-related endophthalmitis after trabeculectomy with mitomycin C, *Ophthalmology* (1996) **103:**650–6.
29. Friedman E, Peyman GA, May DR. Endophthalmitis caused by *Propionibacterium acnes, Can J Ophthalmol* (1978) **13:**50–2.
30. Winward KE, Pflugfelder SC, Flynn HW Jr, et al. Postoperative *Propionibacterium* endophthalmitis: Treatment strategies and long-term results, *Ophthalmology* (1993) **100:**447–51.
31. Zimmerman PL, Mamalis N, Alder JB, et al. Chronic *Nocardia asteroides* endophthalmitis after extracapsular cataract extraction, *Arch Ophthalmol* (1993) **111:**837–40.
32. Wenkel H, Rummelt V, Knorr H, Naumann GO. Chronic postoperative endophthalmitis following cataract extraction and intraocular lens implantation: report on nine patients, *Ger J Ophthalmol* (1993) **2:**419–25.

33. Sawusch MR, Michels RG, Stark WJ, et al. Endophthalmitis due to *Propionibacterium acnes* sequestered between IOL optic and posterior capsule, *Ophthalmic Surg* (1989) **20**:90–2.
34. Busin M, Cusumano A, Spitznas M. Intraocular lens removal from eyes with chronic low-grade endophthalmitis, *J Cataract Refract Surg* (1995) **21**:679–84.
35. Thach AB, Das A, Lopez PF. En bloc capsulectomy in the diagnosis and treatment of refractory, chronic, recurrent pseudophakic endophthalmitis, *Ophthalmic Surg* (1994) **25**:361–4.
36. Owens SL, Lam S, Tessler HH, Deutsch TA. Preliminary study of a new intraocular method in the diagnosis and treatment of *Propionibacterium acnes* endophthalmitis following cataract extraction, *Ophthalmic Surg* (1993) **24**:268–72.
37. Peyman GA, Carroll CP, Raichand M. Prevention and management of traumatic endophthalmitis, *Ophthalmology* (1980) **87**:320–4.
38. Thompson WS, Rubsamen PE, Flynn HW Jr, et al. Endophthalmitis after penetrating trauma: risk factors and visual acuity outcomes, *Ophthalmology* (1995) **102**:1696–701.
39. Alfaro DV, Roth D, Liggett PE. Post-traumatic endophthalmitis: causative organisms, treatment, and prevention, *Retina* (1994) **14**:206–11.
40. Metrikin DC, Wilson CA, Berkowitz BA, et al. Measurement of blood–retinal barrier breakdown in endotoxin-induced endophthalmitis, *Invest Ophthalmol Vis Sci* (1995) **36**:1361–70.
41. Schemmer GB, Driebe WT Jr. Post-traumatic *Bacillus cereus* endophthalmitis, *Arch Ophthalmol* (1987) **105**:342–4.
42. Davey RT Jr, Tauber WB. Post-traumatic endophthalmitis: the emerging role of *Bacillus cereus* infection, *Rev Infect Dis* (1987) **9**:110–23.
43. Alfaro DV, Roth DB, Laughlin RM, et al. Paediatric post-traumatic endophthalmitis, *Br J Ophthalmol* (1995) **79**:888–91.
44. Witherspoon CD, Kuhn F, Owens DS, et al. Endophthalmitis due to *Sporothrix schenckii* after penetrating ocular injury, *Ann Ophthalmol* (1990) **22**:385–8.
45. Dressler S, Berghian S, Frantescu V, et al. The treatment of posttraumatic endophthalmia, *Oftalmologia* (1990) **34**:51–7.
46. Zou Y, Yang W, Li S, Yue L. Primary posterior chamber intraocular lens implantation in traumatic cataract with posterior capsular breaks, *Yen Ko Hsueh Pao* (1995) **11**:140–2.
47. Swerdloff JN, Filler SG, Edwards JE Jr. Severe candidal infections in neutropenic patients, *Clin Infect Dis* (1993) **17** (Suppl 2):S457–67.
48. Smith KG, Ihle BU, Heriot WJ, Becker GJ. Metastatic endophthalmitis in dialysis patients, *Am J Nephrol* (1995) **15**:78–81.
49. Fuller JR, Casswell AG. Endophthalmitis after routine intraocular surgery in an asplenic patient, *J Roy Soc Med* (1995) **88**:475P–6P.
50. Weinstein JM, Elliott J, Tilford RH. Metastatic endophthalmitis due to *Salmonella typhimurium*, *Arch Ophthalmol* (1982) **100**:293–5.
51. Mason W, Igdaloff S, Friedman R, Wright HT Jr. Meningococcal sepsis with endophthalmitis, *Am J Dis Child* (1979) **133**:1151–2.
52. Hull DS, Patipa M, Cox F. Metastatic endophthalmitis: a complication of meningococcal meningitis, *Ann Ophthalmol* (1982) **14**:29–30.
53. Nangia V, Hutchinson C. Metastatic endophthalmitis caused by *Clostridium perfringens*, *Br J Ophthalmol* (1992) **76**:252–3.
54. O'Brart DP, Eykyn SJ. Septicaemic infection with group B streptococci presenting with endophthalmitis in adults, *Eye* (1992) **6** (4):396–9.
55. Greenwald BD, Tunkel AR, Morgan KM, et al. Candidal endophthalmitis after lithotripsy of renal calculi, *South Med J* (1992) **85**:773–4.
56. Al-Hazzaa SA, Tabbara KF, Gammon JA. Pink hypopyon: a sign of *Serratia marcescens* endophthalmitis, *Br J Ophthalmol* (1992) **76**:764–5.
57. De Groot V, Stempels N, Tassignon MJ. Endogenous pneumococcal endophthalmitis after splenectomy: report of two cases, *Bull Soc Belge Ophtalmol* (1992) **243**:147–51.
58. Eliott D, O'Brien TP, Green WR, et al. Elevated intraocular pressure, pigment dispersion, and dark hypopyon in endogenous endophthalmitis from *Listeria monocytogenes*, *Surv Ophthalmol* (1992) **37**:117–24.
59. Snow DG, Eagling EM, Lawrence JD. Bilateral metastatic endophthalmitis as a complication of major burns, *Burns* (1992) **18**:342–4.
60. Ebisuno S, Miyai M. A case of *Klebsiella pneumoniae* endophthalmitis metastasized from prostatitis, *Hinyokika Kiyo* (1994) **40**:625–7.
61. Matsuo T, Nakagawa H, Matsuo N. Endogenous *Aspergillus* endophthalmitis associated with periodontitis, *Ophthalmologica* (1995) **209**:109–11.
62. Graham DA, Kinyoun JL, George DP. Endogenous *Aspergillus* endophthalmitis after lung transplantation, *Am J Ophthalmol* (1995) **119**:107–9.
63. Pettit TH, Olson RJ, Foos RY, Martin WJ. Fungal endophthalmitis following intraocular lens implantation: a surgical epidemic, *Arch Ophthalmol* (1980) **98**:1025–39.
64. Insler MS, Urso LF. *Candida albicans* endophthalmitis after penetrating keratoplasty, *Am J Ophthalmol* (1987) **105**:57–60.
65. Kloess PM, Stulting RD, Waring GO III, Wilson LA. Bacterial and fungal endophthalmitis after penetrating keratoplasty, *Am J Ophthalmol* (1993) **115**:309–16 [published erratum appears in *Am J Ophthalmol* (1993) **115**:548].
66. Samiy N, D'Amico DJ. Endogenous fungal endophthalmitis, *Int Ophthalmol Clin* (1996) **36**(3):147–62.
67. Zarbin MA, Becker E, Witcher J, et al. Treatment of presumed fungal endophthalmitis with oral fluconazole, *Ophthalmic Surg Lasers* (1996) **27**:628–31.
68. Custis PH, Haller JA, de Juan E Jr. An unusual case of cryptococcal endophthalmitis, *Retina* (1995) **15**:300–4.
69. Coats ML, Peyman GA. Intravitreal corticosteroids in the treatment of exogenous fungal endophthalmitis, *Retina* (1992) **12**:46–51.
70. Schulman JA, Peyman GA. Intravitreal corticosteroids as an adjunct in the treatment of bacterial and fungal endophthalmitis: a review, *Retina* (1992) **12**:366–40.
71. Bohigian GM, Olk RJ. Factors associated with a poor visual result in endophthalmitis, *Am J Ophthalmol* (1986) **101**: 332–4.
72. Peyman GA, Raichand M, Bennett TO. Management of endophthalmitis with pars plana vitrectomy, *Br J Ophthalmol* (1980) **64**:472–5.

73. Barza M, Pavan PR, Doft BH, et al. Evaluation of microbiological diagnostic techniques in postoperative endophthalmitis in the Endophthalmitis Vitrectomy Study, *Arch Ophthalmol* (1997) **115:**1142–50.
74. Peyman GA, May DR, Ericson ES, Apple D. Intraocular injection of gentamicin: toxic effects and clearance, *Arch Ophthalmol* (1974) **92:**42–7.
75. May DR, Ericson ES, Peyman GA, Axelrod AJ. Intraocular injection of gentamicin: single injection therapy of experimental bacterial endophthalmitis, *Arch Ophthalmol* (1974) **91:**487–9.
76. Axelrod AJ, Peyman GA, Apple DJ. Toxicity of intravitreal injection of amphotericin B, *Am J Ophthalmol* (1973) **76:**578–83.
77. Axelrod AJ, Peyman GA. Intravitreal amphotericin B treatment of experimental fungal endophthalmitis, *Am J Ophthalmol* (1973) **76:**584–8.
78. Graham RO, Peyman GA. Intravitreal injection of dexamethasone: treatment of experimentally induced endophthalmitis, *Arch Ophthalmol* (1974) **92:**149–54.
79. Graham RO, Peyman GA, Fishman G. Intravitreal injection of cephaloridine in the treatment of endophthalmitis, *Arch Ophthalmol* (1975) **93:**56–61.
80. Koziol J, Peyman G. Intraocular chloramphenicol and bacterial endophthalmitis, *Can J Ophthalmol* (1974) **9:**316–21.
81. Peyman GA, Nelsen P, Bennett TO. Intravitreal injection of kanamycin in experimentally induced endophthalmitis, *Can J Ophthalmol* (1974) **9:**322–7.
82. Nelsen P, Peyman GA, Bennett TO. BB-K8: a new aminoglycoside for intravitreal injection in bacterial endophthalmitis, *Am J Ophthalmol* (1974) **78:**82–9.
83. Bennett TO, Peyman GA. Use of tobramycin in eradicating experimental bacterial endophthalmitis, *Albrecht von Graefes Arch Klin Exp Ophthalmol* (1974) **191:**93–107.
84. Schenk AG, Peyman GA. Lincomycin by direct intravitreal injection in the treatment of experimental bacterial endophthalmitis, *Albrecht von Graefes Arch Klin Exp Ophthalmol* (1974) **190:**281–91.
85. Bennett TO, Peyman GA. Toxicity of intravitreal aminoglycosides in primates, *Can J Ophthalmol* (1974) **9:**475–8.
86. Schenk AG, Peyman GA, Paque JT. The intravitreal use of carbenicillin (Geopen) for treatment of *Pseudomonas* endophthalmitis, *Acta Ophthalmol* (1974) **52:**707–17.
87. Paque JT, Peyman GA. Intravitreal clindamycin phosphate in the treatment of vitreous infection, *Ophthalmic Surg* (1974) **5:**34–9.
88. Daily MJ, Peyman GA, Fishman G. Intravitreal injection of methicillin for treatment of endophthalmitis, *Am J Ophthalmol* (1973) **76:**343–50.
89. Peyman GA, Herbst R. Bacterial endophthalmitis: treatment with intraocular injection of gentamicin and dexamethasone, *Arch Ophthalmol* (1974) **91:**416–18.
90. Peyman GA, Vastine DW, Crouch ER, Herbst RW Jr. Clinical use of intravitreal antibiotics to treat bacterial endophthalmitis, *Trans Acad Ophthalmol Otolaryngol* (1974) **78:**0P862–75.
91. Vlchek JK, Peyman GA. Cephaloridine-induced retinopathy by intravitreal injection: an ultrastructural study, *Ann Ophthalmol* (1975) **7:**903–14.
92. Peyman GA. Antibiotic administration in the treatment of bacterial endophthalmitis: II. Intravitreal injections, *Surv Ophthalmol* (1977) **21:**332,339–46.
93. Stainer GA, Peyman GA, Meisels H, Fishman G. Toxicity of selected antibiotics in vitreous replacement fluid, *Ann Ophthalmol* (1977) **9:**615–8.
94. Vastine DW, Peyman GA, Guth SB. Visual prognosis in bacterial endophthalmitis treated with intravitreal antibiotics, *Ophthalmic Surg* (1979) **10:**76–83.
95. Peyman GA. Aminoglycoside toxicity (letter), *Arch Ophthalmol* (1992) **110:**446.
96. Kasbeer RT, Peyman GA. Intravitreal oxacillin in experimental staphylococcal endophthalmitis, *Albrecht von Graefes Arch Klin Exp Ophthalmol* (1975) **196:**279–87.
97. Peyman GA, Vastine DW, Diamond JG. Vitrectomy in exogenous Candida endophthalmitis, *Albrecht von Graefes Arch Klin Exp Ophthalmol* (1975) **197:**55–9.
98. Peyman GA, Raichand M, Bennett TO. Management of endophthalmitis with pars plana vitrectomy, *Br J Ophthalmol* (1980) **64:**472–5.
99. Peyman GA, Schulman JA. *Intravitreal Surgery: Principles and Practice*, 2nd edn (Appleton & Lange: Norwalk, CT, 1994): 901–5.
100. Peyman GA. A miniaturized vitrectomy system for vitreous and retinal biopsy, *Can J Ophthalmol* (1990) **25:**285–6.
101. De Juan E Jr, Hickingbotham D. Refinements in microinstrumentation for vitreous surgery, *Am J Ophthalmol* (1990) **109:**218–20.
102. Doft BH, Kelsey SF, Wisniewski SR. Additional procedures after the initial vitrectomy or tap-biopsy in the Endophthalmitis Vitrectomy Study, *Ophthalmology* (1998) **105:** 707–16.
103. Peyman GA, Bassili S. A practical guideline for management of endophthalmitis, *Ophthalmic Surg* (1995) **26:**294–303.
104. Kosmin AS, Wishart PK. A full-thickness scleral graft for the surgical management of a late filtration bleb leak, *Ophthalmic Surg Lasers* (1997) **28:**461–8.
105. Zimmer-Galler IE, Santos A, Haller JA, Campochiaro PA. Management of endophthalmitis in a silicone oil-filled eye, *Retina* (1997) **17:**507–9.

Part XI Pediatric Vitreoretinal Surgery

Chapter 44 Pediatric vitreous surgery

Michael T Trese

INTRODUCTION

Some features of pediatric vitreous surgery are different from adult vitreous surgery. Preoperative evaluation and detailed retinal examination must be altered to fit the age of the patient.[1–4] Children require frequent examinations under anesthesia to achieve complete preoperative evaluation. The ocular anatomy is different in the child than in adults because the pars plana is not developed in the premature infant and the vitreoretinal adhesions are strong. The discovery of retinal detachment is frequently delayed, giving rise to proliferative vitreoretinopathy, and often the retinal problems accompany other congenital disorders. In the following sections, we will discuss the management of advanced retinopathy of prematurity (ROP), persistent hyperplastic primary vitreous (PHPV) (renamed persistent fetal vasculature syndrome, PFVS) and congenital retinoschisis.

RETINOPATHY OF PREMATURITY

INDICATIONS

Surgical criteria

ROP has been the subject of much investigation, including the landmark works of Kinsey, Terry and Patz, whose work described this particular retinal problem of premature children.[2,5–7] Fortunately, only a small percentage of eyes progress past stage 3 ROP to stages 4 and 5.[8,9] These eyes develop a progressive retinal detachment that may evolve very rapidly, altering the configuration of the retinal detachment, the surgical approach, the surgical results and the subsequent visual acuities. In the management of advanced ROP, the goal is to reattach the retina and prevent redetachment. The surgical indication that we find helpful is a 4A retinal detachment, which (as defined by the International Classification of Retinopathy of Prematurity) extends 3 clock-hours circumferentially and extends three widths of the ridge posteriorly. In our experience, this type of detachment is likely to progress. This has been confirmed by the findings of the Cryotherapy for Retinopathy of Prematurity Study.[10]

Case selection

Surgical case selection is based upon the clinical impression or visual evoked potential (VEP), testing the confirmation of light perception vision present in the eye (this requires awake VEP testing for children with low vision). If light perception is thought to be present in an eye with retinal detachment, surgical therapy should be considered. Each eye should be considered as an individual event. It is important to realize that retinal detachment in ROP is bilateral in 85% of the cases.[11] Very often when surgery is delayed in one eye because the second eye is not in danger, the eye with delayed surgery develops a much worse visual potential than it would have if an intervention had been performed earlier.

PREOPERATIVE EVALUATION

Examination

Premature infants should be examined according to the recommendations generated from the Cryotherapy for Retinopathy of Prematurity Study.[9] The recommendations suggest that a child of 1500 g dry birthweight should have a retinal examination 4–6 weeks after birth and subsequently every 2 weeks until retinal vascular maturity develops, unless intervening ROP changes would mandate more frequent examinations.

Ancillary testing

We find the VEP to be the most useful ancillary test. The electroretinogram is not helpful in children with retinal detachment. Although ultrasound evaluation provides a two-dimensional picture of the retina, we find it frequently misleading; it does not alter our surgical decision. When there is clinical uncertainty of light perception, we use VEP testing to confirm or rule out light perception vision (although false negative results are possible, depending on the level of patient attention).

Preoperative procedures

If the eye has reached the stage 3 ROP threshold (five contiguous clock-hours of stage 3 or eight non-contiguous clock-hours of stage 3 plus disease), it is treated with peripheral ablation. We perform a confluent laser application to ablate the avascular periphery completely. The indirect laser can be used in either the neonatal intensive-care unit or the operating room. Either topical or general anesthesia is used, depending on the surgeon's preference.

INSTRUMENTATION

In the management of advanced ROP, scleral buckling is used predominantly to treat an effusive retinal detachment (Fig. 44.1). A no. 240 silicone band is used as a buckle, placed around the greatest circle of the eye. This requires a paracentesis and removal of approximately 0.12–0.15 cc of aqueous fluid. This scleral buckle creates a significant anisometropia and requires revision after approximately 3 months. The buckle is secured with 5-0 nylon sutures on a spatulated needle.[12]

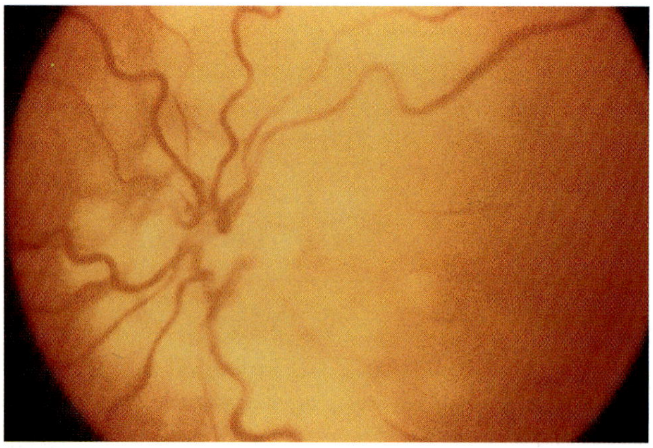

Figure 44.1 *Undulating anterior surface of a predominantly effusive retinal detachment. (Reproduced with permission from Trese MT. Scleral buckling for retinopathy of prematurity.* Ophthalmology *(1994)* ***101:*** *23–6.*[12] *Copyright © 1994, Elsevier Science.)*

Vitrectomy settings

The second useful procedure for advanced ROP is lens-sparing vitrectomy/membrane peeling.[3] This procedure can yield rewarding visual results.[13] Entry is achieved through the pars plicata immediately posterior to the iris root. This entry avoids the lens which never extends beyond the iris root towards the peripheral retina (Fig. 44.2). When the retina touches the lens for more than 6 clock-hours lensectomy–vitrectomy–membrane peeling is necessary. Using either the pediatric sew-on lens or an indirect viewing system, central vitrectomy is performed at a slow cutting rate (300 cuts per minute). Suction is generally applied in small bursts controlled by the foot switch to allow individual bites and thus facilitate removal of less flexible tissue away from the retina and abnormal vessels.

Instruments

The membrane peeling/cutting scissors (MPC) are our preferred instrument for division of epiretinal tissue. This instrument provides small, angled, vertical cutting with a relatively small jaw (compared to the larger scissors) and allows individual or repeated cutting action in the crevices of the convoluted retina in the posterior pole. In addition, these scissors have a vertically movable upper blade on one side of its shaft. One must carefully position the blade to avoid damaging more anterior retinal folds as the blades close and as the posterior dissection approaching the optic nerve is performed. Frequently, during vitreous surgery, folds of retina overlap the disc and these folds must be observed closely to ensure that they are not cut inadvertently as epiretinal tissue. Occasionally, the retina is stretched over the optic nerve so tautly that it cannot be uncovered, even with a meticulous dissection. However, the fold of a dragged retina may flatten with time following surgical intervention.

The surgical approach depends at least in part on the area in which cells are available to form tractional

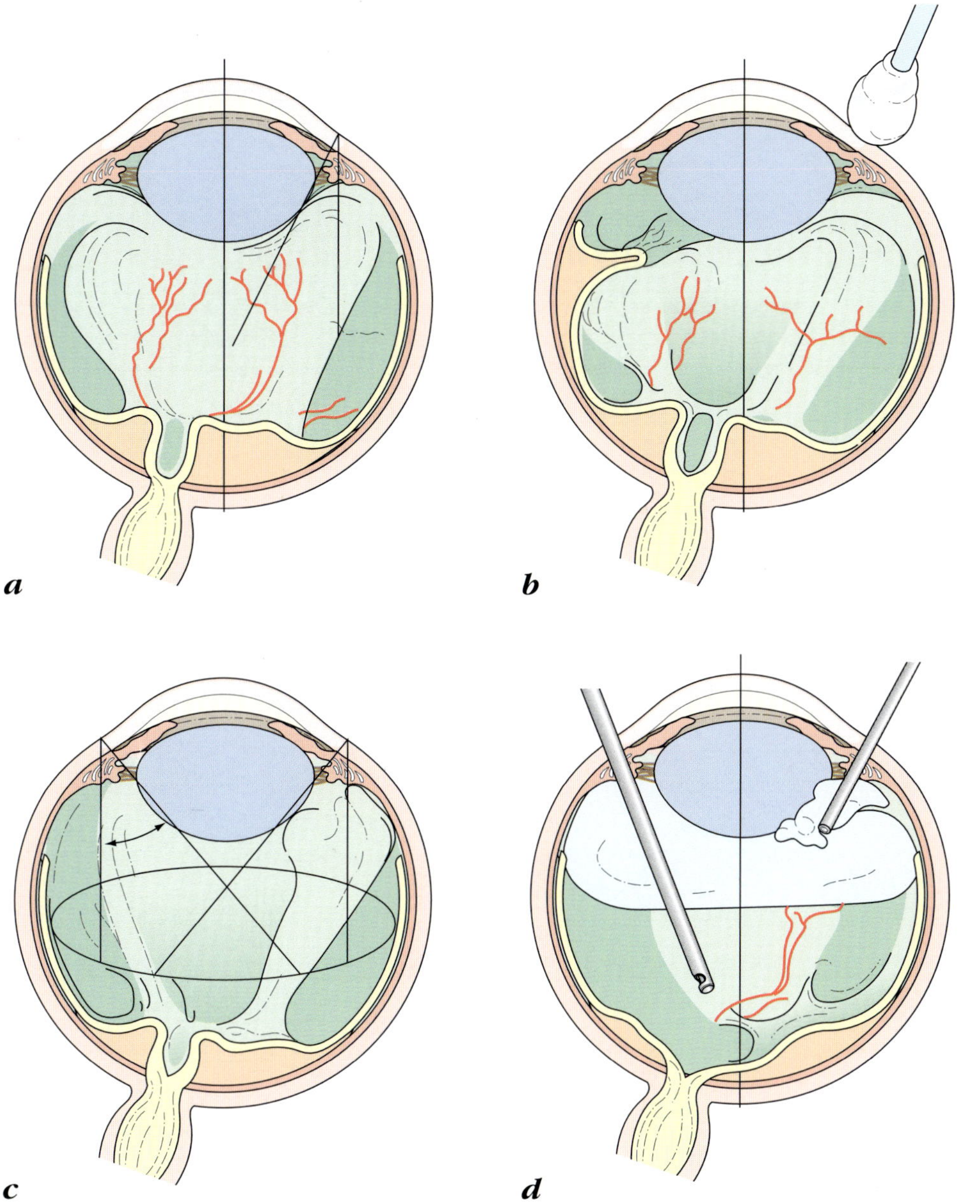

Figure 44.2 *Technique of lens-sparing vitrectomy: (a) retinopathy of prematurity (ROP) tractional detachment of the posterior pole; (b) examination technique to determine whether the lens is clear of adhesions; (c) the plane of influence posterior to which lens-sparing vitrectomy can be performed; (d) injection of air at end of lens-sparing vitrectomy. (Adapted with permission from Peyman GA, Schulman JA.* Intravitreal Surgery: Principles and Practice, *2nd edn. Appleton & Lange: Norwalk, CT, 1994: 381.[34])*

retinal detachment. (Cells are available from the posterior tunica vasculosa lentis in the anterior vitreous cavity or posterior hyaloid system (Fig. 44.3).) At the completion of dissection, a fluid–gas exchange is performed and the child is positioned face down for 24 hours.

Antibiotics, steroids

At the end of surgery, antibiotic is injected subconjunctivally and steroid ointment is placed on the eye. Topical steroids, antibiotic and atropine 1% drops are used postoperatively.

POSTOPERATIVE TREATMENT

Follow-up

The child requires routine pars plana vitrectomy follow-up. These preterm children are in the postoperative period during a critical period of visual development. Therefore, the aid of a pediatric

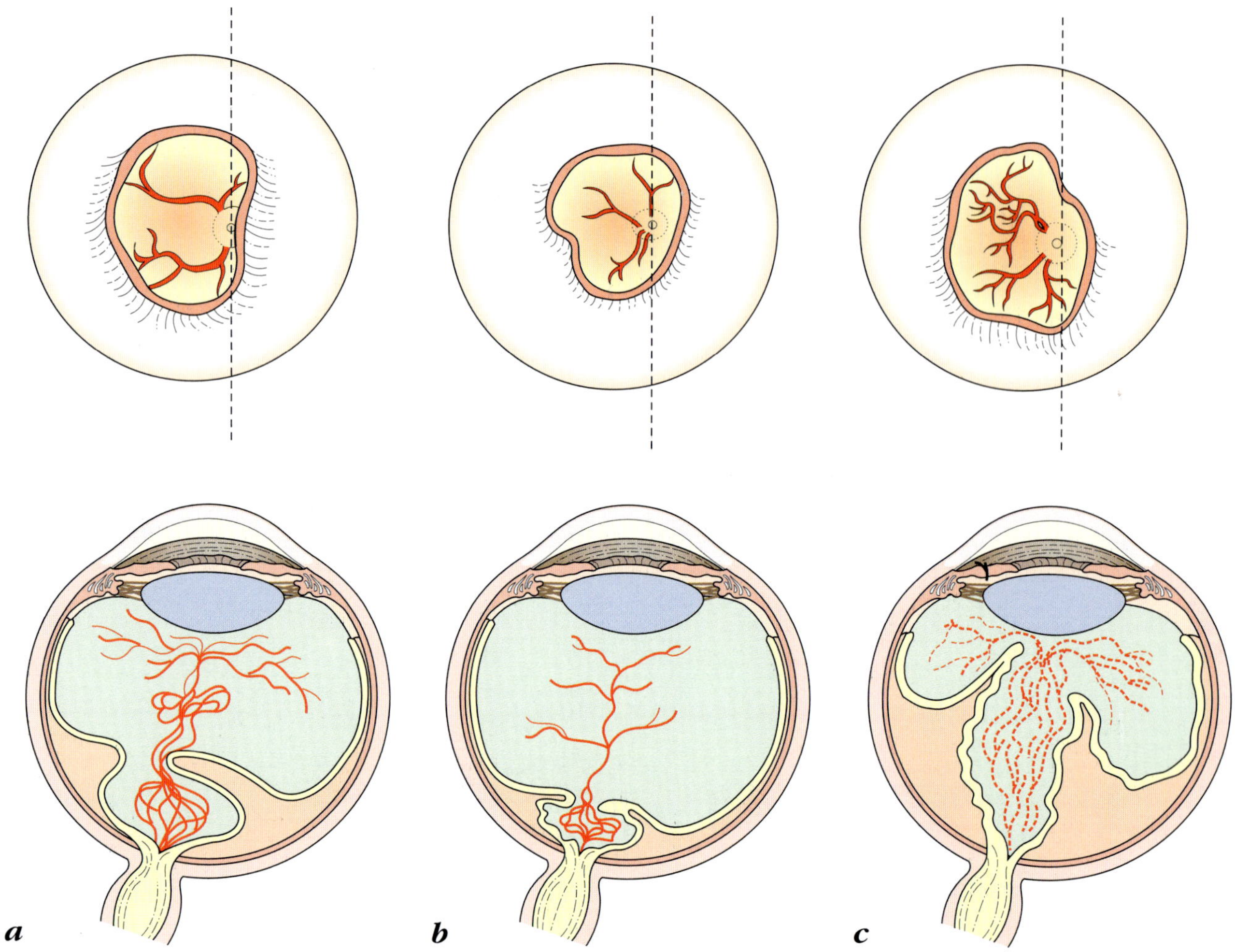

Figure 44.3 *(a) Artist's drawing of a predominantly tractional 4B retinal detachment of ROP with asymmetrical traction by posterior cellular elements (hyaloid vasculature). (b) Symmetrical traction by predominantly posterior cellular elements. (c) Configuration resulting from traction of predominantly anterior cellular elements (tunica vasculosa lentis).*

ophthalmologist is crucial to monitor refractive change and prevent amblyopia. Any evidence of amblyopia should be treated rapidly because amblyopia can occur swiftly and last a lifetime. The eyes should not be occluded beginning on the first postoperative day.

Indications for reoperation

The indication that we have used for reoperation is an eye that has shown improvement in vision followed by a reduction in vision concurrent with a change in retinal anatomy thought to be responsible for the change in vision. Frequently we use autologous plasmin enzyme (a nonspecific protease) in reoperations to help to free residual vitreous from the surface of the retina.[14,15] Autologous plasmin enzyme is a relatively new therapy and has not been used in primary ROP surgery. However, we have found the enzyme helpful in reoperation and may be using it in primary ROP surgery in the future.

SURGICAL RESULTS

Scleral buckling of a predominantly exudative retinal detachment in ROP stages 4A and 4B has approximately a 70% success rate.[3,16] Visual acuity depends in part on the duration and extent of the detachment, the refractive error of the eye and the success of amblyopia therapy.

Success without peripheral ablation

Results of vitreous surgery for ROP depend on presurgical cryotherapy or laser ablation of the peripheral retina. Eyes without adequate peripheral ablation demonstrate approximately a 50% rate of reattachment and only 30% of these reattached eyes have an improvement in vision.[1,17,18]

Visual improvement with peripheral ablation

If eyes have appropriate peripheral ablation (with cryotherapy or preferably laser), 76% show reattachment of at least the posterior pole and 72% of these eyes achieve light perception vision; 48% achieve 20/1900 vision or better; 30% achieve 20/800 vision or better; and 15% achieve 20/300 vision or better. The best vision achieved in one long-term result series was 20/60.[6]

Reoperation

The long-term series mentioned above reported nearly 4 years of follow-up. One-third of the eyes required a second vitreoretinal procedure; however, most of these had undergone only scleral buckling as their initial procedure.[6]

PERSISTENT HYPERPLASTIC PRIMARY VITREOUS (PERSISTENT FETAL VASCULATURE SYNDROME)

INDICATIONS

PHPV recently has been renamed persistent fetal vasculature syndrome (PFVS).[19] This new name emphasizes the importance of both the tunica vasculosa lentis and the persistent hyaloid vasculature. PFVS can be divided into predominantly persistent anterior tunica vasculosa lentis or predominantly persistent posterior hyaloid system. These changes can be accompanied by retinal dysplasia, which is most commonly associated with posterior persistent fetal vasculature.[20] However, we reported a series in which no preoperative determination of which eyes would have significant posterior retinal dysplasia was possible.[21] The pathology usually presents as a small eye with ciliary processes drawn into the retrolenticular tissue. The lens may be cataractous and intimately connected to the retrolental tissue. A retrolental stalk may contain active vasculature attached to the posterior pole and may or may not produce a tractional retinal detachment or a dysplastic retina. In some eyes, this retinal dysplasia can be very marked. Ancillary testing with ultrasound and VEP has been performed to predict the presence or absence of retinal dysplasia. The predictive values of these tests are questionable.

INSTRUMENTATION

The instrumentation used in surgery for PFVS is similar to other pediatric vitrectomy surgery. The entry to the vitreous cavity is very anterior; the pars plicata is the preferred entry site (Fig. 44.4). Anterior entry, sometimes even through the limbus or, preferably, just posterior to the iris root, may be necessary in some cases and allows removal of lens material. The retrolenticular material is then removed to visualize the stalk.

The appearance of the anterior tissue in no way predicts the structure of the posterior pole. Very abnormal-looking anterior structures may conceal a normal posterior pole or very minimal anterior changes may overlie a very distorted and dysplastic posterior pole.

Following removal of the lens material, the size and position of the central stalk can be identified and the stalk structure assessed. The stalk can be diathermized and divided to allow easier manipulation of the anterior tissue.

The ciliary processes must be freed from the abnormal admixed anterior vitreous/posterior lens tissue. This requires both circumferential and radial dissections between the ciliary processes to allow reattachment of the ciliary body, because hypotony is a frequent long-term issue in PHPV (Fig. 44.5). In addition, the retrolenticular tissue may contain unusually dense fibrous plaque requiring dissection and removal. If the fibrous plaque cannot be removed through the pars plana sclerotomy, it is brought to the anterior chamber and removed through a limbal incision.

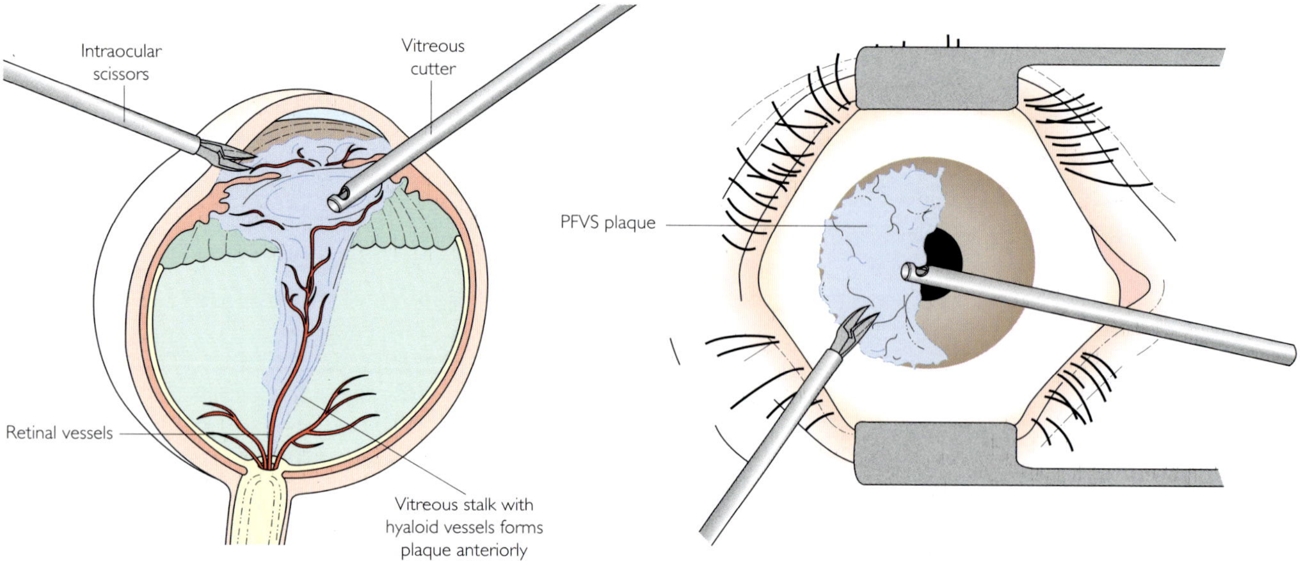

Figure 44.4 *Surgical management of persistent hyperplastic primary vitreous (PHPV). Vitreous cutting instruments are used to remove the lens and retrolenticular material carefully. Anterior incisions of the limbus or pars plicata often are used to avoid the vitreous base and peripheral retina, which may be present anteriorly in PHPV.*

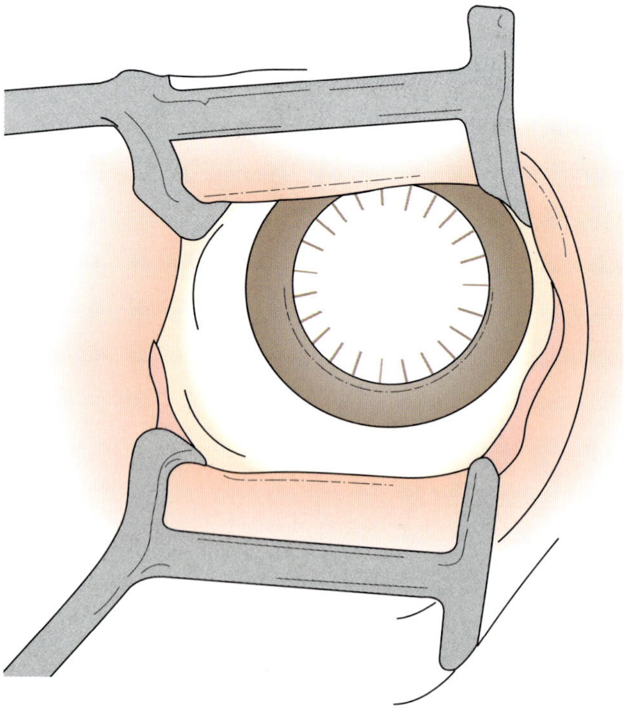

Figure 44.5 *Typical appearance of persistent hyperplastic primary vitreous. An opacified retrolenticular fibrovascular membrane is attached to pulled ciliary processes.*

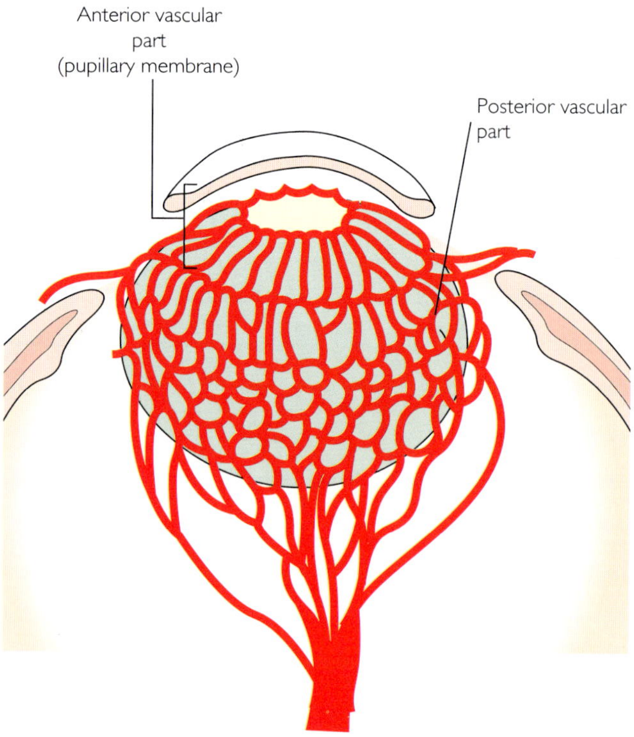

Figure 44.6 *Hyaloid vasculature and primary vitreous shown during embryologic ocular development.*

The posterior dissection is continued following the closure of the limbal wound. The posterior pole is approached using an infusion light pipe and vitreous cutter. Care is taken to remove peripheral vitreous initially. The posterior pole needs to be inspected for the attachment of the stalk at the optic nerve. The retina may be drawn over the optic nerve, producing a tractional detachment at the posterior pole. After completion of vitrectomy, diathermy is used to cauterize the hyaloid vasculature before dissection of the stalk (Fig. 44.6).

POSTOPERATIVE TREATMENT

The postoperative treatment is similar to usual vitrectomy postoperative care. However, unlike adult vitrectomy cases, follow-up also requires intensive amblyopic therapy because frequently there is a very marked anisometropia between these smaller eyes and the normal-sized contralateral eye. During the initial examination under anesthesia, the other eye must be examined completely to be certain that it is normal. Bilateral PHPV/PFVS is an unusual occurrence, according to some authors; it occurs perhaps 10% of the time. Whenever bilateral PFVS is considered, the diagnosis of Norrie's disease also must be entertained. Genetic testing is available to determine if an alteration in the Norrie's disease gene of the X-chromosome is present.

INDICATIONS FOR REOPERATION

Indications for reoperation in PFVS are based on the visual potential of the child. If significant visual function is anticipated, based on retinal structure or the child's function, then reoperation can be considered. If, however, a great deal of retinal dysplasia is present, then a goal is cosmetic appearance, eye growth and comfort of the eye.

SURGICAL RESULTS

Reports of the surgical results in PFVS have been limited to a very few series of patients.[22–25] It is clear, though, from the literature that good visual results (vision better than 20/60) are possible. Achieving good visual outcomes appears to be dependent upon the timing of intervention, the anatomy of the posterior pole, the amount of anisometropia that is present and the refractive management of the patient postoperatively. Preoperatively, we have not been able to determine which tests can predict postoperative function.

CONGENITAL RETINOSCHISIS

Congenital retinoschisis, described by Haas in 1883, involves splitting of the nerve fiber layer with cartwheel-type changes in the central macular area, peripheral schisis cavities and dragging of the optic nerve. These eyes present with decreased vision, strabismus, vitreous hemorrhage and retinal detachment.[26–29] Although congenital retinoschisis was felt to be inherited in an X-linked fashion, many reports have shown both a recessive inheritance pattern as well as some females affected with congenital retinoschisis.[30]

The pathologic features of congenital retinoschisis have been attributed to weakened Mueller pillars, reflected in midretinal changes in the b-wave of the electroretinogram. Recently, however, the gene defect and gene product of congenital retinoschisis have been described. The gene product is a cell-to-cell adhesive protein that is reduced in the diseased retina, allowing splitting of the retina into an anterior and posterior leaflet.[31] The center of the schisis cavity can be filled either with proteinaceous fluid or frank blood. We feel that in congenital retinoschisis, vitreous traction plays a role in the formation of cystic cavities. The vitreous traction combined with the weakness of the intercellular adhesion within the retina contributes to the formation of schisis cavities and inner wall breaks.

There are several challenges in the preoperative evaluation of patients with congenital retinoschisis. First, the child may present in an age group in which a complete office examination is difficult. Secondly, depending on the extent of congenital retinoschisis, the eye may present initially as strabismus or amblyopia. However, eyes with a very extensive intravitreal sheet of membrane in the vitreous are easily diagnosed. Minimal peripheral schisis and foveal schisis are often present in all eyes; peripheral schisis occurs in 50% of eyes and can be associated with amblyopia or strabismus.

Foveal schisis may not be present until the child is 5–8 years of age, although it is sometimes present soon after birth. Therefore, any eye suspected of having congenital retinoschisis must be followed for many years in order to determine if the schisis cavities begin to appear centrally or peripherally. In addition, retinal detachment in congenital retinoschisis can be either rhegmatogenous or tractional. The rhegmatogenous form can be caused by small retinal breaks in the far periphery that can be overlooked easily on office examination. Any eye with rapid progression of the schisis cavity or a new appearance and rapid progression of the schisis cavity should be evaluated to rule out a rhegmatogenous retinal detachment. In addition, if possible, the child should have routine visual fields to assess any significant loss of field, either from full-thickness retinal detachment or extension of the schisis cavity.

INSTRUMENTATION

Instrumentation needed for surgical repair of congenital retinoschisis includes the indirect ophthalmoscope, scleral buckling materials, sophisticated wide-angle viewing systems, both indirect and endolaser photocoagulation, vitreous instrumentation and long-acting gas.[32] The initial decision in the operating room during the examination under anesthesia includes the determination of the diagnosis of congenital retinoschisis and the determination of the presence of retinal detachment, either rhegmatogenous or tractional retinal detachment or both. Rhegmatogenous retinal detachment leads to full-thickness detachment of the retina, often with areas of schisis (inner- and outer wall separation) present in the detached retina. The tractional retinal detachment often is very low-lying, difficult to determine with indirect ophthalmoscopy and frequently detected only when the eye is entered for vitreous surgery. Low-lying tractional retinal detachment is generally posterior to the areas of retinoschisis and is most effectively treated by inner wall retinectomy.[33]

The management of congenital retinoschisis includes scleral buckling, closing outer wall holes and inner wall holes (if possible), and vitreous surgery. The surgical techniques used to repair congenital retinoschisis require standard vitrectomy techniques with the awareness that the peripheral retina may be altered by schisis and, therefore, a two-port vitrectomy technique may be necessary. Surgical repair of congenital retinoschisis in eyes with tractional retinal detachment involves peripheral retinal ablation for 360° with indirect laser photocoagulation, followed by entry into the eye for a two-port vitrectomy system. The infusion light pipe and vitreous cutter on low suction are used to clear the central vitreous cavity, mindful that cortical vitreous may not be peeled off the cysts in the posterior pole, particularly in the foveal area.

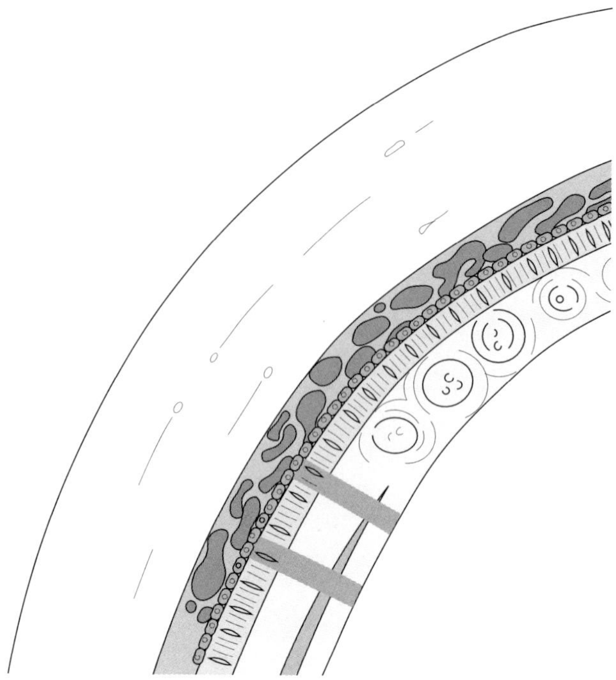

Figure 44.7 *Artist's drawing of laser application to the posterior leaflet of the schisis cavity.*

In the periphery, large retinal vessels in the inner schisis wall are diathermized. These larger vessels are treated one disc diameter anterior to the posterior juncture of the inner and outer wall flap of the schisis cavity, to allow laser photocoagulation on the already damaged inner wall of the schisis cavity. Following this diathermy treatment, scissors are used to create an inner wall retinotomy followed by a fluid–air exchange to flatten the retina. Frequently, the full-thickness retina posterior to the schisis cavity can be seen to flatten at this point.

Photocoagulation is then applied to the posterior edge of the schisis cavity (Fig. 44.7). This management allows flattening of the retina in the posterior pole. Care must be taken to extend laser treatment to the periphery to join the far peripheral laser photocoagulation, which is best done under direct visualization with the wide-angle viewing system. In the phakic eye, the laser probe sometimes must be bent to allow it to course safely behind the crystalline lens. Following flattening of the retina, the outer wall is inspected to see if any outer wall breaks are present. If they are, these breaks are treated with photocoagulation.

In eyes with combined rhegmatogenous schisis retinal detachment, the drainage of subretinal fluid through this outer wall retinal break is achieved first, followed by photocoagulation of the hole. The eye is then filled with a 7–10% mixture of perfluoropropane to allow the prolonged gas fill without concerns of elevated intraocular pressure. In the pediatric population, measurement of intraocular pressure can be difficult and unreliable. The eye is treated like an adult postvitrectomy eye, with examination to ensure that the retina remains attached and that no further rhegmatogenous components are present.

SURGICAL RESULTS

The reported series of eyes with schisis detachment procedures have been small with a 3-year follow-up.[33] Surgical results have shown, however, that retinal reattachment is possible with both improvement in central visual acuity and visual field. Central visual acuity has been noted to return to 20/50 from 20/200 preoperatively in one eye. Visual acuity and visual field improvements were seen with repair of either a rhegmatogenous retinal detachment or a full-thickness tractional retinal detachment when the posterior pole was reattached. As Ferrone points out,[33] vitrectomy in congenital retinoschisis has a somewhat higher failure rate than other vitreous surgeries in children. The eyes require good follow-up with a postvitrectomy examination under anesthesia to detect problems from peripheral retinal breaks or proliferation along the retinal surface.

Pediatric vitrectomy surgery requires the vitreoretinal surgeon to be aware of the special needs of the developing retina, vitreous and visual system. With the application of appropriate surgical techniques and meticulous postoperative care, pediatric vitreous surgery can be rewarding to the patient and the surgeon.

REFERENCES

1. Machemer R. Closed vitrectomy for severe retrolental fibroplasia in the infant, *Ophthalmology* (1983) **90:**436–41.
2. Machemer R. Description and pathogenesis of late stages of retinopathy of prematurity, *Ophthalmology* (1985) **92:**1000–4.
3. Maguire AM, Trese MT. Lens-sparing vitreoretinal surgery in infants, *Arch Ophthalmol* (1992) **110:**284–6.
4. Lightfoot D, Irvine AR. Vitrectomy in infants and children with retinal detachments caused by cicatricial retrolental fibroplasia, *Am J Ophthalmol* (1982) **94:**305–12.
5. Patz A, Kinsey VE. Retrolental fibroplasia: the pediatrician's dilemma, *Pediatrics* (1971) **48:**509–10.
6. Trese MT, Droste PJ. Long-term postoperative results of a consecutive series of stages 4 and 5 retinopathy of prematurity (ROP), *Ophthalmology* (1998) **105:**992–7.
7. Trese MT. Visual results and prognostic factors for vision following surgery for stage V retinopathy of prematurity, *Ophthalmology* (1986) **93:**574–9.
8. Schaffer DB, Johnson L, Quinn GE, et al. Vitamin E and retinopathy of prematurity: follow-up at one year, *Ophthalmology* (1985) **92:** 1005–11.
9. Cryotherapy for Retinopathy of Prematurity Cooperative Group. Multicenter trial of cryotherapy for retinopathy of prematurity: preliminary results, *Arch Ophthalmol* (1988) **106:**471–9.
10. Gilbert WS, Dobson V, Quinn GE, et al. The correlation of visual function with posterior retinal structure in severe retinopathy of prematurity. The Cryotherapy for Retinopathy of Prematurity Cooperative Group, *Arch Ophthalmol* (1992) **110:**625–31.
11. Cryotherapy for Retinopathy of Prematurity Cooperative Group. Multicenter trial of cryotherapy for retinopathy of prematurity: three-month outcome, *Arch Ophthalmol* (1990) **108:**195–204.
12. Trese MT. Scleral buckling for retinopathy of prematurity, *Ophthalmology* (1994) **101:**23–6.
13. Maguire AM, Trese MT. Visual results of lens-sparing vitreoretinal surgery in infants, *J Pediatr Ophthalmol Strabismus* (1993) **30:**28–32.
14. Verstraeten TC, Chapman C, Hartzer M et al. Pharmacologic induction of posterior vitreous detachment in the rabbit, *Arch Ophthalmol* (1993) **111:**849–54.
15. Margherio AR, Margherio RR, Hartzer M, et al. Plasmin enzyme-assisted vitrectomy in traumatic pediatric macular holes, *Ophthalmology* (1998) **105:**1617–20.
16. Greven C, Tasman W. Scleral buckling in stages 4B and 5 retinopathy of prematurity, *Ophthalmology* (1990) **97:**817–20.
17. Trese MT. Surgical results of stage V retrolental fibroplasia and timing of surgical repair, *Ophthalmology* (1984) **91:**461–6.
18. Trese MT. Surgical therapy for stage V retinopathy of prematurity: a two-step approach, *Graefes Arch Clin Exp Ophthalmol* (1987) **225:**266–8.
19. Goldberg MF. Persistent fetal vasculature (PFV): an integrated interpretation of signs and symptoms associated with persistent hyperplastic primary vitreous (PHPV), LIV Edward Jackson Memorial Lecture, *Am J Ophthalmol* (1997) **124:**587–626.
20. Reese AB. Persistent hyperplastic primary vitreous: the Jackson Memorial Lecture, *Am J Ophthalmol* (1955) **40:**317–31.
21. Dass AB, Trese MT. Surgical results of persistent hyperplastic primary vitreous. Presented at the *1995 Annual Meeting of the American Academy of Ophthalmology.*
22. Federman JL, Shields JA, Altman B, Koller H. The surgical and nonsurgical management of persistent hyperplastic primary vitreous, *Ophthalmology* (1982) **89:**20–4.
23. Pollard ZF. Results of treatment of persistent hyperplastic primary vitreous, *Ophthalmic Surg* (1991) **22:**48–52.
24. Karr DJ, Scott WE. Visual acuity results following treatment of persistent hyperplastic primary vitreous, *Arch Ophthalmol* (1986) **104:**662–7.
25. Stark WJ, Lindsey PS, Fagadau WR, Michels RG. Persistent hyperplastic primary vitreous: surgical treatment, *Ophthalmology* (1983) **90:**452–7.

26. Burns RP, Lovrien EW, Cibis AB. Juvenile sex-linked retinoschisis: clinical and genetic studies, *Trans Am Acad Ophthalmol Otolaryngol* (1971) **75:**1011–21.
27. Kraushar MF, Schepens CL, Kaplan JA, Freeman HM. Congenital retinoschisis. In: Bellows JC, ed, *Contemporary Ophthalmology Honoring Sir Stuart Duke-Elder* (Williams & Wilkins: Baltimore, 1972): 265–90.
28. Prosperi L. Congenital hereditary sex-linked retinoschisis, *J Pediatr Ophthalmol Strabismus* (1978) **15:**26–30.
29. Sabates FN. Juvenile retinoschisis, *Am J Ophthalmol* (1966) **62:**683–8.
30. Shastry BS, Hejtmancik JF, Trese MT. Novel missence (R197C) and nonsense (Y89X) mutations in the XLRS1 gene in families with X-linked retinoschisis, *Biochem Biophys Res Commun* (1999) **256:**317–19.
31. Sauer CG, Gehring A, Warneke-Wittstock R, et al. Positional cloning of the gene associated with X-linked juvenile retinoschisis, *Nat Genet* (1997) **17:**164–70.
32. Ashton N, Cook C. Studies on developing retinal vessels: I. Influence of retinal detachment, *Br J Ophthalmol* (1955) **39:**449–56.
33. Ferrone PJ, Trese MT, Lewis H. Vitreoretinal surgery for complications of congenital retinoschisis, *Am J Ophthalmol* (1997) **123:**742–7.
34. Peyman GA, Schulman JA. *Intravitreal Surgery: Principles and Practice*, 2nd edn. Appleton & Lange: Norwalk, CT 1994: 381.

Part XII Surgical Techniques in Viral Retinitis

Chapter 45 Implantation of a sustained-release ganciclovir implant

April Harris, Stephen A Meffert and Mandi D Conway

INTRODUCTION

Cytomegalovirus (CMV) retinitis is the most common opportunistic ocular infection in patients with the acquired immunodeficiency syndrome (AIDS).[1,2] Intravenous ganciclovir was the first treatment shown to be efficacious in the management of CMV retinitis.[3] The drug ganciclovir can be administered in an intravenous solution, via intraocular injection, by surgical implantation of a semipermeable pellet and, most recently, in an oral form. Two other drugs, foscarnet and cidofovir, have also been approved by the US Food and Drug Administration (FDA) for the management of CMV retinitis. Of the three, only ganciclovir is currently available in a sustained-release intraocular delivery device.

Although intravenous ganciclovir, foscarnet and low-dose cidofovir all demonstrate excellent initial activity against CMV retinitis, progression of the disease eventually occurs after 7–8 weeks of therapy.[4,5] Moreover, the former two drugs require a permanent indwelling catheter because frequent administration is required. Many patients must discontinue therapy with ganciclovir and foscarnet because of systemic side-effects, including life-threatening neutropenia and nephrotoxicity, respectively. Less-frequent administration of cidofovir obviates the need for a permanent catheter, but the risk of drug-induced nephrotoxicity requires the adjunctive use of probenecid.[5] In addition, intravenous cidofovir appears to cause anterior uveitis in 26–44% of patients and sight-threatening hypotony in a small number of those patients with uveitis.[6,7]

All three drugs are virustatic, which explains the need for continued maintenance therapy. In fact, progression of the disease is inevitable even while on intravenous maintenance therapy.[8] The main reason is that intraocular drug levels are difficult to achieve with conventional intravenous delivery. Levels may be subtherapeutic for two-thirds of CMV strains while on intravenous ganciclovir maintenance therapy.[9]

Poor ocular bioavailability prompted the use of intravitreal injection of ganciclovir, foscarnet and, more recently, cidofovir in order to treat CMV retinitis. Unfortunately, ganciclovir and foscarnet have short half-lives, necessitating weekly injections. This regimen is poorly tolerated by the patient and risks retinal detachment and endophthalmitis.[10–12] Cidofovir must be administered less frequently, every 6 weeks, but must still be given with probenecid to avoid toxicity to the ciliary body.[13,14] Iritis occurs in 14–26% and irreversible hypotony in 3.8% of patients receiving intravitreal injections of cidofovir.[14,15] Consequently, cidofovir appears to have a narrow therapeutic window compared to ganciclovir when administered locally.[8]

Smith et al tested the first sustained-release device developed for the treatment of CMV retinitis in rabbits in the early 1990s.[16] Because there is no good animal model of CMV retinitis, our knowledge of these devices *in vivo* is based on subsequent clinical trials and case reports. The first sustained-release ganciclovir implants lasted approximately 4–5 months and were successful in delaying the progression of CMV retinitis.[17] Further modifications of the device have extended its therapeutic longevity to 7–8 months. Intravitreal drug concentration with the implant has been shown to average 4.1 μg/ml.[18] This level far exceeds both the therapeutic index and the level of 0.93 μg/ml attained by intravenous ganciclovir therapy.[9]

One of the main drawbacks of this type of local therapy is that other systemic manifestations of CMV are not treated, including CMV in the contralateral eye.[18] Concomitant oral ganciclovir may offer promise in this area, although it is poorly absorbed in the gastrointestinal tract. An ongoing trial is comparing ganciclovir implants alone versus ganciclovir implants plus oral ganciclovir in the treatment of unilateral CMV retinitis.[8]

The comparison of contemporary studies of CMV retinitis to other literature may prove difficult with the recent advent of highly active antiretroviral therapy (HAART). Whitcup et al reported three cases in which antiCMV therapy was discontinued without recrudescence of disease after patients' CD4 counts were elevated on HAART.[19] The same authors also reported resolution of a case of active CMV retinitis in a patient who refused antiCMV medications but was started on HAART. In contrast, Jacobson et al described a series of five patients on HAART with CD4 counts above 195 cells/μl who were diagnosed with new-onset CMV retinitis.[20]

If all the programmed T-cells specific for CMV are lost when the CD4 count drops, then raising the CD4 count with HAART may be ineffective unless antiCMV treatment is also instituted.[19] More patients on HAART need to be monitored before specific recommendations can be made regarding discontinuing antiCMV treatment, although the ganciclovir implant might be useful as either primary or bridge treatment while patients recover their immune function.

INDICATIONS

The ideal candidate for the ganciclovir implant would be an AIDS patient with newly diagnosed unilateral CMV retinitis with no evidence of systemic CMV. Intolerance to intravenous therapy and recurrence of retinitis while on intravenous maintenance therapy are also indications for subsequent local therapy, although the implant is less effective as salvage therapy than as primary therapy (J.P. Dunn, personal communication). Bilateral retinitis and concomitant systemic disease warrant primary intravenous therapy.

Consideration must be given to other pre-existing ocular conditions. Surgical manipulation of the vitreous is inevitable during implantation, therefore, retinal tears must be detected and adequately treated before surgery. Standard contraindications to any form of intraocular surgery, such as severe thrombocytopenia or infection, also should be assessed. Once a patient is considered a suitable candidate for the device, there should be no delay in surgical implantation because it has been shown repeatedly that the time to progression in untreated CMV retinitis is approximately 2–3 weeks.[5,18]

A currently unresolved issue is the use of implants in eyes with retinal detachments repaired with long-term silicone oil tamponade. Ganciclovir is hydrophilic and would not be expected to diffuse into silicone oil. In four silicone oil-filled eyes treated with the ganciclovir implant in the National Eye Institute (NEI) trial, three eyes exhibited no progression of disease with a median follow-up of 4 months. One eye developed reactivation retinitis in a superior location 2 months after implantation. The investigators postulated that the implant may continue to have a therapeutic effect by releasing drug into the fluid portion of the peripheral vitreous base and mobile aqueous component of the inferior vitreous cavity that is present after vitrectomy.[18] In agreement with this theory, Marx et al attempted to minimize the amount of silicone oil used in order to create a larger fluid volume in the vitreous cavity for drug distribution.[21] Further study is needed to evaluate the efficacy of implants in silicone oil-filled eyes.

A ganciclovir implant recently was used successfully to treat a patient with CMV retinitis caused by profound immunosuppression after bone marrow transplantation for myeloproliferative disease. The patient had failed intravenous foscarnet therapy.[22] Given the increasing number of patients being treated with immunosuppressive drugs for a variety of disorders, nonAIDS patients developing CMV retinitis also may be considered candidates for ganciclovir implants. In this select group of patients, only those expected to experience long-term immunosuppression (i.e. CD4+ count less than 50 cells/μl) should be considered for surgical implantation because recovery of immune status is associated with autosuppression of the disease.

PREOPERATIVE EVALUATION

CMV retinitis is a clinical diagnosis. CMV is ubiquitous in the adult population; serologic or urinary titers may not reflect active disease. Careful examination of the retina using indirect ophthalmoscopy, in conjunction with a good clinical history, should be sufficient to make the diagnosis. Analysis of a vitreous biopsy with the polymerase chain reaction may be helpful in an unusual ambiguous case.

Obviously, a full ophthalmologic examination, including best-corrected visual acuity, intraocular pressure measurement and dilated fundus examination, should be completed before surgery is considered. The

Study of the Ocular Complications of AIDS used nine-field fundus photography and demonstrated it to be superior to indirect examination in evaluating the progression of CMV retinitis. This should be considered preoperatively if activity or progression is uncertain.[23]

The patient must be able to tolerate mild intravenous sedation and injection of local anesthetic. General anesthesia is occasionally indicated in cases of dementia or psychological disturbance. Preoperative evaluation by the patient's internist is valuable if there is concern regarding the patient's medical status and ability to tolerate the procedure.

INSTRUMENTATION

The sustained-release ganciclovir implant (Vitrasert, Chiron Vision, Irvine, CA) currently available is 10 mm in length and 3.5 mm in height (Fig. 45.1). The implant consists of a 4.5-mg ganciclovir pellet with a polyvinyl alcohol coating over its entire surface. This polyvinyl alcohol coating is permeable to ganciclovir. A second layer of ethylene vinyl acetate is partially coated over the surface of the pellet. This layer is impermeable to ganciclovir. The tab that extends from the posterior surface of the implant is an extension of the polyvinyl alcohol membrane and is trimmed at the time of surgery to 3 mm.

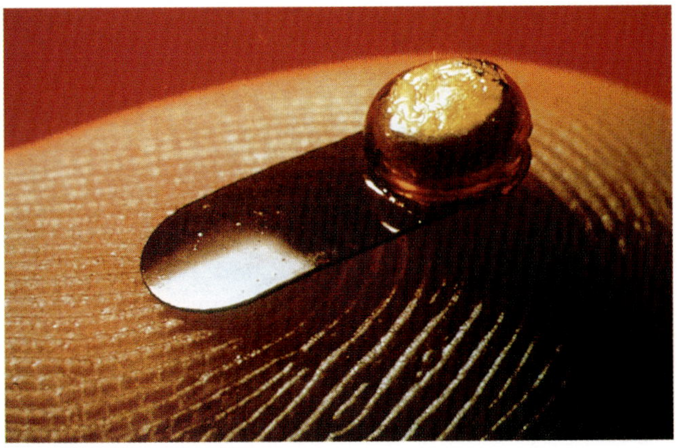

Figure 45.1 *Photograph of sustained-release ganciclovir implant. The device consists of a 4.5-mg ganciclovir implant with a polyvinyl alcohol coating over the pellet that is permeable to ganciclovir. There is a second layer of ethylene vinyl acetate partially coated over the surface of the pellet that is impermeable to ganciclovir. The implant contains between 4.5 and 6.4 mg of drug. The tab that extends from the posterior surface of the implant is trimmed to 3 mm prior to implantation. (Photograph courtesy of Dr Daniel Martin.)*

The pellet may actually contain between 4.5 and 6.4 mg of ganciclovir. Drug is released at a rate of 1.19–1.40 µg/h and, within 24 hours, the mean vitreous drug level of 4.1 µg/ml is achieved.[18,24] Sustained delivery of ganciclovir occurs for approximately 7–8 months.[18]

Standard instrumentation necessary for placement of the implant includes:

- Toothed forceps
- Smooth forceps
- Blunt Westcott scissors
- Vannas scissors
- Lid speculum
- No. 75 blade
- 20-mm microvitreoretinal (MVR) blade
- Bipolar diathermy
- Needle holder
- Double-armed 8-0 nylon suture
- 6-0 or 7-0 Vicryl suture
- Castroviejo calipers
- Automated vitrectomy machine
- Blunt-tipped cannula on syringe with balanced salt solution
- Antibiotic for subconjunctival injection
- Dexamethasone sodium for subconjunctival injection
- Antibiotic–steroid ointment.

SURGICAL PROCEDURE

The implantation of the sustained-release ganciclovir device requires approximately 30–45 minutes. Given the profound immunosuppression in patients with CMV retinitis, placement of the implant should be performed in an operating suite or similar sterile setting. In addition, surgical personnel should wear double gloves and use 'sharps' precautions. The eye receiving the implant should be dilated preoperatively.

A peribulbar or retrobulbar injection must be given in order to achieve adequate anesthesia for the procedure. General anesthesia may be appropriate for the occasional anxious patient or for those unable to cooperate. Approximately 8–10 ml of a standard mixture of equal parts 2% lidocaine and 0.75%

bupivacaine with 150 units of Wydase (hyaluronidase) is prepared.

Ideally, an anesthesiologist is available for the administration and monitoring of mild intravenous sedation just prior to the block and throughout the case.

After adequate local anesthesia has been achieved, the eye is prepped and draped in sterile fashion with particular attention to cleansing the eyelid margins because of the high risk of endophthalmitis in these patients.

The surgeon must prepare the ganciclovir implant before placing it in the eye; the modification is done before the sclerotomy is created, to minimize the risk of infection and potential vitreous loss. A 30-gauge needle is used to puncture the center of the strut approximately 2.0 mm from the edge of the pellet (Fig. 45.2). The top of the strut is then trimmed with blunt Westcott scissors, leaving 0.5 mm between the hole and the superior edge of the strut. Care is taken to avoid creating sharp edges that might erode through the sclerotomy site. An 8-0 double-armed nylon suture is placed through the hole in the strut. It is helpful to perform this maneuver with the operating microscope.

Good exposure without distortion of the globe can be achieved with separate upper and lower Jaffe lid speculums, which reduce the potential for vitreous prolapse.

A stay suture placed in the inferotemporal quadrant of the cornea using 7-0 Vicryl may provide good exposure. Toothed forceps and blunt Westcott scissors are used to make a fornix-based limbal peritomy in the inferotemporal quadrant of the eye. The peritomy should extend the entire length of the quadrant. The conjunctiva and Tenon's capsule may be retracted gently 4–5 mm posteriorly to reveal bare sclera. The scleral bed may be cauterized gently using bipolar diathermy to achieve hemostasis.

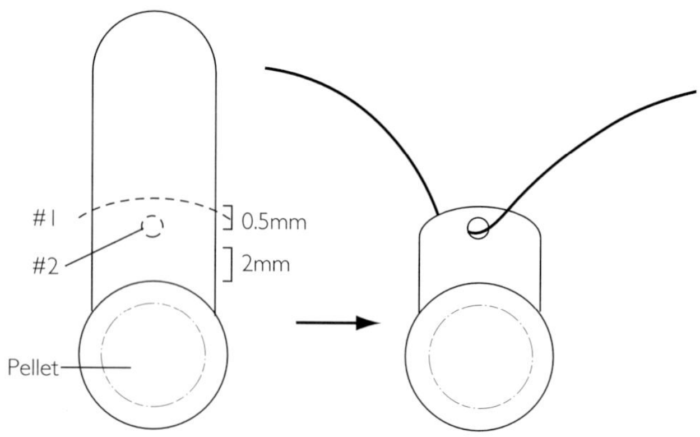

a *b*

Figure 45.2 *(a) Ganciclovir implant prior to modification. Dotted line (1) indicates where the strut is trimmed. Dotted circle (2) shows where the hole is punched with 30-gauge needle. (b) Ganciclovir implant ready for insertion.*

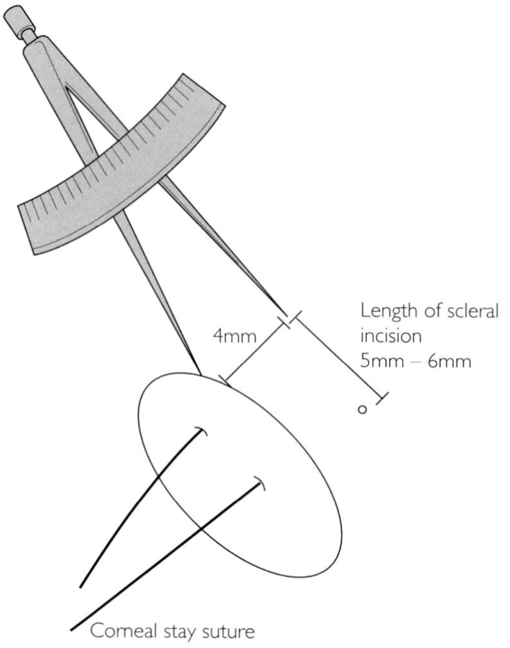

Figure 45.3 *Surgeon's view of the right eye. Castroviejo calipers are used to mark sclera for pars plana incision 4 mm from limbus. Note second indentation mark 5–6 mm away.*

Castroviejo calipers set at 4 mm are used to mark the sclera in the location of the planned pars plana incision. One tip of the calipers is placed at the limbus while the other tip is rotated 90° perpendicular to the plane of the limbus and pressed against the sclera. Two marks, made approximately 5–6 mm apart and parallel to the limbus within the inferotemporal quadrant, guide the sclerotomy location (Fig. 45.3).

After stabilizing the globe with toothed forceps, the sclera is incised with a no. 75 blade at one of the pars plana indentation marks. The no. 75 blade is used to create an incision that extends circumferentially to the second indentation mark (Fig. 45.4). A 5- to 6-mm curvilinear sclerotomy is retracted and a 20-gauge MVR blade passed through the length of the sclerotomy site to ensure complete penetration

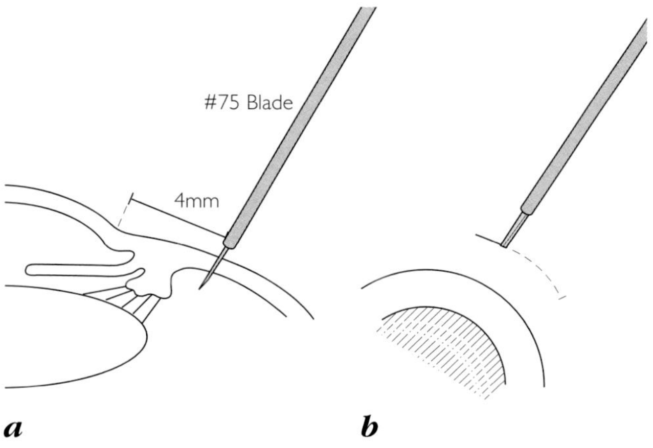

Figure 45.4 *(a) Side view of full-thickness pars plana incision 4 mm from limbus with no. 75 blade. (b) Top view of no. 75 blade engaging sclera.*

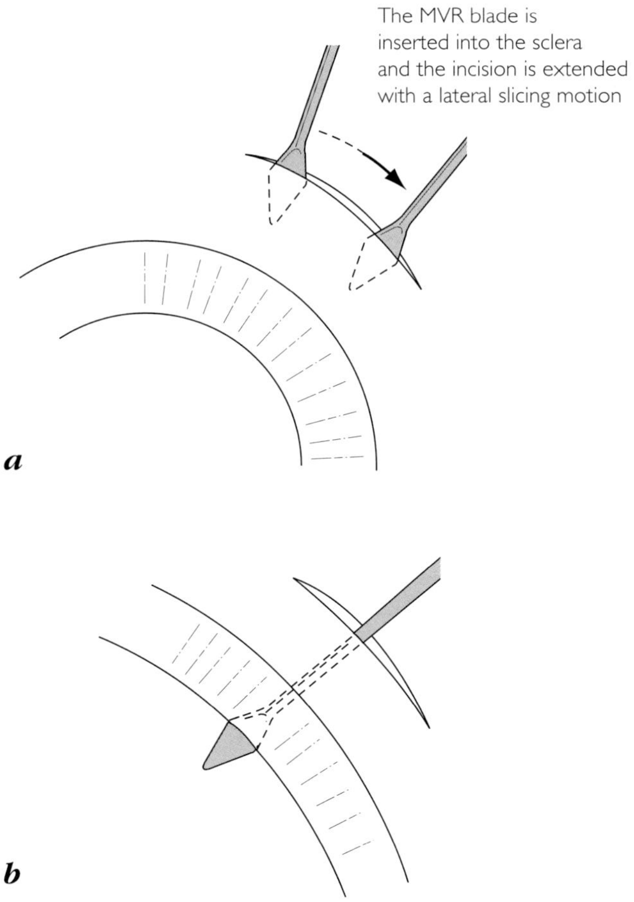

Figure 45.5 *(a) Microvitreoretinal (MVR) blade is slid through the length of the wound. (b) Viewing the tip of the MVR blade through the dilated pupil ensures complete choroidal penetration.*

of the ciliary body (Fig. 45.5). Inevitably, the ciliary body incision is smaller than the scleral incision; this can be rectified by using the MVR blade. It is important to visualize the MVR blade through the pupil in order to avoid incomplete penetration and inadvertent placement of the implant in the suprachoroidal space. Sanborn et al advocate opening the lips of the sclerotomy to ensure that a full-thickness pars plana incision has been made.[25]

After completion of the sclerotomy, a limited external vitrectomy should be performed only on the prolapsed vitreous (Fig. 45.6). Although some surgeons favor mechanical or Weck-cell vitrectomy, automated vitrectomy using a high cutting rate (600 to 750 cuts per minute) and a low aspiration setting (100–150 mmHg) probably causes less traction on the peripheral vitreous. It also allows sample collection for laboratory studies. Only prolapsed vitreous should be removed; do not insert the vitrector into the eye unless it is necessary to remove hemorrhage.

Smooth forceps are used to grasp the implant strut (also called the suture tab) so that the pellet is facing upward to facilitate proper positioning of the implant, with the pellet facing the lens anteriorly and the back of the strut facing the retina posteriorly. As toothed forceps hold open the anterior lip of the sclerotomy, the implant is guided gently into the

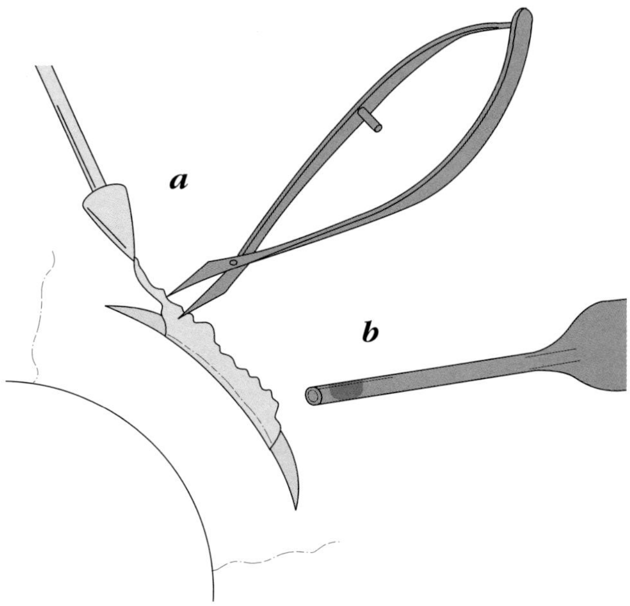

Figure 45.6 *Limited external vitrectomy: (a) mechanical; (b) automated.*

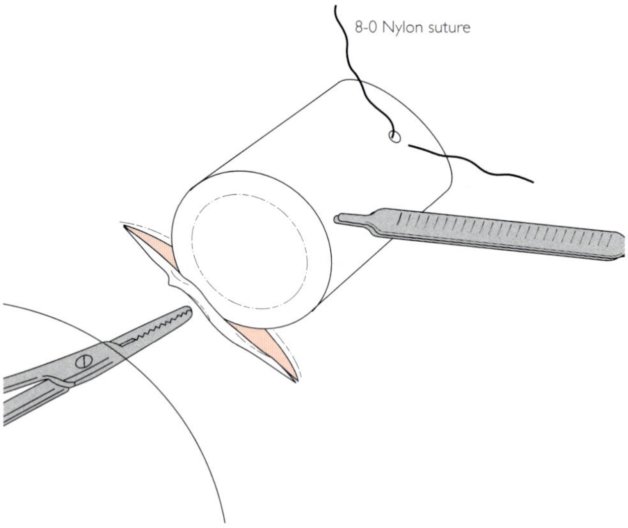

Figure 45.7 *Placement of ganciclovir implant into eye using toothed forceps. Note that the pellet is facing the surgeon.*

vitreous cavity using smooth forceps (with the pellet side toward the cornea) (Fig. 45.7). Care must be taken to avoid brushing the pellet against the sclera or instruments in order to prevent damage to or loss of the coatings responsible for drug delivery.

Once the implant is positioned inside the eye, the preplaced 8-0 nylon suture is used to anchor the implant to the center of the incision. A full-thickness scleral bite is created in the anterior and posterior sclerotomy lips (Fig. 45.8). These must be full-thickness bites to avoid entrapment or exposure of the suture tab in the sclerotomy incision.[26] The two arms of the sutures should be aligned on opposite sides of the incision and tied easily with one triple throw and two single throws. The ends of the knot then are cut long, 3–5 mm, with Vannas scissors. The suture ends are left long so that they may be tucked under the running suture that closes the sclerotomy, to prevent knot erosion through the conjunctiva. The suture should not be tied too tightly because this may induce astigmatism, cause the suture to break or allow the strut to become incarcerated in the wound.

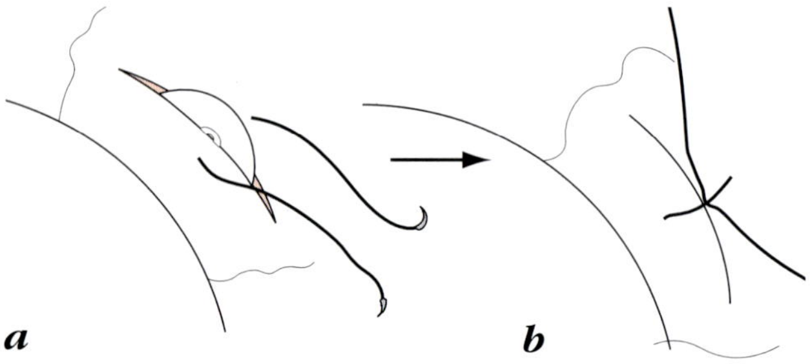

a *b*

Figure 45.8 *(a) Ganciclovir implant positioned in the vitreous cavity. Sutures ends are shown on opposite sides of wound. (b) Anchoring suture is tied and second ends are left long.*

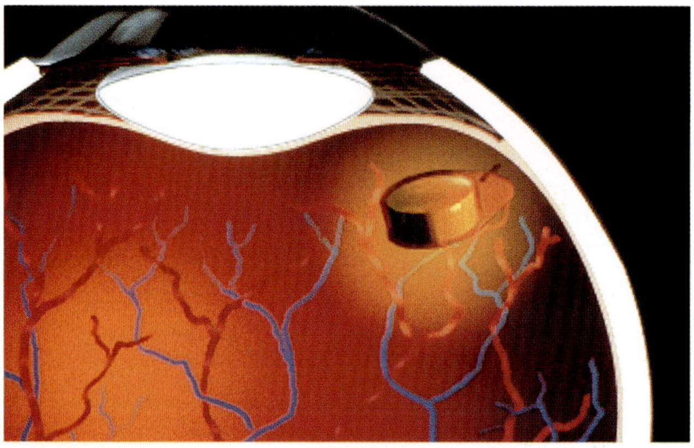

a

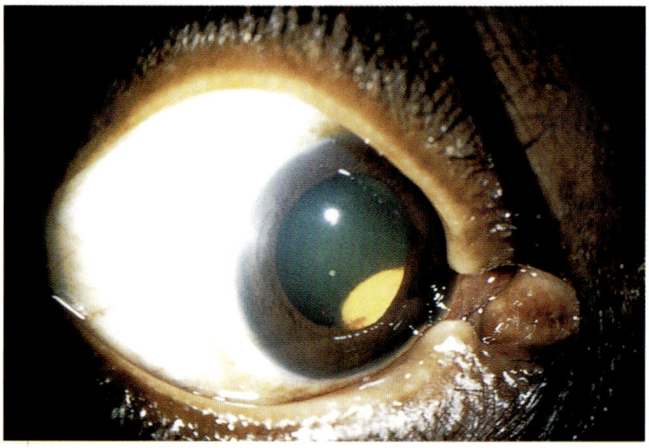

b

Figure 45.9 *(a) Diagram of correctly implanted ganciclovir implant. Notice that the pellet is facing anteriorly, the implantation tab has been shortened to avoid lenticular contact and the medium is clear. (Courtesy of Chiron.) (b) Photograph of a sustained-release ganciclovir implant in the eye. The implant should be visualized behind the lens in the vitreous cavity with the pellet facing anteriorly prior to closing the eye permanently. This is to ensure that the implant has not been placed in the superciliary space. At the end of surgery, the position should be rechecked to ensure that the implant has not moved and there is no retinal detachment.*

After the implant has been secured with the anchoring strut, the eye should be rotated so that the pellet may be visualized in the vitreous cavity (Fig. 45.9). A fiberoptic light source or an indirect ophthalmoscope often is helpful for this maneuver.

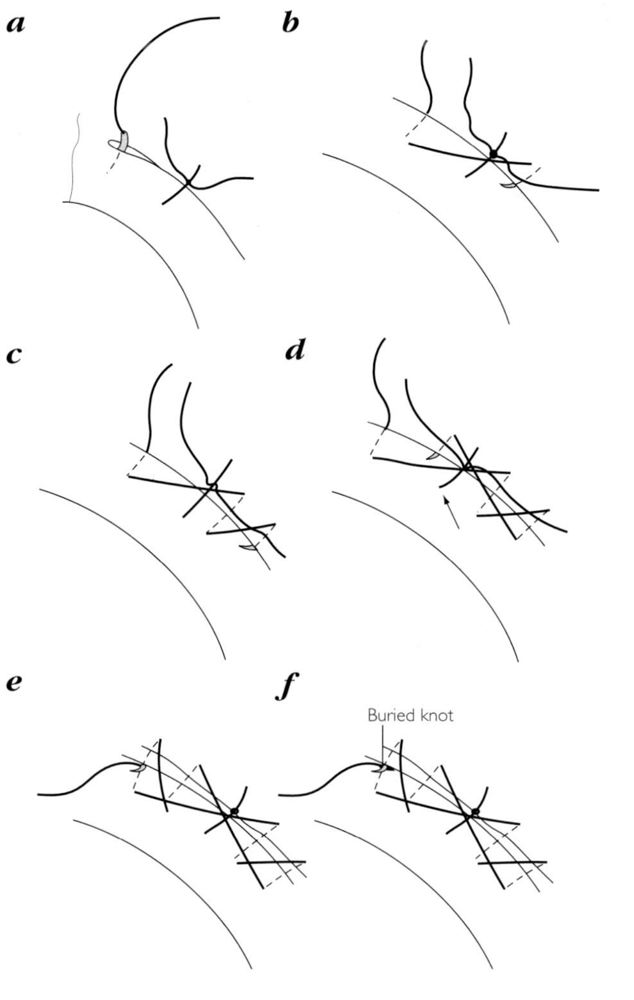

Figure 45.10 *Closure of sclerotomy with single running 8-0 nylon suture. (a) Partial-thickness scleral pass through inside anterior lip of sclerotomy wound. (b) Suture crossing over anchoring suture and starting pass posterior to the incision. (c) Next pass to complete closure at far end of sclerotomy wound. Note that long end of anchoring suture is tucked underneath running suture. (d) Suture direction is reversed and brought back across anchoring suture to start pass posterior to wound. (e) Remaining pass completed. The ends of the suture are opposite each other and inside the wound to allow burial of the knot. (f) Completed running suture. Note that the knot is buried and anchoring suture ends are firmly secured underneath the running suture.*

Once the anchoring suture has been secured, the sclerotomy site can be closed with a running 8-0 nylon suture. There are several different techniques for wound closure. We use a single running suture starting at one end on the inside of the anterior lip of the wound (Fig. 45.10). The sclera can be stabilized with toothed forceps while partial-thickness bites are made. The first pass enters the superior wound edges and exits through the anterior sclera. The running suture then crosses the central anchoring suture and the needle is passed perpendicular to the sclerotomy through both lips of the incision. The surgeon may make two separate bites on either side of the wound or hold the lips of the incision sequentially to complete the scleral pass. Another identical pass is made to close the far end of the sclerotomy site. The suture is brought back across the anchoring suture and another complete pass is made between the anchoring suture and the end of the wound. The running suture is completed by passing the needle through the posterior sclera and exiting from the inside posterior lip across from the initial bite. The suture ends now should be directly opposed. The running suture is tightened by grasping one of the free suture ends while removing slack from the distal suture passes. The suture is tied and cut as described previously, with the knot buried in the wound. Other methods of closure include two figure-of-eight sutures on either side of the anchoring suture or multiple, single interrupted sutures (Fig. 45.11).

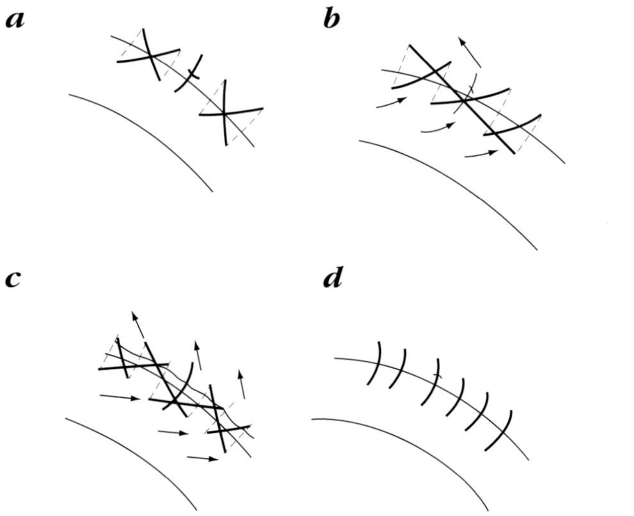

Figure 45.11 *Methods of wound closure. (a) Two 'figure of eight' sutures. (b) Single running suture with three passes up and one back. (c) Single running suture with three passes up and three back. (d) Multiple interrupted sutures.*

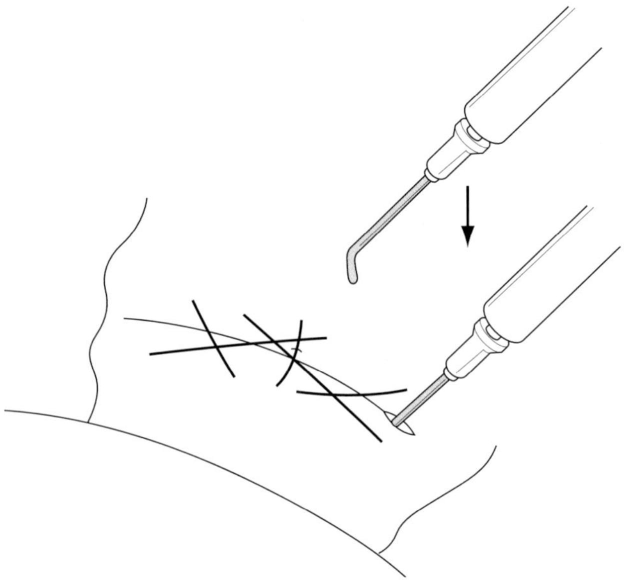

Figure 45.12 *Reformation of the globe with balanced saline solution. Placement of 27- or 30-gauge blunt-tipped cannula in wound prior to tightening sutures.*

Reformation of the globe may be necessary because of the usual loss of some vitreous during surgery. The end of a blunt-tipped 30-gauge cannula is placed through the sclerotomy site to inject sufficient balanced salt solution to restore the globe (Fig. 45.12). The tip of the cannula must be positioned posterior to the strut to avoid disturbing the pellet. Some surgeons advocate using a sharp 27- or 30-gauge needle to inject through a separate site to avoid damaging the sclerotomy site or implant.

After closure of the sclerotomy site, vitreous cutting may be performed again, being cautious about inadvertently cutting the sutures or distorting the wound.

The position of the implant and the condition of the posterior chamber should now be checked with binocular indirect ophthalmoscopy. The implant, if properly positioned, will be visible to the naked eye just behind the lens with rotation of the globe inferotemporally (see Fig. 45.9b).

Finally, the conjunctiva is repositioned and secured with buried interrupted 6-0 and 7-0 Vicryl sutures. The sclerotomy site must be adequately covered by conjunctiva to prevent contact between the lid margins and the sclerotomy wound.

Subconjunctival injections of antibiotics and dexamethasone sodium are administered in the inferior fornix using a 27-gauge needle. A drop of 1% atropine is given before a combination antibiotic–steroid ointment, such as Maxitrol, is placed on the ocular surface. The eye is protected with a soft patch and metal shield.

REPLACING GANCICLOVIR IMPLANTS

The timing and techniques associated with implant replacement are topics of considerable discussion. Standard replacement occurs 6–8 months after implantation of the initial device. The NEI study replaced all implants at 32 weeks.

The first implant is usually placed in the inferotemporal quadrant. Three common approaches to implant exchange have been described in the literature.[27,28] The first approach involves opening the original wound, removing the first device and placing a second one. This procedure appears to work well for the first exchange but continued access through the same incision site may increase the risk of serious complications. Martin et al reported a series of four eyes, three of which developed dense vitreous hemorrhage after receiving a third implant through the same sclerotomy site.[27] Morley et al reported a case in which a patient receiving a third implant at the same site had a wound leak requiring surgical repair with a scleral patch graft.[28] Both authors noted that progressive scleral thinning may occur with repeated exchanges at the same sclerotomy site and that it is prudent to consider a separate location for the third implant.[27,28]

Another approach is to insert the second device next to the first by widening the original incision. The advantage of this technique is that it does not require removal of the first implant. Its disadvantage involves a large pars plana and scleral incision covering a full quadrant of the eye.

The last approach involves the creation of a new site for each subsequent implant. Obviously, available space is a limiting factor in this technique.

A combination of approaches may be required. We usually exchange the device once at the same site and then move on to subsequent sites, beginning inferonasally, for additional implants.

POSTOPERATIVE CARE

On the first postoperative day, the eye should be examined carefully by slit-lamp biomicroscopy to verify the integrity of the sclerotomy site, to ensure adequate conjunctival coverage of the wound and to document the presence of inflammation or vitreous hemorrhage. The intraocular pressure should be measured. The position of the implant and the condition of the retina should be reassessed with indirect ophthalmoscopy. Postoperative topical medications typically include a long-acting dilating agent such as 0.25% hyoscine scopolamine two to three times a day and a broad-spectrum antibiotic such as tobramycin four times a day. Topical steroids such as Pred Forte 1% may be prescribed at the discretion of the surgeon but are usually given four times daily. We like to give Tobradex, an antibiotic–steroid combination, to maximize patient compliance with the drop regimen. It is important to warn the patient of potential signs and symptoms of retinal detachment and endophthalmitis because these complications may occur in the postoperative period.

The patient usually is re-examined after 1 and 3 weeks and the topical medications tapered at the third visit, depending on the clinical examination. Patients should be told to expect a temporary decrease in vision lasting approximately 2–4 weeks because of postoperative astigmatism, inflammation and/or vitreous hemorrhage. Follow-up at 2-week to monthly intervals can be arranged, depending on the patient's condition.

SURGICAL RESULTS

The ganciclovir implant has demonstrated the longest median time (226 days) to progression of CMV retinitis of all FDA-approved treatments for this disease. Left untreated, the median time to progression of CMV retinitis is 15 days.[18] Administration of intravenous ganciclovir, foscarnet or low-dose cidofovir delays the median time to progression to 47, 53 or 64 days, respectively.[4,5] Median time to progression has not yet been successfully delineated in patients receiving high-dose cidofovir, but comparison with ganciclovir implants might be complicated by the recent advancements in AIDS therapy that elevate CD4 counts. The median time to progression with oral ganciclovir is 64 days, which is similar to intravenous therapy.[29]

Oral ganciclovir may be useful as prophylaxis against systemic and contralateral eye disease in patients with implants. This is important, considering that several studies have documented the increased risk of development of CMV retinitis in the fellow untreated eye of those patients with ganciclovir implants. The NEI trial estimated this risk to be 50% over 6 months.[18] The Chiron-sponsored Ganciclovir Implant Study Group (GISG) reported that patients receiving intravenous ganciclovir had half the risk of developing disease in the contralateral eye when compared to patients with implants.[24] In the NEI trial, 13 out of 14 fellow eyes that developed CMV retinitis manifested initial peripheral lesions and ultimately retained 20/25 or better visual acuity throughout the study period.[18] Oral ganciclovir has been shown to provide increased protection to the fellow eye of patients with unilateral disease managed by ganciclovir implant.

Another disadvantage of local therapy is the increased incidence of visceral CMV in patients treated for retinitis with implants as opposed to intravenous therapy. The GISG found that 10.3% of patients with implants developed extraocular disease, versus none receiving systemic therapy. Interestingly, the higher rate of visceral CMV in the implant group did not correlate with increased mortality.[24] Other studies report an even greater percentage of patients (26–31%) developing symptomatic systemic CMV while receiving local treatment with the ganciclovir implant.[17,18] Oral ganciclovir may provide complementary systemic prophylaxis to local therapy.

Visual acuity is decreased temporarily for 2–4 weeks after Vitrasert® implantation. According to the GISG, the disparity in visual acuity between those patients induced with intravenous ganciclovir versus those who received a ganciclovir implant dissipated after 2 weeks and visual acuity levels remained equal throughout the follow-up period of 4 months.[24] The immediate postoperative decline in vision is most often a result of temporary astigmatism induced by the wound and/or transient vitreous hemorrhage derived from the large choroidal incision.[30]

Serious complications of ganciclovir implant surgery include choroidal hemorrhage, cyclodialysis, endophthalmitis, hypotony, hyphema, retinal detachment, retinal tears/holes, severe postoperative inflammation, vitreous hemorrhage, suprachoroidal placement and wound dehiscence.[18,24,31]

The Foscarnet–Ganciclovir Cytomegalovirus Retinitis Trial reported the 6-month cumulative risk of retinal detachment in patients receiving intravenous ganciclovir and foscarnet as 28% and 27%, respectively.[4] The incidence of retinal detachment in eyes receiving ganciclovir implants has been reported as ranging from 11% to 23%.[18,24] Although eyes with ganciclovir implants appear to have a lower incidence of retinal detachment, the NEI trial did note a nonstatistically significant trend toward earlier occurrence of detachments in implant eyes compared to those receiving intravenous therapy. The investigators noticed a correlation between postoperative vitreous detachment and the subsequent development of a retinal detachment. The authors postulated that surgical manipulation of the vitreous might lead to premature posterior vitreous separation that, in turn, can induce retinal tears at the borders of quiescent retinitis.[18] Repair of retinal detachments in patients with CMV retinitis is usually accomplished with vitrectomy and silicone oil tamponade (see Chapter 46).

In the NEI-sponsored ganciclovir implant study, there were no cases of endophthalmitis. However, endophthalmitis was reported in 3 of 177 eyes with ganciclovir implants in the Chiron-sponsored GISG.[24] One case occurred 7 days postoperatively and another 2 months after surgery. The remaining case presented after subsequent cataract extraction and lens implantation. Anand et al reported one case in a series of 30 eyes that developed *Streptococcus pneumoniae* endophthalmitis in the immediate postoperative period.[17]

Vitreous hemorrhage that reduced vision to 5/200 or worse occurred more often after an exchange procedure in the NEI-sponsored trial. In both trials, the vitreous hemorrhages were transient in nature and resolved by 4–6 weeks postoperatively.

SUMMARY

The ganciclovir implant is an important innovation in the treatment of CMV retinitis. It is likely that other sustained-release drug delivery systems will become available and that the cumulative experience with the present device will serve as a guide. Current and future studies with oral ganciclovir and HAART will undoubtedly influence the role of the ganciclovir implant in the treatment of CMV retinitis. At the present time, no other method of drug delivery delays progression of retinitis as long as the ganciclovir implant.

REFERENCES

1. Jabs DA, Enger C, Bartlett JG. Cytomegalovirus retinitis and acquired immunodeficiency syndrome, *Arch Ophthalmol* (1989) **107:**75–80.
2. Hoover DR, Peng Y, Saah A, et al. Occurrence of cytomegalovirus retinitis after human immunodeficiency virus immunosuppression, *Arch Ophthalmol* (1996) **114:**821–7.
3. Felsenstein D, D'Amico DJ, Hirsch MS, et al. Treatment of cytomegalovirus with 9-[2-hydroxy-1-(hydroxymethyl) ethoxymethyl]guanine, *Ann Intern Med* (1985) **103:**377–80.
4. Studies of the Ocular Complications of AIDS Research Group, in collaboration with the AIDS Clinical Trials Group. Foscarnet–Ganciclovir Cytomegalovirus Retinitis Trial 4: visual outcomes, *Ophthalmology* (1994) **101:**1250–61.
5. Studies of the Ocular Complications of AIDS Research Group, in collaboration with the AIDS Clinical Trials Group. Parenteral cidofovir for cytomegalovirus retinitis in patients with AIDS: the HPMPC Peripheral Cytomegalovirus Retinitis Trial, a randomized, controlled trial, *Ann Intern Med* (1997) **126:**264–74.
6. Akler ME, Johnson DW, Burman WJ, Johnson SC. Anterior uveitis and hypotony after intravenous cidofovir for the treatment of cytomegalovirus retinitis, *Ophthalmology* (1998) **105:**651–7.
7. Davis JL, Taskintuna I, Freeman WR, et al. Iritis and hypotony after treatment with intravenous cidofovir for cytomegalovirus retinitis, *Arch Ophthalmol* (1997) **115:**733–7.
8. Kuppermann BD. Therapeutic options for resistant cytomegalovirus retinitis, *J Acquired Immune Defic Syndr Hum Retrovirol* (1997) **14** (Suppl. 1):S13–21.
9. Kuppermann BD, Quiceno JI, Flores-Aguilar M, et al. Intravitreal ganciclovir concentration after intravenous administration in AIDS patients with cytomegalovirus retinitis: implications for therapy, *J Infect Dis* (1993) **168:**1506–9.
10. Ussery FM III, Gibson SR, Conklin RH, et al. Intravitreal ganciclovir in the treatment of AIDS-associated cytomegalovirus, *Ophthalmology* (1988) **95:**640–8.
11. Cantrill HL, Henry K, Melroe NH, et al. Treatment of cytomegalovirus retinitis with intravitreal ganciclovir: long-term results, *Ophthalmology* (1989) **96:**367–74.
12. Diaz-Llopis M, Espana E, Munoz G, et al. High dose intravitreal foscarnet in the treatment of cytomegalovirus retinitis in AIDS, *Br J Ophthalmol* (1994) **78:**120–4.
13. Banker AS, Arevalo JF, Munguia D, et al. Intraocular pressure and aqueous humor dynamics in patients with AIDS treated with intravitreal cidofovir (HPMPC) for cytomegalovirus retinitis, *Am J Ophthalmol* (1997) **124:**168–80.
14. Chavez de la Paz E, Arevalo JF, Kirsch LS, et al. Anterior nongranulomatous uveitis after intravitreal HPMPC (cidofovir) for the treatment of cytomegalovirus retinitis: analysis and prevention, *Ophthalmology* (1997) **104:**539–44. [Published erratum appears in *Ophthalmology* (1997) **104:**1063.]
15. Rahhal FM, Arevalo JF, Munguia D, et al. Intravitreal cidofovir for the maintenance treatment of cytomegalovirus retinitis, *Ophthalmology* (1996) **103:**1078–83.
16. Smith TJ, Pearson PA, Blandford DL, et al. Intravitreal sustained-release ganciclovir, *Arch Ophthalmol* (1992) **110:**255–8.
17. Anand R, Nightingale SD, Fish RH, et al. Control of cytomegalovirus retinitis using sustained release of intraocular ganciclovir, *Arch Ophthalmol* (1993) **111:**223–7.

18. Martin DF, Parks DJ, Mellow SD, et al. Treatment of cytomegalovirus retinitis with an intraocular sustained-release ganciclovir implant: a randomized controlled clinical trial, *Arch Ophthalmol* (1994) **112:**1531–9.
19. Whitcup SM, Fortin E, Nussenblatt RB, et al. Therapeutic effect of combination antiretroviral therapy on cytomegalovirus retinitis (letter), *JAMA* (1997) **277:**1519–20.
20. Jacobson MA, Zegans M, Pavan PR, et al. Cytomegalovirus retinitis after initiation of highly active antiretroviral therapy, *Lancet* (1997) **349:**1443–5.
21. Marx JL, Kapusta MA, Patel SS, et al. Use of the ganciclovir implant in the treatment of recurrent cytomegalovirus retinitis, *Arch Ophthalmol* (1996) **114:**815–20.
22. McAuliffe PF, Hall MJ, Castro-Malaspina H, Heinemann MH. Use of the ganciclovir implant for treating cytomegalovirus retinitis secondary to immunosuppression after bone marrow transplantation, *Am J Ophthalmol* (1997) **123:**702–3.
23. Studies of the Ocular Complications of AIDS Research Group, AIDS Clinical Trials Group. Assessment of cytomegalovirus retinitis: clinical evaluation vs. centralized grading of fundus photographs, *Arch Ophthalmol* (1996) **114:**791–805.
24. Musch DC, Martin DF, Gordon JF, et al. Treatment of cytomegalovirus retinitis with a sustained-release ganciclovir implant, *N Engl J Med* (1997) **337:**83–90.
25. Sanborn GE, Anand R, Torti RE, et al. Sustained-release ganciclovir therapy for treatment of cytomegalovirus retinitis: use of an intravitreal device, *Arch Ophthalmol* (1992) **110:**188–95.
26. Charles NC, Steiner GC. Ganciclovir intraocular implant: a clinicopathologic study, *Ophthalmology* (1996) **103:**416–21.
27. Martin DF, Ferris FL, Parks DJ, et al. Ganciclovir implant exchange: timing, surgical procedure, and complications, *Arch Ophthalmol* (1997) **115:**1389–94.
28. Morley MG, Duker JS, Ashton P, Robinson MR. Replacing ganciclovir implants, *Ophthalmology* (1995) **102:**388–92.
29. Drew WL, Ives D, Lalezari JP, et al. Oral ganciclovir as maintenance treatment for cytomegalovirus retinitis in patients with AIDS, *N Engl J Med* (1995) **333:**615–20.
30. Kertes PJ, Conway MD. *Clinical Trials in Ophthalmology: a Summary and Practice Guide* (Williams & Wilkins: Media, PA, 1998).
31. Virata SR, Kylstra JA. Delayed vitreous hemorrhage after placement of a ganciclovir implant for cytomegalovirus retinitis, *Am J Ophthalmol* (1997) **124:**557–8.

Chapter 46 Surgical repair of retinal detachment associated with viral retinitis

Michael Ip and Jay S Duker

INTRODUCTION

Retinal detachment associated with viral retinitis occurred rarely prior to the onset of the acquired immunodeficiency syndrome (AIDS) epidemic in 1981.[1] Today, viral retinitis caused by cytomegalovirus (CMV) is the most common ocular opportunistic infection found in AIDS patients,[2] and in some urban areas CMV retinitis represents the leading cause of all types of infectious retinitis.

Destruction of the retina by viral infection may lead to retinal breaks that result in retinal detachment in approximately 15–25% of patients with CMV retinitis.[3] Jabs et al reported the cumulative probability of a retinal detachment 1 year following the diagnosis of CMV retinitis to be 50%.[4]

Other types of viral retinitis that may lead to rhegmatogenous retinal detachment include two other members of the herpes family of viruses: herpes simplex (HSV) and varicella-zoster virus (VZV). Both agents have been implicated as a cause of the clinical syndrome known as acute retinal necrosis (ARN).[5] Classically described in healthy, immunocompetent patients, ARN can occur in patients with AIDS and other forms of immunosuppression, such as corticosteroid use, malignancy and chemotherapy.[6]

Although no data are available on the rate of retinal detachment in AIDS patients with ARN, without therapy rhegmatogenous retinal detachment occurs in up to 75% of immunocompetent patients with ARN.[7] A similarly high rate of retinal detachment in immunosuppressed patients with ARN is suggested by several authorities.[5,8] Recently, a distinct clinical entity, the progressive outer retinal necrosis (PORN) syndrome has been associated with VZV retinitis. Seen almost exclusively in the setting of severe immunosuppression associated with AIDS, the rate of retinal detachment is as high as 70%.[9] Other than the herpes family of viruses, retinitis caused by other viruses leads to retinal detachment extraordinarily rarely.

The repair of retinal detachment in the setting of viral retinitis presents unique challenges to the vitreoretinal surgeon. Widespread retinal necrosis often results in multiple posterior breaks. Many of the breaks are small and difficult to localize because of the widespread retinal atrophy and the accompanying alterations in the underlying retinal pigment epithelium.[10] Additional breaks may form in old areas of retinal necrosis following the initial surgical procedure, necessitating reoperation. Reactivation of disease may occur following surgery as well, leading to new areas of necrosis and subsequent redetachment following successful surgery. Finally, the severe inflammation noted most prominently in immunocompetent patients with ARN can produce severe postinflammatory fibrosis and scarring, compromising the anatomic result.[7]

INDICATIONS

The choice of surgical technique is determined by the configuration and complexity of the retinal detachment. However, in AIDS patients, the treatment modality should be tempered by such additional factors as the general health of the patient, status of the fellow eye, visual prognosis of the detached eye and life expectancy. It is important to involve the patient and family in a discussion of whether or not to operate, which treatment modality to use and the realistic expectations of visual recovery.

In macula-sparing retinal detachments caused by CMV retinitis, delimiting laser photocoagulation can be used as an initial treatment.[11] Orellana et al reported a 77% success rate in halting the progression of CMV-related retinal detachments with laser therapy alone.[12] Long-term follow-up in this series of patients was unavailable because the median survival time was 2 months. Other studies with follow-up to 2 years demonstrated that laser treatment prevents the progression of retinal detachment in 48% of patients and reduces the need for surgical intervention.[13] No data are available concerning laser treatment of retinal detachment in ARN, but several studies indicate that prophylactic laser treatment applied to the posterior aspect of involved retina prior to the onset of retinal detachment can reduce the subsequent incidence to 17% or less.[14,15]

In retinal detachment related to CMV without active disease, scleral buckling alone may be attempted if only small, peripheral areas of retina are involved by the retinitis or if an obvious traction-related break can be localized.[12,16] Scleral buckling may be suited particularly to detachments caused by peripheral patches of CMV retinitis anterior to the equator that can be supported fully by scleral indentation. Anecdotally, pneumatic retinopexy does not appear to be a good alternative for the majority of viral-related retinal detachments, although no large series have been published.

Pars plana vitrectomy with silicone oil injection is currently the most widely accepted technique of retinal detachment repair in the setting of viral retinitis.[17–19] This is particularly true when the retinal anatomy is complex with large areas of retinal necrosis, multiple posterior breaks and/or the presence of proliferative vitreoretinopathy (PVR). The majority of cases of viral retinitis with rhegmatogenous retinal detachment are complicated by one or more of these features.

The use of vitrectomy and silicone oil tamponade for retinal detachment repair is generally reserved for rhegmatogenous retinal detachments involving or threatening the macula.[19] Pars plana vitrectomy with silicone oil injection is also the procedure of choice in nearly all monocular patients, including those with small peripheral rhegmatogenous retinal detachments. Finally, patients should have a reasonable life expectancy to warrant the inconvenience and discomfort of surgery.

The use of silicone oil induces 4–7 diopters of hyperopia in phakic patients, often requiring the postoperative use of a contact lens, which may be difficult in certain debilitated patients with AIDS.[18] Cataracts develop in essentially 100% of phakic eyes following the instillation of silicone oil, usually between 6 and 18 months after placement. Additionally, the long-term risks of glaucoma and keratopathy are well known, although less prevalent when silicone oil is used in phakic or pseudophakic eyes.[20] Despite these risks, silicone oil is currently the tamponade of choice. Patients with AIDS tend to have marked systemic morbidity and a shortened life expectancy. The use of silicone oil affords the highest possibility of permanent reattachment in a single operation.[19] In contrast to intraocular gas, return of visual function is rapid and postoperative ambulation is not restricted by face-down positioning. Silicone oil allows a superior view of the retina, both intraoperatively and postoperatively, when compared with a gas tamponade. The use of silicone oil as a permanent tamponade often avoids the necessity of placing a scleral buckle, thus greatly simplifying the procedure.

Elimination of an encircling band also minimizes patient discomfort caused by additional tissue manipulation and minimizes the risk of an accidental needle stick to the surgeon. Garcia et al demonstrated similar reattachment rates for patients undergoing pars plana vitrectomy, silicone oil injection and endolaser with or without scleral buckling for CMV-related retinal detachments.[21] Postoperative visual acuity, final visual acuity and degree of postoperative refractive error did not differ significantly whether or not a scleral buckle was used.

PREOPERATIVE EVALUATION

The diagnosis of viral retinitis is clinical. Ophthalmoscopic examination remains the cornerstone diagnostic test. Each of the three main clinical patterns of viral retinitis-associated retinal detachments (ARN, CMV and PORN) have sufficiently distinguishing clinical characteristics such that, in the majority of cases, a clinical diagnosis can be made. Although the differentiation of these entities is critical for proper medical therapy, generally the surgical approach is not altered on the basis of the etiologic agent alone.

Cytomegalovirus retinitis spreads slowly, classically in one of two patterns.[22] The first pattern is called hemorrhagic and is characterized by broad zones of geographic retinal whitening in close proximity to major retinal blood vessels, with associated retinal hemorrhage. The second pattern is termed brushfire and is characterized by focal granular infiltrates that enlarge slowly across a line, leaving necrotic areas of retina behind. Documented CMV viremia does not confirm the diagnosis of CMV retinitis because the majority of immunosuppressed patients at risk for CMV retinitis demonstrate serological or culture evidence of the virus in body fluids.[23] Polymerase chain reaction (PCR) detection of CMV sequences in aqueous and/or vitreous samples has increased sensitivity but does not confirm unequivocally the diagnosis of CMV retinitis.

Acute retinal necrosis, in contrast to CMV retinitis, classically occurs in immunocompetent patients. Patients present with a triad of posterior segment findings: retinal and choroidal vasculitis, retinal necrosis and vitritis.[24] There is a predilection for the retinal necrosis to involve initially the peripheral retina, with spread to the macula occurring as a late finding. The patches of peripheral retinal necrosis eventually coalesce into broad geographic areas. Vitritis is such a consistent feature of ARN that, in its absence, the diagnosis is suspect. Acute retinal necrosis typically can be differentiated from CMV on the basis of the above-mentioned clinical characteristics, as well as from immune status. When ARN occurs in AIDS patients, the differentiation between the two entities may be more difficult, but ARN patients with AIDS typically have CD4+ counts greater than 60 cells/mm^3 and most have a preceding history of dermatomal herpes zoster or herpes simplex dermatitis.[22]

Serum viral titers to HSV and VZV are generally not helpful in securing the diagnosis because ARN represents a local ocular reactivation of a prior systemic viral infection.[24] Again, PCR detection of viral sequences cannot unequivocally confirm the diagnosis. Fluorescein angiography demonstrates poor retinal perfusion in areas of active retinitis, as well as blockage of the underlying choroidal fluorescence. This is useful in documenting the extent of the infection but the angiographic pattern is not diagnostic.

The PORN syndrome occurs in immunosuppressed patients with a median CD4+ count of 21 cells/mm^3.[9] Characteristic findings include multiple discrete areas of deep retinal opacification that develop in the macula in 33% of patients. There is extremely rapid progression to confluence, resulting in large areas of full-thickness necrosis. The PORN syndrome can be distinguished from CMV retinitis on the basis of multifocality, lack of hemorrhage, absence of vitreous cells and rapid spread. Features that help distinguish PORN from ARN include early involvement of the outer retina, lack of arteritis and absence of significant vitritis. Furthermore, ARN, even in patients with AIDS, typically presents with higher CD4+ counts, as mentioned above.

INSTRUMENTATION

Standard instrumentation required for the repair of rhegmatogenous retinal detachment associated with viral retinitis is discussed elsewhere. The vitrectomy system should provide for cutting, aspiration, illumination and infusion. Capabilities for phacofragmentation should be available if a pars plana lensectomy is required for access to the area of the vitreous base in cases where anterior PVR is prominent. An endophotocoagulation system is required to wall-off areas of necrotic retina and for retinotomies and/or retinectomies. Silicone oil of 5000 or 1000 centistoke (cSt) viscosity should be available, although 5000 cSt silicone oil is generally preferred because it is associated with a lower incidence of glaucoma and is more resistant to emulsification.[25]

SURGICAL TECHNIQUES

The typical surgical approach to viral retinitis-related retinal detachment begins with a standard, bimanual, three-port vitrectomy (Fig. 46.1). Twenty-gauge vitrectomy surgical instruments are used. If a spontaneous posterior vitreous detachment is present, the posterior hyaloid is identified and resected to the posterior margin of the vitreous base. Often, a

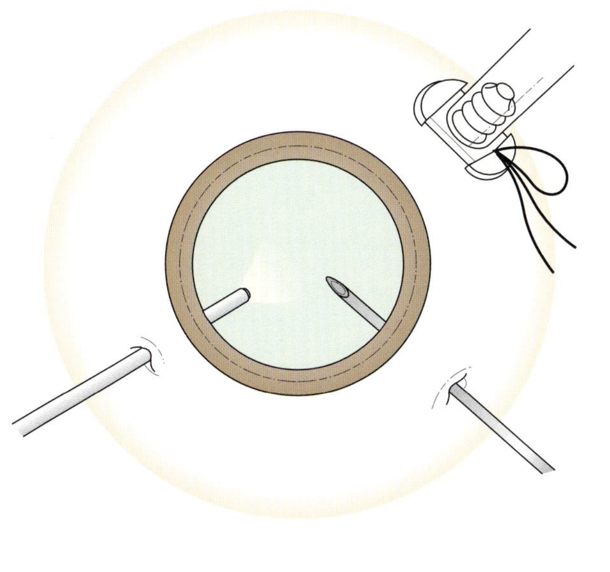

Figure 46.1 *A standard three-port vitrectomy.*

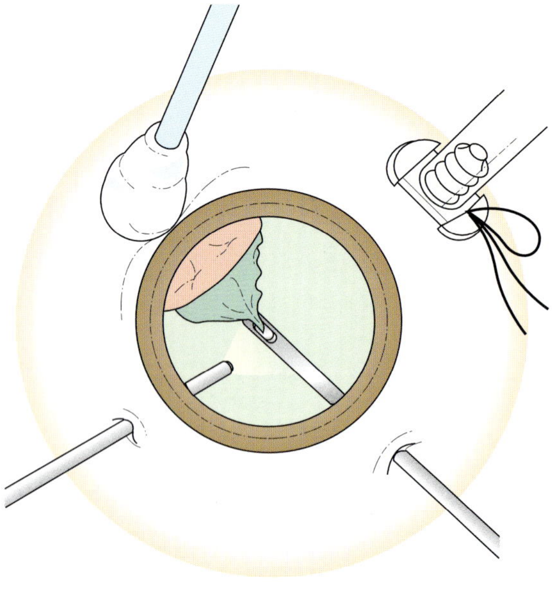

Figure 46.2 *Removal of peripheral vitreous base using scleral depression or wide-field lenses.*

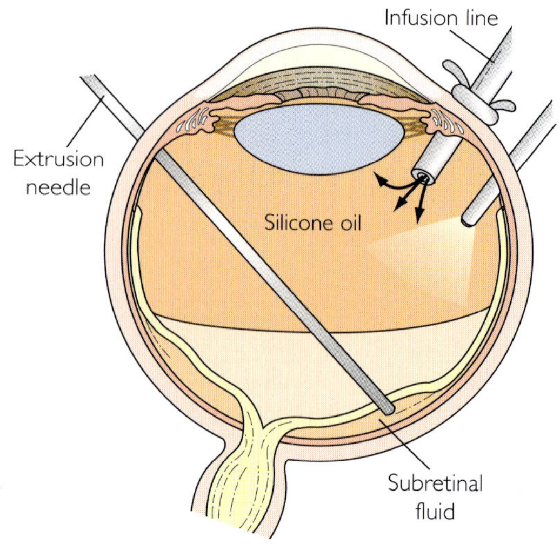

Figure 46.4 *Internal drainage via posterior break using silicone oil–fluid exchange.*

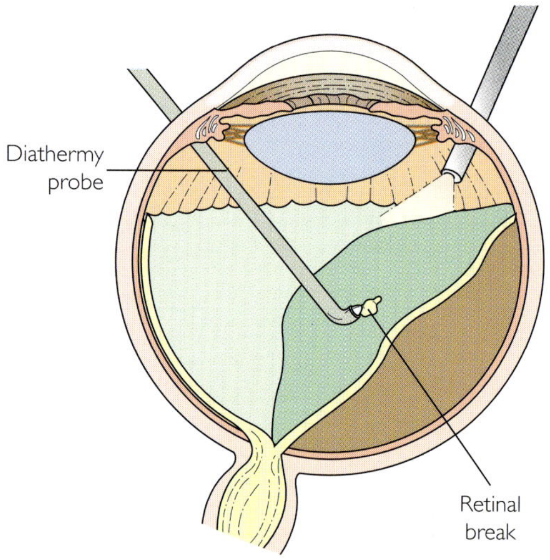

Figure 46.3 *Marking of intraocular breaks with diathermy or bipolar probe.*

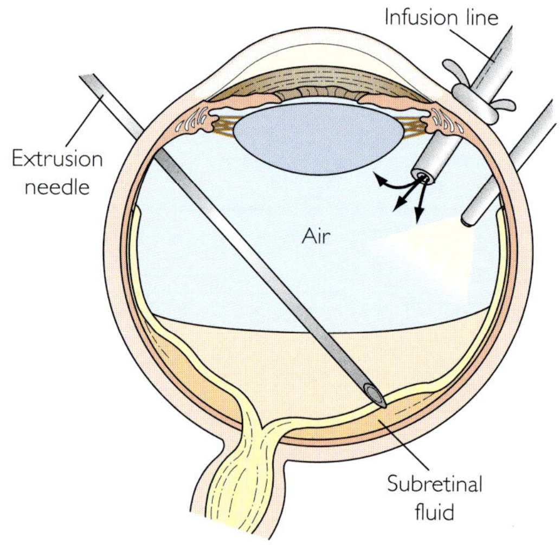

Figure 46.5 *Internal drainage via posterior retinotomy using air–fluid exchange.*

complete posterior vitreous detachment is not present because viral retinitis-related detachments occur in younger age groups. Thus, the posterior hyaloid is engaged with either a soft-tipped cannula or the vitreous cutter and removed from the retinal surface. Removal of as much vitreous cortex as possible is attempted in cases where a posterior vitreous detachment is not possible (Fig. 46.2). Retinal breaks are identified and marked with internal diathermy to facilitate later identification (Fig. 46.3).

Two techniques of internal drainage of subretinal fluid can be employed: air–fluid exchange or direct silicone oil–fluid exchange (Fig. 46.4). Internal drainage is achieved by either placing a soft-tipped extrusion cannula within a pre-existing posterior retinal break or through a retinotomy site created with a diathermy probe in cases where retinal breaks are anterior or difficult to locate (Fig. 46.5). Heavy liquids (i.e. perfluorocarbons) are rarely necessary in these cases and, in the setting of large areas of thin, atrophic retina, can lead to subretinal perfluorocarbon.

Air–fluid exchange is preferable when a pressure-controlled silicone oil pump is unavailable, or when the retina is highly bullous. A flute needle or extrusion needle is placed through a posterior retinotomy into the subretinal space and the subretinal fluid is evacuated as air is forced into the eye under pressure. Following a complete air fill, silicone oil is injected with either a hand injector or a pressure-controlled power injector through a short 20-gauge straight cannula or via the infusion cannula. A power injector is always preferable to hand injection because the proper silicone fill is easier to obtain and, more importantly, it is possible to perform additional intraocular maneuvers (membrane peeling, retinotomy) in the oil-filled eye. The eye is tilted so that the infusion cannula is at the highest point, in order to achieve maximum silicone oil fill (Fig. 46.6). After a complete oil fill, the eye should be re-entered to confirm that the retina remains attached and no additional membrane peeling, laser or retinectomy is necessary.

Alternatively, a direct silicone oil–fluid exchange can be performed. This can be done only with a pressure-controlled silicone oil injector. Such a technique saves the extra step of air–fluid exchange but, in the presence of large amounts of subretinal fluid, can be more time consuming.

After evacuation of all subretinal fluid, argon laser endophotocoagulation then is applied in triple-row fashion along all breaks and zones of retinitis or necrosis (Fig. 46.7). Any silicone oil remaining on the surface of the eye is removed with saline irrigation as the sclerotomies are closed simultaneously in standard fashion.

A lensectomy is needed rarely in these cases unless the cataract is severe enough to preclude an adequate view of the retina. In this setting, lens removal via phacoemulsification from a scleral tunnel is the preferred method because it preserves an intact posterior capsule and allows intraocular lens placement. A foldable acrylic lens can be used; foldable silicone lenses should be avoided. Alternatively, pars plana lensectomy can be performed. The anterior capsule should be kept intact, if at all possible. If an eye is left aphakic, then an inferior peripheral iridectomy must be performed to prevent angle-closure glaucoma and silicone migration into the anterior chamber. In phakic and pseudophakic eyes, peripheral iridectomy is not necessary.

The surgical technique used for the repair of retinal detachment associated with ARN in immunocompetent patients is adjusted for the higher incidence of PVR in these cases. A standard, bimanual, three-port vitrectomy is performed. Removal of as much vitreous cortex as possible is attempted. Posterior epiretinal

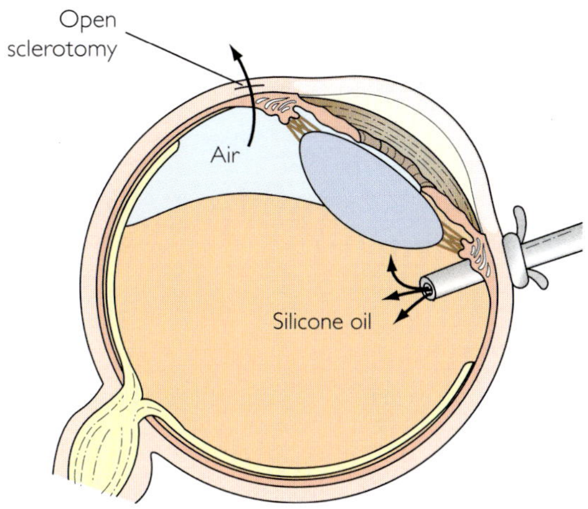

Figure 46.6 *During silicone oil infusion, the eye is tilted so that the nasal sclerotomy is superior in order to maximize silicone fill.*

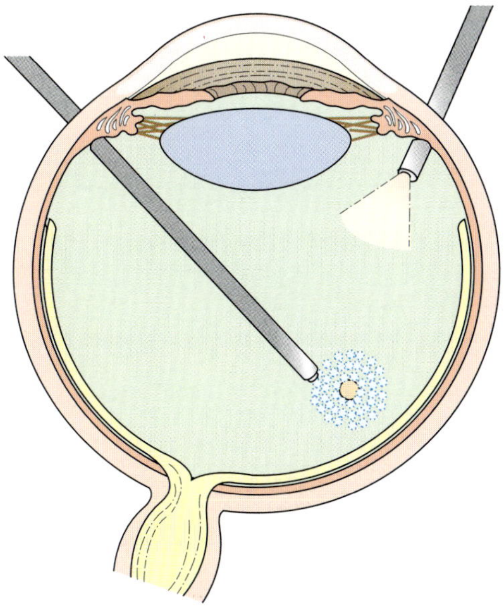

Figure 46.7 *Endophotocoagulation applied in triple-row along retinal breaks and posterior retinotomy.*

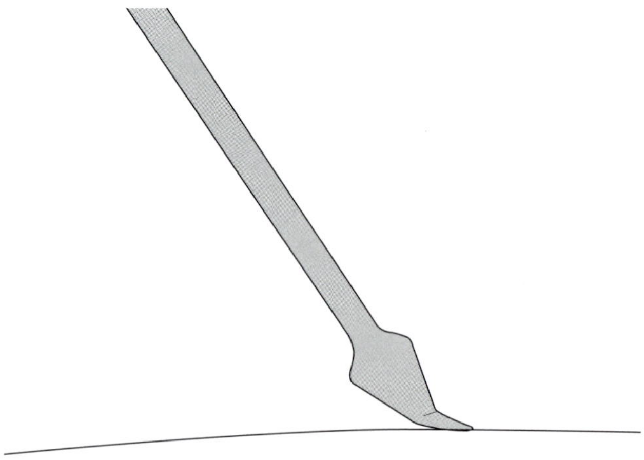

Figure 46.8 *Microvitreoretinal blade, bent at a 45° angle, used for membrane peel.*

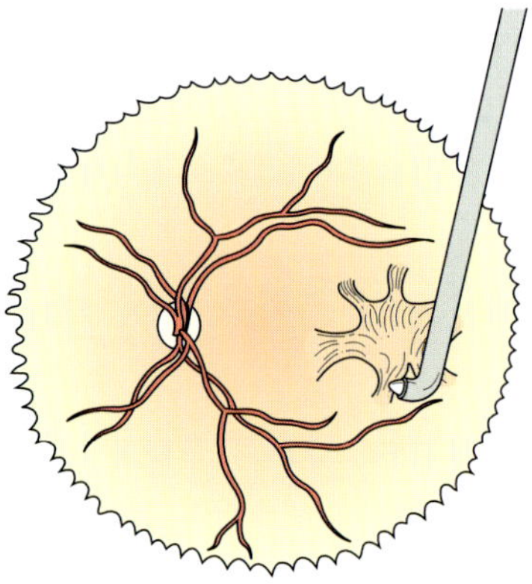

Figure 46.9 *A pick or forceps can be used for membrane peel.*

membranes, if present, are delaminated with a bent microvitreoretinal blade (Fig. 46.8) or with standard picks and forceps (Fig. 46.9).

If anterior PVR is present, pars plana lensectomy may be required to facilitate exposure. Scleral depression with a cotton-tipped applicator may be used to help expose the vitreous base, as well as to stabilize any mobile detached retina. This allows the vitreous cutter and/or retinal picks to be placed in closer proximity to the retinal surface, resulting in maximal removal of vitreous gel and scar tissue.

Once traction from anterior and/or posterior PVR has been released, air–fluid exchange followed by air–silicone oil exchange with endophotocoagulation as described above is performed. If the retina does not flatten with air–fluid exchange, three options are available: adding (or augmenting) a scleral buckle, additional membrane peeling or relaxing retinectomy. Routine use of an encircling scleral buckle in cases of ARN may not be necessary and may lead to a higher incidence of postoperative complications.

SURGICAL RESULTS

The high rate of anatomic success cited in the literature is tempered by the lesser proportion of patients achieving ambulatory vision. However, in recent years, visual results have improved. This may be attributed to earlier intervention, selection of cases without macular or optic nerve involvement, better antiviral therapies and improved surgical technique.

Freeman et al achieved a 100% anatomic success rate in CMV-related detachments treated with vitrectomy and silicone oil.[26] Visual outcome data were limited by a short postoperative follow-up period. Sidikaro reported a 91% anatomic success rate in viral retinitis-related retinal detachment treated by a variety of techniques, including pneumatic retinopexy, scleral buckling and vitrectomy with silicone oil.[27] The visual benefit of surgery was limited in most patients by progression of viral retinitis. Median survival after diagnosis of retinal detachment was 17 weeks.

Jabs et al reported a 70% reattachment rate using vitrectomy with silicone oil as the initial surgical procedure.[4] Visual outcome was disappointing because only 20% of eyes attained ambulatory vision. Median survival time after diagnosis of retinal detachment was 9 months. A 100% reattachment rate was reported by Regillo et al using vitrectomy and silicone oil for viral retinitis-associated retinal detachment.[19] Ambulatory vision was preserved in 75% of patients and was related strongly to a preoperative visual acuity of count fingers or better. More recently, Davis et al evaluated 407 eyes and reported a 73% anatomic success rate with pars plana vitrectomy and silicone oil for retinal detachment secondary to necrotizing retinitis.[18] Sixty-eight percent of eyes achieved ambulatory vision. Despite a large percentage of patients achieving ambulatory vision, a small proportion (12%) of patients had vision of 20/55 or better. Poor final vision may result from a variety of causes, including macular detachment, media opacity, macular retinitis, optic nerve atrophy and silicone oil complications.

Although anatomic reattachment can be achieved in the overwhelming majority of cases using advanced surgical techniques, useful postoperative vision is best correlated with good preoperative visual acuity.[19] Other factors that may be considered include the extent of retinal detachment, presence of active viral infection and overall health of the patient.

Studies examining the results of retinal detachment surgery in ARN patients demonstrate similar findings to those discussed above, in whom the majority of patients were treated for CMV-related detachments. Clarkson et al reported a 70% rate of reattachment using vitrectomy and silicone oil in 1984.[7] Visual function was limited by optic atrophy and macular pucker. In 1988, Blumenkranz et al reported a 100% anatomic success rate, with 5/6 patients achieving ambulatory vision.[28]

More recently, McDonald et al reported reattachment in 89% of eyes treated with vitrectomy and silicone oil.[29] Fifty-six percent of patients achieved ambulatory vision. Poor visual outcome resulted from optic nerve and macular disease. Visual results are perhaps improved in the more recent studies as a result of earlier recognition and awareness of ARN, the use of antiviral therapy, more timely surgical intervention and better surgical technique.

REFERENCES

1. Hennis HL, Scott AA, Apple DJ. Cytomegalovirus retinitis, *Surv Ophthalmol* (1989) **34:**193–203.
2. Schuman JS, Orellana J, Friedman AH, Teich SA. Acquired immunodeficiency syndrome (AIDS), *Surv Ophthalmol* (1987) **31:**384–410.
3. Freeman WR, Quiceno JI, Crapotta JA, et al. Surgical repair of rhegmatogenous retinal detachment in immunosuppressed patients with cytomegalovirus retinitis, *Ophthalmology* (1992) **99:**466–74.
4. Jabs DA, Enger C, Haller J, de Bustros S. Retinal detachments in patients with cytomegalovirus retinitis, *Arch Ophthalmol* (1991) **109:**794–9.
5. Freeman WR, Thomas EL, Rao NA, et al. Demonstration of herpes group virus in acute retinal necrosis syndrome, *Am J Ophthalmol* (1986) **102:**701–9.
6. Chess J, Marcus DM. Zoster-related bilateral acute retinal necrosis syndrome as presenting sign in AIDS, *Ann Ophthalmol* (1988) **20:**431–5.
7. Clarkson JG, Blumenkranz MS, Culbertson WW, et al. Retinal detachment following the acute retinal necrosis syndrome, *Ophthalmology* (1984) **91:**1665–8.
8. Jabs DA, Schachat AP, Liss R, et al. Presumed varicella zoster retinitis in immunocompromised patients, *Retina* (1987) **7:**9–13.
9. Engstrom RE Jr, Holland GN, Margolis TP, et al. The progressive outer retinal necrosis syndrome: a variant of necrotizing herpetic retinopathy in patients with AIDS, *Ophthalmology* (1994) **101:**1488–1502.
10. Holland GN. The management of retinal detachments in patients with acquired immunodeficiency syndrome (editorial), *Arch Ophthalmol* (1991) **109:**791–3.
11. Vrabec TR. Laser photocoagulation repair of macula-sparing cytomegalovirus-related retinal detachment, *Ophthalmology* (1997) **104:**2062–7.
12. Orellana J, Teich SA, Lieberman RM, et al. Treatment of retinal detachments in patients with the acquired immune deficiency syndrome, *Ophthalmology* (1991) **98:**939–43.
13. Davis JL, Hummer J, Feuer WJ. Laser photocoagulation for retinal detachments and retinal tears in cytomegalovirus retinitis, *Ophthalmology* (1997) **104:**2053–61.
14. Han DP, Lewis H, Williams GA, et al. Laser photocoagulation in the acute retinal necrosis syndrome, *Arch Ophthalmol* (1987) **105:**1051–4.
15. Sternberg P Jr, Han DP, Yeo JH, et al. Photocoagulation to prevent retinal detachment in acute retinal necrosis, *Ophthalmology* (1988) **95:**1389–93.
16. Kuppermann BD, Flores-Aguilar M, Quiceno JI, et al. A masked prospective evaluation of outcome parameters for cytomegalovirus-related retinal detachment surgery in patients with acquired immune deficiency syndrome, *Ophthalmology* (1994) **101:**46–55.
17. Chuang EL, Davis JL. Management of retinal detachment associated with CMV retinitis in AIDS patients, *Eye* (1992) **6** (1):28–34.
18. Davis JL, Serfass MS, Lai MY, et al. Silicone oil in repair of retinal detachments caused by necrotizing retinitis in HIV infection, *Arch Ophthalmol* (1995) **113:**1401–9.
19. Regillo CD, Vander JF, Duker JS, et al. Repair of retinitis-related retinal detachments with silicone oil in patients with acquired immunodeficiency syndrome, *Am J Ophthalmol* (1992) **113:**21–7.
20. Federman JL, Schubert HD. Complications associated with the use of silicone oil in 150 eyes after retina-vitreous surgery, *Ophthalmology* (1988) **95:**870–6.
21. Garcia RF, Flores-Aguilar M, Quiceno JI, et al. Results of rhegmatogenous retinal detachment repair in cytomegalovirus retinitis with and without scleral buckling, *Ophthalmology* (1995) **102:**236–45.
22. Kim VY, Duker JS. Ocular manifestations of human immunodeficiency virus, *Semin Ophthalmol* (1996) **11:**93–106.
23. Bloom JN, Palestine AG. The diagnosis of cytomegalovirus retinitis, *Ann Intern Med* (1988) **109:**963–9.
24. Duker JS, Blumenkranz MS. Diagnosis and management of the acute retinal necrosis (ARN) syndrome, *Surv Ophthalmol* (1991) **35:**327–43.
25. Heidenkummer HP, Kampik A, Thierfelder S. Emulsification of silicone oils with specific physicochemical characteristics, *Graefes Arch Clin Exp Ophthalmol* (1991) **229:**88–94.
26. Freeman WR, Henderly DE, Wan LW, et al. Prevalence, pathophysiology, and treatment of rhegmatogenous retinal detachment in treated cytomegalovirus retinitis, *Am J Ophthalmol* (1987) **103:**527–36.
27. Sidikaro Y, Silver L, Holland GN, Kreiger AE. Rhegmatogenous retinal detachments in patients with AIDS and necrotizing retinal infections, *Ophthalmology* (1991) **98:**129–35.

28. Blumenkranz M, Clarkson J, Culbertson WW, et al. Vitrectomy for retinal detachment associated with acute retinal necrosis, *Am J Ophthalmol* (1988) **106:**426–9.

29. McDonald HR, Lewis H, Kreiger AE, et al. Surgical management of retinal detachment associated with the acute retinal necrosis syndrome, *Br J Ophthalmol* (1991) **75:**455–8.

Part XIII Latest Surgical Techniques

Chapter 47 Foveal translocation

Robert J Kraut and Gholam A Peyman

INTRODUCTION

Age-related macular degeneration (ARMD) is one of the leading causes of irreversible vision loss in the USA and worldwide.[1,2] The treatment options for exudative ARMD are limited. Photocoagulation has been shown to reduce the risk of severe vision loss from extrafoveal and juxtafoveal choroidal neovascular membranes.[3,4] However, photocoagulation of subfoveal choroidal neovascularization (CNV) causes immediate, irreversible, severe vision loss.[5,6] Subfoveal surgery for the removal of CNV has been beneficial in patients with presumed ocular histoplasmosis, but not for patients with ARMD.[7–11] Radiation therapy,[12,13] interferon[14,15] and retinal pigment epithelium (RPE) transplantation[16,17] are other modalities that have not been shown to be effective in treating subfoveal CNV secondary to ARMD. Photodynamic therapy (PDT) is a promising experimental treatment for subfoveal CNV. However, a recent report shows a 50% recurrence rate at 4 weeks.[18]

In 1993, Machemer and Steinhorst performed foveal translocation in humans with subfoveal CNV and ARMD.[19] The procedure was first performed in animals and reported by Lindsey et al in 1983[20] and Tiedeman et al in 1985.[21] Because the RPE–Bruch's membrane–choriocapillaris complex is damaged in ARMD, Machemer reasoned that shifting the fovea to an area with healthy RPE would allow visual recovery. Machemer and Steinhorst reported the procedure in three patients with ARMD and recent submacular hemorrhage.

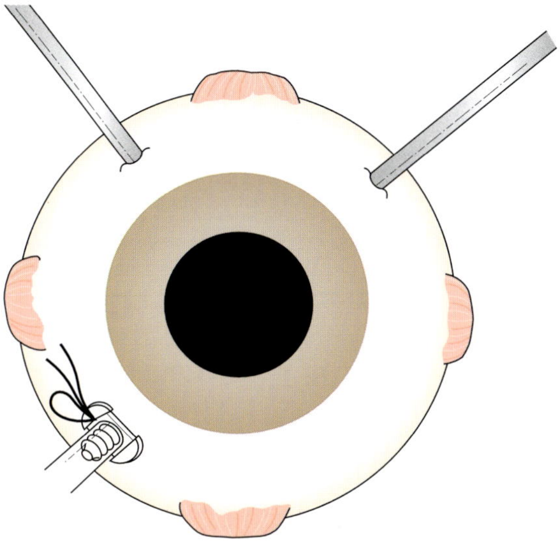

Figure 47.1 *Position of vitrectomy instruments and fiberoptic probe in relation to infusion cannula.*

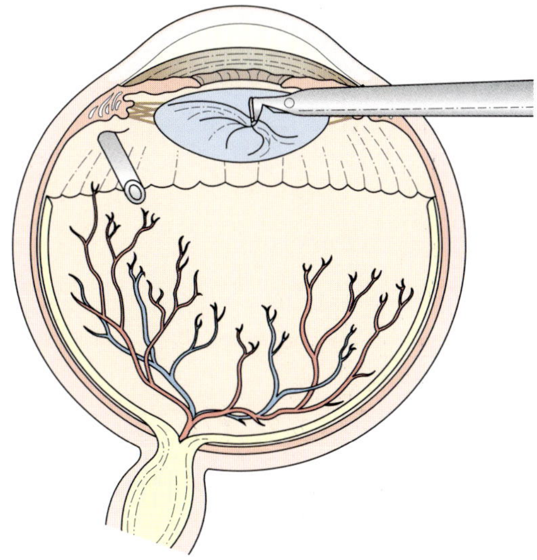

Figure 47.2 *Pars plana lensectomy with port directed posteriorly to preserve anterior capsule.*

TECHNIQUES

After a 360° peritomy was performed, an intravitreal infusion was inserted at the pars plana in the inferotemporal quadrant. Two additional pars plana sclerotomies were made at 10 and 2 o'clock (Fig. 47.1). A lensectomy followed in order to gain access to the peripheral retina (Fig. 47.2). A total retinal detachment

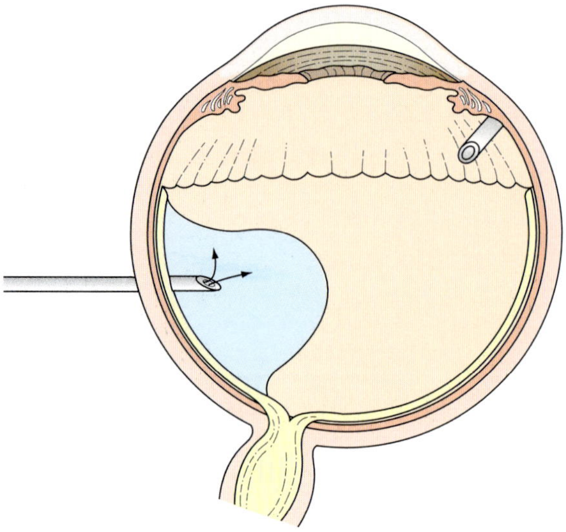

Figure 47.3 *A 27-gauge needle attached to a separate infusion is guided into the subretinal space under direct microscopic visualization. Retinal detachment is created by raising the subretinal infusion bottle while simultaneously lowering the vitreous infusion bottle.*

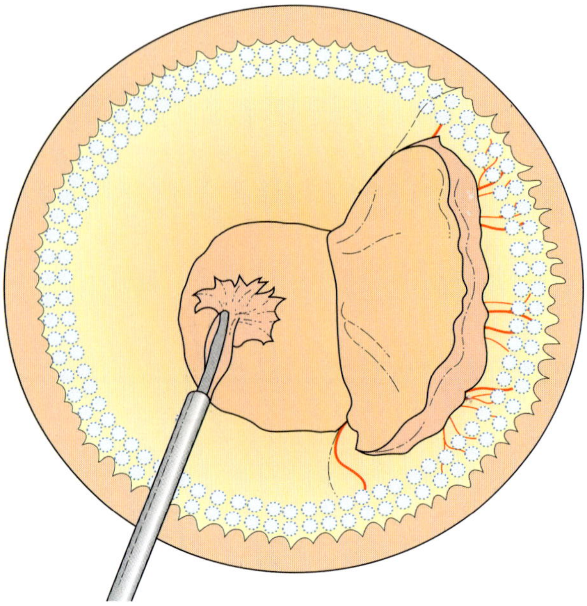

Figure 47.5 *Graphic depiction of the technique for removal of subfoveal choroidal neovascularization with forceps.*

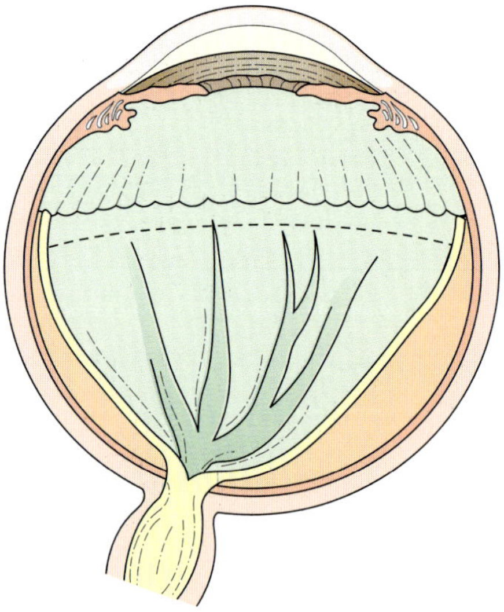

Figure 47.4 *Dotted line indicates the location of incision for anterior retinotomy.*

was created by an exterior approach. A 27-gauge needle attached to a separate infusion line perforated the sclera and choroid and was then held in the subretinal space. If retinal perforation occurred, the needle was retracted and held tangentially to the eye. Once the needle was in the subretinal space, the infusion was started (Fig. 47.3). The subretinal infusion was raised by elevating the bottle as the intravitreal infusion was decreased by lowering the other bottle. This resulted in the formation of a total retinal detachment.

Once the retina had been detached, Machemer and Steinhorst performed a 360° retinotomy with the vitreous cutter (Fig. 47.4) as peripherally as possible. The retina was folded over and the subretinal membrane and blood removed with a pick, scissors or forceps (Fig. 47.5). The retina was unfolded and an air–fluid exchange performed. Use of the original scleral perforation was avoided because of the risk of incarceration. The retina was then rotated clockwise or counter-clockwise by applying suction to the periphery with a soft-tipped flute needle (Fig. 47.6). Machemer and Steinhorst were able to achieve 30–60° of rotation with this technique.

Once the fovea had been repositioned over healthy RPE, the edges of the retinotomy were photocoagulated (Fig. 47.7). A peripheral iridectomy was made and the vitreous filled with silicone oil. The infusion cannula was removed and the sclerotomies closed with 6-0 Vicryl sutures.

In their series of three patients, one improved from 1/200 to 20/60. The other two patients went from 20/200 to 20/400 and 3.5/200, respectively. The latter two patients developed hypotony and proliferative

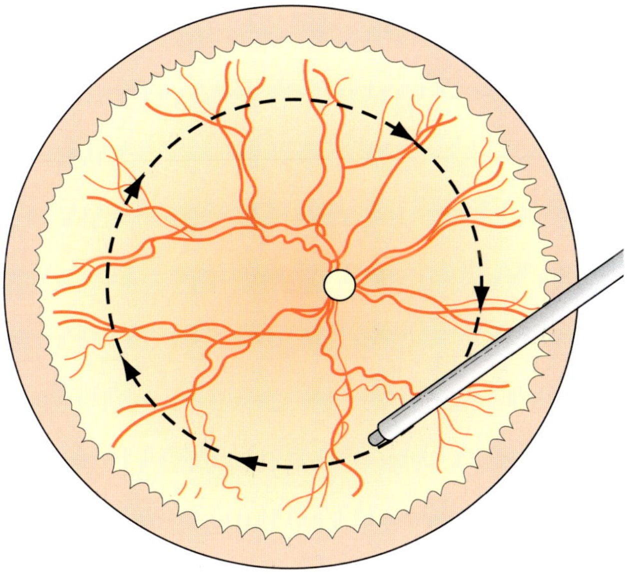

Figure 47.6 *Silicone-tipped needle used to rotate the retina clockwise by applying suction at the edges of the retinotomy.*

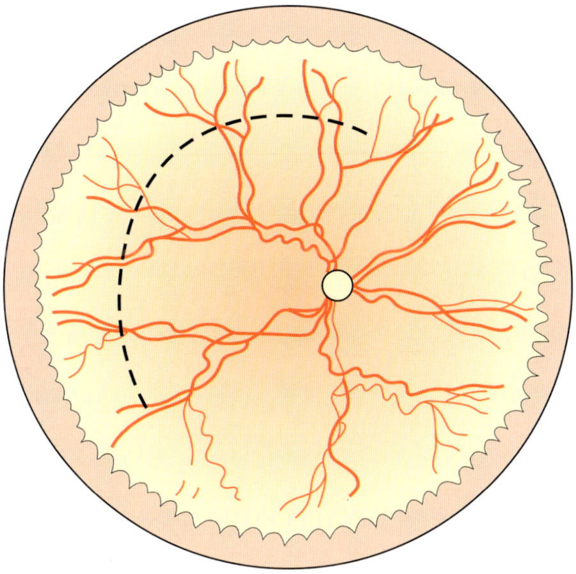

Figure 47.8 *Dotted line indicates the location of incision for 160° retinotomy.*

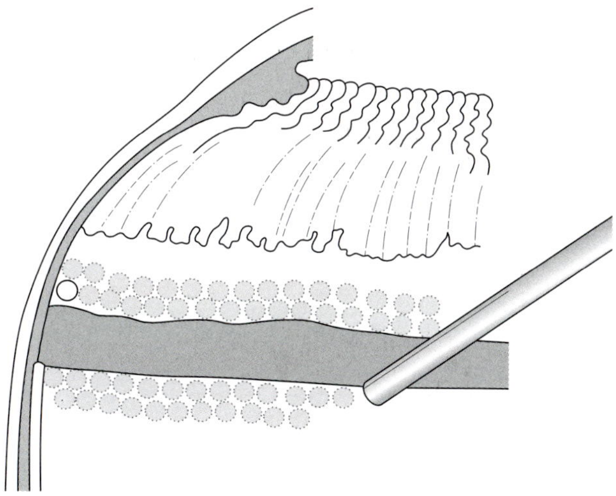

Figure 47.7 *Endolaser being performed along the edges of anterior retinotomy after air–fluid exchange.*

vitreoretinopathy (PVR), necessitating repeat vitrectomy. All three patients developed between 30–60° of excyclotorsion.

Ninomiya et al reported the results of foveal translocation on three patients, two with ARMD and one with myopic degeneration.[22] They modified the technique of Machemer and Steinhorst by performing a retinotomy of less than 180°. They reasoned that a smaller retinotomy would result in a lower incidence of PVR. A total retinal detachment was created by an external approach. The retina was cauterized from anterior to the first bifurcation of the superotemporal arcade circumferentially for 160°, halfway between the disc and the equator from the superonasal to the inferotemporal quadrant (Fig. 47.8). The remainder of the surgery was similar to that of Machemer and Steinhorst.

One patient with ARMD improved from 20/200 preoperatively to 20/20 postoperatively. Another patient with myopic degeneration went from 20/700 to 20/70. The third patient with ARMD went from 20/700 to 20/2000 because the procedure was complicated by retinal detachment and neovascular glaucoma postoperatively. Two of three patients required another surgery to remove an epiretinal membrane. All three developed excyclotorsion, which was tolerated.

Wolf et al[23] published their results performing 360° retinotomy on seven patients with subfoveal CNV secondary to ARMD. Preoperative vision ranged from 20/80 to hand motions. Postoperative vision ranged from 20/100 to 20/400. Only two of the seven had improved vision at six months' follow up. Complications included retinal detachment in three patients, epiretinal membrane in one, and cataract in three.

Eckardt et al[24] reported 360° rotation on 30 eyes. Twenty-two underwent simultaneous oblique muscle

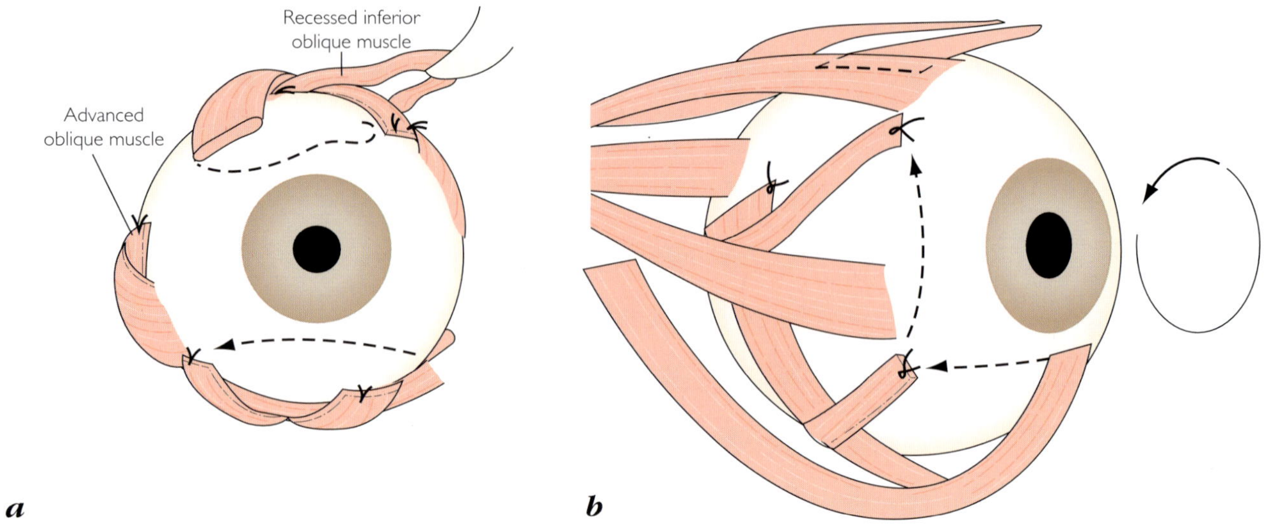

Figure 47.9 *Illustration of torsional muscle surgery to create an excyclotropia in the right eye. The anterior part of the inferior oblique muscle is advanced 12 mm and the posterior part 9 mm, while the anterior and posterior parts of the superior oblique muscle are recessed the same distances. In addition, muscle strips from (a) two opposing rectus muscles or (b) from all four rectus muscles are passed beneath the original muscles and transposed in a clockwise direction and attached at the insertion of the adjoining rectus muscles.*

surgery alone or in combination with surgery on two or four rectus muscles (Fig. 47.9). Seventeen of the 22 also had muscle surgery on the fellow eye. A 12-mm tuck was made in the inferior oblique muscle and a 12-mm recession was performed on the superior oblique muscle. The rectus surgery involved splitting the muscle into 15–17 mm-long and 1.5–2.0 mm-wide strips. Excyclotorsion was created by crossing the strips under the original muscle and moving them in a clockwise (right eye) or counter-clockwise (left eye) direction and refixating them at the insertion of the adjoining rectus muscle.

Sixty percent of these patients achieved reading vision. Six of the eight who did not have muscle surgery developed diplopia and cyclotropia, but only one patient in the muscle surgery group developed these complications. Five patients developed retinal detachment after silicone oil removal, three developed recurrent CNV, and two had subfoveal perfluorocarbon liquid requiring removal.

In 1997, de Juan described a scleral shortening technique to achieve foveal translocation.[25] He reasoned that this technique is less complicated than making large retinotomies and has a lower risk for PVR. After successfully performing the procedure in 14 out of 15 rabbits,[26] de Juan performed the procedure on three patients.[27] A crescent-shaped area measuring 8–10 mm by 12–15 mm was marked at the equator in the superotemporal or inferotemporal quadrant. The sclera in this crescent-shaped area was dissected to remove the external 75% of scleral thickness (Fig. 47.10). A complete pars plana vitrectomy was performed. After an unsuccessful attempt at transscleral subretinal hydrodissection to create a retinal detachment, transretinal hydrodissection through one to three posterior retinotomies was performed successfully. The edges of the sclera were then sutured with 5-0 polyester sutures. An air–fluid exchange was performed and the eye was filled with sulfur hexafluoride or perfluoropropane gas. Superotemporal scleral shortening produced inferonasal foveal translocation, and inferotemporal scleral shortening produced superonasal foveal translocation (Fig. 47.11). The extrafoveal CNV was lasered postoperatively in two of three eyes.

In this three-patient series, one eye improved from 20/126 to 20/70, one eye from 20/200 to 20/70 and the third eye from 20/160 to 20/30 4–6 months postoperatively. Translocation distances were 350, 1500, and 1000 μm, respectively.

The procedure was not without complications. Patient 1 required two additional vitrectomies to reattach the retina. Patients reported gradually improving symptoms of objects being tilted, distorted or magnified. Retinal rotation produced vertical, horizontal and rotatory deviation of the visual axis in the treated eye, explaining the perception of tilted images. Some degree of suppression may have developed because symptoms were noted to improve with time.

Lewis et al[28] reported a prospective study of macular translocation in 10 eyes of 10 patients with subfoveal CNV secondary to ARMD. Preoperative vision ranged from 20/50 to 20/800. Translocation was achieved by means of scleral imbrication, retinal detachment, and partial air–fluid exchange. Three to four 5-0 nylon sutures were placed in a horizontal mattress fashion between the superior and lateral rectus muscles. The sutures were passed 2 mm posterior to the rectus insertion, with 4.5–6.0 mm between the anterior and posterior bites (Fig. 47.12). A 39-gauge cannula was used to inject balanced saline solution into the subretinal space to detach the retina. Additional posterior retinotomies were made to detach the retina from the optic nerve head to the ora serrata in the temporal 180° and inferonasal quadrants (Fig. 47.13). A 60–70% air–fluid exchange was performed without draining subretinal fluid and the patient was placed postoperatively in a sitting position so that the fovea would displace inferonasally; all 10 eyes were followed for six months. Median postoperative foveal displacement was

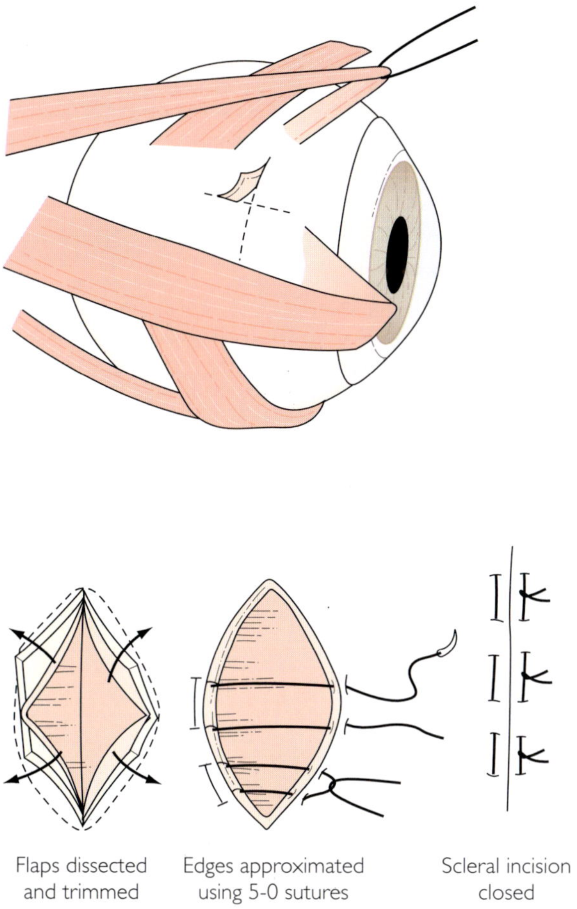

Figure 47.10 *Illustration of scleral shortening technique.*

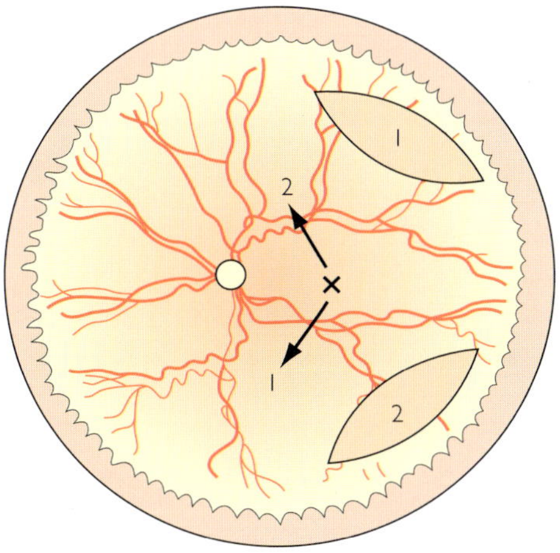

Figure 47.11 *Locations of scleral shortening: superotemporal scleral shortening (area 1) leads to inferonasal foveal translocation (arrow 1) and inferotemporal scleral shortening (area 2) leads to superonasal foveal translocation (arrow 2).*

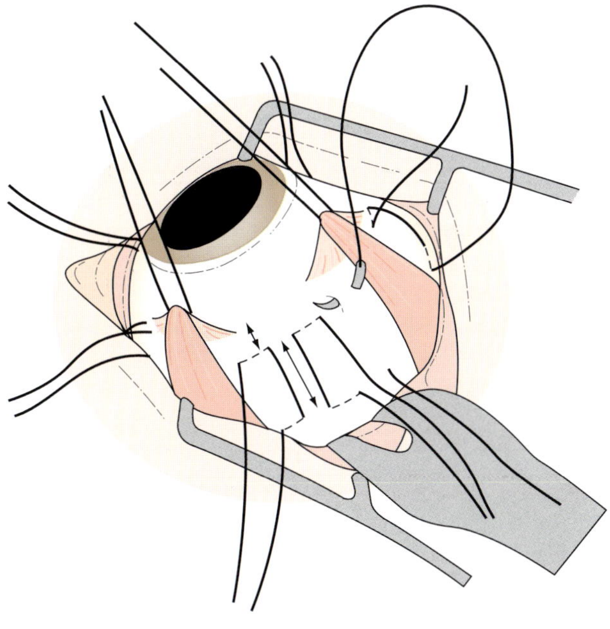

Figure 47.12 *Placement of sutures for scleral imbrication.*

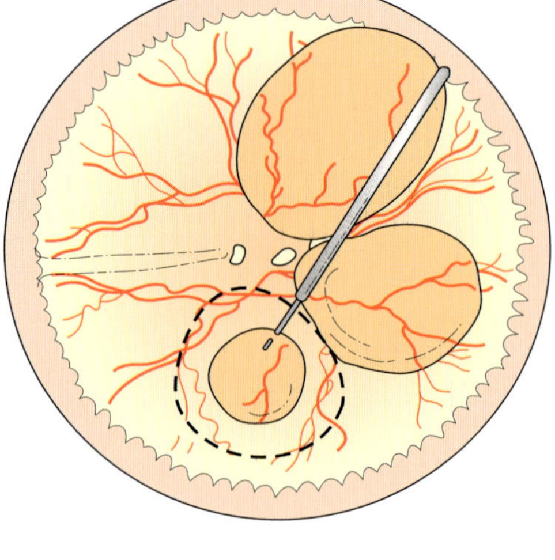

Figure 47.13 *39-Gauge cannula used to inject balanced saline solution into the subretinal space to detach the neurosensory retina from the retinal pigment epithelium.*

1286 µm (range 114–1919 µm). Four patients had improved vision and six had worse; the median vision change was a loss of five letters. Complications included a postoperative foveal fold requiring reoperation in three patients, retinal detachment in one, and persistent image tilt in one patient. The authors advise avoiding detachment of the superior-nasal retina to prevent retinal fold.

Fujikado et al performed de Juan's technique on two patients with myopic subfoveal CNV.[29] Patients improved from 20/150 to 20/20 and from 20/70 to 20/30. Translocation distances were 0.63 and 0.46 disc diameter, respectively. Other visual effects were a hyperopic shift, oblique astigmatism of 6 diopters with an axis parallel to the line of resection, transient diplopia and, in one patient, torsion and aniseikonia. Suppression was documented in the patient with aniseikonia, accompanied by resolution of diplopia.

Ohji et al[30] compared the two techniques (retinotomy and scleral shortening) in a total of ten patients (three with myopic CNV and seven with ARMD).[30] Of the five eyes that underwent retinotomy and relocation, visual acuity improved by three or more lines in two eyes (40%), remained within two lines in two eyes (40%) and worsened by two or more lines in one eye (20%). Final visual acuities improved by three or more lines in two eyes (40%) and worsened by three or more lines in three eyes (60%). Of the five eyes that underwent foveal translocation by scleral shortening, visual acuity improved by three or more lines in two eyes (40%) and remained within two lines in three eyes (60%). Final visual acuity improved in one eye (20%), remained the same in three eyes (60%) and was worse in one eye (20%). The outcomes were comparable to those for surgical removal of CNV.

The eyes that underwent foveal translocation with retinotomy had a translocation distance of 0.5–1.0 disc diameter (average 0.76). Eyes that had translocation by scleral shortening experienced a translocation distance of 0.15–0.7 disc diameters (average 0.53). Greater translocation distance is achieved with retinotomy because the retina can be folded more. This may be advantageous in eyes with large CNV or a large area of RPE atrophy. The scleral shortening technique may be preferred for eyes with smaller CNV, i.e. myopic degeneration; however, translocation distance is harder to predict with this technique.

Complications were more frequent and severe in the retinotomy eyes. Three of five patients developed retinal detachment and two developed PVR postoperatively. The PVR was likely to be caused by the dispersion of RPE cells. Three of five eyes developed macular pucker. Neither PVR nor macular pucker occurred in the scleral shortening group. The most significant complication in this group was astigmatism ranging from 3.25 to 8.5 diopters (average 5.1 diopters). The amount of astigmatism corresponded to the width of the resection. Average astigmatism in the retinotomy group was less than 2 diopters. Visual field constriction was more marked in the retinotomy group.

CONCLUSION

Foveal translocation is a treatment option for patients with subfoveal CNV caused by ARMD or myopic degeneration. Because of the technical difficulty and postoperative complications such as PVR, epiretinal membrane and excyclotorsion, retinotomy and translocation have not been accepted widely. A smaller retinotomy (less than 180°) may result in fewer cases of PVR. Scleral shortening is complicated by the high amount of induced astigmatism, torsion and aniseikonia. However, patients with subfoveal CNV and recent vision loss who are not candidates for laser photocoagulation may be considered for these innovative procedures.

REFERENCES

1. Hyman L. Epidemiology of AMD. In: Hampton GR, Nelson PT, eds, *Age-Related Macular Degeneration: Principles and Practice.* (Raven Press: New York, 1992): 1–35.
2. Klein R, Klein BE, Linton KL. Prevalence of age-related maculopathy: The Beaver Dam Eye Study, *Ophthalmology* (1992) **99:**933–43.
3. Macular Photocoagulation Study Group. Argon laser photocoagulation for senile macular degeneration: results of a randomized clinical trial, *Arch Ophthalmol* (1982) **100:**912–18.
4. Macular Photocoagulation Study Group. Krypton laser photocoagulation for neovascular lesions of age-related macular degeneration: results of a randomized clinical trial, *Arch Ophthalmol* (1990) **108:**816–24.
5. Macular Photocoagulation Study Group. Laser photocoagulation of subfoveal neovascular lesions in age-related macular degeneration: results of a randomized trial, *Arch Ophthalmol* (1991) **109:**1120–31.
6. Macular Photocoagulation Study Group. Laser photocoagulation of subfoveal recurrent neovascular lesions in age-related macular degeneration: results of a randomized clinical trial, *Arch Ophthalmol* (1991) **109:**1232–41.
7. De Juan E Jr, Machemer R. Vitreous surgery for hemorrhagic and fibrous complications of age-related macular degeneration, *Am J Ophthalmol* (1988) **105:**25–9.
8. Thomas MA, Dickinson JD, Melberg NS, et al. Visual results after surgical removal of subfoveal choroidal neovascular membranes, *Ophthalmology* (1994) **101:**1384–96.
9. Holekamp NM, Thomas MA, Dickinson JD, Valluri S. Surgical removal of subfoveal choroidal neovascularization in presumed ocular histoplasmosis: stability of early visual results, *Ophthalmology* (1997) **104:**22–6.
10. Berger AS, Kaplan HJ. Clinical experience with the surgical removal of subfoveal neovascular membranes: short-term postoperative results, *Ophthalmology* (1992) **99:**969–76.
11. Lambert HM, Capone A Jr, Aaberg TM, et al. Surgical excision of subfoveal neovascular membranes in age-related macular degeneration, *Am J Ophthalmol* (1992) **113:**257–62.
12. Finger PT, Berson A, Sherr D, et al. Radiation therapy for subretinal neovascularization, *Ophthalmology* (1996) **103:**878–89.
13. Harino S, Oshima Y, Tsujikawa K, et al. Treatment of age-related subfoveal choroidal neovascularization by low-dose external radiation: a preliminary study, *Nippon Ganka Gakkai Zasshi* (1997) **101:**341–8.
14. Fung WE. Interferon alpha-2a for treatment of age-related macular degeneration (letter), *Am J Ophthalmol* (1991) **112:**349–50.
15. Poliner LS, Tornambe PE, Michelson PE, Heitzmann JG. Interferon alpha-2a for subfoveal neovascularization in age-related macular degeneration, *Ophthalmology* (1993) **100:**1417–24.
16. Algvere PV, Berglin L, Gouras P, Sheng Y. Transplantation of fetal retinal pigment epithelium in age-related macular degeneration with subfoveal neovascularization, *Graefes Arch Clin Exp Ophthalmol* (1994) **232:**707–16.
17. Peyman GA, Blinder KJ, Paris CL, et al. A technique for retinal pigment epithelium transplantation for age-related macular degeneration secondary to extensive subfoveal scarring, *Ophthalmic Surg* (1991) **22:**102–8.
18. Schmidt-Erfurth U, Miller J, Sickenberg M, et al. Photodynamic therapy for subfoveal choroidal neovascularization: clinical and angiographic examples, *Graefes Arch Clin Exp Ophthalmol* (1998) **236:**364–74.
19. Machemer R, Steinhorst UH. Retinal separation, retinotomy, and macular relocation: II. A surgical approach for age-related macular degeneration? *Graefes Arch Clin Exp Ophthalmol* (1993) **231:**635–41.
20. Lindsey P, Finkelstein D, D'Anna S. Experimental retinal relocation, *Invest Ophthalmol Vis Sci* (1983) **24** (Suppl):242.
21. Tiedeman J, de Juan E Jr, Machemer R, et al. Surgical relocation of the macula, *Invest Ophthalmol Vis Sci* (1985) **26**(Suppl):59.
22. Ninomiya Y, Lewis JM, Hasegawa T, Tano Y. Retinotomy and foveal translocation for surgical management of subfoveal choroidal neovascular membranes, *Am J Ophthalmol* (1996) **122:**613–21.
23. Wolf S, Lappas A, Weinberger AW, Kirchhof B. Macular translocation for surgical management of subfoveal choroidal neovascularizations in patients with AMD: first results, *Graefes Arch Clin Exp Ophthalmol* (1999) **237:**51–7.
24. Eckardt C, Eckardt U, Conrad HG. Macular rotation with and without counter-rotation of the globe in patients with age-related macular degeneration, *Graefes Arch Clin Exp Ophthalmol* (1999) **237:**313–25.
25. De Juan E. Macular translocation: techniques and results. *AAO Vitreoretinal Update* (1997) 59–61 (abst). American Academy of Ophthalmology, San Francisco.
26. Imai K, Loewenstein A, de Juan E Jr. Translocation of the retina for management of subfoveal choroidal neovascularization: I. Experimental studies in the rabbit eye, *Am J Ophthalmol* (1998) **125:**635–46.
27. De Juan E Jr, Loewenstein A, Bressler NM, Alexander J. Translocation of the retina for management of subfoveal choroidal neovascularization: II. A preliminary report in humans, *Am J Ophthalmol* (1998) **125:**635–46.
28. Lewis H, Kaiser P, Lewis P, Estafanous M. Macular translocation for subfoveal choroidal neovascularization in age-related macular degeneration: a prospective study, *Am J Ophthalmol* (1999) **128:**135–46.
29. Fujikado T, Ohji M, Saito Y, et al. Visual function after foveal translocation with scleral shortening in patients with myopic neovascular maculopathy, *Am J Ophthalmol* (1998) **125:**647–56.
30. Ohji M, Fujikado T, Saito Y, et al. Foveal translocation: a comparison of two techniques, *Semin Ophthalmol* (1998) **13:**52–61.

Chapter 48 Macular buckle in exudative age-related macular degeneration

Gholam A Peyman, Marta A Recasens and Mandi D Conway

INTRODUCTION

Age-related macular degeneration (ARMD) is implicated as the leading cause of blindness in patients over the age of 65 years.[1] Eighty-five percent of the severe visual loss can be attributed to the exudative form, even though this type only accounts for 15% of ARMD.[2] This exudative neovascular form also has been called 'wet', in contrast to the 'dry' atrophic type that accounts for the majority of the ARMD cases not leading to blindness.

ARMD is the leading cause of choroidal neovascularization in the elderly. The Macular Photocoagulation Study Group (MPS) demonstrated the benefits of laser photocoagulation of classic choroidal neovascularization of juxtafoveal and extrafoveal membranes in ARMD and other disorders.[3] Patients with subfoveal choroidal neovascularization have an especially dismal prognosis, with 64% of eyes losing six or more lines of vision over a 2-year period.[4] The benefits of laser photocoagulation as compared to observation in this group of patients only proved to be superior for contrast sensitivity and reading speed. Treated patients lost an average of three lines of visual acuity immediately and then stabilized, compared to untreated patients who lost an average of two lines of visual acuity at 3 months and then progressively lost more vision.[4–6]

The MPS recommendations are for classic choroidal neovascular membranes (CNVM).[7] Unfortunately, 85% of CNVM cases are occult or ill-defined and many patients with juxtafoveal and extrafoveal CNVM are excluded from the MPS criteria for laser photocoagulation.[8,9] New treatment techniques must be explored to halt the progression of visual loss from the exudative form of ARMD not encompassed in the MPS guidelines.

It has been postulated that there is an engorgement of the choriocapillaris, as demonstrated by differences in density and diameter of choroidal blood vessels of eyes with ARMD when compared with those eyes without ARMD.[10] Friedman et al[11] demonstrated decreased velocity and increased pulsatility of ocular arterial blood flow in eyes with ARMD using color Doppler imaging. These findings support our original hypotheses in search of an alternative treatment for choroidal neovascularization in ARMD.

We agree with the above-cited investigators that there is a relative degree of choroidal congestion or vasodilation under the macula of patients with exudative ARMD.[10] This vascular stagnation may promote growth, exudation and bleeding of CNVM.

In our attempts to reduce the choroidal engorgement, vascular leakage and bleeding found in CNVM of ARMD in patients who are ineligible or unwilling to undergo laser photocoagulation, we apply an external posterior macular buckle. The macular buckle consists of a strip of Gore-Tex (W.L. Gore and Associates, Inc., Flagstaff, AZ) material with an additional 8.5–9-mm piece of silicone sponge buckling material (505T Mira Silicone Sponge, Mira, Inc., Waltham, MA; 5 mm diameter). This produces a scleral indentation at the level of the fovea centered underneath the CNVM, which aids in deturgescing the choroid (Fig. 48.1). A

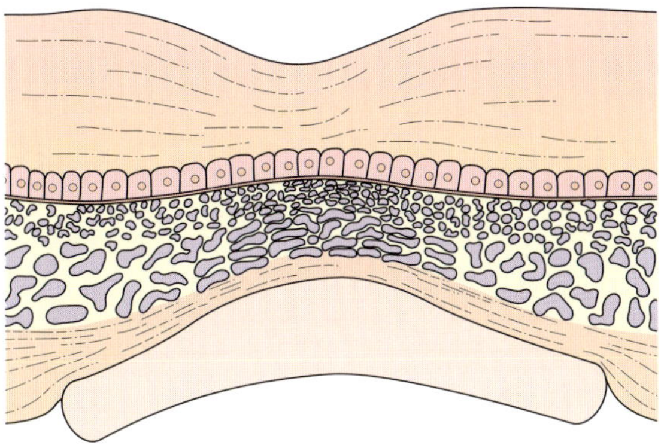

Figure 48.1 *Schematic representation of the indentation produced by the macular buckle underneath the congested choroid.*

preoperative fluorescein angiogram aids in patient selection and intraoperative buckle placement.

All study patients meet the following inclusion criteria:

- Decreased vision/visual perception (decreased visual acuity, metamorphopsia or scotoma) associated with clinical and angiographic evidence of subfoveal or juxtafoveal CNVM.
- Preoperative best-corrected Snellen visual acuity of 20/400 or better.
- Absence of other underlying ocular diseases that would limit visual recovery.
- Confirmation of subfoveal or juxtafoveal classic or ill-defined CNVM by fluorescein angiography and MPS parameters.
- No history of laser photocoagulation to the affected eye.
- Informed consent by the patient of both the Institutional Review Board's and the hospital's specific surgical consent forms.

SURGICAL TECHNIQUE

A 360° peritomy is performed, followed by isolation of the four recti and the inferior oblique muscles with 3-0 silk bridle sutures. The lateral rectus muscle is disinserted from its insertion after a double-armed 6-0 Vicryl suture (Ethicon, Inc., Somerville, NJ) secures its tendon for later reinsertion. The muscle is retracted to expose the macular area. The Gore-Tex strip is marked along one side of its entire length to identify any twisting which may occur during placement. The Gore-Tex strip is threaded through the silicone sponge (8.5–9 mm length of a 505T Mira silicone sponge) and the sponge is centered on the strip. The Gore-Tex strip–sponge unit is passed underneath the inferior rectus and inferior oblique muscles, beginning nasally and ending laterally. The buckle elements are passed under the superior rectus looping from the lateral to the medial aspect of the globe (Fig. 48.2). The buckle is placed behind the macula. Using indirect ophthalmoscopy, the macular indentation produced by the buckle is assessed. The two ends of the buckle are nasal to the two vertical recti muscles and these ends can be used to maneuver the buckle for location and height. Once placement of the macular buckle is confirmed to be indenting the CNVM, the ends of the Gore-Tex strip are sutured to the sclera with 5-0 Mersilene sutures approximately 6 mm from the limbus. The strips are trimmed flush to the globe (Fig. 48.3). The intraocular pressure is assessed using a Schiotz tonometer and if it is greater than 30 mmHg two small Z-shaped relaxing incisions are made in the Gore-Tex strip to release the band tension. This step can be repeated for an optimum intraocular pressure

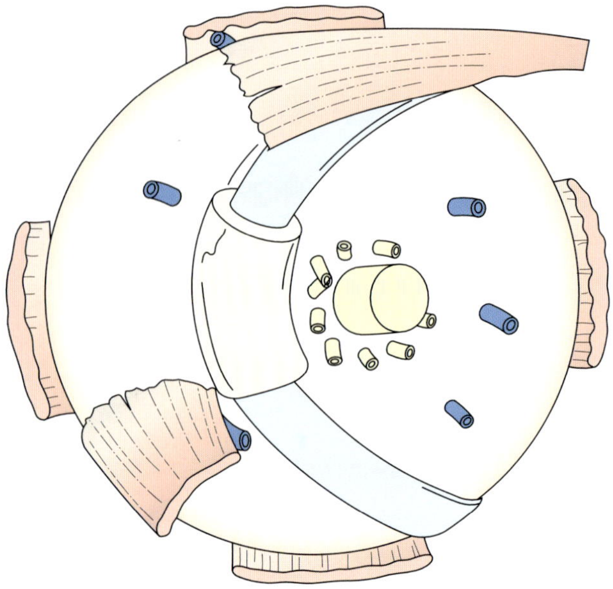

Figure 48.2 *Posterior view of the eye and macular buckle with 8.5–9.0-mm silicone sponge threaded through with a Gore-Tex strip.*

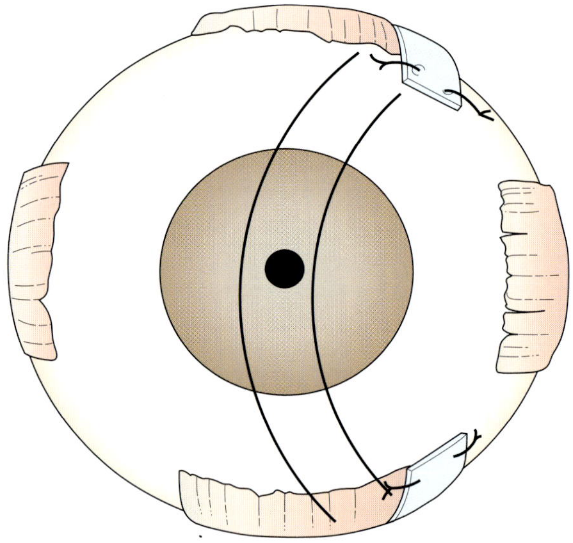

Figure 48.3 *Schematic representation of the macular buckle positioned under the macula and secured to the nasal sclera.*

below 25 mmHg. Adjunctive intraoperative intravenous acetazolamide can be administered in nonallergic patients, if necessary. The position and height of the macular buckle, as well as the perfusion of the central retinal artery, are then reassessed. The lateral rectus muscle is reapproximated to its original insertion. The conjunctival peritomy is closed using interrupted 7-0 Vicryl sutures. Postoperative ocular hypertension can be managed with beta-blockers or oral acetazolamide.

SURGICAL RESULTS

Our results after macular buckle placement in 42 eyes of 42 patients with CNVM secondary to ARMD demonstrate a favorable trend in visual acuity outcomes for patients with subfoveal CNVM. Eyes treated with macular buckle placement were more likely to maintain their preoperative vision compared to retrospective natural history studies.

Of 12 eyes with classic subfoveal CNVM treated with placement of a macular buckle: four (33%) gained two or more lines of Snellen visual acuity; three (25%) gained one line, remained the same or lost one line; and five (42%) lost two or more lines (range +6 to –6 lines). Of 22 eyes with ill-defined subfoveal CNVM treated with macular buckle placement: 12 (54%) gained one line, remained the same, or lost one line; and 10 (46%) lost two or more lines (range +1 to –8 lines). Of the eight eyes with ill-defined juxtafoveal CNVM treated with macular buckle surgery: three (38%) lost between three and six lines of Snellen visual acuity; and five (62%) remained the same (gained one, remained the same or lost one line). The follow-up for the 42 treated eyes ranged from 7 to 76 months (mean of 20.9 months).

Interestingly, 10 eyes (24%) bled subretinally during the follow-up period (average 11.5 months, range 14 days to 27 months), all outside the area of indentation of the macular buckle.

Postoperative complications included: transient elevations in intraocular pressure (managed medically); slippage of the macular buckle toward the optic nerve, producing disc swelling (in one patient, treated with surgical removal of the macular buckle); and suture granulomas (two cases).[12]

Although the results of this novel approach to treating CNVM are promising, further study and continued follow-up are planned.

REFERENCES

1. Hyman L. Epidemiology of eye disease in the elderly, *Eye* (1987) **1:**330–41.
2. Neely K, Bressler NM, Bressler SB. Clinical characteristics, epidemiology, and natural history of age-related macular degeneration, *Ophthalmol Clin North Am* (1993) **6**(2):291–306.
3. Macular Photocoagulation Study Group. Laser photocoagulation of juxtafoveal choroidal neovascularization: five-year results from randomized clinical trials, *Arch Ophthalmol* (1994) **112:**500–9.
4. Macular Photocoagulation Study Group. Laser photocoagulation of subfoveal neovascular lesions of age-related macular degeneration: updated findings from two clinical trials, *Arch Ophthalmol* (1993) **111:**1200–9.
5. Macular Photocoagulation Study Group. Laser photocoagulation of subfoveal neovascular lesions in age-related macular degeneration: results of a randomized clinical trial, *Arch Ophthalmol* (1991) **109:**1220–31.
6. Macular Photocoagulation Study Group. Laser photocoagulation of subfoveal recurrent neovascular lesions in age-related macular degeneration: results of a randomized clinical trial, *Arch Ophthalmol* (1991) **109:**1232–41.
7. Macular Photocoagulation Study Group. Subfoveal neovascular lesions in age-related macular degeneration: guidelines for evaluation and treatment in the Macular Photocoagulation Study, *Arch Ophthalmol* (1991) **109:**1242–57.
8. Moisseiev J, Alhalel A, Masuri R, Treister G. The impact of Macular Photocoagulation Study results on the treatment of exudative age-related macular degeneration, *Arch Ophthalmol* (1995) **113:**185–9.
9. Soubrane G, Coscas G, Français C, Koenig F. Occult subretinal new vessels in age-related macular degeneration: natural history and early laser treatment, *Ophthalmology* (1990) **97:**649–57.
10. Spraul CW, Lang GE, Grossniklaus HE. Morphometric analysis of the choroid, Bruch's membrane, and retinal pigment epithelium in eyes with age-related macular degeneration, *Invest Ophthalmol Vis Sci* (1996) **37:**2724–35.
11. Friedman E, Krupsky S, Lane AM, et al. Ocular blood flow velocity in age-related macular degeneration, *Ophthalmology* (1995) **102:**640–6.
12. Peyman GA, Conway MD, Recasens MA, et al. Use of a macular buckle for exudative age-related macular degeneration. *Ophthalmic Surg Lasers* (1999) **30:**619–30.

Chapter 49 Implant radiotherapy for exudative macular degeneration associated with subretinal neovascularization

Paul T Finger, Ilkka Immonen, Jorge Freire and Gary Brown

INTRODUCTION

The wet form of age-related macular degeneration (ARMD) is the leading cause of severe, irreversible blindness in the western world. Typically, patients with the neovascular form of ARMD are older than 70 years and white, although most other races and ages are affected. Other chorioretinal neovascular disease that could benefit from an effective antiangiogenic treatment include: high myopia, Eales' disease, histoplasmosis and eccentric disciform neovascularization.[1]

Although laser photocoagulation of subretinal neovascularization has been established as the only proven treatment by The Macular Photocoagulation Study (MPS), most (85–90%) eyes with neovascular ARMD are not eligible for laser treatment. Laser-treated maculas usually develop recurrent neovascularization (70% over 5 years) and become legally blind.

Multiple Phase I clinical studies have investigated a range of radiation doses for treatment of neovascular ARMD.[2–9] Most centers have used external beam irradiation because it is readily available and inexpensive. A few centers have investigated temporary surgical implantation of radioactive materials for the treatment of neovascular ARMD. To date: Finger et al. have reported on the use of palladium-103 (^{103}Pd) ophthalmic plaque radiotherapy,[5] Immonen and Freire on strontium-90 (^{90}Sr) applicators[9] and Berta et al. on ruthenium-106 (^{106}Ru).[4] Although none of these groups has performed a prospective, randomized clinical trial to prove whether radiation effectively treats macular degeneration, these Phase I trials have been encouraging.

RADIATION AND ANGIOGENESIS

RADIOBIOLOGY

Radiation is known to induce acute vasculitis followed by slowly progressive vascular closure, which may take years to develop.[10–12] Radiation of a macula containing classic or occult subretinal neovascularization could affect angiogenesis either directly (by destroying neovascular endothelial cells and cytokine-producing macrophages) or indirectly (affecting regulatory genes within cells that produce endothelial growth-regulating cytokines). Commonly employed to prevent aberrant scar formation, low doses have been used to inhibit scar formation known as the cutaneous keloid and more recently to prevent coronary artery stenosis. The experience of Hart et al suggests that radiotherapy may inhibit the scar formation associated with end-stage exudative macular degeneration.[13]

SURGICAL CRITERIA AND CASE SELECTION

The overwhelming majority of Phase I clinical studies employing radiation to treat subretinal neovascularization have used 4–6 MV external beam radiotherapy (EBRT). This is because EBRT is nonsurgical, widely available and inexpensive. Unfortunately, a large number of fractions (days) are required to deliver the dose (e.g. 200 cGy × 10 working days). Plus, this technique also irradiates both eyes, the sinuses and/or the brain (Fig. 49.1).

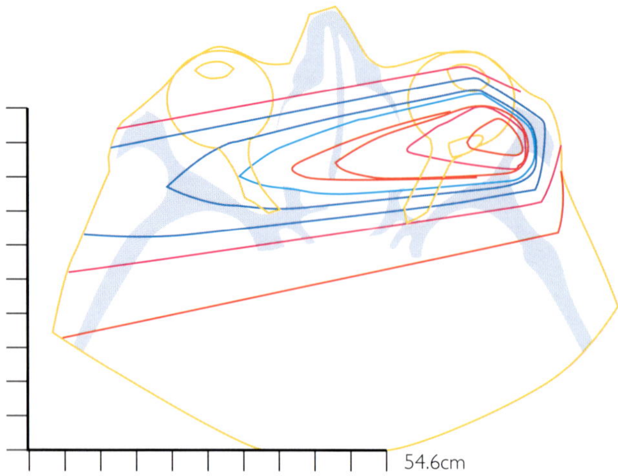

Figure 49.1 *External beam radiotherapy.*

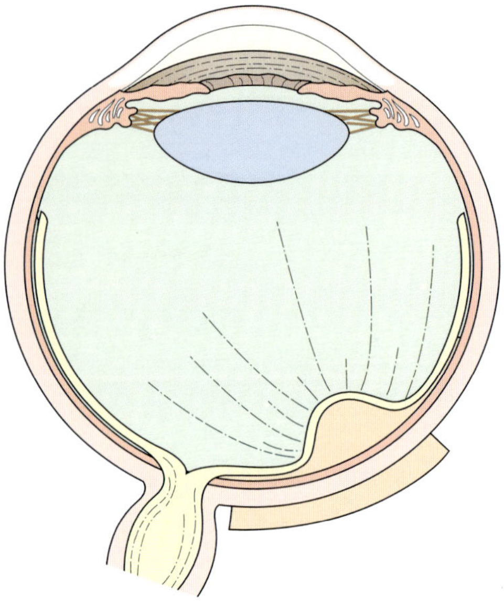

Figure 49.2 *Palladium-103 ophthalmic plaque placed beneath area of subfoveal neovascularization.*

Proton beam therapy (charged-particle external irradiation) also has been used and offers the advantages of being nonsurgical and unilateral. This technique suffers from having to deliver at high dose rates, it can be affected by eye movements and it requires proton facilities that are not widely available.

In contrast, implant radiotherapy or brachytherapy involves placing a radiation source directly beneath the macula. Palladium-103 (^{103}Pd) ophthalmic plaques or strontium-90 (^{90}Sr) applicators have been employed (Figs 49.2 and 49.3). Implant brachytherapy allows a relatively high dose of irradiation over a relatively short duration (1–36 hours). They are both monocular treatments that deliver almost no radiation to the fellow eye, sinuses or brain. Although the involved macula receives a larger dose than with EBRT, most normal ocular structures of the treated eye receive less irradiation with implant radiotherapy.

Case selection involves both patient-specific and disease-specific factors. In general, patients are told of the methods of treatment available at each center. They are told of the number of patients that have been treated with each method and the implications of those facts. The patient's general medical condition is reviewed and discussed with the patient as a factor related to the safety of their surgery. In general, we have found that younger patients with monocular disease have preferred to undergo implant radiotherapy. These patients have expressed concern over having unnecessary irradiation of normal ocular and intracranial structures. A disease-related exclusion factor is the proximity of the neovascular disease to the optic nerve, because it is anatomically difficult to

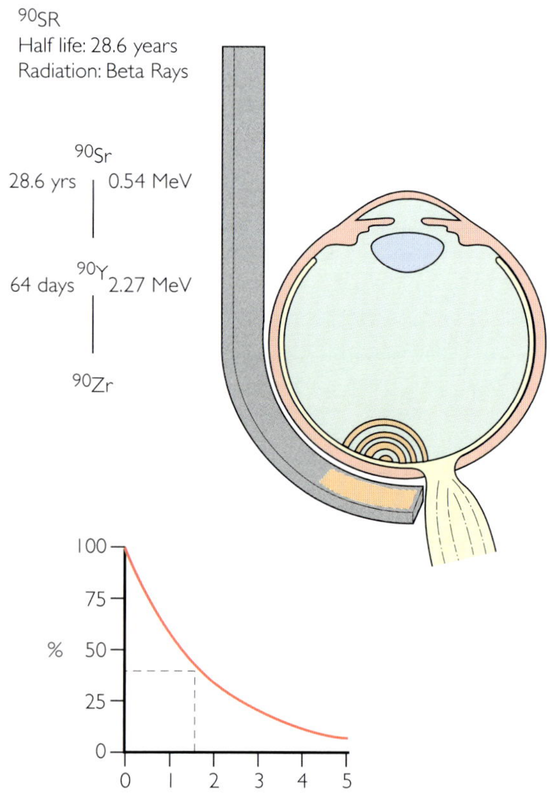

Figure 49.3 *Strontium-90 ophthalmic plaque placed beneath area of subfoveal neovascularization.*

place brachytherapy sources directly beneath juxtapapillary neovascular membranes.

Patients with occult, classic and recurrent neovascular ARMD have been treated. Although a mixture of subtypes can skew the results, a random selection of presentations most closely mimics the general population.

PREOPERATIVE EVALUATION AND MEDICAL CLEARANCE

A complete initial ophthalmic eye examination should be performed on all patients prior to surgery. In order to make treatment results comparable to other centers, it is helpful to perform a refraction using a standardized protocol, such as the Early Treatment of Diabetic Retinopathy Study (ETDRS). Pupillary, ocular motor and slit-lamp examinations are performed, as well as tonometry. Direct, indirect and contact lens ophthalmoscopy techniques are used as necessary. Basal dimensions of the neovascular membranes can be determined by ophthalmoscopy and fundus photography with angiography.

Initially we used the retinal surface as the prescription point for ^{103}Pd plaque radiotherapy. Because of the small size of these lesions, all groups are currently using a standard distance (1.5–2 mm) from the inner scleral surface as the prescription point.

A complete medical survey with clearance for anesthesia was obtained prior to surgery. All patients were determined to be good surgical risks.

INSTRUMENTATION

PALLADIUM-103 EYE PLAQUES

Plaque assembly involves attaching ^{103}Pd seeds (Model 200, Theragenics Corp., Buford, GA) into a 10-mm gold eye plaque (Trachsel Dental Studio Inc., Rochester, MN) with a thin layer of acrylic fixative (Fig. 49.4).[14]

Dosimetric calculations for ^{103}Pd involved a number of assumptions. All seeds were calculated as point sources using the specific dose rate constant, which was aligned perpendicular to the long axis of the seed. Attenuation related to the acrylic fixative was calculated to be 1.4 mm of water.

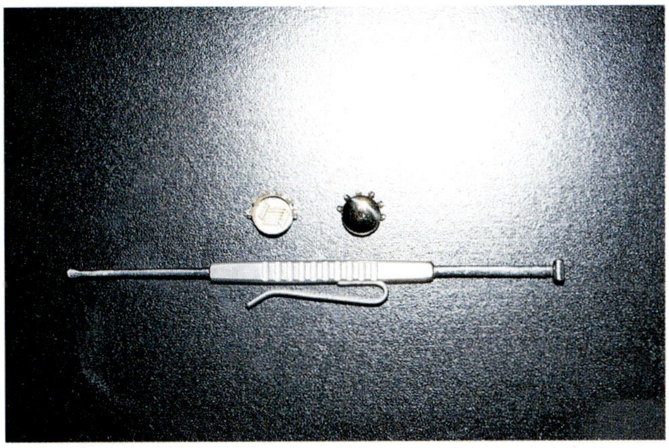

Figure 49.4 *A 10-mm palladium-103 plaque assembly.*

In the ^{103}Pd series, patients were treated at a retinal dose rate of 35–56 cGy/h for a mean treatment duration of 28 hours, which achieved a prescription dose in a range of 1250–2362 cGy.

STRONTIUM-90

Immonen's applicator

Strontium-90 applicators were manufactured for each study. In general, 50% of beta particles are absorbed within 1.5 mm (in tissue). Immonen's round applicator was constructed with an 8-mm active surface (Fig. 49.5). It was calculated to deliver 15 Gy to a depth of 1.75 mm over 54 continuous minutes.

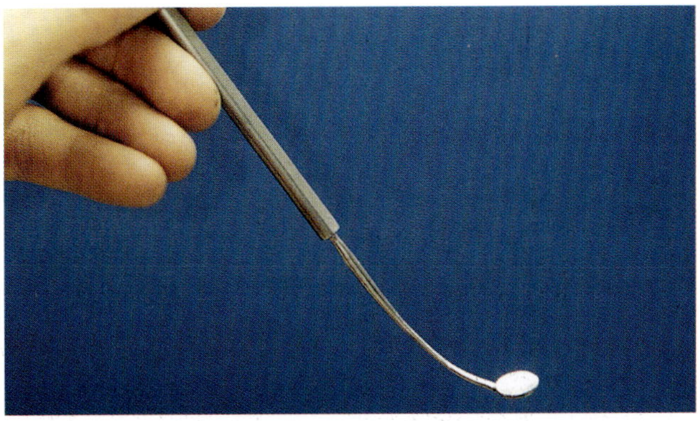

Figure 49.5 *Immonen's round strontium-90 plaque applicator.*

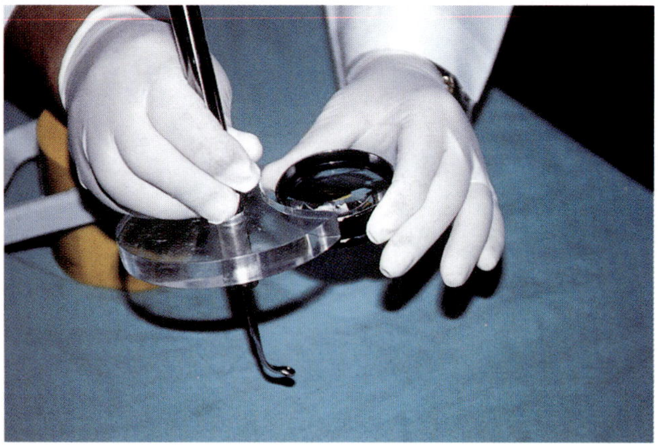

Figure 49.6 *Freire's strontium-90 plaque applicator.*

Freire's applicator

Freire's applicator was constructed as a stainless-steel curved stem with a 6-mm round concave ceramic disc containing 10 mCi of ^{90}Sr (Fig. 49.6). The dose rate was calculated at 1.5 mm depth to deliver 6 cGy per second. The first group of 11 patients was treated with 1000 cGy and the second with 1500 cGy to 1.5 intraocular millimeters. The duration of treatment was 4 minutes 20 seconds for the first group and 6 minutes 40 seconds for the second group. Each treatment was fractionated in 80-second intervals with 1-minute rests between applications (to allow for blood perfusion of the macula).

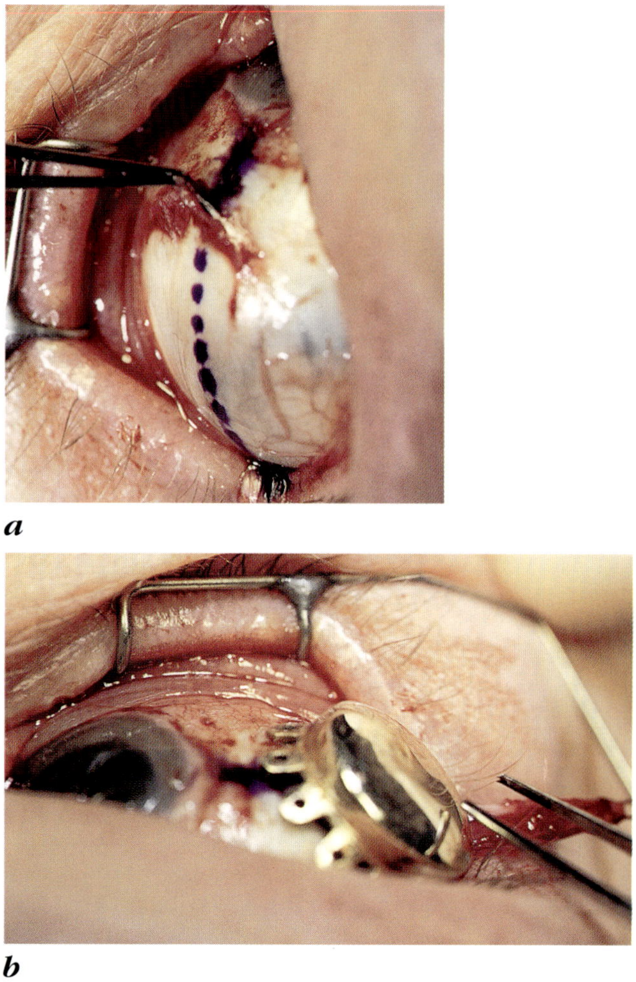

Figure 49.7 *The episcleral line was extended posteriorly (a) and used as a guide for plaque placement (b).*

Radioactive device insertion

Implantation was performed under general (plaque) and local (applicator) anesthesia. Prior to surgery, indirect ophthalmoscopy was used to monitor for a change in the condition of the eye and treatment site. A conjunctival peritomy then was performed around the corneal–scleral limbus. Stevens' scissors were used to open Tenon's fascia. For ^{103}Pd plaque insertion, a line was drawn on the sclera perpendicular to the temporal limbus and toward the insertion of the lateral rectus muscle. The muscle was isolated, locked with a suture, transected and allowed to retract. The episcleral line was extended posteriorly and used as a guide for plaque placement (Fig. 49.7a, b). The plaque was slid into place beneath the macula with its posterior edge against the optic nerve (see Fig. 49.2).

Four episcleral sutures were placed through the suture eyelets to secure the plaque. Indirect ophthalmoscopy with scleral indentation was used to confirm the position of the plaque in relation to the macular target. The lateral rectus muscle was reattached. A lead shield was placed over the eye at the end of the surgery. Plaque removal was performed under local anesthesia without disturbing the lateral rectus muscle.

Strontium-90 applications were performed without disinsertion of the lateral rectus muscle during one surgical procedure (see Fig. 49.3). Treatments involved continuous ophthalmoscopic visualization of the applicator's indentation of the macula. The presence and thickness of the inferior oblique muscle were discounted by all investigators.

Table 49.1 Visual acuity results after brachytherapy for macular degeneration

Author	*Vision*			
	6 months	*12 months*	*18 months*	*24 months*
Finger (^{103}Pd)	13/15 (87%)	6/8 (75%)	6/7 (86%)	3/4 (75%)
Immonen (^{90}Sr)	10/20 (50%)	9/20 (45%)	N/A	5/18 (28%)
Freire (^{90}Sr)	17/22 (77%)	14/22 (64%)	13/22 (59%)	N/A
Mean	40/57 (70%)	29/50 (58%)	19/29 (66%)	8/22 (36%)

COMPLICATIONS AND PROGNOSIS FOR VISION

No radiation-associated complications have been reported as yet. All patients experienced the common side-effects of surgery, including edema, discharge, foreign body sensation and transient diplopia.

A pooled analysis of visual results proved quite interesting (Table 49.1). In this analysis, the authors were asked to quantify how many patients were stable to within two lines of their pretreatment visual acuity. Treated maculas included a mix of classic, occult and previously laser-treated subretinal neovascularization. Although there is a trend toward progressive visual loss at 2 years, some authors have noted a resolution of the exudative component of the ARMD and subsequent atrophy. No radiation retinopathy was noted in the three groups.

On average, stabilization to within two lines of the pretreatment visual acuity was noted in 70% (at 6 months), 58% (at 12 months), 66% (at 18 months) and 36% (at 2 years). The 2-year data are slightly skewed toward the ^{90}Sr results.

It may be important to note that the low-energy photon-emitting ^{103}Pd will deposit relatively less radiation than the beta-particle emitting ^{90}Sr or ^{106}Ru. This may explain why Immonen et al have noted (more or earlier) chorioretinal atrophy within the targeted zone.

CONCLUSIONS

These three studies of brachytherapy for exudative ARMD have all noted resolution of hemorrhages, exudates and subretinal fluid. Despite these positive findings, it has been difficult to assess the clinical effectiveness of low-dose irradiation of neovascular ARMD. This is due in part to the fact that patients with classic and recurrent subfoveal neovascularization suffer earlier visual loss than those with the occult form. Left untreated, patients can suffer intermittent choroidal hemorrhages with fluid and exudate deposition, followed by reabsorption of these components. Depending upon when treatment is given, it is difficult to tell whether the radiation is promoting resolution of these components or if these 'effects' are a natural occurrence. These facts underscore the need for prospective randomized trials.[15–17]

Certain conclusions can be made from this review. Both ^{103}Pd and ^{90}Sr can be used to deliver radiation to the macula. They both provide a unilateral treatment with less irradiation of most normal ocular and intracranial structures. As compared to 6-MV photon external beam radiotherapy, they both deposit more radiation within the targeted macula. Lastly, within the parameters mentioned in this review, low-dose implant radiotherapy has been tolerated by eyes affected by subretinal neovascularization associated with age-related macular degeneration. No complications that might preclude the investigation of this treatment have been noted.

REFERENCES

1. Guyton JS, Reese AB. Use of roengten therapy for retinal diseases characterized by new-formed blood vessels (Eale's disease: retinitis proliferans), *Arch Ophthalmol* (1948) **40:**389–412.

2. Chakravarthy U, Houston RF, Archer DB. Treatment of age-related subfoveal neovascular membranes by teletherapy: a pilot study, *Br J Ophthalmol* (1993) **77:**265–73.
3. Bergink GJ, Deutman AF, van den Broek JF, et al. Radiation therapy for subfoveal choroidal neovascular membranes in age-related macular degeneration: a pilot study, *Graefes Arch Clin Exp Ophthalmol* (1994) **232:**591–8.
4. Berta A, Vezendi L, Vamosi P. Irradiation of macular subretinal neovascularization using ruthenium applicators, *Szemeset (Hung J Ophthalmol)* (1995) **132:**67–75.
5. Finger PT, Berson A, Sherr DA, et al. Radiation therapy for subretinal neovascularization, *Ophthalmology* (1996) **103:**878–89.
6. Berson AM, Finger PT, Sherr DL, et al. Radiotherapy for age-related macular degeneration: preliminary results of a potentially new treatment, *Int J Radiat Oncol Biol Phys* (1996) **36:**861–5.
7. Freire J, Longton WA, Miyamoto CT, et al. External radiotherapy in macular degeneration: technique and preliminary subjective response, *Int J Radiat Oncol Biol Phys* (1996) **36:**857–60.
8. Yonemoto LT, Slater JD, Friedrichsen EJ, et al. Phase I/II study of proton beam irradiation for the treatment of subfoveal choroidal neovascularization in age-related macular degeneration: treatment techniques and preliminary results, *Int J Radiat Oncol Biol Phys* (1996) **36:**867–71.
9. Jaakkola A, Heikkonen J, Tommila P, et al. Strontium plaque irradiation of subfoveal neovascular membranes in age-related macular degeneration, *Graefes Arch Clin Exp Ophthalmol* (1998) **236:**24–30.
10. Chakravarthy U, Biggart JH, Gardiner TA, et al. Focal irradiation of perforating eye injuries, *Curr Eye Res* (1989) **8:**1241–50.
11. Chakravarthy U, Gardiner TA, Archer DB, Maguire CJ. A light microscopic and autoradiographic study of non-irradiated and irradiated ocular wounds, *Curr Eye Res* (1989) **8:**337–48.
12. Flickinger JC, Pollock BE, Kondziolka D, Lunsford LD. A dose–response analysis of arteriovenous malformation obliteration after radiosurgery, *Int J Radiat Oncol Biol Phys* (1996) **36:**873–9.
13. Hart PM, Archer DP, Chakravarthy V. Asymmetry of disciform scarring in bilateral disease when one eye is treated with radiotherapy, *Br J Ophthalmol* (1995) **79:**562–8.
14. Finger PT, Lu D, Buffa A, et al. Palladium-103 versus iodine-125 for ophthalmic plaque radiotherapy, *Int J Radiat Oncol Biol Phys* (1993) **27:**849–54.
15. Brady LW, Freire JE, Longton WA, et al. Radiation therapy for macular degeneration: technical considerations and preliminary results, *Int J Radiat Oncol Biol Phys* (1997) **39:**945–8.
16. Hart PM, Chakravarthy U, MacKenzie G, et al. Teletherapy for subfoveal choroidal neovascularisation of age-related macular degeneration: results of follow up in a non-randomised study, *Br J Ophthalmol* (1996) **80:**1046–50.
17. Stalmans P, Leys A, van Limbergen E. External beam radiotherapy (20 Gy, 2 Gy fractions) fails to control the growth of choroidal neovascularization in age-related macular degeneration: a review of 11 cases, *Retina* (1997) **17:**481–92.

Chapter 50 Therapeutic treatment of non-exudative age-related macular degeneration: a pilot study

R Joseph Olk and Levent Akduman

INTRODUCTION

Clinical and epidemiological studies have demonstrated that the presence of soft drusen is a risk factor for the development of choroidal neovascularization (CNV) in eyes with age-related macular degeneration (ARMD).[1–3] For patients with bilateral drusen, the 3-year risk of developing CNV is estimated to be 13% overall, and 18% for those aged 65 years or older.[3] For patients who have already developed exudative ARMD in the first eye, the risk to the fellow eye approaches nearly 60% at 5 years[4] and increases to nearly 80% at 3 years if the first eye has a retinal pigment epithelial tear.[5]

In order to address the question of whether patients with non-exudative ARMD treated with 810 nm laser macular grid photocoagulation have an improved anatomic and/or visual outcome when compared to the natural history of the disease, a prospective, randomized clinical pilot study was conducted using two different laser intensities (visible burn and subthreshold, invisible lesion) designed to address the following specific effects:

- Reduction/elimination of drusen.
- Improvement/stabilization of visual acuity.
- Reduction/delay in the incidence of CNV.

PATIENTS AND METHODS

Between July 1994 and June 1996, 152 patients (229 eyes) were recruited and entered into the pilot study from four clinical centers: (1) R Joseph Olk, MD and Levent Akduman, MD (St Louis, MO); (2) Keye L Wong, MD, Melvin C Chen, MD and Marc H Levy, MD (Sarasota, FL); (3) Charles A Garcia, MD (Houston, TX); and (4) Lawrence S Morse, MD, PhD (Sacramento, CA).

Eligibility criteria included all of the following:

- Age greater than 50 years.
- Diagnosis of ARMD with at least five large (63 µm or more) soft drusen within 2250 µm of the center of the foveal avascular zone (FAZ) in both eyes (bilateral study arm) or in one eye (unilateral study arm) if the fellow eye had evidence of exudative ARMD.
- Visual acuity of at least 20/63 on the ETDRS (Early Treatment of Diabetic Retinopathy Study) chart in all eligible eyes.

Patients with geographic atrophy could be included, but the total area of geographic atrophy had to be less than one disc area, and the edge of the geographic atrophy had to be no closer than one-half disc diameter (750 µm) from the center of the FAZ.

TREATMENT TECHNIQUE

Eyes were treated with macular grid photocoagulation using the OcuLight® SLx 810 nm diode laser. Eyes received either visible burns or subthreshold (invisible) lesions and were compared to eyes receiving no treatment. Forty-eight laser lesions of 125 µm were applied in four concentric circles outside the FAZ in a scatter or grid pattern between 750 and 2250 µm from the center of the FAZ (Fig. 50.1). Only one laser treatment was applied to each eye throughout the duration of the study.

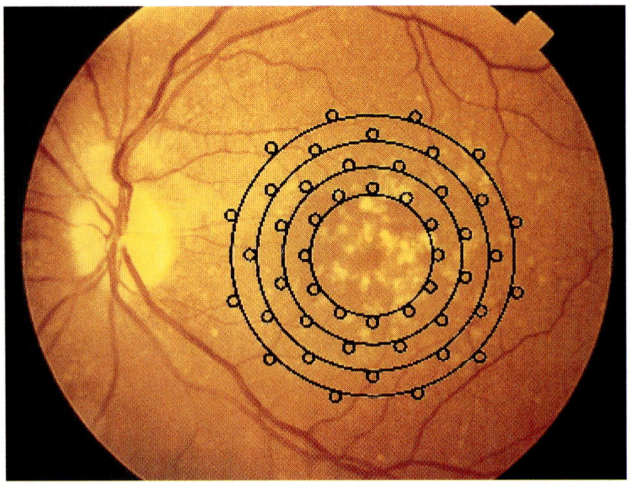

Figure 50.1 *Forty-eight diode laser lesions of 125 µm applied in four concentric circles outside the foveal avascular zone in a scatter or grid pattern between 750 and 2250 µm from the center of the foveal avascular zone.*

RESULTS

The percentage of eyes showing drusen reduction was significantly greater in treated eyes compared to observation eyes ($p < 0.0001$), whether the treatment was with visible or subthreshold laser, at all follow-up time points (Fig. 50.2). At 18 and 24 months after treatment, the percentage of eyes with drusen reduction was comparable in visible and subthreshold laser-treated eyes. At 12 months, reduction of drusen occurred in 62 of 115 treated eyes (53.9%) compared to 7 of 105 (6.7%) observation eyes ($p < 0.0001$). At 24 months, reduction in drusen occurred in 71 of 105 treated eyes (67.6%) compared to 3 of 91 (3.3%) observation eyes ($p < 0.0001$).

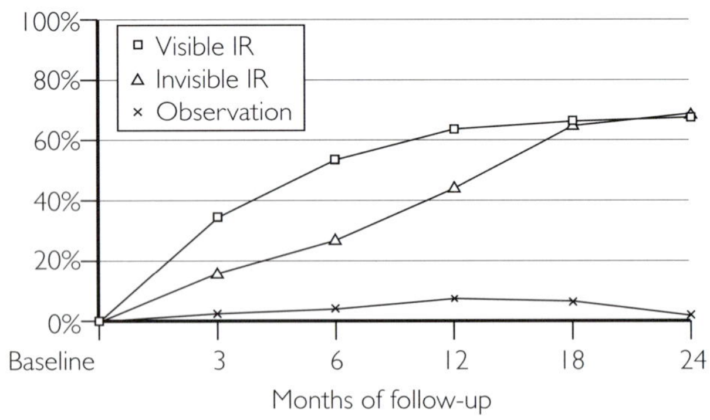

Figure 50.2 *Time course of clinically significant (more than 50%) drusen reduction in eyes treated with visible endpoint (□) and with subthreshold (△) grid photocoagulation vs observation eyes (×). Subthreshold treatment shows the same resorption effectiveness as visible treatment, although at a slower pace.*

In an overall analysis comparing all treated eyes to observation eyes, regardless of the study arm, a greater percentage of eyes receiving laser treatment showed improved visual acuity 12 months and longer after treatment. For example, at 24 months after treatment, 11.4% (12/105) of all treated eyes improved compared to 0% (0/91) of observation eyes ($p < 0.001$).

In analyzing the subset of eyes whose initial visual acuity was 20/32 or worse at entry (i.e. those eyes for which the potential for a two or more line increase exists) at 24 months, 15.4% (10/65) of all treated eyes improved compared to 0% (0/50) of observation eyes. In the bilateral study arm, 41 patients were entered whose treated eye had an initial visual acuity of 20/32 or less. Of these 41 patients, 24.4% (10/41) of the treated eyes showed improvement compared to 0% (0/41) of the observed eyes ($p < 0.002$).

CNV formation was similar in treated and observation eyes through 24 months of follow-up. After 24 months' follow-up, CNV had occurred in a total of 21 eyes. For the 15 unilateral study arm eyes that developed CNV, seven were observation eyes, and the remaining eight were equally divided between visible and subthreshold laser treatment. For the six occurrences of CNV in bilateral study arm eyes, three occurred in observation eyes and three in visible laser-treatment eyes. Remarkably, none of 34 eyes of the bilateral study arm that received subthreshold treatment developed CNV in the first 2 years, compared to three eyes with CNV in the 65 control eyes. This finding is very encouraging but not yet statistically significant. See case examples in Fig. 50.3a and b.

CONCLUSIONS

The results of this clinical pilot study after 24 months of follow-up indicate that infrared (810 nm) diode laser macular grid photocoagulation significantly reduces drusen levels in 67.6% of treated eyes compared to 3.3% of observation eyes ($p < 0.0001$) with one treatment.

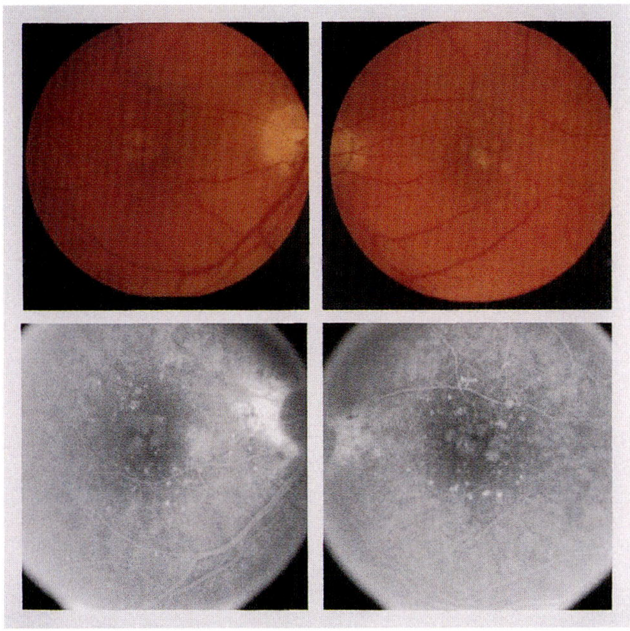

a

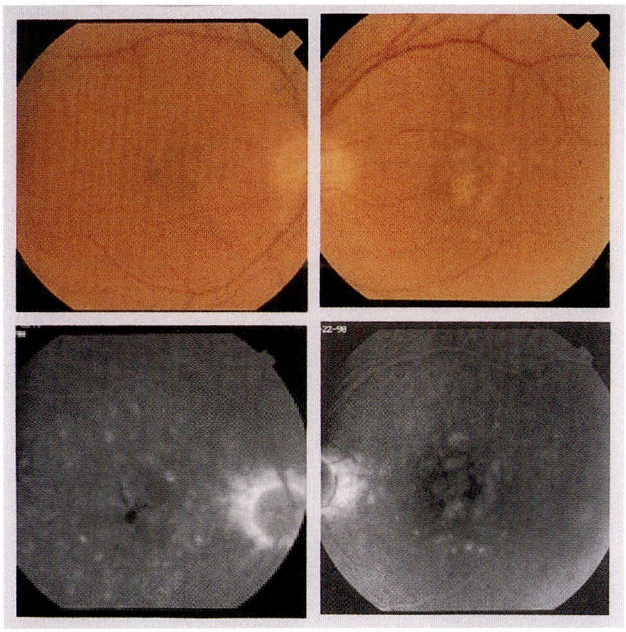

b

Figure 50.3 *(a) A 71-year-old white male with ARMD and bilateral central soft drusen. Visual acuity was 20/40 in his right eye (upper left photo) and 20/32 in his left eye (upper right photo). The right eye was treated with subthreshold laser lesions and the left eye was observed. Bottom photos are the corresponding fluorescein angiograms. (b) At 24 months' follow-up, drusen have resorbed in the treated right eye (upper left photo) and visual acuity was 20/25. Visual acuity in the observed left eye (upper right photo) was 20/50. Bottom photos are late-phase fluorescein angiograms. Note: laser lesions are barely visible on fundus photographs but readily visible on the fluorescein angiograms.*

The vision results at 24 months' follow-up demonstrate that there is a statistically significant improvement of two or more lines in all treated eyes (11.4%) compared to no improvement (0%) in observation eyes ($p < 0.001$). In addition, in the bilateral study arm, 24.4% of treated eyes whose initial visual acuity was 20/32 or less improved, compared to 0% of the observation eyes ($p < 0.002$). This observation is consistent with previous studies[6,7] that show some evidence of perifoveal laser treatment promoting the resolution of foveal drusen and that this coincides with an improvement of vision.

Finally, because the overall results of CNV formation in this pilot study are similar in both observation and treated eyes through 24 months' follow-up, and considering the fact that all complications in the clinical pilot study occurred using visible treatment burns, a larger, multicenter, prospective clinical trial comparing subthreshold (invisible) infrared (810 nm) diode laser macular grid photocoagulation with observation in both unilateral and bilateral eligible eyes with non-exudative ARMD is warranted. A follow-on clinical trial designed to more definitely evaluate the efficacy of subthreshold infrared diode laser treatment – the Prophylactic Treatment of Age-related Macular Degeneration Clinical Trial (PTAMD) – is currently underway.

REFERENCES

1. Smiddy WE, Fine SL. Prognosis of patients with bilateral macular drusen, *Ophthalmology* (1984) **91:**271–7.
2. Bressler SB, Maguire MG, Bressler NM, Fine SL. Relationship of drusen and abnormalities of the retinal pigment epithelium to the prognosis of neovascular macular degeneration, *Arch Ophthalmol* (1990) **108:**1442–7.
3. Holz FG, Wolfensberger TJ, Piguet B, et al. Bilateral macular drusen in age-related macular degeneration: prognosis and risk factors, *Ophthalmology* (1994) **101:**1522–8.
4. Macular Photocoagulation Study Group. Risk factors for choroidal neovascularization in the second eye of patients with juxtafoveal or subfoveal choroidal neovascularization secondary to age-related macular degeneration, *Arch Ophthalmol* (1997) **115:**741–7.

5. Schoeppner G, Chuang EL, Bird AC. The risk of fellow eye visual loss with unilateral retinal pigment epithelial tears, *Am J Ophthalmol* (1989) **108:**683–5.
6. Sarks SH, Arnold JJ, Sarks JP, Walter CJ. Prophylactic perifoveal laser treatment of soft drusen, *Aust NZ J Ophthalmol* (1996) **24:**15–26.
7. Little HL, Showman JM, Brown BW. A pilot randomized controlled study on the effect of laser photocoagulation of confluent soft macular drusen, *Ophthalmology* (1997) **104:**623–31.

Chapter 51 Photodynamic therapy

Darius M Moshfeghi and Gholam A Peyman

INTRODUCTION

Age-related macular degeneration (ARMD) is the leading cause of new blindness in people over age 60 in the Western hemisphere.[1] While many of the patients retain usable vision, 10% of those affected will experience severe visual loss (six or more lines of Snellen acuity).[2] Of these, 25% are caused by atrophy of the retinal pigment epithelium (RPE), choriocapillaris and outer neurosensory retina.[3] There is no treatment currently available for these patients. Exudative ARMD accounts for the remaining 75% of patients who experience severe visual loss, and includes choroidal neovascularization (CNV), disciform scarring, vitreous hemorrhage, pigment epithelial detachments and tears.[3]

The Macular Photocoagulation Study (MPS) evaluated the role of argon and krypton photocoagulation for the treatment of exudative ARMD and noted a small treatment effect that persisted at 5 years.[4] However, the study was hampered by a 50% recurrence of treated vessels, an immediate scotoma following treatment and a limited eligibility group, encouraging the search for alternative therapies.[5] These therapies have included radiation treatment, vitamin supplements, surgical excision of neovascular membranes, macular translocation and photodynamic therapy (PDT).[6–14]

PDT represents an emerging technology for the treatment of neovascular processes affecting the eye and other parts of the body. Specifically, much of the recent ophthalmic work in PDT has been directed at the treatment of the neovascular form of ARMD.[15–17] The basic principle of PDT is the activation of a dye by low-power laser light to induce coagulation of the neovascular vessels. The dye particles absorb the photons and move to a higher energy state, resulting in the creation of an excited oxygen species which damages cell membranes, mitochondria and vascular endothelial cells.[18–23] This can be done with relative ease and safety with regard to the surrounding normal neurosensory retina because of the lower power levels employed in PDT than in photocoagulation.

Photocoagulation depends on the absorption of thermal energy by pigment to achieve a therapeutic effect. This pigment can be located in the tissue of interest or in the surrounding tissue, which results in a transfer of thermal energy to the target tissue. It is not a selective treatment – all tissues exposed to the path of the laser beam will absorb energy if they contain pigment sensitive to the laser wavelength, which results in an unintended yet unavoidable bystander effect. This lack of specificity limits the usefulness of photocoagulation for the treatment of ARMD, especially for juxtafoveal and subfoveal lesions where all of the tissue will either absorb the laser energy or be adjacent to a tissue that absorbs it. Typically, a small spot size (100–200 μm), high power (300–400 mW) and short duration (0.1–0.3 seconds) are employed when using photocoagulation.

PDT, in contrast, relies on large spot sizes (>1000 μm), low powers (10–70 mW) and long duration (10–100 seconds) to achieve its therapeutic effect. The difference is that although a large area of retina is exposed to energy in PDT, there is no thermal effect exerted on the neurosensory tissue. Instead, the laser light acts as a catalyst to activate the photoactive dye within the vessels of interest, inducing occlusion of the vessel and sparing normal surrounding tissue.

PDT is initiated by an intravenous infusion (typically 1–2 mg/kg) of the photodynamic agent into the antecubital vein. This may be performed over 10–15 minutes in the case of suspension preparations or by bolus injection for solution preparations. After administration, 5–15 minutes are allowed to elapse to permit adequate dye delivery to the fundus. Laser energy is then applied to the area of interest with the aid of a fundus contact lens, using the parameters described above. The patient is advised to sit in a light-restricted room for 1 hour after treatment to minimize the possibility of phototoxicity from the dye.

The treatment effect of PDT is not immediately visible to the examiner, in contrast to photocoagulation, which results in an immediate visible thermal burn.[23] Instead, the lesions develop over a period of hours after the application of laser energy to the fundus. Other factors that may affect the efficacy of treatment include intraocular pressure, the region of fundus treated and the total time of exposure to the photodynamic agent.[24]

It has been noted that there is a high rate of recurrence of CNV following treatment with PDT; however, retreatment is possible with PDT. One recent study has demonstrated that caution should be employed when retreating with PDT because of the possibility of damage to overlying photoreceptors.[24]

Presently there are two drugs undergoing multicentered studies in the United States to evaluate their efficacy for treatment of exudative ARMD: Purlytin™ (tin ethyl etiopurpurin (SnET2), Miravant Technologies, Santa Barbara, CA) and Lu-Tex™ (luteium texaphyrin, Alcon Laboratories, Inc., Fort Worth, TX). Visudyne™ (verteporfin, CIBA Vision Corp., Duluth, GA), has recently been approved by the FDA.

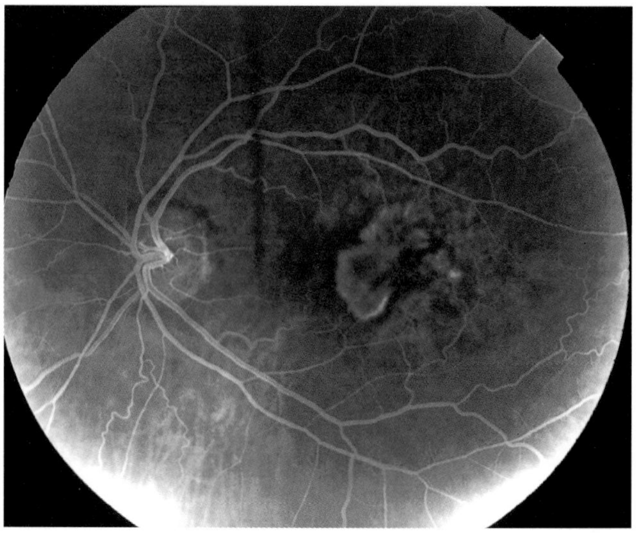

Figure 51.1 *Fundus fluorescein angiogram of a patient with exudative age-related macular degeneration. Note classical subretinal neovascular membrane.*

VERTEPORFIN

Results of verteporfin PDT for the treatment of ARMD were recently reported for both a single session and retreatment as necessary.[25,26] In a nonrandomized, multicenter, open-label clinical trial, five different dosage strategies were employed to test the efficacy of verteporfin PDT in the treatment of subfoveal CNV caused by ARMD. All patients had to demonstrate at least some evidence of classic CNV to be eligible for participation. The verteporfin dose was 6–12 mg/m^2, infusion time ranged from 5–10 minutes, the light dose ranged from 12.5–150 J/cm^2 and the time from start of infusion to laser application ranged from 10–30 minutes.[25] A 689–nm diode laser (Coherent Inc., Palo Alto, CA) at a constant irradiance of 600 mW/cm^2 was used in all patients to activate the dye.

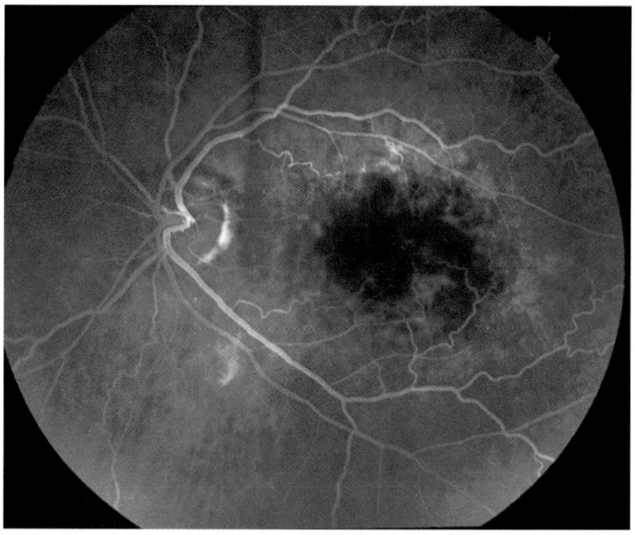

Figure 51.2 *Fundus fluorescein angiogram of the same patient as in Figure 51.1 one week after photodynamic therapy using verteporfin. Note complete closure of neovascular membrane.*

Two outcomes were used to assess efficacy and safety: fluorescein leakage from CNV and stabilization of best-corrected visual acuity at the 12–week follow-up compared to baseline.[25]

At one-week follow-up, all treated patients demonstrated some decrease in the amount of leakage of fluorescein from classical CNV (Figs 51.1 and 51.2), with complete absence of leakage (no CNV within the area of the lesion noted at baseline or beyond the area treated) seen in 52–100% of patients. The results of week 12 analysis showed that lesions demonstrating leakage at week 4 were more likely to have progression (leakage beyond the original borders of CNV) than areas with no leakage at week 4. At week 4 and week 12, those patients treated at 50 J/cm^2 and light application 15 minutes after the start of infusion demonstrated the highest percentage of eyes without leakage (30%).

The results for occult CNV were less clear, with some eyes without pretreatment evidence of occult CNV graded as having progression of occult CNV on follow-up examination. Mean visual acuity change from baseline for all eyes receiving a single treatment at week 12 ranged from –1.6 lines to +0.4 lines.[25]

With respect to safety, results of this study indicated that at the highest light dose tested (150 J/cm^2), verteporfin PDT caused retinal vascular occlusion and marked loss of visual acuity, causing the investigators to discontinue further use of this regimen. The safety and efficacy parameters for verteporfin were determined to be at a light dose greater than 25 and less than 150 J/cm^2.[25]

Thirty-one patients enrolled in the single-treatment study were subsequently enrolled in the retreatment study, which used two of the treatment regimens from the first study: 100 J/cm^2 and light application 20 minutes after the start of infusion of verteporfin, and 50–100 J/cm^2 and light application 15 minutes after the start of infusion.[26] The same angiographic and vision parameters were used to determine outcomes for this study. Results indicated that after one retreatment, most eyes demonstrated an absence of classic CNV leakage at both tested regimens, lack of progression of classic and occult CNV leakage 4 weeks after retreatment, and some evidence of progression of classic CNV leakage 12 weeks after the last treatment. Visual acuity change ranged from –1.0 to +0.2 lines. There was no difference in angiographic or visual acuity changes between the two regimens tested. No significant adverse effects of treatment were associated with retreatment.

In a subsequent study testing the safety of verteporfin PDT retreatment of normal nonhuman primate retina, choroid and optic nerve, retreatment at doses equal to or greater than 12 mg/m^2 was associated with significant adverse effects, including loss of choriocapillaris, loss of photoreceptors and significant optic atrophy.[27] At doses of 6 mg/m^2 and time to laser application (600 mW/cm^2 and fluence of 100 J/cm^2) 20 minutes after the start of infusion, deep retinal whitening was noted in the initial 24 hours following treatment, which usually resolved at 1 week. Mild pigmentary changes and outer photoreceptor damage were noted on histopathologic examination of these specimens 3 weeks after the last retreatment, with some recovery noted 7 weeks following treatment. The optic nerve specimens exhibited spotty loss of axons. This study demonstrated the overall safety of verteporfin for retreatment of normal nonhuman primate retina and choroid at the lower doses and longer latency to treatment times. The authors concluded that the inclusion of the optic nerve in the treatment zone was not advisable under any treatment regimen.[27]

One weakness in this study was that it did not conform to the protocol of the Treatment of Age-related Macular Degeneration with Photodynamic Therapy (TAP) Study Group regimen for time to light application following verteporfin infusion. In the nonhuman primate study, time from start of infusion to initiation of laser treatment was 20 minutes compared with 15 minutes in the TAP study.[27,28] The longer delay in initiation of treatment results in greater dilution of the photosensitizer and may result in a less efficacious treatment and decreased levels of adverse outcomes.[23] Furthermore, the safety results reported in one animal species are not necessarily transferable to humans. Indeed, the authors reported a much higher than expected rate of adverse outcomes in humans tested at the 150 J/cm^2 fluence than they had experienced in primate studies.[25]

The one-year results of the TAP study were published in 1999.[28] The study consisted of two multicenter, double-masked, placebo-controlled randomized trials with identical protocols. Eligible patients had subfoveal CNV from ARMD with the greatest linear dimension of less than 5400 μm and best-corrected visual acuity ranging from 20/40 to 20/200.[28] Verteporfin at 6 mg/m^2 was infused intravenously for 10 minutes, followed by laser activation (689-nm diode laser, 50 J/cm^2, 600 mW/cm^2, 83-second duration, spot size 1000 μm larger than greatest linear diameter of the CNV lesion) 15 minutes after the start of infusion.[28] Patients were evaluated by clinical examination and fluorescein angiography approximately every three months, and retreated at the discretion of the treating ophthalmologist. Of the 609 eyes enrolled in the study (402 treatment, 207 placebo), 94% completed the 12-month follow-up. In the treatment group, 246 (61%) of 402 eyes lost fewer than 15 letters of visual acuity from baseline, compared to 96 (47%) of 207 placebo eyes, a difference that was statistically significant ($P < 0.001$). Subgroup analysis demonstrated the greatest benefit (67% versus 39% losing less than 15 letters of visual acuity, $P < 0.001$) for those eyes with predominantly classic CNV (greater than 50% of the entire lesion being classic CNV before treatment). No significant lasting adverse effects were reported.[28]

In an accompanying editorial, Fine noted that verteporfin represents a welcome addition to the treatment armamentarium against ARMD, particularly for those eyes with evidence of predominantly classic CNV.[29] With US FDA approving verteporfin in early

2000, Margherio and members of the TAP study group recently addressed the socioeconomic impact of PDT on retinal practices.[30] They concluded that of 1000 patients retrospectively reviewed, 99 would have been eligible for photocoagulation under the MPS guidelines, whereas 188 would be eligible for treatment with verteporfin PDT. In the TAP study, the average patient received 3.7 treatments during the one-year follow-up, or approximately every 3 months; for the purposes of this analysis, it was assumed that the average patient would undergo three treatments per year.[28,30] Using these assumptions, they predicted a seven-fold increase in the services provided by retina specialists for patients with predominantly classic CNV resulting from ARMD.[30] If these assumptions prove to be true, there may be a need for restructuring reimbursement for these procedures.

REFERENCES

1. Abdelsalam A, Del Priore L, Zarbin MA. Drusen in age-related macular degeneration: pathogenesis, natural course, and laser photocoagulation-induced regression, *Surv Ophthalmol* (1999) **44:**1–29.
2. Elman MJ, Fine SL. Exudative age-related macular degeneration. In: Ryan SJ, ed, *Retina*, 2nd edn (Mosby Year Book, Inc: St Louis, 1994): 1103–41.
3. Klein R, Klein BE, Jensen SC, Meuer SM. The five-year incidence and progression of age-related maculopathy: the Beaver Dam Eye Study, *Ophthalmology* (1997) **104:**7–21.
4. Macular Photocoagulation Study Group. Five-year follow-up of fellow eyes of patients with age-related macular degeneration and unilateral extrafoveal choroidal neovascularization, *Arch Ophthalmol* (1993) **111:**1189–99.
5. Macular Photocoagulation Study Group. Recurrent choroidal neovascularization after argon laser photocoagulation for neovascular maculopathy, *Arch Ophthalmol* (1986) **104:**503–12.
6. Lewis H, Kaiser PK, Lewis S, Estafanous M. Macular translocation for subfoveal choroidal neovascularization in age-related macular degeneration: a prospective study, *Am J Ophthalmol* (1999) **128:**135–46.
7. De Juan E Jr, Loewenstein A, Bressler NM, Alexander J. Translocation of the retina for management of subfoveal choroidal neovascularization: II. a preliminary report in humans, *Am J Ophthalmol* (1998) **125:**635–46.
8. Mauget-Faÿsse M, Chiquet C, Milea D, et al. Long term results of radiotherapy for subfoveal choroidal neovascularisation in age related macular degeneration, *Br J Ophthalmol* (1999) **83:**923–8.
9. Donati G, Soubrane D, Quaranta M, et al. Radiotherapy for isolated occult subfoveal neovascularisation in age related macular degeneration: a pilot study, *Br J Ophthalmol* (1999) **83:**646–51.
10. Smith W, Mitchell P, Webb K, Leeder SR. Dietary antioxidants and age-related maculopathy: the Blue Mountains Eye Study, *Ophthalmology* (1999) **106:**761–7.
11. Merrill PT, LoRusso FJ, Lomeo MD, et al. Surgical removal of subfoveal choroidal neovascularization in age-related macular degeneration, *Ophthalmology* (1999) **106:**782–9.
12. Finger PT, Berson A, Ng T, Szechter A. Ophthalmic plaque radiotherapy for age-related macular degeneration associated with subretinal neovascularization, *Am J Ophthalmol* (1999) **127:**170–7.
13. Chong NH, Bird AC. Alternative therapies in exudative age related macular degeneration, *Br J Ophthalmol* (1998) **82:**1441–3.
14. Ciulla TA, Danis RP, Harris A. Age-related macular degeneration: a review of experimental treatments, *Surv Ophthalmol* (1998) **43:**134–46.
15. Bressler NM, the TAP Study Group. Photodynamic therapy with verteporfin of subfoveal choroidal neovascularization in age-related macular degeneration (AMD): baseline characteristics and safety in the TAP randomized clinical trials, *Invest Ophthalmol Vis Sci* (1999) **40**(suppl):S401.
16. Slakter J, the VIP Research Study Group. Photodynamic therapy of subfoveal choroidal neovascularization in pathologic myopia with verteporfin: study design and baseline characteristics in the VIP randomized clinical trial, *Invest Ophthalmol Vis Sci* (1999) **40**(suppl):S401.
17. Thomas EL, Rosen R, Murphy R, et al. Visual acuity stabilizes after a single treatment with SnET2–photodynamic therapy in patients with subfoveal choroidal neovascularization, *Invest Ophthalmol Vis Sci* (1999) **40**(suppl):S401.
18. Henderson BW, Dougherty TJ. How does photodynamic therapy work, *Photochem Photobiol* (1992) **55:**145–57.
19. Reed MW, Miller FN, Wieman TJ, et al. The effect of photodynamic therapy on the microcirculation, *J Surg Res* (1988) **45:**452–9.
20. Ben-Hur E, Orenstein A. The endothelium and red blood cells as potential targets in PDT-induced vascular stasis, *Int J Radiat Biol* (1991) **60:**293–301.
21. He DP, Hampton JA, Keck R, Selman SH. Photodynamic therapy: effect on the endothelial cell of the rat aorta, *Photochem Photobiol* (1991) **54:**801–4.
22. Gottfried V, Lindenbaum ES, Kimel S. Vascular damage during PDT as monitored in the chick chorioallantoic membrane, *Int J Radiat Biol* (1991) **60:**349–54.
23. Moshfeghi DM, Peyman GA, Moshfeghi AA, et al. Ocular vascular thrombosis following tin ethyl etiopurpurin (SnET2) photodynamic therapy: time dependencies, *Ophthalmic Surg Lasers* (1998) **29:**663–8.
24. Peyman GA, Kazi AA, Unal M, et al. Problems with and pitfalls of photodynamic therapy, *Ophthalmology* (2000) **107**:29–35.
25. Miller JW, Schmidt-Erfurth U, Sickenberg M, et al. Photodynamic therapy with verteporfin for choroidal neovascularization caused by age-related macular degeneration: Results of a single treatment in a phase 1 and 2 study, *Arch Ophthalmol* (1999) **117**:1161–73.
26. Schmidt-Erfurth U, Miller JW, Sickenberg M, et al. Photodynamic therapy with verteporfin for choroidal neovascularization caused by age-related macular degeneration: Results of retreatments in a phase 1 and 2 study, *Arch Ophthalmol* (1999) **117**:1177–87.
27. Reinke MH, Canakis C, Husain D, et al. Verteporfin photodynamic therapy retreatment of normal retina and

choroid in the cynomolgus monkey, *Ophthalmology* (1999) **106**:1915–23.

28. Treatment of Age-related Macular Degeneration with Photodynamic Therapy (TAP) Study Group. Photodynamic therapy of subfoveal choroidal neovascularization in age-related macular degeneration with verteporfin: One-year results of 2 randomized clinical trials. TAP report 1, *Arch Ophthalmol* (1999) **117**:1329–45.
29. Fine SL. Photodynamic therapy with verteporfin is effective for selected patients with neovascular age-related macular degeneration (editorial), *Arch Ophthalmol* (1999) **117**:1400–2.
30. Margherio RR, Margherio AR, DeSantis ME, TAP Study Group. The socioeconomic impact of photodynamic therapy on retinal practices. *American Academy of Ophthalmology Vitreoretinal Update 1999* (syllabus): 33–35. American Academy of Ophthalmology, San Francisco, CA.

Chapter 52 Transpupillary thermotherapy of choroidal neovascularization

Mark Rivellese and Elias Reichel

INTRODUCTION

Transpupillary thermotherapy (TTT) is a method of delivering radiation to intraocular structures through the pupil. TTT was first described by Oosterhuis et al[1] in 1995 as an adjunct to radiotherapy in the treatment of choroidal melanomas during and after plaque therapy in cases where tumor regression was insufficient. More recently, TTT has been used successfully as a primary treatment for small choroidal melanomas.[2,3] A new and promising application of TTT is for the treatment of subfoveal choroidal neovascularization (CNV) caused by age-related macular degeneration (ARMD).

TECHNIQUES AND PRINCIPLES

TTT is a technique based on the principle of hyperthermia – defined as temperature elevation above normal temperature. Three ranges of temperature can be used for tumor destruction.[4] The low range of 42–44°C does not have a direct destructive effect on cells. This level of hyperthermia potentiates the effects of radiotherapy on choroidal melanoma. In the high range at 60°C and above, hyperthermia results in coagulative necrosis. The intermediate range between 45°C and 60°C induces tumor necrosis without the need for concomitant radiotherapy. In the intermediate range, the coagulative effect seen with higher doses is absent and heat penetration is optimized.[5,6]

Hyperthermia treatment can be applied as either systemic hyperthermia or localized heating. In TTT, the difficulty of delivering hyperthermia to the target tissue is obviated as the anatomy of the eye allows direct access to the posterior segment structures. Thermometry measurements in ocular hyperthermia are invasive and impractical and are not performed. In contrast to cancer treatments in which complete tumor destruction to the last viable cell is required for treatment success, the success in TTT for choroidal neovascularization requires only the occlusion of neovascular vessels, making thermometry readings less important.

For the treatment of CNV, heat energy is delivered slowly to the choroid and retinal pigment epithelium through the pupil using an 810 nm diode laser. The laser is modified for a large spot size of 1.2, 2.0, or 3.0 mm (Iris Medical Instruments, Mountain View, CA). Typical laser parameters used are a duration of 60–70 seconds at power settings of 250–1000 mW.[7] In general, for a 3-mm spot size, the initial power setting is 800 mW and is appropriately reduced for smaller spot sizes by keeping the power density at approximately 10 W/cm^2. Typically, no visible color change is seen at the end of the treatment. Near-infrared irradiation is ideal for use in TTT as tissue penetration is high and absorption by the ocular media is minimized.[8,9] The large diameter of the irradiation beam allows homogeneous treatment of large lesions.[10]

TREATMENT OF AGE-RELATED MACULAR DEGENERATION

ARMD is the most common cause of visual loss in patients over 60 years of age in the United States. The only proven treatment for exudative ARMD is laser photocoagulation of well-defined choroidal neovascular membranes. Approximately 13% of patients with CNV from ARMD are eligible for

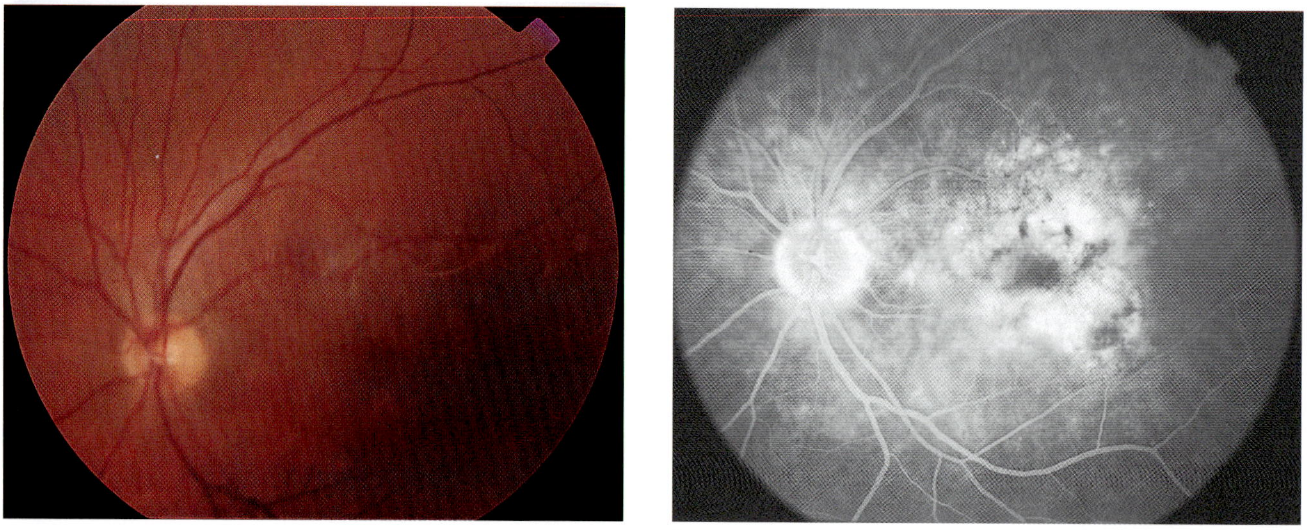

a *b*

Figure 52.1 *(a) An eye with poorly defined choroidal neovascularization before transpupillary thermotherapy. Visual acuity measured 20/100. (b) Corresponding fluorescein angiogram showing diffuse leakage consistent with occult choroidal neovascularization.*

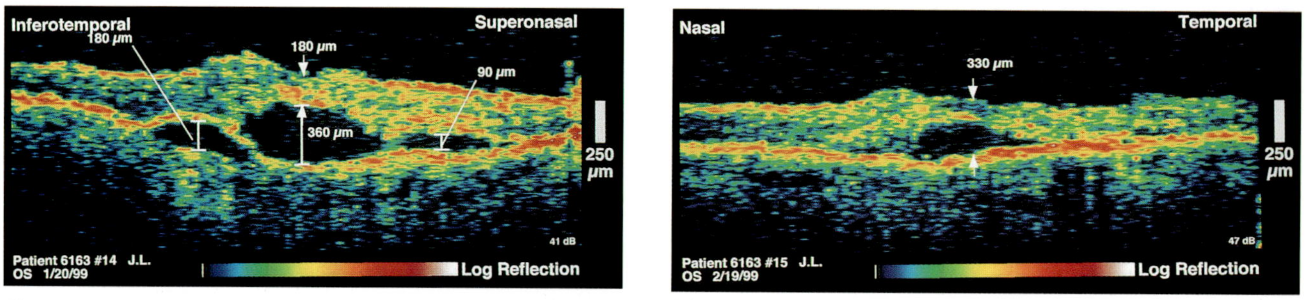

a *b*

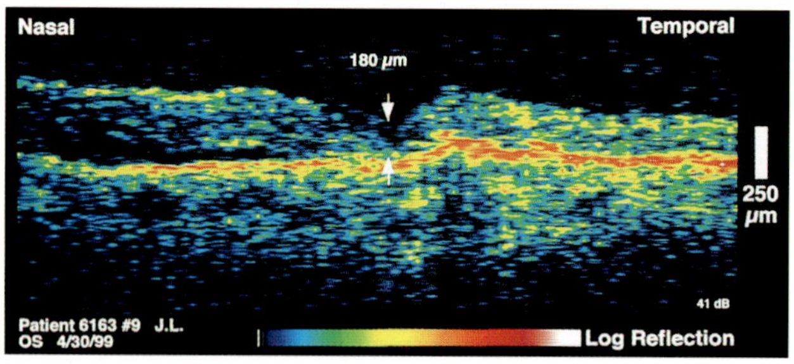

c

Figure 52.2 *(a) Optical coherence tomography of the same eye as in Fig. 52.1 before treatment. Note the retinal thickening, subretinal fluid and retinal pigment epithelial detachment. (b) Optical coherence tomography 1 month after transpupillary thermotherapy. Note the change in retinal thickness and decrease in subretinal fluid. Vision remained 20/100. (c) Optical coherence tomography 3 months after treatment. The central foveal depression can be observed and the subretinal fluid has resolved. Visual acuity measured 20/40.*

treatment according to the criteria of the Macular Photocoagulation Study.[10,11] The absence of an effective therapy for most cases of CNV has prompted the investigation of alternative therapies.

Minimization of collateral tissue damage is the rationale behind photodynamic therapy and indocyanine green-enhanced diode laser treatment. TTT may also minimize the coagulation of surrounding tissues while optimizing deep penetration to the choroid and retinal pigment epithelium. In a pilot study, 16 eyes of 15 patients with subfoveal occult CNV were treated with TTT.[7] Nineteen percent of eyes (3/16) experienced improved visual acuity by two or more lines,

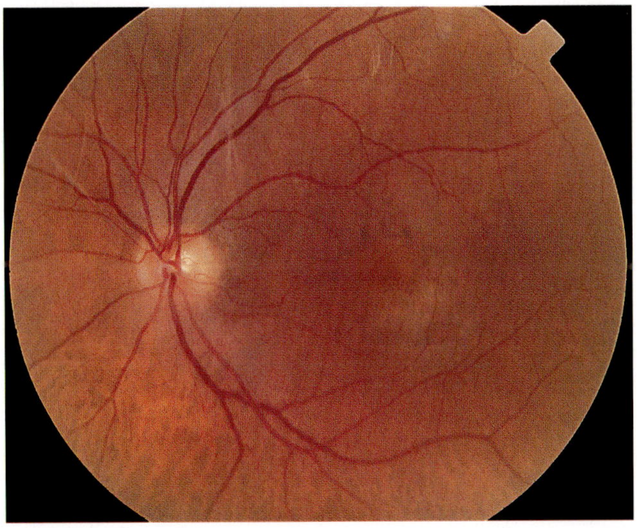

Figure 52.3 *The same eye as in Figs 52.1 and 52.2 three months after treatment.*

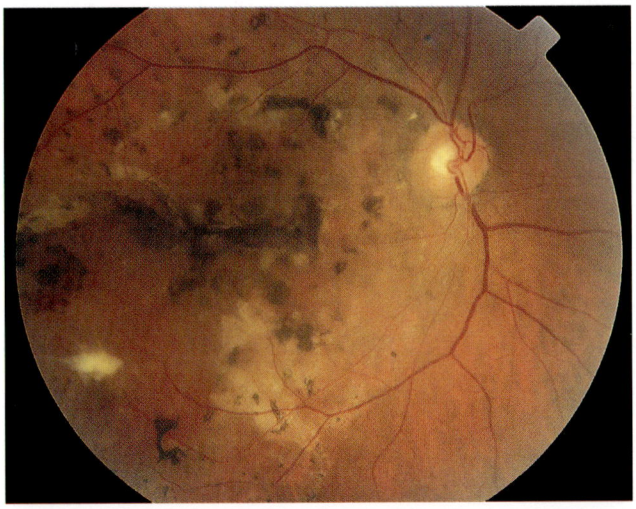

a

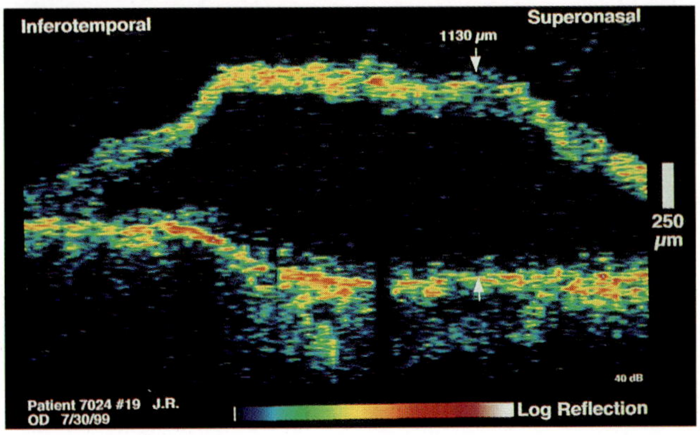

b

56% (9/16) had no change in visual acuity and 25% (4/16) had a decline in visual acuity of two or more lines. Fifteen of 16 eyes (94%) had an improvement in exudation, including three of the four patients who had a decrease in visual acuity. One eye showed persistent subretinal exudation consistent with treatment failure. In less than 1% of treated eyes a small retinal arteriolar occlusion may be observed. These typically reopen and are not associated with permanent loss of vision. Figures 52.1–52.4 show two eyes before and after TTT for subfoveal CNV.

The decreased thermal effect in TTT compared to conventional laser photocoagulation seems to result in less damage to the adjacent retina, a finding which is

Figure 52.4 *(a) An eye before transpupillary thermotherapy. (b) Optical coherence tomography prior to transpupillary thermotherapy. A large serous pigment epithelial detachment is present. (c) Optical coherence tomography 2 months after transpupillary thermotherapy. The serous pigment epithelial detachment has decreased in size. (d) Color photograph taken 2 months after transpupillary thermotherapy.*

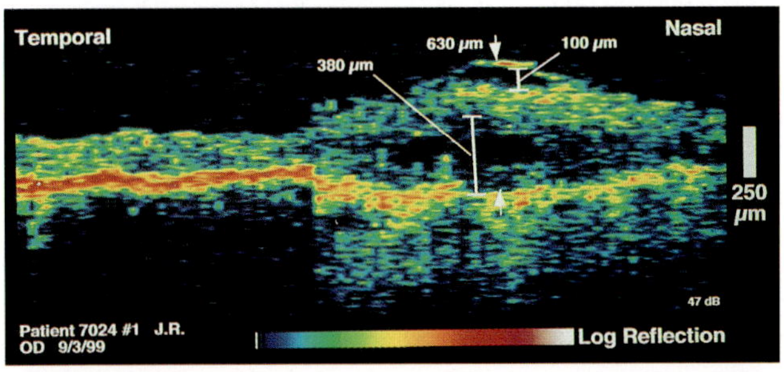

c

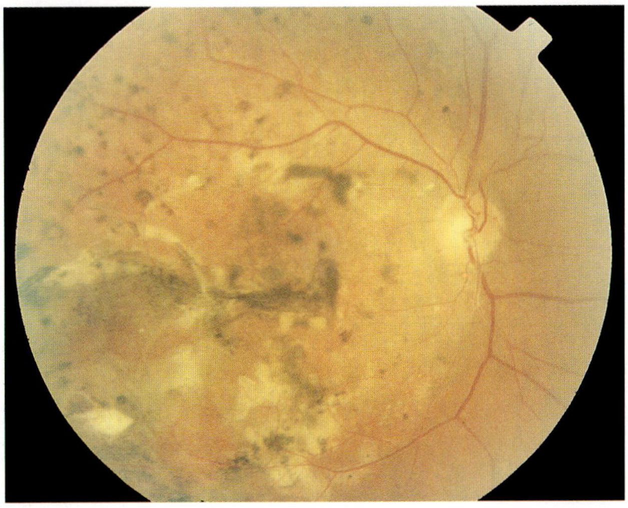

d

important in cases with a subfoveal component to the neovascular complex. The near-infrared wavelength of the diode laser is well suited to treating lesions partially obscured by pigment or hemorrhage. The adjustable spot size is ideal for treating occult CNV that tends to be larger than the 200–500-μm spot size of conventional laser delivery systems. Histologic studies of choroidal melanomas treated with TTT show extensive thrombosis of tumor vessels.[12] A similar mechanism may be responsible for the treatment effect after TTT of CNV in ARMD.

SUMMARY

TTT is a technique based on hyperthermia. The ability selectively to deliver heat energy to the choroid and retinal pigment epithelium make this a viable method for treating subfoveal CNV. The role of TTT for CNV resulting from ARMD has not been determined. However, a small pilot study has provided promising results and warrants further investigation of this technique.

REFERENCES

1. Oosterhuis JA, Journee-de Korver HG, Kakebeeke-Kemme HM, Bleeker JC. Transpupillary thermotherapy in choroidal melanomas, *Arch Ophthalmol* (1995) **113:**315–21.
2. Shields CL, Shields JA, DePotter P, Kheterpal S. Transpupillary thermotherapy in the management of choroidal melanoma, *Ophthalmology* (1996) **103:**1642–50.
3. Shields CL, Shields JA, Cater J, et al. Transpupillary thermotherapy for choroidal melanoma: tumor control and visual results in 100 consecutive cases, *Ophthalmology* (1998) **105:**581–90.
4. Nuijs-Beems EM, Oosteruis JA, Verburg-van der Marel EH, et al. Tumor destruction by intermediate level hyperthermia, *Curr Eye Res* (1990) **9:**771–80.
5. Burgess SE, Chang S, Svitra PP, et al. Effect of hyperthermia on experimental choroidal melanoma, *Br J Ophthalmol* (1985) **69:**854–60.
6. Coleman DJ, Silverman RH, Iwamoto T, et al. Histopathologic effects of ultrasonically induced hyperthermia in intraocular malignant melanoma, *Ophthalmology* (1988) **95:**970–81.
7. Reichel E, Berrocal AM, Ip M, et al. Transpupillary thermotherapy of occult subfoveal choroidal neovascularization in patients with age-related macular degeneration. *Ophthalmology* (1999) **106:**1908–14.
8. Svaasand LO, Boerslid T, Oeveraasen M. Thermal and optical properties of living tissue: application to laser-induced hyperthermia, *Lasers Surg Med* (1985) **5:**589–602.
9. Geeraets WJ, Williams RC, Chan G, et al. The loss of light energy in retina and choroid, *Arch Ophthalmol* (1960) **64:**158–67.
10. Macular Photocoagulation Study Group. Laser photocoagulation of subfoveal neovascular lesions of age-related macular degeneration: updated findings from two clinical trials, *Arch Ophthalmol* (1993) **111:**1200–9.
11. Freund KB, Yannuzzi LA, Sorenson JA. Age-related macular degeneration and choroidal neovascularization, *Am J Ophthalmol* (1993) **115:**786–91.
12. Journee-de Korver HG, Oosterhuis JA, de Wolff-Rouendaal D, Kemme H. Histopathological findings in human choroidal melanomas after transpupillary thermotherapy, *Br J Ophthalmol* (1997) **81:**234–9.

Chapter 53 Development and application of a subretinal semiconductor microphotodiode array

Alan Y Chow, Machelle T Pardue, Gholam A Peyman and Neal S Peachey

INTRODUCTION

Neurosensory systems may be activated artificially by external electrical stimulation. This fundamental feature allowed the development of neuroprosthetics, such as the cochlear implant.[1] The visual system is no exception, and it is well established that electrical stimulation of the retina or occipital cortex has the capacity to induce a visual sensation in human subjects.[2–7] Results obtained from a series of animal studies[8–11] show that a similar outcome may be expected if the stimulating device makes contact with the retina, i.e. near the initial input stage of the visual system. These results raised the possibility of developing a visual prosthetic device analogous to the cochlear implant.

The importance of achieving this goal is underscored by the lack of effective treatments to restore vision compromised by a large number of blinding disorders, including retinitis pigmentosa and macular degeneration. This volume includes chapters describing two strategies toward accomplishing this goal. One approach, which involves stimulation of the inner retina via a device placed into the vitreous cavity, is described in Chapter 54, and is the subject of a recent review.[12] Here, we outline the rationale, surgical techniques and results obtained with a device that is designed to be placed in the subretinal space.[13–15]

The conversion of light energy into neural energy is accomplished by the rod and cone photoreceptors that reside in the outer retina and make up the initial sampling array of the visual system.[16] In contrast to most neurons, photoreceptors respond to stimulation in a graded fashion and without generating action potentials.[16] This feature is relatively simple to replicate with the available semiconductor-based photodiode technology.

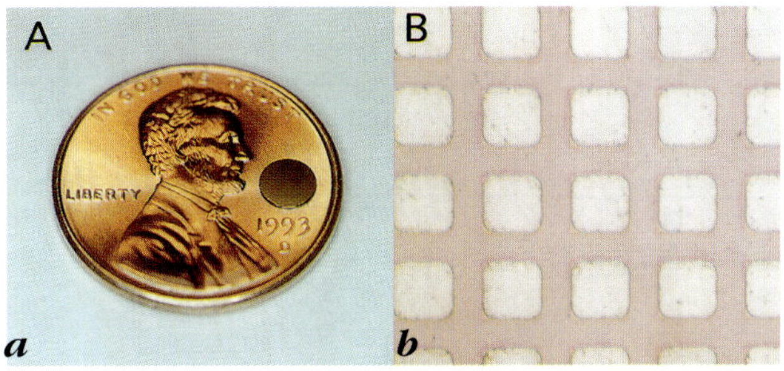

Figure 53.1 *Low- (a) and high- (b) power photographs of the semiconductor microphotodiode array implant.*

In the late 1980s, work was begun to develop a device that would generate current in proportion to the level of incident light. Figure 53.1 presents low- (a) and high- (b) power images of an implant. The higher power image shows that the implant is comprised of a series of microphotodiode subunits electrically separated from one another by a channel stop.[13–15] Here, each of the subunits within an implant has the same polarity, which may be either NiP (negative–intrinsic layer–positive) or PiN (positive–intrinsic layer–negative). In this example, each subunit subtends 20 μm; although this dimension is greater than that of human foveal cones,[17] it would be possible to reduce this dimension by several-fold with present-day fabrication technology. The microphotodiodes originally are fabricated in large wafers; the final diameter is determined when the wafer is cut into 2–3 mm diameter circular discs for implantation.

The implant is intended for use in disorders where the photoreceptors are lost while the remaining retinal layers are relatively spared. This situation is encountered in a wide variety of conditions, including retinitis pigmentosa[18,19] and age-related macular degeneration.[20] In short, the approach involves placing the implant into the subretinal space, and allowing the retina to settle back on top so that the implant is located in the position normally occupied by the photoreceptors. As a result, the light-evoked electrical response of the implant is in close proximity to second-order neurons, particularly the bipolar cells. If these cells could be stimulated electrically by implant activity, the natural behavior of the visual pathway might be relied upon to transmit the signal centrally. One of the features of this response is that the artificial input occurs at an extremely early level, allowing neural processing networks to extract visual information in a relatively normal fashion.

Several initial studies have been carried out in rabbits.[11,21,22] More recently, we have used a cat model.[23,24] In addition to possessing a large eye to accommodate the implant, the cat retina more closely approximates the human retina in having a dual blood supply to the inner and outer retina.

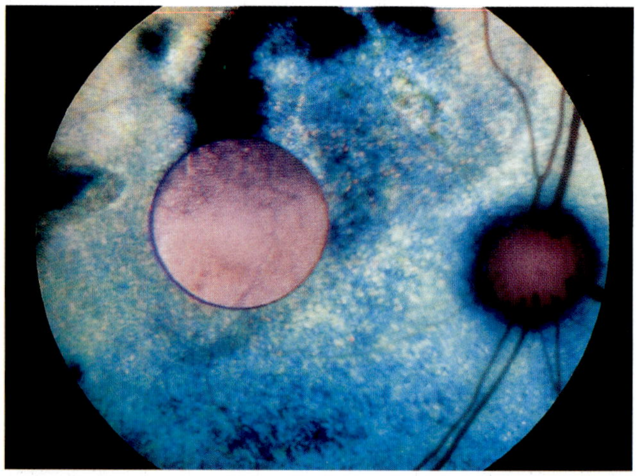

Figure 53.2 *Fundus photograph of a cat taken approximately 3 months after implantation surgery of a microphotodiode array.*

TECHNIQUE

There are certain difficulties that are associated with cat ocular surgery. For example, to gain access to the temporal sclera, it is necessary to remove a portion of the zygomatic arch. In addition, a partial vitrectomy is required to allow free access through the cat vitreous body, which is substantially more viscous and adherent than that of the rabbit. We typically make an approximately 3-mm sclerotomy to provide access to the vitreous cavity, and create a channel between this opening and the implant site through vitrectomy and vitreous replacement with a viscoelastic substance.

A localized separation of the retina is created near the *area centralis* by injecting a small amount of saline into the subretinal space. A retinotomy created near the edge of the bleb allows the implant to be inserted into the subretinal space; in successful operations, the retina will flatten over the implant. Following closure, a 1-week course of topical antibiotics is given.

Ophthalmoscopy and fundus photography are used to evaluate the retina during the postoperative period. Figure 53.2 is a fundus photograph of a cat taken approximately 3 months after placement of an implant into the subretinal space. The pigmentary changes seen in the upper field were induced by the retinotomy and other manipulations carried out during surgery. In most other respects, the overall appearance of the retina is not substantially different from an unoperated eye.

An important consideration concerns how to distinguish any implant-evoked activity from that of the native visual system. This is accomplished by taking advantage of the different spectral sensitivities of the two systems; although vertebrate visual systems respond to light below about 700 nm, the implant responds well into the infrared (IR). As a result, IR stimulation is used to isolate activity of the implant.

Electrophysiological recordings made from an anesthetized cat are shown in Figure 53.3. The

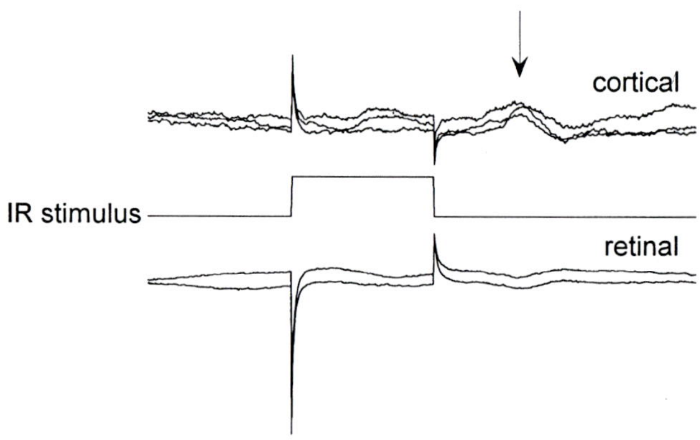

Figure 53.3 *Electrophysiological recordings made at the retinal (lower tracings) and cortical (upper tracings) levels from an anesthetized cat (11 mg/kg ketamine; 2.2 mg/kg xylazine). Recordings were made simultaneously to the presentation of an infrared light-emitting diode stimulus (middle trace) using a pair of differential amplifiers (1–1500 Hz). Several recordings are superimposed for each recording condition. The amplitude of the stimulus trace represents 25 μV for the retinal recordings and 5 μV for the cortical responses.*

middle tracing ('stimulus') represents the 200-ms activation of an IR light-emitting diode. The lower pair of tracings ('retinal') were made using a corneal contact lens electrode and include a prominent negative wave at stimulus onset and an opposite polarity wave at stimulus offset. These components reflect the electrical response of the implant itself, which is a NiP configuration in this example. The upper recordings ('cortical') were obtained from a needle electrode placed over the visual cortex. It is also possible to detect the implant response in the cortical recordings. In addition, a small positive wave (arrow) also is seen following stimulus offset.

When results from different recording sessions are compared, this response is reproducible in amplitude and timing. It is important to note that the polarity of this late wave is the same whether the implant functions in the NiP or the PiN configuration (which lead to opposite polarity implant spikes). Although the results obtained to date suggest that this late wave may represent cortical activation by the implant, recent results indicate that this wave may represent a response of the normal cat retina to IR light.

CONCLUSIONS

In conclusion, we are evaluating the possibility that a subretinal microphotodiode implant may provide the means to activate a retina in which the photoreceptors have been selectively lost. Current efforts are aimed at evaluating the biocompatibility and function of the implant, reducing the size of the implant and building analytic processing into the implant. This work will identify the type of implant that will be most suitable for small-scale human trials.

REFERENCES

1. Balkany T, Hodges AV, Luntz M. Update on cochlear implantation, *Otolaryngol Clin North Am* (1996) **29:**277–89.
2. Brindley GS, Lewin WS. The sensations produced by electrical stimulation of the visual cortex, *J Physiol* (1968) **196:**479–93.
3. Potts AM, Inoue J, Buffum D. The electrically evoked response of the visual system (EER), *Invest Ophthalmol* (1968) **7:**269–78.
4. Carpenter RHS. Electrical stimulation of the human eye in different adaptational states, *J Physiol* (1972) **221:**137–48.
5. Dobelle WH, Mladejovsky MG, Girvin JP. Artificial vision for the blind: electrical stimulation of the cortex offers hope for a functional prosthesis, *Science* (1974) **183:**440–4.
6. Schmidt EM, Bak MJ, Hambrecht FT, et al. Feasibility of a visual prosthesis for the blind based on intracortical microstimulation of the visual cortex, *Brain* (1996) **119:**507–22.
7. Humayun MS, de Juan E Jr, Dagnelie G, et al. Visual perception elicited by electrical stimulation of retina in blind humans, *Arch Ophthalmol* (1996) **114:**40–6.
8. Knighton RW. An electrically evoked slow potential of the frog's retina. I. Properties of the response, *J Neurophysiol* (1975) **38:**185–97.
9. Knighton RW. An electrically evoked slow potential of the frog's retina. II. Identification with PII component of electroretinogram, *J Neurophysiol* (1975) **38:**198–209.
10. Dawson WW, Radtke ND. The electrical stimulation of the retina by indwelling electrodes, *Invest Ophthalmol Vis Sci* (1977) **16:**249–52.
11. Chow AY, Chow VY. Subretinal electrical stimulation of the rabbit retina, *Neurosci Lett* (1997) **225:**13–16.
12. Rizzo JF III, Wyatt J. Prospects for a visual prosthesis, *Neuroscientist* (1997) **3:**251–62.
13. Chow AY. Artificial retina device, US Patent No. 5,016,633, May 21, 1991.
14. Chow AY. Artificial retina device, US Patent No. 5,024,223, June 18, 1991.
15. Chow AY, Chow V. Independent photoelectric artificial retina device and method using same, US Patent No. 5,397,350, March 14, 1995.
16. Dowling JE. *The Retina* (Belknap Press: Cambridge, MA, 1987).
17. Curcio CA, Sloan KR, Kalina RE, Hendrickson AE. Human photoreceptor topography, *J Comp Neurol* (1990) **292:**497–523.
18. Flannery JG, Farber DB, Bird AC, Bok D. Degenerative changes in a retina affected with autosomal dominant retinitis pigmentosa, *Invest Ophthalmol Vis Sci* (1989) **30:**191–211.
19. Santos A, Humayun MS, de Juan E Jr, et al. Preservation of the inner retina in retinitis pigmentosa: a morphometric analysis, *Arch Ophthalmol* (1997) **115:**511–15.
20. Curcio CA, Medeiros NE, Millican CL. Photoreceptor loss in age-related macular degeneration, *Invest Ophthalmol Vis Sci* (1996) **37:**1236–49.
21. Chow AY. Electrical stimulation of the rabbit retina with subretinal electrodes and high density microphotodiode array implants, *Invest Ophthalmol Vis Sci* (1993) **34:**835 (abst).
22. Peyman G, Chow AY, Liang C, et al. Subretinal semiconductor microphotodiode array, *Ophthalmic Surg Lasers* (1998) **29:**234–41.
23. Peachey NS, Toleikis SC, Chow AY. Stimulation of retinal photoreceptor function with arrayed subretinal microphotodiode implants: a pilot study, *Rehab Res Devel Progr Rep* (1994/1995) **32:**249–50.
24. Chow AY, Chow VY, Pardue MT, et al. Retinal and cortical potentials induced by subretinally implanted microphotodiode arrays, *Invest Ophthalmol Vis Sci* (1998) **39:**S565 (abst).

Chapter 54 **Artificial vision**

Mark S Humayun, James D Weiland and Eugene de Juan Jr

INTRODUCTION

Retinitis pigmentosa (RP) and age-related macular degeneration (ARMD) lead to the degeneration of photoreceptors, resulting in a significant visual deficit in the afflicted eye. Research is proceeding to investigate the feasibility of replacing the function of the photoreceptors with an electronic device. The photoreceptors initiate a neural signal in response to light. The experiments to be discussed investigate the possibility of using electrical signals (generated by a retinal prosthesis) to initiate a neural response in the remaining cells of the retina. Results from both animal and human research support the basic retinal prosthesis concept.[1–4]

Specifically, in tests with human volunteers we have used intraocular stimulating electrodes to create the perception of discrete spots of light in eyes with no light perception. Moreover, we were able to create form vision by stimulating the retina through several electrodes. Based on these encouraging results, the current focus is being shifted from feasibility studies to the development of an implantable, electronic device, which will be capable of stimulating the retina at hundreds of individual points.

BACKGROUND

The proposed retinal prosthesis system is shown in Fig. 54.1. A video camera will capture an image and convert it to an electrical signal. The electrical signal will be

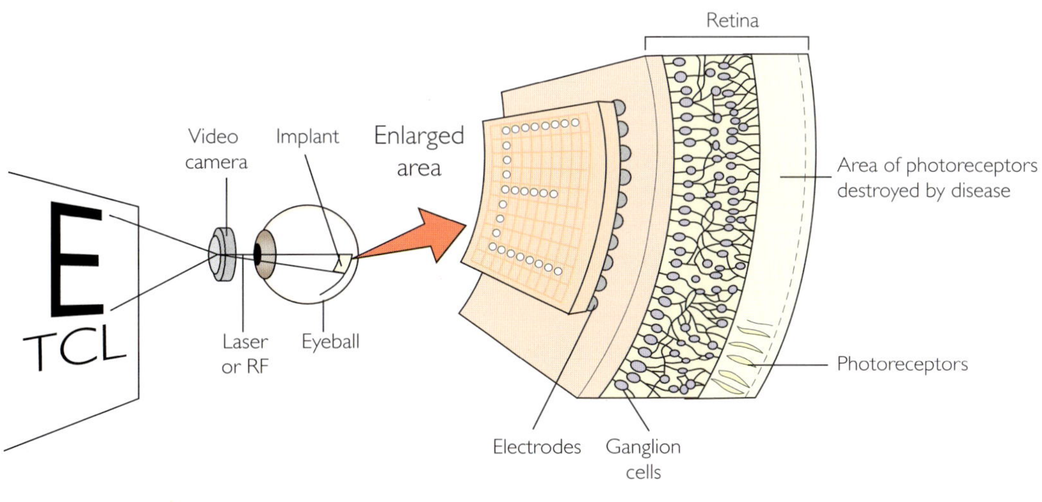

Figure 54.1 *Retinal prosthesis concept. In this artist's rendition, the image of a letter 'E' is captured and sent wirelessly (by laser or radiofrequency) to a retinal implant/chip within the eye. The visual information is decoded and then presented to the retina via controlled electrical pulses through different patterns of electrodes. Each electrode site triggers the perception of a dot of light, which, when viewed as an ensemble, would allow a blind patient with outer retinal degeneration to see the letter 'E'.*

appropriately coded and then sent via telemetry to an implanted receiver. The receiver will decode the signal and generate the desired current pulse pattern for the stimulating array. The engineering of the system, while seemingly daunting, is considered feasible with current technology and is used in today's cochlear implants. There remains the question, 'Will electrical stimulation of the retina result in a usable perception by the individual?'. The remainder of this chapter is dedicated to addressing this question. Although a final answer will not be available until someone is implanted with a retinal prosthesis, animal and human experiments to date have produced encouraging results.

Our approach is analogous to that of the cochlear implant. The cochlear implant electrically stimulates the auditory nerve, bypassing damaged cochlear hair cells, to produce the sensation of sound. Using only six electrical inputs to the auditory nerve, which contains approximately 30 000 fibers, the cochlear implant can produce sound perception with sufficient fidelity to enable a deaf individual to speak on an ordinary telephone. Additionally, cochlear implant patients improve on their ability to hear, with practice. This suggests that the brain can adapt to the reduced input and, with training, restore significant sensory function.

Research in the visual system has shown that reducing visual input to a 25 × 25 array of pixels still allows a good degree of mobility.[5] These are encouraging examples when one considers that a retinal implant will provide input to a system designed to process information from 1 million ganglion cells.

Previous experiments have shown that electrical stimulation of the visual system produces the perception of vision (as opposed to tactile or pain sensation). Stimulation of the visual cortex has been shown to produce phosphenes.[6,7] In our laboratory, human volunteers are evaluated before surgery with electrical stimulation of the globe using a contact lens electrode. The subjects have been able to 'see flashes' when the electrical current is applied. These results make an argument that electrical stimulation will result in excitation of the visual system and may produce a useful percept. The human tests performed in our laboratory will be discussed in more detail to provide direct evidence that electrical stimulation can provide useful vision.

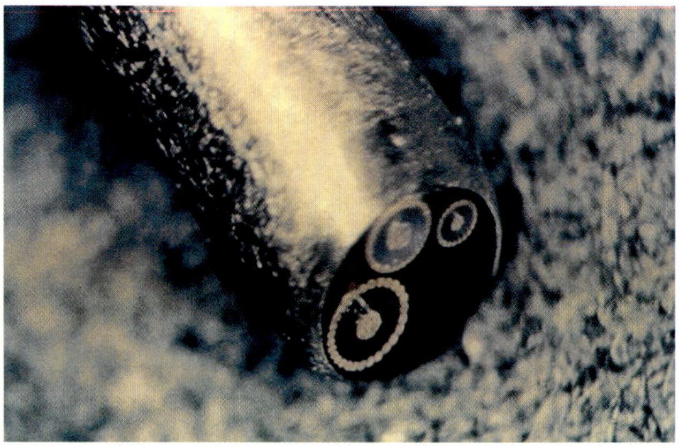

Figure 54.2 *Discrete wire electrode. A photomicrograph of the tip of a compound electrode array is shown. Three concentric electrode sites of different sizes are visible. The electrode material is platinum; the center mantle diameter of the two large electrodes sites measures 100 μm and the smaller mantle diameter measures 50 μm. Also housed with the electrodes is a fiberoptic sleeve, which is not visible because of the reflections from the metal electrode sites. The outer metal cannula is connected to a handpiece. A cable extends from the end opposite the electrode sites to allow connection to the electronics.*

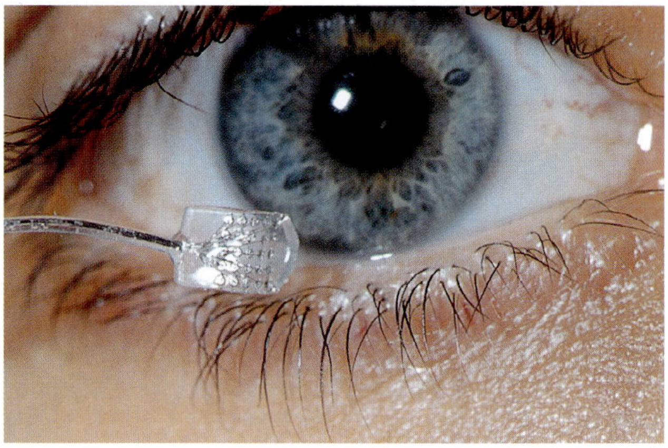

Figure 54.3 *A 5 × 5 array of platinum electrodes in a silicone matrix held near an eye. The side of the square formed by the array is approximately 3 mm. A cable extends from the end opposite the electrode sites to allow connection to the electronics.*

METHODS

Human volunteers (13 with end-stage RP; 2 with ARMD) were tested to assess the perception experienced when a small metal electrode, placed in close proximity to the retina, was used to stimulate the cells of the retina. Two types of electrodes were used. A device consisting of metal wires attached to a handpiece (Fig. 54.2) was used to determine the stimulation threshold, flicker fusion and three-point discrimination. A square array of electrodes (Fig. 54.3) was used to stimulate patterns on the retina. The electrodes were made of platinum. Protocols established for safe stimulation of neural tissue were followed.[8]

Sclerotomies were made similar to those created for a three-port pars plana vitrectomy. To protect optic nerve function, 4% lidocaine was injected near the sclera only at the site of the intended sclerotomies. The stimulating probe(s) and an endoilluminator were placed into the subject's vitreous cavity. A vitrectomy was performed only for the tests using the larger array electrodes. The surgical procedure, including the conversation between the subject and the investigators, was videotaped via a camera and microphone built into the surgical microscope. The video running time was noted to correlate the subject's description of the visual percepts with the electrical stimulation parameters. The stimulating probe was placed close to the retinal surface, without touching it. (We estimate the distance to be 0.5 mm.) Electrical pulses were applied at a rate of 1 Hz or higher. Subjects were asked to describe the size, shape, color and position of any visual perception. Additionally, as the rate of stimulation was increased, the subject was asked to define the point of flicker fusion (i.e. when the electrically elicited visual percept was no longer flashing). Flicker fusion is important because a strobe-like visual input is far less appealing than a stable nonflickering image.

RESULTS

All 15 human subjects were able to perceive phosphenes with electrical stimulation. All but one of these patients were able to localize the position of the stimulating electrode and could track the stimulus as it was moved along the retina. The stimulation threshold varied slightly and was dependent on the proximity of the electrode to the retina and the condition of the retina. Flicker fusion typically occurred between 30 and 40 Hz. Most of the subjects reported seeing a white or yellow flashing light, although some of the subjects saw a black dot surrounded by a white or yellow ring. Some of the results are described below.

A 61-year-old male with RP (no light perception vision) described the phosphene to be as small as the head of a match, indicating that electrical stimulation can be very focal. He also discriminated between two points 435 µm apart, corresponding to 4/200 (crude ambulatory) vision.[1] Tests with a 5 × 5 array yielded the following results:

- When electrodes were stimulated in rows or columns, the patient saw horizontal and vertical lines, respectively.
- When electrodes in a 'U'-shaped pattern were activated, the patient saw the letter 'H'.[2]

Although the patient's responses were not always correct, this investigation is somewhat encouraging for a number of reasons. Firstly, because the stimulating electrode is hand-held and the eye is fully mobile, the movement of the electrodes relative to the retina creates a nonuniform electrical field. Secondly, the tests were conducted for periods of less than 1 hour, which is a relatively short period for the patient to become accustomed to a new mode of visual input. From the cochlear implant experience, we know that usually it takes weeks to begin to use the artificial auditory input. Thirdly, the choice of the letter 'U' was not optimal because it was frequently confused with the letter 'H'. This may have been especially true in our test as our electrodes created a straight horizontal bottom for the letter 'U' rather than the usual slightly curved shape.

For the next patient, we selected a more distinct pattern than the letter 'U'. A 73-year-old female with RP (bare light perception vision) saw lights that outlined the shape of a 'matchbox' when pattern stimulation was applied through electrodes positioned on the perimeter of a square-shaped electrode array. Every electrode on the perimeter of a 3 × 3 electrode array was activated to form this perception. The combination of electrodes that formed the box covered a square area of retina of 1.2 × 1.2 mm. The electrode in the eye, as viewed through the surgical microscope, is shown in Fig. 54.4.

A 52-year-old female with RP (bare light perception vision) described her perception as a firefly, again indicating that the perception produced by electrical stimulation is focused on a small part of the visual field. We were able to map out her visual function by moving the stimulating electrode over the surface of the retina (i.e. akin to dynamic perimetry testing). Stimulation thresholds were lower for macular regions. The phosphene seen by the subject would disappear as the probe was moved peripherally, and then reappear as the probe was moved back into the macula. We believe that this difference in threshold to elicit visual perceptions indicates more

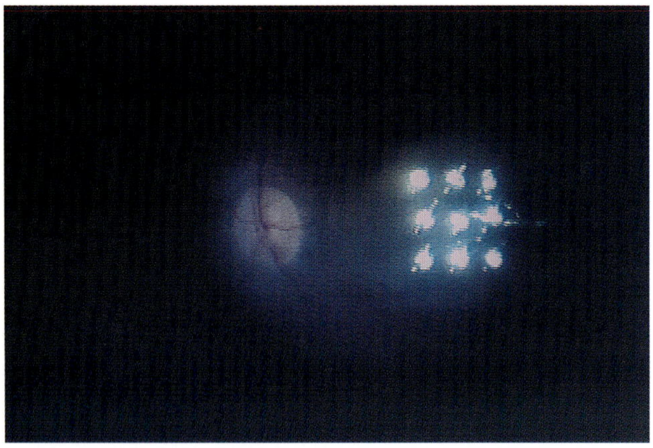

Figure 54.4 *A 3 × 3 array of platinum electrodes in a silicone matrix about to be placed on the retina of a patient with retinitis pigmentosa. The optic disc is visible in the background. When the outside electrodes were activated, the subject saw dots of light that formed the outline of a matchbox. A cable extends from the end opposite the electrode sites to allow connection to the electronics.*

damage in the extramacular region, which had extensive bone-spicule changes.[2]

CONCLUSION

The intraocular prosthesis project has successfully reached each milestone in its development. The most important achievement is the last, wherein tests have shown that blind patients see form vision using this modality. However, before a prototype for human use is widely available, some challenges remain. These include not only hurdles common to all implanted devices, such as ensuring hermetic sealing and avoiding a foreign body reaction, but also other issues specific to an intraocular implant. Two such issues are:

- How to position the array inside a fully mobile eye close enough to the retina to achieve low current requirements but to avoid damaging the retina with the mechanical or electrical effects of the implant.
- How to define a stimulus pattern to generate a usable perception for imagery more complex than a dot or box.

We believe that these challenges are surmountable, making a viable retinal prosthesis a reality in the near future.

REFERENCES

1. Humayun MS, de Juan E Jr, Dagnelie G, et al. Visual perception elicited by electrical stimulation of retina in blind humans, *Arch Ophthalmol* (1996) **114:**40–6.
2. Humayun MS, de Juan E Jr, Greenberg R, et al. Electrical stimulation of the retina in patients with photoreceptor loss, *Invest Ophthalmol Vis Sci* (1997) **38:**S39 (abst).
3. Greenberg RJ. PhD dissertation, Johns Hopkins University (1997).
4. Katona S. Master's thesis, Johns Hopkins University (1997).
5. Cha K, Horch K, Normann RA. Simulation of a phosphene-based visual field: visual acuity in a pixelized vision system, *Ann Biomed Eng* (1992) **20:**439–49.
6. Bak M, Girvin JP, Hambrecht FT, et al. Visual sensations produced by intracortical microstimulation of the human occipital cortex, *Med Biol Eng Comput* (1990) **28:**257–9.
7. Brindley GS, Lewin WS. The sensations produced by electrical stimulation of the visual cortex, *J Physiol* (1968) **196:**479–93.
8. Brummer SB, Robblee LS, Hambrecht FT. Criteria for selecting electrodes for electrical stimulation: theoretical and practical considerations, *Ann NY Acad Sci* (1983) **405:**159–71.

Chapter 55 Mechanical closure of chronic macular holes

Rizwan A Cheema, Gholam A Peyman and Mandi D Conway

INTRODUCTION

In 1991, Kelly and Wendel, reported the first surgical results for closure of full-thickness macular holes, employing pars plana vitrectomy with removal of the posterior hyaloid to relieve vitreomacular traction and complete fluid–gas exchange for prolonged intraocular tamponade to reappose the edges of the macular hole to the retinal pigment epithelium (RPE).[1] Some studies have reported lower success rates in eyes with chronic macular holes as compared with macular holes of recent onset and symptoms.[2,3]

We describe a surgical technique developed by one of us (GAP) of intraoperative mechanical closure of Stages 3–4 full-thickness macular holes in patients with symptoms of chronic macular hole of more than 1 year's duration. This technique is an attempt to close the full-thickness macular hole mechanically as well as stimulate the tissue surrounding the macular hole to release growth factors that induce fibroglial proliferation.

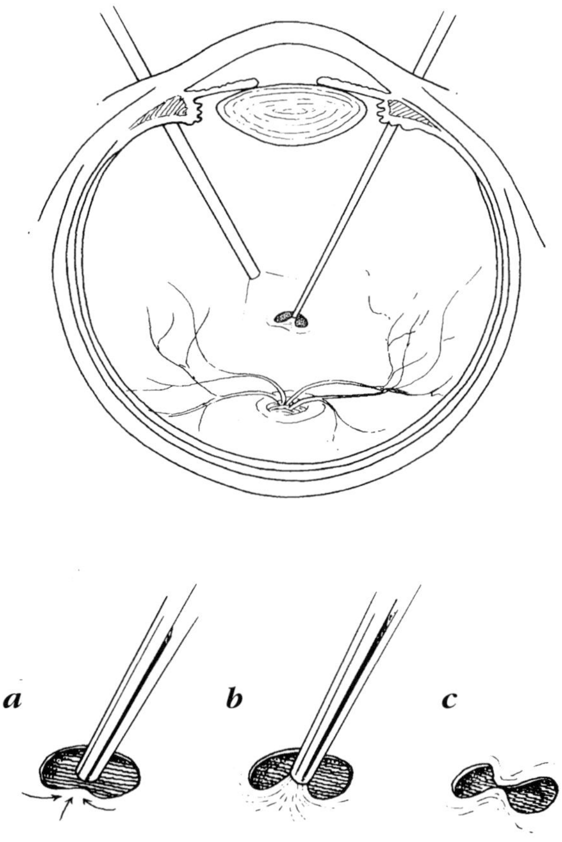

Figure 55.1 *Illustration of the mechanical closure of a macular hole. (a) The 22-gauge hard flute needle is used to approach the edge of the macular hole. (b) The edges of the macular hole are aspirated into the port of the flute needle. (c) The macular hole assumes a dumb-bell shape as its edges are brought together mechanically.*

SURGICAL TECHNIQUE

The surgical procedure consists of pars plana vitrectomy and removal of the posterior hyaloid. The separation and complete removal of the posterior hyaloid are aided by the injection of 1–2 drops of triamcinolone acetonide into the midvitreous cavity before performing core vitrectomy to improve visualization of the cortical vitreous.[4] Mechanical closure of the macular hole is accomplished by using a 22-gauge hard-tipped flute needle to engage the edge of the macular hole (Fig. 55.1a). The edges of the macular hole are then aspirated gently into the port of the flute needle using passive suction, with the height of the infusion bottle 6 inches (15 cm) above the patient's head (Fig. 55.1b). By exerting slight side-to-side movements, the retinal tissue in contact with the needle tip is released. This produces a nipple-shaped configuration of retinal tissue arising from the

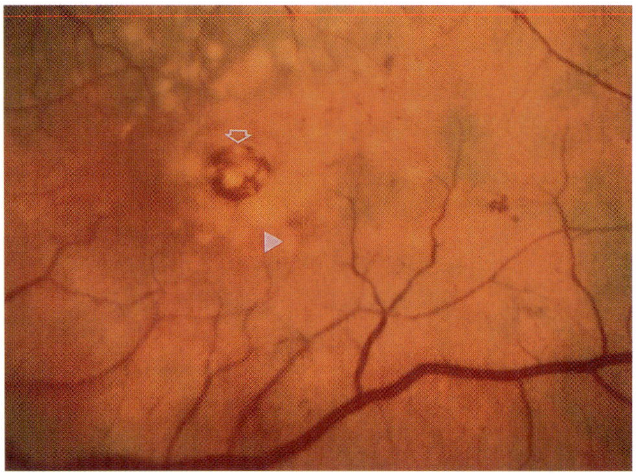

Figure 55.2 *Preoperative color fundus photograph of a left eye showing Stage 3 full-thickness macular hole, soft drusen, and moderate nonproliferative diabetic retinopathy.*

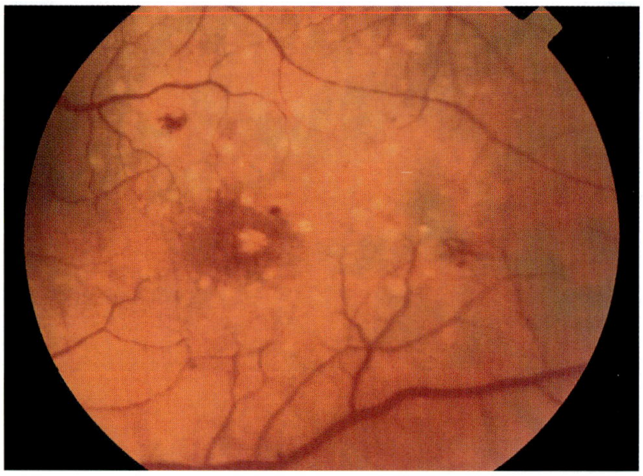

Figure 55.3 *Postoperative color fundus photograph of a left eye showing closed macular hole with fibroglial tissue, age-related macular degenerative changes, and moderate nonproliferative diabetic retinopathy.*

edge of the macular hole, protruding into the middle of the macular hole. When a similar maneuver is performed on the opposite side of the macular hole, the hole assumes a dumb-bell shape rather than a circular configuration (Fig. 55.1c). The retinal engagement into the flute needle may result in punctate hemorrhages visible over the hole margins, as this maneuver is performed. This maneuver can also be performed after air–fluid exchange using minimal air perfusion pressure of 20–30 mmHg. Finally, air in the vitreous cavity is then replaced with a 14% perfluoropropane gas or a 20% sulfur hexafluoride–air mixture. The patient is instructed to maintain strict face down positioning for 1–2 weeks in the postoperative period.

We have successfully closed chronic macular holes employing this surgical technique in five patients (Figs 55.2 and 55.3). Visual and anatomic results in patients with more than 3 months' follow-up are shown in Table 55.1. All five patients have achieved anatomical closure of macular holes with 4/5 achieving visual acuity of 20/50 or better. One patient had visual acuity of counting fingers as a result of a nuclear cataract, for which surgery is planned in the near future.

Table 55.1 Demographic details and visual results of patients who achieved surgical closure of chronic macular holes

Case no.	*Gender*	*Age*	*Stage of macular hole*	*Duration of macular hole (months)*	*Pre-op. VA*	*Result*	*VA at 3 months*	*VA at last FU*	*Comments*
1	F	73	4	26	20/200	Closed	CF	20/40	6 weeks' postoperative pseudophakia
2	F	69	3	17	20/200	Closed	CF	20/50	Pseudophakia
3	F	66	3	13	CF	Closed	CF	CF	NS + 3
4	F	41	3	14	20/200	Closed	20/200	20/40	Pseudophakia
5	F	64	3	12	20/200	Closed	20/80	20/40	Pseudophakia

CF, counts fingers; FU, follow-up; NS, nuclear sclerosis; VA, visual acuity

DISCUSSION

Our surgical technique requires the meticulous evacuation of fluid from the base of the macular hole and bringing the edges of the hole together. This reapposes the neurosensory retina to underlying the RPE, as fibroglial proliferation over a lesser area is required to bridge the gap for closure of the macular hole. The side-to-side motion of the flute needle while releasing the retina may also stimulate fibroglial proliferation needed to bridge the central dehiscence. This modification of surgical technique may provide improved surgical results in anatomic closure of chronic or recurrent macular holes.

REFERENCES

1. Kelly NE, Wendel RT. Vitreous surgery for idiopathic macular holes: results of a pilot study, *Arch Ophthalmol* (1991) **109**:654–9.
2. Ryan EH Jr, Gilbert HD. Results of surgical treatment of recent-onset full-thickness idiopathic macular holes, *Arch Ophthalmol* (1994) **112**:1545–53.
3. Willis AW, Garcia-Cosio JF. Macular hole surgery. Comparison of longstanding versus recent macular holes, *Ophthalmology* (1996) **103**:1811–14.
4. Peyman GA, Cheema R, Conway MD, Fang T. Triamcinolone acetonide as an aid to visualization of the vitreous and the posterior hyaloid during pars plana vitrectomy, *Retina* (2000) (in press).

Chapter 56 Intraoperative visualization of the vitreous and the posterior hyaloid using triamcinolone

Gholam A Peyman, Rizwan A Cheema, Ting Fang and Mandi D Conway

INTRODUCTION

An attached or incompletely separated posterior hyaloid can provide a source of traction in conditions such as macular hole,[1] vitreomacular traction syndrome, and proliferative vitreoretinopathy (PVR), or serve as a scaffold for fibrovascular proliferation in proliferative diabetic retinopathy (PDR). Therefore, complete removal of the vitreous and posterior hyaloid membrane is an important surgical goal in pars plana vitrectomy. Because of the transparency of the vitreous, it is difficult to visualize these structures during pars plana vitrectomy, resulting in incomplete removal of the vitreous and the posterior hyaloid.

In this chapter we describe the use of intravitreal triamcinolone acetonide, a corticoid sterile aqueous suspension, as an aid to visualizing the vitreous. The use of this drug thus assists in the separation of the posterior hyaloid during pars plana vitrectomy.

SURGICAL TECHNIQUE

A standard three sclerotomies are created. A prior core vitrectomy may be performed and 1 or 2 drops of triamcinolone acetonide aqueous suspension (40 mg/ml) are injected with a 20- to 25-gauge needle into the midvitreous cavity. Alternatively, the aqueous suspension may be allowed to stand for 30 minutes, the vehicle separated, the suspension mixed with normal saline and used in a 50% concentration. The white triamcinolone suspension is dispersed into the vitreous cavity with gentle movements of the light pipe and vitrector. The suspension becomes visibly trapped in the gel structure of the vitreous. Active aspiration with a vitrectomy probe or soft cannulated extrusion needle is applied to a maximum of 200–300 mmHg just nasal to the optic disc. The posterior cortical vitreous is seen stretched and elevated from the surface of retina (Fig. 56.1) during this surgical maneuver; the subsequent creation of a posterior vitreous detachment combined with cutting allows infusion fluid to rush into the space created, expanding the posterior hyaloid space. As soon

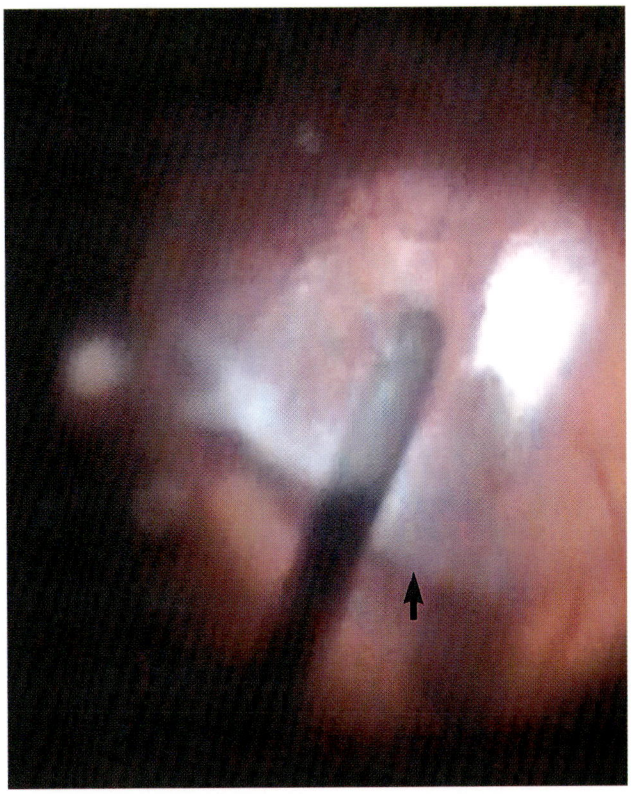

Figure 56.1 *Triamcinolone acetonide delineates the boundary of the posterior hyaloid, which is being separated from the retina by the vitrectomy port. The posterior hyaloid separation is clearly visible (arrow).*

as posterior hyaloid separation occurs, some of the triamcinolone suspended in the midvitreous cavity settles on the dependent retinal surface and can be easily aspirated by suction alone. This confirms complete separation of the posterior vitreous from the retina. The boundary between the posterior cortical vitreous and the fluid-filled posterior hyaloid space is easily visualized because of the different suspension characteristics of triamcinolone in the fluid-filled posterior hyaloid space and the formed gel of the vitreous. Triamcinolone particles in the fluid-filled space are freely mobile, unlike those trapped in the gel structure of the vitreous. This helps in accurate visualization of the posterior hyaloid and vitreous and in the complete removal of the posterior hyaloid and formed vitreous.

DISCUSSION

Triamcinolone is a corticoid with no retinal toxicity in doses of 2–4 mg in vitrectomized and nonvitrectomized eyes.[2,3] The aqueous suspension of triamcinolone in the vitreous provides a good visualization of the vitreous during vitrectomy. The suspension particles are trapped in the gel structure of the vitreous and stand out in contrast to a free-floating suspension of particles of infusion fluid where the vitreous has been removed. This clearly demarcates areas of presence of vitreous and its boundaries during vitrectomy. Residual triamcinolone suspension is removed with the vitreous cutter as the vitrectomy proceeds.

Triamcinolone has no retinal toxicity, and may prevent fibrin syndrome and possibly PVR in the postoperative period because of its inherent anti-inflammatory and antimitotic characteristics.

REFERENCES

1. Johnson RN, Gass JD. Idiopathic macular holes: observations, stages of formation, and implications for surgical intervention, *Ophthalmology* (1988) **95**:917–24.
2. McCuen BW II, Bessler M, Tano Y, et al. The lack of toxicity of intravitreally administered triamcinolone acetonide, *Am J Ophthalmol* (1981) **91**:785–8.
3. Kivilcim M, Peyman GA, El-Dessouky ES, et al. Retinal toxicity of triamcinolone acetonide in silicone-filled eyes, *Ophthalmic Surg Lasers* (in press).

Chapter 57 Retinal vascular diseases

Kamal Kishore and Gholam A Peyman

SURGICAL TREATMENT OF BRANCH RETINAL VEIN OCCLUSION

The ophthalmoscopic findings of an acute branch retinal vein occlusion (BRVO) include superficial flame-shaped hemorrhages, retinal edema and often cotton-wool spots in a sector of retina. The occluded vein is dilated and tortuous, and with time the corresponding artery may narrow and become sheathed. The site of obstruction is almost invariably at an arteriovenous crossing point and is usually located near the apex of the involved retina. The obstruction is caused by thrombosis at the arteriovenous crossing where the artery and vein share a common wall. Compression of the vein by an arteriosclerotic artery may result in turbulent flow, endothelial damage and thrombotic occlusion.[1] At the obstruction site, the artery crosses anterior to the vein in 53–99% of cases. The obstruction involves superotemporal vessels more commonly (63%), probably because of the greater frequency of arteriovenous crossings superiorly.

BRVO usually occurs in patients of middle age or older. Systemic hypertension (65–75%), diabetes (2–13%), atherosclerosis and hyperopia may predispose to BRVO. Patients usually present with a visual field loss corresponding to the involved sector of the retina. Decreased central vision may result from macular hemorrhages, edema or nonperfusion. Hemorrhages and edema resolve over the ensuing several months as collaterals bridging the site of occlusion and horizontal raphe become more apparent. Late sequelae may include retinal and optic disc neovascularization, vitreous hemorrhage, persistent macular edema, macular pigmentary changes, epiretinal membrane and circinate retinopathy caused by leakage of lipid from telangiectatic vessels. Retinal detachment may result from traction-induced holes adjacent to fibrovascular proliferation.

The Branch Vein Occlusion Study Group (BVOS)[2] found that 31% of untreated eyes with greater than five disc diameters of nonperfusion developed neovascularization. Of those eyes with neovascularization, vitreous hemorrhage occurred in 29% of eyes treated with scatter argon-laser photocoagulation compared to 61% of untreated (control) eyes. Only 12% of eyes with vitreous hemorrhage suffered a loss of more than six lines of visual acuity. Even though prophylactic scatter laser treatment of eyes with nonperfusion greater than five disc diameters decreased the incidence of neovascularization from 31% to 19.2%, the study group recommended laser treatment only after the development of neovascularization.

The BVOS also demonstrated beneficial effects of argon-laser grid treatment to edematous parafoveal retina caused by capillary leakage resulting in visual acuity of 20/40 or worse.[3] Treated eyes were more likely to gain two lines of visual acuity (65%) compared with untreated eyes (37%). Additionally, treated eyes were more likely to have 20/40 or better vision at 3 years' follow-up (60% treated, compared with 34% untreated eyes).

Recombinant tissue plasminogen activator (rtPA) is effective in reopening laser-induced BRVO in rabbits.[4] Surgical separation of the retinal vein and artery at the site of arteriovenous crossing by sectioning the common adventitial sheath with microsurgical techniques has been demonstrated in animals, cadaver eyes and one patient with BRVO.[5] This patient had rapid clearing of retinal hemorrhages and macular edema after the procedure, with resultant improvement of visual acuity to 20/25 from the preoperative level of 20/200. The authors of this report[5] noted that the application of this procedure appeared to be limited to arteriovenous crossings near the optic nerve, because vessels at this location appeared to be both large enough and of sufficient strength to tolerate the manipulation associated with creating small cuts between the artery and vein.

REMOVAL OF INTRA-ARTERIAL EMBOLI

Emboli derived from ulcerated atheromatous plaques in the carotid artery are the most common cause of major retinal arterial occlusions. Patients usually experience sudden onset of loss of vision which may be antedated by *amaurosis fugax* in 20–25% of the cases. A field loss is noted if occlusion involves a branch of the central retinal artery. The average age of onset of symptoms is 60 years, and 50–75% of patients with retinal artery occlusion have clinical evidence of carotid artery disease. In younger patients, the emboli are derived usually from damaged heart valves from rheumatic heart disease, congenital anomalies of heart valves or prolapse of the mitral valve (Barlow's syndrome). Ischemic whitening of the retina results, corresponding to the segment supplied by the occluded artery. The fovea may show a cherry-red spot; its absence in central retinal artery occlusion should suggest the presence of choroidal ischemia as well. Narrowing of the artery and segmentation of the blood column occur. Emboli may be visible in the arterial tree.

The major types of emboli are easily recognized. Platelet fibrin emboli are dull, gray-white and elongated, may be single or multiple and are most often lodged at a bifurcation. Cholesterol emboli are yellow, iridescent globules that are often multiple and are seen most often on the temporal side of the fundus. They are often not associated with obstruction of blood flow. Calcific emboli are usually single, solid, white nonrefractile, ovoid or angulated emboli and are found most often near the optic nerve head. They are usually derived from a calcific aortic or mitral valve.

Inner retinal infarction occurs experimentally after complete occlusion of the central retinal artery for 90 minutes. Treatment, therefore, is infrequently beneficial. However, in any patient with a history of occlusion of less than 24 hours, emergency treatment consisting of intermittent massage and/or paracentesis, breathing 95% oxygen and 5% carbon dioxide and administration of intravenous acetazolamide may be helpful. Other modes of therapy that have been employed include the intravenous administration of vasodilators such as papaverine, rtPA and hyperbaric oxygen and infusion of urokinase into the ocular circulation.[6,7]

Peyman and Gremillion[8] reported a case of embolic retinal artery occlusion of 60 hours' duration that was treated by surgical removal of one embolus and direct massage of another, causing fragmentation and distal flow. The surgical technique consisted of a three-port pars plana vitrectomy. An incision into the nerve-fiber layer was made overlying the embolus with the bent tip of a 30-gauge needle. The wall of the artery was incised and the embolus was dislodged into the vitreous cavity. The artery went into spasm and no bleeding was encountered. A similar maneuver was attempted over the embolus in the superior arcade. The embolus was fragmented and appeared to flow distally. The patient's visual acuity improved from counting fingers to 20/200 on the second postoperative day. Mottling of peripapillary pigment epithelium was noted at 3 months.

CENTRAL RETINAL VEIN OCCLUSION

Central retinal vein occlusion (CRVO) is most commonly caused by a thrombus formation in the central retinal vein at the level of the *lamina cribrosa*, where both the central retinal artery and vein share a common adventitial sheath. The inelastic structure of the *lamina cribrosa* causes a narrowing in the central retinal vein, which may be compressed further by pressure from an adjacent sclerotic artery. An intraluminal or intramural thrombus forms, causing occlusion of the central retinal vein, which, by increasing pressure on the venous side, may secondarily reduce arterial flow. Severity of ischemic damage to the retina depends upon the severity of occlusion, rapidity of recanalization and collateral formation and perfusion pressure.

CRVO is seen most commonly in patients of middle age and older. Hypertension is seen in 60% and a history of open-angle glaucoma is present in 40–70%. There is an increased risk of CRVO with diabetes and cardiovascular disease; the risk is decreased with exercise and postmenopausal use of estrogen.

Patients usually present with a variable decrease in vision depending on macular hemorrhage, edema or ischemia. Ischemic CRVO is suggested by extensive hemorrhages and cotton-wool spots, the presence of a relative afferent pupillary defect greater than 0.9 log units, constriction of the peripheral visual field and capillary nonperfusion greater than 10 disc areas on intravenous fluorescein angiogram.[9,10]

The Central Retinal Vein Occlusion Study Group showed that 15% of nonischemic eyes converted to ischemia over 4 months and an additional 19% converted to ischemia over the next 3 years. Thirty-five percent of nonperfused eyes developed 2-clock-hour iris neovascularization (TC-INV) or angle neovascularization (ANV). They also showed that visual acuity of less than 20/200 at presentation was a poor prognostic sign; 54% of such eyes developed TC-INV/ANV.[11] Capillary nonperfusion greater than 30 disc areas was the strongest predictor of neovascularization; 42% of such eyes developed TC-INV/ANV. Prophylactic panretinal photocoagulation did not reduce the incidence of neovascularization. Grid-pattern laser therapy was evaluated for the treatment of macular edema; it reduced angiographic edema but had no beneficial effect on visual outcome.[12]

McAllister and Constable used an argon laser to create chorioretinal anastomosis in 24 eyes with nonischemic CRVO with progressively worsening visual acuity, and achieved success in 33%.[13] Subsequently they reported a 67% success rate in creating a chorioretinal anastomosis with a two-step procedure in which an argon laser was used to break Bruch's membrane with a 50-µm spot of 0.1 second duration and a power level of 2.5–3.0 W. A second spot was then applied at the edge of the vein in an attempt to rupture it. A YAG laser was used at a power level of 3–5 mJ if the argon-laser treatment was unsuccessful.[14] Complications included distal vein occlusion in 21%, minor fibrovascular proliferation in 19%, minor vitreous hemorrhage in 4% and major fibrovascular proliferation in 5%. Other authors have reported a much lower success rate with this procedure.[15,16] Intravitreal and intravenous tPA also have been tried in the treatment of CRVO.[17,18]

Peyman and coworkers attempted to create surgical chorioretinal anastomosis (CRA) in five patients with ischemic CRVO (Figs 57.1 and 57.2).[19] A relative afferent pupillary defect was present in each eye and the ischemic nature of the CRVO was confirmed by an intravenous fluorescein angiogram before surgery. The mean age of patients was 70.6 (range 61–85) years. There were two female and three male patients. Duration of symptoms prior to surgical CRA ranged from 8 days to 4 months. Follow-up ranged from 8 to 20 months (mean 13.4 months).

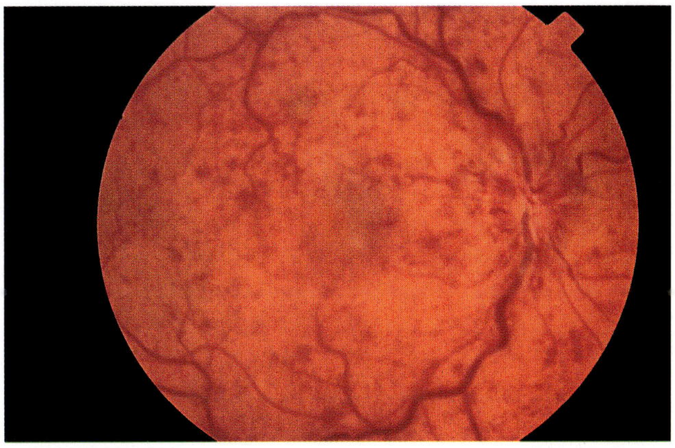

Figure 57.1 *Fundus photograph of the right eye showing characteristic appearance of central retinal vein occlusion.*

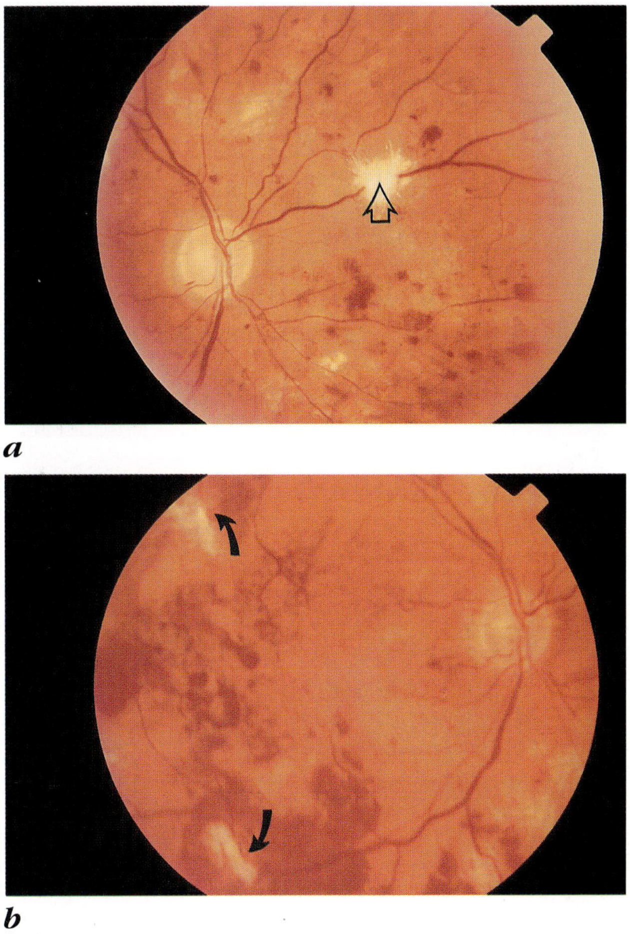

Figure 57.2 *Same eye as in Fig. 57.1 but after surgical chorioretinal anastomosis (CRA). Note nasal CRA sites (a) and temporal CRA sites (b). (Reproduced with permission from Peyman GA, Kishore K, Conway MD. Surgical chorioretinal anastomosis for ischemic central retinal vein occlusion,* Ophthalmic Surg Lasers *(1999)* ***30:*** *605–14.[19])*

Hypotensive general anesthesia was used to maintain a systolic blood pressure of approximately 100 mmHg. Following pars plana vitrectomy, the posterior hyaloid face was removed and slit-like incisions were made with a microvitreoretinal blade adjacent to a major retinal vein in each quadrant. Small pieces of 5-0 Mersilene sutures were positioned over the vein and inserted into these incisions to promote vascularization. Panretinal photocoagulation was applied.

A functioning CRA site was identified by a segment of retinal vein disappearing into the CRA site. Of 16 attempted CRA sites in four eyes (CRA sites could not be evaluated in one eye because of a cataract), 10 sites were functioning. At two sites, the vein seemed to continue through the area of chorioretinal scarring without disruption. Closure of the vein occurred at two sites. The other two sites could not be evaluated, because they were obscured by the proliferation of fibrous tissue. Arteriovenous-shunt formation between the proximal segment of the vein and adjacent artery was noted at one site, which was otherwise functional. Trilaminar flow was not visible at any site; however, this was not a criterion for successful CRA in the study.

Proliferation of glial tissue was noted at all sites. No eye developed rubeosis iridis, angle neovascularization or choriovitreal neovascularization. Two of the eyes were pseudophakic. One eye developed a significant cataract soon after surgery, necessitating cataract extraction. Another eye developed 3+ nuclear sclerosis, but cataract extraction was not recommended because of a poor visual prognosis.

Optic atrophy developed in three eyes. Final postoperative visual acuity was better than preoperative visual acuity in three eyes, remained unchanged in one and was worse in one eye. Secondary procedures included vitreous washout in two eyes, peeling of epiretinal membranes in two eyes, cataract surgery in one eye and repair of traction–rhegmatogenous retinal detachment in one eye.

This pilot study showed that surgical CRA could be established in all eyes by one surgical procedure. The complication rate appears to be high at present but the technique is being refined to minimize these complications.

REFERENCES

1. Frangieh GT, Green WR, Barraquer-Somers E, Finkelstein D. Histopathologic study of nine branch retinal vein occlusions, *Arch Ophthalmol* (1982) **100:**1132–40.
2. Branch Vein Occlusion Study Group. Argon laser scatter photocoagulation for prevention of neovascularization and vitreous hemorrhage in branch vein occlusion. A randomized clinical trial, *Arch Ophthalmol* (1986) **104:**34–41.
3. The Branch Vein Occlusion Study Group. Argon laser photocoagulation for macular edema in branch vein occlusion, *Am J Ophthalmol* (1984) **98:**271–82.
4. Oncel M, Peyman GA, Khoobehi B. Tissue plasminogen activator in the treatment of experimental retinal vein occlusion, *Retina* (1989) **9:**1–7.
5. Osterloh MD, Charles S. Surgical decompression of branch retinal vein occlusions, *Arch Ophthalmol* (1988) **106:**1469–71.
6. De La Paz MA, Patrinely JR, Marines HM, Appling WD. Adjunctive hyperbaric oxygen in the treatment of bilateral cerebro-rhino-orbital mucormycosis, *Am J Ophthalmol* (1992) **114:**208–11.
7. Schmidt D, Schumacher M, Wakhloo AK. Microcatheter urokinase infusion in central retinal artery occlusion, *Am J Ophthalmol* (1992) **113:**429–34.
8. Peyman GA, Gremillion CM Jr. Surgical removal of a branch retinal artery embolus: a case report, *Int Ophthalmol* (1990) **14:**295–8.
9. Hayreh SS, Klugman MR, Beri M, et al. Differentiation of ischemic from nonischemic central retinal vein occlusion during the early acute phase, *Graefes Arch Clin Exp Ophthalmol* (1990) **228:**201–17.
10. The Central Vein Occlusion Study Group. A randomized clinical trial of early panretinal photocoagulation for ischemic central vein occlusion: the Central Vein Occlusion Study Group N report, *Ophthalmology* (1995) **102:**1424–44.
11. The Central Vein Occlusion Study Group. Natural history and clinical management of central retinal vein occlusion, *Arch Ophthalmol* (1997) **115:**486–91.
12. The Central Vein Occlusion Study Group. Evaluation of grid pattern photocoagulation for macular edema in central vein occlusion: the Central Vein Occlusion Study Group M report, *Ophthalmology* (1995) **102:**1425–33.
13. McAllister IL, Constable IJ. Laser-induced chorioretinal venous anastomosis for treatment of nonischemic central retinal vein occlusion, *Arch Ophthalmol* (1995) **113:**456–62.
14. McAllister IL. Laser-induced chorioretinal anastomosis for treatment of perfused central retinal vein occlusion: Technique and updated results, *Vitreoretinal Update 1997*, CD-ROM (© American Academy of Ophthalmology, San Francisco, 1997).
15. Browning DJ. Outcome and complications of laser-induced chorioretinal anastomosis, *Vitreoretinal Update 1997*, CD-ROM (© American Academy of Ophthalmology, San Francisco, 1997).
16. Fekrat S, Goldberg MF, Finkelstein D. Laser-induced chorioretinal venous anastomosis for nonischemic central or branch retinal vein occlusion, *Arch Ophthalmol* (1998) **116:**43–52.
17. Lahey JM, Fong DS, Kearney JM. Intravitreal tissue plasminogen activator for central retinal vein occlusion, *Invest Ophthalmol Vis Sci* (1997) **38**(Suppl): S751 (abst).
18. Elman MJ. Thrombolytic trials for central retinal vein occlusion: results of a pilot study, *Trans Am Ophthalmol Soc* (1996) **94:**471–504.
19. Peyman GA, Kishore K, Conway MD, Surgical chorioretinal venous anastomosis for ischemic central retinal vein occlusion, *Ophthalmic Surg Lasers* (1999) **30:**605–14.

Index

Note: page numbers in *italics* refer to figures and tables